Metabolic, Degenerative, and Inflammatory Diseases of
BONES and JOINTS

Metabolic, Degenerative, and Inflammatory Diseases
of
BONES and JOINTS

HENRY L. JAFFE, M.D.

Consultant Pathologist and Emeritus Director of Laboratories,
Hospital for Joint Diseases, New York, N. Y.
Consultant Pathologist, United Hospitals of Newark,
Newark, N. J.
Honorary Consultant, Armed Forces Institute of Pathology,
Washington, D. C.

1066 Illustrations on 285 Figures

LEA & FEBIGER · *Philadelphia* *1972*

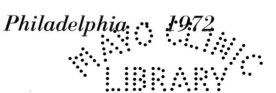

To

Henry W. Frauenthal, M.D.
Founder, Hospital for Joint Diseases
and

To my wife
Clarisse K. Jaffe

Preface

THIS book is intended to present an integrated account of the metabolic, degenerative, and inflammatory diseases of the bones and joints. The clinical findings are given with special attention to their value in narrowing down the diagnostic possibilities pertaining to the various lesions discussed. The roentgenographic appearance presented by a particular lesion is correlated as much as possible with the actual gross pathologic anatomy of the affected area. The microscopic findings are generally coordinated with the gross findings and often also with the roentgenographic reflections of the latter. On the other hand, an effort has been made to avoid distortion of the account as a whole by an excess of histologic detail. The presentations have been guided by the idea that the problems of diagnosis and differential diagnosis raised by skeletal lesions can best be met if, in the interpretation of a given lesion, its clinical, roentgenographic and pathologic features are considered and evaluated together.

In large measure, my personal conceptions of the lesions discussed are based on my own experience. However, due cognizance has been taken of the work of others in the field. Since the pertinent literature is vast, it has not been found feasible to give detailed citations from it. In any event, it is hoped that pathologists, radiologists, and orthopaedic surgeons will find the book useful, and that it will also be of interest to medical colleagues in other specialties who are confronted from time to time by problems relating to diseases involving bones and joints.

Great reliance has been placed on the illustrations, which are arranged on full-page plates to permit the simultaneous display of a number of pictures for purposes of comparison. The accompanying legends give details about each illustration, and many of them embody sufficient clinical information to constitute brief case histories. Actually, though integrated with the text, the illustrations and their legends compose in themselves something like an atlas of the nontumorous skeletal lesions. As to the illustrations, I wish to express my thanks and appreciation to Mr. George R. Struck and to Mr. William S. Cornwell, both of Rochester, New York, for their encouraging interest and valuable suggestions relating to this very important aspect of the book.

A large number of the pictures (especially photomicrographs and also some radiographs) were prepared from the pathologic material which the late Dr. Jakob Erdheim gathered over many years. Professor Erdheim willed the material to Dr. Ernst Freund, who was an associate of Dr. Erdheim in Vienna for about eight years and subsequently worked with me at the Hospital for Joint Diseases for about a year. Shortly before his death, Dr. Freund bequeathed the entire Erdheim collection to me. However, the bulk of the material illustrated in this book is from my own pathology collection. It has always been my practice to roentgenograph significant specimens in order to correlate the gross pathologic findings with the radiographic findings.

Dr. Jacob Kream, who had been Chief Biochemist at the Hospital for Joint Diseases for 11 years and is now Biochemist to the Clinical Center at Montefiore Hospital, wrote most of Chapter 5, which is entitled "Metabolic and Biochemical Considerations." I am greatly indebted to him for his assistance in dealing with this important aspect of skeletal diseases.

For the preparation of many of the gross specimens for photography and detailed study, I am grateful to my former associate, Dr. Golden Selin. The tissue sections from which many of the photomicrographs were made represent the work of my histology technician, Mrs. Rose Afford. Throughout the composition of this book, I have had the unflagging assistance of Miss E. Marion Pilpel, who has worked with me for the past 37 years. Moreover, every chapter of the book has been conscientiously read and typed by Miss Edith Ross, who has also meticulously checked every reference. I am likewise indebted to Miss Ross for her aid in the correction of the galleys and the preparation of the index. I also wish to record my appreciation to The New York Academy of Medicine, whose outstanding library was an indispensable aid to me in my search for pertinent literature.

In 1925, Dr. Henry W. Frauenthal, the Founder of the Hospital for Joint Diseases, appointed me Pathologist and Director of Laboratories, and thus initiated my interest in orthopaedic pathology. The late Dr. Maurice Fishberg, for many years the head of the Department of Pulmonary Tuberculosis at Montefiore Hospital, recommended me to Dr. Frauenthal for the position. It is in part for the sake of perpetuating the memory of Doctors Frauenthal, Erdheim, Freund, and Fishberg that I mention these details of my professional background and career.

Special thanks are accorded to three devoted friends who read parts of the manuscript and offered most helpful suggestions: Dr. Howard D. Dorfman, who succeeded me as Director of Laboratories; Dr. Henry J. Mankin, until recently our Director of Orthopaedics; and Dr. Charles J. Sutro, Consultant Orthopaedist.

I wish to express my gratitude to my colleagues, both at the Hospital for Joint Diseases and at other medical institutions, who so kindly permitted me to draw upon their experience and material relating to individual cases. It is also a pleasure to express my thanks for the friendly interest consistently shown by Mr. Abraham Rosenberg, the former Executive Director of our hospital, and by Mr. Bernard Aronson, currently President of the Board of Trustees, who, with the other Trustees, have been looking forward to the completion of this book. I acknowledge with sincere thanks the patience and cooperation which the publishers have shown during the many years this book was being written.

HENRY L. JAFFE

New York, New York

Contents

Chapter

1

Development and Maturation of Bones and Joints

As is well known, the *bones* and *joints* are derived from the mesenchyme—the pluripotential embryonic connective tissue. With minor exceptions, that part of the mesenchyme which is destined to form the bones gives rise to the latter in one of two ways: (1) It may differentiate into precartilage and then into cartilage, which in turn is replaced by osseous tissue; or (2) it may differentiate into a primitive connective tissue in which osseous tissue forms without the intermediacy of cartilage. Most of the bones are first preformed in cartilage.

In connection with skeletogenesis, a few historical remarks may not be out of place. The idea that cartilage is a forerunner of bone in the embryonic development of the skeleton was already expressed in anatomical writings of the fifteenth and sixteenth centuries. At that time, however, it was mistakenly supposed that all of the bones had cartilage precursors and, furthermore, that they were formed through the direct conversion of the cartilage into osseous tissue. Nesbitt, in 1736, was apparently the first to take issue with these concepts. He postulated that some bones have no cartilage precursors, and that even in the case of those that do have them the cartilage is destroyed in the process of being replaced by bone. It was not until a hundred years later, however, that the correctness of his opinions began to be firmly established.

In 1836, J. Müller demonstrated through histologic studies on lower animal species that bone could be formed from embryonal connective tissue without an intervening cartilage stage. Shortly thereafter, Sharpey proved that certain bones were formed in this way in higher vertebrates, also. In 1858, H. Müller demonstrated microscopically the other important fact relating to embryonal bone formation. He showed that where cartilaginous skeletal tissue does appear as a precursor of bone it is only provisional, and that the osseous tissue which replaces it is a new formation. He did not venture to describe definitely the source and distinctive characteristics of the bone-forming cell, or osteoblast. This description was given by Gegenbaur in 1864. The importance of the osteoclast in the physiologic resorption and remodeling of osseous tissue laid down in the course of bone formation was brought into focus by Kölliker in 1873.

The accumulation of basic knowledge in regard to the development of joints lagged behind that relating to the bones. Indeed, the systematic study by Bernays, published in 1878, was one of the first in this field. He dealt particularly with the knee joint, discussing its development as manifested both in man and in lower animals. The earliest comprehensive presentation of the histology of the fully formed joint was that given by Hammar in 1892, and much of what he stated then has stood the test of time. In 1910, Lubosch attempted to settle many still-disputed or obscure points in relation to articular development and structure. He approached the subject from the point of view of comparative anatomy.

The *bones preformed in cartilage* include those of the extremities, those of the trunk (with the exception of the clavicles), and the bones composing part of the base of the skull. In bones passing through a cartilage stage in their evolution, the mesenchyme differentiates into precartilage and then into cartilage to form the cartilage model of the future bone. In the subsequent course of events, the cartilage model is progressively destroyed and is replaced by osseous tissue. The osteoblasts inaugurating the osteogenesis arise out of the mesenchymal connective tissue coat (the perichondrium) which envelops the cartilage model. For instance, in respect to the tubular bones of the extremities (with the exception of the terminal phalanges), the first evidence of osteogenesis is represented by the appearance of a thin cuff of osseous tissue girdling the midportion of the cartilage model. After the cuff of osseous tissue has been formed, destruction and removal of the cartilage model sets in, proceeding along the lines to be described below. Bones formed in this manner are often denoted as "cartilage-preformed bones," and the process in the course of which the cartilage is destroyed and then replaced by osseous tissue is known as *endochondral ossification*.

The *bones not preformed in cartilage* include those of the cranial vault and most of those of the face. In their evolution, the mesenchyme at the site of their development first gives rise to a membrane of primitive connective tissue rather than precartilage and cartilage. Within this membrane, many of the primitive connective tissue cells differentiate into osteoblasts, which then inaugurate osteogenesis. The bones which evolve in this manner are sometimes denoted as "membrane bones," because they develop through the process of *intramembranous ossification*.

In general, in the evolution of *joints*, the developing bone rudiments are held together by interzones of still-undifferentiated mesenchyme. It is the mesenchyme of the interzones, as well as the neighboring general mesenchyme, that is involved in the formation of the joints. In the course of development of a synovial, or diarthrodial, joint (such as a knee joint), the interzonal mesenchyme is cleared away and the neighboring general mesenchyme is involved in the formation of the joint capsule and any pertinent intra-articular structures. In the evolution of an amphiarthrosis (such as the junction between two vertebral bodies), the interzonal mesenchyme is transformed into a fibrocartilaginous disk which firmly connects the developing bodies. A synarthrosis (such as a cranial suture) results when the mesenchyme between apposed growing bone ends yields almost completely to these ends, so that only a trace of the former separation between them remains.

This chapter is intended to provide merely a general orientation in regard to the development and maturation of the skeleton. Therefore, it will suffice if we limit our presentation to certain representative skeletal parts. Emphasis will be placed on the general sequence of events in the evolution of the part in question, and only essential details will be given on the histologic findings at one stage or another in the development and maturation of the part. In line with the purpose of this chapter, intramembranous bone formation will be described as exemplified in the development of certain of the flat bones of the vault of the skull. Endochondral bone formation will be discussed as illustrated notably in the development of tubular bones of the appendicular skeleton. Some attention will also be devoted to the manner in which the vertebræ develop by way of several ossification centers appearing in separate primordial cartilage masses. Finally, some consideration will be given to the formation of joints, with particular emphasis on diarthrodial (synovial) joints, such as the knee joint.

INTRAMEMBRANOUS BONE FORMATION

At the site of development of the bones of the calvarial vault, the precursive mesenchyme gives rise, as noted, to a primitive connective tissue membrane. The frontal and parietal bones, for instance, develop in this membrane by way of intramembranous ossification. For the frontal bone, which is formed as two halves, a small center of ossification for each half is already manifest early in the ninth week of fetal life. For each parietal bone, such a center appears in the tenth week. In the regions destined to become the centers of ossification, and almost concurrently at various other points in the membranous rudiments of these bones, small groups of cells representing young osteoblasts become differentiated. These cells increase in number, cluster together, and show a tendency to arrange themselves in short irregular strands running in various directions. Constituting a sort of axis for these strands of osteoblasts there are bundles of delicate fibrils, apparently laid down by the osteoblasts and chemically akin to collagen. The fibrils increase in number, become matted together, and form an organic collagenous matrix between the osteoblasts.

Sooner or later, in consequence of certain complex local physicochemical changes, mineral matter (bone salt mineral) comes to be deposited in the organic matrix, and ossification is thus inaugurated. In the course of this, the trabeculæ of non-mineralized organic matrix surrounded by osteoblasts (trabeculæ of osteoid) become converted into trabeculæ of osseous tissue. Within a week or two after the appearance of the original ossification centers for the frontal and parietal bones, osteogenesis is well under way almost throughout the membranous rudiment, or anlage, of these bones (see Macklin, and Inman and Saunders). Specifically, the already mineralized trabeculæ grow by accretion of additional osseous tissue on their surfaces, while at the same time, through further differentiation of osteoblasts in the anlage, additional osteoid trabeculæ are being formed. These osteoid trabeculæ, too, rapidly become mineralized and likewise increase in size. Even at this stage, remodeling of the osseous tissue laid down is already in progress, and some osteoclasts are accordingly present. (See Fig. 1.)

In the course of formation and growth of the osteoid and osseous trabeculæ, some of the surface osteoblasts become entrapped within the substance of the matrix. These embedded osteoblasts constitute the bone cells (the osteocytes), and the space within which each lies in the matrix is called a lacuna. Though they no longer participate in the formation of new bone matrix, the osteocytes serve importantly in the physiologic maintenance of the matrix in which they are embedded. The osteoblasts on the surface of the trabeculæ continue to deposit new collagenous matrix. Since the latter is not instantly mineralized, detailed microscopic study of the trabeculæ will show, between the mineralized matrix and the osteoblasts, a very delicate border zone of matrix which stains more lightly (in hematoxylin-eosin—stained sections) than the mineralized matrix. It seems appropriate to the writer to refer to these delicate border zones as *physiologic osteoid* to contrast them with the wide osteoid borders observed in connection with such pathologic conditions as rickets and osteomalacia.

The osseous trabeculæ formed within the membranous precursor of the bones of the cranial vault increase in number and grow. Gradually, adjacent trabeculæ become contiguous to form an anastomosing lattice-like meshwork of osseous tissue whose spaces are wide and contain rather vascular connective tissue representing the embryonic bone marrow. As the trabeculæ thicken and the intertrabecular marrow spaces become better defined, the embryonal marrow gives place to marrow of a more mature type (red bone marrow). Concomitantly the persisting primitive connective tissue of the membrane becomes condensed on both the external and internal surfaces of the evolving bones to form a periosteal investment for them. Osseous tissue is then also added through the activity of osteoblasts which form from the cells of the deeper layers of the periosteum. However, most of the osseous tissue deposited by the periosteum is first laid down on the external (pericranial) surface of the evolving bones.

By the time of birth of the fetus, the frontal and parietal bones are in juxtaposition at the coronal suture, and the two halves of the frontal bone are still separated by the frontal suture. The two parietal bones are separated in the midline by the sagittal suture, and posteriorly these bones will be found to have grown to meet the occipital bone along the line of the lambdoidal suture. Anteriorly, in the junctional area between the frontal and parietal bones, there is a rather large gap which is filled by fibrous tissue (the anterior, or frontal, fontanel). Also in the median line between the parietal and occipital bones, there is a smaller gap likewise filled by fibrous tissue (the posterior, or occipital, fontanel). The fibrous tissue of the fontanels is continuous with the fibrous tissue filling the linear gaps (the sutures) between the various bones. The periosteum covering the outer surface of these bones (the pericranium) and the periosteum covering their inner surface (the dura mater) blend with the fibrous tissue of the sutures and fontanels.

At birth, the bones of the cranial vault are thin but relatively large in surface area. Growth in thickness occurs through the deposition of additional osseous tissue by the pericranium and dura respectively. However, since the cranial vault expands to accommodate growth of the brain, the accretion of new bone continues to be more active beneath the pericranium than beneath the dura. The fibrous membranes of the fontanels also undergo ossification, so that the bones separated at a fontanel come to meet. The anterior fontanel closes (becomes obliterated) during the second year of postnatal life, but the posterior fontanel is already closed at about 2 months after birth.

In the course of early childhood, the osseous tissue deposited on the pericranial surface becomes compacted to form an outer table. The delimitation of a clear-cut inner table lags somewhat behind, and in any event the inner table is thinner and less conspicuous than the outer. The osseous tissue between the tables remains cancellous, and this cancellous portion of the bones of the cranial vault is denoted as the diploë.

Growth in surface area of the cranial vault occurs through the addition of osseous tissue along the bone margins abutting on the sutures. This growth is slow and

Figure 1

A, Photomicrograph ($\times$ 65) illustrating an early stage of intramembranous ossification. The latter is occurring in the membranous anlage of a parietal bone of a fetus nearing the eleventh week of intra-uterine life. Note that the trabeculæ of newly formed primitive osseous tissue are small and still discrete. Some of them are clearly outlined by osteoblasts, which surround them. The organic matrix of the second trabecula from the left (the dark-staining one) is already well mineralized. Note also, above and to the left, the row of osteoblasts bordering upon a bundle of collagenous fibrils, only faintly discernible at this magnification.

B, Photomicrograph ($\times$ 45) showing the appearance of an evolving parietal bone of a fetus between 16 and 17 weeks of age. The further advance of intramembranous ossification is indicated notably by the increase in number and size of the trabeculæ and by the clear-cut delineation of an outer and an inner periosteal covering membrane. Osteogenesis has been much more lively in relation to the outer membrane (the pericranium) than in relation to the inner membrane (the dura).

C, Photomicrograph ($\times$ 45) illustrating the appearance of a developing parietal bone of a fetus 19 weeks of age. It is to be noted that the inner and outer covering membranes are now well delineated, and that new bone formation continues to be particularly active in relation to the outer covering membrane of the bone. In consequence of anastomosis of contiguous trabeculæ, the osseous tissue now appears as a lattice-like meshwork.

D, Photomicrograph ($\times$ 25) showing the histologic pattern of the parietal bone of a fetus near term. The osseous tissue is now rather compact, but one cannot yet distinguish a clear-cut outer and inner table separated by diploë.

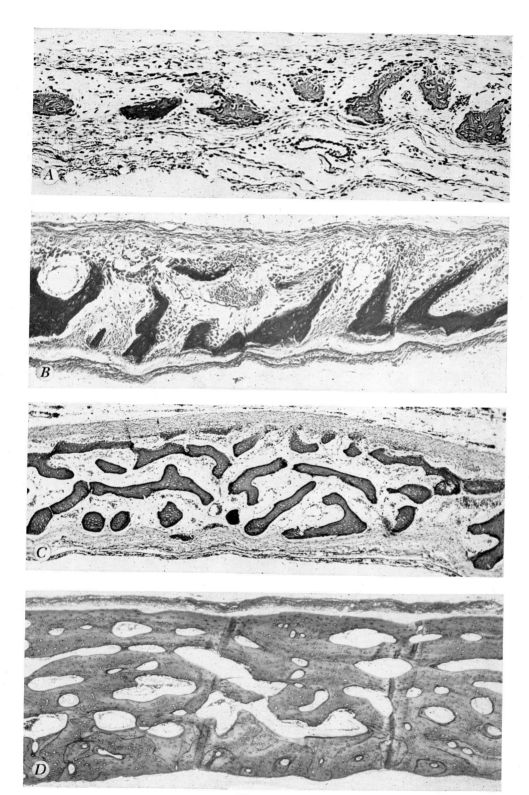

Figure 1

intermittent and continues for about the first 7 years of life. The suture between the two halves of the frontal bone usually disappears at some time between the sixth and tenth years of life, the two halves undergoing osseous fusion. The rest of the sutures of the cranial vault tend to disappear between the ages of 25 and 30 years. However, there is considerable variation both in sequence and in time of completion of the closures, and some sutures may persist, at least in part, even into old age (see Brooks, and Lachman).

In this sketch of the development and maturation of the bones of the cranial vault, details relating to the histologic composition of the osseous tissue being laid down have intentionally been omitted. Here a few general remarks on this point will suffice. In this connection, it is to be noted that the osseous tissue laid down early in the course of development of the frontal and parietal bones is of the nature of nonlamellar (coarse-fibered, or primitive) osseous tissue. The latter is characterized by the fact that its collagenous fibers are mainly coarse and irregularly arranged, and that its cells (the osteocytes) are large, relatively numerous, and not distributed in an orderly fashion. Subsequently, lamellar (fine-fibered, or mature) osseous tissue comes to be laid down. This type of osseous tissue is characterized by the fact that its collagenous fibers are delicate and grouped in orderly layers (lamellæ), and that its bone cells, too, show an orderly arrangement.

Even rather early in fetal life, some lamellar osseous tissue will already be found deposited on the existing nonlamellar osseous tissue. Thus the nonlamellar bone begins to yield to the lamellar. Slowly but surely, in the course of the continual transformation and repeated remodeling undergone by the growing frontal and parietal bones, all the nonlamellar bone comes to be replaced by lamellar bone. Details relating to the histologic features of nonlamellar and lamellar osseous tissue will be found in the chapter dealing with the structure of bone (p. 50).

ENDOCHONDRAL BONE FORMATION

The cartilage models of the bones preformed in cartilage (the bones of the extremities, the trunk, and part of the base of the skull) are well delineated even before the end of the embryonic period. This period extends approximately through the seventh week from the time of ovulation, and the crown-rump length of the embryo is then about 28 to 30 mm. (see Streeter). However, as has long been known, the cartilage models of the bones in question are only precursive structures. That is, in the development of these bones, the cartilage is substantially destroyed and synchronously replaced by osseous tissue. The process of destruction and removal of cartilage and its replacement by osseous tissue (whether this occurs in connection with skeletogenesis or even, for instance, during the repair of a fracture) is commonly denoted as "endochondral bone formation" or "endochondral ossification."

Endochondral ossification of the cartilage models of some bones (the humerus and femur, for instance) already begins shortly after the embryonic period has ended. In the course of the next few weeks (that is, still early in the fetal period), the cartilage models of certain other bones (for example, the metacarpals, metatarsals, and phalanges) begin to show endochondral ossification in their turn. However, there is a range of several weeks in regard to the onset of endochondral ossification in the cartilage models of these bones. In particular, some phalanges begin to ossify several weeks in advance of others, and this also holds true, to a more limited degree, for the various metacarpal and metatarsal bones. Endochondral ossification of the growing cartilage models of yet other bones (the calcaneus and talus) does not begin until late in the fetal period. Still other cartilage models do not present evidence of endochondral ossification for some months or even several years after the birth of the fetus. For example, the cartilage models of the capitate and hamate begin to undergo endochondral ossification about 2 months after birth, the tarsal navicular and middle cuneiform about 14 months, and the patella about 23 months (see Mall, Gray *et al.*, Noback, and Francis and Werle).

For the cartilage models of the long and short tubular bones of the extremities (with the exception of the terminal phalanges), the initial site of endochondral ossification is the midportion of the model. From this "primary ossification center" the endochondral ossification spreads toward the ends of the model. However, the cortex of the evolving tubular bone develops out of the mesenchyme investing the cartilage model, without going through a cartilage stage. That is, the cortex evolves by way of intramembranous ossification rather than by endochondral ossification.

At one or both ends of the evolving bone (depending upon the bone in question), a cartilaginous epiphysis is formed, and sooner or later this, too, develops a center of endochondral ossification. Any center of ossification formed in a bone after the primary center has appeared represents a so-called "secondary center of ossification." For the femur, for instance, the primary center of ossification for the shaft is usually already present by the ninth week of intra-uterine life. The center of ossification for the distal epiphysis of that bone (a secondary center) appears near the end of intra-uterine life and is always present in the full term fetus at birth. On the other hand, the secondary center for the femoral head usually does not appear until the third or fourth month of postnatal life. The secondary center for the greater trochanter is rather likely to be present by the thirtieth month, and that for the lesser trochanter by the eleventh year of postnatal life (see Francis).

DEVELOPMENT OF TUBULAR BONES

The development of the tubular bones of the limbs has received intensive investigation, based on both human and animal material. Anatomists from the turn of the century on have given many detailed descriptions of the morphologic sequence of events relating to the development of the limb bones and particularly the tubular bones (see Bardeen and Lewis, Bardeen, Braus, Streeter, and also Gardner).

In recent years, much light has also been shed on skeletogenesis by *in vitro* tissue culture studies of the developing rudiments of bones and joints (see Fell, Ray *et al.*, Chen, and Sevastikoglou). Concurrently, parallel studies were undertaken in which embryonic skeletal rudiments were removed and grafted or transplanted to one or another site (see Willis, Murray and Huxley, Lacroix, and Felts). All of these experimental studies have shown that the mesenchymal rudiment of a bone or joint exhibits a high degree of developmental autonomy (self-organization) even when removed from its natural environment. Indeed, the general form ultimately attained by a developing bone, bone part, or joint is largely the expression of the pattern of development inherent (or intrinsic) in the skeletogenetic tissue in question. In the total development of a skeletal part, extrinsic influences, such as local compressions and tensions, are subsidiary factors but do come to be reflected to some extent in the final shaping and maintenance of surface detail.

Studies on the morphology of the human embryo have shown that, early in the sixth week of embryonic life, the rudiments of the limb bones are represented merely by vaguely delimited condensations of mesenchyme. Toward the end of the sixth week, the mesenchymal condensations representing the future long tubular bones become more clear-cut, so that they actually suggest these bones. By the end of the seventh week, this is also true in regard to the mesenchymal condensations for the short tubular bones and, incidentally, for the other small bones of the hands and feet as well. The regions of the future joints are also already indicated, being represented by interzones of even less differentiated mesenchyme lying between and blending with the bone rudiments. During the early stages of their development, the latter increase in size through interstitial growth of the component mesenchyme and by additions from the less differentiated neighboring mesenchyme, including that in the interzones.

The Cartilage Model.—As exemplified in relation to an evolving long tubular bone, the mesenchymal condensation at first still merges at its periphery with the surrounding undifferentiated mesenchyme. At this stage, the bone rudiment is composed of a syncytium of cells whose nuclei are oval or round and closely compacted. Gradually, from its center toward the ends, the condensing mesenchyme becomes delimited from the neighboring undifferentiated mesenchyme and is transformed into precartilage. This conversion is associated with the appearance of intercellular matrix, or ground substance, between the previously compacted nuclei. As the precartilage core grows, its more developed central portion begins to be converted into true cartilage and to present rudiments of a perichondrium, while the ends are still precartilage. By further growth and differentiation, a clear-cut cartilage model of the future bone, surrounded by perichondrium, is eventually laid down. It is in the central portion that the cartilage cells are largest and most mature.

The perichondrium arises out of the mesenchymal tissue investing the cartilage model. Even early, the tissue which can justifiably be regarded as perichondrium consists of two layers. The cells of the outer layer are spindle-shaped and present evidence that they are growing into mere fibroblasts. The inner layer is less clearly defined. It is at first a thin mesenchymal syncytium of which the nuclei are large and vesicular while the cell boundaries are not distinct. The inner of the two layers just described possesses osteogenic potentialities, since osteoblasts develop out of the syncytium. The perichondrium becomes vascularized at this stage, but the cartilage model is still entirely avascular. (See Fig. 2.)

Figure 2

A, Photomicrograph ($\times$ 100) presenting an early stage in the delineation of two contiguous short tubular bones. The mesenchymal rudiments of these bones (from the hand of a 7-week embryo) stand out quite clearly, and it can be seen that the mesenchyme in the interior of these rudiments has already been transformed into precartilage.

B, Photomicrograph ($\times$ 11) showing the cartilage models of hand bones of a fetus early in its ninth week. In the midportions of the cartilage models of the phalanges and metacarpals, the cartilage cells are hypertrophic (see *C*). Note also that the metacarpophalangeal joints are well delineated, the interzonal mesenchyme between the contiguous cartilage models having been cleared away, and that each joint space is already closed off by a capsule. In contrast, the joints between the carpal bone models are not yet fully evolved.

C, Photomicrograph ($\times$ 54) depicting in some detail the histologic pattern presented by the proximal phalanx of the middle finger illustrated in *B*. In the midportion of the phalanx, the cartilage cell lacunæ are large, and many of them have become confluent. A very thin layer of osseous tissue is present beneath the perichondrium (periosteum) and bounds the hypertrophic cartilage on each side. Immediately beyond the zone of hypertrophy, the cartilage cell lacunæ appear flattened, and toward each end of the cartilage model, the lacunæ are small and round.

D, Photomicrograph ($\times$ 125) illustrating in histologic detail the midportion of the cartilage model of a metatarsal bone from a fetus 10 weeks old. The subperiosteal cuff of new bone stands out clearly. It surrounds the area in which the cartilage cells are hypertrophic and the intercellular cartilage matrix is calcified. It is to be observed that the cartilage cells become smaller as one moves away from the hypertrophic zone toward the upper and lower ends of the picture.

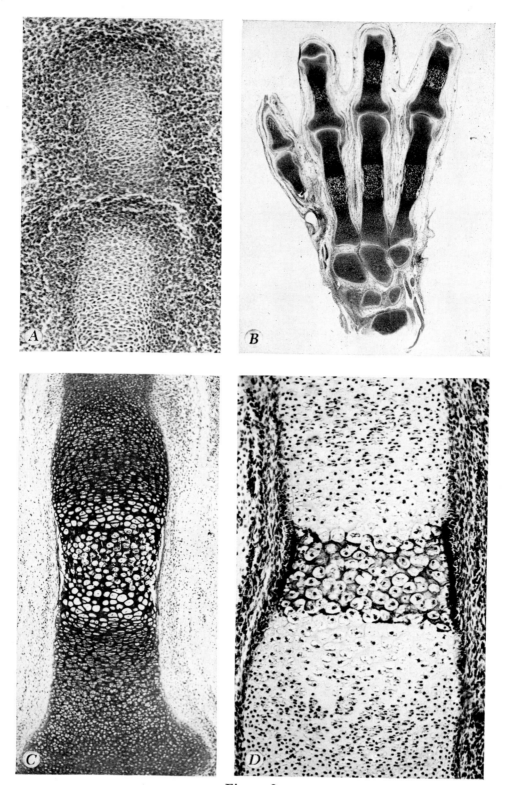

Figure 2

Early Phases of Replacement of the Cartilage Model.—An early indication that the cartilage model of a tubular bone is about to undergo replacement is the appearance of a thin cuff (or girdle) of osseous tissue around its middle. However, even before this happens, the cartilage of the model in the region in question already presents evidences of degeneration. Specifically, the cartilage cell lacunæ appear swollen and in many places confluent, the cartilage cell nuclei show signs of chromatolysis, and the chondromucinous matrix between the degenerating cells manifests calcification. The cuff of osseous tissue laid down around the degenerating cartilage represents the beginnings of the cortex of the evolving bone. This cortical shell develops, by way of intramembranous ossification, from osteoblasts which become differentiated in the inner, or osteogenetic, layer of the perichondrium (or periosteum, as it should now be called). As occurs in connection with intramembranous ossification in general, the osteoblasts increase in number, cluster together, and become arranged about bundles of collagen fibrils which they apparently lay down. The organic collagenous matrix between the osteoblasts becomes mineralized through the deposition of bone salt mineral, and ossification is thus inaugurated in the inner layer of the periosteum.

The formation of the periosteal osseous girdle is rapidly followed by the eruption of vasoformative tissue from the periosteum through the shell of new bone into the cartilage area in process of degeneration. The primitive blood channels enter the degenerating cartilage at many points and carry mesenchymal elements on their walls. The advancing vascular tissue erodes and breaks open the cartilage cell lacunæ. The destruction of the cartilage is facilitated by the accompanying mesenchyme, some of whose cells become chondroclasts and/or osteoclasts. The mesenchyme in question also gives rise to the osseous tissue laid down in the course of endochondral ossification of the model and to the marrow of the evolving bone.

In most long tubular bones, endochondral ossification is inaugurated as soon as the destruction and removal of cartilage in the center of the model is definitely under way. On the other hand, in the phalanges and other short tubular bones, the cartilage in the center of the model is likely to be extensively resorbed before endochondral bone is deposited. In birds, this lag is even more striking and affects

Figure 3

A, Photomicrograph (× 54) illustrating the initiation of endochondral ossification in the cartilage model of a pedal phalanx of a 14-week fetus. The arrow indicates the site of eruption of vasoformative tissue from the periosteum through the subperiosteal shell of new bone into the area in which the cartilage of the model is degenerating. Note that, in the area in question, many of the enlarged cartilage cell lacunæ have fused. As one goes from the hypertrophic zone downward toward the articular end of the model, the cartilage is found relatively more cellular, and the lacunæ are less prominent.

B, Photomicrograph (× 54) depicting the status of endochondral ossification in a manual phalanx (middle phalanx) of a fetus 18 weeks old. The arrow directs attention to the blood vessel in the nutrient canal. It is to be observed that the cartilage in the midshaft region has been cleared away and that a marrow cavity containing the primary bone marrow is now present. Note that the cortical shell has thickened and is increasing in length, in consequence of subperiosteal bone formation. It is apparent that, at each end of the developing shaft, cartilage destruction is in progress and the residual cartilage matrix is calcified.

C, Photomicrograph (× 45) illustrating the histologic pattern presented by a cross section of a tibia from a fetus early in the thirteenth week. There is evidence of active bone formation in relation to the inner layer (cambium layer) of the periosteum, the trabeculæ of new bone rapidly fusing with the cortical bone already present. The arrows direct attention to residual cores of calcified cartilage matrix. These indicate that the trabeculæ of bone present in the marrow cavity, and some of the bone apposed upon the inner surface of the cortex, represent osseous tissue formed in the course of endochondral ossification.

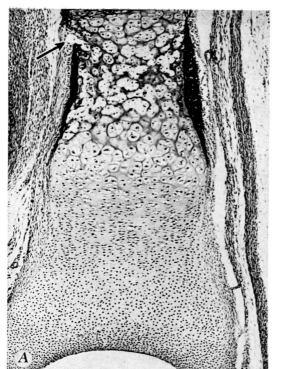

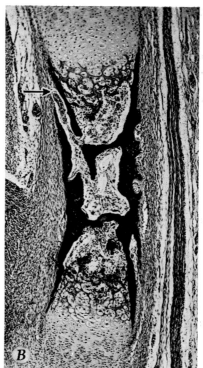

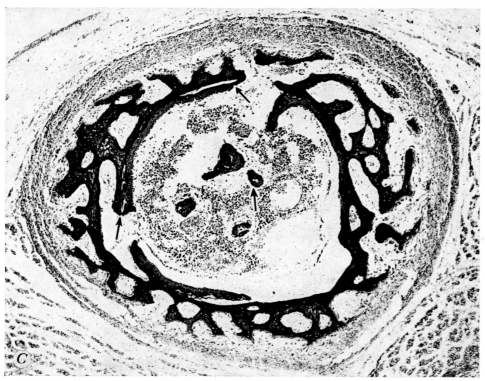

Figure 3

even the long tubular bones. Indeed, very little endochondral bone ever comes to be laid down in bird bones, and the latter are thus more or less hollow tubes created mainly by subperiosteal ossification (see Fell).

As exemplified in the femur of a human fetus, endochondral ossification begins at about the ninth week of intra-uterine life. The osteoblastogenic mesenchyme introduced on the blood vessels gives rise to osteoblasts, and these begin to deposit osseous tissue on the fragments of calcified cartilage matrix remaining at sites where the cartilage is being destroyed. Once started, endochondral ossification spreads from the center toward the ends of the cartilage model. Within about 2 weeks after the onset of endochondral ossification in a long tubular bone, approximately half of the shaft of the cartilage model has undergone this change. The line of advance of the ossification toward each end of the shaft is now represented by a well-defined endochondral growth zone. The cortex, which soon becomes multi-layered, likewise advances toward the epiphysial ends of the model. However, the line of advance of the periosteal ossification at each end is always a little ahead of the frontier for endochondral ossification.

The rapid advance of endochondral ossification toward the epiphysial ends of the cartilage model leaves behind a loose network of endochondral trabeculæ, some of which come to fuse with the already multilayered cortex. However, many of the endochondral trabeculæ are resorbed shortly after they have been formed, so that a marrow cavity is soon established. Those trabeculæ which persist become larger and thicker through the apposition of new bone, though these persisting endo-chondral trabeculæ, too, are subject to resorption and remodeling. Between the trabeculæ, a loose mesenchymal tissue is present which supports the blood vessels. This tissue may be regarded as the primary bone marrow, and it is the progenitor of the blood-forming elements of the marrow which already appear at about the beginning of the fourth month of intra-uterine life. (See Fig. 3.)

The shaft cortex is thickened through the deposition of new trabeculæ of sub-periosteal bone laid down more or less at right angles to the original cortical shell. With the progress of periosteal ossification, many of the ledges of transverse trabec-ulæ fuse in such a way as to enclose cavities containing blood vessels. These cavities constitute the relatively large primary haversian spaces of the evolving cortex.

Figure 4

A, Photomicrograph ($\times$ 45) demonstrating the pattern of the endochondral growth zone at the junction of the lower end of the femoral shaft with the evolving cartilaginous epiphysis in a fetus just past its twelfth week. Note that, from above down, the size of the lacunæ of the cartilage cells increases, and that the hypertrophic cartilage cells in the vicinity of the cartilage-shaft junction are arranged in rows. At the junction, the hypertrophic cartilage cells are being destroyed, and osseous tissue is being deposited on the residual calcified cartilage matrix (see *B*). The cortical shell surrounds the entire band of hypertrophic cartilage. (The inset ($\times$ 8) shows, from above down, the cartilaginous future epiphysis of the bone, the bandlike endochondral growth zone, and a small portion of the shaft abutting on that zone.)

B, Photomicrograph ($\times$ 125) illustrating certain histologic details relating to endochondral ossification occurring at the growth zone of the lower end of a femur in a fetus 16 weeks old. Note that the large and confluent cartilage cell lacunæ are being penetrated by vascular channels, thus exposing intervening cores of calcified cartilage matrix. Osteoblasts are de-positing osseous tissue on these cartilage matrix cores.

C, Photomicrograph ($\times$ 45) illustrating the histologic pattern presented by a cross section of a tibia from a fetus 20 weeks old. Note the relatively large primary haversian spaces in the cortex, and observe that the cortical bone has become more compact (compare with Fig. 3-*C*) on account of fusion of the trabeculæ of bone which had been laid down by the cambium layer of the periosteum.

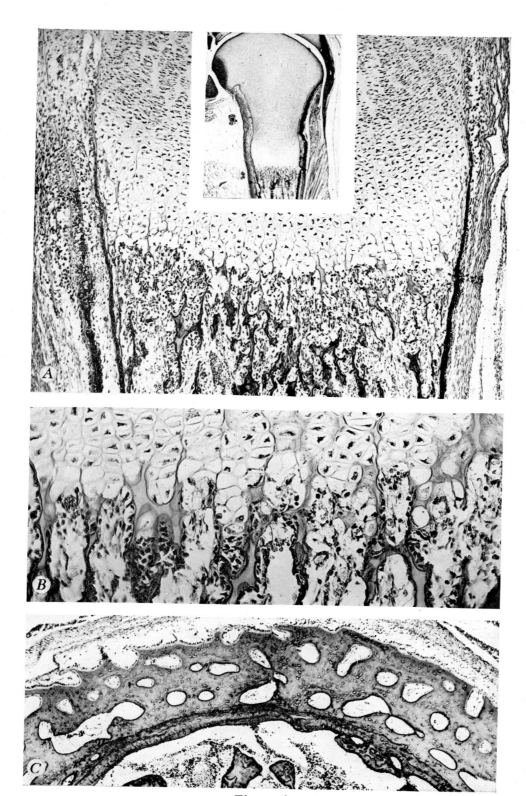

Figure 4

They communicate with the primary marrow cavity internally and the periosteal vessels externally. The marrow cavity of the shaft of the developing tubular bone soon becomes cylindrical in shape. Its sides are slightly concave, however, so that it is narrowest at the center.

Delineation of the Epiphysial Cartilage Plate Regions and Growth of the Shaft.—As endochondral bone formation advances toward each end of the cartilage model, a transverse band of proliferating cartilage becomes more and more clearly defined as the shaft grows in length and as the adjacent cartilaginous epiphysis enlarges. Indeed, the band takes on more and more clearly the aspects of a plate (*epiphysial cartilage plate*) as the contrast between it and the tissue above and below it increases. Both as band and as plate, it constitutes the principal site of longitudinal growth of the developing tubular bone. Wherever formed, the growth plate remains intact between the epiphysis and adjacent bone shaft until longitudinal growth is complete in the area in question. The manner of its subsequent disappearance is described on page 18.

Toward its epiphysial surface, the cartilage cells of the band, or plate, are relatively immature and transversely flattened. Toward its shaft surface, the cartilage cells are hypertrophied and arranged in fairly regular longitudinal columns. The sequence of events by which longitudinal growth progresses in the region of an epiphysial cartilage plate is approximately as follows: The flattened and relatively immature cartilage cells toward its epiphysial surface multiply. The new cells are displaced and move down toward the shaft surface of the plate. As they do so, their lacunæ enlarge and the cells eventually become arranged in longitudinal columns. The cartilage matrix between the cells in columnar arrangement becomes calcified. By the same process as that characterizing the earlier stages of endochondral ossification of the cartilage model, the hypertrophied cartilage cells of the plate area are invaded by vascular channels. Thus, at the junction of the plate with the shaft, blood vessels from the marrow penetrate and evacuate the enlarged cartilage cell lacunæ, many of which have become confluent. The degenerating cartilage cells are destroyed, and some of the calcified cartilage matrix is resorbed. On the remaining spicules of calcified cartilage matrix (the *primary spongiosa*), osteoblasts bordering on the blood vessels then deposit bone matrix, which rapidly becomes mineralized.

The area in which the calcified cartilage matrix of the primary spongiosa acquires its bone covering is called the *zone of provisional calcification* (or *ossification*). That zone is visible even grossly as a narrow yellow line apposed to the shaft surface of the plate. In the continuing process of endochondral ossification at the plate area, new cartilage cells are constantly moving down in mass formation from the more immature portion of the plate toward the zone of cartilage cell destruction and endochondral ossification. As the trabeculæ of bone containing cores of calcified cartilage matrix (the *secondary spongiosa*) are formed at the zone of provisional calcification, they move away from the epiphysial plate. That portion of the shaft into which they extend is known as the metaphysis. (See Fig. 4.)

In the course of the remodeling process (osteoclastic resorption and new bone formation) which is actively going on in the metaphysis, many of the trabeculæ of secondary spongiosa are resorbed before they have extended shaftward for any distance. Some of the trabeculæ which do extend shaftward fuse with, or even become incorporated in, the developing cortex of the bone. It is on this account that tissue sections of fetal bone cortex usually show small inclusions of calcified cartilage matrix at some distance from an epiphysial cartilage plate. (See Dodds, Dodds and Cameron, McLean and Bloom, Follis and Berthrong, Pritchard, and Sissons.)

While the evolving long bone is growing lengthwise internally at the plate regions, the periosteum is aiding in the further development of the cortex. Indeed, as the epiphyses are pushed apart by longitudinal growth of the shaft, the regional perichondrium and/or periosteum is depositing osseous tissue and thus increasing the length of the cortex. The cortical shell actually reaches to the epiphysial cartilage plates and even a little beyond the plates. The covering of the cortical shell in the general vicinity of the plate has been denoted as the "perichondrial zone," and Ranvier's ossification groove ("encoche d'ossification") is located in the zone in question (see Pratt).

Since the cartilaginous epiphysis grows in total mass (including width) and the adjacent epiphysial cartilage plate grows concurrently in width, an adjustment to preserve the basic shape and proportions of the bone end is necessary. In accordance with this need, the ends of the shaft must be continually reduced in width, for otherwise each end of the bone would become unduly bulbous. In this connection, the region of the shaft just below the plate is the site of continual remodeling in consequence of active osteoclastic resorption acting upon both the local spongy trabeculæ and the local cortex. Since the spongy trabeculæ formed in the peripheral zone of the plate tend to amalgamate with the neighboring cortex, it is the osseous tissue in that general area that requires the most active remodeling to ensure the normalization of the contour of the shaft end (see Leblond et al. and Tomlin et al.).

Concurrently with the increase in length of the shaft of a tubular bone, there is an increase in its width, and this is also associated with an increase in thickness of the cortex, particularly in its diaphysial portion. In this connection, the shaft cortex is subjected to continual removal by resorption on its internal surface and to accretion by new bone deposition on its subperiosteal surface. In consequence, not only does the cortex thicken, but those endochondral trabeculæ which had become fused with, and incorporated in, the cortex undergo resorption in the course of the continuous remodeling.

Growth and Ossification of the Cartilaginous Epiphyses.—The epiphyses form from the ends of the cartilage model beyond the epiphysial plate regions. Most tubular bones evolve an epiphysis at each end. Some, such as the phalanges and the metacarpal and metatarsal bones, ordinarily form this structure at one end only. Not long after they are established, the cartilaginous epiphyses are penetrated by canals containing blood vessels. By the third month of intra-uterine life, the epiphyses of many of the long tubular bones already contain at least a few canals of this kind. By the seventh fetal month, the cartilage vessel canals are well developed in all epiphyses of the larger tubular bones. The number of such canals in an epiphysis depends upon the particular one in question. At birth, as many as 15 main canals (excluding branches) are present in the epiphysis of the lower end of the femur. (See Fig. 5.)

Most of the canals enter the epiphysis at right angles to its surface and burrow centripetally. However, they do not break in where tendons and ligaments are attached. They carry blood vessels derived mainly from the inner layer of the adjacent perichondrium, and these nourish the cartilage of the epiphysis. A cartilage vessel canal is lined by connective tissue. It contains one or possibly two arteries and two or at most three distended veins. The present writer has also observed some canals in which the usual arteries and veins were surrounded by a capillary plexus of vessels. As they extend through the epiphysis, the cartilage vessel canals branch only dichotomously. Anastomosis between separate canals occurs very seldom, being found typically only in the head of the humerus, but reunion of the branches of one canal occurs frequently. In older epiphyses, some of the vessel canals enter close to the epiphysial cartilage plate and run parallel with it. They direct a few branches at right angles toward the plate. In this way, intercommunication between the epiphysial and diaphysial blood vessels apparently occurs, though there is not complete agreement on this point (see Langer, Hintzsche, Lexer *et al.*, and Harris).

After vascularization of the cartilaginous epiphysis, months and often years elapse before a center of ossification appears in it. There is no precise time relation between the formation of vessel canals in the cartilage and the initiation of its ossification. Thus, for instance, vessels appear even earlier in the cartilage model of the patella than in that of the lower epiphysis of the femur. An ossification center, however, does not appear in the patella until about the third or fourth year of postnatal life, while in the lower epiphysis of the femur it usually appears somewhat before birth.

The onset of endochondral ossification in the cartilaginous epiphysis of a tubular bone, as in the cartilage model of its shaft, is first indicated by a tiny focus of cartilage cell degeneration, more or less in its center. The site at which ossification begins in the epiphysis is apparently that in which its nutrition is poorest. In this area the cartilage cell lacunæ enlarge and become confluent, the cell nuclei degenerate, and the intercellular matrix calcifies. It is worth noting in this connection that the inception of ossification does not involve regressive disappearance of the cartilage canals. After degenerative changes have taken place in the cartilage cells, their lacunæ are eroded by vascular sprouts growing out of the preformed cartilage canals. Then osteoblasts derived from embryonal connective tissue within the canals deposit osseous tissue upon the residual spicules of calcified matrix, and the epiphysial center of ossification is initiated.

The center continues to grow centrifugally by endochondral ossification. At the same time, the epiphysis as a whole is increasing in size through continued growth of the cartilage surrounding the center, or nucleus, of ossification. Growth of the nucleus is relatively rapid at first but slows down after the center has become fairly large. Between the center of ossification and the joint surface, there is a layer of cartilage which gradually thins as maturity approaches. However, endochondral ossification around the center does not come to a halt until some time after endochondral ossification at the neighboring epiphysial cartilage plate has ceased. The thin coat of persisting cartilage then becomes the definitive articular cartilage. (See Fig. 6.)

Figure 5

A, Photomicrograph ($\times$ 9) showing a knee area of a 16-week fetus. The cartilaginous epiphyses for the lower end of the femur and the upper end of the tibia are well delineated, as is the cartilaginous precursor of the patella. Note that these various structures contain cartilage vessel canals. The latter tend to enter them more or less at right angles to the surface, and it is clear that some canals are extending centripetally.

B, Photomicrograph ($\times$ 4) depicting the histologic pattern presented by the lower end of a femur of an infant 3 months old. The cartilaginous epiphysis reveals a well-developed center of ossification. The light, ringlike zone surrounding the center represents hypertrophic cartilage which is undergoing endochondral ossification. The latter accounts for the continuing centrifugal growth of the epiphysial ossification center. At the junction of the epiphysis and the shaft, one can note a corresponding light zone of cartilage representing the evolving epiphysial cartilage plate area, where longitudinal growth of the bone shaft occurs— likewise through endochondral ossification. (See also Figs. 6-*A* and *B*.)

C, Photomicrograph ($\times$ 9) showing the histologic pattern presented by the lower end of a femur of a child 3 years old. The epiphysial center of ossification is relatively large, and now there is only a narrow border of cartilage surrounding it. Endochondral ossification is still evident around the periphery of the center, but growth of the center as a whole has slowed down. Above the ossification center for the epiphysis, one can see the clearly delimited epiphysial cartilage plate, where endochondral ossification is still active. (See also Figs. 6-*C* and *D*.)

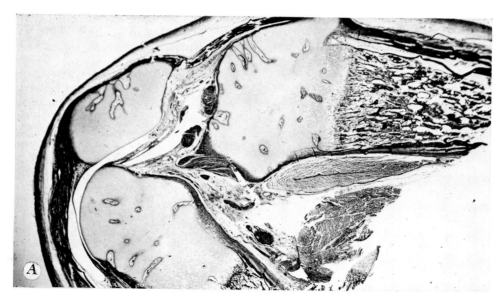

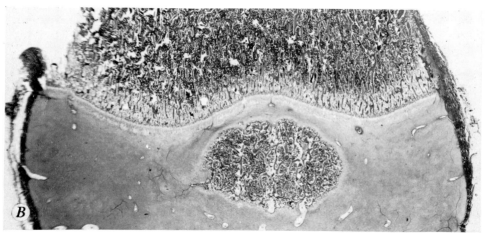

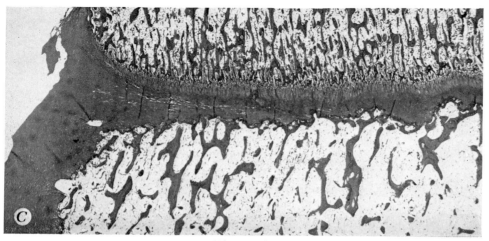

Figure 5

Many vertebrates, even low ones, develop cartilaginous epiphyses or their homologues. However, in most genera below mammals, centers of ossification do not appear in these structures. Nevertheless, in several groups of reptiles, notably lizards, the epiphyses are highly developed, and many of them ossify (see Lubosch).

Fusion of Epiphysis with Shaft.—After the epiphysis has developed a clear-cut center of ossification, the epiphysial cartilage plate stands out as a real disk between the epiphysis and the adjacent part of the shaft. With increasing age, the plate tends to become thinner. In any long bone, even during the period of active growth, it is never more than a few (1 to 3) millimeters thick. This thickness varies from bone to bone. Furthermore, it is different at opposite ends of the same bone. The plate is always thicker at the more actively growing end of the bone—for instance, at the lower end of the femur than at the upper end, and at the upper end of the tibia than at the lower. When pressure is made against the end of a long bone to separate the epiphysis from the diaphysis, the plate remains with the former. This is also so when, in children, an epiphysis has been traumatically avulsed.

Fusion of the ossified epiphysis with the shaft is associated with the disappearance of the intervening plate. Some time before the latter is obliterated, proliferative activity ceases in it, and the plate becomes "closed." In the process of closure,

Figure 6

A, Photograph showing the cut surface of the lower end of a femur from an infant 3 months old. Note the center of ossification for the lower femoral epiphysis, and the epiphysial cartilage plate which is being delimited between it and the shaft. Extending transversely along the junction of the shaft with the epiphysis, the zone of provisional calcification is faintly visible (see arrows). The photomicrograph shown in Figure 5-B was prepared from a histologic tissue section made from this specimen.

B, Roentgenograph representing the specimen shown in A. The zone of provisional calcification stands out particularly well on the right as a delicate radiopaque line between the epiphysis and the shaft.

C, Photograph showing the cut surface of the lower end of a femur from a child 3 years old. The epiphysial cartilage plate now stands out clearly between the shaft and the epiphysis, whose center of ossification has become fairly large but is still surrounded by a border of proliferating cartilage. The photomicrograph shown in Figure 5-C was prepared from a histologic tissue section made from this specimen.

D, Roentgenograph representing the specimen illustrated in C. The epiphysial cartilage plate stands out as a radiolucent zone between the shaft and the epiphysis. The relatively radiopaque zone at the end of the shaft is the area in which the cores of calcified cartilage matrix extending from the plate have been clothed by osseous tissue in the course of endochondral ossification.

E, Photograph illustrating the cut surface of the lower end of a femur from a boy 12 years of age. Note that the epiphysial cartilage plate is thinner than it is in C, and that it is undulated. These appearances are related to the fact that endochondral ossification at the plate has slowed down.

F, Roentgenograph prepared from the specimen illustrated in E. In conformity with the slowing down of endochondral ossification, the radiolucent zone representing the plate area is now quite narrow. Furthermore, as compared with D, the end of the shaft in the vicinity of the plate does not show a conspicuous zone of radiopacity, such as would indicate lively endochondral ossification at that site.

G, Photograph showing the cut surface of the lower end of a femur from a boy 15 years of age. Note that the plate is very thin and quite undulate and is apparently interrupted in some places. These appearances reflect the fact that the plate is well on the way toward obliteration. (Compare with E.)

H, Roentgenograph prepared from the specimen illustrated in G. The plate area is no longer represented by a clear-cut radiolucent zone traversing the epiphysis-shaft junction completely, though traces of it are still visible (see arrow).

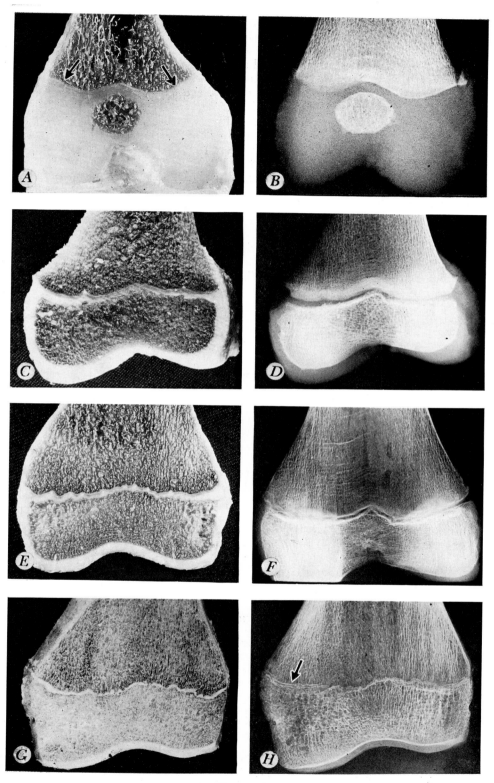

Figure 6

the cells of the plate become irregularly disposed, the intercellular matrix becomes calcified, proliferation on its diaphysial surface comes to an end, and this surface is now lined by trabeculæ of bone. Blood vessels from the shaft invade the closed plate, disrupting it into small islands of cartilage entirely surrounded by bone. The residual fragments of plate are slowly "squeezed out of existence" by the process of creeping replacement. The spongy trabeculæ of the epiphysis then become fused with those of the shaft, and finally all remnants of the cartilage plate disappear. The epiphysis and diaphysis are now firmly synostosed. Final maturation of the epiphysis is associated with termination of endochondral growth on the deep surface of the articular cartilage and the closing off of this surface by arches of spongy bone constituting the bony end plate. As already noted, this occurs only after the epiphysial cartilage plate has disappeared.

After this, a "fusion line" (sometimes denoted as the "epiphysial scar") may mark the former site of the plate. This line is recognizable in the x-ray picture as a narrow, transverse zone of increased density. It represents a number of spongy trabeculæ which run across the bone more or less at right angles to the longitudinally directed trabeculæ. The fusion lines are observed most clearly in the long tubular bones of the lower extremity (see Cope). At the lower end of the femur and at the upper end of the tibia, fusion lines frequently persist until late in life. The present writer has observed the persistence of fusion lines in both ends of the femur and in the upper end of the tibia even in cases in which these bones have undergone severe atrophy in consequence of inactivity. It is of some interest that the sites of persisting fusion lines in man are the sites which in the rat manifest late disappearance of the epiphysial cartilage plate (see Dawson).

Finally, it should be noted that the lines marking the sites of epiphysial fusion should not be confused with the "lines of arrested growth due to disease," to which Harris has devoted so much attention. In children who have had bouts of severe illness, the metaphyses of long bones may show, in the x-ray picture, multiple transverse lines (the so-called Harris lines) representing periods of arrested growth. These lines are also visible grossly and can be demonstrated in tissue sections as transverse trabeculæ. The longitudinal trabeculæ in the area have become atrophic, and they are also sparser than they would normally be (p. 66). (See Figs. 7 and 19.)

DEVELOPMENT OF VERTEBRAE

The components of the vertebral column develop from mesenchymal cells which migrate from both sides toward the midline. These cells become aggregated in clusters at intervals along and about the notochord. The individual cell aggregates

Figure 7

A, Photomicrograph ($\times$ 6) demonstrating the status of the epiphysial cartilage plate at the upper end of a radius from a girl 17 years old. Toward the left, the plate is still intact, though under higher magnification (see B) it is clear that endochondral ossification has already ceased in this area and that the shaft surface of the plate is being closed off by osseous tissue. Toward the right (see C) the degenerating plate has been breached in several places, and at the extreme right, synostosis has already taken place between the epiphysis and the shaft.

B, Photomicrograph ($\times$ 30) illustrating in greater detail the histologic appearance presented by that part of the epiphysial cartilage plate shown in A which is inactive but not yet disrupted.

C, Photomicrograph ($\times$ 30) illustrating in greater detail the area shown on the extreme right in A. The fragment of epiphysial cartilage plate shown is calcified, and trabeculæ of osseous tissue span the area where the plate has been destroyed.

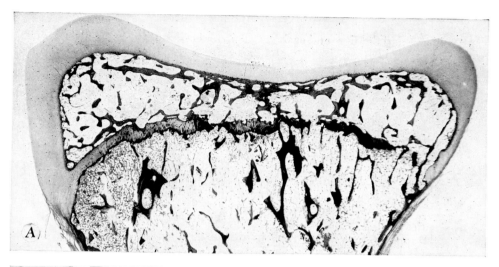

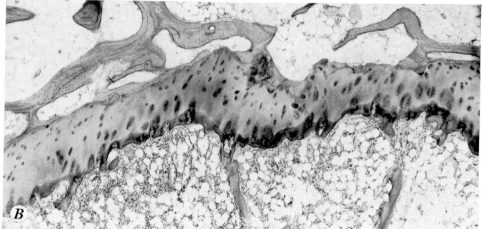

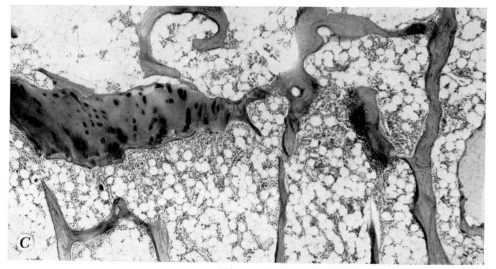

Figure 7

increase in size and density, and each mesenchymal cell mass becomes the rudiment for the body (or centrum) of a vertebra. Soon after the centrums take shape, paired mesenchymal concentrations extend dorsally and laterally from them to surround the neural tube. The mesenchymal concentrations in question thus establish the rudiments for each neural arch, the ribs in the thoracic region, and the rib homologues in the other parts of the column. (See Bardeen, Williams, Wyburn, and also Sensenig.)

The mesenchymal rudiments for the evolving vertebral bodies are soon converted into precartilage and then into cartilage, and shortly afterward the rudiments for the neural arches and any associated ribs undergo these changes. The cartilaginous model of a vertebra is at first a unit, presenting no lines of demarcation between the body and the neural arch and not even a clear-cut delimitation between the body and the adjacent rib rudiments. However, after endochondral ossification sets in, the rib cartilages in the thoracic region do become clearly set off from the vertebræ through the delimitation of the future costovertebral and costotransverse joints.

Except in the cervical region of the column, endochondral ossification of the cartilage model of a vertebra usually begins somewhat earlier in the vertebral body than in its arch. By the thirteenth week of intra-uterine life, the cartilage models of all the thoracic and lumbar vertebræ already show a well-developed ossification center for the body of the vertebra and a center on each side of the cartilaginous neural arch. On the other hand, by the eleventh week of intra-uterine life, the neural arches of the evolving cervical vertebræ already have an ossification center on each side. However, the centers for the bodies of the various cervical vertebræ do not begin to make their appearance until 2 or 3 weeks later, at the earliest.

In the course of chondrification and ossification of the mesenchyme which forms the body of the vertebra, the segment of notochordal tissue which had become encased within the ossification center undergoes obliteration. Indeed, the disappearance of the segments of notochord within the vertebral bodies is already well under way during the second month of intra-uterine life. Nevertheless, the notochordal tissue between the developing bodies (that is, in the areas in which the intervertebral disks appear) persists for some time in the nucleus pulposus of the

Figure 8

A, Photomicrograph ($\times$ 12) illustrating the histologic appearance of a transversely sectioned thoracic vertebra from a fetus 14 to 15 weeks old. The cartilaginous model of the vertebral body presents vessel canals and a well-developed ossification center. On the left, a cartilaginous neural arch with its center of ossification is to be observed. The corresponding neural arch for the right side is incomplete because the block of tissue from which the section was prepared was cut off-center. Posteriorly, the two neural arch centers are advancing to surround the spinal canal, and both neural arches are advancing laterally to form transverse processes. Note also on the left the cartilaginous end of a rib and the corresponding costovertebral joint.

B, Photomicrograph ($\times$ 30) illustrating the histologic appearance (in longitudinal section) of several developing thoracic vertebræ, likewise from a fetus in its fourteenth to fifteenth week. The centers of ossification for the vertebral bodies stand out clearly, as do the intervertebral disks. In one of the intervertebral disks (see arrow), one can see a remnant of the notochord, the histologic details of which are shown in C. (The block of tissue from which the section was prepared had been cut off-center, and this fact accounts for the lack of symmetry in the illustration.)

C, Photomicrograph ($\times$ 125) showing in detail the fragment of notochord indicated by the arrow in B. Above and below, the notochordal tissue extends into the cartilage of the adjacent bodies.

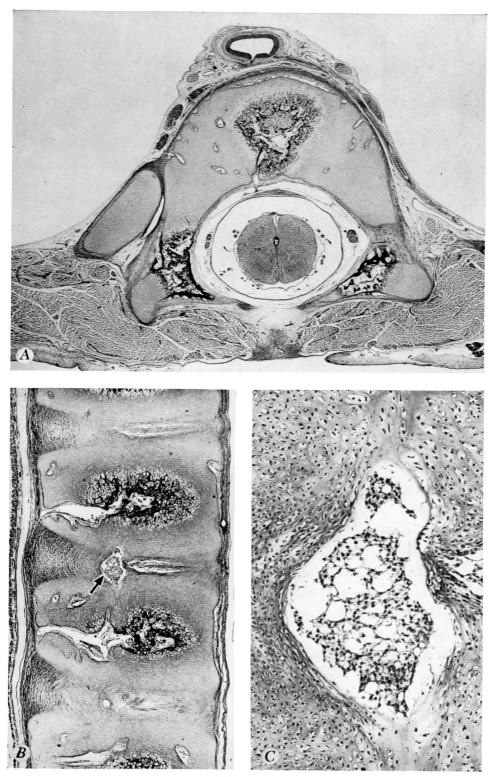

Figure 8

23

disks. At its cranial end the notochord becomes substantially obliterated in the course of development of the base of the skull in the vicinity of the foramen magnum. However, remnants of notochordal tissue not infrequently persist in relation to the pharyngeal surface of the base of the skull and on the cranial aspect of the base (or possibly even within the bone) in the vicinity of the spheno-occipital synchondrosis. In the sacrococcygeal region the notochord is continued into the tail end of the embryo. In this region, too, the notochord undergoes regression and involution, but it is not unusual for notochordal remnants to persist, especially in and about the end of the coccyx—a fact which explains the relatively high incidence of chordomas in the sacrococcygeal region (see Jaffe).

The center of ossification for the body of the vertebra enlarges, and at the same time the center for each half of the neural arch also grows. Posteriorly, the two centers for the arch advance to surround the spinal canal. Ventrally, they advance toward the ossification center for the body, and laterally they extend outward to form the transverse processes. (See Fig. 8.)

At birth, all the vertebræ, with the possible exception of the last sacral and the first coccygeal, already consist largely of osseous tissue. However, cartilage is still to be found along the line of junction of each side of the neural arch with the vertebral body, and in the spinous, transverse, and articular processes. Also, a plate of hyaline cartilage, representing the analogue of an epiphysial cartilage plate of a tubular bone, covers the upper and lower surface of each body. Longitudinal

Figure 9

A, Photomicrograph ($\times$ 8) showing part of the lower portion of the ninth thoracic vertebral body and part of the upper portion of the tenth, along with part of the corresponding intervertebral disk, from a male 16 years old. The arrows direct attention to the epiphysial (secondary) centers of ossification for the upper and lower margins, respectively, of these bodies. Note that the thin plate of cartilage (appearing dark) which separates the centers of ossification from the main part of each vertebral body is continuous with the cartilage which covers the surfaces of these adjacent bodies. Note also that the cartilage between these secondary centers and the vertebral bodies proper is in the process of being disrupted. For a three-dimensional gross view of the marginal ringlike epiphysial centers of ossification developing around the upper and lower borders of each vertebral body, see *C*.

B, Photomicrograph ($\times$ 8) showing part of the lower portion of the twelfth thoracic and the upper portion of the first lumbar vertebral body, along with part of the corresponding intervertebral disk, from a male 20 years old. The epiphysial centers of ossification are no longer distinguishable as such, having fused with the corresponding bodies, and the intervening cartilage plates have been destroyed. The arrows direct attention to the smoothly arched contour of the lower and upper margins, respectively, of the two adjacent vertebral bodies. This arched area represents the bony marginal ridge (see *D*), which is an important site of anchorage for the annulus fibrosus.

C, Photograph of a macerated segment of vertebral column from a female 14 years of age illustrating the appearance of the epiphysial centers of ossification of thoracic vertebral bodies at that age. The ossification centers around the upper and lower margins of the vertebral body appear as beaded circlets of osseous tissue. In the course of the next few years, the contiguous bony foci of each circlet would have fused to form a solid bony ring, and the latter would have fused with the vertebral body in consequence of destruction of the cartilage between the ringed epiphysis and the body.

D, Photograph of a macerated first lumbar vertebra from a male 20 years of age. The intervertebral disk tissue has been completely removed by the maceration, so that the entire superior surface of the body is exposed. In the central part of the picture, the finely porous spongiosa of the body is revealed. One sees, extending around the periphery of the body, the arched bony marginal ridge, which is more prominent and wider anterolaterally than posteriorly.

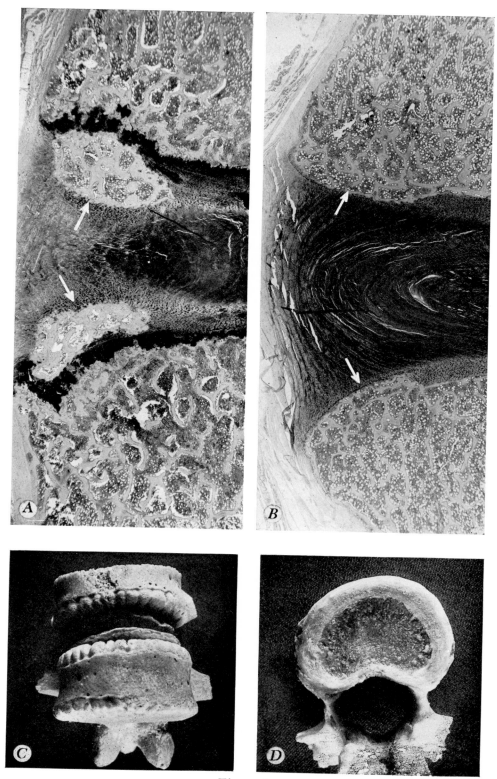

Figure 9

growth of the vertebral body occurs through endochondral ossification at these plates. Growth in length of the developing processes likewise takes place through endochondral ossification. However, growth in width and/or thickness of the body and the processes occurs through intramembranous ossification—that is, through the deposition of bone by the periosteum.

Bony union of the osseous components of a vertebra begins during early childhood. It occurs through obliteration of the synchondrosis between the ossification center for the body and each of the paired ossification centers for the neural arch. Posteriorly, the two ossification centers for the neural arch fuse, and the ossification extends into the cartilaginous model of the spinous process. However, in the case of the neural arches of the sacral vertebræ and the posterior arch of the atlas, fusion with the corresponding ossification centers of the body does not take place until late in childhood and sometimes not at all.

In the young child, the thin plate of hyaline cartilage which covers the upper and lower surface of each vertebral body terminates at its periphery in a thick ring of cartilage. Each ring of cartilage (the cartilaginous marginal ridge) is set in a groove which extends around the upper and lower border of the developing vertebral body. At some time between the seventh and ninth year, a number of foci of endochondral ossification appear in each cartilaginous marginal ridge, and the epiphysial centers of ossification (secondary centers) for the vertebral body are thus established. As the individual foci of ossification enlarge, they fuse and form (by about the twelfth year) a continuous osseous ridge around the upper and lower margins of the vertebra. For the next few years, each osseous marginal ridge remains separated from the vertebral body proper by a thin plate of cartilage.

However, by the time the subject is 14 or 15 years of age, the cartilage plate between each marginal ridge and the vertebral body proper comes to be disrupted by invading blood vessels. In time, the intervening cartilage plates are completely destroyed, and bony fusion of the osseous marginal ridge with the vertebral body takes place. This does not, of course, occur simultaneously in all vertebræ. In the lumbar vertebræ, in particular, the synostosis of the marginal ridges with the rest of the vertebral body is sometimes not complete before the age of 25.

Like its cartilaginous predecessor, the ringlike osseous marginal ridge is more prominent along the anterior margin of the body than laterally and posteriorly.

Figure 10

A, Photomicrograph ($\times$ 25) showing, in the longitudinal plane, the histologic appearance of a knee area from a fetus 8 weeks old. The joint capsule is well delineated anteriorly, though not yet posteriorly, and one of the cruciate ligaments stands out clearly. The synovial mesenchyme is loose-meshed, but no clear-cut joint space is visible yet between the femur and tibia. This is so because the section runs through the midportion of the joint area rather than through the periphery, where, at this age, liquefaction of the synovial mesenchyme to form the articular cavity is already under way in its progress toward the interior.

B, Photomicrograph ($\times$ 25) showing an ankle and the rear part of a foot from the same fetus whose knee area is illustrated in *A*. Note that the cartilage models of the bone parts shown are still separated only by narrow strands of interzonal mesenchyme in which cavitation has not yet taken place.

C, Photomicrograph ($\times$ 20) showing, in the longitudinal plane, the histologic appearance of a knee area from a fetus 10 weeks old. Note that the articular cavity is well developed, that the capsule is complete and lined by a synovial membrane, and that the menisci are well formed. Since the section was cut far off-center, only a small fragment of the cartilage model of the patella is apparent.

D, Photomicrograph ($\times$ 30) illustrating a metacarpophalangeal joint of a fetus 21 weeks old. Note the well-formed joint capsule and articular cavity and the infoldings of synovial membrane somewhat suggestive of menisci in their architecture.

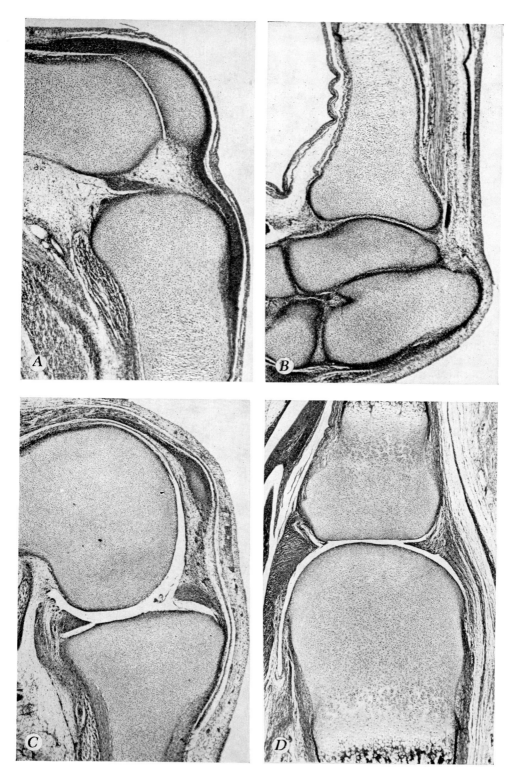

Figure 10

At any rate, the marginal ridge serves as the most important site of anchorage for the annulus fibrosus of the intervertebral disk. Furthermore, the anterior longitudinal ligament fuses with the outer fibers of the annulus and is thus firmly anchored to the upper and lower margins of the vertebral body at its ridge-cortex junctions. (See Fig. 9.)

DEVELOPMENT OF JOINTS

In its finished form, a joint is essentially a bridged space between two or more bones. The bones may be so joined that the resulting articulation is rigid (a synarthrosis), somewhat movable (an amphiarthrosis), or freely movable at least in one plane (a diarthrosis).

A *synarthrosis* is characterized not only by its immobility but by the complete absence of a joint space and by the sparsity of the intermediary tissue. Indeed, in the formation of a synarthrosis, all but a vestige of the tissue originally connecting the bones is gradually replaced by the encroaching bone ends. Such joints are well exemplified in the sutures of the skull. At the sutures, the margins of the adjacent bones are virtually in contact, being separated merely by a thin fibrous membrane known as the sutural ligament. During early adult life, many of the sutures even become obliterated in consequence of osseous fusion of the adjacent bones (see Pritchard *et al.*).

In the formation of an *amphiarthrosis*, the mesenchyme between the developing bones is converted into fibrous tissue which, in turn, tends to become fibrocartilage. In such a joint there is again no genuine articular space and no capsule or synovial membrane, but some motion is nevertheless possible. The most important amphiarthroses are the joints between the vertebral bodies, where the junctures are made by the intervertebral disks. Such a disk consists of two hyaline cartilage plates, the nucleus pulposus, and the annulus fibrosus. The plates (one covering each of the apposed vertebral bodies) are sites of endochondral bone growth and correspond to the epiphysial cartilage plates of the tubular bones. The nucleus, which occupies the interior of the disk, is semigelatinous, contains some collagen fibers, and, in a young subject, may, as indicated, still show remnants of the notochord. The annulus fibrosus is a thick ring of highly collagenous fibrous tissue which surrounds the nucleus. Its fibers are anchored to the cartilage plate and the marginal ridge of each adjacent vertebral body and also blend with the fibers of the longitudinal ligament (see Peacock, and Walmsley).

In accordance with its potentiality for free motion, a *diarthrosis* possesses a clear-cut articular cavity. The latter is lined by synovial membrane and is delimited by a fibrous capsule which is attached to the bone ends of the joint beyond their articular cartilages. In addition, a diarthrosis may have accessory intra-articular structures, such as menisci and/or ligaments.

The site where a diarthrodial (or synovial) joint is to appear between developing bone rudiments is marked by a well-defined interzone of still-undifferentiated mesenchyme. The evolutionary changes involved in the formation of the joint take place in this interzonal mesenchyme and in the general mesenchyme neighboring upon the area in question. The central portion of the interzonal mesenchyme becomes loose-meshed, while the general mesenchyme neighboring on the rudimentary bone ends becomes vascularized. That portion of the general mesenchyme which is adjacent to the loose-meshed interzonal mesenchyme becomes continuous with the latter. Together they constitute the so-called synovial mesenchyme.

The joint capsule is formed through condensation of the outer portion of the general (or extrablastemal) mesenchyme. The joint space begins to form near the periphery of the synovial mesenchyme and advances centripetally. The ultimate single space is constituted through confluence of many smaller cavities which become manifest as that mesenchyme continues to loosen and (apparently) liquefies. In a knee area, for instance, an articular cavity begins to form at about the seventh week of intra-uterine life (that is, by the end of the embryonic period). Once started, the development of the cavity progresses very rapidly. Indeed, practically all of the diarthrodial joints already present well-delineated articular cavities by the time the fetus is about 10 weeks old. In any case, the synovial mesenchyme gives rise to the synovial membrane and to menisci and/or ligaments in joints which develop these structures. (See Fig. 10.)

As the synovial mesenchyme recedes and the joint space forms, the convex cartilaginous end of the articulation is etched out before the apposed concave or flat end. Further development of the joint during the fetal period consists largely of maturation of structures already differentiated. Thus the subsequent modeling of the apposed convex and concave surfaces of the joint seems to proceed independently. The depth of the concavity (as exemplified at the hip joint) is the result not so much of yielding of this end to the convexity as of deepening of the hollow by growth and extension of its margin, or lip. At the same time, the capsule becomes more collagenous, and, if the joint possesses menisci and ligaments, the latter, too, become more collagenous. Synovial villi are to be observed by about the third month of fetal life. In the interphalangeal joints, in particular, short, infolded projections of synovial membrane, somewhat analogous to menisci, are to be observed extending from the capsule into the joint space. (See Lubosch, Haines, O'Rahilly, and also Gardner.)

REFERENCES

BARDEEN, C. R.: Studies of the Development of the Human Skeleton, Am. J. Anat., *4*, 265, 1905·
————: The Development of the Thoracic Vertebræ in Man, Am. J. Anat., *4*, 163, 1905·
————: Early Development of the Cervical Vertebræ and the Base of the Occipital Bone in Man, Am. J. Anat., *8*, 181, 1908.
BARDEEN, C. R., and LEWIS, W. H.: Development of the Limbs, Body-Wall and Back in Man, Am. J. Anat., *1*, 1, 1901.
BERNAYS, A.: Die Entwicklungsgeschichte des Kniegelenkes des Menschen, mit Bemerkungen über die Gelenke im Allgemeinen, Morphol. Jahrb., *4*, 403, 1878.
BRAUS, H.: Gliedmassenpfropfung und Grundfragen der Skeletbildung. I. Die Skeletanlage vor Auftreten des Vorknorpels und ihre Beziehung zu den späteren Differenzierungen, Morphol. Jahrb., *39*, 155, 1909.
BROOKS, S. T.: Skeletal Age at Death: The Reliability of Cranial and Pubic Age Indicators, Am. J. Phys. Anthropol., *13*, 567, 1955.
CHEN, J. M.: Studies on the Morphogenesis of the Mouse Sternum. II. Experiments on the Origin of the Sternum and its Capacity for Self-Differentiation *in vitro*, J. Anat., *86*, 387, 1952.
COPE, Z.: Fusion-lines of Bones, J. Anat., *55*, 36, 1920.
DAWSON, A. B.: The Age Order of Epiphyseal Union in the Long Bones of the Albino Rat, Anat. Rec., *31*, 1, 1925.
DODDS, G. S.: Osteoclasts and Cartilage Removal in Endochondral Ossification of Certain Mammals, Am. J. Anat., *50*, 97, 1932.
DODDS, G. S., and CAMERON, H. C.: Studies on Experimental Rickets in Rats. I. Structural Modifications of the Epiphyseal Cartilages in the Tibia and Other Bones, Am. J. Anat., *55*, 135, 1934.
FELL, H. B.: The Osteogenic Capacity *in vitro* of Periosteum and Endosteum Isolated from the Limb Skeleton of Fowl Embryos and Young Chicks, J. Anat., *66*, 157, 1932.
————: Skeletal Development in Tissue Culture. Chapt. XIV in *The Biochemistry and Physiology of Bone*, edited by G. H. Bourne, New York, Academic Press, Inc., 1956.
FELTS, W. J. L.: Transplantation Studies of Factors in Skeletal Organogenesis. I. The Subcutaneously Implanted Immature Long-bone of the Rat and Mouse, Am. J. Phys. Anthropol., *17*, 201, 1959.
FOLLIS, R. H., JR., and BERTHRONG, M.: Histochemical Studies on Cartilage and Bone. I. The Normal Pattern, Bull. Johns Hopkins Hosp., *85*, 281, 1949.

FRANCIS, C. C.: The Appearance of Centers of Ossification from 6 to 15 Years, Am. J. Phys. Anthropol., *27*, 127, 1940.

FRANCIS, C. C., and WERLE, P. P.: The Appearance of Centers of Ossification from Birth to 5 Years, Am. J. Phys. Anthropol., *24*, 273, 1939.

GARDNER, E.: Osteogenesis in the Human Embryo and Fetus. Chapt. XIII in *The Biochemistry and Physiology of Bone*, edited by G. H. Bourne, New York, Academic Press, Inc., 1956.

——————: Comparative Arthrology, Lab. Invest., *8*, 1160, 1959.

GEGENBAUR, C.: Ueber die Bildung des Knochengewebes, Jenaische Ztschr. Med. u. Naturwissensch., *1*, 343, 1864, and *3*, 206, 1867.

GRAY, D. J., and GARDNER, E.: Prenatal Development of the Human Knee and Superior Tibiofibular Joints, Am. J. Anat., *86*, 235, 1950.

GRAY, D. J., GARDNER, E., and O'RAHILLY, R.: The Prenatal Development of the Skeleton and Joints of the Human Hand, Am. J. Anat., *101*, 169, 1957.

HAINES, R. W.: The Development of Joints, J. Anat., *81*, 33, 1947.

HAMMAR, J. A. H.: *Bidrag till Ledgangarnes histologi*, Upsala, E. Berling, 1892.

——————: Ueber den feineren Bau der Gelenke, Arch. mikr. Anat., *43*, 266 and 813, 1894.

HARRIS, H. A.: The Vascular Supply of Bone, with Special Reference to the Epiphysial Cartilage, J. Anat., *64*, 3, 1929.

——————: *Bone Growth in Health and Disease*, London, Oxford University Press, 1933.

HINTZSCHE, E.: Untersuchungen an Stützgeweben. I. Über die Bedeutung der Gefässkanäle im Knorpel nach Befunden am distalen Ende des menschlichen Schenkelbeines, Ztschr. mikr.-anat. Forsch., *12*, 61, 1927.

——————: Untersuchungen an Stützgeweben. II. Über Knochenbildungsfaktoren, insbesondere über den Anteil der Blutgefässe an der Ossifikation, Ztschr. mikr.-anat. Forsch., *14*, 373, 1928.

INMAN, V. T., and SAUNDERS, J. B. DE C. M.: The Ossification of the Human Frontal Bone. With Special Reference to its Presumed Pre- and Post-Frontal Elements, J. Anat., *71*, 383, 1937.

JAFFE, H. L.: *Tumors and Tumorous Conditions of the Bones and Joints*, Chapt. 26, Philadelphia, Lea & Febiger, 1958.

KÖLLIKER, A.: *Die normale Resorption des Knochengewebes und ihre Bedeutung für die Entstehung der typischen Knochenformen*, Leipzig, F. C. W. Vogel, 1873.

LACHMAN, E.: The Life History of Cranial Vault Sutures as Revealed in the Roentgenogram, Am. J. Roentgenol., *79*, 721, 1958.

LACROIX, P.: *The Organization of Bones.* (Translated from the Amended French Edition by S. Gilder), Philadelphia, The Blakiston Co., 1951.

LANGER, C.: Über das Gefässsystem der Röhrenknochen, Denkschr. k. Akad. Wissensch. Wien, Math.-Naturw. Classe I, *36*, 1876.

LEBLOND, C. P., WILKINSON, G. W., BÉLANGER, L. F., and ROBICHON, J.: Radio-autographic Visualization of Bone Formation in the Rat, Am. J. Anat., *86*, 289, 1950.

LEXER, E., KULIGA, P., and TÜRK, W.: *Untersuchungen über Knochenarterien*, Berlin, A. Hirschwald, 1904.

LUBOSCH, W.: *Bau und Entstehung der Wirbeltiergelenke*, Jena, G. Fischer, 1910.

MACKLIN, C. C.: The Skull of a Human Fetus of 43 Millimeters Greatest Length, Contrib. Embryol., *10*, 57, 1921.

MALL, F. P.: On Ossification Centers in Human Embryos Less Than One Hundred Days Old, Am. J. Anat., *5*, 433, 1906.

McLEAN, F. C., and BLOOM, W.: Calcification and Ossification. Calcification in Norma Growing Bone, Anat. Rec., *78*, 333, 1940.

MÜLLER, H.: Ueber die Entwickelung der Knockensubstanz nebst Bemerkungen über den Bau rachitischer Knochen, Ztschr. wissensch. Zool., *9*, 147, 1858.

MÜLLER, J.: Abhandl. preuss. Akad. Wissensch. Berlin, Physik.-Math. Classe, 1836.

MURRAY, P. D. F., and HUXLEY, J. S.: Self-Differentiation in the Grafted Limb-Bud of the Chick, J. Anat., *59*, 379, 1925.

NESBITT, R.: *Human Osteogeny Explained in Two Lectures*, London, T. Wood, 1736.

NOBACK, C. R.: The Developmental Anatomy of the Human Osseous Skeleton During the Embryonic, Fetal and Circumnatal Periods, Anat. Rec., *88*, 91, 1944.

O'RAHILLY, R.: The Development of Joints, Irish J. M. Sc., Sixth Series, 456, 1957.

PEACOCK, A.: Observations on the Postnatal Structure of the Intervertebral Disc in Man, J. Anat., *86*, 162, 1952.

PRATT, C. W. M.: The Significance of the "Perichondrial Zone" in a Developing Long Bone of the Rat, J. Anat., *93*, 110, 1959.

PRITCHARD, J. J.: A Cytological and Histochemical Study of Bone and Cartilage Formation in the Rat, J. Anat., *86*, 259, 1952.

PRITCHARD, J. J., SCOTT, J. H., and GIRGIS, F. G.: The Structure and Development of Cranial and Facial Sutures, J. Anat., *90*, 73, 1956.

RAY, R. D., MOSIMAN, R., and SCHMIDT, J.: Tissue-Culture Studies of Bone, J. Bone & Joint Surg., *36-A*, 1147, 1954.

SENSENIG, E. C.: The Early Development of the Human Vertebral Column, Contrib. Embryol., *33*, 21, 1949.

SEVASTIKOGLOU, J.: The Early Stages of Osteogenesis in Tissue Culture, Acta orthop. scandinav., Suppl. *33*, 1, 1958.

SHARPEY, W.: in Quain, R.: *Elements of Anatomy*, 5th ed., London, Taylor, Walton, and Maberly, 1848. (*See* Vol. I, p. cxlvii.)

SISSONS, H. A.: Experimental Determination of Rate of Longitudinal Bone Growth, J. Anat., *87*, 228, 1953.

STREETER, G. L.: Developmental Horizons in Human Embryos (Fourth Issue): A Review of the Histogenesis of Cartilage and Bone, Contrib. Embryol., *33*, 149, 1949.

TOMLIN, D. H., HENRY, K. M., and KON, S. K.: Autoradiographic Study of Growth and Calcium Metabolism in the Long Bones of the Rat, Brit. J. Nutrition, *7*, 235, 1953.

WALMSLEY, R.: The Development and Growth of the Intervertebral Disc, Edinburgh M. J., *60*, 341, 1953.

WILLIAMS, L. W.: The Later Development of the Notochord in Mammals, Am. J. Anat., *8*, 251, 1908.

WILLIS, R. A.: The Growth of Embryo Bones Transplanted Whole in the Rat's Brain, Proc. Roy. Soc. London s.B, *120*, 496, 1936.

WYBURN, G. M.: Observations on the Development of the Human Vertebral Column, J. Anat., *78*, 94, 1944.

Chapter

2

Chronology of Postnatal Ossification and Epiphysial Fusion

A CENTER of ossification which appears as the first one in the cartilaginous precursor of a bone (whether in fetal or postnatal life) is ordinarily denoted as a *primary center* of ossification. Primary ossification centers appearing postnatally are well exemplified by those which develop for the carpal and tarsal bones. However, in regard to the latter it should be noted that the primary centers for the calcaneus and talus are usually already present in the full term neonate at birth. An ossification center which develops for an epiphysis of a bone is usually denoted as an *epiphysial center*. At birth, a full term neonate ordinarily shows an ossification center in the cartilaginous epiphysis for the lower end of the femur and commonly also in that for the upper end of the tibia. In any event, it can be assumed that a fetus is at least full term if it shows, at birth, centers of ossification for the calcaneus, the talus, and the lower epiphysis of the femur.

Under normal circumstances, the centers of postnatal ossification display a certain regularity in respect to date and sequence of appearance. This regularity is more conspicuous in the epiphysial than in the primary centers. Indeed, in early childhood the primary centers may vary relatively widely in their chronology and evolution among different subjects, in accordance with the influence of such factors as sex, genetic background, general nutrition, and general health. However, since the number of the more regular (that is, the epiphysial) centers is much greater than that of the primary centers, the greater variability of the latter is more or less absorbed (statistically) in the larger tendency toward chronologic consistency. Also, in any subject the time and sequence of appearance of the centers, and of fusion of the epiphysial centers with the bone shafts, are practically the same for both sides of the body. That is, the chronology of the postnatal ossification is, on the whole, bilaterally symmetrical. Indeed, in regard to the right versus the left hand and wrist, for instance, accumulated evidence seems to indicate that in a particular subject the divergencies in the over-all maturation pattern on the two sides are so minor as to be negligible in the evaluation of the skeletal status from roentgenographs (see Roche).

Since the advent of roentgenography, the latter has been used with increasing frequency in the study of the postnatal chronology of these processes. This method has supplemented, and now predominates over, that of direct anatomic investigation, by means of which the earliest data in this field were accumulated. Roentgenography has facilitated the collection of relatively large series of observations on the bones of growing infants, children, and young people of known age, sex, and health status. In consequence, sets of normal values (standards) have been established which represent the progress of postnatal ossification in large numbers of carefully and repeatedly measured subjects of good or very good economic status on adequate and well-balanced diets (see Todd, Francis and Werle, Pyle and Sontag, Francis, Pyle and Hoerr, Acheson, and Greulich and Pyle).

The data collected by these various workers deal with the chronology of ossification mainly as it occurs in relation to limb bones. In contrast to the postnatal centers for the vertebræ and ribs, for instance, those for the extremities are easily visualized roentgenographically. Since, furthermore, the limbs show a wealth of both primary and epiphysial centers appearing over a wide range of the growth period, the chronology of ossification in the extremities can safely be held to represent that in the skeleton as a whole. In fact, the general skeletal status is well reflected even by conditions pertaining to the hand and wrist alone. In this connection, however, one must consider the chronology of the appearance of all the primary and epiphysial centers, along with the time of fusion of the relevant epiphyses with the bone shafts.

FACTORS INFLUENCING THE CHRONOLOGY

The Factor of Sex.—A sex difference in the chronology of ossification is already so definite as to be measurable in the latter part of fetal life. Indeed, from the seventh fetal month on, females are slightly in advance of the males in respect to this chronology (see Pryor, and Hill). In the full term neonate, the difference in favor of the female is already clear-cut (see Menees and Holly, and Christie). This difference becomes accentuated in the course of infancy and childhood. Indeed, the whole program of postnatal ossification of the primary and epiphysial centers, as well as fusion of epiphyses with the bone shafts, is run off earlier in the female than in the male.

By the end of the fifth year, the advance of the female over the male has increased, so that for many ossification centers it now amounts to a year or more. For centers appearing from 6 to 15 years, the sex difference becomes even more accentuated, amounting to more than two years for certain centers. In respect to the subsequent fusion of the ossified epiphyses with the bone shafts, the sex difference in favor of females amounts, on the average, in many skeletal regions to two or three years and, in some, even to four. It is plain from all this why, in presenting data on the postnatal chronology of the appearance of centers of ossification and fusion of epiphyses, the two sexes must be considered separately. (See Tables 1 to 4.)

The Factor of Kinship.—The time and order of appearance of ossification centers are evidently influenced by heredity. For instance, it has been found that twins (identical), siblings, cousins, and unrelated children ranked in that descending order in respect to similarity of their ossification patterns (see Reynolds). It has also been noted that sets of uniovular triplets resembled each other minutely in regard to mode and rate of ossification (see Buschke). In a set of identical quadruplets studied by Pryor, there was an almost complete correspondence concerning the sequence of appearance of the ossification centers for the wrist and hand. He also found evidence, on studying the sequence of carpal ossification in quadruplets, triplets, and twins, that there are genetic factors operating along mendelian lines in the causation of normal variations in this respect. Thus, in his opinion, it is not merely by chance that we find the same variations in the sequence of carpal ossification in several members of a family. However, a study of monozygous triplets has shown that the genetic pattern of ossification of an individual triplet may nevertheless be modified by certain environmental and metabolic factors (see Sontag and Reynolds).

In respect to kinship between man in general and the anthropoids, it is interesting to note the finding of Vallois that in a gorilla of 6 months the postnatal centers of ossification were at almost exactly the same stage as in man at the same age. He believes that the probable reason for this is the particularly close correspondence between the gorilla and man as to limb proportions.

Table 1.—Time Order of Ossification of Centers in the Limbs of Females from Birth to 5 Years+

Centers	Francis and Werle Present in 20% of Cases (Months)	Pyle and Sontag Mean (Months)	S.D.	Greulich and Pyle Mean (Months)	S.D.
Calcaneus	Birth				
Talus	Birth				
Femur, distal	Birth	Birth			
Tibia, prox.	Birth	0.1			
Cuboid	Birth	0.4			
Humerus, head	Birth	0.9			
Capitate	2	2.3	2.1		
Hamate	2	2.5	2.3		
Cuneiform, lat.	2	3.8	4.4		
Femur, head	3	3.7	1.6	3.6	1.6
Humerus, capitulum	3	4.1	3.6	4.4	2.5
Tibia, distal	3	3.4	1.4	3.7	1.4
Humerus, greater tuber.	4	6.6	3.3	6.5	2.9
Fibula, distal	6	9.3	2.6	8.7	2.8
Radius, distal	6	10.8	4.4	9.5	4.2
Toe (1), distal phal.	7	10.6	2.8	9.4	3.0
Finger (3), prox. phal.	7	10.4	3.1	9.8	2.9
Finger (4), prox. phal.	7	11.1	3.2	10.7	3.3
Finger (2), prox. phal.	8	11.0	3.0	10.6	3.1
Finger (1), distal phal.	8	12.8	5.0	11.6	4.2
Toe (3), prox. phal.	8	12.2	3.8	11.2	3.6
Toe (3), middle phal.	9				
Toe (4), prox. phal.	9	13.6	3.8	12.4	3.8
Cuneiform, medial	9	16.7	8.5	15.6	6.8
Metacarpal (2)	10	12.8	3.7	12.0	3.2
Toe (2), middle phal.	10				
Toe (4), middle phal.	10				
Metacarpal (3)	10	14.2	4.0	13.4	3.4
Toe (2), prox. phal.	10	14.1	3.8	13.2	3.6
Triquetrum	10	23.6	13.7	21.0	13.7
Metacarpal (4)	11	16.0	4.1	15.1	4.0
Finger (5), prox. phal.	11	15.2	4.2	14.0	3.8
Finger (4), middle phal.	12	15.8	4.8	14.9	4.7
Finger (3), middle phal.	12	15.9	4.9	14.7	4.6
Metacarpal (5)	13	17.2	4.7	16.5	4.7
Finger (2), middle phal.	13	17.3	5.2	16.4	4.6
Metacarpal (1)	14	20.3	5.3	18.1	4.7
Toe (1), prox. phal.	14	20.3	5.5	18.1	4.2
Toe (5), prox. phal.	14	21.3	4.8	20.1	5.4
Finger (3), distal phal.	14	20.2	3.9	17.6	4.5
Finger (4), distal phal.	14	19.9	5.9	17.8	4.8
Navicular, foot	14	25.8	11.1	21.4	9.8
Cuneiform, middle	14	21.3	7.6	19.1	6.6
Metatarsal (1)	14	20.1	3.3	19.2	3.4
Finger (1), prox. phal.	15	21.6	5.1	20.0	5.1
Finger (5), middle phal.	15	24.9	7.9	22.1	7.5
Finger (2), distal phal.	17	25.8	6.9	23.4	5.8
Finger (5), distal phal.	17	25.5	7.0	22.8	5.8
Metatarsal (2)	19	25.8	6.1	24.0	4.7
Toe (5), distal phal.	21				
Metatarsal (3)	22	29.1	6.4	28.6	4.6
Patella	23	34.8	8.5	29.1	7.3
Lunate	24	34.6	14.2	34.3	13.5
Toe (3), distal phal.	24	32.8	7.7	32.8	8.2
Toe (4), distal phal.	24	30.7	7.9	28.9	6.9
Fibula, prox.	24	32.6	9.3	33.0	11.2
Femur, greater troch.	24	29.8	6.4	29.0	5.2
Toe (2), distal phal.	26	35.5	7.3	35.1	8.4
Metatarsal (4)	26	34.0	7.2	33.2	7.2
Metatarsal (5)	29	38.6	8.4	38.5	8.5
Trapezium (greater multang.)	32	47.0	14.8	47.3	14.2
Humerus, medial epic.	33	41.3	9.9	43.2	12.2
Radius, prox.	36	47.5	12.1	48.7	13.9
Trapezoid (lesser multang.)	36	48.3	14.8	49.2	11.6
Scaphoid (navicular, hand)	38	47.8	12.3	50.9	11.8
Ulna, distal	54	63.2	15.3	69.4	13.0
Toe (5), middle phal.	60+				
Calcaneus, epiphysis	60+	63.7	11.8	60.0	10.6

Table 2.—Time Order of Ossification of Centers in the Limbs of Males from Birth to 5 Years+

Centers	Francis and Werle Present in 20% of Cases (Months)	Pyle and Sontag Mean (Months)	S.D.	Greulich and Pyle Mean (Months)	S.D.
Calcaneus	Birth				
Talus	Birth				
Femur, distal	Birth	Birth	0.1		
Tibia, prox.	Birth	0.1	0.3		
Cuboid	Birth	0.5	0.7		
Humerus, head	Birth	0.7	0.8		
Capitate	2	2.4	1.8		
Hamate	2	3.4	2.2		
Cuneiform, lat.	2	4.4	4.3		
Femur, head	3	4.4	2.0	4.5	1.8
Humerus, capitulum	3	6.3	4.3	7.1	4.4
Tibia, distal	3	3.9	1.5	4.3	1.8
Fibula, distal	6	12.5	4.1	12.1	4.2
Humerus, greater tuber.	7	11.4	7.2	12.3	7.0
Radius, distal	7	13.0	4.7	12.8	5.1
Triquetrum	10	27.3	15.9	29.6	16.3
Finger (3), prox. phal.	11	16.2	5.3	15.5	4.0
Toe (1), distal phal.	11	16.8	5.6	15.9	5.8
Finger (2), prox. phal.	12	17.3	5.0	16.5	4.3
Finger (4), prox. phal.	12	17.7	5.4	17.2	4.8
Finger (1), distal phal.	12	18.4	6.2	18.6	6.8
Toe (3), prox. phal.	13	19.5	5.2	18.6	4.7
Metacarpal (2)	13	17.9	5.1	18.1	5.5
Cuneiform, medial	13	21.9	9.9	24.7	10.5
Toe (4), prox. phal.	14	21.0	5.1	20.3	5.1
Toe (2), prox. phal.	14	22.2	5.8	20.9	5.2
Toe (3), middle phal.	14				
Metacarpal (3)	15	21.1	6.4	20.4	5.2
Toe (2), middle phal.	15				
Finger (5), prox. phal.	15	22.2	5.6	21.4	5.3
Toe (4), middle phal.	16				
Metacarpal (4)	16	23.6	7.1	23.0	6.3
Finger (2), middle phal.	18	26.9	7.5	25.8	6.4
Finger (3), middle phal.	18	24.9	7.6	23.8	6.0
Finger (4), middle phal.	18	24.9	7.8	24.2	5.9
Metacarpal (5)	18	26.0	8.0	25.7	7.3
Toe (1), prox. phal.	20	29.9	5.8	27.8	5.4
Cuneiform, middle	20	28.4	11.2	28.8	8.7
Finger (3), distal phal.	21	27.8	6.4	27.6	6.2
Finger (4), distal phal.	21	28.3	7.0	27.9	6.5
Navicular, foot	21	33.4	13.5	30.7	13.5
Toe (5), prox. phal.	21	32.0	5.9	31.0	7.0
Metacarpal (1)	22	29.8	7.3	31.6	8.7
Metatarsal (1)	22	27.7	4.7	28.7	4.9
Finger (1), prox. phal.	23	34.8	7.9	32.4	7.5
Finger (5), middle phal.	24	40.3	11.7	39.0	9.8
Lunate	24	46.0	19.3	42.4	19.0
Metatarsal (2)	26	33.4	6.8	34.2	6.9
Finger (2), distal phal.	29	37.0	7.9	37.3	7.9
Finger (5), distal phal.	29	37.4	7.4	37.2	8.9
Metatarsal (3)	35	41.5	7.9	41.2	8.0
Fibula, prox.	35	47.0	11.8	45.2	12.1
Femur, greater troch.	37	42.6	7.6	42.1	9.8
Patella	37	51.9	11.6	46.0	11.4
Metatarsal (4)	39	48.7	9.0	46.9	7.9
Toe (5), distal phal.	40				
Toe (3), distal phal.	43	53.5	11.2	53.2	14.0
Toe (4), distal phal.	43	51.2	10.1	50.9	12.8
Metatarsal (5)	44	53.6	10.6	53.0	9.9
Toe (2), distal phal.	44	57.0	11.4	57.9	13.3
Radius, prox.	46	63.5	17.2	65.3	14.8
Trapezium (greater multang.)	50	64.3	19.7	67.0	19.2
Scaphoid (navicular, hand)	52	60.1	14.1	66.0	15.2
Trapezoid (lesser multang.)	56	64.4	15.2	68.7	15.5
Humerus, medial epic.	62	73.6	17.5	72.7	14.9
Ulna, distal	66	82.4	10.6	82.5	14.0
Toe (5), middle phal.	60+				
Calcaneus, epiphysis				88.6	11.5

Influence of Race.—There are no findings which can be regarded as definitive in respect to the chronology of appearance of the postnatal centers and epiphysial fusion as influenced by race.   However, it has been reported by Dommisse and Leipoldt that the rate of ossification of the carpal centers in colored children (of South Africa) is, in general, several months in advance of the rate in European children.   A similar and even more striking acceleration of the ossification rate was shown for the lower ulnar and radial epiphyses by the colored children they studied. In regard to epiphysial fusion, the studies by Sidhom and Derry on Egyptian adolescent boys and by Galstaun on Indian and Anglo-Indian adolescent girls suggest that the fusions occur somewhat earlier in these adolescents than in those of English or European stock.   On the other hand, there are also reports suggesting that racial differences may be responsible for the relative retardation in skeletal development observed in children in certain parts of the world when comparisons are made with American standards.   However, it is quite likely that these differences are largely (or, at least, in part) attributable to such factors as inadequate diet, endemic illnesses, and other unfavorable environmental influences (see Greulich).

Influence of Illness and Nrutition.—Numerous studies have indicated that protracted illness during childhood disturbs the sequence of postnatal ossification. Indeed, the disturbance is reflected earliest, and often solely, in the ossification centers, though, of course, it may also influence height, weight, bodily maturity, and even mental expansion.   Sick children show a lag in the ossification rating proportionate to the duration and intensity of the constitutional disturbance created by the illness, and when convalescence is completed the rating advances again.   Gastrointestinal difficulties, even when so well controlled that there is no

Table 3.—Time Order of Ossification of Centers from 6 to 15 Years (Mainly in the Limbs)

	Female				Male			
	Francis Present in 20% of Cases		Present in 50% of Cases†		Francis Present in 20% of Cases		Present in 50% of Cases†	
Center	Yr.	Mo.	Yr.	Mo.	Yr.	Mo.	Yr.	Mo.
Calcaneus, epiphysis					6	2	7	3
Olecranon	6	8	7	8	8	8	9	11
Talus, epiphysis	6	10	7	11	8	0	9	3
Pisiform	7	1	8	2	9	10	10	11
Humerus, trochlea	7	2	8	3	8	4	9	8
Femur, lesser troch.	7	7	9	2	9	4	11	4
Sesamoids, flex. hall. brev.	8	2	9	0	10	4	11	6
Humerus, lat. epic.	8	3	9	2	10	5	11	6
Metatarsal (5), prox.	8	7	9	8	11	0	12	0
Tibia, tubercle	9	0	9	8	10	10	11	9
Ilium, ant. inf. spine*	9	3	11	6	13	4	14	5
Sesamoid, flex. poll. brev.	9	4	10	5	11	8	12	11
Rib (1), tubercle	10	0	12	1	13	3	14	3
Coracoid, angle	11	3	12	2	13	10	14	8
Thor. vert. (1), trans. proc.	11	4	12	2	13	4	14	5
Acromion	11	4	12	4	13	5	14	5
Ilium, crest	12	0	12	10	13	5	14	5
Ischium, tuber.*	13	2	15	0	15	0		
Clavicle, medial	14	6			15+			

*Provisional
†Estimated by the writer on the basis of Francis's data

Table 4.—*Chronology of Fusion of Epiphyses of the Limb Bones and a Few Others* (From data of Flecker)

Epiphysis	May Occur as Early as				Occurs in at Least 50% by	
	Yr.	Mo.	Yr.	Mo.	Yr.	Yr.
	(Female)		(Male)		(Female)	(Male)
Humerus, conjoint upper	15	9	16	0	17	18
Humerus, conjoint lower	13	4	14	7	13	16
Humerus, medial epic.	10	0	12	0	14	16
Ulna, olecranon	13	10			14	16
Radius, prox.	13	10	14	0	14	16
Radius, distal	15	11	17	3	18	19
Ulna, distal	15	0	17	3	17	19
Metacarpal (1)	13	0	14	0	15	18
Metacarpal (2)	14	9	16	0	16	18
Metacarpal (3)	14	9	16	0	16	18
Metacarpal (4)	14	9	16	0	16	18
Metacarpal (5)	14	9	16	0	16	18
Finger (1), prox. phal.	13	8	14	0	15	17
Finger (2), prox. phal.	13	8	14	0	15	18
Finger (3), prox. phal.	13	8	14	0	14	18
Finger (4), prox. phal.	14	9	14	0	14	18
Finger (5), prox. phal.	13	0	14	0	14	18
Finger (2), middle phal.	13	8	14	0	16	17
Finger (3), middle phal.	14	9	15	11	18	17
Finger (4), middle phal.	14	9	14	0	16	17
Finger (5), middle phal.	14	9	14	0	16	17
Finger (1), distal phal.	13	8	14	0	13	17
Finger (2), distal phal.	14	9	14	0	14	17
Finger (3), distal phal.	14	9	14	0	14	16
Finger (4), distal phal.	14	9	14	0	14	17
Finger (5), distal phal.	15	6	14	0	15	17
Femur, prox.	13	4	14	0	14	17
Femur, greater troch.	14	4	15	10	14	16
Femur, distal	14	0	16	0	17	19
Tibia, prox.	14	0	16	0	15	18
Fibula, prox.	14	0	16	0	17	19
Tibia, distal	13	0	14	9	14	17
Fibula, distal	14	10	15	0	14	17
Calcaneus, apophysis	12	10	14	6	14	17
Metatarsal (1)	14	0	15	0	14	17
Metatarsal (2)	14	0	15	2	14	17
Metatarsal (3)	14	0	15	2	14	17
Metatarsal (4)	14	0	15	2	14	17
Metatarsal (5), distal	14	0	15	2	14	17
Toe (1), prox. phal.	14	0	15	0	14	17
Toe (2), prox. phal.	14	0	15	0	14	17
Toe (3), prox. phal.	14	0	15	0	14	17
Toe (4), prox. phal.	14	0	15	0	14	17
Toe (5), prox. phal.	14	0	15	0	14	17
Toe (2), middle phal.	12	10	15	0	15	17
Toe (1), distal phal.	13	0	15	0	15	17
Toe (2), distal phal.	12	10	15	0	13	15
Toe (3), distal phal.	12	10	15	0	13	15
Toe (4), distal phal.	12	10	15	0	15	15
Clavicle					18	
Acromion					17	17
Innominate, fusion 3 centers	10	6	13	7	13	15
Ilium, crest	17	1			21	21
Ischial tuber.					21	20

4

retardation in body length, nevertheless also tend to retard the chronology of ossification. Even acute illness of short duration may exert some effect on the appearance of the centers of ossification, but on the whole the latter are not easily influenced by an acute illness (see Francis, and Sontag and Lipford).

Protracted undernutrition likewise has a retarding effect on the chronology of ossification of the postnatal centers. In a pertinent study by Dreizen *et al.*, the mean time of appearance for each of the ossification centers of the hand and wrist of chronically undernourished infants and children was found to be delayed in every instance, when the evaluations were compared with the age standards in the Greulich-Pyle atlas (see Tables 1 and 2). Delay in the advent of ossification was somewhat greater for boys than for girls, and was much more pronounced in relation to the centers for the carpals than in relation to the metacarpal and phalangeal epiphyses. In both sexes the delay in the ossification of the distal epiphysis of the ulna greatly exceeded that of the distal epiphysis of the radius.

Children suffering from chronic undernutrition show not only a delay in the time of appearance of the postnatal ossification centers but also an aberration in the seasonal cycle of postnatal ossification in comparison with that for adequately nourished children. In particular, while in healthy children the appearance of ossification centers of the hand reaches its maximum in the spring, in undernourished children the rate is highest in the summer (see Dreizen *et al.*). The explanation for this may be that the undernourished children are likely to come closer to meeting the minimum requirements for calcium, phosphorus, and vitamin D during the summer season. Even in healthy and otherwise well-nourished children, the ossification rating is influenced by available mineral and vitamin D. Of two normal subjects of the same age, the more rapidly growing subject was found to require proportionately more of these if his rating was to keep pace with that of a subject otherwise equivalent but growing more slowly (see Francis).

Influence of Endocrine Disturbances.—Disordered functioning of the glands of internal secretion profoundly affects the chronology of postnatal ossification and epiphysial fusion (see Mellman *et al.*). *Hypothyroidism* and *hypopituitarism* setting in during childhood result in delayed appearance and retarded growth of the centers of postnatal ossification, retarded bone growth at the epiphysial cartilage plates and at the synchondroses and sutures, and persistence of these structures well beyond the age when they would normally disappear. On the other hand, *precocious puberty* is associated with abnormal acceleration of skeletal development, as indicated by premature times of appearance of the primary and epiphysial ossification centers. Because of accelerated endochondral ossification at the epiphysial cartilage plates in cases of pubertas praecox, growth in height is accelerated for some time, but, since the epiphyses are likely to fuse prematurely, the final height of the subject may be below average. Further details relating to the influence of the endocrine glands on the chronology of postnatal ossification and epiphysial fusion will be found in the chapters dealing with the skeletal reflections of disordered functioning of these various glands.

CENTERS APPEARING IN THE LIMBS FROM BIRTH TO 5 YEARS+

Table 1 (on females) and Table 2 (on males) have been constructed from data compiled for this age period by Francis and Werle, Pyle and Sontag, and Greulich and Pyle. It should be noted that the figures of Francis and Werle represent the age when a given center was present in 20 per cent of the cases, while the figures given by Pyle and Sontag and by Greulich and Pyle represent the age when it was present in 50 per cent. Thus, in using the standards of Francis and Werle, one should bear in mind that "the stated age of appearance for each center is that date when it may be expected to appear in a healthy child with a satisfactory environment." That is, their figures represent the ideal (applying to children superior in physical and economic status) rather than the mean, as do the figures of Pyle and Sontag, and Greulich and Pyle.

In the tables the reader will find, next to the mean age given for each center by Pyle and Sontag and by Greulich and Pyle, the corresponding standard deviation in months for that center, as they calculated it from their data. Pyle and Sontag state that, within ±1 standard deviation from the mean age in months for any given center of ossification, approximately 68 per cent of the children will have acquired that center. If 1 S.D. in months is subtracted from the 50 percentile age value for that center (Pyle and Sontag figures), it appears that the age value obtained corresponds very closely to the 20 per cent value given for the center by Francis and Werle.

If the various centers are considered in sheaves or groups, and not individually, as to their time of appearance, they have a value as maturity determinators, with due regard, of course, for the influence upon them of constitutional health, general nutrition, and the intake and utilization of minerals and vitamin D. It is common practice to give the skeletal age rating of a child on the basis of the center most recently ossified, even though other centers of that sheaf may not yet be evident. Thus, in order that a child receive an ossification rating of one year, he need have only one center of that age group or sheaf ossified, and may even lack some centers of an earlier age group.

If an infant has some temporary interruption of growth just before the 11-month centers are due to ossify, these may be held back for months, even though the disturbance of general health is of brief duration. If, by the time the infant is 12 months old, normal health has returned, the normal schedule of appearance of centers is resumed and the 12-month centers ossify on time. Under these circumstances, the infant would be given an ossification rating of one year, though this rating should be qualified by mention of the evidence for previous disturbance. Indeed, even failure of all the centers comprised in one sheaf to appear at the scheduled age is not an adequate reason for assuming that the sheaf next due to ossify will likewise be delayed in appearance or be deficient in number. In other words, though appearance of a given center or sheaf may be delayed for months or even years if it has missed its proper time, centers or sheaves due at subsequent ages may appear promptly at the expected time. The skeletal age rating, then, becomes that indicated by the latest sheaf represented.

CENTERS APPEARING FROM 6 TO 15 YEARS (MAINLY IN THE LIMBS)

Table 3 lists, for the 6 to 15 year period, the ages of appearance of centers of ossification in the limbs (including some for the more important sesamoids) and in a few other body areas. This table was constructed from the data presented by Francis for this age period and covers both males and females. It should be noted that the first age listed after each center for each sex represents the actual figure given by Francis to show when the center was present in 20 per cent (the eightieth percentile) of his subjects. This age figure stands, he says, for "the date at which the center may be expected to appear in a healthy child in a satisfactory environment."

It was felt by the present writer that it would be desirable also to have for each center an age figure corresponding to the time when the center could be expected to be present in 50 per cent of the same subjects (the 50 percentile). Therefore, he has estimated the 50 percentile age level mathematically for each center on the basis of the detailed data for each center which Francis gives in his article. These

50 percentile estimates are listed in the second column after each center in the table. The writer obtained these estimates by mathematical interpolation. Hence, they do not have, of course, the same foundation as the figures obtained from actual observations. Nevertheless, they seem to be sufficiently accurate to supply a working conception of the fiftieth percentile level. It was thought that even estimated values on the fiftieth percentile for the 6 to 15 year period would be useful, because Tables 1 and 2, dealing with the period from birth to 5 years, give actual figures for the fiftieth percentile, as well as those for the twentieth percentile.

CHRONOLOGY AS AN INDEX OF MATURATION

The statistical results of studies of the chronology of postnatal ossification and epiphysial fusion are useful in appraising the skeletal age of subjects from birth to adulthood. The skeletal age of a given subject signifies the chronological age which is the norm for subjects presenting a corresponding degree of skeletal maturation in statistical groups of cases from which developmental standards have been derived.

As already indicated, children who are in good health show considerable regularity in respect to the order in which ossification centers appear postnatally. Particularly detailed attention has been given to the hand and wrist in regard to the order in which ossification begins in the carpals and in the epiphyses of the phalanges and metacarpals; the sequence of changes in shape undergone by the individual ossification centers as they develop; and the order in which the epiphyses eventually fuse with the shafts. If there are any irregularities in the chronology of ossification in the hand and wrist, these are more likely to appear in relation to the ossification centers for the carpal bones than in relation to those for the epiphyses of the phalanges and metacarpals.

At any rate, in healthy children the sequence of ossification of the carpals, except for the scaphoid (navicular), is rather consistent and is the same for the two sexes. That sequence is: capitate, hamate, triquetrum, lunate, trapezium (greater multangular), trapezoid (lesser multangular), and pisiform. The scaphoid center tends to appear before that of the trapezium, particularly in males. In females, the scaphoid either closely precedes or closely follows the trapezoid. However, since the centers of ossification for the scaphoid, trapezium, and trapezoid usually appear within one to three months of each other, their variability creates no great practical problem in the assessment of skeletal age.

In any event, normal children usually show sufficient consistency in respect to the appearance and growth of the various ossification centers of the hand and wrist, so that one can assign to the part in question a single skeletal age based on acknowledged standards for comparison (see Greulich and Pyle). However, children who have suffered from severe illness or prolonged nutritional inadequacies are very likely to show aberrations in regard to the ossification centers of the hand and wrist. Thus, if a febrile or other illness occurs at about the time when a center for a carpal bone or for an epiphysis is due to appear, that center often fails to appear on schedule. After the child has recovered from the illness, the next center of ossification due to appear (and perhaps one or two of those due subsequently) usually shows up at about the proper time and before the one whose ossification was disturbed puts in a belated appearance.

If the x-ray films of the hand and wrist of a child show significant aberrations from the standards in regard to the ossification centers, additional films taken some months later permit one to obtain a record of the skeletal status at two points of time. The second film will then indicate the extent to which the disordered chronology has been corrected. However, genetic differences give rise to differences in the rate of growth and development of children, even when the latter are adequately nourished and not handicapped by serious illnesses. There are early maturing and late maturing strains in our population, in addition to the great majority who are intermediate in this respect. That is, the skeletal status of an early maturing child will be distinctly more advanced than that of a more slowly developing child of the same age. Even children of the same sex and age in different parts of the same country may show differences in physical growth and development. All these factors must be taken into consideration when one is evaluating the skeletal status of an individual subject on the basis of a recognized standard.

Buehl and Pyle have correlated the appearance of certain centers of ossification with evidence of maturity as indicated by the menarche. They found that, in two thirds of their girls (healthy, normal subjects), ossification began in the crest of the ilium within 6 months of the menarche. Fusion of the epiphysis for the distal phalanx of the second finger occurred shortly after the menarche in the majority of their group. In their male subjects, the center for the crest of the ilium appeared later than in females, and the authors think that the time of appearance of this center might possibly indicate a point in the maturation cycle of the male which is comparable to the point reached by the female at the time of the menarche. Simmons and Greulich studied the skeletal age of girls 7 to 17 years of age in relation to the time of appearance of the menarche. They found that, on the whole, an early menarche tended to be correlated with an advanced skeletal age in relation to the chronological age, and a late menarche with a retarded skeletal age.

FUSION OF EPIPHYSES

Table 4 lists the time of fusion of the epiphyses of the limb bones and a few others, and brings out very well the sex differences in fusion of the epiphyses listed. The figures given in this table have been selected from Table LXI (covering also many other epiphysial fusions) in the article by Flecker. They represent his own data only, as compiled from his roentgenographic observations. In making the table from his x-ray films, he has adopted an all-or-none policy. Specifically, he is averse to noting degrees of fusion, as some other workers have done, and simply regards an epiphysis as unfused until all roentgenographic evidence of the epiphysial plate has disappeared. Figure 6 (p. 19) illustrates the development and growth of an epiphysial ossification center (the one for the lower end of the femur) and progress toward fusion of that epiphysis with the bone shaft, in the course of which the epiphysial cartilage plate will disappear. Figure 7 (p 21.) illustrates the histologic findings relating to an epiphysial cartilage plate which is no longer functioning and which has already disappeared in some places. It is well known, of course, that a transverse linear radiopaque line marking the site of fusion of the epiphysis and shaft may persist well into adult life. However, this line (the so-called epiphysial scar) is composed of osseous tissue and hence need cause no confusion.

In the part of Table 4 where the age is given in years only, the year refers to the last birthday. The figures of Flecker apparently represent the time of fusion of epiphyses much more accurately than those given by Stevenson. The latter's compilation was based on the findings in a relatively small number of skeletons, which, furthermore, represented mainly males and mainly older adolescents and young adults. It should be noted, however, that Flecker's data on fusion can be regarded only as a supplement to, and not as a direct continuation of, the figures on the appearance of the centers of ossification given in Tables 1, 2 and 3. To note only one point, his data, though based on large numbers of cases, represent mainly hospital patients, in contrast to the data in Tables 1, 2, and 3, which represent findings under good conditions of health and nutrition.

There has been a lack of studies dealing with the time elapsing between the cessation of endochondral bone growth at the various epiphysial cartilage plates and the fusion of the relevant epiphyses with the adjacent bone shafts. Directing their attention to this question, Moss and Noback investigated the temporal course of epiphysial fusion of the phalanges of the hand by means of closely spaced serial roentgenographs. They report that the total elapsed time from the onset to the completion of fusion of all 15 digital epiphyses of the hand had a mean value of approximately 13 months, with a range of 8.5 to 18 months.

Much of the work on epiphysial fusion has been done with the aim of applying it to age determination of adolescent and postadolescent subjects. The possibility of such calculations is based upon the relative constancy of the sequence of fusion of certain of the more important epiphyses. Though the time of onset and completion of the series of fusions is influenced by sex, the chronological relation of the individual fusions to each other is not much influenced by this. In attempting to determine the age on the basis of fusion in an individual case, one really ought to know the status of many epiphyses. For this purpose, the bones of the hand and wrist, foot and ankle, knee, and os coxæ (the innominate bone) probably ought to be roentgenographed, so that one would have a general picture of the fusion status in the case as a whole. A comparison with the average findings as noted in Table 4 would then make a relative evaluation of the individual status possible.

REFERENCES

ACHESON, R. M.: The Oxford Method of Assessing Skeletal Maturity, Clinical Orthopaedics, *10*, 19, 1957.

BUEHL, C. C., and PYLE, S. I.: The Use of Age at First Appearance of Three Ossification Centers in Determining the Skeletal Status of Children, J. Pediat., *21*, 335, 1942.

BUSCHKE, F.: The Radiological Examination of the Skeletons of Triplets, J. Hered., *26*, 391, 1935.

CHRISTIE, A.: Prevalence and Distribution of Ossification Centers in the New-born Infant, Am. J. Dis. Child., *77*, 355, 1949.

DOMMISSE, F. H., and LEIPOLDT, C. L.: The Ossification of the Carpal Centres in Coloured Children, South African M. J., *10*, 713, 1936.

DREIZEN, S., SNODGRASSE, R. M., WEBB-PEPLOE, H., and SPIES, T. D.: The Retarding Effect of Protracted Undernutrition on the Appearance of the Postnatal Ossification Centers in the Hand and Wrist, Human Biol., *30*, 253, 1958.

DREIZEN, S., SNODGRASSE, R. M., DREIZEN, J. G., and SPIES, T. D.: Seasonal Distribution of Initial Appearance of Postnatal Ossification Centers in Hand and Wrist of Undernourished Children, J. Pediat., *55*, 738, 1959.

FLECKER, H.: Time of Appearance and Fusion of Ossification Centers as Observed by Roentgenographic Methods, Am. J. Roentgenol., *47*, 97, 1942.

FRANCIS, C. C.: The Appearance of Centers of Ossification from 6 to 15 Years, Am. J. Phys. Anthropol., *27*, 127, 1940.

————: Factors Influencing Appearance of Centers of Ossification During Early Childhood, Am. J. Dis. Child., *57*, 817, 1939; Factors Influencing Appearance of Centers of Ossification During Early Childhood. II. A Comparative Study of Degree of Epiphysial Ossification in Infancy Under Varying Conditions of Diet and Health, Am. J. Dis. Child., *59*, 1006, 1940.

FRANCIS, C. C., and WERLE, P. P.: The Appearance of Centers of Ossification from Birth to 5 Years, Am. J. Phys. Anthropol., *24*, 273, 1939.

GALSTAUN, G.: Some Notes on the Union of Epiphyses in Indian Girls, Indian M. Gaz., *65*, 191, 1930.

GREULICH, W. W.: A Comparison of the Physical Growth and Development of American-born and Native Japanese Children, Am. J. Phys. Anthropol., n.s. *15*, 489, 1957.

GREULICH, W. W., and PYLE, S. I.: *Radiographic Atlas of Skeletal Development of the Hand and Wrist*, 2nd ed., Stanford, Stanford University Press, 1959.

HILL, A. H.: Fetal Age Assessment by Centers of Ossification, Am. J. Phys. Anthropol., *24*, 251, 1939.

MELLMAN, W. J., BONGIOVANNI, A. M., and HOPE, J. W.: The Diagnostic Usefulness of Skeletal Maturation in an Endocrine Clinic, Pediatrics, *23*, 530, 1959.

MENEES, T. O., and HOLLY, L. E.: The Ossification in the Extremities of the New-born, Am. J. Roentgenol., *28*, 389, 1932.

Moss, M. L., and Noback, C. R.: A Longitudinal Study of Digital Epiphyseal Fusion in Adolescence, Anat. Rec., *131*, 19, 1958.

Pryor, J. W.: Differences in the Time of Development of Centers of Ossification in the Male and Female Skeleton, Anat. Rec., *25*, 257, 1923.

————: Time of Ossification of the Bones of the Hand of the Male and Female and Union of Epiphyses with the Diaphyses, Am. J. Phys. Anthropol., *8*, 401, 1925.

————: Bilateral Symmetry as Seen in Ossification, Am. J. Anat., *58*, 87, 1936.

————: Ossification as Additional Evidence in Differentiating Identicals and Fraternals in Multiple Births, Am. J. Anat., *59*, 409, 1936.

————: Normal Variations in the Ossification of Bones Due to Genetic Factors, J. Hered., *30*, 249, 1939.

Pyle, I., and Sontag, L. W.: Variability in Onset of Ossification in Epiphyses and Short Bones of the Extremities, Am. J. Roentgenol., *49*, 795, 1943.

Pyle, S. I., and Hoerr, N. L.: *Radiographic Atlas of Skeletal Development of the Knee*, Springfield, Charles C Thomas, 1955.

Reynolds, E. L.: Degree of Kinship and Pattern of Ossification. A Longitudinal X-ray Study of the Appearance Pattern of Ossification Centers in Children of Different Kinship Groups, Am. J. Phys. Anthropol., n.s. *1*, 405, 1943.

Roche, A. F.: Lateral Comparisons of the Skeletal Maturity of the Human Hand and Wrist, Am. J. Roentgenol., *89*, 1272, 1963.

Sidhom, G., and Derry, D. E.: The Dates of Union of some Epiphyses in Egyptians from X-ray Photographs, J. Anat., *65*, 196, 1931.

Simmons, K., and Greulich, W. W.: Menarcheal Age and the Height, Weight, and Skeletal Age of Girls Age 7 to 17 Years, J. Pediat., *22*, 518, 1943.

Sontag, L. W., and Lipford, J.: The Effect of Illness and Other Factors on the Appearance Pattern of Skeletal Epiphyses, J. Pediat., *23*, 391, 1943.

Sontag, L. W., and Reynolds, E. L.: Ossification Sequences in Identical Triplets. A Longitudinal Study of Resemblances and Differences in the Ossification Patterns of a Set of Monozygotic Triplets, J. Hered., *35*, 57, 1944.

Stevenson, P. H.: Age Order of Epiphyseal Union in Man, Am. J. Phys. Anthropol., *7*, 53, 1924.

Todd, T. W.: *Atlas of Skeletal Maturation*, St. Louis, The C. V. Mosby Co., 1937.

Vallois, H. V.: L'ossification des os des membres chez le Gorille du point de vue comparatif, Compt. rend. Soc. de biol., *133*, 69, 1940.

Chapter

3

Gross and Histologic Structure of Bones

THE earlier chapters gave a general account of the progress of skeletal development in the embryo and fetus, as exemplified in certain representative skeletal
parts, and also traced the course of postnatal growth and maturation of bones. In
the present chapter, some consideration will be given to the general architecture
of bones as skeletal units, but the principal emphasis will be placed upon the histologic organization of bone as a tissue—that is, upon osseous tissue *per se*.

Despite the obvious differences in size and shape, most of the bones have certain
gross structural features in common. These include a delimiting shell, or cortex
(substantia compacta). The extent and thickness of the latter vary with the type of
bone in question, and the thickness may even be different in different parts of the
same bone. Within the cortical shell there are varying amounts of a more or less loose-
meshed spongy, or cancellous, osseous tissue (substantia spongiosa). In the cavities
between the anastomosing trabeculæ of the spongiosa, there is myeloid and/or fatty
marrow. In a normal adult, most of the myeloid (blood-forming) marrow resides
in the bones of the trunk, though some is also present in the calvarium and in the
upper ends of the humeri and femora.

Except where they articulate with other bones and are covered by cartilage, or
at the sites of direct insertion of tendons and ligaments, bones are enveloped by a
thin connective tissue membrane known as the periosteum. The nourishment of
the cortical bone is supplied in part by numerous capillaries and arterioles which
enter it from the periosteum. These small periosteal vessels permeate the cortex
through its system of vessel canals (to be described below) and ultimately reach
the interior of the bone. However, the main blood supply for the bone marrow
and spongiosa comes from larger vessels which penetrate the bone cortex at certain
sites. In relation to a long tubular bone, for instance, the latter vessels include the
main nutrient artery (and sometimes an accessory nutrient artery), entering the
shaft at a site well away from its ends, and the so-called epiphysial-metaphysial
arteries, which penetrate the cortex at each end of the bone. In general, veins
and venules accompany the arteries and arterial channels. The nerve fibers which
accompany the blood vessels entering the bone are mainly vasomotor. In regard
to the presence and distribution of lymphatics in the cortex and medullary cavity
of bones, there is still much controversy.

Bone as a tissue (osseous tissue) is essentially a specialized connective tissue. It
consists of collagen fibrils of a distinctive type, cells with numerous ramifying
processes (osteocytes), cement substance (mainly mucopolysaccharides), and
mineral matter (mainly hydroxyapatite), which contributes the characteristic hardness to the tissue. The collagen fibrils (which are collected into fiber bundles)
and the osteocytes are embedded in the cement substance. The crystals of mineral
matter are not in the cement substance *per se* but have a specific orientation to the
collagen fibrils. In a bone of a normal adult, osteoblasts (the cells which take part
in the formation of osseous tissue) are present only in sparse numbers and usually

as flattened, inactive cells. Osteoclasts (the cells which participate in the resorption of osseous tissue) are very sparse and really do not represent cells indigenous to normal and mature osseous tissue.

Mainly on the basis of the arrangement and character of the fiber bundles and the osteocytes (bone cells), osseous tissue may be subclassified into: *nonlamellar* (coarsely bundled, coarse-fibered, woven) bone and *lamellar* (finely bundled, fine-fibered, stratified) bone. In nonlamellar bone the collagen fiber bundles are thick and irregularly arranged, and the osteocytes are prominent, numerous, and not distributed in an orderly fashion. In lamellar osseous tissue the collagen fiber bundles are grouped into stratified layers, or lamellæ, and the bone cells too (though smaller and less numerous than in nonlamellar bone) show an orderly arrangement.

Phylogenetically, woven, or coarse-fibered, bone is the older and more primitive osseous tissue, and indeed it is sometimes also denoted as "primitive bone." Onto-genetically, too, the first osseous tissue to appear in human skeletogenesis is of this variety. In fact, during the early part of intra-uterine life, practically all the osseous tissue present in the fetus is likely to be woven, or coarsely bundled. However, later in fetal life, finely bundled, or lamellar, osseous tissue appears and the woven, or nonlamellar, begins to yield to it. By the fourth year of postnatal life, the lamellar bone has so largely replaced the nonlamellar that hardly any of the latter remains in the normal human skeleton. As to lower mammals, there is a good deal of variation among the different species in regard to the rapidity with which the lamellar osseous tissue replaces the nonlamellar. Furthermore, some of the lowest vertebrates even retain nonlamellar bone for their adult skeleton.

GENERAL ARCHITECTURE OF BONES

In respect to general architecture, bones may be grouped as: tubular (long and short), short (cuboidal), flat, and irregular.

Tubular Bones.—These bones include the humerus, radius, ulna, femur, tibia, and fibula (the *long* tubular bones), and also the metacarpals, metatarsals, and pha-langes (the *short* tubular bones). In most textbooks on human anatomy, all these bones are classed as long bones rather than as tubular bones, the short ones among them sometimes being denoted as miniature long bones. The writer prefers the designation "tubular bones" because the term "tubular" stresses their distin-guishing gross anatomic feature—a more or less hollow tubelike bone shaft. It is to indicate the fact that the *shaft* (diaphysis) is long in some tubular bones and short in others that they are subclassified as long and short tubular bones.

The shaft of a tubular bone (a tibia, for instance) consists of a cortex of compact osseous tissue outlining a tubular cavity (the medullary, or major marrow, cavity). The cortex is thickest in the midportion of the shaft and tapers toward the ends of the bone, where it is usually rather thin. As to the cancellous osseous tissue of the bone shaft, this is rather loose-meshed in texture and meager in quantity in the midportion as compared with the shaft ends. Indeed, in certain long tubular bones (the fibula, for instance) and in the short tubular bones, cancellous osseous tissue may be practically absent in the midportion of the shaft. As a rule, the ends of a tubular bone are broader and thicker than the adjacent parts of the shaft, which itself tends to flare somewhat. This is particularly striking in regard to the lower end of the femur and the upper end of the tibia. The principal exception to the rule is represented by the terminal phalanges, whose distal ends tend to taper. The end of a tubular bone which has formerly had an epiphysis (that is, an end of an adult tubular bone) seems to be more appropriately designated as an *epiphysial bone end* than, in the customary fashion, as an epiphysis, since the epiphysis as such has already fused with the shaft. The spongy, or cancellous, osseous tissue in the interior of the epiphysial end of an adult tubular bone blends with the spongiosa at the corresponding shaft end (the *metaphysis*).

The honeycomb pattern of the spongiosa is created by anastomosing bars, or trabeculæ, of osseous tissue. As a rule, the marrow present in the spaces of the spongiosa at the ends of adult tubular bones is yellow, or fatty, marrow. In the proximal ends of the femur and humerus, however, small foci of red marrow are commonly still found until very late in life. In the diaphyses of adult tubular bones, the major marrow cavity again shows mainly yellow, or fatty, marrow, since the latter progressively replaces the red (blood-forming) marrow present in the diaphysis at birth (see Hashimoto). If the marrow and other soft tissues occupying the honeycomb spaces of the spongiosa are macerated, one notes that adjacent spaces open into each other through small lacunæ in the walls of the trabeculæ outlining the spaces. (See Fig. 11.)

Short Bones.—The short bones comprise those of the carpus and tarsus, the sesamoids, and certain anomalous or supernumerary bones (such as accessory tarsal naviculars). They are denoted as short bones because their main dimensions are not strikingly unequal, as are those of the tubular bones. They are sometimes also referred to as "epiphysioid bones." This name is based on the fact that they tend to ossify in the manner of epiphyses. That is, their ossification proceeds from a center in the interior of the cartilaginous precursor of the bone, the center enlarging centrifugally as in epiphyses. However, in relation to the talus and calcaneus in particular, some subperiosteal cortical bone is laid down, these bones thus differing to some extent from the other tarsal bones in respect to their pattern of development. At any rate, the bulk of the various short bones is made up of spongy osseous tissue, and, where they are not covered by articular cartilage, they are enclosed by only a thin cortical shell. Furthermore, their spongy osseous tissue is, on the whole, decidedly close-meshed, and the constituent trabeculæ are relatively thick.

Flat Bones.—The bones usually placed in this category include the ribs, sternum, scapulæ, and many of the bones of the cranium. These bones are distinguished as much by the fact that they are thin (in part or throughout) and possess relatively little spongiosa as by actual flatness. The flat bones of the cranial vault present the architecture of an inner and outer table, or plate, of cortical bone separated by a thin layer of spongy osseous tissue (the diploë), whose marrow spaces show numerous vascular channels. In the ribs and sternum, the cortex is by no means so thick and compact as the cortical tables of the calvarial bones, and the spongiosa is also more loose-meshed and contains considerable red (myeloid) marrow. The construction of the hard palate resembles that of the calvarial bones to a great degree. On the other hand, the lacrimal bone, the roof of the orbit, and part of the body

Figure 11

A, Roentgenograph of a longitudinal section of approximately the lower third of a femur, cut in the frontal plane, from a woman 60 years of age. Note that the cortex tapers as it approaches the epiphysial end of the bone, and that the most prominent spongy trabeculæ run in the long axis of the bone—that is, in the direction in which the strain and pressure involved in function are greatest. The spongiosa is most condensed in the region of the articular end of the bone. Note also the faint transverse line (see arrows) marking the site of fusion of the distal femoral epiphysis with the bone shaft.

B, Photograph showing the gross appearance of the femur illustrated in *A*, after the specimen had been freed of all its soft tissue by maceration. The details of the architecture of the spongy bone in the region indicated by the arrows are shown in *C*.

C, Photograph (enlargement of the area marked out in *B*) revealing the details of the honeycomb pattern presented by the spongiosa, and the elaborate intercommunications among the marrow spaces outlined by the bony trabeculæ.

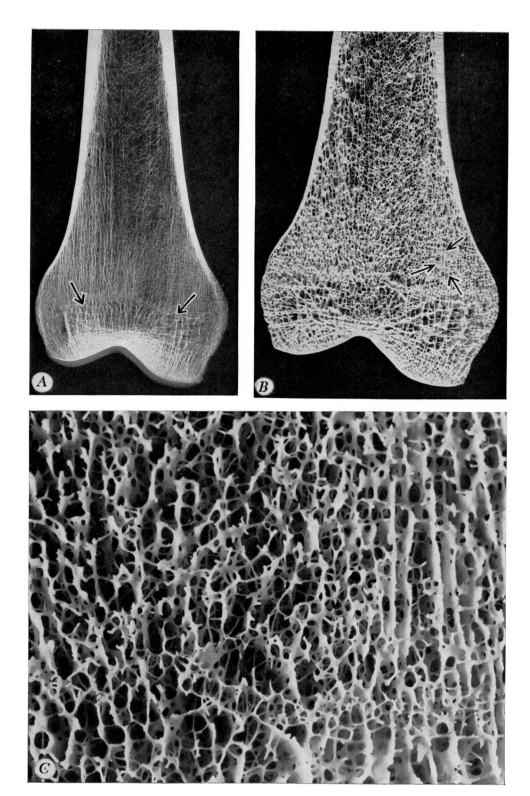

Figure 11

47

of the scapula have no spongiosa at all. These areas consist solely of a few closely compacted flakelike sheets of osseous tissue. A similar architecture is revealed by the sinus walls of the ethmoid bone (actually a so-called irregular bone).

Irregular Bones.—These include the innominate bones, some of those of the skull, and all those of the vertebral column. Though one part or another of an irregular bone may resemble a short bone or a flat bone, an irregular bone as a unit does not fit into any of the categories already discussed. Thus, if one considers the vertebræ, it becomes apparent that the body of a vertebra resembles a short bone, while much of the arch has the gross configuration of a flat bone. A vertebral body consists almost entirely of spongy osseous tissue, the delimiting cortical shell, where present, being very thin. Indeed, the upper and lower surfaces of a vertebral body, centrally to the corresponding marginal ridge, are devoid of cortex. In these regions the cartilage of the pertinent intervertebral disk is apposed directly upon condensed spongiosa. In contrast to the vertebral body, with its thin cortical shell and abundant loose-meshed spongiosa, the vertebral arch has a rather thick cortex (especially in some places) and a relatively sparse and thick-meshed spongiosa. (See Fig. 12.)

HISTOLOGIC TYPES OF OSSEOUS TISSUE

In recent years, use of the techniques of microradiography and autoradiography, and explorations in the fields of electron microscopy and histochemistry have greatly increased our knowledge of the histologic organization of osseous tissue (see Fitzgerald, Engfeldt, Glimcher, Robinson and Watson, Rutishauser and Majno, and Pritchard). Yet it is reassuring to note how much detailed and basic information had already been amassed in regard to the structure of bone by the earlier histologists, who used relatively simple tissue techniques and based their interpretations on what they saw through the light microscope (see von Ebner, Gegenbaur, Gebhardt, Weidenreich, Heuler, and Jaffe). The following general presentation of the histologic types of bone represents observations for which the light microscope is quite adequate, provided that properly prepared tissue sections are available.

As already indicated, the primary constituents of osseous tissue are: collagen

Figure 12

A, Photograph of the sectioned and macerated carpal bones (of an adult) demonstrating their gross internal architecture. The bulk of these short bones (pisiform, upper left) is composed of spongy osseous tissue, and in many of them the spongiosa is quite close-meshed.

B, Photograph of the sectioned and macerated cuboid (left) and the cuneiforms from the foot of an adult demonstrating their gross internal architecture. These short bones, too, are composed substantially of more or less close-meshed spongy bone. (*A* and *B* adapted from Triepel.)

C, Roentgenograph of a longitudinal section of a thoracic vertebral body from a middle-aged adult. That the bulk of the osseous tissue is spongy bone and that a well-developed cortical shell is lacking anteriorly (left) and posteriorly is clearly apparent. What might be taken to be cortex superiorly and inferiorly represents somewhat more closely set spongy bone which had been in apposition to the cartilage plates of the corresponding intervertebral disks (see *D*).

D, Photograph (enlarged) showing the gross architectural details of the spongiosa of a thoracic vertebral body. Note the striking honeycomb pattern of the sectioned body, revealed by maceration of all the soft tissues. The spongy trabeculæ are somewhat more close-set superiorly and inferiorly than in the central portion of the body. The absence of a significant cortical shell anteriorly (left) and posteriorly is also apparent.

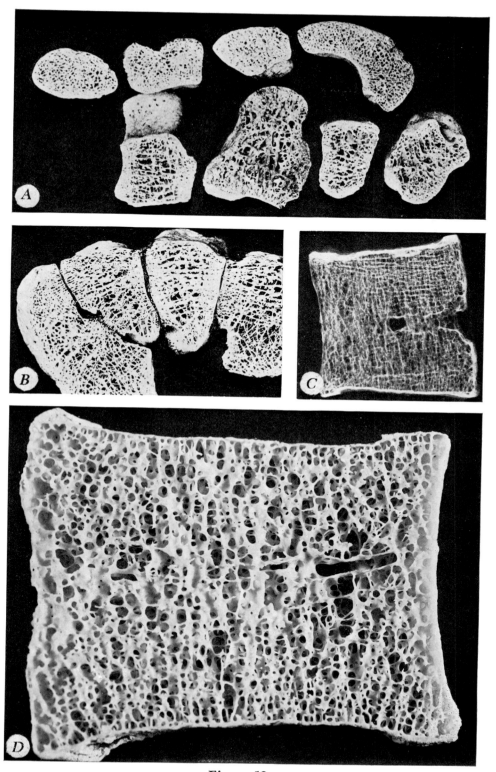

Figure 12

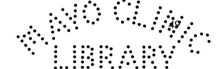

fibers, cement substance, mineral matter, and osteocytes with ramifying processes. This is true whether the osseous tissue is of the nonlamellar or of the lamellar type, or represents a mixture of the two types. Nonlamellar bone (coarsely bundled, coarse-fibered, or woven bone) is the type of osseous tissue first laid down in mammalian skeletogenesis. In human skeletogenesis it is gradually replaced by lamellar bone (finely bundled, fine-fibered, or stratified bone), the replacement starting well before birth of the fetus. Already by early childhood, the osseous tissue of human bones is very largely of the lamellar type.

Nonlamellar (Coarse-fibered) Bone. — The histologic structure of coarse-fibered osseous tissue is well exemplified in the long tubular bones of rather young fetuses. In a femur from a fetus even 5 months of age, the coarse-fibered type of osseous tissue still predominates, but some of the fine-fibered variety is already present with it. On microscopic examination of cross sections prepared from the shaft of such a bone, the cortex reveals the presence of numerous relatively large haversian (vascular) spaces. If cross sections taken at different levels of the shaft are compared, it will be observed that these spaces are larger toward the ends of the shaft cortex than in its midportion, and again larger, on the whole, near the outer, or periosteal, surface of the cortex than near its inner, or endosteal, surface. The osseous tissue immediately surrounding the spaces is bordered by osteoblasts, which are particularly numerous in relation to the newly formed bone beneath the periosteum.

If suitable staining methods and other technical procedures are used, it can be demonstrated clearly that much of the osseous tissue in the femoral cortex of a young fetus is characterized by the coarseness of its fiber bundles and the irregularity of their arrangement. Specifically, this tissue consists of bundles of thick fibers interlacing at random through the cement substance and interspersed with numerous irregularly disposed osteocytes. Especially near the periosteum, one may observe some particularly coarse fibers (Sharpey fibers) extending from the periosteum into the osseous tissue (see Müller, and Kölliker).

As to the osteocytes in coarse-fibered bone (compared with those of lamellar bone), it will be apparent even in sections stained with hematoxylin and eosin that they are large and numerous and that the cell lacunæ are quite prominent. By methods directed especially toward study of the cell processes and canaliculi of these osteocytes, it will also be found that the processes are few, short, and thick, and the canaliculi short and wide. The bone cells are particularly numerous in the most recently formed coarse-fibered osseous tissue—that beneath the periosteum.

Where endochondral ossification is in progress at the epiphysial-diaphysial junctions of a long tubular bone of a young fetus, the osseous tissue first deposited on the calcified cartilage matrix of the growth zones is likewise of the coarse-fibered variety. However, the arrangement of the fiber bundles of this endochondrally formed coarse-fibered bone is by no means so haphazard as it is in the coarse-fibered bone laid down by the periosteum in connection with the formation of cortical bone. The lines of separation between the cores of calcified cartilage matrix and the coarse-fibered osseous tissue deposited on these cores are irregular and correspond in many respects to the cement lines (p. 61) of mature bone. At sites of active endochondral bone formation, osteoblasts are again prominent on the surfaces of the newly deposited osseous tissue. (See Fig. 13.)

Replacement of the Nonlamellar by Lamellar Bone. — A cross section through the shaft of a long tubular bone from a fetus near term (or from a neonate) will show that the vascular spaces (vessel canals) of the cortex have already decreased considerably in diameter. By appropriate techniques it can also be demonstrated that the fiber bundles and cells of the osseous tissue present immediately around

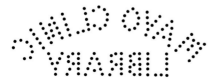

the vessel canals are disposed more regularly than they were during early fetal life. That is, the osseous tissue now being laid down by the osteoblasts on the walls of the vessel canals is of the lamellar type. However, deep to the lamellar bone which outlines the vessel canals, some coarse-fibered osseous tissue is still present. Furthermore, the osseous tissue newly deposited under the periosteum is to a considerable extent still of the coarse-fibered variety in the fetus near term. On the other hand, at sites of endochondral ossification the osseous tissue being laid down at this time is already largely of the lamellar type.

The substitution of the lamellar for the nonlamellar osseous tissue in the growing shaft cortex, for instance, does not involve to any notable extent the resorption of the nonlamellar bone by osteoclasts (p. 70). Instead, the substitution takes place gradually and insidiously, the nonlamellar bone undergoing "creeping replacement," in the course of which it is resorbed ("choked" or "squeezed," as it were, out of existence) and replaced by the lamellar bone.

Since less and less nonlamellar and more and more lamellar osseous tissue is being laid down after the replacement has once begun, the osseous tissue of human bones becomes increasingly lamellar in character. However, even in an adult, some coarse-fibered bone is still to be found, for instance, in the tooth sockets, near cranial sutures, at sites of attachment of tendons and ligaments, and in the bony capsule of the labyrinth of the ear.

In relation to pathologic conditions, coarse-fibered bone may be observed at any age. In the repair of a bone fracture, it replaces the cartilaginous callus before it is replaced in turn by lamellar osseous tissue. Bone laid down beneath a periosteum irritated by trauma or infection, for instance, is also of the nonlamellar type and likewise tends to be replaced by lamellar bone. In an osteogenic sarcoma appearing in an adolescent or even in an adult, much of the tumor bone may have the pattern of coarse-fibered osseous tissue. In short, whenever, in postnatal life, new bone is being formed rapidly, and not in the course of normal reconstruction of bone, it is usually first laid down as nonlamellar (coarse-fibered) bone, though it, too, may later be replaced by lamellar bone.

Lamellar (Fine-fibered) Bone.—As already pointed out, one of the main distinctions between nonlamellar and lamellar osseous tissue resides in the size and arrangement of the fiber bundles. In nonlamellar (coarsely bundled, coarse-fibered, or woven) bone, the fiber bundles are thick and interlace and cross each other more or less at random. On the other hand, in lamellar (finely bundled, fine-fibered, or stratified) bone, the fiber bundles are much more delicate, and the general pattern of the fiber arrangement is strikingly uniform and regular. In particular, the fiber bundles seem to be arranged in parallel or concentric layers, or sheets (lamellæ)— an appearance which results from the differences in the directional orientation of the fibers in the successive layers. This "laminated" composition of lamellar bone is more apparent than real, since the individual lamellæ are not actually composed of isolable and independent thin layers, as the name and optical impression suggest (see Pritchard).

From about the fourth year on, under normal conditions the osseous tissue of the cortex of a long tubular bone is almost entirely of the lamellar variety. By the eleventh year, the cortex of such a bone already shows its fully evolved lamellar architecture (see Heuler). Indeed, the shaft cortex of the femur of an adult offers the full scope of the microscopic architecture of lamellar cortical bone. In regard to spongy bone, the full range of the lamellar organization is also well exemplified by the conditions existing in a femur, since some of the spongy trabeculæ of that bone are thick and others are thin. In view of the extent to which the lamellæ of adult cortical bone are oriented to the vessel canals, it seems necessary to describe these canals before discussing in detail the arrangement and fibrillar structure of the lamellæ. (See Fig. 14.)

CORTICAL BONE: THE VESSEL CANALS

As seen through the microscope under relatively low power, one of the most prominent features of the cortex of a long tubular bone of an adult is the system of narrow canals (*vessel canals*) by which it is permeated. Through these canals, which carry capillaries and postcapillary veins, blood circulates between the periosteum and the bone marrow (see Morgan, and Nelson *et al.*). A very narrow vessel canal may contain only a capillary. Vessel canals of greater caliber may contain an arteriole, one or more venules, and even a vascular capillary plexus. Occasional nerve fibers probably accompany the larger blood vessels of the canals, but it is difficult to demonstrate them. The presence of lymphatic channels in these vessel canals is a controversial matter, but there seems to be increasing evidence that some of the numerous lymphatic vessels of the periosteum do traverse the cortex to enter the medullary cavity (see Smith *et al.*). An occasional inactive, flattened osteoblast is to be seen apposed to the osseous tissue outlining the canals. Furthermore, large canals may contain a few primitive cells of supporting connective tissue.

Haversian Canals.—In human cortical bone the haversian canals are definitely the dominant channels for blood vessels. In cross section the canals appear round or oval and range from about 25 to 125 microns in diameter, the average being about 50 microns. Under normal conditions the widest canals are those nearest the medullary cavity. The so-called haversian systems, or osteons, are composed of the canals with their blood vessels and the concentric lamellæ which surround the canals (p. 58).

While the general direction of the haversian canals is longitudinal, they do not pursue a straight course for more than short distances. As seen in a longitudinal section or ground disk, the canals of the cortex appear as a continuous anastomosing and ramifying network. At intervals of one or a few millimeters, they give off branches. These may come off almost at right angles, obliquely, or in an arch. In

Figure 13

A, Photomicrograph ($\times$ 125) showing in cross section (from above down) the periosteum and outermost portion of the developing cortex of a femur from a fetus 16 weeks of age. One can distinguish between the outer, or fibrous, layer of the periosteum and its inner, or cambium, layer. Osseous tissue is being laid down by the actively functioning osteoblasts in the cambium layer. Even under this relatively low magnification, it can be seen that the osteoblasts which become surrounded by, or entrapped in, bone matrix become the osteocytes of the newly formed bone. The latter is loose-meshed, still almost entirely of the nonlamellar type, and surrounds relatively large haversian spaces. These are bordered by osteoblasts which diminish the size of the spaces as they lay down additional new bone.

B, Photomicrograph ($\times$ 125) showing a small area of rib cortex and overlying periosteum from a child $2\frac{1}{2}$ years of age. The periosteum no longer presents a clear-cut cambium layer. Immediately beneath the periosteum the osseous tissue is of the nonlamellar type, as is evident from the large numbers and haphazard arrangement of the osteocytes. However, layers of osseous tissue of the lamellar type (see arrows) are apposed against the nonlamellar bone, though separated from the latter by cement lines.

C, Photomicrograph ($\times$ 125) illustrating the appearance, under polarized light, of the same field as that shown in *B*. The fiber bundles in the nonlamellar bone are distributed in haphazard fashion, showing no orderly arrangement. In the narrow borders of lamellar bone, on the other hand, the fiber bundles run a rather orderly course.

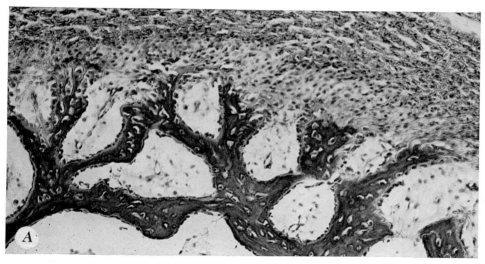

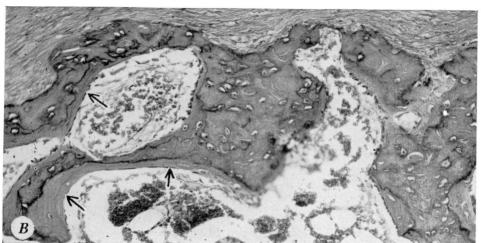

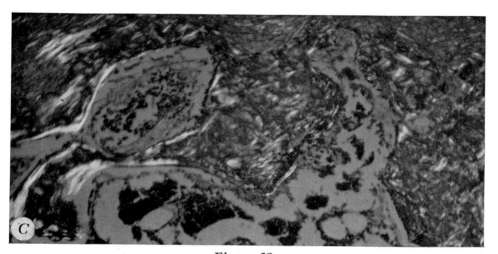

Figure 13

any case, the branches join adjacent haversian canals or branches of such canals. Also, a haversian canal itself may terminate by joining an adjacent canal or by becoming a communicating channel between two such canals.

The communicating channels between the longitudinal trunk canals are almost invariably branches of the latter. These branches are often designated erroneously as Volkmann canals (see below). Actually, in normal bone there are few communicating canals of the type described by Volkmann. The haversian canals near the surface of the cortex connect with the canals of the circumferential (ground) lamellæ. The latter canals open onto the external surface of the bone, while the haversian canals in the innermost portion of the cortex lead into the medullary cavity.

Canals of the Circumferential Lamellae (Ground Lamellae).—Since, in cortical bone of man, the layers of outer and inner ground lamellæ (circumferential lamellæ) are always extremely thin and sometimes almost negligible, special vessel canals are necessarily few and may be absent in these layers. In animals, such as the dog, sheep, and cow, in which ground lamellæ are highly developed, the latter show a relatively large number of vessel canals. In these animals, canals in the ground lamellæ are of two kinds—circumferential and radial. Those which run circumferentially lie compressed between ground lamellæ, while the radial type cross the lamellæ transversely. The radial channels appear to be perforating the ground lamellæ, but actually the latter weave over and under them.

Volkmann Canals.—The Volkmann canals are new and abnormal channels which appear almost solely in the course of pathologic resorption of bone by vessels growing out from already existing vessel canals (see Volkmann, and Jaffe). In its earliest form, a Volkmann canal appears as a short, irregular fine crack radiating from a haversian canal or one of its branches. Its progress is associated with demineralization of the bone along its path. The crack gradually grows longer. It also increases in width, the increase beginning at the base, which is at the haversian canal or one of its channels of communication. An elongated triangular passage is thus produced. The borders of the Volkmann canal at this stage are irregular

Figure 14

A, Photomicrograph ($\times$ 100) showing, in cross section (unstained frozen section), part of the shaft cortex of a long tubular bone of an infant 12 weeks of age. From above downward, one notes large haversian spaces beneath the periosteum, and then the smaller haversian canals, some of which are already surrounded by concentric lamellæ of fine-fibered bone. Thus, for the cortex as a whole, lamellar systems are not yet well developed and, indeed, much of the osseous tissue between the haversian canals is still of the coarse-fibered (non-lamellar) type.

B, Photomicrograph ($\times$ 20) illustrating the histologic pattern of an unstained ground disk of the shaft cortex of a femur from a male child 2 years of age. Even under this low magnification it can be seen that the osseous tissue is already well organized into haversian systems composed of lamellæ of fine-fibered bone. Study of the section under higher magnification would reveal that much of the osseous tissue between the haversian systems is also already of the lamellar type.

C, Photomicrograph ($\times$ 10) illustrating the histologic pattern of an unstained ground disk section prepared from the cortex of a femoral shaft from a woman 35 years old. The definitive organization of the cortex into closely set haversian systems of lamellar bone is apparent. Between the haversian systems, small fragments of interstitial lamellar bone are discernible, and thin layers of outer and inner ground lamellæ are visible on the outer and inner surfaces, respectively, of the cortex. (The writer is indebted to Dr. Ellis R. Kerley, Orthopaedic Pathology Section, Armed Forces Institute of Pathology, for the ground disk sections from which *B* and *C* were prepared.)

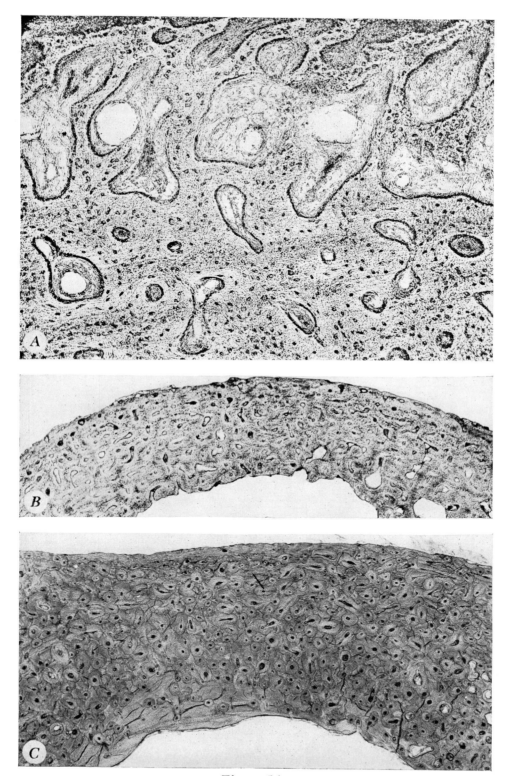

Figure 14

and toothed. The channel becomes vascularized, but the vessel is preceded by a wedge of connective tissue which seems to play a part in opening the crack (see Pommer). As the Volkmann canal grows, the toothed contour smooths out and the space may become as wide as an ordinary haversian canal or even wider.

Briefly, then, the principal difference between a haversian canal or its branches on the one hand and a Volkmann canal on the other may be stated as follows: A haversian canal results from a concentric deposition of bone lamellæ about a pre-existing blood vessel. A Volkmann canal, on the other hand, results from a canalization of fully formed bone by new vessels which perforate the existing lamellæ tangentially, obliquely, or at right angles to the long axis of the bone. To be correctly designated as a Volkmann canal, a channel should fulfill these conditions and these only. (See Fig. 15.)

CORTICAL BONE: ARRANGEMENT AND STRUCTURE OF THE LAMELLÆ

In a long tubular bone of an adolescent or an adult, the fiber bundles of the osseous tissue of the cortex appear on microscopic examination to be arranged in more or less parallel or concentric layers, or sheets—lamellæ. Actually, as already noted, the lamellæ are not structurally independent units of osseous tissue. The impression of their being so in microscopic tissue sections represents something of an optical illusion, for the lamellæ cannot really be separated from each other. The "lamellar" appearance is created by differences in the general directional orientation of the fiber bundles in the visualized successive layers, or strata.

When prepared specifically for the study of its lamellar architecture, the cortex of a femur, for instance, reveals diversified arrangements of its lamellæ. A large proportion of the latter surround the haversian vessel canals and their branches and are known as *haversian lamellæ*. A *haversian system* (or *osteon*) is composed of a haversian canal with its encircling layers of more or less concentric lamellæ. The *circumferential lamellæ*—those on the periosteal and endosteal surfaces of the cortex—run parallel to these surfaces and are also known as the outer and inner *ground lamellæ* respectively. In the interstices between the haversian systems,

Figure 15

A, Photomicrograph (× 100) of an unstained ground disk illustrating in cross section the histologic pattern of an area of shaft cortex from a femur of an adult. Note the roundish haversian canals surrounded by more or less concentric lamellæ of osseous tissue. The canals and their pertinent lamellæ make up the haversian systems (osteons). Interspersed between the osteons one can note irregular fragments of lamellar osseous tissue—the interstitial lamellar bone (see arrows).

B, Photomicrograph (× 100) of an unstained ground disk illustrating the vessel canal systems as they appear in a longitudinal section of cortical bone. Note the branching and communicating channels which interconnect the adjacent haversian canals (see arrows).

C, Photomicrograph (× 35) prepared from an unstained frozen section of adult human cortical bone to illustrate perforating canals of Volkmann. The bone was the site of an osteomyelitis, and the inflammatory process extending along the haversian canals had resulted in bone resorption and enlargement of the diameter of these canals. The large, irregular space in the upper part of the picture is the result of coalescence of several modified haversian canals. A number of Volkmann canals extend downward and outward from the enlarged haversian space. These are the result of canalization of preformed osseous tissue by blood vessels appearing in connection with the inflammatory process.

D, Photomicrograph (× 100) showing a toothed Volkmann canal connecting two enlarged haversian canals. The illustration was prepared from an unstained frozen cross section of tibial cortex from a dog affected with osteoporosis resulting from severe calcium deprivation.

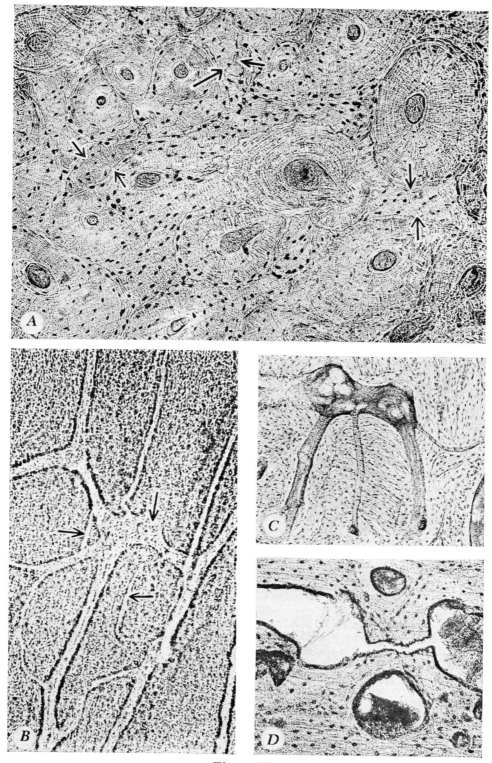

Figure 15

there are irregular fragments of lamellar osseous tissue, and the lamellæ of these fragments are denoted as the *interstitial lamellæ*.

The proportion and distribution of the haversian, interstitial, and ground lamellæ will be found to vary to a certain extent even in different segments of a given complete cross section of the shaft cortex of a bone. At different levels of the shaft, cross sections of the cortex may show even greater differences in these respects. Furthermore, if one compares cross sections of several different tubular bones at the same level (the bones having been taken from the same person), the arrangement of the different kinds of lamellæ in the cortex will manifest even wider variations in detail. In cortical bone in which osteons are numerous in relation to the interstitial lamellæ, the static tensile strength of the bone is greater than when that proportion is reversed (see Evans and Riolo).

Haversian Lamellæ.—As noted, these are arranged in systems (*haversian systems*) and the latter constitute the most important structural component of cortical bone. Each system is composed of a ringlike aggregation of lamellæ about a haversian canal. Where one canal is branching to anastomose with another, there is a break in the circle. Here the lamellæ may embrace two haversian systems and the anastomosing channel between them. As viewed in cross section, the size and shape of the haversian systems show considerable variety because of the reconstruction of the osseous tissue which is constantly taking place. As to shape, most haversian systems appear fairly round or only slightly ovoid in cross section. Upon actual count, it appears that in human cortical bone the average haversian system shows between 8 and 15 lamellæ. Sometimes only 4 or 5 are present; sometimes 18 to 22 may be counted. The thickness of the individual lamellæ varies but is usually between 6 and 9 microns. In general, it may be said that when there is a wide vessel canal the surrounding ring of lamellæ is likely to be narrow. It is the systems with canals of medium size that have the thickest lamellar bands. If the canal is small, the number of encircling lamellæ is again rather meager.

Interstitial Lamellae.—The irregular fragments of osseous tissue in the interstices between the haversian systems represent persisting remnants from haversian systems which have been broken up in the course of the continual, slow reconstruction which normally goes on even in mature bone. Because of the interstitial position of such bone fragments, their lamellæ are denoted as interstitial lamellæ. The latter are of the same thickness as the haversian lamellæ. (In rare instances, in

Figure 16

A, Photomicrograph (× 100) illustrating in cross section the histologic architecture of an area of cortex from a tibial shaft of a middle-aged woman. The bone had been decalcified in nitric acid and stained rather heavily with hematoxylin. A number of haversian systems, made up of haversian canals and surrounding lamellæ, stand out clearly. The fragments of interstitial bone between the haversian systems are also clearly demonstrated, as are the cement lines which separate the haversian systems and/or interstitial bone fragments.

B, Photomicrograph (× 75) showing a layer of outer ground (circumferential) lamellæ on the surface of a ground disk section of tibial cortex (see arrows). Note that, except for the direction they take, the appearance of these lamellæ is not different from that of the haversian lamellæ.

C, Photomicrograph (× 75) showing inner ground (circumferential) lamellæ (see arrows) present on the medullary surface of the cortex in the same tissue section used for *B*.

D, Photomicrograph (× 100) showing the histologic pattern of femoral cortical bone from a boy 15 years of age, as seen under polarized light. It is the difference in orientation of the fiber bundles in successive layers that creates the alternating light and dark bands apparent through the analyzing prism.

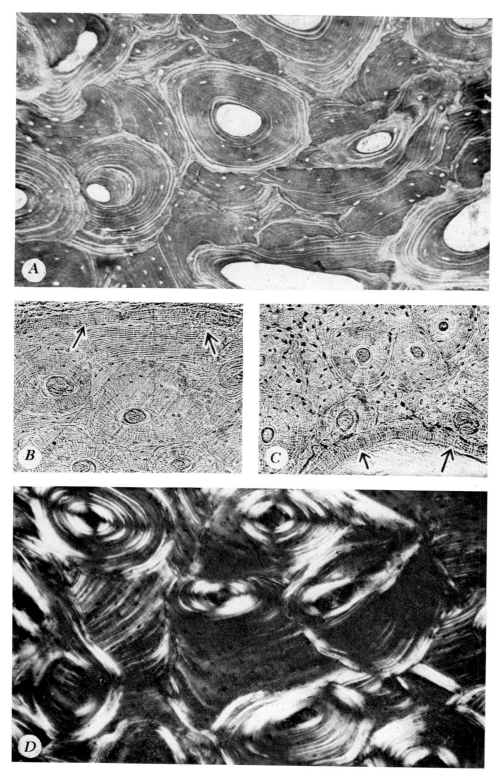

Figure 16

adult cortex one also finds, between the haversian systems, an occasional small nest of typical coarse-fibered bone.)

Circumferential (Ground) Lamellae.—The layers of the outer ground lamellæ are deposited by the periosteum as rings around the zone of the cortex containing the haversian and interstitial lamellæ. The inner ground lamellæ are deposited by the endosteum and encircle the marrow cavity. Inner ground lamellæ are found only in relation to the shaft cortex of tubular bones, and then only where spongiosa is absent and the cortex abuts upon the marrow. In man, neither the inner nor the outer system of ground lamellæ is prominent, though the former is always more so than the latter. Even when it is relatively well developed, however, the outer system does not exceed 900 microns in diameter. The thickness of an individual ground lamella is about the same as that of a haversian lamella. (See Fig. 16.)

Fibrillar Structure of the Lamellae.—As already indicated, the collagen fibrils of osseous tissue are set in a cement substance now commonly interpreted as a protein-polysaccharide complex (mainly mucopolysaccharides). Together, the fibrils and cement substance make up the organic matrix of the ground substance of osseous tissue. The mineral matter of the ground substance is present in the form of bone salt crystals (mainly hydroxyapatite). While some of the crystals seem to lie against the surface of the collagen fibrils, most of the crystals are apparently within the fibrils. The individual collagen fibrils are visible only with the aid of the electron microscope. Small groups of these fibrils represent the smallest fiber units discernible with the light microscope under high magnification. Aggregates of such fiber units constitute the fiber bundles of osseous tissue, and these can be recognized relatively easily with the light microscope. When viewed with the electron microscope, the collagen fibrils show an axial periodicity, or banding. The banded pattern of the fibrils and certain other details relating to the chemical nature of the collagen fibrils, cement substance, and mineral matter of osseous tissue are discussed in Chapter 5.

To demonstrate the fiber structure of bone satisfactorily with the light microscope, one may use ground disks of undecalcified cortical bone, or cortical bone which has been decalcified (preferably in a 10 per cent solution of hydrochloric acid) and then sectioned on the freezing microtome or sectioned after being embedded in paraffin. If a suitably prepared and silver-stained cortical cross section is examined with the light microscope under high magnification, the individual haversian lamellæ present a stippled appearance. The dots are very closely compacted and represent cross sections of bundles of fibrils. In longitudinal sections of cortical bone prepared and examined in the same way, the fiber bundles composing the lamellæ have considerable length and give the tissue section a serially striated appearance. It is because the collagen fibers are argentophil and the cement substance in which they are embedded is argentophobe that silver-stained sections show the fiber bundles nicely. However, since the collagen fibers are closely packed within a given lamella, the argentophobe cement substance does not stand out nearly so well between the fibers and between the individual lamellæ as in the fiber-free cement lines which demarcate individual haversian systems and fragments of interstitial lamellar bone from each other (see below).

The arrangement of the fibrils in an individual haversian lamella is complex and has been variously interpreted (see Smith). That groups of fibrils make up primitive fiber bundles which in turn are aggregated into thicker fiber bundles is clear. Apparently the fibrils within a bundle intertwine, and there is evidence that in addition the individual fiber bundles are twisted spirally. It has also been reported that the mass of fiber bundles constituting a haversian lamella usually winds clockwise around the haversian canal in one lamella and counterclockwise in the next. However, the obliquity of the fiber direction apparently varies in adjacent lamellæ. Furthermore, some of the fibers of each lamella enter the immediately adjacent lamellæ and thus produce interlocking between neighboring fiber bundles (see Weidenreich, and also von Ebner, and Gebhardt).

In successive lamellæ the direction of the fiber bundles may vary through any angle from 0 to 90°, the stratification being most clearly apparent when the angle is large. It is the differences in optical effect caused by this alternating orientation of the fiber bundles in successive layers that give rise to the "lamellar" appearance, although, as already noted, there are no actual lamellæ in the sense of separate layers of osseous tissue. With the polarizing microscope, the lamellation is even more evident, because the degree of rotation of the beam of polarized light varies from 0 to 90° as the direction of the fibers changes from parallel to right angles to the direction of the incident light. The successive lamellæ thus appear as alternating light and dark bands when viewed through the analyzing prism. (See Fig. 17.)

Cement Lines.—While individual lamellæ are not isolable or independent of each other, groups of them making up a fragment of interstitial bone or part or all of a haversian system do constitute more or less independent units of osseous tissue. Indeed, the haversian systems and interstitial fragments of bone in the cortex are set off from each other or are themselves partitioned by well-defined straight, smoothly curved, or indented lines—the cement lines. The latter are relatively wide zones of cement substance similar to the cement substance in which the collagen fibrils of the individual lamellæ are embedded.

Adult cortical bone is thus actually composed of innumerable irregular fragments of lamellar osseous tissue held together at the cement lines, and to a lesser degree this is true of spongy bone, also. The union at the cement lines is dependent mainly upon interlocking of the adjacent pieces of osseous tissue. In fact, tissue sections of bone which have not been properly processed very often show structural artifacts due to separation or splitting of the tissue at the cement lines. Thus, the union of the bone fragments at the cement lines is not so firm as the union of two individual lamellæ through the intertwining of some of their fibrils. Structures corresponding to the cement lines between the haversian systems and interstitial bone fragments are also present in the inner and outer ground lamellæ. Their course is naturally concentric with that of the circumference of the bone.

The straight or smoothly curved cement lines are more or less parallel. They mark resting stages in the process of progressive but intermittent new bone deposition and are often denoted as "resting lines." The irregularly indented cement lines indicate sites of new bone deposition against a surface which had been the site of active bone resorption, and are denoted accordingly as "reversal lines." On the average, a cement line is thinner than a lamella, but the two may be of about the same thickness. The cement lines are nonfibrillar. It is interesting to note how strictly, as a rule, these lines bar communication between neighboring fragments of osseous tissue. Only infrequently does one find even bone cell processes and canaliculi traversing them. The cement lines permit one to judge the degree of reconstructive activity taking place in the osseous tissue. When this activity is very lively (as, for instance, in Paget's disease), reversal cement lines are numerous. In the outer ground lamellæ, cement lines are a useful indicator of the rhythmic growth and cessation of growth of periosteal lamellar bone. (See Figs. 17-C and D, and also 21-A.)

The Lamellar Architecture of Subhuman Cortical Bone.—If certain requirements are satisfied, it is often possible to decide whether a given fragment of bone cortex comes from a human bone or a bone from some other mammal, and, in the latter case, perhaps even a specific mammal. In studies aiming at such differentiation, cross sections of cortex prepared as ground disks or as frozen sections made after decalcification are usually employed. Even small fragments of cortex suffice, provided that the entire thickness of the cortex is included.

In the evaluation of the histologic picture presented by cortical tissue sections, the age of the subject is an important factor to be considered. Furthermore, the comparisons are most likely to be valid if, in addition, they relate to the same bone in the different subjects (that is, if a femur is compared with another femur) and if the specimens being contrasted have been taken more or less at the same level of the bone in question (see Kenyeres and Hegyi, Petersen, and Jaffe).

For instance, cortical cross sections of corresponding bones of mature rats, guinea pigs, and rabbits reveal pronounced differences in the arrangement and proportional representation of the lamellæ. The rat tibia shows a strikingly thick layer of outer ground (circumferential) lamellæ, while the haversian lamellæ are few and the inner ground lamellæ are also meager. In contrast, the tibia of a guinea pig shows a relatively thin layer of outer ground lamellæ and a thick layer of inner ground lamellæ, but more haversian lamellæ. A section through the tibia of a rabbit shows still better development of the haversian lamellæ at the expense of the outer and inner ground lamellæ.

A cross section of cortex from a long tubular bone of a cloven-hoofed animal, such as a goat or cow, likewise presents an architecture easily distinguishable from that of a corresponding human bone. In these animals, too, circumferential lamellæ are extremely prominent. Some cloven-hoofed animals also show a fair number of lamellæ arranged in haversian systems, but there is a striking lack of interstitial lamellar bone and cement lines. In the dog, the haversian lamellæ are still more highly developed, but the haversian systems are not so large nor so irregular as those of human cortical bone. The cortex of a long tubular bone of a horse shows a lamellar architecture which resembles that of human cortex even more closely. In any case, a feature which tends to distinguish human bone from that even of other high forms of mammals is the rather random arrangement of the lamellar components in the compacta. Indeed, in human cortex there is usually a considerable amount of interstitial lamellar bone interspersed between the haversian systems, which themselves are of irregular size. However, this guide is by no means infallible. (See Fig. 18.)

Figure 17

A, Photomicrograph ($\times$ 400) illustrating the collagen fiber bundles of lamellar bone. The section was prepared from a block of femoral shaft cortex and had been stained by the Bielschowsky silver stain method. The center of the picture is occupied by part of a haversian system, cut transversely, and the latter is bordered by some additional lamellar bone. The collagen fiber bundles are argentophil and hence stand out as closely compacted, dark-staining dots. The cement substance in which the numerous fibers are embedded is argentophobe and, being relatively meager in comparison with the fibers, does not stand out well.

B, Schematic representation of a haversian system, intended to indicate that the fiber bundles in adjacent lamellæ run in contrasting directions (after Gebhardt). However, the directional changes from lamella to lamella are not nearly so clear-cut as the diagram suggests.

C, Photomicrograph ($\times$ 65) of a fragment of cortical bone, intended to demonstrate cement lines. After decalcification the tissue had been sectioned on the freezing microtome and stained with a silver stain. Since cement substance is argentophobe, the cement lines do not take the silver stain and hence stand out as white lines.

D, Photomicrograph ($\times$ 100) showing a small fragment of cortical bone cut after it had been decalcified and embedded in celloidin, the section being stained with hematoxylin and eosin. By contrast with their appearance in *C,* the cement lines are dark when so stained.

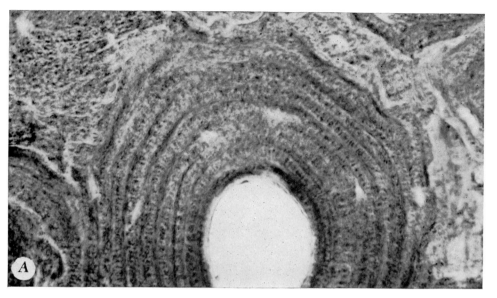

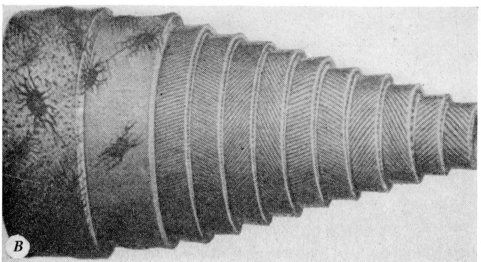

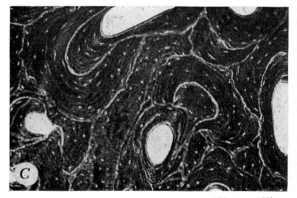

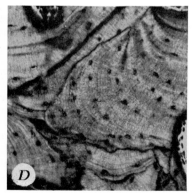

Figure 17

SPONGY BONE

As already indicated, spongiosa constitutes most of the osseous tissue of the tarsal and carpal bones and of such other skeletal regions as the bodies of the vertebræ and the ends of long tubular bones. The spongy bone is composed of thin osseous plates which cross each other more or less at right angles, so as to mark out spaces which contain the marrow. The delimiting walls are often thicker and longer in one axis than in the other. They show numerous fine apertures through which there is communication between the marrow spaces. These features of spongy bone do not stand out prominently unless the specimen is cleared of all its soft contents by maceration. (See Figs. 11 and 12.)

The general architectural arrangement of spongiosa is such as to give this bone region strength without undue weight. Furthermore, if one examines the spongiosa of a number of different bones, it will be observed that the thickest and strongest spongy trabeculæ run through the structure in that direction in which the strain and pressure involved in function are greatest (see Amstutz and Sissons).

On *microscopic examination* of a suitable preparation of the spongiosa of mature bone, it can be seen that those lamellæ of a spongy trabecula which border upon a marrow space are arranged somewhat concentrically around this space. Between

Figure 18

A, Photomicrograph ($\times$ 35) illustrating the histologic pattern presented by a cross section (unstained frozen section) of part of a tibial cortex from a young rat. Note the thick layer of outer ground (circumferential) lamellæ, traversed radially by some vessel canals, and the sparsity of haversian systems.

B, Photomicrograph ($\times$ 18) illustrating the histologic pattern presented by a cross section (unstained ground disk) of part of a femoral cortex from a goat 6 months of age. Note that practically the entire thickness of the cortex is made up of circumferential lamellæ, and that almost no haversian systems are present. The direction of the vessel canals is mainly circumferential, these canals lying between almost evenly spaced layers of circumferential lamellæ. When examined under higher magnification, numerous vessel canals running at right angles to the circumferential canals can be seen to interconnect the latter.

C, Photomicrograph ($\times$ 18) illustrating the histologic pattern presented by a cross section (unstained ground disk) of the femoral cortex of a mature dog (greyhound). Note the presence of a relatively prominent layer of circumferential lamellæ and vessel canals on the outer surface of the cortex and the sparsity of haversian systems in this region. However, deep to the latter, numerous haversian systems (haversian canals and surrounding lamellæ) are intermingled with lamellar osseous tissue still disposed circumferentially.

D, Photomicrograph ($\times$ 11) illustrating the histologic pattern presented by a cross section (unstained ground disk) of tibial cortex from a beef. The outer half (more or less) of the cortex is composed almost solely of circumferential lamellæ and vessel canals disposed mainly circumferentially between layers of these lamellæ. Further inward there is a zone showing numerous closely set haversian systems, and deep to that zone there is a thin layer of inner ground (circumferential) lamellæ.

E, Photomicrograph ($\times$ 12) illustrating the histologic pattern presented by a cross section (unstained ground disk) of femoral cortex from a boy 15 years of age. There is a striking contrast between the lamellar architecture of the subhuman bone cortices illustrated and the cortex in this specimen of human bone. In man, the fully evolved cortex is composed largely of lamellar bone organized into haversian systems, between which there are fragments of interstitial lamellar bone. Since the subject represented by the bone in this illustration was 15 years of age, one can still note thin but distinct layers of outer and inner circumferential lamellæ. In a fully mature human subject, these zones of circumferential lamellæ are even less prominent. (The writer is indebted to Dr. Ellis R. Kerley, Orthopaedic Pathology Section, Armed Forces Institute of Pathology, for the ground disk sections from which *B, C, D,* and *E* were prepared.)

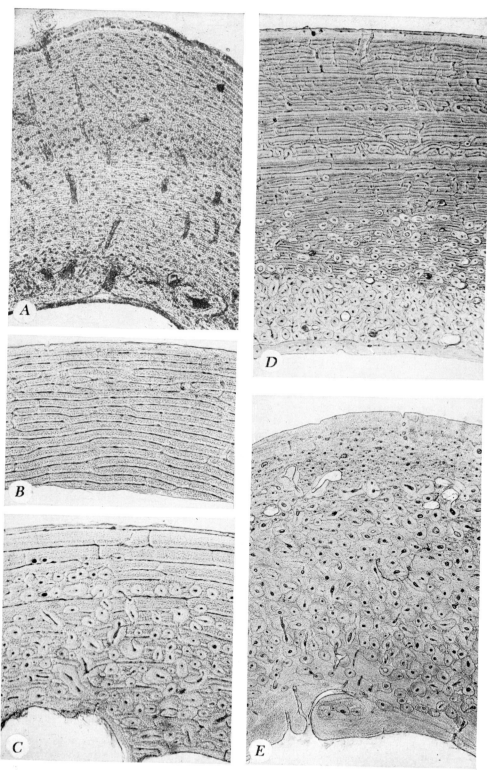

Figure 18

these layers of delimiting lamellæ, a number of juxtaposed fragments of osseous tissue are to be noted. The latter are tiny, angular pieces of bone whose own lamellæ frequently run diagonally to those bordering the marrow surfaces of the trabecula. Study discloses also that it is unusual for vessel canals to be present in the spongy trabeculæ. In the large thick trabeculæ in which such canals are occasionally found, the latter are surrounded by concentrically arranged lamellæ, such as are characteristic of haversian systems. In regard to the details of the histologic organization of the various constituents of spongy bone (fibers, cement substance, cement lines, osteocytes, etc.), there are no basic differences between spongy and cortical osseous tissue.

Fusion Lines and Lines of Arrested Growth.—These lines, to which brief reference has already been made on page 20, stand out well in roentgenographs of the bone part. If a bone showing one or the other of the lines in question has been appropriately sectioned, they can also be identified from their gross and microscopic appearance, though not so easily as from the x-ray picture.

A *fusion line* marks the site of synostosis between a fully evolved epiphysis and the neighboring shaft end after the intervening epiphysial cartilage plate has disappeared. In an adult, fusion lines are most likely to be present and can be observed most clearly in the long tubular bones of the lower extremity. In the knee area, in particular, they are not unusual even in elderly persons.

The line in question is created by some spongy trabeculæ extending across the bone more or less at right angles to the longitudinally directed trabeculæ. The line does not represent a structural abnormality but rather the counterpart of a structural feature normally present late in the course of maturation of the bone. In particular, the horizontally directed trabeculæ which make up the fusion line correspond in location to those bony trabeculæ of the maturing epiphysis which had been present as a thin layer of bone abutting upon the epiphysial cartilage plate before the latter ceased functioning and underwent destruction. In any event, it is erroneous to interpret a fusion line as the residuum of the epiphysial cartilage plate or as a "scar" remaining after the plate has disappeared. (See Figs. 11-*A* and *B*, and 19-*A* and *B*.)

Figure 19

A, Photomicrograph ($\times$ 5) showing, in longitudinal section, part of the upper end of the humerus of an adolescent boy. The epiphysial cartilage plate has become wavy, as it normally does when endochondral bone formation slows down prior to destruction and disappearance of the plate. Above the plate (see arrows) there is a stratum of osseous tissue which extends across the almost completely ossified epiphysis. After the plate disappears and the epiphysis fuses with the shaft, the site of this stratum becomes the site of the transverse trabeculæ representing the fusion line.

B, Photomicrograph ($\times$ 4) showing, in longitudinal section, part of the upper end of a femur of a boy 19 years of age. The epiphysial cartilage plate has completely disappeared, and the capital epiphysis (above) is synostosed with the neck of the femur (below). The transverse trabeculæ representing the fusion line are indicated by the arrows.

C, Roentgenograph of the lower end of a femur removed at autopsy from a female child $2\frac{1}{2}$ years of age who died shortly after a surgical intervention undertaken to relieve a hydrocephalus of long duration. Note the two transverse lines of relative radiopacity (lines of arrested growth) extending across the metaphysis slightly beyond the epiphysial cartilage plate.

D, Photograph of the lower end of the femur shown in *C*, cut in the frontal plane. The line of arrested growth nearer the epiphysial cartilage plate is indicated by the arrows.

E, Photomicrograph ($\times$ 3) showing two rows of trabeculæ disposed in an irregularly transverse pattern and representing the lines of arrested growth seen in *C* and *D*.

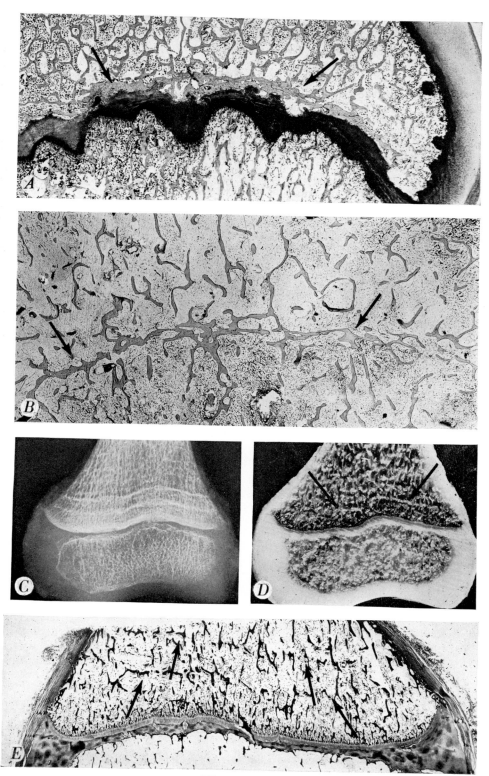

Figure 19

In contrast to fusion lines, *lines of arrested growth* represent aberrations in the general architecture of the spongy bone. These lines (the so-called Harris lines) stand out best in the metaphyses of the long tubular bones. Here, such a line is represented in the x-ray picture by a delicate, more or less transverse stripe of relative radiopacity. In children who have had repeated bouts of illness, the metaphyses of the long tubular bones may show multiple transverse stripes, or lines. These mark the periods during which the illnesses have caused a diminution or arrest of the normal sequences of endochondral bone formation at the epiphysial cartilage plates.

In consequence of an illness (even a relatively mild one of short duration), proliferation of the cartilage cells on the metaphysial side of the plate slows down or ceases, and a layer of osseous tissue comes to be deposited against the plate in a horizontal plane. When the depressing effect of the illness on endochondral ossification ceases and the latter resumes its normal course, the bone which had been deposited against the plate moves shaftward and comes to appear in the x-ray picture as the horizontal stripe, or stratum, of radiopacity. In a case in point, if the lower end of a femur, for instance, is removed and sectioned in its long axis, lines of arrested growth can also be visualized on gross inspection. Tissue sections prepared from pertinent areas will also demonstrate that the lines in question are created by bony trabeculæ extending transversely across the bone. The longitudinally directed trabeculæ between those which run transversely are usually relatively sparse and atrophic. (See Fig. 19-C, D, and E.)

OSTEOCYTES, OSTEOBLASTS, OSTEOCLASTS

Osteocytes.—As is well recognized, osteocytes are derived from osteoblasts. Specifically, they arise from osteoblasts which have become entrapped in the bone matrix during the formation of osseous tissue. The osteocytes lie in so-called bone cell lacunæ and have processes which extend into canaliculi representing prolongations of these lacunæ. As observed in tissue sections, the osteocytes usually do not completely fill their lacunæ, but this appearance represents an artifact due to shrinkage which occurs in the course of processing of the tissue. As to their function, it is probable that the osteocytes help to maintain the vitality (structural and metabolic integrity) of the bone matrix by facilitating the exchange of materials between the tissue fluids and the matrix by way of their canalicular systems. Death of the osteocytes in an area of osseous tissue is followed by disorganization of the fibrillar structure of the local bone matrix and eventually by disintegration and/or resorption of the devitalized osseous tissue.

In bone of the nonlamellar type, the osteocytes are large, relatively numerous, and irregularly distributed, and their processes (which anastomose freely with the processes of neighboring osteocytes) are few and rather short. Being derived from osteoblasts, newly formed osteocytes still show many of the nuclear and cytoplasmic features of active osteoblasts. (An active osteoblast tends to present a large hyperchromatic nucleus, considerable basophilic cytoplasm, numerous rod-shaped mitochondria, a large Golgi apparatus, and a moderate amount of glycogen. It also gives evidence of alkaline phosphatase activity.) On the other hand, in the mature osteocytes of lamellar bone, the cytologic properties in question are much less conspicuous, and phosphatase activity may not be exhibited at all.

In bone of the lamellar (in contrast to the nonlamellar) type, the osteocytes are relatively few and also smaller, but have many more processes. These osteocytes are located between the lamellæ or near their borders and lie in flattened or ovoid lacunæ. In longitudinal sections of lamellar bone, the lacunæ appear much more elongated than they do in cross sections. The tubules (canaliculi) issuing from the lacuna of each mature osteocyte are numerous and delicate and branch freely. These canaliculi, too, contain processes which represent protoplasmic extensions from the bone cells. (See Fig. 20.)

The canaliculi extend between the fibrils of adjacent lamellæ and communicate with the canaliculi of neighboring lacunæ. Through such anastomoses, a network of passages is established which permits the circulation of tissue fluid throughout a fragment of lamellar bone roughly delimited by cement lines. As noted above, only few canaliculi traverse cement lines. Therefore, the fragments of interstitial lamellar bone, relatively isolated as they are from haversian canals, periosteum, and marrow cavity alike, are the most poorly nourished portions of compacta. Indeed, even in otherwise normal cortical bone, the interstitial osseous tissue has a low level of vitality as judged on the basis of absence of cells in some lacunæ and/or poor staining of those still present. In addition, it is to be observed that, as the vitality of the osseous tissue diminishes further, the bone cell lacunæ increase in size and the arrangement of the fibers in the neighboring lamellæ becomes disordered. All these various histologic criteria of slow decadence and death of osseous tissue presuppose, of course, that the changes observed in a particular tissue section do not represent artifacts produced by faulty technique in the processing of the tissue (see Jaffe and Pomeranz, Rutishauser and Majno, Sherman and Selakovich, and Frost).

Osteoblasts.—The rapidly evolving skeleton of a young fetus shows numerous osteoblasts at all sites of intramembranous and endochondral bone formation. In relation to a developing long tubular bone, for instance, osteoblasts are abundant in the cambium, or inner, layer of the periosteum, where they participate in the formation of the cortex by way of intramembranous ossification. They are also abundant in the interior of the evolving bone, where they lay down spongy osseous tissue in the wake of destruction and replacement of the cartilage during endochondral ossification. (See Figs. 1-*A*, 4-*B*, and 13-*A*.) In the older fetus, as the pace of skeletogenesis slows down, osteoblasts are no longer so abundant as in the young fetus, though they are still numerous. In particular, they are now less prominent in the inner layer of the periosteum and in the vessel canal spaces of the developing cortex, though they are still conspicuous at sites of endochondral ossification and on the surfaces of already formed spongy trabeculæ which are being remodeled.

Osteoblasts are mononuclear cells whose size and shape are related to their functional activity. They are always oriented to the surfaces of bone matrix and rarely show mitotic division figures. An osteoblast which is dormant, or resting, is a relatively small, flat or elongated cell with a correspondingly flattened nucleus. On the other hand, an osteoblast which is participating actively in the formation of bone matrix is usually about 20 to 30 microns in diameter, tends to be cuboidal or columnar in shape, and usually has a rather large, roundish nucleus oriented to one end of the cell. Delicate cytoplasmic processes may be found extending from the cell body of an active osteoblast, and some of these processes apparently anastomose with the processes of neighboring osteocytes.

The large size and eccentric location of the nucleus of an actively functioning osteoblast have already been mentioned. The nucleus is poor in chromatin and contains one or several nucleoli. The cytoplasm of the actively functioning osteoblast is strongly basophilic. In the cytoplasm abutting upon the nucleus, a large clear area (the juxtanuclear vacuole) may be observed. This represents the site of the Golgi apparatus, which is usually destroyed by fixation. Scattered through the cytoplasm, except in the region of the juxtanuclear vacuole, there are numerous short thick rods (mitochondria). The cytoplasm also contains small amounts of glycogen, some fine granules (apparently representing glycoprotein), and a scattering of sudanophilic (lipid) granules. Functioning osteoblasts show a moderate degree of phosphatase activity in the cytoplasm and relatively little in the nucleus (see Pritchard, and Tonna and Pillsbury).

In postnatal life, as skeletal maturation proceeds and the individual bones attain their full development, osteoblasts in the sense of actively functioning bone-forming cells are sparse. Not only does the number of osteoblasts diminish as skeletal maturation proceeds, but such osteoblasts as are still present are much smaller than the active osteoblasts of the fetus. Furthermore, these small osteoblasts are functionally dormant, or inactive, and thus no longer show the cytochemical features characterizing active osteoblasts. Nevertheless, in response to normal wear and tear or to pathologic stimuli, the dormant (or resting) and relatively sparse osteoblasts in the inner layer of the periosteum, on the walls of the vessel canals of the cortex, on the walls of the spongy trabeculæ, and in the supportive reticulum of the bone marrow may become rejuvenated into active osteoblasts.

That functioning osteoblasts are actively secreting cells is strongly indicated by their morphological and cytochemical features as described above. They produce and secrete most if not all of the material essential for the production of the organic matrix of osseous tissue. In particular, they elaborate the various protein molecules out of which the collagen fibrils of bone are formed (Carneiro and Leblond). They are also concerned with the formation of the mucopolysaccharides or with their precursors. The mucopolysaccharides are present as the "cement substance" between the collagen fibrils. The osteoblasts also secrete phosphatases and other enzymes, as well as various other substances, apparently including hexose phosphates. In Chapter 5, some consideration is given to the chemical nature of the organic matrix of bone and the possible mechanisms by which the matrix becomes mineralized through the deposition of crystals of hydroxyapatite and thus converted into osseous tissue.

Osteoclasts.—Osteoclasts are large multinuclear cells characteristically found on or near—that is, oriented to—osseous tissue which is in the process of resorption. They are ephemeral cells which develop rapidly, function for a few days at most, and then begin to degenerate. Some degenerating osteoclasts are phagocytosed *in situ*, while others (since osteoclasts are ameboid) may leave the local scene by entering neighboring capillaries and be swept into the circulation.

Figure 20

A, Photomicrograph ($\times$ 50) of a cross section of cortical bone prepared as a ground disk and impregnated with silver to demonstrate lacunæ and canaliculi. The lacunæ stand out as black dots, and the canaliculi are barely perceptible as filamentous threadlike structures.

B, Photomicrograph ($\times$ 600) showing the details in an area from A which is not too heavily blackened by the silver. Note the canaliculi streaming out from the lacunæ, and the anastomoses between the canaliculi of neighboring lacunæ.

C, Photomicrograph ($\times$ 150) showing, in a conventional tissue section, a small area from a femoral cortex in cross section. The patient was a woman 36 years of age who died of cardiac failure associated with rheumatic endocarditis and terminal pulmonary infarction. Note that osteocytes are largely absent from the bone cell lacunæ of the interstitial osseous tissue in the center of the picture. In the upper part of the picture, on the other hand, where haversian systems are present, most of the bone lacunæ contain osteocytes. The absence of osteocytes from the interstitial lamellar bone is to be related to the fact that the latter is normally the least well nourished part of the compacta.

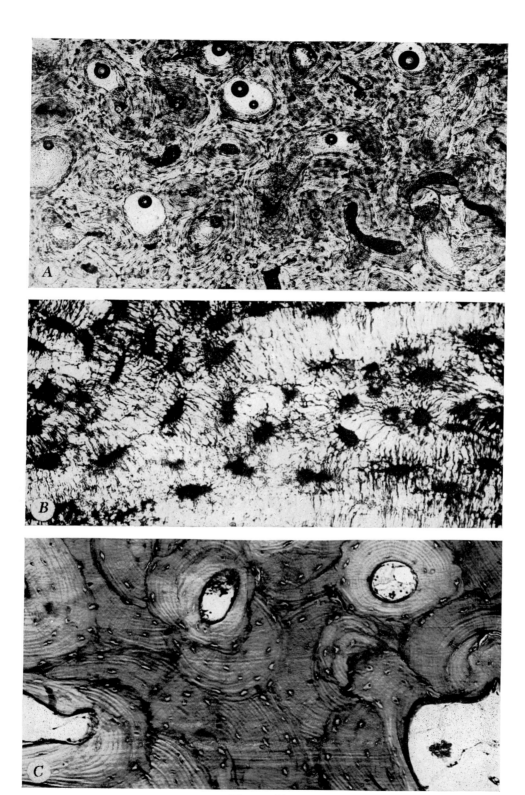

Figure 20

Though the fact that osteoclasts play a part in bone resorption has long been recognized, there is still much about them that remains obscure and intriguing. For instance, there is general agreement that the osteoclasts arise through fusion of mononuclear cells, but there is no unanimity of opinion in regard to the identity of the precursor cell. Some hold that osteoclasts are formed through the fusion of osteoblasts, while others claim that they are formed by fusion of osteocytes freed from the matrix in the course of dissolution of the ground substance. It is possible that osteoblasts in particular do participate in the formation of osteoclasts, but the idea that the latter arise mainly by fusion of the so-called wandering cells (macrophages) still seems the most plausible to the present writer. Concerning the manner in which osteoclasts function in bone resorption, there are many details which remain to be settled, but a brief consideration of the possible mechanism will be given below.

Osteoclasts vary a good deal in respect to their size and the number of nuclei they contain. Most of them measure about 30 to 50 microns in their longest diameter and have about 10 to 20 nuclei. An occasional osteoclast measures as much as 100 microns or even more in its longest dimension and may have as many as 100 nuclei or more. Such large osteoclasts undoubtedly represent the result of fusion of smaller ones into a single syncytial mass. At the other extreme, one encounters osteoclasts which are only about 20 microns in their longest dimension and have 2 or 3 nuclei. Osteoclasts also vary in shape, some being flattened and spread along the surface of the neighboring osseous tissue, while others are more or less roundish and oriented to pits, or hollows (Howship's lacunæ), on the surface of the osseous tissue.

In appropriately stained sections, the cytoplasm of actively functioning osteoclasts appears somewhat oxyphilic and presents numerous granules and some fine vacuoles. The nuclei are roundish and vesicular and usually show one or two nucleoli. In degenerating osteoclasts the cytoplasm is rather pronouncedly oxyphilic, the vacuoles are more numerous and larger, and the nucleoli are pyknotic; in frankly degenerated cells the nuclei are often in a state of karyolysis. Within the cytoplasm of functioning osteoclasts, one may occasionally also observe vacuoles containing one or more degenerating osteocytes, the latter having been phagocytosed by the osteoclast during the disintegration of the local osseous tissue in the course of its resorption.

Under favorable technical conditions, an osteoclast may show a striated, or "brush," border along the surface where the cell is in contact with the osseous tissue bounding a Howship's lacuna. The direction of the striations of the brush border is roughly perpendicular to the surface of the subjacent bone. Opinions differ as to what makes up the border, some holding that it represents merely a fringe of collagenous fiber bundles freed from the ground substance, while others hold that the border is produced by fringed projections of the cytoplasm of the osteoclast. However, evidence seems to favor the idea that the border is made up of both of these components and is the result of intermeshing of exposed collagenous bone fibers with projections from the cytoplasm of the osteoclast. In the region of brush borders, one can occasionally also observe tiny vacuoles, and it has been deduced that these represent secretion from the osteoclasts.

The biological mechanisms underlying bone resorption and the part which the osteoclast plays in these processes are by no means fully understood. Nor is it clear what stimulates their formation through the fusion of precursor cells. However, no one maintains any longer that where the osteoclast is at work it removes or "chews out" the bone without the occurrence of any preliminary changes in the local osseous tissue. Indeed, there is mounting evidence that while, or just before, an area of osseous tissue is resorbed to form a Howship's lacuna (resorption lacuna), the ground substance of the area in question is modified. (See Fig. 21.)

Though the sequence of events occurring in the ground substance in the course of bone resorption is not settled, it appears that the bone salt crystals are freed from the collagenous fibrils, the latter become disorganized, and the cement substance between the fibrils loosens. The changes in the cement substance and the fibrils probably occur through the agency of specific enzymes which modify (and depolymerize) the macromolecular structure of the mucopolysaccharides and collagen respectively. It is possible that the osteoclasts either directly secrete the enzymes involved or are implicated in some other way in their elaboration. Whether the liberated bone salt crystals are dissolved locally (by acids or other substances possibly secreted by the osteoclasts) or are swept away intact into the tissue fluid is still a matter of conjecture. There are also indications that, at sites of resorption, osteoclasts may actually take up some of the mineral crystals. In any event, it is only after disintegration of the ground substance has set in that this substance begins to be nibbled away (phagocytosed) by the osteoclasts, and that resorption pits (Howship's lacunæ) are formed. Under high power, one can note even with the light microscope some collagen fibers extending into a Howship's lacuna, and observe that the immediate margin of the lacuna stains somewhat differently from the osseous tissue at some distance from the margin. (See Kölliker, Arey, Jaffe, Hancox, Barnicot, Heller-Steinberg, Cameron and Robinson, Kroon, and also Tonna.)

In the normal course of skeletogenesis, osteoclasts participate actively in the remodeling of the osseous tissue which is laid down. The cells are relatively much more numerous in the skeleton of a young fetus than in that of an older fetus. While osteoclasts are also to be found in connection with postnatal growth and maturation of the bones, they become less and less numerous as the child develops, and in later childhood they are concentrated mainly at sites of active endochondral ossification. Osteoclasts are also to be observed where bone resorption is going on in pathologic states. In cases of Paget's disease and hyperparathyroidism, for instance, they are likely to be very numerous and widely distributed over the skeleton. They may also be found at sites of local bone damage or disease, as, for example, in areas of bone repair following a fracture or at sites of revascularization of a focus of aseptic bone necrosis.

Finally, it must be emphasized that the osseous tissue of a bone may be resorbed or become diminished in amount even without the agency of osteoclasts. There can be no doubt that, in the pronounced destruction of the skeleton which occurs, for instance, in connection with multiple myeloma, osteolytic carcinoma metastases, and leukemia, osteoclasts play an insignificant role at most. In these conditions it is the expansive growth of the tumor tissue against the osseous tissue that, directly or indirectly, causes the extensive bone resorption. On the other hand, bones may become rarefied or waste away through loss of osseous tissue, because new bone deposition does not keep pace with the continual loss resulting from metabolic turnover. Thus again, osteoclasts play hardly any part in the loss of bone substance encountered with postmenopausal osteoporosis or inactivity atrophy, for in these states there is a negative balance between bone resorption occurring in the course of the metabolic turnover and compensatory new bone deposition.

PERIOSTEUM AND ENDOSTEUM

Periosteum.—The periosteum is a membrane-like coat of connective tissue which substantially covers the outer surface of a bone and links or unites the latter with the surrounding soft parts. On the whole, it is a relatively thin membrane— considerably thinner in the young infant than in the adult. Also, it is by no means so intimately adherent to the bone in the young subject as in the adult. Indeed, under normal conditions in an adult, the periosteum is so firmly adherent that one encounters great difficulty in detaching or stripping an area of it as a distinct membrane. The periosteum does not extend over the surface of the articular cartilage (or cartilages) of a bone, stopping at the site of reflection of the joint capsule, with which it fuses. Where tendons, ligaments, and fasciæ fuse with the periosteum, the latter may be quite thick and usually has a tendinous sheen.

The periosteum is a rather vascular tissue. Large numbers of small capillaries leave it to enter the vessel canals of the underlying cortex, and postcapillary veins emerge from the cortex to enter the periosteum. The latter also contains numerous lymph vessels, which accompany the larger vascular channels. To some extent, the attachment of the periosteum to the bone is brought about by the blood vessels entering the cortex and by some strands of connective tissue which accompany them. In addition, some connective tissue fibers or fiber bundles enter the cortex independently and are incorporated in its ground substance. These penetrating fibers are known as Sharpey fibers. At sites such as tuberosities, the linea aspera, and the anterior surface of the patella, great numbers of coarse connective tissue fibers may be found to have entered the bone, and in such sites the periosteum no longer exists as a distinct membrane. In these areas, as already noted, the osseous tissue takes on the character of coarse-fibered bone, and the line along which the periosteum would normally continue is indicated by a thick band of calcified fibers. (See Fig. 22.)

In respect to its *histologic structure*, the periosteum may be regarded as consisting fundamentally of two layers. The inner (osteoblastogenic) layer is most clearly defined during embryonic and fetal life. The outer (fibrous) layer is often subdivided into two parts because of the presence of numerous elastic fibers in its deeper portion. The latter portion, in consequence, is often designated as the fibroelastic layer.

On the whole, the outer portion of the fibrous layer is rather collagenous and poor in cells. It is the most vascular portion of the periosteum. It also has some fat cells but only a few elastic fibers. Some of its collagen fibers are continuous with those in the interior of adjacent muscles, and where tendons blend with this portion of the periosteum the latter is highly collagenous. Pacinian corpuscles have been noted in it where it comes into contact with muscles. In addition, the outer

Figure 21

A, Photomicrograph (× 65) illustrating osteoclasts in Howship's lacunæ (see arrows) in bone from a case of Paget's disease. Note also the numerous irregularly indented cement lines ("reversal lines"). These mark the sites of new bone deposition against surfaces where resorption by osteoclasts had taken place.

B, Photomicrograph (× 400) showing a large Howship's lacuna (or two adjacent lacunæ) containing two osteoclasts possibly about to fuse. The osteoclast toward the left is apparently evacuating a bone cell lacuna and phagocytosing the osteocyte in it. There is a faint suggestion of a "brush" border at the bone-osteoclast junction. The osteoclast toward the right appears to be in an early stage of degeneration.

C, Photomicrograph (× 400) showing an osteoclast in a Howship's lacuna. The "brush" border stands out plainly (see arrows), and, toward the lower left, an osteocyte is apparently being drawn out of its lacuna.

D, Photomicrograph (× 400) showing an osteoclast in a Howship's lacuna. Its cytoplasm is granular and presents numerous fine vacuoles.

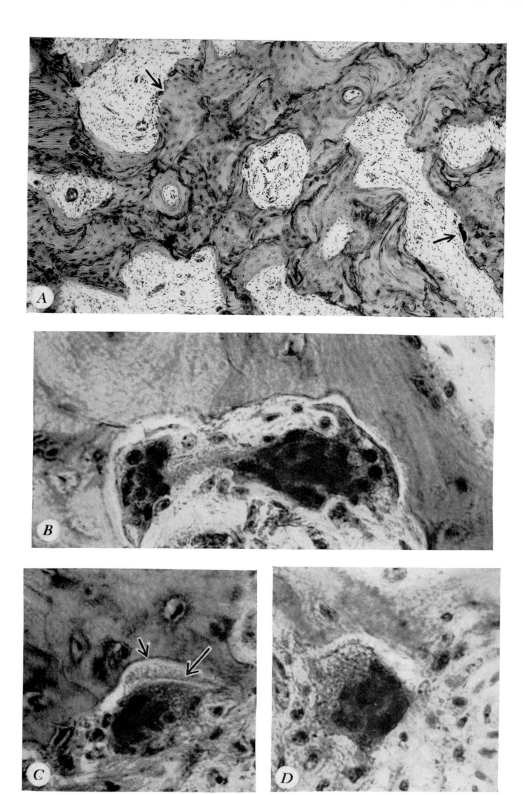

Figure 21

fibrous layer of the periosteum has a rich supply of nerve filaments, some of which accompany the blood vessels as they enter the cortex but most of which terminate in the deeper (fibroelastic) part of the fibrous layer (see Miskolczy). This part is relatively poor in blood vessels but particularly rich in elastic fibers, which are abundantly distributed through its connective tissue component. The latter is even more collagenous and poorer in cells than the connective tissue of the fibrous layer. Where tendons become inserted in the periosteum, the tendon fibers usually lose themselves in its fibroelastic portion.

In adults, an inner (osteoblastogenic) layer no longer exists as a distinct component of the periosteum, having fused with the outer layer. Indeed, even in childhood, it is no longer easy to distinguish it as a separate layer. At best—that is, during fetal life—the inner layer never constitutes more than a small part of the thickness of the periosteum. At that time, this layer consists mainly of rather loose vascular connective tissue entirely devoid of elastic fibers. Its deep surface contains numerous osteoblasts arranged more or less like epithelial cells. This stratum of osteoblasts, known as the cambium (in analogy with the cambium of the bark of a tree), disappears even before the inner layer of the periosteum merges with the outer layer. However, even in an adult, some osteoblasts are still present in the periosteum near the bone, although they are now merely drawn-out dormant cells, indistinguishable from ordinary fibroblasts. Whenever periosteal activity is restimulated, the dormant osteoblasts undergo reviviscence into functioning osteoblasts to resume their osteogenic activity.

Endosteum.—Theoretically, the endosteum may be defined as the lining of the interior of a bone. In regard to a long tubular bone, for instance, it may be conceived as the lining of the main marrow cavity, the marrow spaces of the spongiosa, and in a sense even the haversian canals of the cortex. It is true that, particularly in fetal life, a layer of functioning osteoblasts more or less lines these surfaces of such a bone. However, neither at that time nor later is the so-called endosteum a clearly defined and detachable membrane like the periosteum. Indeed, in a normal adult, the various interior surfaces of a bone do not even show a sheet of functioning osteoblasts, such as might vaguely suggest an endosteal lining. At this stage, the term "endosteum" can be applied only to the cells of the supporting connective tissue reticulum of the marrow which are apposed to the inner surface of the cortex, to the spongy trabeculæ, and to the walls of the haversian canals. The cells of this reticulum have osteogenic potentialities and may be interpreted

Figure 22

A, Photomicrograph ($\times$ 54) showing, in cross section, part of the cortex of a femur and its covering periosteum from a fetus 16 weeks old. The periosteum is composed of two easily distinguishable layers. Even under this relatively low magnification, it can be noted that the inner (cambium) layer of the periosteum is very cellular and that its component osteoblasts are actively laying down new bone.

B, Photomicrograph ($\times$ 45) showing, in cross section, part of the cortex of a tibia and its covering periosteum from a fetus 34 weeks old. Note that already the inner layer of the periosteum is much less prominent than in A and shows up only as a very narrow zone containing some osteoblasts.

C, Photomicrograph ($\times$ 80) illustrating Sharpey fibers (see arrows) which are penetrating and being incorporated into the osseous tissue beneath the periosteum.

D, Photomicrograph ($\times$ 100) showing the site of the attachment of a ligament directly into bone. Note that at this site a periosteal layer is absent and that, where the connective tissue fibers of the ligament become incorporated into the osseous tissue, there is a broad, dark-staining, calcified zone.

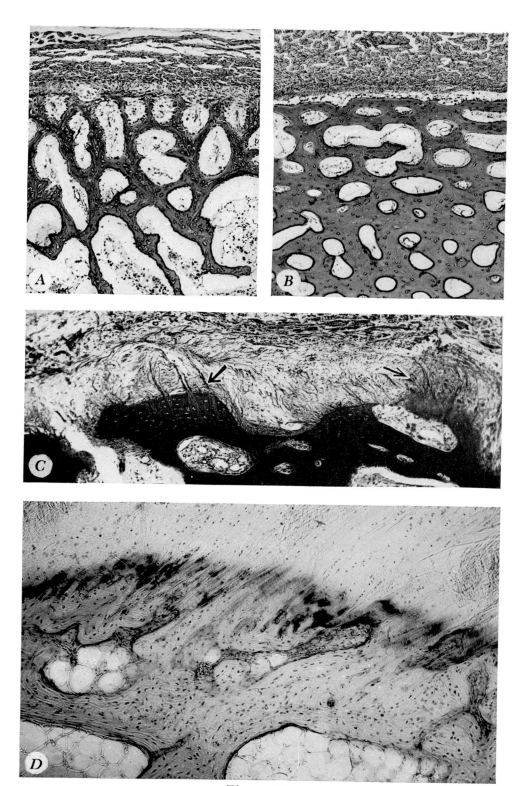

Figure 22

as resting osteoblasts. In fact, they become converted into active osteoblasts under the stress of such emergencies as fractures, or under other conditions involving the reconstruction of mature osseous tissue.

REFERENCES

AMSTUTZ, H. C., and SISSONS, H. A.: The Structure of the Vertebral Spongiosa, J. Bone & Joint Surg., *51–B*, 540, 1969.

AREY, L. B.: The Origin, Growth and Fate of Osteoclasts and their Relation to Bone Resorption, Am. J. Anat., *26*, 315, 1919–1920.

AXHAUSEN, G.: Ueber die durchbohrenden Gefässcanäle des Knochengewebes (Volkmann'sche Canäle), Arch. klin. Chir., *94*, 296, 1911.

BARNICOT, N. A.: The Local Action of the Parathyroid and other Tissues on Bone in Intracerebral Grafts, J. Anat., *82*, 233, 1948.

CAMERON, D. A., and ROBINSON, R. A.: The Presence of Crystals in the Cytoplasm of Large Cells Adjacent to Sites of Bone Absorption, J. Bone & Joint Surg., *40-A*, 414, 1958.

CARNEIRO, J., and LEBLOND, C. P.: Role of Osteoblasts and Odontoblasts in Secreting the Collagen of Bone and Dentin, as Shown by Radioautography in Mice Given Tritium-Labelled Glycine, Exper. Cell Res., *18*, 291, 1959.

VON EBNER, V.: Über den feineren Bau der Knochensubstanz, Sitzb. k. Akad. Wissensch., *72*, 1, 1875.

ENGFELDT, B.: Recent Observations of Bone Structure, J. Bone & Joint Surg., *40-A*, 698, 1958.

EVANS, F. G., and RIOLO, M. L.: Relations between the Fatigue Life and Histology of Adult Human Cortical Bone, J. Bone & Joint Surg., *52–A*, 1579, 1970.

FITZGERALD, P. J.: In *X-ray Microscopy and Microradiography (symposium)*, edited by V. E. Cosslett, A. Engström and H. H. Patee, Jr., New York, Academic Press, Inc., 1957, p. 49.

FROST, H. M.: *In Vivo* Osteocyte Death, J. Bone & Joint Surg., *42-A*, 138, 1960.

GEBHARDT, F. A. M. W.: Über funktionell wichtige Anordnungsweisen der gröberen und feineren Bauelemente des Wirbelthierknochens. I. Allgemeiner Theil. (Zweiter Beitrag zur Kenntnis des funktionellen Baues thierischer Hartgebilde.), Arch. Entwicklungsmechanik, *11*, 383, 1901; Zweite Hälfte: Theoretischer Theil, Arch. Entwicklungsmechanik, *12*, 167, 1901; II. Spezieller Teil. 1. Der Bau der Haversschen Lamellensysteme und seine funktionelle Bedeutung, Arch. Entwicklungsmechanik, *20*, 187, 1905–1906.

GEGENBAUR, C.: Ueber die Bildung des Knochengewebes, Jenaische Ztschr. Med. u. Naturwissensch., *1*, 343, 1864, and *3*, 206, 1867.

GLIMCHER, M. J.: Molecular Biology of Mineralized Tissues with Particular Reference to Bone, Rev. Mod. Physics, *31*, 359, 1959.

————: Specificity of the Molecular Structure of Organic Matrices in Mineralization. P. 421 in *Calcification in Biological Systems*, edited by R. E. Sognnaes, Washington, D. C., American Association for the Advancement of Science, 1960.

HANCOX, N.: The Osteoclast. Chapt. VIII in *The Biochemistry and Physiology of Bone*, edited by G. H. Bourne, New York, Academic Press, Inc., 1956.

HASHIMOTO, M.: The Distribution of Active Marrow in the Bones of Normal Adult, Kyushu J. M. Sc., *11*, 103, 1960.

HELLER-STEINBERG, M.: Ground Substance, Bone Salts, and Cellular Activity in Bone Formation and Destruction, Am. J. Anat., *89*, 347, 1951.

HEULER, K. M.: Besteht eine Korrelation zwischen Alter und Knochenstruktur? Ztschr. Zellforsch. u. mikr. Anat., *7*, 41, 1928.

JAFFE, H. L.: The Structure of Bone, Arch. Surg., *19*, 24, 1929.

————: The Vessel Canals in Normal and Pathological Bone, Am. J. Path., *5*, 323, 1929.

————: Methods for the Histologic Study of Normal and Diseased Bone, Arch. Path., *8*, 817, 1929.

————: Hyperparathyroidism (Recklinghausen's Disease of Bone), Arch. Path., *16*, 63 and 236, 1933. (See discussion relating to osteoclastic activity.)

JAFFE, H. L., and POMERANZ, M. M.: Changes in the Bones of Extremities Amputated Because of Arteriovascular Disease, Arch. Surg., *29*, 566, 1934.

KENYERES, B., and HEGYI, M.: Unterscheidung des menschlichen und des thierischen Knochengewebes, Vrtljschr. gerichtl. Med., *25*, 225, 1903.

KÖLLIKER, A.: Ueber die grosse Verbreitung der "perforating fibres" von Sharpey, Würzburg. naturwissensch. Ztschr., *1*, 306, 1860.

————: *Die normale Resorption des Knochengewebes und ihre Bedeutung für die Entstehung der typischen Knochenformen*, Leipzig, F. C. W. Vogel, 1873.

————: *Handbuch der Gewebelehre des Menschen*, Vol. 1, Leipzig, Wilhelm Engelmann, 1889.

KROON, D. B.: The Bone-Destroying Function of the Osteoclasts (Koelliker's "Brush Border"), Acta anat., *21*, 1, 1954.

MACEWEN, W.: *The Growth of Bone. Observations on Osteogenesis*, Glasgow, James Maclehose and Sons, 1912.

MISKOLCZY, D.: Über die Nervenendigungen der Knochenhaut, Ztschr. Anat., *81*, 638, 1926.

MORGAN, J. D.: Blood Supply of Growing Rabbit's Tibia, J. Bone & Joint Surg., *41-B*, 185, 1959.

MÜLLER, H.: Ueber Sharpey's durchbohrende Fasern im Knochen, Würzburg. naturwissensch. Ztschr., *1*, 296, 1860.

NELSON, G. E., JR., KELLY, P. J., PETERSON, L. F. A., and JANES, J. M.: Blood Supply of the Human Tibia, J. Bone & Joint Surg., *42-A*, 625, 1960.

PETERSEN, H.: Die Organe des Skeletsystems, in *Handbuch der mikroskopischen Anatomie des Menschen*, Vol. 2, edited by W. v. Möllendorff, Berlin, Julius Springer, 1930.

POMMER, G.: Über den Begriff und die Bedeutung der durchbohrenden Knochenkanäle, Ztschr. mikr.-anat. Forsch., *9*, 540, 1927.

PRITCHARD, J. J.: A Cytological and Histochemical Study of Bone and Cartilage Formation in the Rat, J. Anat., *86*, 259, 1952.

————: General Anatomy and Histology of Bone. Chapt. I in *The Biochemistry and Physiology of Bone*, edited by G. H. Bourne, New York, Academic Press, Inc., 1956.

ROBINSON, R. A., and WATSON, M. L.: Crystal-Collagen Relationships in Bone as Observed in the Electron Microscope. III. Crystal and Collagen Morphology as a Function of Age, Ann. New York Acad. Sc., *60*, 596, 1955.

RUTISHAUSER, E., and MAJNO, G.: Physiopathology of Bone Tissue: The Osteocytes and Fundamental Substance, Bull. Hosp. Joint Dis., *12*, 468, 1951.

SHERMAN, M. S., and SELAKOVICH, W. G.: Bone Changes in Chronic Circulatory Insufficiency. A Histopathological Study, J. Bone & Joint Surg., *39-A*, 892, 1957.

SMITH, J. W.: The Arrangement of Collagen Fibres in Human Secondary Osteones, J. Bone & Joint Surg., *42-B*, 588, 1960.

SMITH, R. J., SAGE, H. H., MIYAZAKI, M., and KIZILAY, D.: The Relationship of Lymphatics to Bone, Bull. Hosp. Joint Dis., *21*, 25, 1960.

TONNA, E. A.: Osteoclasts and the Aging Skeleton: A Cytological, Cytochemical and Autoradiographic Study, Anat. Rec., *137*, 251, 1960.

TONNA, E. A., and PILLSBURY, N.: Mitochondrial Changes Associated with Aging of Periosteal Osteoblasts, Anat. Rec., *134*, 739, 1960.

TRIEPEL, H.: *Die Architekturen der menschlichen Knochenspongiosa*, Munich and Wiesbaden, J. F. Bergmann, 1922.

VOLKMANN, R.: Zur Histologie der Caries und Ostitis, Arch. klin. Chir., *4*, 437, 1863.

WEIDENREICH, F.: Knochenstudien. I. Teil. Über Aufbau und Entwicklung des Knochens und den Charakter des Knochengewebes, Ztschr. Anat., *69*, 382, 1923.

————: Knochenstudien. II. Teil: Über Sehnenverknöcherungen und Faktoren der Knochenbildung, Ztschr. Anat., *69*, 558, 1923.

Chapter

4

Structure of Joints, Bursae Mucosae, and Tendon Sheaths

THE individual bones of the skeleton are joined to each other in various ways. Some of the resulting junctures, or articulations, are rigid (synarthroses), others are somewhat movable (amphiarthroses), and still others are freely movable (diarthroses). From a structural point of view, joints are also distinguished on the basis of the type of tissue which particularly characterizes the junctional area. On this basis, the various articulations are classified as: (1) fibrous joints, (2) cartilaginous joints, and (3) synovial joints. In regard to the joints, it is the synovial joints, and in particular their anatomic components, that will mainly concern us in this chapter. The bursae mucosae and tendon sheaths will receive only brief consideration.

FIBROUS JOINTS

In *fibrous joints* the apposed bony surfaces are fastened together by intervening connective tissue. The fibrous junctures may be grouped into syndesmoses and sutures. A *syndesmosis* is a fibrous articulation in which the uniting fibrous tissue (much more abundant than in a suture) constitutes: (1) an interosseous ligament, as in the distal tibiofibular articulation, or (2) an interosseous membrane, as in the attachment of the shaft of the radius to that of the ulna. *Sutures* are found only in the skull. From the point of view of mobility, they are synarthroses, since they are rigid. There are several varieties of sutures, differing in detail as to the way in which the apposed parts of the bones are coapted to one another. The enumeration and description of these varieties belong in the province of descriptive anatomy.

The sutures of the vault of the skull play a crucial role in the expansion of the cranial cavity. If one examines calvaria, it appears that until about the eighth year of life their sutural connective tissues are sites of active new bone formation permitting expansive growth of the bones which they bind. In this sense (that is, as sites of bone growth), these tissues are analogous to the epiphysial cartilage plate regions of tubular bones, although the bone formed in sutures is always of the connective tissue variety. After growth ceases in them, the apposed bone surfaces approximate each other more and more closely. Now only a trace of the connective tissue remains between them. Microscopic examination will disclose that the pericranium and dura (the equivalents of periosteum) are not interrupted at the sutures. The residual connective tissue between the bones at a suture contains blood vessels which enter it from the diploic spaces. Decades later, even this vestige of sutural connective tissue may disappear, and the calvarial parts previously separated by the sutures then undergo bony union—that is, synostosis.

CARTILAGINOUS JOINTS

The *cartilaginous joints* are of two types—symphyses and synchondroses. In *symphyses* the adjacent bony surfaces are connected by a disk, or plate, of tissue which arises by chondrification of the mesenchyme between two separate bone rudiments which were themselves originally cartilaginous. Subsequently, much of this tissue undergoes regression into fibrocartilage or fibrous connective tissue. Usually, however, the disk (or plate) still retains some hyaline cartilage, though only where it is apposed to the bone. Symphyses are best exemplified in the connection between two vertebral bodies or between the pubic bones. Such joints are neither completely fixed nor freely movable, and are hence amphiarthroses. In *synchondroses* the tissue joining the bone parts has, from the first, been hyaline cartilage. This tissue is a remnant of the continuous cartilaginous mass in which the articulated bony parts were formed. The type of articulation in question is exemplified by the cartilaginous connection (epiphysial cartilage plate) between the epiphysis (or epiphyses) and the diaphysis of any growing tubular bone. Since this is a rigid connection, it is also a synarthrosis. When the epiphysial cartilage plates disappear (by the end of the growth period), these synchondroses become obliterated, and bony union (synostosis) occurs between the previously articulated bone parts. The tissue changes by which epiphysial cartilage plates are destroyed and the synostosis occurs have been described in a previous chapter (p. 18).

Symphyses.—The pubic bones are connected by a disk—the *pubic symphysis*. In adults this disk is composed essentially of fibrous or fibrocartilaginous tissue, though next to the bone there is hyaline cartilage. It contains no nucleus pulposus, but instead, there is a slitlike cleft in the center of the fibrocartilaginous plate. This is not a genuine articular cavity but merely the result of regressive tissue changes. The pubic symphysis has a special interest because of the pathologic changes appearing in it in the course of pregnancy and childbirth. It seems appropriate to make brief mention of these pathologic changes here, since they will not be discussed again. (See Fig. 23.)

As noted, the symphysis pubis contains a slitlike cleft in its central portion. As the subject grows older, the cavity within the symphysis pubis in males and also in nulliparous females consistently undergoes enlargement merely in consequence of the normal mechanical influences exerted on the symphysis during the subject's ordinary activities. During the latter part of pregnancy and during childbirth, the pubic symphysis is, of course, subjected to a striking increase of functional and mechanical influences. These lead to widening and conspicuous irregularity of the original cavity in the symphysis, and to the appearance of other slitlike spaces in the disk which are irregular and usually multiple. Some of these new spaces extend transversely across the disk, while others may parallel the direction of the original cavity of the disk. In addition, slitlike spaces may be found even beneath the ligaments binding the pubic bones. Multiparous females come to show still more pronounced changes, including degeneration of cartilaginous portions of the symphysis pubis, leading eventually to the development of a local osteoarthritis. Thus the gross anatomic appearances and particularly the microscopic findings relating to a given symphysis pubis of an adult permit one to judge whether the subject was a male, a nulliparous female, or a parous female (see Eymer and Lang, Haslhofer, Sutro, and also Boland).

Let us now consider the amphiarthroses between the vertebral bodies. These articulations are of strategic importance in the architecture and functioning of the vertebral column. The vertebral bodies are joined by the *intervertebral disks* and by the anterior longitudinal ligament and, less importantly, by the posterior longitudinal ligament. For gross examination of the articulating surfaces of two apposed vertebral bodies, the intervertebral disk must be entirely removed by maceration. Then it will be seen: (1) that each of these surfaces presents around its margin a ringlike, bony elevation—the epiphysial ring, or marginal ridge, and (2) that the rest of each surface is composed of somewhat closely compacted spongy bone, which, although it is not a genuine bony end plate, has been designated by Schmorl as the "Schlussplatte." When the disk is in its normal position, each of the relatively compact spongy surfaces of the apposed vertebral bodies is covered by a thin plate of hyaline cartilage. These cartilage plates are actually parts of the intervertebral disk. The rest of this structure—the disk proper—consists of a relatively soft, more or less central tissue mass (the nucleus pulposus) and a larger, densely fibrous, indeed tendinous, outer part (the annulus fibrosus, or lamellosus).

The tissue constituting the nucleus has an exceedingly delicate fibrous network, a highly fluid matrix, and a profusion of cells in its meshes. During life, this nucleus is under rather high pressure, and especially in young persons it possesses considerable turgor. Consequently, if an intervertebral disk from a young subject is sectioned longitudinally, the nucleus immediately protrudes above the surface of the surrounding annulus fibrosus, or lamellosus. Sometimes the nucleus shows a small, irregular space. However, this is not a true joint cavity, such as one finds in diarthrodial (synovial) joints. Instead, it is apparently related to desiccation or degeneration in this region during life, or it is due merely to the shrinkage involved in the preparation of the tissue for examination. Some of the fibers of the nucleus merge above and below with the cartilage plates, and elsewhere with the surrounding and encapsulating annulus fibrosus.

This annulus consists of dense fibrous tissue arranged in a series of more or less concentric lamellae. The fibrous lamellae extend from one vertebral surface to the opposite one in wide curves, and are attached mainly to the neighboring epiphysial rings, or marginal ridges. In front and behind, they fuse with the anterior and posterior longitudinal ligaments respectively. Internally they merge, of course, with the plates of hyaline cartilage covering the central portions of the articulating surfaces of the vertebral bodies. The tissue composing the annulus is made up of dense, coarse connective tissue fibers with little matrix between them. (See Fig. 24–A.) We have become increasingly aware of the frequency with which the

Figure 23

A, Photomicrograph (× 5) illustrating the general histologic architecture of the symphysis pubis in an adult male. The subject, a salesman by occupation, died of bronchopneumonia at the age of 60 years. Since the slitlike cleft in the symphysis pubis does not extend through the entire thickness (or depth) of the symphysis, only a faint suggestion of a cleft is visible in the upper part of the picture. (The posterior surface of the symphysis is at the upper part of the picture, as it is in the other illustrations on this page.)

B, Photomicrograph (× 5) showing the general histologic architecture of the symphysis pubis from another elderly male. In this case, death was due to arteriosclerotic heart disease. The slitlike cleft in this symphysis pubis is clearly apparent.

C, Photomicrograph (× 5) illustrating the histologic appearance of the symphysis pubis area from the case of a multiparous female who died at the age of 52 from peritonitis following intestinal perforation. Note the disruption of the symphysis as a whole; the extension of the central cavity beyond the limits of the pubic bones; and the presence, in the right half of the picture, of islands of cartilage within the substance of the pubic bone. These changes indicate that, in this multiparous female, advanced changes of osteoarthritis have developed at the articulation in question. (The illustrations in this figure, and several others in this chapter, were made from specimens removed at autopsy by Dr. Charles J. Sutro when he was studying the pathologic anatomy of various joints during his tenure [1934–1936] as an Orthopaedic Research Fellow in the Department of Pathology under the author's direction.)

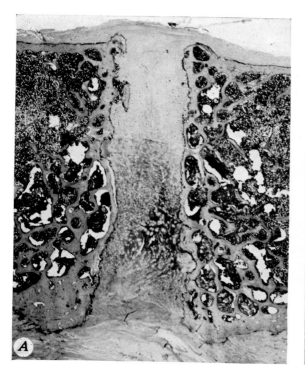

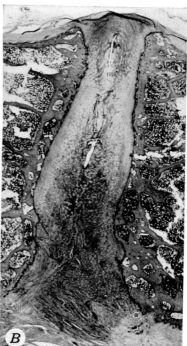

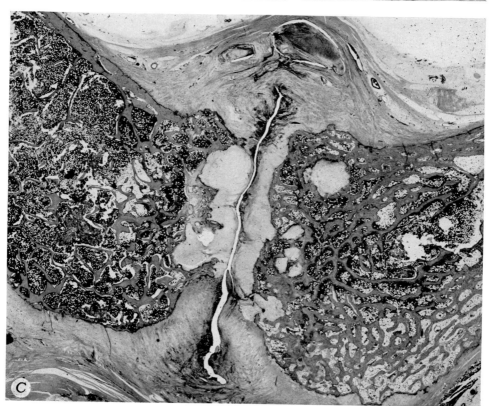

Figure 23

83

intervertebral disks undergo degenerative changes, especially in later life. The details relating to the regressive pathologic changes occurring in the intervertebral disks are discussed in the section dealing with spondylosis deformans (p. 762).

SYNOVIAL JOINTS

Synovial joints, also known as diarthroses, are capable of free motion, and this may be very ample. It is this type of joint that articulates the tubular bones of the extremities and that we usually have in mind in speaking of joints in general. These "true" joints are distinguished by the presence of a joint space. This is closed off by a capsule which holds the bone ends together and into whose formation ligaments and tendons enter. This ligamentous capsular tissue is lined by synovial membrane. Where the bone ends articulate, they are covered by cartilage, which in most diarthroses is smooth and hyaline. Such portions of the bone ends as are not covered by cartilage but are nevertheless included within the limits of the capsule are covered at least by synovial membrane. In some synovial joints the articular space is divided, completely or incompletely, by a disk or by menisci. The periphery of these intra-articular structures is continuous with the capsule.

There are a number of varieties of synovial joints, differing in regard to the kind of motion possible in each. In hinge joints (ginglymi) and pivot (trochoid) joints, movement takes place only around one axis, although within this limit its range may be considerable. In *hinge joints* the plane of motion is forward and backward, as in a hinge. A perfect example of this type of articulation is an interphalangeal joint. The knee and ankle joints are less characteristic of this type, as they allow a slight degree of rotation or side-to-side movement in certain positions. In *pivot joints* the movement is limited to rotation. The joint is formed by a pivot-like process turning within a ring (as in the proximal radio-ulnar articulation) or by a ring rotating on a pivot (as in the articulation of the odontoid process of the axis with the atlas).

In other synovial joints, movement is biaxial. It may proceed around two horizontal axes at right angles to each other, as in a *condyloid articulation* ex-

Figure 24

A, Photograph showing, in transverse section, the cut surface of an intervertebral disk from the lumbar region of the spine of a man 34 years of age. The concentric lamellae visible in the outer portion of the disk constitute the annulus fibrosus, or annulus lamellosus. Much of the nucleus pulposus, which lies within the interior of the disk, has been lost in the course of sectioning the latter. Below the disk and to each side of it, a facet joint (formed by the inferior and superior articular processes of two adjacent vertebrae) is apparent.

B, Photomicrograph ($\times$ 10) showing the general architecture of a facet joint—a diarthrosis in which motion is limited to gliding of its surfaces upon each other. The joint surfaces are covered by hyaline cartilage. The bony end plate beneath each of the articular cartilages is normally very thick, as is apparent in the picture. On the left side of the picture, one can see the capsular ligament of this vertebral synovial joint. The capsular tissue is dense fibrous tissue. On its inner surface it shows synovial membrane with a small amount of subsynovial fat. At the right side of the picture, the dark-staining tissue closing off the joint represents ligamentum flavum.

C, Photomicrograph ($\times$ 20) illustrating the general histologic architecture of a synovial joint as represented by an interphalangeal joint of a finger. The articular capsule on the left side of the picture shows a wedgelike fold of synovial membrane protruding from its inner surface into the joint space.

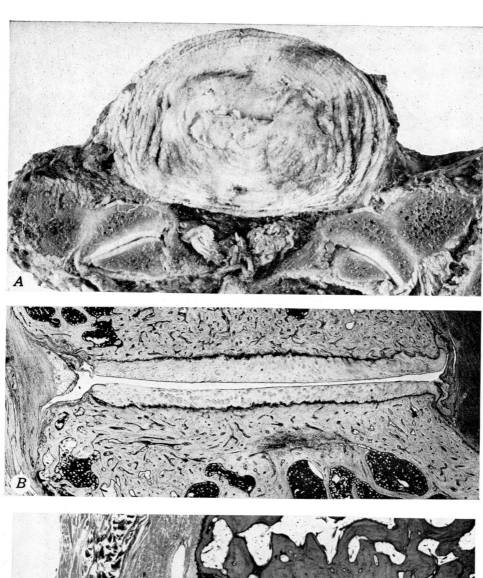

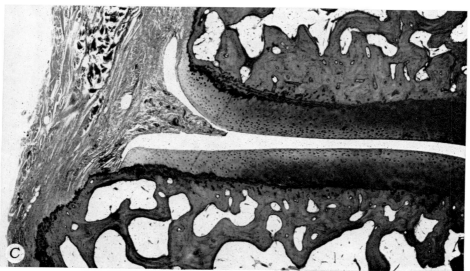

Figure 24

emplified by the wrist joint. Or the biaxial movement may take place along axes which may not be vertical or horizontal but are nevertheless at right angles to each other. This is the case in the *saddle joint* at the carpometacarpal articulation of the thumb.

A synovial joint which is formed by the reception of a globular head into a cuplike cavity is known as a *ball-and-socket joint* (enarthrosis). In such an articulation (for instance, the hip or shoulder joint), the distal articular surface is capable of motion along an indefinite number of axes which have one common center. *Plane*, or *gliding*, *joints* (arthrodia) are a form of diarthrosis in which both apposed articular surfaces tend to be flat and in which the only motion possible is a limited gliding movement of these surfaces upon each other. Many articulations, including notably those between the articular processes of the vertebrae, are of this type. (See Fig. 24.)

We shall now consider the structure of the various anatomical components of synovial joints. (See also the monograph by Barnett *et al.*)

ARTICULAR CARTILAGE

The articulating surfaces of the bone ends of diarthrodial joints are normally covered by hyaline cartilage. The extent of this cartilage on each bone end corresponds in general to the area of functional contact between the apposed bones. However, this cartilage does not become definitive articular cartilage in the sense of an anatomic structure until the skeletal part which it covers has completed its growth. The reason for this is that, up to the end of the growth period, endochondral bone formation is still taking place to some extent along the deep surface of the cartilage. The completion of endochondral bone formation on the deep surface of the cartilage is signalized by the appearance of a narrow zone of calcification which, in the definitive articular cartilage, represents the calcified zone of that cartilage. The latter abuts on and meshes with the underlying subchondral bone—the bony end plate. Thus, if a thin vertical section of hyaline articular cartilage of a young adult is inspected with the naked eye, it will be seen that, toward the joint surface, the cartilage appears translucent, while further down against the bony end plate it presents a cloudy appearance. In an x-ray picture the outlines of the bones entering into the formation of the joint are determined mainly by the immediately subchondral bone (the bony end plates). Indeed, under normal conditions the articular cartilages are radiolucent except for their deeply situated calcified zones, which abut on the corresponding bony end plates. At its periphery, the articular cartilage fuses with the joint capsule and with the periosteum. Even for the same joint, the position of the line on which these tissues meet varies somewhat in different persons. The immediate region of the fusion is also precisely the site at which exostoses develop in connection with arthritis—for instance, of the hypertrophic variety.

Normal articular cartilage is devoid of blood vessels, lymphatics, and nerves. The cartilage cells receive their nourishment by means of diffusion of tissue fluids through the intercellular substance. The chief source of nutriment for the articular cartilage is the synovial fluid, though the cartilage apparently also receives some nourishment by diffusion from the blood coursing through the vessels in the adjacent subchondral bone.

Color and Thickness.—The *color* of the cartilage covering the bone ends of diarthrodial joints varies with the age of the subject. In a young child the cartilage is essentially white but is likely to have a bluish tinge. In a young adult the cartilage (which is now definitive articular cartilage) appears white and glossy and is somewhat compressible. In an adult of middle age, the color of the articular cartilage has usually shifted to yellowish white, and the cartilage feels firmer and less compressible than in a young adult. With further advance in age (even in the absence of gross pathologic changes), the articular cartilages tend to take on a yellowish brown tinge and to become less resilient—that is, even more resistant to pressure.

The *thickness* of articular cartilage is by no means the same on all articular surfaces or on corresponding surfaces in different persons. It is also not necessarily uniform over any one articular surface. Thus, in the hip it is greater at the margins of the acetabulum than at the bottom of the fossa, while in the head of the femur it is greater at the convexity than at the margins. In the knee the cartilage of the patella is ordinarily much thicker than that covering the other bones of this joint. Except in special locations (such as on the patella, where it is particularly thick, and on the phalanges, where it is particularly thin), the thickness of normal articular cartilage in adults is usually about 2 or 3 mm. On the patella it may reach 5 or 6 mm., and on the phalanges it is usually not more than 1 mm.

On the whole, the principal points which seem to be of interest in relation to the thickness of articular cartilage are: (1) that it is generally greater in large joints than in small ones; (2) that it tends to be relatively greater in joints or in parts of joints in which there is considerable functional pressure (notably in the joints of the lower extremity as compared with the upper); (3) that it seems to be increased by friction and by scissor action on the cartilage and by pronounced functional lateral displacement due to tangential forces; (4) that in general it is less in smoothly fitting joints than in poorly adapted ones; (5) that its amount tends to be decreased by nonuse of the joint; and (6) that in old age the articular cartilages of an individual person are likely to be somewhat thinner than they were during middle life.

It also seems worth noting that a period of active exercise, particularly in young adults, may result in swelling of the articular cartilages of the exercised joints, though this subsides after a brief period of rest. It is held that the swelling is due to the imbibition of fluid by the cartilage cells and the cartilage matrix (see Ekholm and Ingelmark).

Histologic Structure.—On microscopic examination, articular cartilage is found to be composed of cells (chondrocytes) which are embedded in an intercellular matrix. The cartilage matrix consists essentially of collagenous fibrils set in a homogeneous ground substance. Apart from its high water content (about 75 per cent), the ground substance in which the fibrils are set consists in large measure of mucopolysaccharides, and specifically of chondroitin sulfate A along with some chondroitin sulfate C. In the articular cartilages of elderly persons, small amounts of keratosulfate may also be present. Because the refractive index of the collagen fibrils and ground substance is similar, the fibrils are not visible in sections stained with hematoxylin and eosin and examined with the light microscope. It is generally believed that the chondrocytes of the articular cartilage elaborate both the mucopolysaccharides and the fibrils of the intercellular matrix.

In a stained tissue section which includes the entire thickness of the articular cartilage of a large joint of an adult, microscopic examination will reveal a tendency toward stratification and arrangement of the cartilage cells into four roughly distinct zones. The first three are set apart from each other by differences in the slant and grouping of their cells. The fourth zone, the deepest, is further distinguished from the others by the presence of calcium in the intercellular matrix.

The most superficial of the four zones is the narrow *gliding*, or *tangential*, zone. The cells of the latter are flattened and lie parallel to the articular surface. Incidentally, this portion of the cartilage was formerly misinterpreted as a continuation, in modified form, of the synovial membrane of the joint.   Beneath the gliding zone there is the somewhat broader *transitional zone*.   Its cartilage cells are less flattened (or are even roundish), and may appear clumped into groups. The third zone, or the *radial zone*, is by far the broadest.   The total thickness of a particular cartilage is largely determined by the thickness of this zone.   Where the radial zone is well developed, it takes up about two-thirds of the depth of the cartilage.   Its cells are flattened laterally and arranged in more or less short rows vertical or somewhat radial to the surface of the cartilage.   Finally, apposed to the bony end plate (subchondral bone cortex), there is the irregular *calcified zone*, which, as noted, stands out by virtue of calcification of its matrix.   It is delimited from the radial zone by a wavy line, along which the calcareous material is rather concentrated.   The arrangement of its cells is like that in the radial zone.   In the transition region between them, there are sometimes cells lying partly in one zone and partly in the other.   Below the delimiting wavy line of the calcified zone, there may be one or more other calcium lines running parallel to it for various distances. Thus, in places a set of parallel calcareous striations becomes manifest in the calcified zone.   However, in other places within the latter, the calcium is diffusely distributed through the matrix or is concentrated only here and there around cells. The calcified zone is set off from the bony end plate by cement lines, analogous to those between fragments of osseous tissue.

Although its details vary, the stratification and cellular arrangement described above are well-recognized features of the histology of articular cartilage in general. On the whole, the division into zones is more clearly evident in animals than in man.   The columnar arrangement of the cells in the radial zone stands out much more distinctly in the dog and cat, for instance, than in man.   Furthermore, in man the cellular arrangement of the first three zones is manifested most clearly in the articular cartilages of large joints.   In certain of the smaller joints of adults, the arrangement of the cartilage cells may suggest that found in the larger joints but usually does not present it plainly.   Again, in a growing person the stratification into four zones is not found even in a large joint if the cartilage covering the end of the bone in question is still manifesting evidence of endochondral bone formation on its deep surface.

That *collagen fibrils* are present in the intercellular matrix of articular cartilage has been known for a long time (see Tillmanns and also Nykamp).   For the demonstration of the fibrils, special methods (including phase-contrast microscopy and/or electron microscopy) are necessary, since, in normal hyaline cartilage stained with hematoxylin and eosin, the fibrils, as already noted, are completely masked by the cartilage ground substance.   The course and disposition of the collagenous fibrils of the articular cartilage have received much study.   It is clear that these fibrils are grouped into fiber bundles.   However, there are differences of opinion in regard to the pertinent details.   The concept which prevailed for a long time and which still has much in its favor can be outlined as follows: Many of the fiber bundles are arranged in loops whose summits reach the gliding zone and whose ends are anchored in the calcified zone.   On or near the surface of the cartilage—that is, in the gliding zone—the fiber bundles run horizontally for short distances.   This was already maintained in 1898 by Hultkrantz on the basis of his studies of the direction taken by mechanically induced splits in the superficial layers of the cartilage.   In particular, he held that in this region the fibrils are numerous and closely compacted into small bundles, but are not arranged in any systematic way in relation to the cartilage cells.   The more firmly the intercellular ground substance knits the tangential fibrils of the gliding layer together, the smoother and glossier is the surface of the cartilage.   So far as function is concerned, this layer is apparently resistant to vertically directed pressure, and particularly adapted for smooth rolling of the apposed surfaces against each other. The presence of some elastic fibers in the gliding layer has long been known, and had already been mentioned by Hammar.

The direction of the fibrils in the transitional zone is very difficult to discern. Van der Stricht was apparently the first to suggest that in this zone the fibrils, which in the gliding layer were parallel to the surface, arch down on their way into the radial zone, in which they run perpendicular to the surface. Furthermore, Benninghoff and others have reported that some of the fibrils do not reach the radial zone but terminate as fibrillar nests around the cells of the transitional zone. They also held that many of the fibrils which do reach the radial zone end there in the same way (that is, as fibrillar nests about cells in the radial zone), while other fibrils continue down and become anchored in the calcified zone, as already stated. (See Fig. 25.)

The course and disposition of the collagenous fiber bundles in the articular cartilage as outlined above have been questioned particularly by MacConaill. The latter holds that, at the free surface of the articular cartilage, there is an exceedingly thin layer of cartilage matrix devoid of collagenous fibrils. He reported that the collagenous fiber bundles lying immediately beneath the surface layer are present as an anastomosing and interlacing network, within whose interstices the cartilage cells lie singly or in groups. Moreover, he contended that the main direction of the fiber bundles is oblique, and not vertical or radial, as proposed by Benninghoff. It may well be that the reported differences in the predominant course of the collagen fibers of articular cartilage are to be related to the age of the subject and the presence or absence of mild degenerative changes on the surface of the cartilage. Certainly in an older subject the direction of the fibers in the articular cartilage is predominantly radial or vertical rather than oblique or horizontal (see Trueta and Little, and Silberberg et al.).

Fibrous (Dehyalinized) Articular Cartilage.—Wherever articular cartilage lacks hyalin or has become dehyalinized, the fibrillar substratum of its ground substance becomes easily detectable. The cartilage in such areas may be designated as fibrocartilage. Grossly, such cartilage is distinguishable from the hyaline variety by its tendinous sheen and by the recognizable striations that its surface may present.

Even where the cartilage is otherwise hyaline (as notably in joints of extremities), the fibrillar nature of the tangential layer may be apparent normally at the periphery of the cartilage. As already noted, this marginal fibrous cartilage enters into combination with the capsule of the joint at its angle of reflection and with the edge of the periosteal cuff. It is held (for instance, by Benninghoff) that at its periphery the gliding layer of hyaline joint cartilage is fibrous, because in this region there is no vertical functional pressure and the cartilaginous tissue is subjected merely to transverse pull. In some of the joints whose cartilage comes nearest to being exclusively hyaline, areas other than the periphery may also be more or less fibrous. Among these are: (1) the region immediately surrounding the fovea of the head of the femur; (2) the juncture of the labium with the hyaline cartilage covering the rest of the articular fossa of the scapula and of the innominate bone; and (3) the point where the cruciate ligaments radiate into the cartilage of the knee joint.

There are certain diarthrodial joints (for instance, the temporomandibular and sternoclavicular joints) in which the fibrous aspect of the articular cartilage is very conspicuous. "Fibrous" articular cartilage is found in large amounts mainly in joints in which the apposed bone ends are separated by thick fibrous disks which completely divide the articular space. The hindrance of contact between the joint ends favors the extensive dehyalinization which makes this "fibrousness" predominate. The cartilage may be fibrous through the transitional zone and even down into the radial zone. In fact, in the temporomandibular joint, only a small remnant of the articular cartilage, close to the bone, retains its hyaline character. In the outer, or more superficial, portion of the cartilage, the collagen fiber bundles tend to have a parallel direction in relation to the surface. If the radial zone becomes de-hyalinized, most of its fiber bundles, originally perpendicular, collapse and come to take a more or less oblique course in relation to the surface of the cartilage. Distributed among the collagen fiber bundles there are elastic fibers, and these are most abundant near the surface of the fibrous articular cartilage (see Miles and Dawson). Fibrous articular cartilages also have a calcified zone. Furthermore, they are anchored to the underlying bony end plate in exactly the same way as are hyaline cartilages.

Dehyalinization is likewise the mechanism by which cartilage that is normally hyaline becomes "fibrous" under pathologic conditions. It is apparent even on gross examination that fibrous cartilage yields to pressure much more easily than does that of the hyaline variety. When the fibrils of hyaline articular cartilage have once become demasked through dehyalinization, they are revealed even in a section stained with hematoxylin and eosin.

Anchorage of the Articular Cartilage to the Bony End Plate.—The *bony end plate*, upon which the articular cartilage rests, is the layer of osseous tissue which seals off the marrow cavity of a bone in the region of a joint. In most human bones this plate is thin, consisting mainly of the arches of spongy trabeculae which curve around just below the articular cartilage. These arches are usually no thicker than the trabeculae themselves. In the case of certain human bones, the bony end plate is so thick that it virtually constitutes a subchondral bone cortex. The latter has a highly complex architecture and is penetrated by numerous vessel canals which may extend up to the cartilage. In the larger hoofed animals, the plate is almost always of this thick dense type. In human bones the plate may be thicker in some parts of a given articular surface than in others. Thus, in the middle regions of articular fossae (for example, the acetabular area of the innominate bone), it is much thicker than it is below the cartilage of the apposed convex head. Also, below the subchondral cortex of such fossae, the trabeculae are particularly broad and the spongy spaces quite narrow—presumably in adaptation to functional pressure.

Figure 25

A, Photomicrograph ($\times$ 100) demonstrating the histologic structure of articular cartilage and the underlying bony end plate. The deep-lying calcified zone of the articular cartilage and the interdigitation of that zone with the arched trabeculae of spongy bone (constituting the bony end plate) are clearly apparent. Above the calcified zone, one can discern the almost columnar arrangement of the cartilage cells making up the wide radial zone. Above the latter, one can note an area in which the cartilage cells are more numerous but irregularly distributed—the transitional zone. At the surface of the articular cartilage, the nuclei of the cartilage cells tend to be somewhat flattened, and this area represents the tangential, or gliding, zone of the cartilage.

B, A schematic representation illustrating the course and disposition of the collagen fiber bundles in the intercellular matrix of the articular cartilage. As indicated in the text, many of the fiber bundles take the form of loops whose ends are anchored in the calcified zone and whose summits reach the tangential zone. On turning down from the tangential zone, some of the fibrils terminate as fibrillar nests around cells in the transitional and radial zones, thus failing to reach the calcified zone, while still other fibrils continue down and are anchored in the calcified zone.

C, Photomicrograph ($\times$ 250) showing a vascular channel extending up from the sub-chondral spongiosa and penetrating the calcified zone of the cartilage. Though the articular cartilage receives most of its nutriment from the synovial fluid, the deeper portion of the cartilage also receives some from capillaries extending to it from the spongiosa.

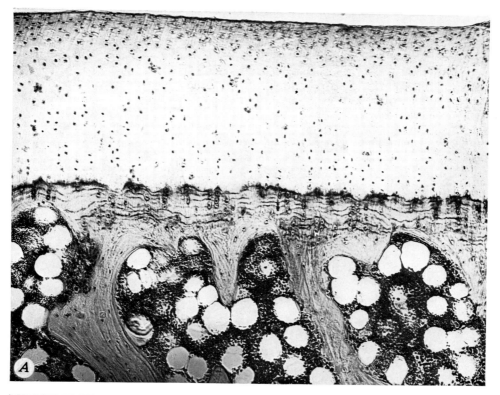

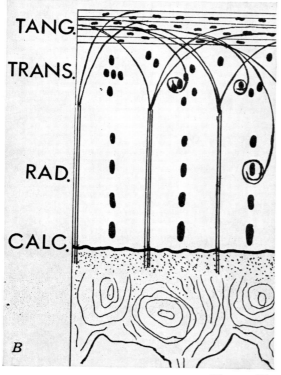

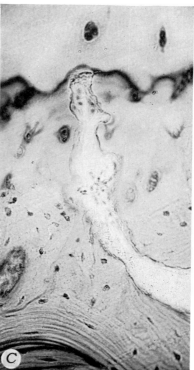

Figure 25

91

Projections from the deepest, or calcified, zone of articular cartilage fill in the wavy and toothed indentations on the surface of the bony end plate. In consequence of the interlocking of the two tissues, the cartilage is firmly anchored to the bone underlying it. In fact, even if the joint end of the bone is macerated, residua of the calcified cartilage zone remain, so that the surface of the bony end plate is still more or less smooth. In spite of this intimate interlocking, the individual fibrils of the cartilage do not intertwine with those of the bone, being separated from the latter by cement lines. Nevertheless, the connection between the cartilage and bone is so firm that a break is less likely to occur in the region of interlocking than below it. This region of interlocking is the site at which growth, reconstruction, or pathologic processes are most active in the articular end of a bone. That is, new endochondral bone may be deposited there after resorption has occurred.

ARTICULAR CAPSULE

The capsule of a diarthrodial joint is a somewhat yielding envelope of connective tissue. It is attached to the bone ends of the joint somewhere beyond the articulating surfaces, and closes off the joint space. At the site of attachment to the bone, the collagenous fibers of the capsule are anchored in the osseous tissue along a calcified zone which is continuous with the calcified zone of the articular cartilage. Essentially, an articular capsule is composed of a thin inner coat (the synovial membrane) and a relatively thick and toughly fibrous outer layer (the fibrous capsule). The outer fibrous layer, which largely determines the thickness of the articular capsule, acquires its characteristic texture from the ligaments and tendons which terminate in it. Indeed, where the fibrous layer of the capsule does not include such structures, the capsule as a whole is much attenuated. In such thin places it may consist mainly of synovial membrane which is covered merely by the para-articular soft parts. Furthermore, in such places there may be communication between the main joint cavity and an adjacent bursa mucosa, the lining membrane of the bursa (its synovial membrane) being continuous with the synovial membrane lining the articular capsule. In addition to the capsular ligament, which may or may not have special bands, there may be other ligaments connecting the bones. These accessory ligaments may lie outside of the capsule or, like the cruciate ligaments of the knee joint, be intracapsular.

Where it is well developed, the outer portion of the capsule is found, on *microscopic examination,* to consist of fibrous tissue varying in cellularity. In places it may be so densely and evenly collagenous, and relatively so poorly supplied with cells, as to have a true tendinous quality. Elsewhere it is more richly cellular and more like ordinary connective tissue. In either case, the fibrous elements are arranged mainly along the axes of tension, though there are also some connective tissue bundles running vertically or radially to these axes.

The capsule of a joint is richly supplied with blood vessels, lymphatic vessels, and nerves. All these structures are arranged in plexuses, or networks, and all penetrate from the fibrous portion of the capsule almost to the inner surface of the synovial membrane. Many of the nerve endings bulge into small corpuscles. In the synovial membrane the capillaries are quite numerous and tend to run parallel to its surface. At the site of mergence of the capsule with the margin of the articular cartilage, delicate capillary loops extend into the latter. These are part of the vascular border of the joint, which was denoted long ago by Hunter as the "circulus articuli vasculosus."

Synovial Membrane.—As noted, it is the outer coat that gives the capsule its distinctive structural qualities as a tough, fibrous envelope for the joint. As a site of articular disease, however, the inner coat—the synovial membrane—is the more important. In principle, this membrane is a thin but distinct and detachable highly vascular lining covering the inner surface of the articular capsule. Furthermore, synovial membrane covers any intra-articular ligaments or tendons present in a diarthrodial joint. It also covers any intracapsular bone parts where these parts are clothed by periosteum or perichondrium but not by articular cartilage. In certain articulations, large masses of fat covered by attenuated synovial membrane may protrude into the joint space. In the infrapatellar region of the knee joint, there is a particularly prominent pad of this kind. Moreover, the synovial membrane has a tendency to form small sleevelike synovial folds which may project inward for short distances between the apposed articular cartilages (see Grant).

Where present as a distinct and detachable lining on the inner surface of the capsule, the synovial membrane is found to consist of two layers—a thin intimal (surface) layer and a deeper subintimal layer. Under these conditions the intimal layer has a poorly defined surface coat consisting of cells of various shapes and only two or three cells deep at most. Beneath these covering cells there is a loose meshwork of connective tissue, some of whose collagenous fibers are interspersed among the surface cells. When present as a distinct layer, the subintimal portion of the synovial membrane may vary nevertheless (even from place to place) in respect to its histologic structure. In particular, it may be composed of loose connective tissue or more fibrous connective tissue, or in places the subintimal layer may consist essentially of fat. The subintimal layer merges on its deep surface with the fibrous coat of the capsule, and, where the subintimal layer is highly collagenous, it may not be clearly demarcated from the tough, fibrous part of the capsule.

In certain locations and under certain circumstances, the synovial membrane may be greatly attenuated and usually fails to present distinct intimal and subintimal layers. Thus, in relation to intra-articular ligaments (for instance, the cruciate ligaments of the knee joint) and tendons entering into the capsule of a joint (for instance, the quadriceps tendon of the knee joint), one may be unable to discern two distinct layers. Also, under these conditions the cells on the surface of the synovial membrane will be found sparse and flattened, and the deeper portion of the membrane may not be distinguishable from the ligament or tendon in question. (See Fig. 26.)

The *villi* are projections which may form on the surface of the synovial membrane. When the latter is otherwise entirely normal, villi are not to be found except in special regions, such as the niches between large fat folds. Even there they are usually so small as to be visible only microscopically. Such tiny villi are nearly always nonvascular protrusions (often branching) from the synovial membrane. They are likely to show considerable variation in the details of their shape and arrangement. They are composed of collagenous fibrils and covered with cells which in places are compacted into groups. The surface cells may be arranged in such a way as to suggest a lining, but there is no specialized lining layer of cells. It is quite common to find the tips of these villi either completely necrotic or in stages of disintegration. Villi forming on the surface of an otherwise normal synovial membrane probably represent a response to strictly local disturbing conditions, appearing, for instance, in response to trauma or the accumulation of irritative debris.

As a result of chronic low grade irritation and/or inflammation of the synovial membrane, villus formation is likely to be so abundant that most of the synovial surface of the capsule is covered by villous projections. Under such circumstances the villi vary widely in size, shape, and composition. As to structure, some may be merely narrow or plump stalked folds of fat covered by synovial membrane. Most, however, are highly vascular villous projections of the membrane itself. These are more consistently delicate and frequently quite long, sometimes protruding far into the joint cavity. Striking villous proliferation of the synovial membrane occurring as a feature of inflammatory and degenerative arthritis is illustrated in the chapters devoted to those conditions (pp. 779 and 735).

Finally, it should be noted that the synovial membrane does not cover the articular cartilages of the joint nor such intra-articular structures as disks and menisci, if these are present. The deeper, or subintimal, layer of the synovial membrane merges with the periosteum covering those bony components of the joint which lie within the capsule. At the margins of the articular cartilages, the merged periosteum and subintimal layer of the synovial membrane becomes continuous with the margin of the articular cartilage by way of a transitional fibrocartilaginous zone. The intimal layer of the synovial membrane overlaps the periphery of the articular cartilage for a very short distance, thins out, and merges with the margin of the cartilage.

For a long time it was held that the surface cells of the synovial membrane were specialized lining cells, and that the synovial lining of the joint capsule was thus a serous membrane. This opinion has been superseded by the idea that the synovial membrane represents a specialized connective tissue (see Hueter, Hammar, and also Sigurdson). In addition, the current conception is that, even when the surface cells seem to constitute a lining layer for the synovial membrane, they do not differ intrinsically from the other indigenous cells of the membrane. The cells of the intimal layer of the membrane, and particularly those on the surface, secrete the sticky mucoid substance present in the synovial fluid (see Vaubel, and Ropes and Bauer). These cells also possess phagocytic capacity, as do the resting wandering cells which may be present in small numbers about the blood vessels of the synovial membrane.

As to the precise position of synovial membrane among connective tissues, the findings obtained by Vaubel are of interest. Judging from their manner of growth in tissue cultures, he concluded that the cells of the synovial membrane are much

Figure 26

A, Photomicrograph ($\times$ 10) showing part of the articular surface and capsule of the upper end of a humerus and revealing the manner in which the capsule inserts itself into the bone just beyond the articular cartilage. Note that the thick collagenous fibers of the capsule are anchored in the bone beyond the cartilage. The anchorage is achieved by penetration of a zone of calcification which covers the local bone in the region of insertion of the capsule. The calcified zone in question is a continuation of the calcified zone of the articular cartilage. The subject was a man 59 years of age who died of multiple myeloma. Normally in a man of this age, the intertrabecular marrow spaces in the upper end of a humerus contain mainly fatty marrow, but in the present picture the dark-staining material in the intertrabecular spaces represents myeloma cells.

B, Photomicrograph ($\times$ 110) illustrating the general histologic architecture of synovial membrane of the knee joint in an area in which, deep to the intimal layer, the tissue is composed largely of simple fat. Note that the cells at the surface of the membrane are few in number and present no clear-cut arrangement in relation to that surface. Immediately beneath the surface of the membrane, numerous thin-walled capillaries are to be noted. The tissue came from the knee joint of a boy 13 years of age on whom an amputation of the lower extremity had been done because of an osteogenic sarcoma in the shaft of the tibia, definitely below the site of attachment of the capsule of the knee joint.

C, Photomicrograph ($\times$ 110) illustrating the general histologic pattern of the synovial membrane from another area of the same knee joint. In this area of the membrane, the immediate subintimal layer is composed largely of collagenous fibrous tissue.

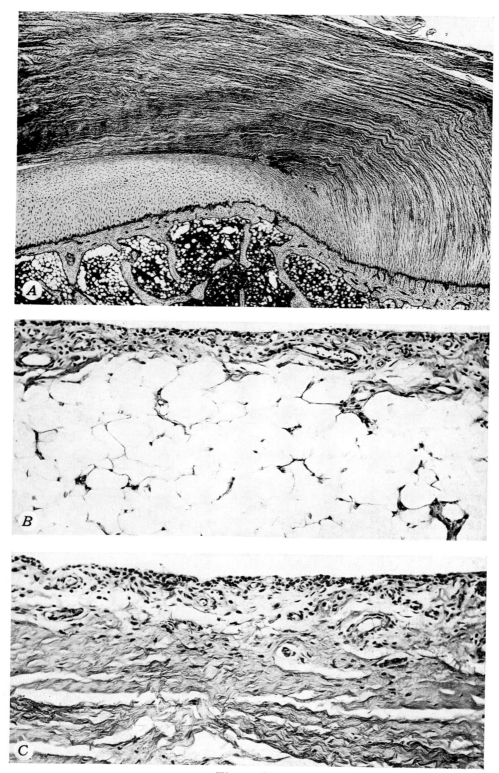

Figure 26

closer to chondroblasts and osteoblasts than they are to ordinary fibroblasts. This observation is in harmony with the fact that bone, cartilage, and synovial membrane have a common origin in the mesenchyme from which the skeleton is formed. It is also in accord with the familiar experience that, under pathologic conditions, cartilage and also bone may develop in the synovial membrane as a result of metaplasia.

SYNOVIAL FLUID (SYNOVIA)

The synovial fluid is the viscid mucoid lubricant of joints, and its alternate name (synovia) is derived from its suggestive resemblance to the white of an egg. Normal human synovial fluid is clear and slightly yellow as a rule, and ordinarily there is only a thin film of it spread over the surfaces outlining the articular cavity. Indeed, an articulation even as large as the human knee may, if normal, yield as little as a few drops of synovia when the joint is opened. In any event, the amount obtainable under these circumstances does not often exceed 1 cc. The quantity recoverable from a normal ankle joint is somewhat greater, on the average, than that recoverable from the knee joint. Thus the amount of synovial fluid obtainable from normal human joints may vary somewhat from joint to joint. Moreover, there may be slight differences in viscosity and even in color of the fluid. This has been demonstrated in respect to synovia obtained from various joints of a slaughtered animal. There are also indications (based on experimental studies) that exercise of a joint results in a slight and temporary increase in its synovial fluid (see Ekholm and Norbäck), while prolonged bed rest seems to favor a reduction.

It seems appropriate to regard the synovial fluid as a dialysate of blood plasma to which a mucoid substance (secreted by the synovial cells) is added as the plasma constituents diffuse through the tissue spaces of the synovial membrane to enter the articular cavity (see Ropes *et al.*, and Bauer *et al.*). It is, of course, the presence of the mucoid substance (hyaluronic acid) in the synovial fluid that distinguishes the latter from other body fluids (for instance, pleural fluid and peritoneal fluid) also representing dialysates of blood plasma. The idea that the mucoid substance is a product of the synovial cells is supported by the observation that synovial cells growing in tissue culture media elaborate, among other materials, a mucin-like substance, while dying synovial cells apparently do not produce this substance (see Vaubel).

Current conceptions of the *chemical composition* and *cytological components* of human synovia have been derived mainly from work on synovia of animal joints. This indirect approach has been necessitated by the fact that individual human joints from which it is possible to collect enough fluid for analysis are *ipso facto* abnormal. In such joints the synovia has become diluted by somewhat modified blood serum and admixed with various types and amounts of blood cells which have transuded into the joint cavity. The resultant synovial fluid should be clearly distinguished from the normal lubricant of joints—the synovia. Furthermore, though synovia is in all likelihood entirely comparable to the normal lubricant of bursae mucosae and tendon sheaths, it is again not of the same composition as the secretions which accumulate in these structures when they are inflamed. Therefore, information obtained by study of such fluids, too, is not directly applicable to synovia.

Human synovial fluid is slightly alkaline. In respect to glucose, nonprotein nitrogen, and uric acid, the content (concentration) is approximately the same in the synovial fluid as in the blood plasma. The content of chloride and bicarbonate is higher in the synovial fluid than in the plasma. However, the concentrations of sodium, potassium, calcium, and magnesium are lower in the synovial fluid, apparently because of the latter's low protein content. Not only is the protein content very much lower in synovial fluid than in blood plasma, but the proportion of albumin to globulin is very much greater in the synovial fluid than it is in the plasma. The basis ordinarily given for these differences in the protein content and the type of protein predominating is that the synovial membrane is not highly permeable to the plasma proteins, and since albumin has a lower molecular weight than globulin, more of the albumin diffuses through (see Ropes *et al.*, and Ropes and Bauer).

As determined by these investigators, the synovial fluid of man contains relatively few nucleated cells. In a rather large series of specimens of synovia obtained at autopsy from human knee joints free of disease, they found that the cell counts ranged from 13 to 180 nucleated cells per cubic millimeter, the average content being 63 cells. The cells present were polymorphonuclear leukocytes, lymphocytes, monocytes, clasmatocytes, and synovial cells. Monocytes (mononuclear phagocytes) predominated, and the proportion of lymphocytes was also high. The number of polymorphonuclear leukocytes was found to be relatively small. If any red blood cells are present in otherwise normal synovial fluid, they generally represent contamination occurring in the course of aspiration of the fluid.

The number of nucleated cells in human synovial fluid is low in comparison with what it is in cattle and dogs, for instance. The average number of nucleated cells per cubic millimeter of synovia in the knee joint was 246 for cattle (see Davies) and 963 for dogs (see Warren *et al.*), while, as already indicated, the comparable average value reported for the knee joint fluid of man was 63 cells. It has been suggested that this difference may be due to the fact that the cell counts made on human synovial fluid usually represented values obtained at the time of death on subjects who had been inactive and confined to bed, while the cell counts on the synovial fluid of animals were made just after the latter had been slaughtered. Furthermore, even in the same animal there may be considerable variation in the cell content from joint to joint. For instance, Davies found that in cattle the average number of cells in the fluid of the ankle joint was 194 per cu. mm., in the temporomandibular joint 1,337, and in the atlanto-occipital joint 783, while, as already noted, the cell content of the knee joint in cattle averaged 246 cells per cubic millimeter.

Since most of the cells in the synovial fluid are capable of phagocytosis, it is reasonable to suggest that their chief function is the removal of the debris which appears in joints under normal use. To a great extent, this debris consists of minute particles of articular cartilage which have been rubbed off in the course of articular function. It may also include some bits of synovial membrane.

Various enzymes have also been found to be present in the synovial fluid. In that obtained from oxen, the presence of lipase, diastase, and protease has been demonstrated (see Podkaminsky). The synovial fluid also shows *alkaline* phosphatase activity. In man, its value is generally lower in the synovial fluid than in the blood plasma. In certain cases of arthritis, *acid* phosphatase has also been demonstrated in synovial fluid obtained from knee joints (see Kream *et al.*). Moreover, the acid phosphatase content in the synovial fluid in cases of *inflammatory* arthritis of various types appears to be higher than in the synovial fluid obtained from cases of *noninflammatory* (degenerative) arthritis (see Lehman *et al.*).

An interesting review of the historical aspects of synovia has been authored by Rodnan *et al.*

INTRA-ARTICULAR DISKS AND MENISCI

In man, the only joints in which disks or menisci are regularly found are the temporomandibular, sternoclavicular, wrist (inferior radio-ulnar), and knee joints.

In addition, a disk is not infrequently found in the acromioclavicular joint. Phylogenetically, menisci are semilunar vestiges of complete disks which apparently once entirely separated the bone ends of joints in which menisci are now present. Most studies of these intra-articular structures have centered upon the menisci of the knee joint. Indeed, the latter have been intensively investigated in regard to: (1) their presence or absence in different animal species, and (2) the influence of the manner of function of the joint upon their shape and upon the details of their structure (see Retterer, and also Fénis). Detailed comparative studies on the disk of the temporomandibular joint in man and other mammals have also been carried out (see Baecker, and also Choukas and Sicher). Comparative studies of the sternoclavicular and acromioclavicular joints in relation to the presence and the anatomic condition of intra-articular disks in subjects of various ages have also been made (see DePalma, and also Ramotowski).

In the sternoclavicular and temporomandibular joints in man, a complete disk usually divides the articular space into two chambers. The disk is a more or less circular pad of highly collagenous connective tissue located between the bone ends of the joint and attached at its periphery to the articular capsule. In the knee joint of man, two menisci in the form of semilunar, or cresent-shaped, intra-articular pads of collagenous connective tissue are normally present. The menisci are located marginally—one on the lateral and the other on the medial aspect of the joint. In addition to being attached at their outer margins to the articular capsule, both menisci are attached anteriorly and posteriorly to the tibia. (See Fig. 27.)

As a very rare anomaly in the knee joint, one may encounter an extremely large single disk (showing a central defect) instead of two marginally located menisci. This single disk may divide the articular space completely, as in some more primitive animal groups, such as the Amphibia. A more common anomaly, however, is that consisting of abnormal development of one of the menisci (nearly always the lateral meniscus). Under these circumstances the abnormal meniscus is discoid in shape. The writer has also observed a case in which, in both knee joints, each lateral

Figure 27

A, Photograph of a sternoclavicular joint sectioned to show the intra-articular disk which divides the cavity. The specimen came from a man who was 50 years of age and who died of peritonitis secondary to acute gangrenous appendicitis. Above and to the left, the articular end of the clavicle is visible. Below and to the left, a small portion of the cartilaginous end of the first rib, abutting on the manubrium of the sternum, can be seen.

B, Photomicrograph (× 2) showing the large, wedge-shaped intra-articular disk of a sternoclavicular joint. The disk occupies the joint cavity almost completely and separates the bones entering into the formation of the joint. Note the extensive fraying of the lower end of the disk. This represents a degenerative change. The subject was a 67 year old woman whose death was due to a carcinoma of the cervix which had extensively metastasized locally.

C, Photomicrograph (× 6) illustrating a focus of bone formation within the lateral meniscus of a knee joint of a man 22 years of age. The meniscus was rather large and discoid in shape and contained several discrete foci of bone formation. As might be expected, these foci of ossification developed in the more peripheral part of the meniscus—the part which normally contains blood vessels.

D, Photomicrograph (× 30) of a meniscus of a knee joint from a guinea pig. The meniscus was sectioned in the long (horizontal) plane. The anterior half of the meniscus shows the presence of trabeculae of bone and also of intertrabecular myeloid marrow. The inner margin of the meniscus in the area in which bone is present still shows a narrow rim of hyaline cartilage.

E, Roentgenograph of the knee joint areas of an adult guinea pig. Note the wedge-shaped intra-articular radiopacities (see arrows) representing foci of bone formation in the menisci.

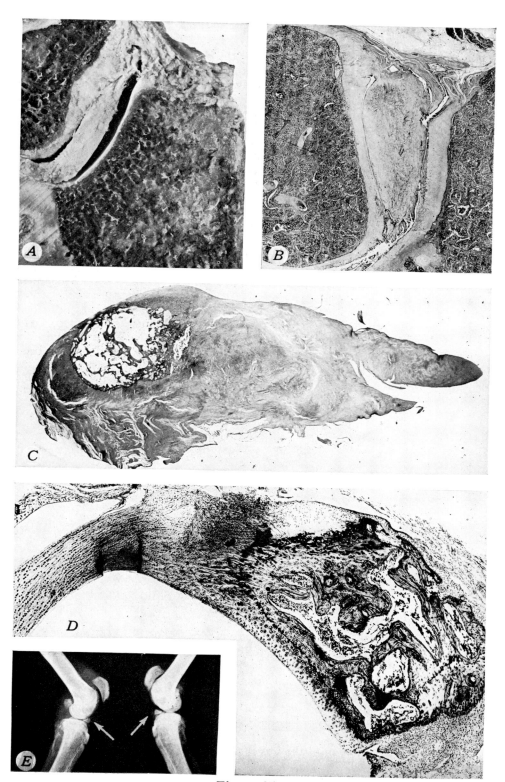

Figure 27

meniscus was so large as to cover completely the corresponding articular surface of the tibia. In this connection, it is interesting that, as pointed out by Fénis, in the knees of the types of bats that show only incomplete formation of menisci, the lateral meniscus is the one still present. Furthermore, in the knee of man, the lateral meniscus is the one which normally attains the larger size.

The menisci are more or less pearly white at birth. Early in life, however, even before puberty, they often undergo changes in color, becoming yellowish or yellowish brown, and in advanced age they may appear brownish. These changes in color are associated with a progressive degeneration within the substance. In a human joint, as already indicated, the periphery of the disk or the outer margin of each meniscus is attached more or less intimately to the capsule. Histologically, the disks and menisci in man consist predominantly of collagenous connective tissue which is interspersed with some elastic fibers. In the vicinity of the capsule, the disks and menisci contain some bloated cells near their surfaces—cells which somewhat resemble cartilage cells. In the core of the disks and menisci, the tissue is more strictly fibroelastic in character. Its fiber bundles do not run parallel, as they do in tendon, but interlace at acute angles. In the menisci, most of the fibers are disposed obliquely in the direction of the long axis of the meniscus. Some fiber bundles take a radial course, and these are disposed mainly along the blood vessels penetrating these structures at the periphery. Because of the presence of the bloated cells mentioned above, the tissue constituting the disks and menisci in man was formerly regarded as fibrocartilage, but this idea has definitely been superseded by the conception that it represents fibroelastic connective tissue (see Apolant). The junctional tissue at the site of attachment of a disk or meniscus to the joint capsule is a rather loose, vascular connective tissue, and not highly collagenous fibroelastic connective tissue.

The blood supply of these structures has been studied most intensively in relation to the menisci of the knee joint. Henschen, in 1928, discussed the distribution of the blood vessels in the menisci of the knee joint and reviewed the previous pertinent work. More or less in conformity with others, he found: (1) that the anterior and posterior quarter segments of each meniscus contain blood vessels which penetrate almost to the inner margin, and (2) that in the adult the middle two quarters of the meniscus show blood vessels only along the margin in the immediate vicinity of the attachment of the meniscus to the capsule. Thus the bulk of this middle region of the meniscus is avascular. The extent of the *avascular area* in the midsection of each meniscus increases with the age of the subject. In the newborn, blood vessels penetrate this portion of the meniscus to about one half of its width, while in the adult they extend inward only to about one sixth of its width (see Davies and Edwards). The various intra-articular disks (temporomandibular and sterno-clavicular) are vascularized mainly in the peripheral area, the major portions of these disks being avascular.

The blood vessels penetrate the menisci where the latter are attached to the capsule, extend inward radially, and terminate within the menisci as capillary loops. In regard to the vessels themselves, it is important to note that in all age categories, including childhood, it is common to encounter sclerosis of the walls of some of the blood vessels which are penetrating the menisci (or disks) and also of some of the blood vessels (both capillaries and venules) of the adjacent synovial membrane and even of vessels in the articular capsule. The reason for the sclerosis of the pericapsular, capsular, and synovial blood vessels (capillaries and venules) is unknown. In the opinion of the writer, the sclerotic thickening of the walls of some of the small blood vessels in the synovial membrane and capsular and peri-capsular tissues is as much an element of the inherent structure of these vessels as is the striking thickness of the vessels in the ovaries and uterus in all age groups. That is, it has no pathologic significance by itself. Indeed, the writer has long been cognizant of the fact that, in relation to the synovial membrane and capsular tissues in general, unless one is aware that the presence of thick-walled capillaries and venules represents a normal aspect of the histologic structure, such findings may be misinterpreted as indications of a disease process. More recently, considerable attention has been devoted to the details of the histologic structure of the blood vessels of joints (see Lang, and Elmore *et al.*).

Ossification and Calcification.—Ossification (*bone formation*) within the substance of a human meniscus occurs very rarely; in fact, only a few instances have been recorded (see Burrows, and also Watson-Jones and Roberts). In the course of a large experience with menisci of the human knee joint examined after they had been removed at surgery, the writer has encountered only a single instance of bone formation in these structures. On the other hand, in the rat, mouse, and guinea pig, for instance, the menisci of the knee normally develop islands of hyaline cartilage after birth. Later, the cartilage, especially in the anterior half of each meniscus, is largely replaced by osseous tissue. Between the bony trabeculae, lymphoid marrow appears. As the animal grows older, the osseous tissue constituting these islands of bone becomes more mature and consequently more lamellar in its histologic structure.

Observations along these lines were already recorded by Retterer in 1905, but lost to sight for a long time. They were subsequently confirmed by the writer and reported at a meeting of the New York Pathological Society in 1932 (see Jaffe). The normal presence of islands of bone in the menisci of rodents is now common knowledge, and a number of pertinent detailed reports have been published (see Harris, and also Pedersen). It is to be doubted, however, that there is any phylogenetic correlation between those extremely rare instances of intrameniscal ossification observed in man and the normal occurrence of islands of bone in the menisci of rodents. That is, a focus of bone in a meniscus of a human knee probably does not represent a vestigial structure.

In contrast to ossification, calcification (*calcium deposition*) in the menisci of the knee joint is not unusual. The writer has encountered several instances in which the calcification was limited to the menisci of one knee joint and there was no evidence of calcification of the articular cartilages even of that knee. Whether these instances of isolated meniscal calcification represent a "forme fruste" of so-called "pseudogout" or "chondrocalcinosis articularis" is still to be established (see Bundens *et al.*). In the latter conditions the articular cartilages and also intra-articular disks and menisci of many joints may be found calcified (see McCarty and Haskin, Moskowitz and Katz, and also Ahlgren).

In cases of idiopathic articular chondrocalcinosis (so-called pseudogout), there may be a long history of aching pains in various joints (most often the knee joints), interspersed with acute attacks of articular pain. Furthermore, it has been demonstrated that, in the synovial fluid and articular cartilages in these cases, the calcific material consists of crystals having the composition of calcium pyrophosphate dihydrate. The underlying cause of idiopathic articular chondrocalcinosis (so-called pseudogout syndrome) is obscure. There are indications to the effect that the condition may have a hereditary basis, but the findings bearing on this point are not as yet conclusive. Be that as it may, it seems worth noting that analogous calcifications are not infrequently encountered in cases of hyperparathyroidism, often in association with hyperuricemia (see Bywaters *et al.*, and also Vix).

BURSAE MUCOSAE AND TENDON SHEATHS

Bursae Mucosae.—The human body contains large numbers of bursae mucosae distributed in many different localities. They are found notably under the skin

8

over bony prominences (the *subcutaneous bursae*), beneath the deep fascia (the *subfascial bursae*), and between tendons and muscles (the *subtendinous bursae*). They serve to facilitate the play between the tissues which they separate. Bursae mucosae are saccular, rather thin-walled connective tissue structures. They are usually completely closed off and contain a small quantity of viscid fluid resembling synovia. The inner surface of a bursa is lined by a thin layer of tissue akin to the synovial membrane of joints. In some bursae the space may be subdivided by partitioning walls into several compartments. Furthermore, when situated in the neighborhood of a joint, the bursal lining is continuous with the synovial lining of the joint capsule through an aperture in the capsular ligament.

Bursae mucosae form in consequence of the coalescence of pre-existing minute spaces in loose connective tissue. As they develop, their walls become differentiated from the rest of the connective tissue by their greater density. A number of bursae already appear during fetal life. Thus the subacromial bursa may begin to form as early as the third fetal month, and was found present in about 72 per cent of 200 fetuses ranging from 3 months to full term (see Black). However, the vast majority of bursae mucosae evidently form only after birth. These appear in response to functional irritation or friction, but whether this is necessarily true of those forming before birth is still open to question. The importance of these factors in the development of bursae is further made clear by pathologic findings. It has been observed, for instance, that a bursa almost invariably develops over an abnormal bony prominence, such as an osteocartilaginous exostosis, where it constitutes a so-called *exostosis bursata*.

Tendon Sheaths.—Over part of its length, a tendon is likely to be completely or partially surrounded by a sheath. The latter varies in the definiteness with which it stands out from the neighboring tissues. Tendon sheaths, like joint capsules, are composed of two coats. The inner coat is thin and in other ways, too, resembles synovial membrane. On the other hand, the outer coat of a tendon sheath (unlike that of a joint capsule) is usually also rather thin, though occasionally it is thickened to some extent by ligamentous tissue. Tendons running in "osteofascial" tunnels are partially surrounded by sheaths whose walls are relatively thick. These are so much like bursae mucosae that they might be so regarded. Between the tendon and its sheath there is a small amount of lubricant resembling synovia. The sheath and the lubricant together apparently act as a buffer where the tendon would otherwise rub against bone or ligament.

Many aspects of the structure of tendon sheaths in relation to tendons were delineated by Mayer. He noted that, whether or not it completely encircles the tendon, the sheath nearly always forms a closed sac. He also described the various reflections of the inner lining of the sheath onto the tendon. In relation to certain tendons, this lining folds inward from the floor of the sheath to form a long, resilient, mesentery-like membrane of connective tissue—the *mesotendon* (or mesotenon). The latter carries blood vessels and attaches itself to the nonfrictional surface of the tendon along a longitudinal line known as the *hilus*. On reaching the tendon, the mesotendon spreads out over the surface of the latter, forming the *epitenon*. At the hilus it also enters the tendon, and sends vascular connective tissue strands (the *endotendineum*, or endotenon) between the tendon bundles. When there is no fully developed mesotendon, it is represented nevertheless either by a shorter membrane at each end of the sheath or merely by some delicate strands of connective tissue. The mesotendon is continuous with the fatty areolar tissue (*paratenon*) surrounding the tendon above and below the sheath, and thus helps to close off the latter as a sac.

The microscopic structure of a tendon sheath need not be presented here in detail, since its inner layer (by far the more important) is analogous to synovial membrane histologically as well as grossly. Thus, like synovial membrane, this layer has some relatively cellular areas and others which are poorly cellular and more closely bound to the underlying fibrous coat. Furthermore, in some portions of a tendon sheath, as in a joint capsule, there may be small amounts of fatty areolar tissue interposed between the two coats.

As already noted, the tendon sheath is highly vascular and, by way of the mesotendon, sends blood vessels into the tendon which enter the latter at the hilus. The tendon sheath also contains nerves and lymphatics. The efferent lymph channels drain into the regional lymph nodes (see Ssawwin). In addition to receiving a supply of blood through the mesotendon, the tendon receives some also from the muscle at one end and from the periosteum or bone at the other end where it is attached to these latter structures. It is also to be noted that the paratenon communicates with the neighboring connective tissues, including perimysium, perineurium, and adventitia of blood vessels.

REFERENCES

AHLGREN, P.: Chondrocalcinosis and Bony Changes, Nord. med., *73*, 309, 1965.

APOLANT, H.: Über Faserknorpel, Berlin Thesis, 1890.

BAECKER, R.: Zur Histologie des Kiefergelenkmeniskus des Menschen und der Säuger, Ztschr. mikr.-anat. Forsch., *26*, 223, 1931.

BARNETT, C. H., DAVIES, D. V. and MacCONAILL, M. A.: *Synovial Joints. Their Structure and Mechanics*, Springfield, Charles C Thomas, 1961.

BAUER, W., ROPES, M. W. and WAINE, H.: The Physiology of Articular Structures, Physiol. Rev., *20*, 272, 1940.

BENNINGHOFF, A.: Form und Bau der Gelenkknorpel in ihren Beziehungen zur Funktion. II. Der Aufbau des Gelenkknorpels in seinen Beziehungen zur Funktion, Ztschr. Zellforsch. u. mikr. Anat., *2*, 783, 1925.

BLACK, B. M.: The Prenatal Incidence, Structure and Development of Some Human Synovial Bursae, Anat. Rec., *60*, 333, 1934.

BOLAND, B. F.: Separation of Symphysis Pubis, New England J. Med., *208*, 431, 1933.

BUNDENS, W. D., JR., BRIGHTON, C. T. and WEITZMAN, G.: Primary Articular-Cartilage Calcification with Arthritis (Pseudogout Syndrome), J. Bone & Joint Surg., *47-A*, 111, 1965.

BURROWS, H. J.: Two Cases of Ossification in the Internal Semilunar Cartilage, Brit. J. Surg., *21*, 404, 1934.

BYWATERS, E. G. L., DIXON, A. ST. J. and SCOTT, J. T.: Joint Lesions of Hyperparathyroidism, Ann. Rheumat. Dis., *22*, 171, 1963.

CHOUKAS, N. C. and SICHER, H.: The Structure of the Temporomandibular Joint, Oral Surg., *13*, 1203, 1960.

DAVIES, D. V.: The Cell Content of Synovial Fluid, J. Anat., *79*, 66, 1945.

DAVIES, D. V. and EDWARDS, D. A. W.: The Blood Supply of the Synovial Membrane and Intra-articular Structures, Ann. Roy. Coll. Surgeons England, *2*, 142, 1948.

DEPALMA, A. F.: The Role of the Disks of the Sternoclavicular and the Acromioclavicular Joints, Clinical Orthopaedics, *13*, 222, 1959.

EKHOLM, R. and NORBÄCK, B.: On the Relationship between Articular Changes and Function, Acta orthop. scandinav., *21*, 81, 1951.

EKHOLM, R. and INGELMARK, B. E.: Functional Thickness Variations of Human Articular Cartilage, Acta Soc. med. upsalien., *57*, 39, 1952.

ELMORE, S. M., MALMGREN, R. A. and SOKOLOFF, L.: Sclerosis of Synovial Blood Vessels, J. Bone & Joint Surg., *45-A*, 318, 1963.

EYMER, H. and LANG, F. J.: Anatomische Untersuchungen der Symphyse der Frau im Hinblick auf die Geburt und klinische Deutung der Befunde, Arch. Gynäk., *137*, 866, 1929.

DE FÉNIS, F.: Note sur la formation et la disparition des ménisques intra-articulaires du genou, Bull. et mém. Soc. anthropol., series 6, *9*, 19, 1918.

GRANT, J. C. B.: Interarticular Synovial Folds, Brit. J. Surg., *18*, 636, 1931.

HAMMAR, J. A.: Ueber den feineren Bau der Gelenke. I. Die Gelenkmembran, Arch. mikr. Anat., *43*, 266, 1894.

————: Ueber den feineren Bau der Gelenke. II. Der Gelenkknorpel, Arch. mikr. Anat., *43*, 813, 1894.

HARRIS, H. A.: Calcification and Ossification in the Semilunar Cartilages, Lancet, *1*, 1114, 1934.

HASLHOFER, L.: Anatomische und mikroskopische Untersuchungen der Gelenke des Beckenringes, mit besonderer Berücksichtigung der Veränderungen durch Schwangerschaft und Geburt, Zentralbl. Gynäk., *54*, 2317, 1930.

HENSCHEN, K.: Arterielle Gefässversorgung der Menisken des Kniegelenkes, Arch. klin. Chir., *152*, 144, 1928.

HUETER, C.: Zur Histologie der Gelenkflächen und Gelenkkapseln, mit einem kritischen Vorwort über die Versilberungsmethode, Arch. path. Anat., *36*, 25, 1866.

HULTKRANTZ, W.: Ueber die Spaltrichtungen der Gelenkknorpel, Anat. Anz., Suppl. *14*, 248, 1898.

JAFFE, H. L.: Comparative Anatomy of the Semilunar Cartilages of the Knee: Normal Presence of Bone in the Menisci of Some Animals, Arch. Path., *15*, 599, 1933.

KREAM, J., LEHMAN, M. A., KAMBOLIS, C. and BROGNA, D.: The Clinical Significance of Synovial Fluid Acid Phosphatase Levels, Clin. Chem., *9*, 482, 1963.

LANG, J.: Die Gelenkinnenhaut, ihre Aufbau- und Abbauvorgänge, Jahrb. Morphol. u. mikr. Anat., *98*, 387, 1958.

LEHMAN, M. A., KREAM, J. and BROGNA, D.: Acid and Alkaline Phosphatase Activity in the Serum and Synovial Fluid of Patients with Arthritis, J. Bone & Joint Surg., *46-A*, 1732, 1964.

MacCONAILL, M. A.: The Movements of Bones and Joints. 4. The Mechanical Structure of Articulating Cartilage, J. Bone & Joint Surg., *33-B*, 251, 1951.

MAYER, L.: The Physiological Method of Tendon Transplantation. I. Historical; Anatomy and Physiology of Tendons, Surg. Gynec. & Obst., *22*, 182, 1916.

McCARTY, D. J., JR. and HASKIN, M. E.: The Roentgenographic Aspects of Pseudogout (Articular Chondrocalcinosis), Am. J. Roentgenol., *90*, 1248, 1963.

MILES, A. E. W. and DAWSON, J. A.: Elastic Fibres in the Articular Fibrous Tissue of Some Joints, Arch. Oral Biol., *7*, 249, 1962.

MOSKOWITZ, R. W. and KATZ, D.: Chondrocalcinosis (Pseudogout Syndrome), J.A.M.A., *188*, 867, 1964.

NYKAMP, A.: Beitrag zur Kenntniss der Structur des Knorpels, Arch. mikr. Anat., *14*, 492, 1877.

PEDERSEN, H. E.: The Ossicles of the Semilunar Cartilages of Rodents, Anat. Rec., *105*, 1, 1949.

PODKAMINSKY, N. A.: Über Fermente in der Synovia und deren Bedeutung, Arch. klin. Chir., *165*, 383, 1931.

RAMOTOWSKI, W.: Morphology of the Acromioclavicular Articulation Cartilages, Folia morphol., *6*, 253, 1955.

RETTERER, E.: Des ménisques interarticulaires du genou du Cobaye et du Rat, Compt. rend. Soc. biol., *58¹*, 44, 1905.

RODNAN, G. P., BENEDEK, T. G. and PANETTA, W. C.: The Early History of Synovia (Joint Fluid), Ann. Int. Med., *65*, 821, 1966.

ROPES, M. W., ROSSMEISL, E. C. and BAUER, W.: The Origin and Nature of Normal Human Synovial Fluid, J. Clin. Invest., *19*, 795, 1940.

ROPES, M. W. and BAUER, W.: *Synovial Fluid Changes in Joint Disease*, Cambridge, Harvard University Press, 1953.

SCHMORL, G.: Über bisher nur wenig beachtete Eigentümlichkeiten ausgewachsener und kindlicher Wirbel, Arch. klin. Chir., *150*, 420, 1928.

SIGURDSON, L. A.: The Structure and Function of Articular Synovial Membranes, J. Bone & Joint Surg., *12*, 603, 1930.

SILBERBERG, R., SILBERBERG, M., VOGEL, A. and WETTSTEIN, W.: Ultrastructure of Articular Cartilage of Mice of Various Ages, Am. J. Anat., *109*, 251, 1961.

SSAWWIN, V. J.: Abführende Lymphgefässe der Synovialsehnenscheiden der Extremitäten des Menschen, Anat. Anz., *80*, 119, 1935.

SUTRO, C. J.: The Pubic Bones and their Symphysis, Arch. Surg., *32*, 823, 1936.

TILLMANNS, H.: Ueber die fibrilläre Structur des Hyalinknorpels, Arch. Anat. u. Physiol., Anat. Abteil., p. 9, 1877.

TRUETA, J. and LITTLE, K.: The Vascular Contribution to Osteogenesis. II. Studies with the Electron Microscope, J. Bone & Joint Surg., *42-B*, 367, 1960.

VAN DER STRICHT, O.: Recherches sur le cartilage hyalin, Arch. biol., *7*, 1, 1887.

VAUBEL, E.: The Form and Function of Synovial Cells in Tissue Cultures, J. Exper. Med., *58*, 63, 1933.

VIX, V. A.: Articular and Fibrocartilage Calcification in Hyperparathyroidism: Associated Hyperuricemia, Radiology, *83*, 468, 1964.

WARREN, C. F., BENNETT, G. A. and BAUER, W.: The Significance of the Cellular Variations Occurring in Normal Synovial Fluid, Am. J. Path., *11*, 953, 1935.

WATSON-JONES, R. and ROBERTS, R. E.: Calcification, Decalcification, and Ossification, Brit. J. Surg., *21*, 461, 1934 (see p. 492).

Chapter

5

Metabolic and Biochemical Considerations*

THE subject matter to be discussed in this chapter includes: (1) the human nutritional requirements in respect to calcium and phosphorus; (2) the absorption and excretion of calcium and phosphorus; (3) the chemical composition of bone (that is, of the osseous tissue) in regard to both its organic matter and its inorganic (mineral) matter; (4) the physicochemical conditions which govern the formation and/or precipitation of the crystals of bone mineral; (5) the humoral and local factors involved in the mineralization of the bone collagen, the principal constituent of the organic matter of osseous tissue; (6) the mechanism of action and the role of parathyroid hormone, thyrocalcitonin, and vitamin D in the exchange of calcium and phosphorus between the bone and the internal environment, or fluid matrix, of the body (that is, the intercellular fluids and blood) in the maintenance of metabolic homeostasis in respect to these minerals; and (7) the normal values and the values considered to be abnormal for serum calcium, inorganic phosphorus, and alkaline and acid phosphatase, to serve as a basis of reference for comparison with the values encountered in various metabolic skeletal disorders. "Phosphorus" as used in this discussion does not imply its presence in biological systems in its elemental form (P). Phosphorus rather is present in the forms of phosphate ion (for example, sodium or calcium phosphate), or in the form of phosphoric acid esters which are bound to simple organic molecules (for example, hexose phosphates) or complex organic molecules (for example, phospholipids and nucleoproteins). The terms "inorganic phosphorus" and "phosphate ion" (or phosphate) are therefore used interchangeably.

NUTRITIONAL REQUIREMENTS FOR CALCIUM AND PHOSPHORUS

Since large amounts of calcium and phosphorus are needed to ensure the proper postnatal growth and mineralization of the bones, it is natural that the demands of the organism in respect to these minerals per kilo of body weight should be particularly high during infancy and childhood. As the subject grows older, the daily calcium and phosphorus requirements per kilo of body weight decrease. In the adult, the requirements have usually diminished to the amounts needed for the proper metabolic maintenance of the bones (and other tissues)—that is, to amounts which compensate for (or counterbalance) that which is lost daily in the course of endogenous metabolism. Indeed, despite the disparity in body weight between the adult and the infant, an adult under ordinary conditions will be in metabolic balance, so far as calcium and phosphorus are concerned, if the total daily intake of these minerals is equivalent to that which is required daily by the infant and/or young child. Pregnancy and lactation, of course, make additional demands on the

* This chapter was written in collaboration with Dr. Jacob Kream (formerly Chief of the Section of Chemistry of the Hospital for Joint Diseases), who also prepared the line drawings appearing in the chapter. Dr. Kream is now Biochemist to the Clinical Center, Montefiore Hospital and Medical Center, New York City.

organism for calcium and phosphorus. Under all conditions, the nutritional requirement for calcium (and to a lesser degree for phosphorus) is influenced by the intake
of vitamin D. Within the limits of physiological safety, vitamin D favors the
absorption of calcium from the small intestine, and it seems likely that at the same
time it improves the absorption of phosphorus.

Sources of Calcium and Phosphorus.—For man, the best natural sources of
calcium are milk and milk products. Lesser but still good sources of calcium include:
eggs (mainly the yolk) and such green leafy vegetables as cabbage and lettuce.
Certain green leafy vegetables, such as spinach, are not satisfactory nutritional
sources of calcium despite a fairly high calcium content, since much of the calcium
present is in the form of an oxalate, which is not readily utilized by the body. In
connection with some of the cereals, it is a high phytic acid content that reduces
the availability of the calcium, since that acid forms an insoluble compound with
the calcium. Meat, of course, has a low calcium content—about 10 mg. per 100 g.
Cow's milk, in contrast, has a calcium content of 1.1 g per quart.

On the other hand, meat is a good source of phosphorus, its phosphorus content
averaging about 175 mg. per 100 g. However, some of the best sources of phosphorus
are certain cheeses (notably Cheddar), nuts, bread (particularly whole wheat
bread), and also milk. The phosphorus content of cow's milk is about 93 mg. per
100 g, a quart of milk thus supplying about 0.88 g of phosphorus.

When necessary, the maintenance needs in respect to calcium and phosphorus
can also be supplied (at least in part) through the administration of various salts
of these minerals. In particular, humans are capable of utilizing inorganic and
organic salts of calcium, such as the carbonate, citrate, phosphate, lactate, and
gluconate. Therapeutically, such salts are sometimes administered as supplements
to the diet. Furthermore, the drinking water, especially in limestone regions, may
contain a substantial amount of calcium in the form of dissolved calcium bicarbonate. In fact, such a source may contain as much as 100 mg. of calcium per liter
and be an effective supplement to the daily calcium intake of man and animals of
the region.

Requirements of the Infant.—For the healthy infant receiving cow's milk, a total
daily calcium intake of about 0.6 to 0.8 g (approximately 125 to 150 mg. per kilo
of body weight) would amply satisfy the calcium requirements and provide a
liberal margin of safety. Such an infant is in positive calcium balance to the extent
of about 40 mg. of calcium per kilo a day: that is, the infant stores this amount
of calcium daily (see Stearns). If an infant is receiving milk in quantities sufficient
to meet its needs for calcium, its needs for phosphorus (about 95 mg. per kilo of
body weight) will also be satisfied.

In connection with the calcium and phosphorus needs of the infant, it seems
worth noting that the calcium content of cow's milk is about four times as high as
that of human milk. Specifically, there are approximately 128 mg. of calcium in
100 ml. of cow's milk compared with 30 mg. in the same amount of human milk.
However, an infant ordinarily absorbs only about 30 per cent of the calcium in
cow's milk, while it absorbs about 60 per cent of that in mother's milk (see Telfer).
Thus the lower calcium content of human milk is partially compensated by the
greater availability of the calcium in question. The phosphorus content of cow's
milk is about six times as high as that of human milk. There are approximately
100 mg. of phosphorus in 100 ml. of cow's milk compared with 16 mg. in the same
amount of human milk. However, an infant ordinarily absorbs only about 20 per
cent of the phosphorus in cow's milk compared with 50 per cent of that in mother's
milk. Thus the lower phosphorus content of human milk (like its lower calcium
content) is partially compensated by a higher percentage of absorption or utilization.

The features of human milk which may contribute to this include a lower casein, a higher lactose, and a relatively higher lactalbumin content in comparison with cow's milk. There are also differences between human and cow's milk in respect to phosphoproteins (other than casein), phospholipids, and neutral fats. For example, human milk contains larger quantities of the triglyceride olein. However, though mother's milk thus has a number of over-all advantages over cow's milk for human infants, the fact remains that, for the same total amount of milk consumed daily, the infant receiving cow's milk is still absorbing more calcium and phosphorus than the breast-fed infant, because of the higher concentration of these minerals in cow's milk.

Requirements During Childhood and Adolescence.—It appears that a child 3 years of age requires daily about 70 mg. of calcium and about 80 mg. of phosphorus per kilo of body weight. By the time the subject reaches 16 years of age, the calcium requirement has decreased to about 12 mg. and the phosphorus requirement to about 35 mg. per kilo of body weight.

As expressed in terms of total daily requirement, the optimum calcium intake for children between 3 and 10 years of age is about 1.0 g per day. Indeed, in a child about 7 or 8 years of age, a calcium intake of less than 0.45 g per day is likely to be associated with a negative calcium balance. That is, the total calcium excreted (by way of the stool, urine, and sweat) will be likely to exceed the amount ingested. For older children and adolescents, the optimum calcium intake is somewhat greater than 1.0 g daily. In general, during childhood and adolescence the calcium requirements are met or exceeded by the amounts derivable from one quart of milk supplemented by the calcium contained in the rest of the diet, if the latter is otherwise adequate.

As for phosphorus requirements, for a child about 8 years of age, a minimum total of about 0.7 g of phosphorus daily is needed to avoid a negative phosphorus balance. In order to allow for proper growth of bones, teeth, and muscles in the child and leave a margin of safety, however, the daily phosphorus intake should probably be at least 1.0 g. This would amply allow for a storage of about 10 mg. of phosphorus per kilo of body weight per day (see Sherman, and Sherman and Hawley).

Requirements of the Adult.—Under ordinary conditions, the need of adults for calcium is somewhat less, in terms of total daily intake, than that of children. To avoid calcium deficiency—that is, to maintain themselves in calcium balance— adults should have a minimum daily calcium intake of about 0.45 to 0.55 g. If the generally advised margin of safety of 50 per cent is allowed, the so-called "standard requirement" of calcium for a normal adult is about 0.7 to 0.8 g daily. Thus an average adult is able to maintain himself in calcium balance on a daily intake of about 10 mg. per kilo of body weight. As to the phosphorus requirement, the average human adult must take in at least 0.88 g of phosphorus daily if equilibrium is to be maintained in regard to this mineral. This figure represents nearly twice the corresponding total minimal calcium requirement. However, so many of the foods—including, notably, meat—which are eaten for their energy value contain phosphorus that there is always less danger of a phosphorus than of a calcium deficiency.

Requirements During Pregnancy and Lactation.—As already noted, pregnancy and lactation impose special demands on the organism for calcium and phosphorus. The total daily calcium requirement rises to at least 1.5 g during the latter part of pregnancy and even to 2.0 g or more during lactation. The total daily phosphorus requirement during pregnancy is about 2.5 g. On a calcium and phosphorus intake of this order (assuming that the vitamin D intake is also adequate), a pregnant female tends to be in positive calcium and phosphorus balance. Of the calcium and phosphorus retained under these circumstances, the excess above that utilized by the fetus is stored in the maternal skeleton, with the exception of about 15 to 20 per cent of the retained phosphorus. This portion of the retained phosphorus is metabolically active, in that it participates in the body's cellular intermediary metabolism of carbohydrate, fat, protein, and nucleic acids.

Actually, the fetal demands for calcium are not very large until after the twenty-eighth week. This is evident from the fact that, whereas in the twenty-eighth week the skeleton of the fetus contains approximately 5.5 g of calcium, at term it contains about 30 g. During the last two months of pregnancy, the amount of calcium being retained by the mother is sufficient not only to meet the greatly increased fetal demands but also to anticipate to a certain extent the additional drain which will begin with lactation (see Coons and Blunt). If the calcium and/or phosphorus intake of the pregnant female is inadequate for the fetal demands, the store of these elements in the mother's bones is drawn upon.

When lactation begins, the calcium and phosphorus balances usually become negative even if large amounts of these minerals are ingested. Near the end of lactation, if the mother is well nourished and receives an adequate vitamin D supplement, both calcium and phosphorus may even again be stored in the maternal organism. Usually, however, the mother does not regain equilibrium in respect to calcium and phosphorus for several months after the cessation of lactation, and sometimes the negative balance in regard to these minerals persists for as long as a year after lactation has stopped. A woman who has nursed her infant for many months may finally lose as much as one-fifth of her calcium store. However, this loss is only a temporary depletion and is usually not associated with any physiologic disturbances or roentgenographically detectable changes in the bones (see Morse and Furness).

ABSORPTION OF CALCIUM AND PHOSPHORUS

The Mobilization of Calcium and Phosphorus from Ingested Food.—The ordinary diet usually contains both organically bound and inorganic calcium and phosphorus compounds. Interestingly enough, however, foods contain relatively little calcium phosphate as such. In plant tissues, for instance, calcium is commonly present as salts of such weak acids as carbonic, lactic, citric, tartaric, and malic, and only to a small extent as calcium phosphate. In certain plants, some of the calcium also exists in the form of calcium oxalate and phytate. In such foods as milk, much of the calcium is bound to protein in the form of a calcium caseinate complex, while smaller amounts are bound to lactalbumin and lactoglobulin. Some calcium phosphate and other salts of calcium are undoubtedly also present in milk. As for phosphorus, most of this in animal and plant tissues and also in milk exists as esters and other organic compounds of phosphoric acid (both relatively simple and complex). These include such derivatives of phosphoric acid as hexose and pentose phosphates, phospholipids, nucleoproteins, and phosphoproteins. The casein of milk, for example, is a phosphoprotein.

The calcium and phosphorus in the ingested food are made available for absorption mainly by being mobilized from compounds such as those mentioned above. The digestive enzymes accelerate the liberation of calcium bound to proteins and of phosphoric acid from the various organic compounds. The relative acidity of the contents of the stomach, the duodenum, and the proximal part of the jejunum is instrumental in keeping in solution the salts of calcium and phosphorus ingested, or formed during digestion, in these parts of the alimentary canal. Indeed, calcium and phosphorus become available for absorption mainly in the form of inorganic salts which are partially or completely ionized. As actually absorbed, most of the calcium and phosphorus is probably in the form of calcium and phosphate ions. However, absorption is not merely a passive physical process of diffusion but rather a process in which the cells, too, participate actively. A small amount of calcium and phosphorus may be absorbed in other than ionic form; thus, some of the organic phosphate esters present in the food may be absorbed directly—that is, without an initial splitting off of the phosphoric acid. Also, in the course of absorption, some phosphate is transformed into organic phosphate esters or similar compounds, and some of these may likewise be absorbed as such. There is evidence that glucose, for example, must be phosphorylated before it can be absorbed. This phosphorylation takes place in the cells of the intestinal mucosa (see Beck). Furthermore, there is little doubt that some calcium is also absorbed in the form of nonionized but soluble complexes—for instance, as calcium citrate.

Sites of Absorption.—The calcium contained in the food is largely made available for absorption in the upper part of the small intestine, while the phosphorus contained in the food is largely made available for absorption in the lower part of the small intestine. Furthermore, most of the absorption of both calcium and phosphorus actually takes place in the upper and lower parts, respectively, of the small intestine. Some calcium and phosphorus is discharged and/or secreted into the small intestine with the various digestive juices, and much of this *endogenous* calcium and phosphorus is reabsorbed. There are some indications that small amounts of phosphorus may also be absorbed from the large intestine (see Bergeim), but it is doubted that any absorption of calcium takes place from that part of the gut (see Nicolaysen, and Nicolaysen *et al.*). (See Fig. 28.)

It is fortunate that, in the main, the absorption of calcium and of phosphorus tends to take place at different levels of the small bowel, for otherwise large amounts of insoluble calcium phosphate might be formed in the intestinal canal. The probable consequence of formation of such salt in excess would be decreased absorption of both calcium and phosphorus. The reason for this is that calcium phosphate, having a low solubility except in a highly acidic medium, is absorbed less and less easily as it passes down the intestinal canal, since the contents of the latter become increasingly alkaline. One may assume that, on absorption from the intestine, the calcium and phosphorus enter the blood of the portal system. From there they reach the blood of the general circulation and also the other body fluids. It appears that the lymphatic route, too, plays some role in bringing these substances from the intestinal canal into the general circulation.

Although there is probably no absorption of calcium or phosphorus from the *stomach*, it is in the stomach that much of the calcium of the food is brought into solution and thus made available for absorption. The hydrochloric acid of the gastric juice renders the gastric contents acid, the pH being about 2.0. In consequence, certain of the calcium salts of weak organic acids present in the food are readily converted by the hydrochloric acid of the gastric juice into free organic acids, thus liberating calcium ions. Some protein digestion, too, takes place in the stomach. Therefore a certain amount of calcium bound to proteins is also liberated and also tends to be transformed into soluble salts. Furthermore, some basic calcium phosphate, which is soluble only with difficulty, may be present in the food that is being digested. If the latter remains in the stomach long enough to permit effective action of the hydrochloric acid upon any such calcium phosphate present, much of this salt, too, will be brought into solution.

On the other hand, in regard to the phosphorus, it is important to note that, except as an agent for effecting solution of calcium phosphate or other phosphates, the gastric juice probably plays no important role in liberating phosphorus from the various esters of phosphoric acid. Phosphatases which split these esters are present in the gastric secretion in small amounts. However, they probably find the high acidity of the gastric contents unfavorable for their activity. The action of the proteolytic enzymes in the gastric juice on phosphoproteins may liberate small amounts of phosphorus. In any event, in the stomach the tendency toward the formation of calcium phosphate (which would be very difficult to dissolve, especially in the small intestine) is fortunately slight.

In contrast to the stomach, the *duodenum* and the *jejunum* are essential for the absorption of calcium. The calcium entering this part of the gut in the form of soluble and largely ionized salts is probably mainly absorbed before the intestinal contents become alkaline. However, though the various alkaline intestinal digestive juices tend to neutralize the hydrochloric acid in the material discharged from the stomach, the intestinal contents normally remain slightly acid for a considerable distance down the alimentary canal (see McClendon *et al.*). This fact is attributable to the formation of organic acids (such as lactic acid) through the action of bacteria upon the intestinal contents and to the acidity resulting from carbon dioxide and carbonic acid formation. This continued acidity of the intestinal contents tends to keep the calcium salts soluble and absorbable.

The absorption of calcium from the upper part of the small intestine is further facilitated because the phosphate ions are released only gradually from the organic esters of phosphoric acid contained in the food. Indeed, it is in the *ileum* that the ingested phosphorus is largely made available for absorption, and most of the actual absorption of the available phosphorus takes place in that part of the intestine. The liberation of the phosphate ions occurs through the activity of phosphatases present in large amounts in the pancreatic juice and in the succus entericus. These enzymes do not hydrolyze the phosphoric acid esters well except in a medium whose pH lies near or on the alkaline side of neutrality. The optimal activity of the intestinal phosphatases apparently takes place at a pH of 9.0 to 10.0. Since the pH of the medium in much of the small intestine remains well below that required for

Figure 28

Diagrammatic representation illustrating the absorption and excretion of calcium and phosphorus and also the exchange of these minerals, under normal conditions, between the bone and soft tissues and their internal fluid environment (the plasma of the blood and the interstitial fluids). The diagram shows in particular the conditions obtaining in a normal adult weighing 70 kilos who is in calcium and phosphorus equilibrium and who is ingesting daily 0.8 g of calcium and 1.0 g of phosphorus. Under the conditions represented, the subject excretes in the feces 0.65 g of calcium and 0.30 g of phosphorus, and excretes in the urine 0.15 g of calcium and 0.70 g of phosphorus. That there can be a dermal loss of calcium is also shown, but it is assumed that the subject has not been sweating heavily and that this loss is therefore negligible. The solid heavy arrows extending horizontally from the schematized gastrointestinal tract into the plasma compartment indicate that the absorption of calcium is greatest in the duodenum and upper part of the jejunum and that the absorption of phosphorus is greatest in the lower part of the jejunum and in the ileum. The dotted arrows extending across from the plasma compartment into the gastrointestinal tract direct attention to the fact that endogenous calcium and phosphorus are excreted into the intestinal tract as constituents of the various digestive juices. The small solid arrows extending into the plasma compartment from the schematized kidneys call attention to the reabsorption of calcium and phosphate taking place in the renal tubules from the glomerular ultrafiltrate. Note that, in addition to showing the exchange of calcium and phosphorus between the plasma and interstitial fluid, and between the interstitial fluid and bone and soft-tissue compartments, the diagram indicates the total normal amounts of calcium and phosphorus in each of these compartments. Of course, the diagram does not show the actual proportions of each of these compartments to the others in respect to their content of calcium and phosphorus. For example, to be in the proper proportion, the bone compartment would have to be many hundred times larger than it appears in the drawing.

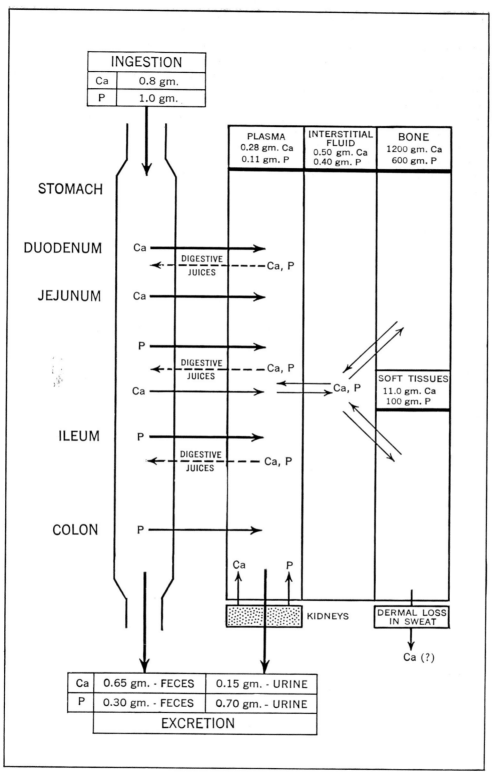

Figure 28

the most effective action of the phosphatases, the tendency toward the production of local high concentrations of phosphate ion is reduced, and consequently the formation of poorly soluble calcium phosphate is minimized. If it were not for these facts, much of the calcium and the phosphorus ingested would probably fail to be absorbed. If the pH of the intestinal contents approaches or lies distinctly on the alkaline side, such calcium ions as are still in the intestinal canal become largely combined with phosphate and carbonate ions to form poorly soluble and hence poorly absorbable basic calcium phosphate and calcium carbonate. In addition, some of the phosphate ions may be combined with still unassimilated magnesium ions to form poorly soluble magnesium phosphate, and hence fail to be absorbed.

Factors Influencing the Absorption of Calcium and Phosphorus.—Mention has already been made of the fact that vitamin D, when available in adequate and physiologic amounts, improves the absorption of calcium and apparently also of phosphorus. Thus the adaptation to a relatively low calcium intake which is achieved, for instance, by inhabitants of certain tropical countries is apparently due to their exposure to abundant sunshine, which ensures the endogenous synthesis of large amounts of vitamin D and hence improves the absorption of whatever calcium is ingested (see Malm). Increasing evidence is accumulating to the effect that, under physiologic conditions, parathyroid hormone, too, promotes the intestinal absorption of calcium and phosphorus. The possible mechanism of action of vitamin D and parathyroid hormone in this connection is considered elsewhere (p. 138).

There are various other factors which may influence the absorption of calcium and/or phosphorus. As is well known, calcium present in foods in the form of oxalate, and calcium and phosphorus in combination with phytates (inositol hexaphosphate) are not readily absorbed. Moderate quantities of easily digested fats in the diet tend to promote an acid intestinal medium, which is favorable to the absorption of calcium. Also, the products of fat digestion provide substances which may enhance the absorption of calcium. However, when fats are present in excess in the gastrointestinal contents, they tend to hinder the absorption of calcium. This interference is due to the combination of fatty acids with the calcium in the bowel to form insoluble calcium soaps which pass out with the stool. For instance, in idiopathic steatorrhea there is a disturbance in gastrointestinal function, manifested in very fatty stools and hence in diminished absorption of calcium. Certain proteins (particularly those which yield large amounts of the amino acid lysine during intestinal digestion) also tend to diminish the absorption of calcium from the gut. This effect seems to be due to the fact that lysine forms a poorly soluble complex with calcium (see Wasserman et al.).

A proper ratio of calcium to phosphorus in the diet is another important factor in the absorption of these minerals. Milk, which may be considered a sound basis for good nutrition, has a Ca:P ratio of about 1.2:1. On the basis of a satisfactory absolute intake of the minerals in question, a satisfactory proportion of calcium to phosphorus in the diet is generally held to be represented by a calcium:phosphorus ratio of 1.5:1 to 2:1 (for the infant), about 1:1 (for the older child), and about 1:1 to 1:1.5 (for the adult). In the event of a decided abnormality in the Ca:P ratio in the diet, both calcium and phosphorus may be lost to the body, mainly through failure of absorption. For instance, when there is a great excess of calcium and a subnormal or even normal amount of phosphorus, some of the phosphorus which would have been absorbed in the lower part of the small intestine is made unavailable, because it combines with the surplus calcium to form the poorly soluble calcium phosphate. On the other hand, a distorted ratio representing a low calcium-high phosphorus intake creates less difficulty, because much of the calcium is absorbed high up in the small intestine and hence is no longer available to combine lower down with phosphorus to form the poorly soluble calcium phosphate (see Shohl and Wolbach). Disordered absorption due to a disturbed calcium:phosphorus ratio can be rectified to some extent by regulation of the vitamin D intake.

It has also been shown experimentally in animals that, when more or less soluble salts of certain metals, such as strontium, magnesium, beryllium, aluminum, and iron, are added to the diet in great excess, they interfere with the absorption of phosphorus. Specifically, these salts tend to render the phosphorus in the diet unabsorbable by combining with it to form poorly soluble or insoluble phosphates. In consequence, rachitoid bone lesions akin to those of low-phosphorus rickets are likely to appear. Thus the addition of excesses of metallic salts has effects similar to those of a high calcium-low phosphorus rachitogenic diet, the metal added acting in the same way as an excess of calcium. It is interesting to note, however, that vitamin D (which can correct or ameliorate the rachitogenic effects of an abnormally high ratio of calcium to phosphorus in the diet) is futile against rachitoid lesions caused by the feeding of excesses of the metallic salts in question here. It should also be pointed out that, if the bones of the animals are ashed, they may show traces or larger amounts of the particular metal used in the experiment (see Jacobson).

EXCRETION OF CALCIUM AND PHOSPHORUS

Ordinarily, calcium and phosphorus are excreted from the body mainly in the urine and feces. It also appears that under conditions of heavy sweating there is considerable loss of calcium through the skin. However, in the absence of visible sweating the daily dermal loss of calcium is small and not easily measurable (see Malm). The dermal loss of phosphorus even under conditions of heavy sweating is negligible.

The calcium and phosphorus present in the urine is of endogenous origin. That is, it represents calcium and phosphorus from the body pool.* On the other hand, the calcium and phosphorus eliminated in the feces represent a mixture of: (1) such amounts of ingested calcium and phosphorus as, for one reason or another, had failed to be absorbed and had merely passed down along the gastrointestinal canal, and (2) such amounts of calcium and phosphorus as had been discharged or secreted into the gastrointestinal canal with the various digestive juices (including the saliva and bile) and which had not been reabsorbed as they passed along the canal. Thus some of the calcium and phosphorus in the feces is also endogenous, since it, too, came from the body pool.

Fecal Excretion.—In respect to a healthy adult on a mixed diet, it is difficult to arrive at a representative figure which would express what proportion of the calcium and phosphorus in a 24-hour fecal sample is unabsorbed dietary calcium and phosphorus and what proportion is endogenous—that is, calcium and phosphorus which

---

* The body pool (metabolic pool) of calcium and phosphorus may be defined as that portion of the body's calcium and phosphorus which is active in metabolic chemical transformations. The pool for calcium and phosphorus comprises the calcium and phosphorus in the intracellular fluid (the fluid within the cells) and the calcium and phosphorus in the extracellular fluids (blood and interstitial fluid). These minerals may be present in various forms, such as calcium ions, calcium proteinate, phosphate ions, organic phosphate esters, etc. Certain of these forms are exchangeable —that is, they pass in and out of the intracellular and extracellular portions of the pool. Contributors to the pool are: the calcium and phosphorus entering the body in the course of intestinal absorption; the calcium and phosphorus available from the various soft tissues of the body; and the calcium and phosphorus available from the mineral salt of the bones. The most important contributor to the body pool is, of course, the store of calcium and phosphorus in the bones. It is assumed that the size of the metabolic pool in respect to calcium and phosphorus is normally maintained at a steady state through a "dynamic equilibrium" between the pool and the various sources contributing to it. (See Fig. 28.)

came from the body pool. The difficulty arises from the great number of variables (the age of the subject, the amounts of calcium and phosphorus ingested and absorbed, the amounts of these minerals in the various digestive juices, etc.). For instance, in an adult the total amount of the various digestive juices entering the gastrointestinal canal per day is believed to range between 8 and 11 liters. In regard to calcium in particular, it has been estimated that these juices may contain as much as 1,100 mg. of this mineral per day, the calculated average figure being about 760 mg. (see Nicolaysen, and Malm). Studies carried out with the aid of radiocalcium (^{45}Ca) place the total daily amount of calcium in the digestive juices definitely below these estimates. In any event, these latter studies seem to indicate that about 15 per cent of the daily fecal output of calcium is endogenous—that is, calcium of digestive juice origin that had not been reabsorbed (see Bronner *et al.*).

In the absence of significant dermal loss of calcium which is associated with heavy sweating, the greater part of the total calcium eliminated daily by a normal adult appears in the feces, while the greater part of the total phosphorus eliminated daily appears in the urine. Under these circumstances, the calcium in the feces usually constitutes about 70 to 75 per cent of the total daily output, and the calcium in the urine about 25 to 30 per cent. Of the total daily output of phosphorus, on the other hand, only about 30 per cent is in the feces and about 70 per cent in the urine. However, fluctuations in these proportions occur. Thus, should the calcium ingested on any one day be in a form not readily absorbable, the proportion of fecal to urinary calcium will tend to rise above the figures given. Conversely, the ingestion of calcium in a very readily absorbable form will tend to increase both the amount and the proportion of calcium excreted in the urine. There is, indeed, a reciprocal relationship between the amount of calcium and phosphorus absorbed from the gastrointestinal canal and the amount excreted or lost in the feces. That is, anything that improves the absorption of these minerals necessarily decreases their fecal excretion, and vice versa.

A normal adult on a diet containing an amount of calcium and phosphorus below the minimal requirement will tend to excrete more of these elements than he ingests —that is, the subject will be in negative balance in regard to them. A normal adult on a test diet providing a total calcium intake of 110 mg. daily will excrete 263 mg. of calcium daily (63 in the urine and 200 in the feces). The consequent negative calcium balance will be 153 mg. daily (see W. Bauer *et al.*). It must be borne in mind, however, that the results of calcium and phosphorus balance studies which involve a diet low in calcium but which extend over only a few days are necessarily of limited significance in relation to the total picture of the metabolism of these minerals. Indeed, such large losses of calcium do not continue if the test period is prolonged. Much more often than not, an otherwise normal adult on a low-calcium diet soon begins to conserve his calcium, so that the large initial losses shown in short-time balance studies do not continue, although equilibrium may not be entirely regained.

This conservation occurs mainly at the expense of the fecal excretion of calcium, which becomes sharply curtailed if the intake continues at the low level. This reduced fecal excretion of calcium is due apparently in large measure to better utilization (increased absorption) of the dietary calcium, and possibly also to a somewhat greater reabsorption of the endogenous calcium entering the gastrointestinal tract with the digestive juices. It may also be pointed out here that, in a general way, whatever abnormally increases the elimination of calcium from the body over protracted periods also increases that of phosphorus. The synchronous loss of the two substances is due to the fact that the body draws largely upon the stores of these minerals in the bones, where they are present together as constituents of the complex mineral salt of the osseous tissue. The phosphorus in the various soft tissues (about 25 per cent of the total body phosphorus) is less readily depleted, since in these tissues the phosphorus is mainly in the form of phosphate esters and hence relatively unavailable.

Urinary Excretion.—Both calcium and phosphorus are filtered through the renal glomeruli. Of the total calcium in the plasma, only about 60 per cent is filterable. This filterable (more specifically, the ultrafilterable) fraction is composed mainly of calcium in ionic form, and includes a small amount of soluble nonionized calcium (for example, calcium citrate). In an adult with a total plasma calcium of 10 mg. per 100 ml. and a total plasma protein concentration of about 7.0 per cent, the ionized calcium constitutes approximately 5.3 mg. per 100 ml., and the soluble nonionized filterable calcium complexes about 1.3 mg. per 100 ml. The nonfilterable fraction of the plasma calcium is present mainly in the form of calcium bound to protein. For further details, see page 154.

In regard to the phosphorus in the blood of an adult, it is to be noted that the plasma contains about 3.5 mg. per 100 ml. of inorganic phosphorus and that practically all of this is filterable. This inorganic phosphorus is present almost entirely in the form of ions of orthophosphoric acid. At a plasma pH of 7.4, these phosphate ions are present as $HPO_4^=$ and $H_2PO_4^-$ in an approximate ratio of 4:1 respectively. In addition, there is about 0.5 mg. per 100 ml. of soluble filterable organic phosphoric acid esters (hexose phosphates, etc.) in the plasma. The nonfilterable fraction of the plasma phosphorus is composed mainly of phosphorus bound to phospholipids.

Normally, most of the calcium and phosphorus filtered through the renal glomeruli is reabsorbed in the proximal renal tubules. Naturally, those portions which are not reabsorbed are excreted in the urine. The daily urinary excretion of calcium is about 100 to 125 mg., while the daily urinary excretion of phosphorus is about 800 mg., though it may vary over a wide range.

In a normal adult weighing about 70 kilos and having a body surface of about 1.7 square meters, approximately 180 liters of fluid are filtered daily through the renal glomeruli. Dissolved in this fluid (the plasma ultrafiltrate) are the various substances which have been filtered through the glomeruli (calcium, inorganic phosphorus, glucose, urea, etc.). Since the daily urinary output of a normal adult ranges between 1 and 2 liters, it is obvious that almost all of the water of the plasma ultrafiltrate is reabsorbed as it passes along the renal tubules. In regard to calcium, it is to be noted that between 9.0 and 12.5 g are filtered through the glomeruli in the course of a day. However, somewhat more than 99 per cent of the filtered calcium is reabsorbed in the proximal renal tubules, so that the amount of calcium actually excreted daily in the urine is relatively small, totaling, as already stated, about 100 to 125 mg. In the absence of disordered renal function, a rise in the calcium content of the plasma is associated with a proportional increase in the urinary excretion of calcium, and a fall in the calcium content of the plasma with a decrease in the urinary excretion of calcium.

With a daily glomerular flow of 180 liters, the amount of inorganic phosphorus filtered through the glomeruli is approximately 8.0 g. However, only about 90 per cent of this filtered phosphorus is usually reabsorbed in the proximal renal tubules. Thus the daily urinary excretion of inorganic phosphorus is much higher than that of calcium, approximating, as noted, 800 mg. This figure varies widely with the dietary intake of phosphorus. It is also influenced by the fact that a greater proportion of dietary phosphorus than of dietary calcium is absorbed.

As already noted, parathyroid hormone increases the urinary excretion of calcium and phosphorus by improving the intestinal absorption of these minerals. This hormone also mobilizes calcium and phosphorus from the stable fraction of the bone salt mineral, and, on this account, too, an increased amount of calcium and phosphorus is consequently filtered through the renal glomeruli. Furthermore, it is believed that parathyroid hormone also has a direct action on the kidney insofar as the urinary excretion of phosphorus is concerned. In particular, it seems to decrease the reabsorption of phosphate ion from the proximal renal tubules, so that a larger proportion of the phosphorus filtered through the glomeruli passes out in the urine.

The diminished proximal tubular reabsorption of inorganic phosphorus is probably related to the accumulation of phosphate in the cells of the tubules themselves—an effect which may be induced by parathyroid hormone. It has been reported that inhibition of respiration and phosphorylation in the mitochondria of rabbit kidney cortex occurs after the *in vivo* administration of parathyroid hormone. This inhibition correlates with the increased amounts of calcium and inorganic phosphorus which are found in the whole kidney and in mitochondria (see Cohn *et al.*). There is evidence to support the fact that the phosphaturic effect of parathyroid hormone may also be due to an increased rate of secretion of inorganic phosphorus by the distal renal tubules. Thus the observed increase in urinary inorganic phosphorus as mediated by parathyroid hormone may be the result of both a decrease in proximal tubular reabsorption of phosphate ion and an increase in distal tubular secretion of this substance.

Recent investigations of the role of cyclic AMP (adenosine 3′,5′ monophosphate) as a mediator of hormone action has implicated this substance in the primary action of parathyroid hormone on the kidney. Cyclic AMP is a mononucleotide of adenylic acid with the phosphate group diesterified at carbones 3′ and 5′ of the ribose moiety to form a cyclic phosphate. In this form, it is less subject to acid and alkaline hydrolysis and is not attacked by many phosphatases and diesterases, although it can be enzymatically hydrolyzed (and therefore inactivated) to 5′-AMP (5′ adenosine monophosphate) by a rather specific magnesium requiring phosphodiesterase found in cells.

Cyclic AMP was first isolated as a heat-stable factor which was necessary for the activation of liver phosphorylase as a result of studies on the mechanism of action of epinephrine and glucagon in the breakdown of glycogen (glycogenolysis) in the liver. This heat-stable factor was subsequently shown to be cyclic AMP. This substance was shown to be synthesized in cells from ATP (adenosine triphosphate) by a magnesium-requiring enzyme—adenyl cyclase (see Sutherland *et al.*). From this developmental work was formulated the idea of the two-messenger system for hormone action. According to this scheme, a hormone secreted as a result of the stimulation of a specific endocrine gland acts as the first messenger and travels to other cells where it interacts with specific target cells (effector cells). This interaction may be with specific recognition sites on the cell membrane of the target cell. The primary action of the hormone is then to stimulate adenyl cyclase (which is bound to the inner surface of the cell membrane and probably has a structural relationship to the recognition site of the outer surface) which in turn catalyzes the formation of cyclic AMP from ATP. Cyclic AMP then acts as a second messenger within the interior of the cell, where it may stimulate the synthesis of steroid hormones and/or enzymes, and effect changes in cell membrane permeability, etc. Thus, cyclic AMP may act as the intracellular agent which sets off the various physiological responses originally initiated by the hormone itself. This scheme therefore affords a working hypothesis which explains how a peptide hormone may initiate an intracellular response in a target cell without necessarily entering the cell itself. Furthermore, the action of the hormone secreted by the endocrine gland (first messenger) can be modulated by the action of extracellular inactivators, and the cyclic AMP produced in the cell (second messenger) can as well be modulated by being acted upon by the specific intracellular phosphodiesterase. The mechanisms by which cyclic AMP exerts its intracellular effects have not been definitely established. However, it has been observed that cyclic AMP is able to stimulate a class of enzymes (protein kinases) which are found in a wide variety of tissue cells—muscle, liver, brain, and adipose tissue. The specific protein kinases in turn catalyze the phosphorylation by ATP of certain proteins within the cell (casein, protamine and/or histone, and phosphorylase kinase). The phosphorylated proteins, some of which are activated enzymes, have significant metabolic roles within the cell. Therefore, all of the wide effects elicited by cyclic AMP could be mediated through the stimulation of the protein kinases. There is also evidence that cyclic AMP might not be the sole second messenger within the cell, and that other intracellular cyclic nucleotides may be present and may act in a similar capacity.

Since the first reports of the role of cyclic AMP as a mediator of the action of epinephrine on glycogenolysis in liver, this substance has been implicated in the mechanism of action of a variety of hormones, both peptide (protein-like) and non-peptide hormones. (See Sutherland et al., Sutherland and Robison, Robison et al., and also Butcher.)

Specifically with regard to the action of parathyroid hormone on the kidney, an increase in the urinary excretion of cyclic AMP has been observed in parathyroidec-tomized rats immediately after the start of an infusion of parathyroid hormone or after a single injection of this hormone. Furthermore, an increase in urinary cyclic AMP occurs within 5–10 minutes after the administration of parathyroid hormone, and precedes the usual phosphaturia. The effect seems to be specific for parathy-roid hormone, although vasopressin also has an effect but at higher doses. It has been reported that parathyroid hormone and vasopressin activate adenyl cyclase in the kidney, but at different receptor sites. Parathyroid hormone acts primarily in the cortex, consistent with the action of this hormone on calcium and phosphorus transport in the proximal renal tubules, while vasopressin stimulates adenyl cyclase primarily in the medulla, consistent with the effect of this hormone on sodium transport and water permeability in the collecting tubules of the medulla (see Chase and Aurbach). That cyclic AMP can mimic the action of parathyroid hormone is demonstrated by the fact that a single injection of this substance into the renal ar-tery of a dog results in the prompt onset of a phosphaturia.

In man, an increase in urinary cyclic AMP has been observed after the administra-tion of parathyroid hormone; hyperparathyroid subjects show significant increases in the urinary excretion of cyclic AMP; and finally, subjects with pseudohypo-parathyroidism demonstrate a defective renal excretion of cyclic AMP after the administration of parathyroid hormone. Consequently, parathyroid hormone may act at receptor sites in the renal cortex (possibly in the proximal renal tubules themselves) to stimulate adenyl cyclase, which in turn catalyzes an increase in the rate of synthesis of cyclic AMP, thus mediating a series of events affecting other renal cortical enzymes, etc. These metabolic changes could induce an intracellular accumulation of phosphate ion and result in a reduction in tubular resorption, finally producing a phosphaturia. Cyclic AMP has also been implicated as a second mes-senger in the stimulatory action of parathyroid hormone on bone resorption, and it may also be involved in the inhibitory action of calcitonin (thyrocalcitonin) on bone resorption (p. 144).

THE ORGANIC MATTER OF BONE

The composition, by weight, of a sample of normal adult cortical bone (free of adherent soft parts and thoroughly defatted) is about 5 to 10 per cent water, 25 to 30 per cent organic matter, and 65 to 70 per cent inorganic matter. The bone salt mineral which constitutes nearly all of the inorganic matter of osseous tissue has

9

the crystalline structure of an apatite. Though this has been recognized for a long time, there is not yet complete agreement on the exact nature of this apatite.

In regard to the *organic matter*, it is known that most of this is contributed by the so-called organic matrix of the osseous tissue, and only a small fraction is derived from its cellular elements (mainly osteocytes). The organic matrix consists largely of protein in fibrillar form, but includes a small amount of interfibrillar cement substance (the ground substance) in which the fibrils are embedded. A small amount of intercellular fluid (tissue fluid) is also present in the ground substance, and this fluid acts as a medium for the exchange of dissolved substances between the blood and the osseous tissue. The protein composing the fibrils of the organic matrix is collagen, while the ground substance of the matrix consists mainly of various mucopolysaccharides. For the most part, these mucopolysaccharides are not in chemical combination with the collagen. However, certain specific mucopolysaccharides are apparently so combined, and these mucopolysaccharide-collagen combinations may constitute active centers (nucleation centers) where crystal formation of bone salt mineral is initiated. Certain mucopolysaccharides have also been implicated as control mechanisms, in that they may cover nucleation sites on the collagen and thus prevent mineralization. In recent years the chemical composition of the organic matter of connective tissue, including that of bone, has been the subject of intensive investigation, and many comprehensive reviews have also been published (see Meyer, Kulonen, Eastoe, Piez and Likens, Glimcher, and Seifter and Gallop).

The Collagen of Osseous Tissue.—Collagen, the protein constituent of the various connective tissues of the body, comprises about 20 to 25 per cent of the total protein of the body. About 40 per cent of the body's total collagen is in the bones, and collagen makes up about 90 to 95 per cent, by weight, of the dry, fat-free organic matter of bone. In bone (as in the other connective tissues), collagen is present in the form of fibrils. The individual fibrils are bunched into small fiber units, which in turn are aggregated into bundles of collagen fibers. The individual fibrils are too small to be visible under the light (optical) microscope. However, under high magnification the light microscope will already reveal the small fiber units and will show the larger fiber bundles clearly if appropriate staining methods and other technical aids are used in the preparation and study of the tissue sections (see Fig. 17). On the other hand, the electron microscope reveals certain structural details even in regard to the individual collagen fibrils.

The chemical structure of collagen can appropriately be described in respect to: (1) the fundamental structural units of the collagen molecule (namely, its composition in terms of amino acids); (2) its macromolecular structure (that is, the manner in which its constituent amino acids are linked together to form the collagen macromolecules); and (3) its fibrillar structure (the specific manner in which the collagen macromolecules aggregate to form fibrils). As to its amino acid composition, collagen is poor in the aromatic amino acids (such as tyrosine and phenylalanine) and poor or altogether lacking in certain other amino acids essential to protein metabolism in man (such as methionine, tryptophane, and cystine). On the other hand, collagen is rich in glycine and also contains relatively high concentrations of the amino acids proline, hydroxyproline, alanine, and lysine, among others. Collagen also contains a small proportion of hydroxylysine (about 1 per cent). It seems particularly interesting in this connection that hydroxylysine apparently occurs in collagen alone among the various body proteins, and that hydroxyproline (present in the proportion of about 10 per cent of the total amino acid residues in collagen) is apparently not to be found in any other protein except elastin. In addition, most purified collagens of vertebrates contain about 0.6–2 per cent carbohydrates (identified as D-glucose and D-galactose).

The amino acid molecules of collagen are linked to one another by means of peptide linkages, or bonds. The linked amino acids tend to form long polypeptide chains.* It is believed that each collagen macromolecule (tropocollagen) is composed of three such polypeptide chains, arranged in a helical (screw-like) array about one another in a very specific fashion, so that certain amino acid residues in each chain have a definite spatial relationship to certain amino acid residues in the other chains. Cross linkages between juxtaposed amino acids of each of the polypeptide chains constituting the collagen macromolecule apparently hold the latter together. The collagen macromolecule has a molecular weight of about 300,000, is rodlike in shape, and measures about 14 A in diameter and about 2,900 A in length. (An angstrom, A, is a unit of length equal to 1/10,000 of a micron or 1/10,000,000 of a millimeter.)

Each of the three individual chains of the tropocollagen molecule has a molecular weight of about 100,000 and contains about 800 amino acid residues. In respect to the relative proportions of each of their constituent amino acids, two of the polypeptide chains are almost identical, while the third is different. Denaturation of collagen (for example, by boiling in slightly acidic or neutral water) will convert it to gelatin. The formation of gelatin does not involve the rupture of peptide bonds, but instead involves the rupture of certain of the cross linkages of the tropocollagen molecule. Specific selective chemical procedures have demonstrated that the polypeptide chains of the tropocollagen macromolecule can be degraded to smaller polypeptide fragments. These fragments (molecular weights averaging about 25,-000) are considered to represent structural subunits of the intact polypeptide chain (molecular weight 100,000). The nature of the groupings on the polypeptide chains of tropocollagen responsible for the cross linkages between chains, and the linkages of the subunits within a particular chain have been investigated. One type of linkage which might account for both cross linking and subunit linking involves the amino acids aspartic acid and tyrosine linked to one another via a glucose or galactose molecule. Certain amino acid residues of glutamic acid, lysine, and hydroxylysine have also been proposed as providing a means of cross linking in the tropocollagen molecule. Recently, evidence has been obtained suggesting that the initial step in the formation of cross linkages in tropocollagen is the conversion of peptide-bound lysine to an aldehyde derived from the epsilon amino group of this amino acid. The aldehyde group can then react with other groups on the adjacent polypeptide chain to form cross linkages. The conversion of the epsilon amino group of lysine to an aldehyde group is said to be catalyzed by a specific enzyme. Such an enzyme has actually been demonstrated in bone and certain other tissues. It is of interest to note that this enzyme is inhibited by the lathyrogenic compound

---

* In regard to protein structure, amino acids are linked together in the protein molecule by chemical reaction of the alpha amino group of one amino acid with the carboxyl group of another amino acid. This reaction can be summarized as follows:

$$\begin{matrix} NH_2 & & COOH & & NH_2 & H & COOH \\ | & & | & & | & | & | \\ R-C-COOH & + & H_2N-C-R^1 & \longrightarrow & R-C-C-N-C-R^1 & + & H_2O \\ | & & | & & | \quad \| \quad \quad | \\ H & & H & & H \quad O \quad \quad H \end{matrix}$$

The resulting chemical bond $\left(\begin{matrix} & H \\ & | \\ -C-N-C- \\ \| \\ O \end{matrix} \right)$ is called a peptide bond, and the resulting

compound is called a dipeptide. If additional amino acids then combine with the free amino group and the free carboxyl group of the dipeptide, a more complex polypeptide is formed and eventually protein molecules are elaborated.

beta-aminopropionitrile, which has been known to interfere with cross linking in collagen. Beta-aminopropionitrile or similar agents, when administered to animals, cause a condition known as lathyrism (osteolathyrism). This compound also occurs naturally in the sweet pea (*Lathyrus odoratus*), and when large amounts of this plant are consumed by humans or by animals, lathyrism is known to occur. The condition is characterized by mesenchymal deformities, loss of tensile strength in the tissues, and a severe increase in the solubility of collagen. The collagen produced in this condition has thus failed to undergo maturation because of the defective cross linking induced by the lathyrogenic compound.

As to its fibrillar structure, numerous macromolecules, polymerized or linked together in a highly specific fashion, both from side to side and from end to end, enter into the formation of each fibril of collagen. The individual fibrils are of variable length and may be 3,000 to 5,000 A in diameter. When visualized by means of the electron microscope, native collagen fibrils from decalcified bone will display closely approximated dark double crossbands running at right angles to the long axis of the fibril at intervals of about 640 to 700 A. These major crossbands reflect the high degree of structural regularity of the individual fibril. That is, the banding is a manifestation of the characteristic distribution of chemical groupings in a regular repeated pattern along the length of the fibril. The regular repeated distribution of chemical groupings also manifests itself in variations in electron density, and it is this that produces the series of alternating light and dark cross-striations along the fibril. The chemical groupings responsible for the observed fine band structure are believed to be regions (varying between 10 to 100 A along the length of the macromolecule) which contain polar (charged) amino acid groups that alternate with regions containing nonpolar (noncharged) amino acid groups. Specifically, it is the staggered arrangement of the macromolecules by almost $\frac{1}{4}$ of their length of 2,500 to 2,800 A that gives the collagen fibril the observed axial repeat period of 640 to 700 A. This characteristic organization of the macromolecules in the collagen fibrils also becomes evident when studied by means of x-ray diffraction techniques. The patterns obtained by these techniques have the same fundamental repeat period as that seen under the electron microscope. The collagen fibrils, as described above, being highly ordered aggregates of macromolecules, can be considered to be crystalline in nature. (See Fig. 29.)

During the biosynthesis of collagen, the polypeptide chains are formed on polyribosomes (large ribonucleoprotein structures) within the fibroblasts of mesenchymal tissue, and particularly fibroblasts of the bone-forming mesenchymal tissue. During the synthesis of these polypeptide chains, the individual constituent amino acids are introduced into specific positions along the chain. It is of interest that, while the important structural amino acid proline is directly incorporated into the polypeptide chain, the equally important structural amino acid hydroxyproline is not itself incorporated. Certain proline residues of a microsomal RNA-bound polypeptide of smaller size (protocollagen) are hydroxylated to hydroxyproline by a specific enzyme. In this form, the protocollagen (now containing proline as well as hydroxyproline residues) is incorporated into the larger polypeptide chain of tropocollagen. The hydroxylation of proline to hydroxyproline requires vitamin C (ascorbic acid). This vitamin is therefore necessary for the synthesis of collagen. Scorbutic animals lack the ability to synthesize adequate amounts of collagen because of the failure of the hydroxylating mechanism that converts proline to hydroxyproline. It is believed that the hydroxylysine amino acid residues of the polypeptide chains are formed from lysine residues by a similar mechanism.

Once the polypeptide chains are fully formed within the fibroblast, three chains are joined by cross linkages to form the 3-stranded helical tropocollagen macromolecule (molecular weight 300,000). The fully formed tropocollagen macromolecules are then secreted by the fibroblasts into the matrix, where they are randomly dispersed. They then align themselves end to end and side to side (by means of intermolecular cross linkages) in the specific staggered arrangement to form native collagen fibrils with an axial repeat period of 640 to 700 A.

The fact that, under normal *in vivo* conditions, the collagen of osseous tissue comes to have bone salt mineral deposited on or within its fibrils must reflect some feature in its chemical composition which distinguishes it from the collagen of the other connective tissues. Apparently the calcifiability of bone collagen is related to its molecular structure, and specifically to the manner in which the constituent amino acids are grouped and oriented in the molecules, and possibly also to the manner in which the molecules are linked to form the collagen macromolecules. More particularly, it appears that the calcifiability of bone collagen may be related to its organization at the submacromolecular level, the macromolecular level, and the fibrillar level.

Specifically, there is evidence that the calcifiability of the collagen fibril of bone is attributable in part to certain amino acids which constitute end groups of the polypeptide chains of the macromolecules. As a result of their position, they may provide amino end groups for the binding of the phosphate and/or calcium ions from the tissue fluid circulating between the newly formed collagen fibrils. It is possible that the development of bone mineral crystals is initiated in this way. However, the amino acid groups of collagen apparently do not represent the exclusive components of the nucleation centers of the organic matrix. In regard to the specific arrangement of the macromolecules in the collagen fibrils of bone, the observed axial repeat period of 640 to 700 A is also in some way related to their calcifiability.

The Ground Substance of Osseous Tissue.—As mentioned previously, the ground substance consists mainly of mucopolysaccharides* but also includes a small amount of intercellular (interstitial) fluid. The mucopolysaccharides found in bone

---

* Mucopolysaccharides are found in all forms of connective tissue and not only in the ground substance of bone (and of cartilage). A particular mucopolysaccharide is characterized by the chemical composition of its repeatable structural unit which exists in a highly polymerized state. The fundamental compounds found as constituents of the structural units of mucopolysaccharides are: uronic acids (D-glucuronic acid or L-iduronic acid), a hexose (galactose), acetylated hexosamines (N-acetyl-D-galactosamine or N-acetyl-D-glucosamine), and sulfuric acid (as sulfate groups esterified at carbons 4 or 6 of the acetylated hexosamine). Of the mucopolysaccharides isolated from connective tissues in general and from certain body fluids (synovial fluid, vitreous humor, etc.), those which have been most extensively studied in regard to their chemical structures are hyaluronic acid, chondroitin sulfate A, chondroitin sulfate B, chondroitin sulfate C, chondroitin, keratosulfate, heparin, and heparitin sulfate. The mucopolysaccharides found in bone include chondroitin sulfate A and keratosulfate. Chondroitin sulfate A, in addition to having been isolated from bone, has also been obtained from cartilage and cornea. Chondroitin sulfate B, on the other hand, has been isolated from skin, tendon, heart valves, aorta, and ligaments, but is absent from cartilage and bone. Chondroitin sulfate C is found in cartilage, in tendon, and in the sclera of the eye.
Chondroitin sulfates A and C both contain D-glucuronic acid, N-acetyl-D-galactosamine and sulfate ester groups (esterified at carbon 4 of the hexosamine in chondroitin sulfate A, and at carbon 6 of the hexosamine in chondroitin sulfate C). Chondroitin sulfate B, however, contains L-iduronic acid instead of D-glucuronic acid, N-acetyl-D-galactosamine, and sulfate groups (esterified at carbon 4 of the hexosamine). This substance, like heparin, has high anticoagulant activity. Hyaluronic acid is composed of D-glucuronic acid, N-acetyl-D-glucosamine (instead of N-acetyl-D-galactosamine), and is without sulfate groups. Finally, keratosulfate is a polymer containing galactose, N-acetylglucosamine, and sulfate groups. The cellular mechanisms concerned with the biosynthesis of mucopolysaccharides in fibroblasts are quite complex. They involve a class of enzymes designated as uridyl transferases which function to convert glucose (by way of a compound called uridinediphosphoglucose) to the various uronic acids, acetylated hexosamines, and finally to the fully formed mucopolysaccharides and protein-polysaccharides. The biosynthetic steps are regulated at different stages by insulin, thyroxin, and growth hormone.

include chondroitin sulfate A, keratosulfate, and other sulfated and nonsulfated mucopolysaccharides of still undetermined chemical structure. Though some still maintain that these mucopolysaccharides exist in an amorphous state, the prevailing view is that they are highly organized, possessing a definite macromolecular structure though not a true crystalline structure. The interstitial fluid of the ground substance may be freely circulating or may exist as a gel (that is, in a semifluid, water-rich, colloidal phase).

The concentration of mucopolysaccharide in bone is low (about 0.5 per cent by weight). It exists in osseous tissue in the form of a mucopolysaccharide-protein complex (proteinpolysaccharide). The biological significance of the mucopolysaccharides of the ground substance is little understood. By special staining techniques (for example, metachromatic staining with toluidine blue) the mucopolysaccharides of the ground substance can be shown to give a positive staining reaction after decalcification. This phenomenon (metachromasia) is attributed to the highly polymerized state of the native mucopolysaccharides in the ground substance and the presence of negatively charged groups (sulfate groups) in the mucopolysaccharides.

The mucopolysaccharides of the ground substance of fully formed bone are therefore highly polymerized. When bone mineral is being deposited or resorbed, there is a rapid loss in metachromatic staining of the mucopolysaccharides, indicating a loss in the degree of polymerization. This change in staining reaction, in conjunction with the use of other staining techniques (for example, the Hotchkiss periodic acid-fuchsin sulfite stain), seems to suggest that the property of calcifiability of the

Figure 29

A, Diagrammatic representation of the structure of a collagen macromolecule as proposed by Rich and Crick. The macromolecule is conceived as consisting of three separate polypeptide chains which coil clockwise (*i.e.* in a right-handed helix) about a central major axis. In addition (though this is not illustrated), each of the three polypeptide chains actually has a minor coil arrangement of its own, running counterclockwise as it gradually twists around the major axis.

B, Diagrammatic representation of a part of the macromolecule shown in *A*, enlarged to illustrate the distribution of the amino acid residues of the polypeptide chains in relation to the major axis. The residues are represented as black circles in polypeptide chain number 1, as clear circles in polypeptide chain number 2, and as circles with central dots in polypeptide chain number 3. As to the spacing of the amino acid residues in the polypeptide chains, note, for example, that the distance between two such residues in chain number 1 is 3.1 angstrom units. The amino acid composition of each polypeptide chain includes about 33 per cent glycine residues, and investigations of the amino acid sequence of these chains indicate that glycine is in every third position along the chain.

C, Schematic representation of a specific aggregation state of the collagen macromolecules in a portion of a collagen fibril. A tropocollagen molecule is depicted by an arrow 2,560 A in length, whose head is a filled-in triangle and whose tail is an unfilled circle. In the collagen fibril, the macromolecules are polymerized head to tail longitudinally and are staggered $\frac{1}{4}$ of their length with respect to adjacent macromolecules. This particular aggregation state of the macromolecules in the collagen fibril gives the latter the characteristic banding expressed in the 640 A axial repeat pattern. In particular, the head-to-tail joining of the polymerized collagen macromolecules results in an accumulation of chemical groupings at intervals of 640 A at right angles to the long axis of the collagen fibril, and produces these dark bands as illustrated in the reconstructed collagen fibrils. In addition, this diagram demonstrates the fine band structure of the fibril. (This diagrammatic illustration has been adapted from the one presented by Glimcher.)

D, An electron micrograph ($\times$ 26,000) revealing the actual crossbanding of collagen fibrils of lamellar bone. (Reproduced from Rutishauser and Majno, and enlarged.)

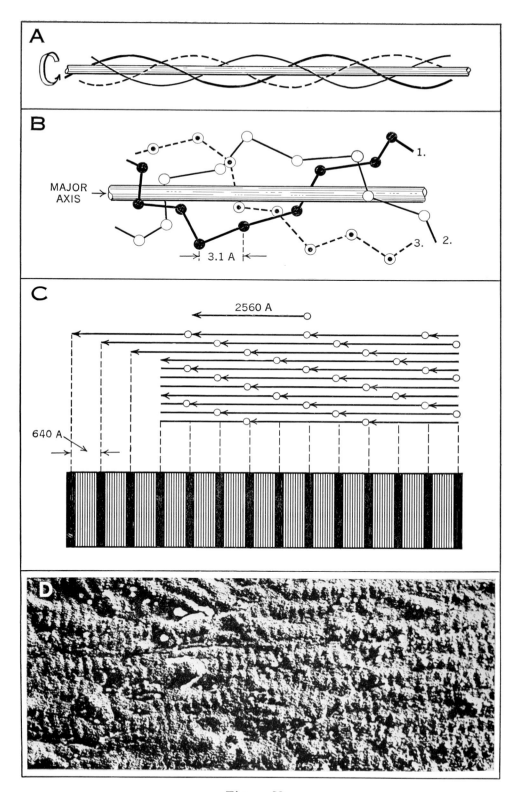

MAJOR
AXIS

1.

3.

2.

3.1 A

2560 A

640 A

Figure 29

bone collagen is also dependent in some way upon the state of polymerization of the mucopolysaccharides of the ground substance. Since the mucopolysaccharides found in bone are also found in connective tissues that do not calcify, the particular relationship of the mucopolysaccharides of the ground substance of bone to the calcifiability of the collagen is probably again to be related to the macromolecular structure of the pertinent mucopolysaccharides and the manner in which these mucopolysaccharides are arranged with respect to the nucleation centers of the collagen (p. 135).

THE INORGANIC MATTER OF BONE

After a given sample of normal, mature, cortical bone has been freed of all adherent soft tissue and thoroughly defatted, it can be determined that, as already noted, approximately 5 to 10 per cent of the weight of the sample represents water, about 25 to 30 per cent organic matter, and about 65 to 70 per cent inorganic matter. These values are obtained through estimations of progressive weight loss occurring in the course of dehydration of the sample, followed by treatment with hot alkali, and then ashing at controlled temperatures. As given for samples of cortical bone, these values (representing weight in grams per 100 g of sample) must not be applied uncritically to osseous tissue in general. In regard to cancellous bone, for instance, thorough defatting and dehydration are difficult to achieve, and there are, of course, significant differences in compactness and/or density between cancellous and cortical bone. Furthermore, even under normal conditions and in the same subject, there are differences in the degree of mineralization of bone samples taken from different sites.

Thus, expressions of bone composition achieve greater analytical significance if they are given in terms of weight of constituents per unit volume of osseous tissue. If the results of chemical analyses of bone are expressed in terms of volume, it becomes apparent that the amount of organic matter remains relatively constant as the amount of inorganic matter increases. Such analyses will also show that the water content of the bone sample decreases as the amount of mineral matter increases. This implies that, as more bone mineral is deposited in the matrix of osseous tissue, the water molecules are displaced, and the spaces which had been occupied by them become occupied by bone mineral (see Robinson).

Elementary Composition.—In regard to the inorganic matter of bone, it is recognized that the bone salt mineral has the crystalline form of an apatite. However, before discussing the chemical composition and architecture of this apatite, it seems worth considering the inorganic matter of bone in respect to its elementary composition. In this connection, chemical analysis demonstrates that the mineral fraction of osseous tissue consists mainly of the following ions: calcium, phosphate, hydroxyl, carbonate, and citrate, with smaller amounts of sodium, magnesium, potassium, chloride, and fluoride. In addition, certain other elements may be found in trace amounts, as, for instance, strontium and lead. A representative elementary analysis of a single sample of dry, fat-free bovine cortical bone is given in the following table, the values having been reconstructed from the analytical findings of Armstrong and Singer (see McLean and Urist).

As illustrated in the table, calcium constitutes approximately 27 per cent of the dry, fat-free weight of the bone specimen analyzed. The cations present in relatively smaller amounts are magnesium, sodium, potassium and strontium. The sodium present in bone undoubtedly constitutes a reserve store which can become partially available to the body fluids in times of need—that is, whenever sodium depletion of the body fluids occurs. Likewise, some of the magnesium in the inorganic matter

Composition of Dry, Fat-free Bovine Cortical Bone

	Per Cent*	mEq/g†
Cations:		
Calcium (Ca⁺⁺)	26.70	13.32
Magnesium (Mg⁺⁺)	0.436	0.358
Sodium (Na⁺)	0.731	0.318
Potassium (K⁺)	0.055	0.014
Strontium (Sr⁺⁺)	0.035	—
Total	—	14.01
Anions:		
Phosphorus	12.47	—
as PO_4	—	12.06
Carbon dioxide	3.48	—
as CO_3	—	1.58
Citric acid	0.863	—
as Cit	—	0.138
Chloride (Cl⁻)	0.077	0.022
Fluoride (F⁻)	0.072	0.038
Total	—	13.84
mEq. cations / mEq. anions	—	1.01
mmoles Ca / mmoles P	—	1.656
Nitrogen	4.92	

* Grams of constituent per 100 g of dry, fat-free bovine cortical bone.

† In the present connection, a milliequivalent (mEq.) may be simply defined as the atomic or molecular weight in milligrams of the particular ion (cation or anion) divided by its valence. Calculation in terms of milliequivalents permits the direct addition of all the anions and cations, since these are expressed as "combining weights."

of the bone also becomes available to the body fluids in the case of magnesium deficiency.

Of the anionic constituents, it is phosphorus and carbonate that make up the major portion. Of the anions, citric acid possibly plays a role in the processes of bone resorption and calcium transport. Its role will be discussed in greater detail elsewhere. The most significant information that one derives from an examination of these data is the fact that the calculated millimole calcium:phosphorus ratio of 1.656 corresponds very closely to the theoretical ratio of 1.667 for these minerals in hydroxyapatite. That is, these figures for calcium and phosphorus derived from the elementary analysis lend support to the idea that the bone salt mineral very likely corresponds in crystalline form to that of a hydroxyapatite.

Crystal Structure of the Bone Mineral.—The individual crystals of bone mineral are so small that the electron microscope is needed for their visualization. Some observers have described the crystals as having the shape of hexagonal tablets. Crystals of this shape have been reported as measuring 300 to 500 A (angstrom units) in length, about 250 A in width, and 85 to 100 A in thickness (see Robinson). Others have described the crystals as being rodlike or hexagonal prisms measuring about 50 A in diameter and of various lengths. Reported differences in regard to the shape of the individual crystals may very well be due to differences in their position when visualized. For example, a tablet-like crystal might be interpreted as a rod if viewed in relation to its edge. In any event, the crystals are oriented to the long axis of the collagen fibrils and also have a special relation to the cross-banding of the fibrils as observed under the electron microscope (see Fig. 30).

Much of our knowledge of the structure of these crystals has been derived from the analysis of x-ray diffraction patterns obtained by the study of purified mineral samples of bone.* By comparing diffraction patterns of crystals of bone mineral with those of samples of synthetic or naturally occurring crystals of known composition, it has been established that the structure of the crystalline mineral of bone is essentially that of an apatite—a form of hydroxyapatite—$Ca_{10}(PO_4)_6(OH)_2$. It should be emphasized that hydroxyapatite as represented is not the formula of a molecule, but represents only the ratios of all the constituent ions of the mineral phase in terms of the smallest whole numbers.

The structure of the pure hydroxyapatite crystal may be best understood in terms of its "unit cell." It should be pointed out in this connection that the term "unit cell" merely designates the arrangement of the ions of the bone mineral crystal in three-dimensional space. The unit cell therefore can be conceived as the smallest expression of the arrangement of the ions in relation to one another which is found as a repeatable unit throughout the crystal. Imaginary lines connecting these ions outline the unit cell. When these lines are extended through the crystal structure, they create a three-dimensional repeatable figure called the *crystal lattice*.

The ions which delineate the unit cell in three-dimensional space are components of the crystal structure of hydroxyapatite. In a cross-sectional representation running perpendicular to its long axis, this crystal may be considered as being composed of a series of adjacent hexagons with sides in common. A calcium ion is present at each intersection of every hexagon and is thus shared among three adjacent hexagons. At the center of each hexagon there are two superimposed

---

* A monochromatic x-ray beam (an x-ray beam composed of a single wave length of radiant energy or composed of a group of rays of closely related wave lengths) is passed through a sample. When a photographic film is placed near the sample, it is possible to obtain a "diffraction pattern" on the photographic plate. Analysis of the pattern permits one to measure the angles between the incoming x-ray beam and the outgoing (diffracted) beams. Consequently, it is possible to obtain data relevant to the arrangement of the atoms within the crystal, the distances between the atoms in the crystal, and the type of atoms themselves.

Figure 30

A, Electron micrograph ($\times$ 80,000) of part of a reconstituted collagen fibril at an early stage of *in vitro* calcification. Note the periodic distribution, both longitudinally and transversely, of the small, dense particles which represent crystals of bone mineral. The apatite crystals are developing at nucleation centers in the fibril, the centers occurring at regular intervals. The nucleation sites correspond to the intraperiod fine structure of the fibril. (This illustration is an enlarged reproduction of a print kindly contributed by Dr. M. J. Glimcher.)

B, Electron micrograph ($\times$ 100,000) showing the regular periodic arrangement of apatite crystals in avian embryonic subperiosteal bone. The mineralization is at a very early stage, and the mineral crystals are developing at the nucleation centers within the collagen fibrils. Note the general similarity of this *in vivo* pattern of mineralization at the nucleation centers to the *in vitro* pattern shown in *A*. (This illustration is a slightly enlarged reproduction of a print kindly contributed by Dr. S. Fitton Jackson. See Proc. Roy. Soc. London, s.B., *146*, 270, 1957.)

C, Electron micrograph ($\times$ 225,000) showing crystals of bone mineral distributed along loose collagen fibrils of fish bone. Note that the long axes of the apatite crystals correspond more or less to the long axes of the collagen fibrils. (I am grateful to Dr. Glimcher for permission to reproduce this illustration, which, like *A*, was used in his article in *Calcification in Biological Systems*, see references.)

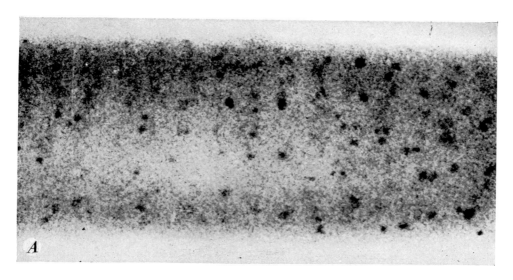

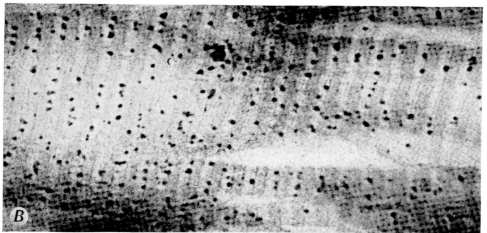

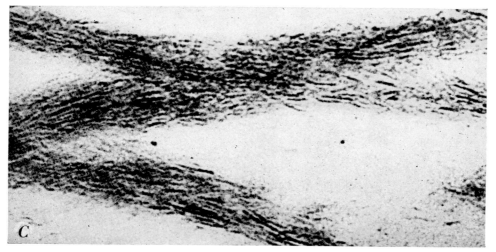

Figure 30

127

hydroxyl ions. Three of the six calcium ions forming the hexagon share one hydroxyl ion, the other three sharing the other hydroxyl. Each calcium ion has phosphate ions specifically oriented around it. In addition, there is a screw axis running spirally around the columns of hydroxyl ions, calcium and phosphate ions being symmetrically arranged with respect to this screw axis.

If one then connects the points corresponding to the hydroxyl ions, one obtains the so-called unit cell, which can be described as a diamond-shaped parallelogram with angles of $120°$ and $60°$ at the intersections. When this parallelogram is extended into the third dimension (the long axis of the crystal), one obtains, as the unit cell in three-dimensional space, a six-sided prism. The dimensions of this prism have been calculated by means of x-ray diffraction studies and found to have the following unit cell dimensions in angstrom units: $a = 9.432$, $b = 9.432$, and $c = 6.881$. The c axis is oriented in the long dimension of the crystal of hydroxyapatite.

In summary, therefore, when a diagram of the lattice of a pure crystal of hydroxyapatite is viewed parallel to the c axis, one can visualize columns of calcium and phosphate ions arranged at the intersections of the hexagons, and columns of hydroxyl ions at the intersections of the parallelograms representing the unit cells. These columns of hydroxyls run through the center of each hexagon. This appearance has been described as a sort of honeycomb arrangement of ions, oriented in the long axes of the crystals. What has been described above can be said to represent a relatively simple picture of the crystal structure of hydroxyapatite.

As noted, a bone cell crystal is composed of fundamental repeatable units. The weight of each individual unit cell corresponds to the formula weight of hydroxyapatite—$[Ca_{10}(PO_4)_6(OH)_2$, formula weight = 1,004]. For example, in a crystal of bone mineral 500 A in length, about 250 A wide, and 100 A thick, there will be about 23,400 unit cells, each with a formula weight of approximately 1,000. (See Fig. 31.)

It should be pointed out that the diffraction pattern of bone mineral, although close to that of synthetic hydroxyapatite, is not absolutely identical with the latter pattern. It is known, for example, that many discontinuities may appear in the structure of a single bone mineral crystal as it grows. These discontinuities may then permit the introduction of impurities into the crystal structure. It is also possible, conversely, that the impurities may produce the observed discontinuities. In addition, substitutions may occur in some of the unit cells. (For example: sodium may substitute for calcium, fluoride may substitute for hydroxyl, and also perhaps carbonate may substitute for phosphate.) These replacements may occur by the introduction of the substituting ions during the process of unit cell formation, or by exchange after the crystals are formed. It is to be emphasized, however, that there are differences of opinion concerning the substitution of ions in the unit cells. In particular, it is possible that certain of the ions mentioned may actually be merely adsorbed onto the surfaces of the crystals of hydroxyapatite instead of being substituted in the unit cell. Citrate, being too large a molecule to fit into the unit cell of hydroxyapatite, is adsorbed, or bound, onto the surface of the crystals. Some of the adsorbed citrate molecules may actually be combined with calcium as a complex, while others may exist as citrate ion, some of the adsorbed citrate being dissolved with great difficulty from powdered bone, the rest being more readily soluble.

It should not be assumed that the only type of calcium phosphate in bone mineral exists as hydroxyapatite. An amorphous (noncrystalline) form of calcium phosphate has also been found in bone, and is considered to be another phase of bone mineral, separate and distinct from hydroxyapatite. The physiological significance of the amorphous form of calcium phosphate is as yet unclarified. However, it is known that the first mineral formed in bone is amorphous, but decreases with aging of the bone as the content of crystalline hydroxyapatite increases. There is evidence that the amorphous calcium phosphate is not a direct precursor of hydroxyapatite; instead, the former is mobilized and dissolved in the fluids permeating the bone, and the calcium and phosphate ions are subsequently reassembled (together with hydroxyl ions) on the collagen matrix to form hydroxyapatite.

THE FORMATION AND DEPOSITION OF BONE MINERAL

The formation and deposition of bone mineral will be considered in relation to: (1) the physicochemical state of the calcium and phosphorus in the various body fluids and (2) certain special characteristics of the organic matrix of bone which seem to favor the deposition of bone mineral.

The Physicochemical State of Calcium and Phosphorus in the Body Fluids.— Bone mineral may be regarded as representing a solid phase of certain forms of calcium phosphate, the mineral having a relatively low solubility in the fluid which bathes it. In fact, a sort of equilibrium may be said to exist between the bone mineral (that is, the calcium phosphate of the solid phase) and the calcium and phosphate ions of the fluid bathing the mineral.

As already stated, about 50 per cent of the calcium in the plasma is in the form of calcium ion, and almost all of the inorganic phosphorus is in ionized form. The calcium and phosphate ions of the plasma are diffusible and therefore rapidly exchangeable with the corresponding ions in the intercellular fluids and, in this connection, of course, with the intercellular fluid bathing the bone mineral. Thus, changes in the concentrations of calcium and phosphate ions in the plasma will be reflected in changes in the concentrations of these ions in the fluid bathing the bone, and vice versa. Accordingly, since the concentrations of calcium and phosphate ions in the plasma "mirror" the concentrations of these ions in the other circulating body fluids, it is the plasma that has been most extensively studied as representing a humoral system involved in mineralization of bone.

The relationship between dissolved ions (in this instance, the calcium and phosphate ions) and a solid phase (in this instance, the calcium phosphate composing the bone mineral) can be described in terms of an "ion product." Simply expressed, the ion product is the arithmetical value obtained by multiplying the values for the concentration of each individual ion in solution which is in equilibrium with the particular solid phase that results when these ions interact.* If bone and the sur-

* For example, let us consider the compound calcium hydrogen phosphate ($CaHPO_4$), a salt with a low solubility in aqueous solutions at pH values above 5.5. If this salt is present as a solid phase in a solution containing Ca^{++} and $HPO_4^=$, the conditions at equilibrium can be described as follows: $Ca^{++} + HPO_4^= \rightleftharpoons CaHPO_4$. In addition, the ion product at equilibrium may be written as: $[Ca^{++}] \times [HPO_4^=] = K_{s.p.CaHPO_4}$. At equilibrium, the value for $K_{s.p.}$ which is obtained by multiplying the molar concentration (moles per liter of solution) of Ca^{++} and $HPO_4^=$ is denoted as the ion product constant, or the solubility product constant for $CaHPO_4$. Thus the value for $K_{s.p.}$ is a constant at a given temperature which represents the ion product at concentrations of the ions at which the rates of solution and precipitation of the salt are equal. It thus defines the conditions present at equilibrium. Stated in other words, if the ion product of the molar concentrations exceeds the value for $K_{s.p.}$, precipitation of $CaHPO_4$ will occur. If the value for the ion product is less than the $K_{s.p.}$, no precipitation will occur. It is obvious that the value of $K_{s.p.}$ may be raised through an increase in the concentration of Ca^{++} or $HPO_4^=$, or both. When precipitation occurs, the value of the ion product will be restored to the value of $K_{s.p.}$. The ion product as described above is valid for salts in which the ions are present in equimolar amounts, where 1 mole of the salt dissociates. The law of mass action requires that when an ion is present in a salt in numbers greater than 1, its molar concentration must be raised to the power corresponding to the number of ions in the formula of this salt. For example, the ion product constant of tricalcium phosphate $[Ca_3(PO_4)_2]$ is calculated as follows: $[Ca^{++}]^3 \times [PO_4^=]^2 = K_{s.p.Ca_3(PO_4)_2}$. The method of calculating this product should thus be compared with the calculation for $CaHPO_4$ as outlined above.

rounding fluids are to be treated as such a physicochemical system, one should be able to calculate a value for the ion product constant of calcium and phosphate ions in the plasma (and therefore in the fluid bathing the bone). This value would define the product of the concentrations of calcium and phosphate ions that would have to be attained in these fluids before mineralization could occur.

Attempts to determine such a solubility product constant have been largely unsuccessful, because the solubility product must be referred to a known homogeneous solid phase in order to be meaningful. The bone mineral does not meet this requirement, since it is not homogeneous itself, being composed of hydroxyapatite and a number of other ions which are adsorbed onto the surface of the mineral. In addition, other soluble ions are present in the tissue fluids which may modify the

Figure 31

A, Diagrammatic representation of a mature, tabular, hexagonal crystal of hydroxyapatite of bone. If we consider this crystal as being approximately 500 A in length, 250 A in width, and 100 A in thickness, then this diagram magnifies the size of the crystal about 2,000,000 times. As present in bone, the hydroxyapatite crystals naturally vary somewhat in size and relative dimensions—that is, in the ratios of length to width to thickness. In the diagram, the stippled area, whose front face is delimited by the letters ABCD, represents part of a cross-sectional segment through the crystal.

B, Diagrammatic representation of part of the cross-sectional segment of the crystal marked out in *A*, as viewed from its front face, which is here designated as A′B′C′D′. As illustrated, the crystal may be conceived as being composed of a series of adjacent hexagons with sides in common, a calcium ion being present at each intersection of every hexagon. By means of heavy lines in the center of the diagram, one face of a *unit cell* is illustrated in relation to these hexagons. These lines form a parallelogram with a hydroxyl ion at each of its four corners. The stippled area on the left represents a unit cell as extended into the third dimension, or the so-called *C* axis. The broken lines forming adjacent parallelograms represent the crystal lattice.

C, Diagrammatic representation of a single unit cell indicating, in a simplified conceptual form, the distribution of its constituent calcium, phosphate, and hydroxyl ions. Actually, the ions in question are larger than represented in proportion to the unit cell as a whole, completely filling the cell. In addition, the pattern of their arrangement in relation to one another is more complex. Furthermore, the ions have not been represented in their true relative dimensions. In any event, the prime purpose of this illustration is to demonstrate that each unit cell has a molecular weight which can be accounted for by the formula weight for hydroxyapatite—$Ca_{10}(PO_4)_6(OH)_2$. In the latter connection, it is to be noted that certain of the calcium and phosphate ions lie completely within this unit cell, while others are shared by it with adjacent unit cells. Note that the shared calcium and phosphate ions are represented in the diagram as lying at the periphery of the various sides of the unit cell. Actually, however, half of each of these atoms lies within the interior of the unit cell, and the other half is shared with only one other adjacent unit cell. The composition of the unit cell is accounted for as follows: (1) 6 calcium ions lie completely within the unit cell, and 8 additional calcium ions are shared equally among adjacent unit cells. Thus, as shown, this unit cell contains 6 whole calcium ions and 8 "half" calcium ions, giving a total of 10 calcium ions. (2) In regard to the phosphate ions, 2 lie completely within the unit cell and 8 are shared equally with adjacent unit cells. Thus there are 2 whole phosphate ions and 8 "half" phosphate ions, or a total of 6 phosphate ions. (3) As to the hydroxyl ions which form the corners of the unit cell, though only 8 ions are indicated in the diagram, there are actually 16 ions—2 superimposed on each other at each corner. Each of these hydroxyl ions is shared by 8 adjacent unit cells, and therefore one eighth of each of these superimposed hydroxyl ions can be said to lie within the unit cell represented, the total thus accounting for 2 hydroxyl ions. When the weight of all these ions is totalled, a figure is obtained which corresponds to the formula weight of hydroxyapatite—namely, 1,004. It has been estimated by Robinson that a crystal of the size illustrated in *A* (500 × 250 × 100 angstrom units) contains about 23,400 unit cells.

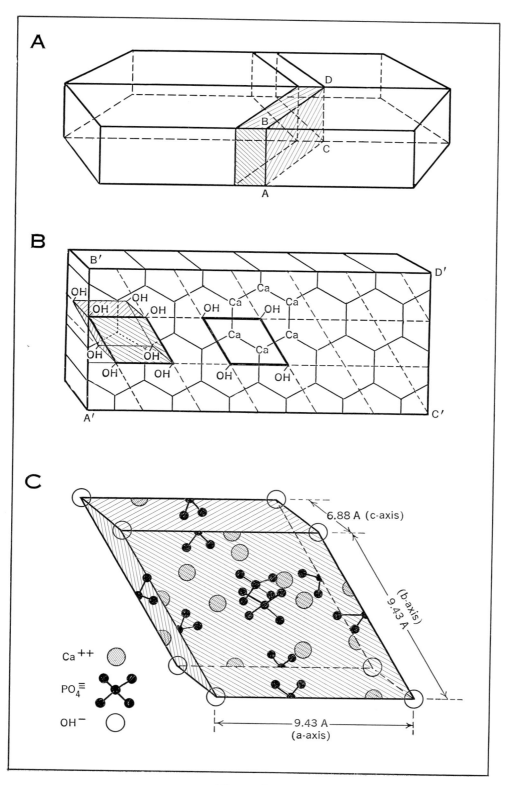

A

B

C

Ca^{++}

PO$_4^{\equiv}$

OH$^-$

6.88 A (c-axis)

(b-axis) 9.43 A

9.43 A (a-axis)

Figure 31

131

calculated $K_{s.p.}$ for the pure salt (that is, some form of calcium phosphate) and its dissociated ions. Another difficulty is attributable to the fact that the calcium and phosphate in the bone mineral on the one hand and in the fluid surrounding the mineral on the other are influenced by certain biological factors (for example, the action of vitamin D and parathyroid hormone). Therefore, the relationship between the calcium and phosphate ions in the bone mineral and those in the fluid bathing the bone is not that of a simple physicochemical equilibrium between insoluble calcium phosphate and a solution of calcium and phosphate ions.

The chemical composition of the particular solid phase which may be in direct equilibrium with the dissolved calcium and phosphate ions in the tissue fluids has been intensively investigated. For example, solubility products have been determined after equilibration of synthetic hydroxyapatite or bone powder with fluids (such as serum, plasma, or aqueous solutions) containing calcium and phosphate ions in various concentrations. These *in vitro* experiments were intended to shed light on *in vivo* conditions in respect to the bone salt and the fluids bathing the mineral. However, these experiments have yielded relatively little information in regard to the *in vivo* physicochemical equilibrium between the tissue fluids and the particular solid phase, mainly because the experimental conditions did not permit one to be sure that true equilibrium had been attained.

In vitro experiments have also been conducted on slices of rachitic cartilage immersed in solutions of calcium and phosphate ions. By varying the relative concentrations of these ions (varying the ion product), it is possible to attain an ion product which will result in mineralization (calcification) of the rachitic cartilage. The minimum ion product at which mineralization will occur has been referred to as the "biological end point." Investigations utilizing this experimental procedure were directed toward determining whether it is the ion product constant (solubility product constant) for $CaHPO_4$ or that of $Ca_3(PO_4)_2$ that is critical for *in vitro* mineralization.

The results obtained seem to indicate that at pH values above 7.2 it is the ion product constant for $CaHPO_4$ that is a determining factor in such mineralization. It should be emphasized that, since these results have been obtained with *in vitro* systems, they are probably not completely relevant to *in vivo* conditions. Nevertheless, they are consistent with certain *in vivo* observations. It is known, for instance, that $HPO_4^=$ (divalent or secondary phosphate) is the major form of inorganic phosphorus existing in the plasma and tissue fluid under normal conditions, while $PO_4^≡$ (trivalent or tertiary phosphate) represents only 0.004 per cent of the total inorganic phosphorus in these fluids. Consequently, $PO_4^≡$ is present in concentrations so low that its contributions to any type of equilibrium are negligible. Support for the concept that the ion product of calcium and inorganic phosphorus in the plasma plays an important role in mineralization is supplied by the biochemical findings relating to the concentration of these substances in the blood plasma in cases of rickets (see Howland and Kramer). In this connection it has been observed that the magnitude of the arithmetical product of the total serum calcium and inorganic phosphorus (both expressed in milligrams per 100 ml.) is of diagnostic significance in directing attention to the presence or absence of rickets in young children.* For example, the serum or plasma of nonrachitic children usually gives a calcium $\times$ inorganic phosphorus value well above 40 (the normal value for adult serum or plasma). On the other hand, the serum or plasma of

---

* In the absence of concurrent changes in the concentration of plasma proteins, changes in the concentration of total calcium in the serum or plasma are attributable to variations in the concentration of calcium ion. Since, within the physiologic range of blood pH, $HPO_4^=$ is the major form of inorganic phosphorus, the determination of total inorganic phosphorus in serum or plasma is essentially a determination of the concentration of $HPO_4^=$.

rachitic children usually gives a calcium $\times$ inorganic phosphorus value below 40—a value which is not high enough to support the mineralization of bone at a normal rate. These facts, taken together with the fact that the total serum calcium very often varies inversely with the total inorganic phosphorus, lend additional support to the idea that these constituents might bear a solubility product relationship to each other.

The Role of the Organic Matrix and Specific Enzymes in Mineralization.—As already indicated, there seems to be an ion product constant (probably that for $CaHPO_4$) which is critical for the deposition of bone mineral. Normally, however, the ion product of Ca^{++} and $HPO_4^=$ in the plasma and intercellular fluids has a value which makes these fluids undersaturated in respect to these ions. Since, under normal conditions, mineralization of the organic matrix of bone and cartilage nevertheless occurs, it seems reasonable to deduce that certain local mechanisms, also, are operative at sites of mineralization (see Gutman, also Fleish and Neuman, and Follis).

Such a local mechanism was first postulated by Robison and evolved from the observation that functionally active osteoblasts and cartilage cells elaborate the enzyme alkaline phosphatase. That is, this enzyme appears in cartilage which is undergoing the hypertrophic changes known to precede mineralization of its matrix, and in osteoid (that is, uncalcified matrix of osseous tissue) which has been laid down in the vicinity of actively proliferating osteoblasts. The significance of the appearance of alkaline phosphatase at these sites is related to the fact that this enzyme is capable of catalyzing the hydrolysis of various organic esters of phosphoric acid, resulting in an increase in the concentration of phosphate ion in the tissue fluid. The increased concentration of these ions, if great enough, could cause supersaturation of the local tissue fluid, leading to the precipitation of calcium phosphate at the sites being mineralized.

The requirements for the functioning of the alkaline phosphatase mechanism just mentioned are: (1) At sites of mineralization there must be enough calcium and phosphate ions in the intercellular tissue fluid so that rather small increases in phosphate ion will favor the precipitation of calcium phosphate; and (2) there must be a sufficient amount of organic phosphate esters in the tissue fluids so that their hydrolysis by alkaline phosphatase will increase the local concentration of phosphate ions enough to precipitate calcium phosphate. It should be noted that the concentration of organic phosphate esters in both the plasma and intercellular tissue fluid is normally very low (approximately 0.5 mg. per 100 ml., expressed as organic phosphorus). In order to overcome this difficulty, Robison expanded his concept concerning local enzyme action. He proposed the existence, at sites of mineralization, of a *multienzyme system* whose integrated action could result in the local synthesis of organic phosphate esters which in turn could be rapidly hydrolyzed by the alkaline phosphatase (a component of this multienzyme system) to produce significant quantities of phosphate ion.

It is known that glycogen and alkaline phosphatase accumulate in the hypertrophic cells of cartilage whose matrix is soon to be mineralized in preparation for so-called endochondral ossification of the cartilage. Furthermore, the glycogen content of the hypertrophic cartilage cells decreases as mineralization of the cartilage matrix proceeds. From these observations it is reasonable to deduce that the accumulation of glycogen and its utilization (through metabolic breakdown) are involved in the process of mineralization of cartilage matrix. Since the enzyme phosphorylase is partially responsible for the breakdown of glycogen to hexose phosphates, its activity assumes an important role in this scheme.

In addition, a good deal of information already exists in regard to other enzymes and intermediate compounds involved in the metabolism of glycogen in biological

10

systems. In one phase of the metabolism of glycogen (the glycolytic phase, or glycolytic cycle), a number of different organic phosphate esters are produced as glycogen is converted to lactic acid. Most of the enzymes and intermediate compounds involved in this process have been shown to be present in calcifying cartilage as well as in other tissues. At least one of these intermediates (glucose-1-phosphate) is readily hydrolyzed by alkaline phosphatase, producing glucose and phosphate ions. Cartilage therefore possesses a multienzyme system (probably identical with the glycolytic phase as found in other tissues) which is involved in the metabolism of glycogen, producing intermediate organic phosphate esters, some of which are acted on by alkaline phosphatase. Furthermore, it has been well established that certain steps of the glycolytic phase are reversible; that is, the synthesis of glycogen also occurs. Consequently, a mechanism is provided for the accumulation of glycogen in cartilage cells prior to the initiation of calcification of the cartilage matrix.

There is little doubt that the operation of this system (and the part which phosphatase plays in it) is somehow involved in mineralization. However, the emphasis has shifted away from the idea that the particular function of the alkaline phosphatase is to liberate, and thereby make available, additional phosphate ions through enzymatic hydrolysis of organic phosphate esters formed in the course of glycolysis. On the other hand, the belief is growing that the importance of alkaline phosphatase as well as the other enzymes of the glycolytic cycle relates instead to the elaboration or the organization of the macromolecular structure of the collagen and/or mucopolysaccharides of the organic matrix of bone and cartilage before the matrix is calcified. Indeed, it has been known for many years that alkaline phosphatase is concerned in some way with the biosynthesis of many fibrous proteins. In this respect, phosphatase is plentiful in cells engaged in protein synthesis (for example, in teeth, hair, bone marrow, and epithelial cells of the small intestine). In addition, vitamin C-deficient guinea pigs display significant decreases in cellular alkaline phosphatase, and at the same time display defective collagen formation. Finally, phosphatases have been found in close association with nucleic acids in cell nuclei and in the cytoplasm of cells, substantiating the idea that they have a role in protein synthesis. Therefore, the enzymes involved in the synthesis of the collagen and/or mucopolysaccharides help create macromolecules of specific structure. The ability of the collagen of the organic matrix to attract or bind calcium and/or phosphate ions seems to be related to the amino acid structure of tropocollagen and to the specific manner in which these macromolecules are oriented in the collagen fibrils (see Rich and Crick, Glimcher, and Neuman and Neuman).

In connection with the mineralization of the collagen, it is now believed that calcium and phosphate ions (and the other component ions of the unit cell of hydroxyapatite) are first bound to form primordial crystal nuclei of bone mineral. This process has been termed "nucleation," and the sites on the collagen fibrils where this occurs are known as "nucleation centers." These centers are composed of chemical groupings, or aggregates, bearing a strict, uniform, three-dimensional relationship to one another. In a sense, such centers may be compared to those groupings on the surfaces of enzymes which are responsible for the binding of specific substrates during enzyme action.

As has already been pointed out, when native collagen fibrils from decalcified bone are visualized by means of the electron microscope, one can observe, at intervals of 640 to 700 A, closely approximated double crossbands running at right angles to the long axis of the individual fibrils. These axial repeat bands represent a physical manifestation of the specific manner in which the reactive chemical groupings of the macromolecules are distributed along the long axis of the collagen fibrils. Therefore it seems reasonable to assume that the nucleation centers might be located in the region of the crossbands delineating the 640 to 700 A axial repeat pattern of the fibrils. Indeed, the examination of electron micrographs of reconstituted collagen fibrils which had been subjected to various degrees of *in vitro* calcification has demonstrated that the first crystals of mineral do appear in the axial repeat bands (see Fig. 30A and B).

There are some indications that the mucopolysaccharides of the ground substance may also be implicated in mineralization of the organic matrix. Indeed, some workers have maintained that this mineralization is determined by the presence of a collagen-mucopolysaccharide complex rather than by the collagen alone. However, this has not been proved. On the other hand, there is some evidence suggesting that certain of the mucopolysaccharides may actually inhibit mineralization of the collagen fibrils. This inhibition is believed to occur either by direct blocking of the nucleation centers of the collagen fibrils or by binding of the calcium ions to the mucopolysaccharides so that these ions are unavailable to the collagen nucleation sites. As already noted, certain chondroitin sulfates are found among the mucopolysaccharide constituents of the ground substance of bone. The sulfate groups of these chondroitin sulfates bear negative charges, and consequently are capable of strongly binding calcium ions. Changes in the staining characteristics of the mucopolysaccharides during mineralization of the organic matrix seem to indicate that depolymerization of mucopolysaccharides takes place during mineralization of the collagen. In other words, as the mucopolysaccharides are depolymerized (or broken down), their inhibitory action in mineralization is abolished.

Additional evidence relating to the possible implication of the mucopolysaccharides of the ground substance in mineralization has been furnished by the results of studies of the ground substance of normally nonmineralizing tissue. For example, experiments have been conducted which have demonstrated that, whereas native collagens of tissues such as rat tail tendon, pig skin, and calf skin did not mineralize *in vitro* even though the fibrils in question had an axial repeat period of 640 to 700 A, these fibrils were subsequently able to mineralize if the tissues were first treated by procedures designed to depolymerize or extract the mucopolysaccharides of the ground substance. Along similar lines, it has been observed that *in vitro* mineralization may occur in collagen fibrils which have been extracted away from normally nonmineralizing connective tissue and which have subsequently been reconstituted so that they have a 640 to 700 A axial repeat period. Thus, if inhibitory mechanisms attributable to specific mucopolysaccharides are operative under *in vivo* conditions, these mucopolysaccharides may constitute a "control" mechanism for the mineralization of the collagen of the newly formed matrix of bone and an inhibitory mechanism by which the collagen of normally nonmineralizing connective tissue is prevented from mineralizing at all.

In *summary*, our present knowledge of the sequence of events involved in the mineralization of newly formed organic matrix of bone may be outlined as follows: Phosphate ions, along with calcium ions, from the intercellular tissue fluid possibly are bound by reactive amino acid end groups at the nucleation sites of the collagen fibrils. In addition to these ions, other ions from the tissue fluid (hydroxyl ions, for instance) are bound at the same time, and the various ions are so oriented to one another in a specific spatial relationship that they form the unit cell structure for hydroxyapatite. The nucleus for the formation of hydroxyapatite is provided by a small number (possibly only three or four) of these unit cells, their formation being denoted as "nucleation."

After nucleation has once started, crystal growth proceeds upon the crystal nuclei, provided an adequate amount of calcium and phosphate ions is available from the tissue fluids that bathe the organic matrix. The growing crystals orient themselves with their long axis to the long axis of the fibrils. At a certain point, cessation of crystal growth occurs through the mediation of mechanisms which are still unknown. When the collagen fibrils are fully mineralized, they are found to be heavily impregnated with crystals of hydroxyapatite. The mechanism of nucleation as described is not the only one that can be formulated. For example, since the presence of pyrophosphoric acid ($H_4P_2O_7$), or pyrophosphate, has been demonstrated in bone, the question arises whether these ions are also bound by reactive free amino groups at the nucleation sites. Adenosine triphosphate (ATP) has been shown to accumulate in calcifying cartilage in the course of glycolysis. Since ATP contains an active pyrophosphate group in its molecule, it has been postulated that ATP is involved in a "transphosphorylation" reaction with the free amino groups resulting in a direct transfer of pyrophosphate onto the nucleation sites. The fixation of pyrophosphate may be followed by its combination with calcium, thus leading to nucleation and the formation of bone mineral. There are, however, conflicting views about the role of pyrophosphate in the process of mineralization. Indeed, some investigators claim that this substance in certain forms may actually induce an *inhibition* of collagen matrix mineralization. Pyrophosphate is also one of the products formed during the adenyl cyclase-mediated conversion of ATP to cyclic AMP (p. 116). In this connection, there is evidence implicating pyrophosphate as an inhibitor of parathyroid hormone-induced bone resorption, this phenomenon occurring because of the inhibition by pyrophosphate of the hormonally induced activation of adenyl cyclase. Lower cellular levels of cyclic AMP (a mediator of bone resorption) result.

CALCIUM AND PHOSPHORUS HOMEOSTASIS

The term "homeostasis" refers to the regulatory biological mechanisms by which the internal environment (or fluid matrix) of the body is maintained in a relatively steady state. The internal environment is represented by the blood and the various interstitial (intercellular) tissue fluids, including the gel-like tissue fluid permeating the ground substance of the osseous tissue.

In the homeostasis of calcium and phosphorus, one important factor is the constant adjustment of the calcium and phosphorus levels of the blood (through fecal and urinary excretion) in adaptation to the absorption into the blood stream of dietary and/or endogenous calcium and phosphorus from the gastrointestinal tract. Another essential mechanism is the continuous exchange of calcium and phosphorus between the mineral matter of the osseous tissue and the blood, mediated through the interstitial fluid permeating the ground substance of the osseous tissue. Furthermore, the maintenance of homeostasis involves not only the physiologic exchange of these minerals between the bone and its interstitial fluid, and in turn between the latter and the blood, but also the actual replenishment of the mineral stores of calcium and phosphorus by new deposition (especially in the bones), in compensation for any unusual and prolonged drain upon these stores. (See Fig. 28.) In the regulation of the homeostasis of calcium and phosphorus, parathyroid hormone, vitamin D, and calcitonin (thyrocalcitonin) play important roles.

It should be emphasized that over 98 per cent of the body's total store of calcium and 70 to 75 per cent of its total store of phosphorus are in the bones. In an adult male weighing 70 kilos, the skeleton contains about 1.1 kilos (approximately 2.4 pounds) of calcium and about 0.6 kilos (approximately 1.3 pounds) of phosphorus.

As noted, the mineral matter is present in the form of submicroscopic crystals of a complex salt of calcium and phosphate having the nature of an apatite. The mineral crystals lie on or within the collagen fibrils, and they are generally described as having the shape of hexagonal tablets. The small size and flat shape of the crystals give them a relatively large surface area. Since there are approximately 2.75

kilos of apatite crystals in the skeleton of an adult male weighing 70 kilos, it has been estimated that the total surface area of the bone crystals in such a person exceeds 100 acres (see Neuman and Neuman). One may estimate that, in a crystal which measures $500 \times 250 \times 100$ A, about 15 per cent of the constituent unit cells are oriented to the surface of the crystal. The ions which are adsorbed onto the surface of the crystal, those immediately below the surface, and those in solution in the hydration shell (the shell of fluid surrounding the crystal) constitute the labile and readily exchangeable ions. In regard to the labile ions, it is to be noted that since they participate freely in ion transfer they represent exchangeable or reactive ions. That is, these labile ions are involved in the maintenance of direct physico-chemical equilibrium between the bone mineral and its fluid environment. However, the ions which are structural constituents of the crystals themselves (that is, the ions which make up the unit cell lattice of the crystals of hydroxyapatite) are exchangeable at a much slower rate. Their exchange is mediated largely by parathyroid hormone, which may induce dissolution of apatite crystals directly and/or by stimulating the formation of osteoclasts. Calcitonin, by its antagonistic action to parathyroid hormone-induced resorption of bone mineral, also must be considered to play a significant role in the exchange of ions between the crystals of hydroxyapatite and the fluid environment. Thus the ion exchange which is involved in the maintenance of the direct physicochemical equilibrium of calcium and phosphorus is not to be confused with what occurs at sites of active osteoclastic resorption, in the course of which there is wholesale focal dissolution of bone crystals and also removal of the local organic matrix.

It is estimated that of the 1,100 g (more or less) of calcium in the skeleton of an adult, only about 5 g is readily exchangeable calcium (see G. Bauer *et al.*). It has also been calculated that, under physiologic conditions, all or practically all of the 0.28 g of calcium in the plasma of an adult is exchanged every minute with equal amounts of calcium in the intercellular fluid and in turn with corresponding amounts of labile calcium in the bones. The exchange of phosphate ion within and between the fluid compartments of the body and between the interstitial fluid and bone is also constantly taking place, and probably occurs at the same rapid rate as the exchange of calcium. Thus, in an adult in whom the absorption and excretion of calcium and phosphorus are in balance, there is a rapid and constant exchange in respect to these minerals between the mineral matter of bone and the fluid compartments of the body. As noted, this exchange occurs without participation of osteoclasts and hence without detectable histologic changes in the osseous tissue or in the levels of calcium and phosphorus in the plasma.

The transfer of ions between the bone mineral and the tissue fluid and blood is undoubtedly influenced by the bone cells (osteocytes) of the organic matrix. In particular, the osteocytes help to maintain the vitality (structural and metabolic integrity) of the organic matrix. They do this by facilitating, through their canalicular systems, the exchange of materials between the tissue fluids and the matrix. The tubules (canaliculi) issuing from the lacuna of each osteocyte are numerous and delicate and branch freely. These canaliculi contain processes which represent protoplasmic extensions from the bone cells. The canaliculi of the osteocytes extend between the collagen fibrils of the organic matrix and communicate with the canaliculi of neighboring lacunae. Through such anastomoses, a network of passages is established which permits the circulation of tissue fluid through the cement substance of the organic matrix in which the collagen fibrils (and the bone crystals oriented to them) are embedded. Variations in the composition of the tissue fluid permeating the cement substance influence the amount of calcium and phosphorus available from the mineral crystals to the fluid compartments of the body.

The Role of Parathyroid Hormone, Vitamin D, and Calcitonin (Thyrocalcitonin). —Biologically active extracts prepared from bovine parathyroid glands first became available about 1925 (see Collip). Such extracts (including original commercially available "parathormone") were, by present standards, impure preparations. The isolation of a homogeneous parathyroid hormone polypeptide from bovine parathyroid glands was first reported in 1961 (see Rasmussen and Craig). Parathyroid hormone preparations now available are considered to be absolutely pure.

Bovine parathyroid hormone is a single-chain polypeptide containing about 83 amino acid residues with a molecular weight of 8500. Recently, its amino acid sequence, as well as its structure, have been elucidated. It is of interest to note that if this polypeptide is subjected to mild acid hydrolysis, a smaller 20-amino acid polypeptide which still possesses significant parathyroid hormone activity can be isolated from the hydrolysate. The pure bovine hormone has both bone mineral mobilizing activity and renal phosphaturic activity. Therefore there is now no support for the view that the parathyroid glands secrete separate parathyroid hormones—one of which has exclusively bone mineral mobilizing activity, the other possessing exclusively phosphaturic activity. In addition, the pure hormone has been shown to be devoid of any hemodynamic action on the kidney (that is, the phosphaturic effect of the hormone is not due to any effect upon the rate of renal glomerular filtration of phosphate ion). A pure parathyroid hormone polypeptide has also been isolated from porcine glands (molecular weight 9600–11000) and from human parathyroid adenomas (molecular weight about 8500). The amino acid sequence and other chemical properties of the pure bovine hormone have been elucidated, and a model for its structure has been proposed (see Hawker *et al.*, Potts *et al.*, and also Arnaud *et al.*).

Vitamin D, on the other hand, is a nonprotein substance of relatively low molecular weight. By virtue of its chemical structure and properties, it is related to certain naturally occurring sterol precursors (provitamins) which in themselves have no vitamin D activity. For example, upon being irradiated with ultraviolet light (especially radiation at wave lengths of 290–320 nm), ergosterol (a sterol present in yeast) and 7-dehydrocholesterol (a sterol present in, and synthesized by, many tissues of man) are converted to vitamin D_2 (ergocalciferol) and vitamin D_3 (cholecalciferol), respectively. Of the 10 or so different compounds (having structures similar to that of vitamin D_2 and D_3) with antirachitic activity, vitamins D_2 and D_3 are the most important. Vitamins D_2 and D_3, while differing in certain aspects of their chemical structures, nevertheless both possess high antirachitic potency *in vivo*. In nature, the human organism secures vitamin D either by absorbing it from foods which contain it (oily fish, oysters, cod liver oil, etc.), or by synthesizing it within the body in consequence of exposure of the skin to the ultraviolet rays of the sun. In regard to the *in vivo* synthesis of vitamin D, the ultraviolet rays of the sun either: (1) activate the provitamins (for example, 7-dehydrocholesterol) contained in the skin and notably in the sebaceous glands, or (2) penetrate the capillaries beneath the epidermis and activate the provitamins in the blood. Ingested vitamin D (which occurs in nature in an esterified form) requires bile in order to be absorbed from the gastrointestinal tract. After absorption, vitamin D is apparently transported in the blood plasma bound to an alpha-2 globulin. Cholecalciferol (vitamin D_3) as such is apparently not the biologically active form; recent investigations have indicated that the biologically active form is a more polar compound (a compound more soluble in aqueous systems) identified as 25-hydroxycholecalciferol (see Blunt *et al.*). This active metabolite, sometimes called the "circulating" or "hormonal" form of vitamin D_3, can be synthesized in the liver by means of the enzymatic hydroxylation of vitamin D_3 (see Ponchon and DeLuca, and also Ponchon *et al.*). 25-Hydroxycholecalciferol is more active than vitamin D_3 in curing rickets in rats. In vitamin D-deficient rats, 25-hydroxycholecalciferol is also more active than vitamin D_3 in inducing bone resorption and in increasing the transport of calcium across the intestinal mucosa. It is of interest that subjects with familial vitamin D-resistant rickets (that is, where no renal disease and no dietary vitamin D insufficiency can be demonstrated) who have been found to lack the ability to enzymatically convert cholecalciferol to 25-hydroxycholecalciferol respond satisfactorily to treatment with this more active form of vitamin D_3.

More recent evidence indicates that 25-hydroxycholecalciferol may be converted in tissues to at least 2 more metabolites which are more polar than the parent compound. This conversion can take place in bone, intestinal mucosa, kidney, and liver (see Cousins *et al.*). Furthermore, the still-partially characterized more polar metabolites of 25-hydroxycholecalciferol represent forms (possibly target tissue forms) which may be tissue-generated regulatory metabolites of vitamin D_3 (p. 143).

The structures of vitamin D_3 and 25-hydroxycholecalciferol, as well as the *in vivo* metabolic events leading to the synthesis of the active metabolites of this vitamin, may be depicted as follows:

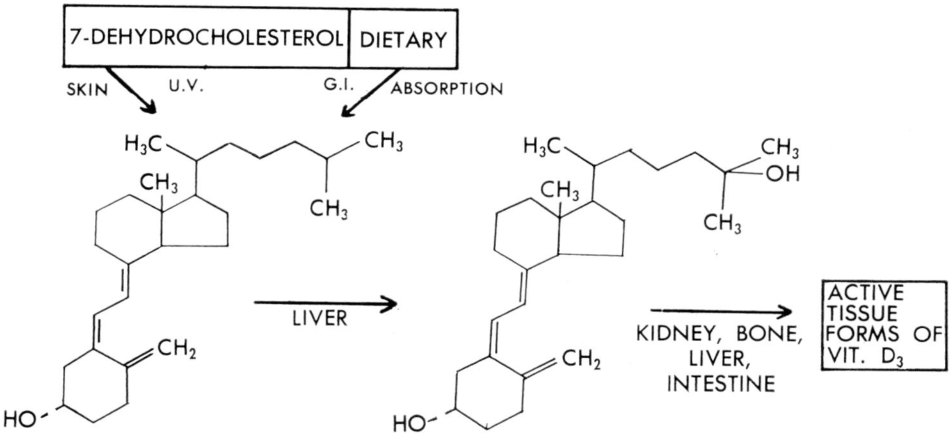

| 7-DEHYDROCHOLESTEROL | DIETARY |

SKIN   U.V.   G.I.   ABSORPTION

LIVER →   KIDNEY, BONE, LIVER, INTESTINE → ACTIVE TISSUE FORMS OF VIT. D_3

CHOLECALCIFEROL (VITAMIN D_3)   25-HYDROXYCHOLECALCIFEROL (ACTIVE CIRCULATING FORM OF VIT. D_3)

The structures of these compounds as shown in the diagram differ from those which are presented in many textbooks, since it is now known that they are closer to the actual configurations of these vitamins (see Orten and Neuhaus).

The discovery of a second peptide hormone involved in calcium and phosphorus metabolism has contributed greatly to our understanding of the nature of the homeostatic control of calcium and phosphorus. *Calcitonin* (thyrocalcitonin) is essentially a hypocalcemic hormone, although it also causes hypophosphatemia (lowers serum inorganic phosphorus), and at high doses has been reported to cause phosphaturia. In its hypocalcemic effects, calcitonin can be said to have an action which is antagonistic to that of parathyroid hormone.

The action of calcitonin is not related to any competitive inhibition of the activity of parathyroid hormone molecules, but is related to its direct effect upon bone mineral. It has now been established that calcitonin exerts an inhibitory action upon bone resorption. (For further details, see p. 144.)

Suggestive evidence for the existence of calcitonin was first reported in 1961 by Munson. The calcitonin concept, however, was fully developed in that same year by Copp and his co-workers, and was based mainly upon observations of the fall in levels of serum calcium in dogs during the perfusion of their thyroid and parathyroid glands with hypercalcemic blood. A hypercalcemic stimulus applied directly to the thyroid-parathyroid complex by way of the thyroid artery produced a sharp drop in serum calcium level. This effect could also be demonstrated, but to a lesser extent, in parathyroidectomized animals, indicating that the drop in serum calcium was not due to an inhibition of secretion of parathyroid hormone. Furthermore, when the perfusate collected from the thyroid vein was injected intravenously into recipient intact dogs, a similar fall in serum calcium was observed. The amounts injected were, of course, too small to produce a hypercalcemia in the recipient dogs, and therefore no inhibition of parathyroid hormone secretion could be involved. (See Copp *et al.*, and Munson *et al.*)

None of these early experiments using the dog could distinguish between the thyroid and the parathyroid glands as the source of calcitonin because of their close anatomical relationship and common blood supply. In fact, at that time it was believed that the parathyroid glands secreted a hypercalcemic hormone (parathyroid hormone) as well as a hypocalcemic hormone (calcitonin). However, further work proved that it was indeed the thyroid gland that secreted calcitonin. Some of the substantiating facts were: (1) the discovery of hypocalcemic activity in mammalian thyroid extracts; (2) rats with intact thyroid glands were much better protected against hypercalcemia than were thyroidectomized animals (due to the presence of the hypocalcemic hormone in thyroid tissue); (3) perfusion experiments using goats and pigs, in which there is an anatomical separation of the thyroids and parathyroids (including separation of blood supply), led to decisive evidence that it was the thyroid gland only that produced calcitonin in response to the hypercalcemic perfusion of the thyroids separately.

Calcitonin is produced by the inter- or parafollicular cells of the thyroid gland (sometimes called the "light" cells or "C" cells). It should be noted that the ultimobranchial body in chickens and dogfish contains hypocalcemic activity at concentrations greater than that found in rat thyroid glands. While the ultimobranchial cells are quite different histologically from the calcitonin-producing cells of the thyroid, there is evidence that the two cell types have the same embryological origin. In mammals, the ultimobranchial tissue invades the thyroid gland during embryological development, while in lower vertebrates (fish, birds, reptiles, etc.), the ultimobranchial bodies remain as distinct entities. Calcitonin has been found in all mammalian thyroids studied, including those of man.

Calcitonin has been isolated in pure form from porcine thyroid glands. It appears to be a single-chain polypeptide consisting of 32 amino acid residues with a molecular weight of about 3600. Its amino acid sequence and its structure have been elucidated, and its chemical synthesis has been reported. Isolation of human thyrocalcitonin has also been accomplished, but its amino acid composition differs considerably from that of the porcine hormone. Porcine calcitonin, when administered to man in low doses, is capable of lowering serum calcium levels.

So closely interrelated are the functions of parathyroid hormone and vitamin D that they may be regarded as components of an integrated synergistic system in the homeostasis of calcium and phosphorus. The role of calcitonin, in contrast, may be considered the "control" hormone that antagonizes the action of parathyroid hormone and vitamin D on bone.

Both parathyroid hormone and vitamin D are involved in the regulation of: (1) the absorption of calcium and phosphorus from the gastrointestinal tract; (2) the urinary excretion of calcium and phosphate ions; and (3) the exchange of calcium and phosphate ions between bone mineral and the extracellular fluids. While the underlying mechanisms by which parathyroid hormone and vitamin D exert their physiological action at these three sites are not fully understood, much progress has been made in recent years in elucidating their action at cellular and subcellular levels. It is known that the administration of parathyroid hormone and/or vitamin D tends to raise the citrate content of bone, blood plasma, and other body fluids. Since normally the citrate content of bone is about 0.86 per cent by weight, a major portion of the citrate found in body fluids originates in the skeleton. Moreover, these substances may enhance the concentration of citrate in the body fluids by mobilization of bone citrate during the process of mineral resorption. However, the absolute increase that is observed in the citrate content in bone and other tissues after the administration of this hormone or vitamin seems to indicate that a direct cellular mechanism exists.

Parathyroid hormone and vitamin D may enhance the citrate content of tissues (and consequently body fluids) by their ability to initiate a more rapid conversion of pyruvate to citrate in the tricarboxylic acid cycle (Krebs cycle, or citric acid cycle). In contrast, there is evidence to suggest that tissue citrate might accumulate because of the inhibitory action of these substances on certain sequential enzyme systems which operate in the tricarboxylic acid cycle beyond the formation of citrate (for example, isocitric dehydrogenase), or that parathyroid hormone or vitamin D may limit the availability of certain coenzymes (for example, nicotinamide adenine dinucleotide phosphate) necessary for the activation of the enzymes involved in the metabolism of citrate. In consequence, an increase in the amount of citrate tends to occur in the lumen of the gastrointestinal tract, and on this account the absorption of calcium (and secondarily of phosphate) may be increased. This increase might be mediated by the ability of citrate to bind calcium ion as a soluble, but unionized, complex and thus bring poorly soluble calcium phosphate into solution. The formation of calcium citrate may provide a vehicle for the transport of calcium across the intestinal mucosa and thereby enhance its absorption. Evidence of the role of citrate may be deduced from: the ameliorating effects of orally administered sodium citrate on experimentally induced rickets in rats; the reduced concentration of citric acid in the bones of rachitic rats as compared with normal controls; and the observation that rachitic children show reduced levels of plasma citrate, the levels rising in the course of treatment with vitamin D (see Talmage and Elliott, Harrison and Harrison, and Rasmussen). As noted, both parathyroid hormone and vitamin D are capable of inducing an increase in bone citrate, which could conceivably bring insoluble bone mineral into solution.

It is now apparent that the effects of parathyroid hormone and vitamin D upon tissue citrate levels is one manifestation of their fundamental action at both a cellular and a subcellular level. Parathyroid hormone, at times working synergistically with vitamin D, may have a profound action on every cell in the body, probably involving the cell membrane, certain subcellular structures (for example, mitochondria), and possibly the cell nucleus itself.

There is a large body of literature covering the biochemical observations that have been made concerning the cellular and subcellular effects of parathyroid hormone and vitamin D.* Attempts have been made to correlate all of these data, so that a unified concept might be formulated to explain the action of these substances on all cells of the body, including those of the gastrointestinal mucosa, bone, and kidney tubules. One such concept of parathyroid hormone action explained all the aspects in terms of its ability to enhance the transport of phosphate ions into various tissue cells. Membrane transport of phosphate was considered to be a primary action of the hormone, while calcium transport was secondary, being cou-

---

* See *The Parathyroid Glands: Ultrastructure, Secretion, and Function*, edited by P. J. Gaillard, R. V. Talmage, and A. M. Budy, Chicago, The University of Chicago Press, 1965; *Parathyroid Hormone and Thyrocalcitonin (Calcitonin)*, edited by R. V. Talmage and L. F. Bélanger, New York, Excerpta Medica Foundation, 1968; and the F. Raymond Keating, Jr., Memorial Symposium—Hyperparathyroidism, 1970, in Am. J. Med., *50*, 557, 1971.

pled to the transport of phosphate (see Neuman). In this respect it had also been demonstrated that calcium could be taken up by isolated mitochondria mainly as a phosphate salt and deposited as an amorphous precipitate (not hydroxyapatite) in granules in these structures. This translocation was believed to be driven by energy derived from *oxidative phosphorylation** in the mitochondria themselves, stimulated in some way by parathyroid hormone (a subcellular effect). Subsequent observations, however, led to the conclusion that, at a cellular and subcellular level, parathyroid hormone stimulated two distinct metabolic processes—one for phosphate ion transport and the other for calcium ion transport. In summary: (1) The uptake of calcium by mitochondria was not stimulated by parathyroid hormone and/or vitamin D, but was dependent upon an energy source such as ATP (produced during oxidative phosphorylation) and magnesium ions. (2) Both parathyroid hormone and vitamin D stimulated the release (efflux) of calcium phosphate from mitochondria. However, when vitamin D alone was added to mitochondria isolated from the tissues of parathyroidectomized vitamin D-deficient rats, a stimulation of the release of calcium was observed; added parathyroid hormone acted synergistically with vitamin D. The hormone alone also stimulated the release of calcium from mitochondria, but only if the mitochondria had been isolated from rats receiving vitamin D. In the absence of vitamin D, parathyroid hormone had no effect, even at high concentrations. Obviously, the presence of vitamin D was required for the action of parathyroid hormone. (3) Unlike the calcium-release system noted above, which is absolutely vitamin D-dependent, the uptake (influx) of phosphate ions into mitochondria was shown to be completely independent of vitamin D, because parathyroid hormone acted independently (but requiring magnesium ions) to stimulate phosphate ion influx. There was also evidence that parathyroid hormone interacted in some manner with the chain of oxidative phosphorylation (see DeLuca and Sallis). These findings reaffirm the fact that, in many aspects of their action at cellular and subcellular levels, parathyroid hormone and vitamin D may be regarded as component parts of an integrated system. Moreover, there seems to be a distinct parallelism between the effects observed at a subcellular level and those observed on the animal organism itself.

Thus parathyroid hormone, by virtue of its highly specific effect on cellular and subcellular metabolism, exerts a profound influence upon the transport of calcium, magnesium, and phosphate ions across cell and mitochondrial membranes, seeming to modify membrane permeability. The exact way in which the hormone stimulates a series of metabolic events within the cell, itself being unable to enter the cell, can be rationalized in terms of our present knowledge. Parathyroid hormone acts at the cell membrane to stimulate adenyl cyclase within the cell, resulting in increased amounts of cyclic AMP (p. 116). Cyclic AMP in turn may induce and/or regulate cellular and subcellular metabolism so that modifications in cell membrane permeability, among other changes, occur. Vitamin D is also involved in this

---

* Oxidative phosphorylation takes place in nearly all aerobic cells—in nucleated cells the enzymes catalyzing the reactions involved in this process being located in the inner membrane of the mitochondria. Pairs of hydrogen atoms (or their equivalent electrons), derived from the oxidation of intermediate compounds of the tricarboxylic acid cycle, flow down a multimembered chain of electron-carrier enzymes of successively lower energy level until they reduce molecular oxygen to form water. During this process, about 40 per cent of the total free energy released is conserved in the form of the phosphate-bond energy of adenosine triphosphate (ATP) molecules which are synthesized by phosphorylation of adenosine diphosphate (ADP). The formation of ATP, coupled with the electron-carrier chain (actually a complex series of oxidation-reduction systems), is the process designated as oxidative phosphorylation. It represents an aerobic mechanism by which cells conserve part of the energy released during cellular metabolism. (For greater detail, see Lehninger.)

transport system and acts synergistically with parathyroid hormone. In addition, vitamin D seems to be an absolute requirement for the proper functioning of this integrated system in calcium ion transport.

In recent years, investigation of the metabolism of vitamin D and its role in calcium ion transport has led to a clarification of the mechanism of its action at a cellular and subcellular level. Vitamin D (specifically, 25-hydroxycholecalciferol) induces the synthesis of a calcium-binding protein in the cells of the intestinal mucosa. For example, the administration of vitamin D_3 to rachitic chicks leads to an increased formation of a calcium-binding factor which can be isolated from the intestinal mucosa and identified as a specific protein. The enhanced gastrointestinal absorption of calcium observed in the rachitic chicks after treatment with vitamin D_3 occurs simultaneously with the appearance of the calcium-binding protein (see Wasserman and Taylor). In addition, rachitic rats show a decreased amount of calcium-binding protein, particularly in the duodenal tissue of the intestinal mucosa (where most of the calcium is absorbed). Treatment of these rats with vitamin D_2 or D_3 results in a significant rise in the content of calcium-binding protein in this tissue (see Kallfelz et al.).

The exact mechanism by which vitamin D induces the synthesis of the calcium-binding protein has not yet been fully elucidated, but there are suggestions that it may act at sites in the cell nucleus itself. Much of the evidence supporting this concept has been obtained by observing the effects of actinomycin D on the action of vitamin D. Actinomycin D is an antibiotic which is frequently used in the study of the basic mechanisms of protein synthesis within the cell. This substance has been shown to block the cytoplasmic synthesis of proteins by interfering with the synthesis of mRNA (messenger ribonucleic acid) in the cell nucleus. The synthesis of specific mRNA molecules is directed and controlled by genetic DNA (deoxyribonucleic acid). Thus, mRNA, carrying the specific "transcribed" genetic message from DNA in respect to protein synthesis, in turn "translates" the genetic message and thus directs the synthesis of specific proteins in the cell. The injection of actinomycin D into rats completely prevents both the rise in serum calcium and the increase in calcium transport in the small intestine by suppressing the actions of vitamin D. From this evidence it may be concluded that the action of vitamin D, in inducing the synthesis of a specific calcium-binding protein, could be on the genetic apparatus of the cell, since actinomycin D prevents the synthesis of cellular proteins and at the same time prevents the full expression of vitamin D action. Vitamin D, when administered to vitamin D-deficient or rachitic rats, also stimulates the incorporation of tritium-labeled orotic acid into the nuclear RNA of intestinal mucosa. Since orotic acid is a metabolic precursor of certain pyrimidine bases of cellular nucleic acids, vitamin D can be said to have stimulated the metabolism of nuclear RNA. Thus, vitamin D influences DNA-directed RNA synthesis in the cell nucleus, possibly by increasing the rate of synthesis of the messenger RNA responsible for the elaboration of the specific calcium-binding protein.

In order to exert its biological effect of inducing the synthesis of a calcium-binding protein in the cells of the intestinal mucosa, vitamin D_3 must be enzymatically converted in the liver to 25-hydroxycholecalciferol, its metabolically active form. The more polar metabolites of 25-hydroxycholecalciferol produced in bone, intestinal mucosa, and kidney may represent the true biologically active compounds in these target tissues themselves. (p. 139.) One of these polar metabolites has been isolated from the blood plasma of hogs and has been identified as 21,25-dihydroxycholecalciferol. This compound has been found to have biological action in the mobilization of bone mineral, while having only a slight effect on intestinal calcium absorption. Furthermore, it has recently been established that another metabolite, identified as 1,25-dihydroxycholecalciferol, is produced in the kidneys of rachitic chicks, and is, in fact, considerably more active than vitamin D_3 in the stimulation of intestinal calcium transport.

In summary, the major function of vitamin D_3 or its active metabolite is the induction of the biosynthesis of a calcium-binding protein essential to the transport of calcium across the intestinal mucosa. This action is *independent* of the action of parathyroid hormone at this site. Vitamin D_3—more specifically, 25-hydroxy-cholecalciferol (or certain of its tissue metabolites)—also increases bone resorption, producing a rise in serum calcium. The mechanism involved is still uncertain, but may entail a stimulation of a calcium-binding factor affecting the calcium transport system, analogous to that occurring in the intestinal mucosa. Some of the actions of parathyroid hormone, its effect on the resorption of bone mineral, and probably its effect on the intestinal absorption or transport of calcium are not fully expressed in vitamin D-deficient animals. Therefore, parathyroid hormone appears to be dependent on vitamin D for its action on bone and the intestinal mucosa. As to the kidney, vitamin D probably has an action on the renal transport of calcium. This may be deduced from the fact that 25-hydroxycholecalciferol is metabolized to more polar metabolites in this organ. Thus, since the conversion of 25-hydroxy-cholecalciferol also occurs in the two known primary targets of vitamin D (bone and intestine), the kidney might also be a primary target organ. Concerning the renal excretion of phosphate ion, the situation is quite different. Apparently, para-thyroid hormone or its second messenger, cyclic AMP, can exert its phosphaturic action on the kidney without requiring vitamin D. Therefore, parathyroid hormone and vitamin D act synergistically in the stimulation of bone resorption and in the enhancement of calcium absorption in the intestine. However, the roles played by each are quite different: Parathyroid hormone may be considered to alter cell membrane permeability to calcium, while vitamin D may be involved in an intracellular transport system for calcium by virtue of its ability to induce the synthesis of a calcium-binding protein. The manner in which the two substances induce these intracellular events is again quite different: Parathyroid hormone acts at cell membranes through the mediation of cyclic AMP, while vitamin D (specifically, its active tissue metabolites) acts directly within the cell to influence protein synthesis, and probably is not involved with cyclic AMP action. The role of citrate, if any, as a mediator of calcium ion transport is now vague. However, this substance may still function in some capacity as a vital component of the cell membrane transport system or as an extracellular transport agent for calcium ion—for example, from bone to extracellular fluid. As to the process of bone resorption, emphasis has shifted toward a consideration of citrate (as citric acid) as one of many acidic sub-stances (including lactic, succinic, and carbonic acids) produced during parathyroid hormone-regulated cellular metabolism in bone. Many believe that these acids may be important in the solubilizing of bone mineral (p. 148).

The mode of action of parathyroid hormone and vitamin D has already been discussed. Regarding the primary action of calcitonin (thyrocalcitonin) on bone, evidence to date indicates that it inhibits all phases of bone resorption. The manifestation of its action on the animal organism is a lowering of the serum cal-cium and inorganic phosphorus. Calcitonin lowers the serum calcium levels in normal and in hypercalcemic subjects, being most marked when bone resorption is previously stimulated by parathyroid hormone, vitamin D, or vitamin A. In its inhibitory action on bone resorption, and consequently its production of a hypo-calcemia, calcitonin has an effect which is opposite to that of parathyroid hormone and vitamin D. However, both calcitonin and parathyroid hormone produce a hypophosphatemia as well as a phosphaturia. Calcitonin produces its hypophos-phatemic effect by inhibiting the release of calcium phosphate from bone mineral; parathyroid hormone stimulates resorption and consequently produces a hypercalcemia which manifests itself in an increase in the plasma calcium ion concentration and a decrease in the phosphate ion concentration, in accordance with solubility product requirements. The phosphaturic action of both parathyroid hormone and calcitonin on the kidney undoubtedly plays a part in their induction of hypophosphatemia. The mechanisms by which parathyroid hormone acts on the kidney to induce phosphaturia are well known; in contrast, the manner in which calcitonin exerts its effect on the kidney to induce phosphaturic action is not clear. Calcitonin exerts its hypocalcemic and hypophosphatemic effects in parathyroidectomized animals. Therefore its action cannot be related to any inhibition of parathyroid hormone secretion or inactivation of the hormone. Moreover, the results following the administration of both calcitonin and parathyroid hormone (separately or in combination) to parathyroidectomized rats indicate that competitive inhibition of parathyroid hormone molecules by calcitonin is also not a factor.

Calcitonin is effective in lowering the serum calcium when administered to rats which have been either nephrectomized or have had their gastrointestinal tracts excised. Thus the kidney and gastrointestinal tract, both of major importance in calcium metabolism in the animal organism, are not important factors in the action of calcitonin. Evidence that the sole action of calcitonin is its suppression of bone resorption was first obtained from in vivo kinetic studies, and confirmed by in vitro bone culture investigations employing purified preparations from humans and from animals. It has also been reported that human calcitonin caused a lowering of the serum inorganic phosphorus and magnesium when administered to the rat.

An important action of parathyroid hormone and calcitonin on the animal organism is related to the urinary excretion of hydroxyproline. This amino acid is a constituent of the collagen of bone and other connective tissues (p. 118). All animals excrete a small amount of hydroxyproline in the urine. For example, on a collagen (gelatin)-free diet, a normal human adult excretes about 50 mg. of low molecular weight hydroxyproline peptides daily. Most of the hydroxyproline excreted is thus in a bound form, with very little present as free. The hydroxyproline normally excreted in the urine is considered to be derived from the metabolic breakdown of mature collagen in the body. Thus, when there is an active synthesis and breakdown of collagen in the body (as during growth), the urinary excretion of hydroxyproline will increase. An increase in urinary hydroxyproline is also observed in many diseases of bone in which there is either an increase in the metabolic turnover of bone matrix collagen (as in Paget's disease) or an increase in bone matrix collagen breakdown (as in hyperparathyroidism). Parathyroid hormone, stimulating bone collagen breakdown, will result in an increase in urinary hydroxyproline, while calcitonin, inhibiting bone resorption and bone collagen breakdown, will result in a decrease in urinary hydroxyproline. Calcitonin also prevents parathyroid hormone-induced hydroxyprolinuria.

Very little is known about the actions of calcitonin at cellular and subcellular levels. It has been reported that this hormone causes a decreased release of citrate into the tissue culture medium of a system employing embryonic mouse calvaria (an effect on citrate opposite to that observed with parathyroid hormone and vitamin D). Calcitonin, when administered to vitamin D-deficient rats, still causes a hypocalcemia and a hypophosphatemia. Thus it can be said that its physiologic action, unlike that of parathyroid hormone, is independent of vitamin D. Recent evidence suggests that calcitonin, like parathyroid hormone, may act at the membrane of bone cells to activate adenyl cyclase and thus stimulate the intracellular synthesis of cyclic AMP. Cyclic AMP acting as a second messenger could initiate a series of intracellular events, resulting in an inhibition of bone resorption. Since the actions of calcitonin are antagonistic to those of parathyroid hormone at a cellular level, both hormones acting independently of one another, it can be deduced that the recognition or receptor sites at the cell membrane are distinct and different. Other findings have implicated cyclic AMP as a stimulator of calcitonin secretion under *in vivo* conditions. Accordingly, the activation of an adenyl cyclase system in the "C" cells of the thyroids may result in an increase in cyclic AMP, which then may act to enhance calcitonin secretion.

Parathyroid hormone, vitamin D, and thyrocalcitonin have a profound effect upon cellular metabolism of such a nature that they markedly influence the exchange, transport, and cellular and intracellular accumulation of calcium and phosphate ions. Therefore the maintenance of *extracellular homeostasis* of calcium and phosphorus is in a sense a reflection of the effects of parathyroid hormone, vitamin D, and thyrocalcitonin (in its action on bone resorption) in the regulation of *cellular homeostasis* in respect to these minerals. (See Rasmussen.) At an organ or tissue level, extracellular calcium homeostasis is regulated by: (1) the excretion of calcium by the kidney, controlled principally by parathyroid hormone (possibly functioning synergistically with vitamin D); (2) the absorption of calcium from the gastrointestinal tract, controlled by vitamin D and parathyroid hormone; and (3) the exchange of calcium between bone mineral and the extracellular fluids, controlled primarily by parathyroid hormone (functioning synergistically with vitamin D) and secondarily by thyrocalcitonin.

As already stated, of the total amount of calcium ion which is filtered through the renal glomeruli daily in a normal adult, about 99 per cent is reabsorbed by the epithelium of the proximal renal tubules, the remainder being excreted in the urine. The reabsorption of this calcium appears to be under the control of the parathyroid hormone, through its action on the renal tubular epithelium. That is, the parathyroid hormone, through its effect on the kidneys, tends to conserve calcium by returning practically all of it from the glomerular filtrate to the blood.

However, in the hyperparathyroid state (clinical hyperparathyroidism or that following the administration of adequate amounts of parathyroid hormone), the daily urinary excretion of calcium tends to rise sharply above the normal level. In addition, it is well known that in the hyperparathyroid state the concentration of calcium in the plasma is increased, the increase relating primarily to the calcium ion fraction. This increased concentration of calcium in the plasma represents, in the main, calcium which has been mobilized from the bone through the mediation of the parathyroid hormone. As a result of the increased concentration of calcium ions in the plasma, the amount of calcium ion present in the glomerular filtrate is increased.

It is true that in the hyperparathyroid state the total tubular reabsorption of calcium ion from the glomerular filtrate is increased. Nevertheless, the capacity of the tubular epithelium to reabsorb the additional calcium is not great enough to prevent an increase in the urinary excretion of calcium. On the other hand, decreases in plasma levels of calcium which occur in the hypoparathyroid state result in a decrease in the urinary excretion of calcium. This is due largely to a decrease in the amount of calcium ion which is filtered through the renal glomeruli. Thus the urinary excretion of calcium is reduced in the hypoparathyroid state, despite the fact that the tubular reabsorption of calcium is probably also decreased. The role played by parathyroid hormone and vitamin D in the intestinal absorption of calcium has already been discussed. Vitamin D, when administered in high (non-physiologic) doses, has the ability by itself to mobilize calcium from bones by increasing bone resorption. The increases in plasma levels of calcium ion thus produced by vitamin D alone may in turn result in an increase in calcium excretion by the kidney.

In regard to the effect of parathyroid hormone on the bones, it has long been recognized that, in an animal receiving this hormone, histologic examination of the bones will show the presence of numerous osteoclasts, associated with evidences of lively osteoclastic resorption (see Jaffe and Bodansky, Bodansky *et al.*, and Jaffe *et al.*). Analogous histologic changes in the bones are produced by the administration of very large doses of vitamin D (see Soeur).

Opinions still differ as to whether the osteoclasts are derived through fusion of osteoblasts, osteocytes, or macrophages. In this connection it is contended, for instance, that the administration of parathyroid hormone modifies the tricarboxylic acid cycle in osteoblasts (in such a way that citric acid tends to accumulate in them) and concomitantly promotes the conversion of such osteoblasts into osteoclasts (see Walker). We now know that the ability of parathyroid hormone to increase the conversion of osteoblasts into osteoclasts is a result not only of its action on the tricarboxylic acid cycle, but also of its action on a host of metabolic events within these cells. The formation of osteoclasts as a result of parathyroid hormone administration is presently considered to be a direct action of this substance on the cellular metabolism of osteoblasts and osteocytes, so that an increased conversion of these cells to osteoclasts occurs. It is of interest that, in contrast, thyrocalcitonin apparently has a cellular action which results in the stimulation of osteoblast formation and a decrease in osteoclasts. These changes have been interpreted by some as evidence that this hormone may be capable of stimulating bone formation in addition to its primary action (that is, its inhibition of bone resorption or calcium release from bones). Perhaps the most profound action of parathyroid hormone on osteoblasts is its effect on RNA synthesis. Following a single injection of parathyroid extract in young rabbits, there is observed a *stimulation* of RNA synthesis in osteoclasts and an *inhibition* of RNA synthesis in osteoblasts. Since RNA is so intimately involved in cellular protein synthesis, these findings can be interpreted as meaning that protein synthesis in osteoclasts is stimulated secondarily to the stimulation of RNA synthesis, while the reverse is true in the osteoblasts (that is, inhibition of RNA synthesis in turn results in a depressed protein synthesis). In support of this contention, it has been reported that parathyroid hormone does indeed suppress the synthesis of collagen by osteoblasts.

Irrespective of their mode of derivation, it seems clear that the functioning of osteoclasts as bone resorbers is associated with secretory activity on the part of these cells. The specific nature of the secretions elaborated by the osteoclasts and the manner in which osteoclastic resorption is effected have still not been fully clarified. However, it has been suggested: (1) that osteoclasts secrete acidic substances (p. 144) which have the ability to dissolve bone mineral, or substances (citrate) which have the ability to complex calcium and which are therefore capable of mobilizing calcium from the bone salt; (2) that the osteoclasts secrete enzymes (for example, collagenases and/or hyaluronidases) which are capable of depolymerizing the collagen and/or the mucopolysaccharides of the organic matrix of bone, bone mineral being released in consequence of this depolymerization; and (3) that the osteoclasts are capable of secreting complexing substances, acids, and depolymerizing enzymes. Thus, there are various conceptions of the processes by which the bone mineral is dissolved or liberated and the organic matrix altered at sites of osteoclastic resorption.

However, it is now generally accepted that the formation of resorption defects (Howship's lacunae) at these sites is necessarily preceded by focal demineralization and/or focal alteration of the organic matrix of the osseous tissue where osteoclastic resorption is taking place. The current concept of bone resorption by osteoclasts thus presents a complete contrast to the old concept, whose notable protagonist was Pommer. His interpretation had been that, at sites of osteoclastic resorption, the osteoclasts removed the mineralized organic matrix as a unit, the osseous tissue in process of resorption not having undergone any preliminary alterations. The present writer's own histologic findings relating to bone resorption (in various pathologic skeletal conditions) had led him long ago to reject the Pommer concept and to suggest mechanisms of resorption more in line with the current interpretation (see Jaffe). In confirmation of these interpretations, recent studies have demonstrated that bone cells (identified as osteoclasts) contain a group of hydrolytic enzymes which act optimally at an acid pH (pH 4.0–5.0). These *acid hydrolases* have been shown to be associated with cytoplasmic particles identified as lysosomes. The functions of these lysosomal acid hydrolases are probably related to their ability to degrade the organic matrix of bone during the process of bone resorption. Among the enzymes identified as components of the acid hydrolases are those degrading mucopolysaccharides and their derivatives (hyaluronidase, beta-glucuronidase, acetylglucosaminidase, and beta-galactosidase); acid phosphatases (acid phenylphosphatase and acid beta-glycerophosphatase); proteolytic enzymes (cathepsin); and enzymes degrading nucleic acids (deoxyribonuclease and ribonuclease). In addition, lysosomes may also contain a protease which is able to degrade native collagen. The enzymes (acid hydrolases) are normally contained within a restricting lysosomal membrane (that is, they are within the lysosomes themselves), so that in this condition they are not available to attack the substrates of the bone matrix. However, when parathyroid extract (or pure parathyroid hormone) is added to an *in vitro* bone culture of mouse embryo calvaria, resorption lacunae develop in the tissue, and at their edges numerous osteoclasts can be visualized. The development of the resorption cavity is accompanied by a release into the culture medium of several lysosomal acid hydrolases. Another important observation is that, with the release of the enzymes during resorption, one can also demonstrate a release into the culture fluid of organic acids (lactic and citric) as well as calcium (as ^{45}Ca) and phosphate ions. (See Vaes.)

From these and other observations, it is possible to formulate a working hypothesis for parathyroid hormone-stimulated bone resorption in which the lysosomal enzymes are the agents that actually resorb the organic matrix of bone by virtue of their ability to degrade the constituents of this matrix. The sequence of events may be visualized as follows: (1) Parathyroid hormone stimulates the formation of osteoclasts and also stimulates the intracellular metabolism (probably glycolysis) of the osteoclasts, so that an increased synthesis, or activation, of lysosomal acid hydrolases results, in addition to an increase in organic acids (lactic and citric). (2) The lysosomal enzymes are then extruded from the osteoclasts and are solubilized in the extracellular fluid around the resorption zone. The organic acids which are also released from the osteoclasts supply hydrogen ions which, by their action, solubilize the bone mineral. The organic matrix which is uncovered is degraded by the acid hydrolases. The hydrogen ions supplied by the organic acids not only function to solubilize bone mineral, but also lower the pH of the extracellular fluid around the resorption zone, so that the acid hydrolases act maximally in their digestion of the uncovered organic matrix. (3) The residues, or fragments, resulting from the initial extracellular digestion are then ingested by the osteoclasts, through a process of endocytosis, where they are subjected to a further intracellular degradation (inside digestive vacuoles) by the action of the lysosomal acid hydrolases and acids.

The metabolic activity of *osteoblasts* has been demonstrated in the synthesis of the components of the organic matrix of bone (collagen and mucopolysaccharides). Moreover, recent evidence suggests that resting osteoblasts may have a role in calcium homeostasis, in that calcium exchange across their membranes has been shown to occur, resulting in intracellular calcium accumulation and release. *Osteocytes* have intracellular characteristics and structures which suggest that they too may be metabolically active. In this respect the capacity to synthesize protein and mucopolysaccharides has been attributed to osteocytes. In addition, lysosomes containing acid hydrolases have been described in these cells. It is also said that osteocytes have the ability to accumulate and release calcium (that is, they are active in the exchange of calcium with the extracellular fluid environment). Thus the ability to resorb bone mineral has also been attributed to osteocytes, and consequently they are considered to have a role in calcium homeostasis.

The homeostasis of calcium and phosphorus in the body fluids is therefore regulated by the activity of two hormones—parathyroid hormone secreted by the parathyroid glands, and thyrocalcitonin secreted by specialized cells of the thyroid glands. These two hormones have antagonistic actions: Parathyroid hormone tends to raise the calcium ion levels of the fluids, while thyrocalcitonin tends to lower the concentration of this ion. Of the two hormones, parathyroid hormone probably is more important. Under normal conditions, there is a basal secretion of both of these hormones, the effect of which is to maintain the constancy of calcium levels in the extracellular fluids. The secretion of the two hormones is markedly influenced by the concentration of calcium ion in the blood perfusing the glands in question. Recently it has been demonstrated that the concentration of magnesium ion in the blood can also influence the secretion of parathyroid hormone and calcitonin. An increase in calcium or magnesium ion, or an increase in the total calcium plus magnesium, depresses the secretion of parathyroid hormone by the parathyroid glands (and by parathyroid tissue *in vitro*), and at the same time stimulates the secretion of calcitonin by the "C" cells of the thyroid glands. Conversely, a decrease in the level of these ions stimulates the secretion of parathyroid hormone while decreasing the secretion of calcitonin. In most animals, parathyroid hormone probably is more important than calcitonin in respect to calcium homeostasis. However, since calcitonin plays an important part in the regulation of bone resorption, especially that which is induced by parathyroid hormone, it could be said to have a significant role in the control of unexpected episodes of hypercalcemia, as, for example, in clinical hyperparathyroidism. The action of the two hormones has been compared to the action of insulin and glucagon in the regulation of blood glucose. Insulin (secreted by the beta cells of the pancreatic islets of Langerhans) is hypoglycemic in action, and is the principal hormone involved in this regulation, while glucagon (secreted by the alpha cells) is hyperglycemic in action and provides a fine adjustment. (See Copp.)

The mechanisms by which calcium ion controls the hormonal secretions of these glands have not been fully elucidated. *In vitro* organ culture experiments using bovine parathyroid glands have demonstrated that an inverse relationship exists between the concentration of calcium ion in the fluid medium and protein synthesis in the glands (as measured by the incorporation of added radioactive amino acids into cellular proteins). In addition, these experiments have demonstrated that the amount of parathyroid hormone released into the culture medium bears an inverse relationship to the concentration of calcium ion, magnesium ion, or calcium plus magnesium ion. Therefore it can be deduced that a lowering of the calcium ion (or magnesium ion) concentration of the fluids bathing the parathyroid glands will stimulate both the synthesis of parathyroid hormone by the glands and its release into the fluid medium. Increasing the calcium ion (or magnesium ion) concentration will have an opposite effect on both hormone synthesis and release. Similar findings have been reported using porcine parathyroid slices. In addition, these studies have suggested that calcitonin added to the fluid medium may actually stimulate parathyroid hormone secretion even in the presence of high calcium ion concentrations in the medium (under which conditions parathyroid hormone secretion is usually partially inhibited). It is known that the parathyroid hormone that exists in the parathyroid glands (before secretion) is different immunologically

11

from the secreted parathyroid hormone that circulates in the blood, although both forms have biological activity. Recently it has been demonstrated that porcine parathyroid tissue has an enzyme system that degrades (inactivates) parathyroid hormone in the *presence of calcium,* and in the absence of calcium converts parathyroid hormone from the form found in the glands to the secreted form found in the blood. These findings therefore suggest an additional mechanism by which the calcium ion concentration may regulate parathyroid hormone release.

For many years the evidence regarding the effects of calcium ion on parathyroid hormone secretion was presumptive, since no methods were available for the direct measurement of circulating levels of this hormone. The development of bioassays provided a method for such studies, but the methods were limited in their sensitivity, and were of doubtful specificity. A major advance was made with the introduction of radioimmunoassay methods for the estimation of peptide hormones. These methods, which employ tracer hormones labelled with radioactive iodine, and also employ specific antibodies which bind these hormones, do not measure biological activity, but instead measure the actual concentrations of a hormone in biological fluids in terms of mass per unit volume. For example, insulin in plasma can be detected at the level of the "nanogram" (1 nanogram $= 10^{-9}$ grams). A radioimmunoassay for insulin in human blood plasma was first introduced by Yalow and Berson in 1959, and subsequently methods were developed for the assay of other peptide hormones, such as growth hormone, glucagon, ACTH, parathyroid hormone, and calcitonin. Utilization of radioimmunoassay methods in basic investigation has now provided direct proof for the relationship of hormone secretion to the levels of calcium in the blood. For example, increased amounts of parathyroid hormone can be detected in the blood of subjects in whom a hypocalcemia has been induced. On the other hand, a hypercalcemia can be shown to lead to reduced levels of this hormone in the blood. Similar studies employing radioimmunoassay methods for the detection of circulating levels of thyrocalcitonin in the blood have demonstrated that the levels of this hormone, increased during hypercalcemia, subsequently fall as the calcium ion concentration is decreased. Whereas methods have been developed for the assay of parathyroid hormone levels both in human blood plasma and in the blood plasma of animals, such as hogs and sheep, no successful methods for the assay of thyrocalcitonin in human plasma have as yet been described. As a consequence, the direct measurement of blood levels of this hormone has been restricted to animals, such as rabbits, hogs, and cows. Thus, the development of radioimmunoassay methods has permitted the direct examination of the control and dynamics of parathyroid hormone and calcitonin secretion.

Radioimmunoassay procedures for parathyroid hormone and calcitonin have also been used in the study of pathologic conditions. For example, blood serum from hyperparathyroid subjects contains significantly more immunoassayable parathyroid hormone than blood serum from normal subjects, and serum from subjects with idiopathic hypoparathyroidism has no detectable hormone. (See Berson and Yalow.)

The normal functional adaptation of the parathyroid glands and the calcitonin-secreting cells of the thyroid to variations in calcium ion concentration in the blood represents a self-regulating process. That is, under physiologic conditions, the level of the calcium ion concentration of the blood influences the secretion of parathyroid hormone and thyrocalcitonin, and is influenced in turn by the two hormones. In particular, the self-regulatory process takes the form of a negative "feedback" mechanism when an elevated blood calcium leads to a decrease in parathyroid gland secretion, and takes the form of a positive "feedback" because of the increased thyrocalcitonin secretion by the thyroids. When the calcium ion concentration in the blood is reduced, and the secretory activity of the parathyroid glands is increased, the self-regulatory process takes the form of a positive "feedback" mechanism. A reduction in the calcium ion concentration in the blood leads to a decreased secretion of thyrocalcitonin by the thyroids, and is therefore considered a negative "feedback." (See Fig. 32.) The terms negative and positive "feedback," as used above, adequately describe the response of the parathyroid glands and the calcitonin-producing cells of the thyroids in respect to the correction of particular metabolic situations (calcium depletion or calcium excess).

Recently the homeostasis of calcium ions in the body fluids has been considered in terms of *cybernetics* or *control-system theory*. In applying this theory to the action of the parathyroid glands (the same principles can be applied to the calcitonin-producing cells of the thyroids), it is again the calcium ion concentration in the blood plasma that is the stimulus to which these glands respond. In general terms, the condition being regulated (calcium ion concentration in particular) activates the regulatory mechanism (parathyroid gland secretion in particular) feeding back information about the output to an earlier stage in order to influence the action of the glands and thereby control the output. In terms of cybernetic theory, this is an example of a *negative feedback*, and is so considered, whether the parathyroid glands respond by an increase in secretion or by a decrease in secretion of parathyroid hormone. In other words, in cybernetic theory the deviation from normal is called the *error*, and the term *negative feedback* refers to a reduction of this error. With respect to calcium ion, this negative feedback may operate to correct a concentration which is either too high or too low. A system such as this (there being many similar systems in living organisms) is called a *closed-cycle system* or a *servo system*. (See McLean and Urist.)

In the absence of the parathyroid glands, plasma levels of calcium can be maintained only at approximately 7.0 mg. per 100 ml. Since this level is achieved through the physicochemical equilibrium that exists between the labile bone mineral and the extracellular fluids (interstitial fluid and blood), it is not regulated by any "feedback" mechanism. In the presence of the parathyroid glands, plasma calcium values will be maintained at the normal level of approximately 10 mg. per 100 ml. This normal level is attained mainly through the mobilizing effect of the parathyroid hormone on the stable mineral (apatite crystals) of the bone, and is regulated by a "feedback," as described above. Thyrocalcitonin, by its inhibitory effect on bone resorption, also plays a role in maintaining normal calcium levels.

SERUM CALCIUM, INORGANIC PHOSPHORUS, PROTEIN, AND PHOSPHATASE VALUES

When one is dealing with a disorder involving the skeleton, the values for serum calcium, inorganic phosphorus, protein, and alkaline and acid phosphatase activity frequently offer important diagnostic information. In this section we shall give figures indicating the range of these values, without relating aberrations from the normal values to specific diseases. That is, the values (both normal and abnormal) to be given here are intended mainly to serve as a basis of reference for comparison with the values encountered in various skeletal disorders to be discussed in subsequent chapters.

In evaluating the clinical significance of the serum calcium level in a given case, one must pay attention not only to the calcium value but also to the values for the inorganic phosphorus and the proteins of the serum. For instance, it is a well-known fact that the calcium and inorganic phosphorus may be reciprocally related in such a way that, at times, an increase in the inorganic phosphorus is associated with a reduction in the calcium, and vice versa. This reciprocal relation is one to be

Figure 32

   A series of diagrams illustrating the regulatory action of the parathyroid and thyroid glands in relation to calcium homeostasis.

   A, Diagrammatic representation of the normal state.   There is equilibrium between the calcium of the labile bone mineral and the calcium of the interstitial fluid and the plasma, so that the total calcium in these three compartments is maintained at the normal levels— 5.0 g, 0.50 g, and 0.28 g, respectively.   Since the total plasma calcium level is normal (10.0 mg. per 100 ml.), one can assume that the concentration of the calcium *ions* in the plasma is also normal.   The calcium ions influence the parathyroid glands in such a way that the secretory output of parathyroid hormone (PTH) is at a normal level.   This influence (normal "feedback") is indicated by the wavy arrow.   Under these conditions, the circulating parathyroid hormone acts on the stable bone mineral (apatite), the kidney, and the gastrointestinal tract so that an adequate amount of calcium is retained, and an adequate amount is excreted to maintain normal calcium levels in the plasma and interstitial fluids, and therefore also in the labile bone mineral. The role played by the thyroid gland in calcium homeostasis is also illustrated.   The parafollicular cells of this gland secrete calcitonin (thyrocalcitonin—TCT), whose effect is antagonistic to the effect of parathyroid hormone on stable bone mineral.   Unlike parathyroid hormone, calcitonin acts on bone mineral and inhibits resorption, and its effect is therefore hypocalcemic.   In the normal state, there is probably a basal secretion of calcitonin (controlled by the levels of calcium ion) which contributes to the maintenance of normal calcium homeostasis.

   B, Diagram showing the adjustment of parathyroid activity that occurs during calcium depletion of the plasma, the interstitial fluid, and consequently the labile bone mineral.   A drop below the indicated normal value in the calcium concentration of the plasma and, in particular, in the calcium ion concentration provides a stimulatory action to the parathyroid glands, thus acting as a positive "feedback," so that an increased secretion of parathyroid hormone results.   The increased level of circulating parathyroid hormone acts on the stable bone mineral, causing an increased mobilization of calcium.   It also affects the kidney by increasing the reabsorption of calcium from the renal tubules, and consequently the urinary excretion of calcium is initially reduced. However, it should be borne in mind that, as the calcium depletion is rectified, the urinary excretion of calcium will increase as a result of the hypercalcemic effect of parathyroid hormone.   Furthermore, parathyroid hormone influences the gastrointestinal tract to increase the absorption of calcium, and thereby tends to reduce the fecal excretion.   All of the actions of the parathyroid hormone are directed toward supplying the plasma and the interstitial fluid with increased amounts of calcium.   Hence, the lowered levels of calcium in these fluids tend to be restored to normal, with replenishment of the labile bone calcium.   The levels of calcium ion in the plasma in this condition provide a negative "feedback" to the calcitonin-producing cells of the thyroids, so that there is decreased secretion of calcitonin.   The inhibitory effect of this hormone on the resorption of bone mineral is thereby minimized.

   C, Diagram representing a condition which is the reverse of the one illustrated in *B*.   The increased concentration of calcium ion in the plasma depresses parathyroid activity (acts as a negative "feedback").   In consequence, there is a reduction in the secretion of parathyroid hormone.   This reduction in turn causes an initial increase in the urinary and fecal excretion of calcium, as well as a decreased mobilization of calcium from the bone mineral.   However, as the calcium excess is rectified, the urinary excretion of calcium will decrease.   The hypercalcemia acts as a positive "feedback" stimulus to the calcitonin-secreting cells of the thyroids, thus increasing the secretion of thyrocalcitonin (an effect opposite to that observed with respect to the secretion of parathyroid hormone by the parathyroid glands).   The increased amount of circulating calcitonin inhibits bone resorption to a greater extent.   Thus, the supply of calcium from the stable bone mineral is further reduced.   Ultimately, as the calcium levels of the fluids decrease, the secretion of parathyroid hormone will increase, while the secretion of calcitonin will decrease.

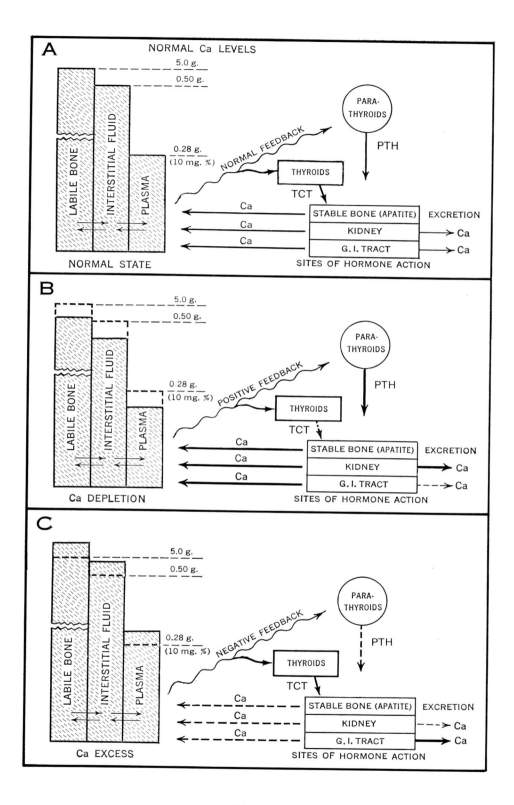

Figure 32

expected theoretically, and it is observed clinically and experimentally under certain conditions. For example, the hypocalcemia encountered as a result of advanced renal disease can be considered as a secondary effect related to the retention in the plasma of inorganic phosphorus (hyperphosphatemia) because of impaired renal excretion. As to the calcium-protein interrelationship, since about half of the total serum calcium is bound to protein (and particularly to the albumin fraction), a decrease in the serum protein concentration (especially of the albumin fraction) lowers the serum calcium value, other factors remaining the same. On the other hand, borderline increases in serum calcium values are occasionally observed in cases in which the serum protein (particularly the serum albumin fraction) is elevated.

Serum Calcium.—In regard to the calcium in the serum (or plasma), it is to be noted that this is present in two forms—diffusible and nondiffusible. The diffusible portion (about 60 to 65 per cent of the total calcium) is mainly calcium in ionic form, but includes a small amount of nonionized diffusible compounds (mainly calcium citrate, calcium bicarbonate, and calcium phosphate). More specifically, about 80 per cent of the diffusible calcium is in ionic form, and about 20 per cent consists of various nonionized diffusible compounds. The nondiffusible portion consists almost entirely of calcium bound to the protein of the serum—calcium proteinate. Of the protein-bound calcium, about 80 per cent is bound to the serum albumin and about 20 per cent to the serum globulin. The following schema is intended to illustrate the approximate proportions of the different forms of calcium in the serum of a normal adult whose total serum calcium level is 10 mg. per 100 ml.

Schema Illustrating Calcium Partition

(Approximate Proportions)

Total Serum Calcium 10.0 mg. per 100 ml.	
Diffusible Ca. 6.6	Nondiffusible Ca. 3.4
Ionized Ca. 5.3	(Ca. Proteinate) Albumin Fraction 2.7
Nonionized Ca. Compounds 1.3	Globulin Fraction 0.70

The procedures for determining only the diffusible fraction and/or the ionized calcium of the serum are not well adapted to general clinical use. However, the diffusible serum calcium fraction may be estimated in a given case by determining the total calcium of the cerebrospinal fluid, since, in general, the two values are roughly equivalent, provided the protein content of the cerebrospinal fluid is not much above the normal limit of 40 mg. per 100 ml. Furthermore, as to the ionized calcium in the serum, one can calculate its approximate concentration by using the formula derived by McLean and Hastings or the nomogram based upon it. The ionized fraction of the total serum (or plasma) calcium can now be directly determined by bioassay, ultracentrifugation, ultrafiltration, and by potentiometric measurements employing specific calcium ion electrodes. The results obtained by these methods agree surprisingly well with the results obtained by calculations using the McLean-Hastings formulations.

When the calcium level of the serum is determined by a standard clinical biochemical method, the result obtained represents the total value—that is, a composite of all the forms of calcium making up both the diffusible and the nondiffusible fractions. In ascertaining the calcium content of the serum, one is accounting for all but a trace of the calcium in the blood. Most of this trace represents calcium lost to the serum in the process of clot formation; if the cellular elements of the blood contain any calcium, the amount is negligible (at most 0.1 to 0.2 mg. per 100 ml. of whole blood).

As determined in the morning after a fast of about 12 hours, practically all *normal calcium values* of human blood serum fall within the following limits: *adults*, 9.5 to 10.5 mg. per 100 ml.; *children*, 10.0 to 11.5; and *neonates* and *other infants*, 10.5 to 12.0.   It should also be noted that these individual values remain practically the same from morning to morning. Because of the strict homeostatic regulation of the concentration of calcium ion in the body fluids, the serum calcium value of a normal subject remains relatively constant throughout the course of the day.

A definite *hypocalcemia* is represented by a value 1.0 mg. or more below the low normal limits just indicated—that is, by the following values: *adults*, 8.5 mg. or less per 100 ml.; *children*, 9.0; and *infants*, 9.5.   Correspondingly, a definite *hypercalcemia* is represented by a value 1 mg. or more above the high normal limits— that is, by the following values: *adults*, 11.5 mg. or more per 100 ml., and *children*, 12.5 mg. or more.   These delimiting values for serum calcium can be stated in this rather dogmatic fashion if methods are employed which are accurate within 0.3 to 0.4 mg. per 100 ml. (see Bodansky and Jaffe, Gutman *et al.*, and Jaffe and Bodansky).   The following graph shows the range of normal serum calcium values in the different age groups and also indicates for each of these groups the critical values for hypo- and hypercalcemia.

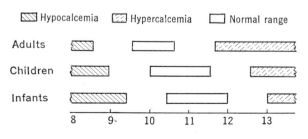

Mg. calcium per 100 ml. serum

Serum Inorganic Phosphorus.—It should be understood, first of all, that the term "serum inorganic phosphorus" as used in clinical medicine usually refers only to the phosphate ions of the serum. As a matter of fact, the serum inorganic phosphorus constitutes only a portion of the total serum phosphorus. Practically all *normal* serum inorganic phosphorus values for *adults* fall between 2.5 and 4.0 mg. per 100 ml.; for *children*, between 4.5 and 5.5, and for *infants*, between 5.5 and 6.5. Except perhaps in infants, values only 0.5 mg. below the normal lower limit in the various age groups may already indicate the presence of *hypophosphatemia*, and values 1.0 mg. or more above the normal upper limit may be stated to indicate a *hyperphosphatemia*.   As has already been mentioned, the calcium and inorganic phosphorus of the serum are reciprocally related in such a way that an increase in the phosphate ion is associated with a reduction in the calcium, and vice versa.

The following graph depicts the range of normal serum inorganic phosphorus values in the different age groups and also indicates for each of these groups the critical values for hypo- and hyperphosphatemia.

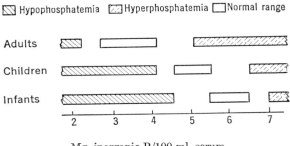

Mg. inorganic P/100 ml. serum

Serum Proteins.—In *adults* the *normal values* for total serum protein, as determined by chemical methods, tend to fall between 6.5 and 7.5 g per 100 ml., the albumin fraction being between 4 and 5 g and the globulin fraction between 2 and 3 g. A total protein value significantly below 6 g is to be interpreted as representing a *hypoproteinemia*, and a value significantly above 8 g as representing a *hyperproteinemia*. The protein values must be viewed in relation to the calcium values, because, as already pointed out, a considerable proportion of the serum calcium is combined with the proteins, most of this combination being with the albumin fraction. Thus a decrease in the serum protein, due to a decrease particularly in the albumin fraction, is associated with a decrease in the serum calcium, other factors remaining the same.

For clinical purposes, the proportions of the albumin and globulin fractions and, in particular, the proportions of the various globulins making up the globulin fraction are now commonly estimated by electrophoretic methods—especially by electrophoresis on paper and on cellulose acetate. Discrepancies exist between values determined by chemical means and those determined by electrophoresis. However, the values obtained by electrophoretic methods are generally considered to be more accurate. The following table gives the normal range of values for the various serum proteins as obtained by electrophoresis.

Electrophoretic Distribution of Human Serum Proteins

	% of Total Protein	*G/100 ml. Serum*
Albumin	52–68	3.8 –5.0
Alpha-1 globulin	2–6	0.15–0.45
Alpha-2 globulin	5–11	0.4 –0.8
Beta globulin	8–16	0.65–1.15
Gamma globulin	10–22	0.8 –1.6

Serum Alkaline Phosphatase.—As is well known, the enzyme alkaline phosphatase, normally present in relatively small amounts in the serum, acts optimally at a pH of 9.5. As determined by the Bodansky method, the *normal values* for serum alkaline phosphatase activity for *adults* range between 1.5 and 3.5 units per 100 ml. of serum and average about 2.6 units. In fact, the normal values lie so strictly within this range that any value even very slightly above 4.0 units may be suspected of being abnormal. For *children* the normal values lie between 5 and 14 units and average about 7.7 units. In children, since the normal range is so wide, values near the upper limit of the normal range should already arouse attention, and values of 18 units or more are to be considered clearly abnormal. For *infants* not more than a few months of age, normal values lie between 10 and 20 units, and values between 20 and 25 units are not necessarily abnormal, though they deserve special attention. (See Bodansky, Bodansky and Jaffe, and Jaffe and Bodansky.)

For alkaline phosphatase as determined by the method of King and Armstrong, most *normal values* for *adults* lie between 5 and 10 units per 100 ml. of serum and average about 8 units (see King and Armstrong). In adults, values above 13 are considered to be abnormal. For *children*, values of 10 to 25 units, with an average of about 20 units, are obtained by this method. Within the normal range the values obtained by the Bodansky method are roughly about one third as high as those obtained by the King-Armstrong method. However, in the abnormal range, this relationship no longer holds, the Bodansky values rising very much more steeply than the King-Armstrong values. Thus, when dealing with abnormally high alkaline phosphatase values, one cannot convert a value obtained by the Bodansky method into a King-Armstrong value, or vice versa, by simply multiplying or dividing, respectively, by 3.

Acid Phosphatase.—The enzyme acid phosphatase acts optimally at a pH of 5.0. The serum normally shows extremely low acid phosphatase activity—in fact, much lower than alkaline phosphatase activity. As determined by the Bodansky acid phosphatase method, the *normal range* of values for serum acid phosphatase (for children and adults of both sexes) can be stated as lying between 0.1 and 0.4 units per 100 ml. As determined by the Gutman method (an adaptation of the King-Armstrong method for alkaline phosphatase), the corresponding normal values lie between 0.5 and 3.0 units (see Gutman and Gutman). About 90 per cent of hospitalized subjects without prostatic disease show values within the indicated normal ranges by both methods. Acid phosphatase values which are slightly elevated sometimes raise diagnostic problems. In particular, this problem may present itself in cases showing very high *alkaline* phosphatase values. The suspected elevation of the acid phosphatase value in these cases may not be due to an actual increase in acid phosphatase but may be due to the presence of such large amounts of alkaline phosphatase that some alkaline phosphatase activity becomes measurable even at a pH of 5.0—the optimum pH of the acid phosphatase.

As to the practical measurement of serum acid phosphatase levels, it has been well documented that the Gutman and Gutman method has a relatively low specificity for prostatic acid phosphatase. On the other hand, the acid phosphatase methods which are modifications of the Bodansky alkaline phosphatase method have a relatively high specificity for prostatic acid phosphatase. In addition, the acid phosphatase which is present in the erythrocytes of the blood readily acts on phenyl phosphate (the substrate used in the method of Gutman and Gutman), whereas it does not act on beta glycerophosphate, the substrate used in the Bodansky acid phosphatase method. Therefore, unless special modifications are introduced (for example, the tartrate inhibition method of Fishman and Lerner), the analysis of serum obtained from hemolyzed blood by the Gutman method may result in misleading elevated acid phosphatase values.

For purposes of comparison and reference, the following table is given to show the normal range of alkaline and acid phosphatase values for adults, as determined by the methods most frequently used.

Résumé of Serum Alkaline and Acid Phosphatase Methods

Method	Substrate	Adult Normal Range (units/100 ml.) Alkaline	Acid
Bodansky	beta glycerophosphate	1.5 –3.5 2.2 –8.6*	0.1–0.4 0 –1.0*
King-Armstrong	phenyl phosphate	5.0 –10	0.5–3.0†
Bessey-Lowry	p-nitrophenyl phosphate	0.85–2.0	0.1–0.23
Huggins-Talalay	phenolphthalein phosphate	5–15	3–10

* Shinowara, Jones, and Reinhart modification of the Bodansky method.
† Gutman and Gutman modification of the King-Armstrong method.

REFERENCES

ARNAUD, C. D., JR., TENENHOUSE, A. M., and RASMUSSEN, H.: Parathyroid Hormone, Ann. Rev. Physiol., 29, 349, 1967.

BAUER, G. C. H., CARLSSON, A., and LINDQUIST, B.: Accretion Rate of Bone Salt in Osteoporosis Studied by Means of P³², Acta med. scandinav., 158, 139, 1957.

————: Bone Salt Metabolism in Humans Studied by Means of Radiocalcium, Acta med. scandinav., 158, 143, 1957.

BAUER, W., ALBRIGHT, F., and AUB, J. C.: Studies of Calcium and Phosphorus Metabolism. II. The Calcium Excretion of Normal Individuals on a Low Calcium Diet, also Data on a Case of Pregnancy, J. Clin. Invest., 7, 75, 1929.

BECK, L. V.: Organic Phosphate and "Fructose" in Rat Intestinal Mucosa, as Affected by Glucose and by Phlorhizin, J. Biol. Chem., 143, 403, 1942.

BERGEIM, O.: Intestinal Chemistry. V. Carbohydrates and Calcium and Phosphorus Absorption, J. Biol. Chem., 70, 35, 1926.

————: Intestinal Chemistry. VII. The Absorption of Calcium and Phosphorus in the Small and Large Intestines, J. Biol. Chem., 70, 51, 1926.

BERSON, S. A., and YALOW, R. S.: Clinical Applications of Radioimmunoassay of Plasma Parathyroid Hormone, Am. J. Med., 50, 623, 1971.

BLUNT, J. W., DeLUCA, H. F., and SCHNOES, H. K.: 25-Hydroxycholecalciferol. A Biologically Active Metabolite of Vitamin D₃, Biochemistry, 7, 3317, 1968.

BODANSKY, A.: Phosphatase Studies. II. Determination of Serum Phosphatase. Factors Influencing the Accuracy of the Determination, J. Biol. Chem., 101, 93, 1933.

BODANSKY, A., BLAIR, J. E., and JAFFE, H. L.: Serum Calcium and Phosphorus of Guinea Pigs After Administration of Single and Repeated Doses of Parathormone, Proc. Soc. Exper. Biol. & Med., 27, 708, 1930.

BODANSKY, A., and JAFFE, H. L.: Parathormone Dosage and Serum Calcium and Phosphorus in Experimental Chronic Hyperparathyroidism Leading to Ostitis Fibrosa, J. Exper. Med., 53, 591, 1931.

————: Phosphatase Studies. III. Serum Phosphatase in Diseases of the Bone: Interpretation and Significance, Arch. Int. Med., 54, 88, 1934.

————: Phosphatase Studies. V. Serum Phosphatase as a Criterion of the Severity and Rate of Healing of Rickets, Am. J. Dis. Child., 48, 1268, 1934.

BRONNER, F., HARRIS, R. S., MALETSKOS, C. J., and BENDA, C. E.: Studies in Calcium Metabolism. The Fate of Intravenously Injected Radiocalcium in Human Beings, J. Clin. Invest., 35, 78, 1956.

BUTCHER, R. W.: Role of Cyclic AMP in Hormone Actions, New England J. Med., 279, 1378, 1968.

CHASE, L. R., and AURBACH, G. D.: Parathyroid Function and the Renal Excretion of 3′5′-Adenylic Acid, Proc. Nat. Acad. Sc., U.S., 58, 518, 1967.

————: Renal Adenyl Cyclase: Anatomically Separate Sites for Parathyroid Hormone and Vasopressin, Science, 159, 545, 1968.

COHN, D. V., BAWDON, R., and ELLER, G.: The Effect of Parathyroid Hormone in Vivo on the Accumulation of Calcium and Phosphate by Kidney and on Kidney Mitochondrial Function, J. Biol. Chem., 242, 1253, 1967.

COLLIP, J. B.: The Parathyroid Glands, Medicine, 5, 1, 1926.

COONS, C. M., and BLUNT, K.: The Retention of Nitrogen, Calcium, Phosphorus, and Magnesium by Pregnant Women, J. Biol. Chem., 86, 1, 1930.

COPP, D. H.: Parathyroid Hormone, Calcitonin and Calcium Homeostasis. A Summary, in *Parathyroid Hormone and Thyrocalcitonin (Calcitonin)*, edited by R. V. Talmage and L. F. Bélanger, New York, Excerpta Medica Foundation, p. 25, 1968.

COPP, D. H., DAVIDSON, A. G. F., and CHENEY, B.: Evidence for a New Parathyroid Hormone Which Lowers Blood Calcium, Proc. Canad. Fed. Biol. Soc., *4*, 17, 1961.

COUSINS, R. J., DELUCA, H. F., and GRAY, R. W.: Metabolism of 25-Hydroxycholecalciferol in Target and Nontarget Tissues, Biochemistry, *9*, 3649, 1970.

DELUCA, H. F., and SALLIS, J. D.: Parathyroid Hormone: Its Subcellular Actions and Its Relationship to Vitamin D, in *The Parathyroid Glands: Ultrastructure, Secretion, and Function*, edited by P. J. Gaillard, R. V. Talmage, and A. M. Budy, Chicago, The University of Chicago Press, p. 181, 1965.

EASTOE, J. E.: The Organic Matrix of Bone. Chapt. IV in *The Biochemistry and Physiology of Bone*, edited by G. H. Bourne, New York, Academic Press, Inc., 1956.

FISHMAN, W. H., and LERNER, F.: A Method for Estimating Serum Acid Phosphatase of Prostatic Origin, J. Biol. Chem., *200*, 89, 1953.

FLEISH, H., and NEUMAN, W. F.: Mechanisms of Calcification: Role of Collagen, Polyphosphates, and Phosphatase, Am. J. Physiol., *200*, 1296, 1961.

FOLLIS, R. H. JR.: Calcification of Cartilage. In *Calcification in Biological Systems*, edited by R. E. Sognnaes, Washington, D.C., American Association for the Advancement of Science, p. 245, 1960.

GLIMCHER, M. J.: Molecular Biology of Mineralized Tissues with Particular Reference to Bone, Rev. Mod. Physics, *31*, 359, 1959.

————: Specificity of the Molecular Structure of Organic Matrices in Mineralization. In *Calcification in Biological Systems*, edited by R. E. Sognnaes, Washington, D.C., American Association for the Advancement of Science, p. 421, 1960.

————: The Role of the Macromolecular Aggregation State and Reactivity of Collagen in Calcification. In *Macromolecular Complexes*, edited by M. V. Edds, Jr., The Ronald Press Co., p. 53, 1961.

GUTMAN, A. B.: Current Theories of Bone Salt Formation, with Special Reference to Enzyme Mechanisms in Endochondral Calcification, Bull. Hosp. Joint Dis., *12*, 74, 1951.

GUTMAN, A. B., TYSON, T. L., and GUTMAN, E. B.: Serum Calcium, Inorganic Phosphorus and Phosphatase Activity in Hyperparathyroidism, Paget's Disease, Multiple Myeloma and Neoplastic Disease of the Bones, Arch. Int. Med., *57*, 379, 1936.

GUTMAN, E. B., and GUTMAN, A. B.: Estimation of "Acid" Phosphatase Activity of Blood Serum, J. Biol. Chem., *136*, 201, 1940.

HARRISON, H. E., and HARRISON, H. C.: Physiology of Vitamin D. In *Bone as a Tissue*, edited by K. Rodahl, J. T. Nicholson, and E. M. Brown, Jr., New York, The Blakiston Division, McGraw-Hill Book Co., Inc., p. 300, 1960.

HAWKER, C. D., GLASS, J. D., and RASMUSSEN, H.: Further Studies on the Isolation and Characterization of Parathyroid Polypeptides, Biochemistry, *5*, 344, 1966.

HOWLAND, J., and KRAMER, B.: Calcium and Phosphorus in the Serum in Relation to Rickets, Am. J. Dis. Child., *22*, 105, 1921.

JACOBSON, S. A.: Bone Lesions in Rats Produced by the Substitution of Beryllium for Calcium in the Diet, Arch. Path., *15*, 18, 1933.

JAFFE, H. L.: The Resorption of Bone. A Consideration of the Underlying Processes Particularly in Pathologic Conditions, Arch. Surg., *20*, 355, 1930.

JAFFE, H. L., and BODANSKY, A.: Experimental Fibrous Osteodystrophy (Ostitis Fibrosa) in Hyperparathyroid Dogs, J. Exper. Med., *52*, 669, 1930.

————: Diagnostic Significance of Serum Alkaline and Acid Phosphatase Values in Relation to Bone Disease, Bull. New York Acad. Med., *19*, 831, 1943.

————: Serum Calcium: Clinical and Biochemical Considerations, J. Mt. Sinai Hosp., *9*, 901, 1943.

JAFFE, H. L., BODANSKY, A., and BLAIR, J. E.: Fibrous Osteodystrophy (Osteitis Fibrosa) in Experimental Hyperparathyroidism of Guinea-Pigs, Arch. Path., *11*, 207, 1931.

KALLFELZ, F. A., TAYLOR, A. N., and WASSERMAN, R. H.: Vitamin D-Induced Calcium Binding Factor in Rat Intestinal Mucosa, Proc. Soc. Exper. Biol. & Med., *125*, 54, 1967.

KING, E. J., and ARMSTRONG, A. R.: A Convenient Method for Determining Serum and Bile Phosphatase Activity, Canad. M.A.J., *31*, 376, 1934.

KULONEN, E.: Recent Advances in the Chemistry of Collagen. In *Connective Tissue in Health and Disease*, edited by G. Asboe-Hansen, Copenhagen, E. Munksgaard, p. 70, 1954.

LEHNINGER, A. L.: *Biochemistry, The Molecular Basis of Cell Structure and Function*, New York, Worth Publishers, 1970. (See Chapters 15–18.)

MALM, O. J.: *Calcium Requirement and Adaptation in Adult Men*, Oslo, Oslo University Press, 1958.

McClendon, J. F., Culligan, L. C., Gydesen, C. S., and Myers, F. J.: Relative Length of the Intestine is More Important than the Character of the Food in Determining the Hydrogen Ion Concentration of Intestinal Contents, J. Biol. Chem., *41*, (Scientific Proceedings XIII, *v.i.*), 1920.

McLean, F. C., and Hastings, A. B.: The State of Calcium in the Fluids of the Body. I. The Conditions Affecting the Ionization of Calcium, J. Biol. Chem., *108*, 285, 1935.

McLean, F. C., and Urist, M. R.: *Bone: Fundamentals of the Physiology of Skeletal Tissue*, 3rd ed., Chicago, The University of Chicago Press, p. 64, 1968.

Meyer, K.: The Chemistry of the Ground Substances of Connective Tissue. In *Connective Tissue in Health and Disease*, edited by G. Asboe-Hansen, Copenhagen, E. Munksgaard, p. 54, 1954.

Morse, K. T., and Furness, F. N. (editors): Calcium and Phosphorus Metabolism in Man and Animals with Special Reference to Pregnancy and Lactation, Ann. New York Acad. Sc., *64*, 279, 1956.

Munson, P. L.: In *The Parathyroids*, edited by R. O. Greep and R. V. Talmage, Springfield, Illinois, Charles C Thomas, p. 94, 1961.

Munson, P. L., Hirsch, P. F., Brewer, H. B., Reisfeld, R. A., Cooper, C. W., Wästhed, A. B., Orimo, H., and Potts, J. T., Jr.: Thyrocalcitonin, Recent Progr. Hormone Res., *24*, 589, 1968.

Neuman, W. F.: The Influence of Parathyroid Hormone on the Cellular Exchange and Transport of Phosphate, in *The Parathyroid Glands: Ultrastructure, Secretion, and Function*, edited by P. J. Gaillard, R. V. Talmage, and A. M. Budy, Chicago, The University of Chicago Press, p. 175, 1965.

Neuman, W. F., and Neuman, M. W.: *The Chemical Dynamics of Bone Mineral*, Chicago, The University of Chicago Press, 1958.

Nicolaysen, R.: Untersuchungen über die Kalkausscheidung bei Hunden. Ein Beitrag zur Physiologie des Kolons, Skand. Arch. Physiol., *69*, (suppl.), 1934.

Nicolaysen, R., Eeg-Larsen, N., and Malm, O. J.: Physiology of Calcium Metabolism, Physiol. Rev., *33*, 424, 1953.

Olson, E. B., and DeLuca, H. F.: 25-Hydroxycholecalciferol: Direct Effect on Calcium Transport, Science, *165*, 405, 1969.

Orten, J. M., and Neuhaus, O. W.: *Biochemistry*, 8th ed., St. Louis, C. V. Mosby Co., p. 779, 1970.

Piez, K. A., and Likins, R. C.: The Nature of Collagen. II. Vertebrate Collagens. In *Calcification in Biological Systems*, edited by R. E. Sognnaes, Washington, D.C., American Association for the Advancement of Science, p. 411, 1960.

Pommer, G.: Ueber die Osteoblastentheorie, Arch. path. Anat., *92*, 296, 1883.

Ponchon, G., and DeLuca, H. F.: The Role of the Liver in the Metabolism of Vitamin D, J. Clin. Invest., *48*, 1273, 1969.

Ponchon, G., Kennan, A. L., and DeLuca, H. F.: "Activation" of Vitamin D by the Liver, J. Clin. Invest., *48*, 2032, 1969.

Potts, J. T., Jr., Aurbach, G. D., and Sherwood, L. M.: Parathyroid Hormone: Chemical Properties and Structural Requirements for Biological and Immunological Activity, Recent Progr. Hormone Res., *22*, 101, 1966.

Rasmussen, H.: Parathyroid Hormone. Nature and Mechanism of Action, Am. J. Med., *30*, 112, 1961.

————: Ionic and Hormonal Control of Calcium Homeostasis, Am. J. Med., *50*, 567, 1971.

Rasmussen, H., and Craig, L. C.: Isolation of a Parathyroid Polypeptide from Acetic Acid Extracts of Bovine Parathyroid Glands, J. Biol. Chem., *236*, 1083, 1961.

Rich, A., and Crick, F. H. C.: The Structure of Collagen, Nature, *176*, 915, 1955.

Robinson, R. A.: An Electron-microscopic Study of the Crystalline Inorganic Component of Bone and Its Relationship to the Organic Matrix, J. Bone & Joint Surg., *34-A*, 389, 1952.

————: Chemical Analysis and Electron Microscopy of Bone. In *Bone as a Tissue*, edited by K. Rodahl, J. T. Nicholson, and E. M. Brown, Jr., New York, The Blakiston Division, McGraw-Hill Book Co., Inc., p. 300, 1960.

Robison, G. A., Butcher, R. W., and Sutherland, E. W.: Adenyl Cyclase as an Adrenergic Receptor, Ann. New York Acad. Sc., *139*, 703, 1967.

————: Cyclic AMP, Ann. Rev. Biochem., *37*, 149, 1968.

Robison, R.: *The Significance of Phosphoric Esters in Metabolism*, New York, New York University Press, 1932.

Rutishauser, E., and Majno, G.: Physiopathology of Bone Tissue: The Osteocytes and Fundamental Substance, Bull. Hosp. Joint Dis., *12*, 468, 1951.

Seifter, S., and Gallop, P. M.: The Structure of Proteins, in *The Proteins: Composition, Structure, and Function*, 2nd ed., Vol. IV, edited by H. Neurath, New York, Academic Press, p. 238, 1966.

SHERMAN, H. C.: *Calcium and Phosphorus in Foods and Nutrition*, New York, Columbia University Press, 1947.

SHERMAN, H. C., and HAWLEY, E.: Calcium and Phosphorus Metabolism in Childhood, J. Biol. Chem., *53*, 375, 1922.

SHOHL, A. T., and WOLBACH, S. B.: Rickets in Rats. XV. The Effect of Low Calcium-High Phosphorus Diets at Various Levels and Ratios upon the Production of Rickets and Tetany, J. Nutrition, *11*, 275, 1936.

SOEUR, R.: De l'effet de l'ergostérol irradié sur l'os, Arch. internat. méd. expér., *6*, 365, 1931.

STEARNS, G.: The Significance of the Retention Ratio of Calcium:Phosphorus in Infants and in Children, Am. J. Dis. Child., *42*, 749, 1931.

————: Human Requirement of Calcium, Phosphorus and Magnesium, J.A.M.A., *142*, 478, 1950.

STOHS, S. J., ZULL, J. E., and DeLUCA, H. F.: Vitamin D Stimulation of [³H] Orotic Acid Incorporation into Ribonucleic Acid of Rat Intestinal Mucosa, Biochemistry, *6*, 1304, 1967.

SUTHERLAND, E. W., RALL, T. W., and MENON, T.: Adenyl Cyclase. I. Distribution, Preparation, and Properties, J. Biol. Chem., *237*, 1220, 1962.

SUTHERLAND, E. W., ØYE, I., and BUTCHER, R. W.: The Action of Epinephrine and the Role of the Adenyl Cyclase System in Hormone Action, Recent Progr. Hormone Res., *21*, 623, 1965.

SUTHERLAND, E. W., and ROBISON, G. A.: The Role of Cyclic-3′,5′-AMP in Responses to Catecholamines and Other Hormones, Pharmacol. Rev., *18*, 145, 1966.

TALMAGE, R. V., and ELLIOTT, J. R.: Removal of Calcium from Bone as Influenced by the Parathyroids, Endocrinology, *62*, 717, 1958.

TELFER, S. V.: Mineral Metabolism in Infancy. Part I. The Mineral Constituents of Human Milk and of Cow's Milk, Glasgow M. J., *113*, 246, 1930.

————: Mineral Metabolism in Infancy. Part II. The Utilization of the Mineral Elements in Human Milk, Glasgow M.J., *114*, 10, 1930.

————: Mineral Metabolism in Infancy. Part III. The Substitution of Cow's Milk for Human Milk in Infant Feeding, Glasgow M.J., *114*, 265, 1930.

VAES, G.: The Role of Lysosomes and of Their Enzymes in the Development of Bone Resorption Induced by Parathyroid Hormone, in *Parathyroid Hormone and Thyrocalcitonin (Calcitonin)*, edited by R. V. Talmage and L. F. Bélanger, New York, Excerpta Medica Foundation, p. 318, 1968.

WALKER, D. G.: Citric Acid Cycle in Osteoblasts and Osteoclasts. A Histochemical Study of Normal and Parathormone-Treated Rats, Bull. Johns Hopkins Hosp., *108*, 80, 1961.

WASSERMAN, R. H., COMAR, C. L., and NOLD, M. M.: The Influence of Amino Acids and other Organic Compounds on the Gastrointestinal Absorption of Calcium[45] and Strontium[89] in the Rat, J. Nutrition, *59*, 371, 1956.

WASSERMAN, R. H., and TAYLOR, A. N.: Vitamin D_3-Induced Calcium-Binding Protein in Chick Intestinal Mucosa, Science, *152*, 791, 1966.

YALOW, R. S., and BERSON, S. A.: Assay of Plasma Insulin in Human Subjects by Immunological Methods, Nature, *184*, 1648, 1959.

————: Immunoassay of Endogenous Plasma Insulin in Man, J. Clin. Invest., *39*, 1157, 1960.

Chapter

6

Osteogenesis Imperfecta

OSTEOGENESIS imperfecta is a relatively uncommon disease whose most striking and characteristic clinical feature is fragility of the bones, although the disorder is not limited to the skeleton. The condition may be inherited from either parent or may appear *de novo* as a mutation, and it is transmitted as an autosomal dominant mendelian character. The disease complex comprising the various manifestations of osteogenesis imperfecta apparently has its basis in defectiveness of the mesenchyme in general. The bone fragility in particular is ascribed to an inadequacy of the bone-forming mesenchyme and, more specifically, to an inadequacy of the osteoblasts derived from it. Certainly the osseous tissue laid down in the course of the formation and growth of the bones is both meager in quantity and poor in quality. The basic aberration of the osseous tissue formed relates to its collagen (the principal constituent of the organic matrix), the collagen being not only deficient in amount but poorly organized, and apparently also anomalous in respect to its chemical composition. One of the abnormalities pertinent to the collagen macromolecule seems to relate to a deficient rate of incorporation of the amino acid proline (see Summer).

In addition to bone fragility, the disease complex includes slate blue sclerae, abnormalities of the teeth (notably of the dentin), progressive deafness, hyperlaxity of joints, and thinness of the skin due to maldevelopment of the corium. These various manifestations, too, reflect the basic mesenchymal abnormality as expressed in the connective tissues in general.

Nomenclature.—Osteogenesis imperfecta has long been recognized as a clinical entity. Vrolik was apparently the first to use the term "osteogenesis imperfecta." He applied it to the cases in which the disorder was already present at birth. The clinical aspects of the disease in older subjects had been discussed previously by Lobstein under the name of "osteopsathyrosis idiopathica" (idiopathic fragility of the bones). Other names under which the condition has been described include "fragilitas ossium," "periosteal dysplasia," "brittle bones," and "brittle bones and blue sclerae." On the whole, the name "osteogenesis imperfecta" seems the best, since it emphasizes the idea that the characteristic fragility of the bones has its basis in defective or imperfect osseous tissue. Furthermore, that term has the advantage of being equally applicable to the early and the late cases, emphasizing, as it does, the underlying factor common to the two types.

CLINICAL CONSIDERATIONS

Cases of osteogenesis imperfecta are commonly subclassified into two main clinical groups: (1) *osteogenesis imperfecta fetalis* (or *congenita*), in which the fetus is usually born dead and at best has a very poor prognosis for life, and in which fractures (usually very numerous) are already present at birth, and (2) *osteogenesis imperfecta tarda* (or *tardiva*), in which the fetus is born apparently normal, manifests

162

fractures only after birth (and perhaps even none until after the first decade), and has a much better prognosis for life, many of these subjects outgrowing their bone fragility. However, not all cases fit neatly into one or the other of these two categories. Thus an infant may be born with only a few fractures, survive into adult life despite many new ones, and then begin to show a decrease in bone fragility. Conversely, the affected infant, though born without any fractures, may develop large numbers of them very soon after birth and succumb during infancy or early childhood.

Osteogenesis Imperfecta Fetalis.—In the usual case of osteogenesis imperfecta fetalis, the infant is small and underweight, even if not premature. Its skin is soft, thin, and delicate, and the hair on the head is abundant. The crown of the head is rather large, but the face is small, the nose and mouth are well formed, and the tongue is not enlarged. The abdomen tends to protrude abnormally. The limbs are short, drawn in toward the trunk, and nearly always very crooked because of deformity of the long bones. The lower extremities are often curved in such a way that the soles of the feet tend to face each other. On palpation, the crown of the head is almost certain to reveal abnormal softness of the calvarial region. In fact, bone deficiency may be so extreme in this region that the calvarium is represented by a yielding structure which is either substantially nonosseous or contains only small islands of bone. Even when a fairly bony skull cap can be felt, the sutures and fontanelles are found exceptionally wide, but the calvarium may nevertheless yield to pressure almost as if it were parchment. Along the ribs, one may feel numerous nodosities which represent fractures in various stages of healing. If not born dead, such an infant, at least in the past, usually survived for only a few weeks or months, then succumbing to shock or intercurrent infection. In an occasional instance, even a rather severely affected infant survives to reach late childhood or even adult life, although fractures have continued to occur and the skeleton is badly deformed.

On *roentgenographic examination* of the skeleton of a severely affected neonate or very young infant, one usually finds, as would be expected, large numbers of healed or healing fractures, particularly of the ribs and major long bones. The latter appear stunted, and their shafts are usually found curved and broadened. The general meagerness of the osseous tissue is most strikingly revealed in the thinness of the cortices of the bones. The fracture lines are usually more or less transverse to the long axis of the bone, and the fracture fragments are seldom displaced. Each rib may have so many transverse fractures that it may appear "pleated" in the *x*-ray picture. The bones of the vertebral column will be found highly porotic, and the calvarium will show the presence of smaller or larger numbers of wormian bones.

The postnatal centers of ossification make their appearance in approximately normal sequence in an affected infant who continues to survive. Though these centers enlarge, they appear porotic because of their deficiency in osseous tissue. The epiphysial-diaphysial junctional zones show no widening of the epiphysial cartilage plates. If the affected infant survives into early or middle childhood, some of the bones (particularly those of the lower extremities) are likely to present a "multiloculated" appearance in the *x*-ray picture. (See Figs. 33 and 34.)

Osteogenesis Imperfecta Tarda.—The usual case of osteogenesis imperfecta tarda is probably best typified in an older child, adolescent, or adult subject who presents skeletal deformities from previous fractures and still undergoes occasional ones, but who is no longer in much danger of succumbing to the disease. The subject's fractures may not have started to take place until the latter part of the first year, or even not until some years after birth. In cases in which the appearance of fractures is delayed, the presence of blue sclerae may be the first obvious indication that one is dealing with osteogenesis imperfecta.

The person affected is likely to be somewhat short in stature, mainly because of skeletal deformities but sometimes also because of actual shortness of the long bones of the lower extremities. The configuration of the head may be abnormal, in consequence of protuberance of the temporal regions or of the frontal or occipital region, but the calvarium is no longer soft, as it is in the affected neonate. More obvious now are the deformities which result from alterations in the long bones (particularly those of the lower extremities) and also to some extent from curvature of the vertebral column. The deformations of the long bones arise chiefly from the healing of repeated fractures into positions of malalignment. The curvatures of the vertebral column are due mainly to laxity of its ligaments, though partial or total collapse of one or more vertebrae may also play a role. (See Scherr.)

As to the fractures, inquiry will reveal that most of them have occurred in the shafts of the long bones of the lower extremities, though some may also have taken place in those of the upper extremities. Among the other bones in which fractures are likely to have occurred are the clavicles, mandible, and ribs. In the average case there is a history of about 10 or 12 fractures, most of which have taken place within a period of a few years. Furthermore, the incidence of fractures is likely to have decreased as the subject approached adulthood. In some cases, however, the subject has already undergone as many as 50 fractures or even more, and the tendency toward them seems to abate much more slowly. While not spontaneous, the fractures occur after very slight provocation (such as a mere muscle pull). The fractures are striking in that: (1) They are almost always simple transverse or oblique breaks; (2) they are associated with but little pain, apparently because the periosteum is not torn through; (3) they tend to heal with remarkable rapidity, though the callus formed is ordinarily not excessive; and (4) they are not likely to recur at sites of previous fractures.

On *roentgenographic examination* of an affected older child, adolescent, or adult, the long bones usually show abnormally thin cortices (though not necessarily along the whole length of the shaft) and thin, sparse spongy trabeculae arranged in wide

Figure 33

A, Photograph of an infant (2 months of age) affected with osteogenesis imperfecta fetalis. The condition had already been recognized at birth, and the infant died at the age of 4 months. Note the characteristic bowing deformities of the lower extremities—the result of multiple fractures of the long bones of these limbs. X-ray examination of the skeleton also revealed many fractures of other bones.

B, Roentgenograph of part of the sternal aspect of the thoracic cage from a case of osteogenesis imperfecta fetalis. The fetus was full term at birth and died 2 days later. The ribs show transverse fracture lines extending more or less at right angles to their long axes. In several of the ribs, multiple fracture lines are present, giving these ribs the appearance of being "pleated" (see also *C* and *D*).

C, Roentgenograph of part of the vertebral aspect of the thoracic cage from the case mentioned in *B*. Note that multiple fractures are also present in the shafts of the ribs posteriorly.

D, Roentgenograph showing the appearance of some of the bones of a lower limb from the case mentioned in *B*. Note that the center of ossification for the lower epiphysis of the femur is present, as is to be expected in a full term neonate. Note also the deformity of the tibia and, in particular, the broadened outline of the bone, the striking thinness of the cortex, and the presence of a line representing an almost completely healed fracture.

E, Roentgenograph showing part of the calvarium of the infant illustrated in *A*. Note, in the upper left-hand part of the picture, numerous small islands of radiopacity. These represent foci of calvarial ossification which have not yet fused to form a bone unit, as they would normally have done. Such unfused islands of calvarial bone constitute the basis for the so-called wormian bones.

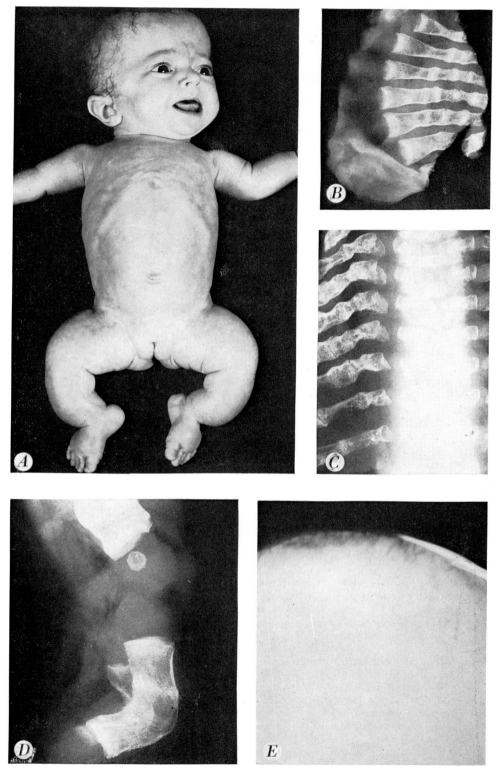

Figure 33

meshes, especially at the epiphysial bone ends. Furthermore, the long bones (especially of the lower extremity) present narrowed shafts which are often found very curved. This curvature is usually ascribable to fractures and infractions, even though evidence of fractures of recent occurrence may be lacking. The bony epiphyses may appear somewhat enlarged and deformed. The bones of the vertebral column may appear porotic, and some vertebral bodies may even show partial collapse. Occasionally, even the pelvis may be deformed and its outlet contracted. The calvarium (posteriorly and laterally in particular) is likely to present the pattern of a mosaic of so-called wormian bones (p. 172).

While healing of the fractures in osteogenesis imperfecta is not ordinarily associated with *excessive callus* formation, this does take place once in a great while. The observed instances occurred in cases of osteogenesis imperfecta tarda, and the site of the exuberant callus was usually a femur. On the basis of the roentgenographic picture, such a focus of massive callus, especially if it is very radiopaque, might be misinterpreted as an osteogenic sarcoma (see Brailsford, Baker, Fairbank and Baker, Banta *et al.*, and Schwarz). However, in some of the reported instances, the roentgenographic shadow cast seems to the writer to be more suggestive of myositis ossificans than of hyperplastic callus. Klenerman *et al.* have reported two cases of osteogenic sarcoma occurring in subjects affected with osteogenesis imperfecta. They suggested that the tumors in those cases arose spontaneously and were not related to the underlying osteogenesis imperfecta.

Extraskeletal Manifestations.—The principal extraskeletal manifestations entering into the syndrome of osteogenesis imperfecta and bearing a genetic relationship to the bone fragility are slate or gray-blue sclerae, progressive deafness, and hyperlaxity of joints (see Key). Many other extraskeletal abnormalities occurring less often but still possibly associated genetically with the disorder have also been recorded (see McKusick).

The *blue sclerae* are found in practically all surviving subjects affected with bone fragility and are usually already manifest early in childhood. The blueness is due to the fact that the sclerae are less dense (and possibly thinner) than in normal persons and therefore more translucent. The *progressive deafness* is also a very common manifestation, though not so common as the blue sclerae. Usually it does not set in much before adulthood, by which period the fractures may have ceased

Figure 34

A, Roentgenograph showing the right femur, tibia, and fibula from a case of osteogenesis imperfecta in a female infant 7 months of age. The disorder was already clearly manifest at birth. The bones present the characteristic bowing deformity, and the tibia in particular shows two clearly recognizable transverse infractions or fractures without displacement. The cortices of the bones are extremely thin. Note that the centers of ossification for the lower epiphysis of the femur and the upper epiphysis of the tibia are well formed, though they, too, manifest osteoporosis.

B, Roentgenograph depicting the status of the bones of the pelvis and lower extremities of the child mentioned in *A* as they appeared when she was 6 years of age. Because of the deformities, the child had never walked. Note the multiloculated (honeycombed) appearance presented by the femora, for instance. Such roentgenographic findings in cases of osteogenesis imperfecta have led Fairbank to subclassify these cases as instances of osteogenesis imperfecta cystica.

C, Roentgenograph of the right upper extremity of the infant, 7 months of age, to whom reference has been made in *A*. The phalanges and metacarpal bones show osteoporosis but are not deformed. The radius and ulna show healing fractures through their shafts.

D, Roentgenograph showing the upper extremity illustrated in *C* as it appeared when the subject had reached the age of 6.

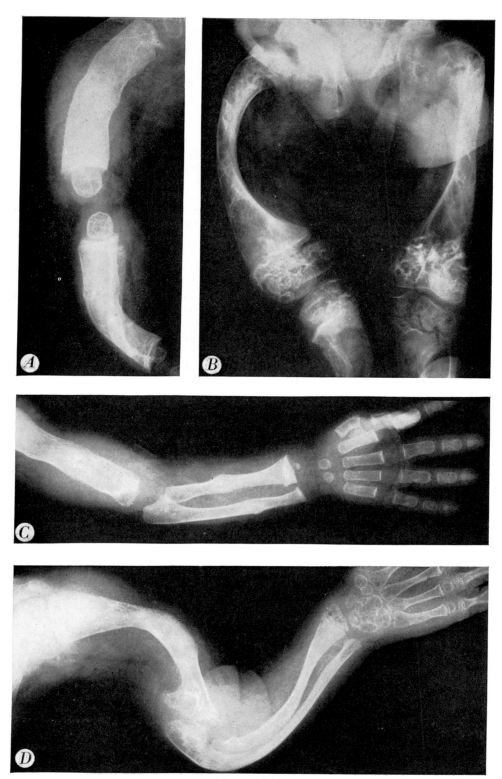

Figure 34

to occur. In many cases it seems clearly to result from otosclerotic disease of the osseous labyrinth. This is not surprising in view of the fact that, at autopsy, infants with osteogenesis imperfecta already show some changes in this structure. In some cases, however, there is nerve deafness in addition. Concerning the *hyperlaxity of joints,* our information is much less precise than in respect to the blue sclerae and the progressive deafness. It evidently results from laxity of the articular ligaments and articular capsules, and predisposes to sprains and dislocations. It is, of course, not nearly so striking as the hypermobility of joints which constitutes so prominent a feature of the Ehlers-Danlos syndrome. The latter, on the other hand, is not associated with fragility of the bones, though certain skeletal aberrations do appear in connection with it. (See Fig. 35.)

Clinical Laboratory Findings.—The serum calcium and serum inorganic phosphate values are normal in osteogenesis imperfecta. The serum alkaline phosphatase value ought theoretically to be subnormal, in accordance with the deficiency in the deposition of osseous tissue which is characteristic of the disorder. Actually, however, we have found it to be approximately normal unless healing fractures are present. In the presence of such fractures, the serum alkaline phosphatase is likely to be moderately elevated above the normal (see Bodansky and Jaffe). In regard to the absorption and excretion of calcium and phosphorus, it has been reported that in affected children, although the absorption of these minerals is satisfactory, their retention is clearly subnormal (see Stevenson and Cuthbertson, and Hansen). Others have found no aberration in the calcium and phosphorus metabolism of either children or adults affected with the disorder (see Aub and Farquharson).

PATHOLOGIC FINDINGS

Osteogenesis Imperfecta Fetalis.—The skeletal abnormalities presented by neonates and young infants affected with the so-called fetal form of osteogenesis imperfecta have been the subject of a number of detailed studies. The earlier contributions dealt mainly with the gross pathologic aberrations and the microscopic

Figure 35

A, Photograph of a man 29 years of age who presents very gross deformity of the skeleton in consequence of osteogenesis imperfecta tarda. The subject appeared normal at birth and suffered his first fracture (through the right tibia) when he was 4 months of age. Subsequently, that tibia and other bones underwent many fractures, and scoliosis also developed. The subject never walked, and he became deaf during adult life. (This photograph is reproduced from the article by Bell in the *Eugenics Laboratory Memoirs,* No. 24, 1928.)

B, Photograph of a deformed tibia and fibula from the case of a girl 16 years of age whose lower extremities were amputated through the lower third of the thighs because these limbs were so badly deformed that the subject could not walk. There had been multiple fractures of these and many other bones since early childhood. A pronounced scoliotic deformity had resulted in telescoping of the chest into the abdomen, so that the lower costal border on each side was in close contact with the iliac crest. The histologic architecture of the cortex of the tibia in this case is illustrated in Figure 37-*B.*

C, Photograph of the deformed skeleton of a man who apparently had suffered from osteogenesis imperfecta and who was believed to have been 45 years old at the time of his death. This illustration is reproduced from an article by Hektoen (Am. J. M. Sc., *125,* 751, 1903). Though some doubts are expressed in that article that the condition actually represented osteogenesis imperfecta, the appearance of the calvarium (see *D*) strongly supports that diagnosis.

D, Photograph of the skull from the case cited in *C* showing the numerous wormian bones composing the cranium. The relatively large cranial vault is made up of 172 such bones.

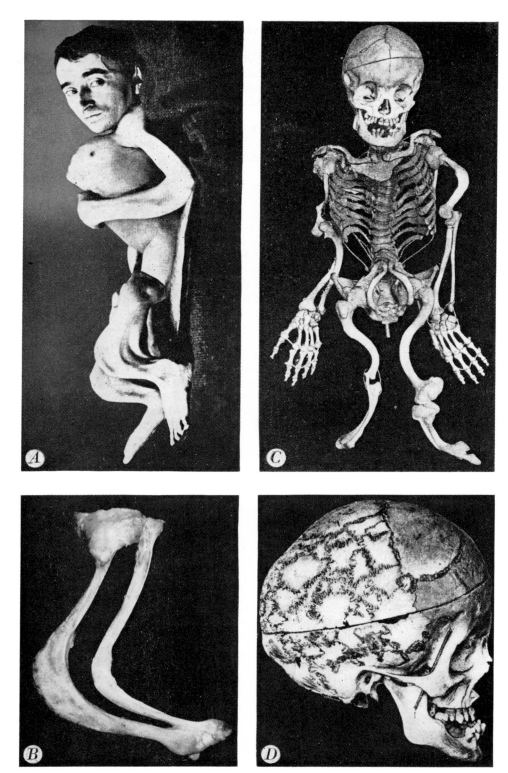

Figure 35

findings as revealed by the conventional histologic techniques (see Stilling, Harbitz, Jeckeln, and also Gruber). In some of the more recent studies, the skeletal tissues were investigated with the aid of histochemical procedures and such biophysical techniques as microradiography, polarized light, and x-ray diffraction (see Follis, and Engfeldt *et al.*).

The findings obtained in these various ways have reinforced each other in pointing up the nature of the basic defect insofar as the bones are concerned. They converge to show that this defect resides in disordered osteoblastic activity. This is reflected particularly in the collagen of the organic bone matrix, the collagen being deficient in amount, poorly organized, and apparently also anomalous in respect to its chemical composition. On the other hand, it has become evident that where the organic matrix has undergone mineralization the crystal structure of the bone mineral (apatite) is not abnormal. Furthermore, the mineral crystals are oriented to the collagen fibrils, as in normal bone.

As to the *gross changes*, it has already been indicated that the *calvarium* (and especially its vault) is likely to be extremely abnormal. At best in these cases, it is only a thin shell of osseous tissue. The individual bones are separated by abnormally wide sutures and large fontanelles. In other instances it may be represented merely by a fibrous connective tissue membrane containing tiny islands of bone. In contrast, the floor of the cranial cavity and the facial bones are relatively only mildly involved.

The gross changes in the *long bones* of the affected infants are very conspicuous. If a long bone (for instance, a tibia or femur) from a case in which the changes are of average severity is sectioned longitudinally, the bone is found to cut very easily and to have a very thin cortex except at sites of fracture. In the medullary cavity the spongy trabeculae are very sparse. At sites of fractures the medullary cavity may contain blood clots, and there may be endosteal or periosteal callus—fibrous, cartilaginous, or bony, in accordance with the time which has elapsed since the occurrence of the fracture or fractures. At the epiphysial-metaphysial junctions the cartilage is sharply delimited from the shaft, as in normal neonates or infants. However, the amount of osseous tissue present at these junctions is exceedingly sparse, and it is not unusual to find infractions at the juxta-epiphysial junctions. The epiphysial cartilage plates themselves show nothing abnormal. Furthermore, the long bones of the affected infant usually show such centers of epiphysial ossification as would be present in the corresponding bones of a normal infant of the same age, though these centers may be somewhat small and are certainly not so densely osseous as they should be.

As to *other skeletal parts*, it should be noted first that the clavicles are likely to present rather numerous fractures in various stages of healing. Many ribs (sometimes all of them) may be found fractured—often in many places. Their cortices, too, will be found very thin if the ribs are cut open. The changes in the vertebral column are also concordant with those in other skeletal regions. Thus there may be fractures through the vertebral arches. Furthermore, in consequence of the sparsity of spongy trabeculae in the ossification centers for the vertebral bodies, some of these centers may be compressed and the vertical height of the corresponding bodies hence be somewhat reduced. In an affected infant, the pelvis ordinarily shows no striking changes. However, in cases of extreme severity it may undergo lateral compression because of the insufficiency of the constituent osseous tissue. The metacarpals and metatarsals have not received much study, but such examinations as have been made of them indicate that in them, too, the cortex is thin and the spongy bone meager.

On *microscopic examination*, a long bone of an affected neonate will show that in its epiphyses the appearance of the cartilage cells, intercellular matrix, and cartilage vessel canals is approximately normal. Furthermore, at the epiphysial-metaphysial junctions or around a center of ossification developing in an epiphysis, the proliferation of the cartilage cells preparatory to endochondral ossification proceeds in a regular and orderly fashion. However, though tongues of calcified cartilage matrix are prepared for the deposition of bone upon them, the tissue laid down on these calcified cartilage matrix cores and presumably representing bone is peculiar and meager. Plump osteoblasts are not present on the surface of the deposited bone; the surface cells (modified osteoblasts) appear drawn out and spindled. In sections treated with hematoxylin and eosin, the deposited material stains blue, since it is strongly basophilic. The cells embodied in this peculiarly modified osseous tissue lie in lacunae and appear to be osteocytes. Altogether, the tissue deposited on the calcified cartilage cores at all sites of endochondral ossification has the histologic appearance of very primitive or immature fiber bone.

On microscopic examination, the shaft cortex of an affected long bone is found to be abnormally thin and spongified, except where it reveals the secondary effects of fracture. Furthermore, the cortical osseous tissue still consists entirely (or almost entirely) of fiber bone of rather primitive character, although, in the shaft cortex of a long bone from a normal fetus, considerable lamellar osseous tissue would already be present. Where there are no fractures, the periosteal covering of the shaft cortex is well delineated, showing a clear-cut outer fibrous and inner cambium layer. Indeed, the inner layer may even be more prominent than it would be if the fetus were normal. However, though this inner layer is likely to be quite cellular, relatively few of the cells in question have the configuration of plump, actively functioning osteoblasts. Osteoclasts, too, are rather sparse. (See Fig. 36.)

A neonate or young infant manifesting osteogenesis imperfecta fetalis may already show some abnormalities in the *osseous labyrinth* (see Weber, and Meyer). These aberrations probably underlie the progressive deafness not uncommonly manifest in more long-lived subjects with osteogenesis imperfecta. The unerupted *teeth*, too, like the genuine osseous structures, may show abnormalities. In particular, there is a deficiency of the mesodermal part of tooth formation, while the ectodermal part is not directly impaired. Hence the formation of dentin is usually abnormal, while the formation of enamel is usually affected only indirectly (see Rushton, and Roberts and Schour).

The *viscera* do not appear to undergo any important alterations and are usually found developed in accordance with the infant's age. Aberrations in the *glands* of *internal secretion* (mainly increases in size) have been reported rather frequently (see Fahr). It may perhaps be safely stated that there is a slight tendency toward precocity in the development of these glands which accounts for their enlargement. However, it is not yet clear how these deviations are related to the disease. Some observers have also remarked upon the presence, in neonates and infants showing the disease, of pronounced calcification of the arteries of the extremities and even cerebral hemorrhage following upon the rupture of a blood vessel (see Johansson).

Osteogenesis Imperfecta Tarda.—As already noted, adolescents and young adults still presenting osteogenesis imperfecta in active form are no longer in much danger of succumbing to it. On this account, relatively little anatomic material from such cases has been available for study. However, a fairly clear conception of the skeletal alterations present in these cases can be built up on the basis of: (1) inferences to be drawn from the roentgenographs of the entire skeleton in such subjects; (2) findings in the bones in the occasional instances in which an affected extremity has been amputated because of gross and inconvenient distortions; and (3) study of the few available museum skeletons of adults who had been gravely deformed by the disease in question but died from some other cause.

Looser examined the tibiae of the amputated deformed legs of a 17 year old patient who, since the age of $1\frac{1}{2}$ years, had undergone 50 fractures in various parts of the body. The tibiae under discussion were found curved and recurved like corkscrews and also showed infractions and fractures. In each tibia, on longitudinal section, the cortex appeared very thin throughout—in some places as thin as parchment. The periosteum showed nothing striking on the whole. The medullary cavity was expanded in many places and the marrow quite fatty throughout. The spongy trabeculae at the ends of the bones were thin, wide-meshed, and lined by flattened osteoblasts. Resorptive processes (partly expressed by the presence of osteoclasts) were not excessive anywhere. The epiphysial cartilage plates were still present. They were somewhat wavier than they would normally be. Endochondral ossification at these plates was not active, but in view of the age of the patient this is not surprising.

The skeleton described by Hektoen—that of a subject about 45 years old—reveals the extent to which deformation (especially of the long bones and the vertebral column) may go before the disease comes to a standstill. It also reveals, to a very pronounced degree, the peculiar calvarial abnormalities which persist even into adult life. In the case in question, the posterior and lateral regions of the cranial vault were composed of a mosaic of wormian bones, and some bones of this kind were found also in the vertical and orbital portions of the frontal region. In all, there were 172 wormian bones. They were generally star-shaped, and their interlacing processes traced on the external surface of the calvarium an extensive pattern of delicate inlaid work consisting of small flat bone islands separated by sutures. The pronounced recession of the face, also observed, was ascribed by Hektoen to the defective evolution of the teeth and consequent underdevelopment of the jaws.

The writer has examined anatomically the amputated lower extremities from a case of osteogenesis imperfecta in a girl 16 years of age. The limbs were so badly deformed as to make ambulation impossible, and the amputations (through the lower third of each thigh) had been done on this account. As was to be expected, the histologic architecture of the cortical bone was by no means so glaringly abnormal as it is in an affected infant. In particular, some of the osseous tissue was of the lamellar (fine-fibered) type. However, a good deal of it was still of the nonlamellar (coarse-fibered) type. In this connection it should be emphasized that in a normal subject, by the age of 4, the cortex of a bone already consists

Figure 36

A, Photomicrograph ($\times$ 18) showing part of a rib of a somewhat premature stillborn neonate with osteogenesis imperfecta. Note the presence of a recent fracture at the costochondral junction, the sparsity of spongy trabeculae in that region, and the meagerness of the cortical bone.

B, Photomicrograph ($\times$ 65) showing the status of endochondral ossification at an epiphysial-diaphysial junction (lower end of tibia) from a case of osteogenesis imperfecta in a full term neonate who died 2 days after birth. Note that the cartilage cells are lined up in columns as they normally would be, that the cartilage matrix in the vicinity of the junctional area is calcified, and that cores of calcified cartilage matrix extend into the bone shaft. On the other hand, only a meager amount of osseous tissue has been deposited on these cores. (Compare with Fig. 4-*B*, which represents the status of endochondral ossification at an epiphysial-diaphysial junction in an unaffected fetus of only 16 weeks.)

C, Photomicrograph ($\times$ 65) illustrating the histologic architecture of the cortex of a rib from a case of osteogenesis imperfecta fetalis in a fetus stillborn near term. Note that the cortical bone in question is composed entirely of nonlamellar osseous tissue and that the amount of osseous tissue is very meager. This picture corresponds to what one would observe in a rib cortex from an unaffected fetus of about 10 weeks. (Compare with Fig. 3-*C*, which represents the status of a tibial shaft cortex from a fetus of about 12 weeks.)

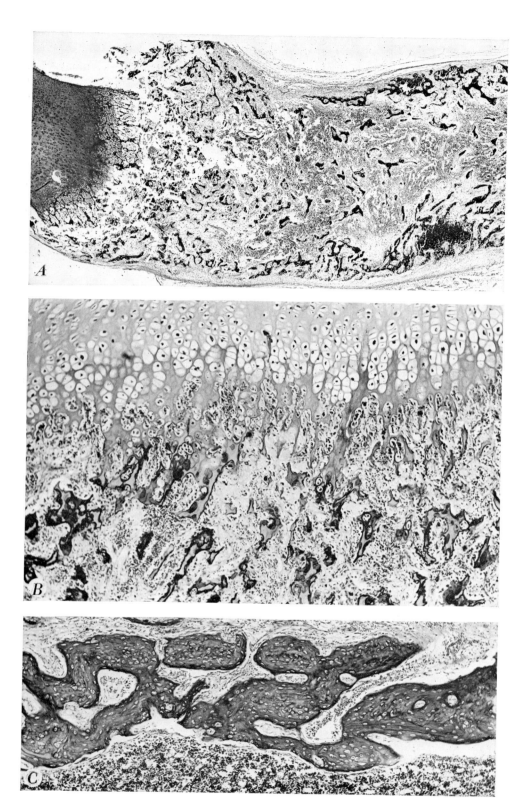

Figure 36

entirely of lamellar osseous tissue. Furthermore, in the 16 year old girl in question, the cortical bone failed to show the full organization of the osseous tissue into haversian systems which is already so conspicuous in the cortical bone of normal adolescents and young adults. (See Fig. 37.)

GENETIC AND PATHOGENETIC ASPECTS

It has been known for a long time that in cases of osteogenesis imperfecta it is often possible to trace the condition back in the family of the subject. In fact, recognition of a hereditary basis for the bone fragility dates from about 1788 (see Ekman). The next important step in our knowledge of the genetic aspects of the disorder was not made until 1896. At that time, Spurway showed that victims of hereditary bone fragility also present hereditary blue sclerae. Since then, evidence has also accumulated to the effect that bone fragility may be genetically linked with progressive deafness and hyperlaxity of joints. Thus Bell, who made a statistical study of the inheritance of blue sclerotics, found that, of 400 subjects presenting this condition, approximately 60 per cent had an associated liability to fracture, 60 per cent had an associated otosclerosis, and 44 per cent suffered from all three defects. The data on hyperlaxity of joints were not found sufficient to permit evaluation of that aspect of the disease in the present connection. Other workers evaluating groups of affected families have reached the same conclusions as to the relative incidence of these various aspects of the disorder (see Fuss, and Hills and McLanahan).

In any event, as noted, the disease complex is inherited as an autosomal dominant. In particular, it is clear that, if a male or female subject suffering from osteogenesis imperfecta survives into adult life and becomes a parent, the offspring are very likely to present blue sclerae, either alone or in combination with one or more of the following: bone fragility, progressive deafness, and hyperlaxity of joints. However, the offspring of a person affected with osteogenesis imperfecta may show bone fragility by itself. Holcomb reports on a family tree in which he traced osteogenesis imperfecta through five generations and found it manifested consistently as bone fragility alone. On the other hand, the child of a parent who presents merely blue sclerae may show blue sclerae alone or blue sclerae and bone fragility, perhaps in association with deafness or hyperlaxity of joints.

Furthermore, it should be noted in regard to the genetic aspects of the disorder that an isolated instance of fetal or delayed osteogenesis imperfecta may crop up as a mutation in a family whose pedigree over several generations reveals no evi-

Figure 37

A, Photomicrograph ($\times$ 100) showing the histologic architecture of part of the cortex of a tibia from a case of osteogenesis imperfecta in a child $3\frac{1}{2}$ years of age. Note that considerable amounts of primitive (nonlamellar) osseous tissue are still present, and that no well-organized haversian systems are to be observed. Normally, in a subject 3 years of age, nonlamellar osseous tissue is no longer present in the cortex of a long tubular bone. (Compare with Fig. 14-A and B.)

B, Photomicrograph ($\times$ 100) illustrating the architecture of the cortex of a tibia from the case of an affected girl 16 years of age whose deformed leg bones are shown in Figure 35-B. Note that even at this age the cortex fails to show the normal organization into haversian systems composed of lamellar osseous tissue. Note also that a considerable amount of the cortical bone still consists of nonlamellar (primitive) osseous tissue. (Compare with Fig. 18-E.)

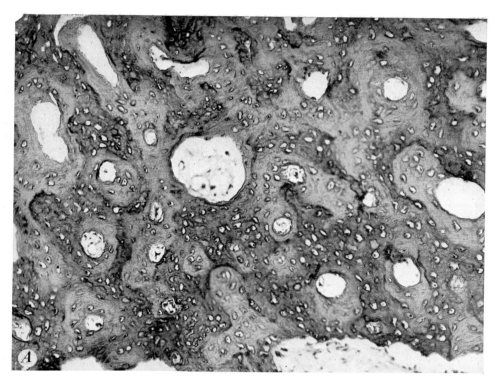

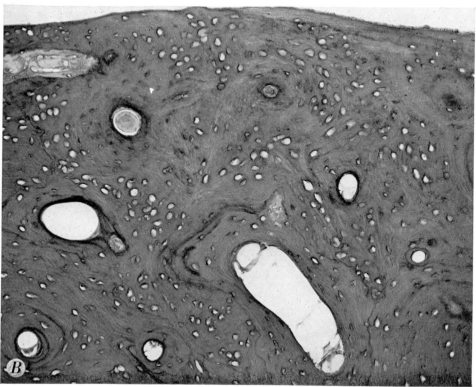

Figure 37

dences of the disease. It is, of course, these isolated instances that constitute the point of departure for new series of cases in descendants of the affected subjects. Conditions similar to osteogenesis imperfecta in man have also been described as occurring in various animals (see Inderbitzin, Scott *et al.*, and Lettow and Dämmrich).

The pathogenetic basis for the various manifestations of osteogenesis imperfecta has long been related to a hereditary inferiority of the mesenchyme. Bauer (one of the early proponents of this conception) held that all the connective tissues which arise from the mesenchyme are inferior in the condition in question. That is, he maintained that the abnormality involves not only the calcified connective tissue (the osseous tissue) but also the various other connective tissues. He stated that in the nonskeletal supporting connective tissue the fibroblasts are small and the intercellular fibrils tend to be too short and to run a crooked course. In the latter relation, Follis has shown that in cases of osteogenesis imperfecta fetalis the corium of the skin is strikingly defective in respect to the formation of collagen. In particular, he noted that in the corium the expected transformation of reticulum fibrils into collagen fibers fails to take place. All evidence thus indicates that the fundamental aberration underlying the disease relates to the defectiveness of formation, organization, and chemical composition of the body's collagen.

REFERENCES

Aub, J. C., and Farquharson, R. F.: Studies of Calcium and Phosphorus Metabolism. XV. In Various Metabolic and Bone Diseases, J. Clin. Invest., *11*, 235, 1932.

Baker, S. L.: Hyperplastic Callus Simulating Sarcoma in Two Cases of Fragilitas Ossium, J. Path. & Bact., *58*, 609, 1946.

Banta, J. V., Schreiber, R. R. and Kulik, W. J.: Hyperplastic Callus Formation in Osteogenesis Imperfecta Simulating Osteosarcoma, J. Bone & Joint Surg., *53-A*, 115, 1971.

Bauer, K. H.: Über Osteogenesis imperfecta. Zugleich ein Beitrag zur Frage einer allgemeinen Erkrankung sämtlicher Stützgewebe, Deutsche Ztschr. Chir., *154*, 166, 1920.

————: Über Identität und Wesen der sogenannten Osteopsathyrosis idiopathica und Osteogenesis imperfecta. Zugleich ein Beitrag zur Konstitutionspathologie chirurgischer Krankheiten, Deutsche Ztschr. Chir., *160*, 289, 1920.

Bell, J.: Blue Sclerotics and Fragility of Bone. *Eugenics Laboratory Memoirs*, No. 24, London, Cambridge University Press, 1928.

Bodansky, A., and Jaffe, H. L.: Phosphatase Studies. III. Serum Phosphatase in Diseases of the Bone: Interpretation and Significance, Arch. Int. Med., *54*, 88, 1934.

Brailsford, J. F.: Osteogenesis Imperfecta, Brit. J. Radiol., *16*, 129, 1943.

Ekman, O. J.: Descriptio et casus aliquot osteomalaciae, Upsala, J. Edman, 1788.

Engfeldt, B., Engström, A., and Zetterström, R.: Biophysical Studies of the Bone Tissue in Osteogenesis Imperfecta, J. Bone & Joint Surg., *36-B*, 654, 1954.

Fahr, T.: Über Osteogenesis imperfecta, Virchows Arch. path. Anat., *261*, 732, 1926.

Fairbank, T.: *An Atlas of General Affections of the Skeleton*, Edinburgh & London, E. & S. Livingstone Ltd., 1951.

Fairbank, H. A. T., and Baker, S. L.: Hyperplastic Callus Formation, with or without evidence of a Fracture, in Osteogenesis Imperfecta, Brit. J. Surg., *36*, 1, 1948.

Follis, R. H., Jr.: Maldevelopment of the Corium in the Osteogenesis Imperfecta Syndrome, Bull. Johns Hopkins Hosp., *93*, 225, 1953.

————: Histochemical Studies on Cartilage and Bone. III. Osteogenesis Imperfecta, Bull. Johns Hopkins Hosp., *93*, 386, 1953.

Fuss, H.: Die erbliche Osteopsathyrose, Deutsche Ztschr. Chir., *245*, 279, 1935.

Gruber, G. B.: Zur Kenntnis und Kritik der Osteogenesis imperfecta congenitalis, Virchows Arch. path. Anat., *316*, 317, 1949.

Hansen, A. E.: Influence of Viosterol and Parathyroid Extract on Mineral Metabolism in Osteogenesis Imperfecta, Am. J. Dis. Child., *50*, 132, 1935.

Harbitz, F.: Ueber Osteogenesis imperfecta, Beitr. path. Anat., *30*, 605, 1901.

Hektoen, L.: Anatomical Study of a Short-limbed Dwarf, with Special Reference to Osteogenesis Imperfecta and Chondrodystrophia Foetalis, Am. J. M. Sc., *125*, 751, 1903.

Hills, R. G., and McLanahan, S.: Brittle Bones and Blue Scleras in Five Generations, Arch. Int. Med., *59*, 41, 1937.

HOLCOMB, D. Y.: A Fragile-Boned Family. Hereditary Fragilitas Ossium, J. Hered., *22*, 105, 1931.

INDERBITZIN, A.: Über Anosteoplasia congenita beim Kalbe, Virchows Arch. path. Anat., *269*, 665, 1928.

JECKELN, E.: Systemgebundene mesenchymale Erschöpfung. Eine neue Begriffsfassung der Osteogenesis imperfecta, Virchows Arch. path. Anat., *280*, 351, 1931.

JOHANSSON, S.: Ein Fall von Osteogenesis imperfecta mit verbreiteten Gefässverkalkungen, Acta radiol., *1*, 17, 1921.

KEY, J. A.: Brittle Bones and Blue Sclera. Hereditary Hypoplasia of the Mesenchyme, Arch. Surg., *13*, 523, 1926.

KLENERMAN, L., OCKENDEN, B. G. and TOWNSEND, A. C.: Osteosarcoma Occurring in Osteogenesis Imperfecta, J. Bone & Joint Surg., *49-B*, 314, 1967.

KNAGGS, R. L.: *The Inflammatory and Toxic Diseases of Bone*, Bristol, John Wright and Sons, Ltd., 1926.

LETTOW, E., and DÄMMRICH, K.: Beitrag zur Klinik und Pathologie der Osteogenesis imperfecta bei Junghunden, Zentralbl. Veterinärmed., *7*, 936, 1960.

LOBSTEIN, J. F.: *Traité d'anatomie pathologique*, Paris, F. G. Levrault, Vol. II, p. 204, 1833.

LOOSER, E.: Ueber Osteogenesis imperfecta tarda, Verhandl. deutsch. path. Gesellsch., *9*, 239, 1905.

McKUSICK, V. A.: *Heritable Disorders of Connective Tissue*, St. Louis, The C. V. Mosby Company, 1956.

MEYER, M.: Über Osteogenesis imperfecta congenita der Labyrinthkapsel, Ztschr. Hals-, Nasen- u. Ohrenh., *26*, 297, 1930.

RIESENMAN, F. R., and YATER, W. M.: Osteogenesis Imperfecta. Its Incidence and Manifestations in Seven Families, Arch. Int. Med., *67*, 950, 1941.

ROBERTS, E., and SCHOUR, I.: Hereditary Opalescent Dentine (Dentinogenesis Imperfecta), Am. J. Orthodontics, *25*, 267, 1939.

RUSHTON, M. A.: The Structure of the Teeth in a Late Case of Osteogenesis Imperfecta, J. Path. & Bact., *48*, 591, 1939.

SCHERR, D. D.: A Severely Deformed Patient with Osteogenesis Imperfecta at the Age of Fifty-four, J. Bone & Joint Surg., *46-A*, 159, 1964.

SCHWARZ, E.: Hypercallosis in Osteogenesis Imperfecta, Am. J. Roentgenol., *85*, 645, 1961.

SCOTT, P. P., McKUSICK, V. A. and McKUSICK, A. B.: The Nature of Osteogenesis Imperfecta in Cats, J. Bone & Joint Surg., *45-A*, 125, 1963.

SPURWAY, J.: Hereditary Tendency to Fracture, Brit. M. J., *2*, 844, 1896.

STEVENSON, G. H., and CUTHBERTSON, D. P.: Blue Sclerotics and Associated Defects. A Study of Four Families with Notes on their Mineral Metabolism, Lancet, *2*, 782, 1931.

STILLING, H.: Osteogenesis imperfecta. Ein Beitrag zur Lehre von der sogenannten fötalen Rachitis, Arch. path. Anat., *115*, 357, 1889.

SUMMER, G. K.: Oral Proline Tolerance in Osteogenesis Imperfecta, Science, *134*, 1527, 1961.

VROLIK, W.: *Tabulae ad illustrandam embryogenesin hominis et mammalium, tam naturalem quam abnormem*, Amsterdam, G. M. P. Londonck, 1849.

WEBER, M.: Osteogenesis imperfecta congenita der Labyrinthkapsel, Ztschr. Hals-, Nasen- u. Ohrenh., *25*, 345, 1930.

Chapter

7

Osteopetrosis

OSTEOPETROSIS is a relatively rare inborn disorder centered in the skeleton. The bones are abnormally heavy and compact, and appear radiopaque on x-ray examination. Because the bones tend to be brittle, some subjects suffer from repeated pathologic fractures. The condition is inheritable and is commonly transmitted as an autosomal recessive trait. In most instances of osteopetrosis, the skeletal aberration is already pronounced at birth. In these cases the affected neonate is often stillborn, and if born alive the infant usually does not survive for more than a few months. These early and severe expressions of osteopetrosis represent its so-called "malignant" form. In less severe expressions of this form of the disorder, the victim may even survive into early childhood. However, there are some cases of osteopetrosis in which the disease gives rise to so little clinical difficulty that the patient reaches adulthood (or perhaps middle life) before its presence is discovered. In these cases the disease may first come to light when an x-ray picture of a skeletal area is taken in connection with the occurrence of a fracture or for some other reason. These very mild expressions of osteopetrosis represent the so-called "benign" form of the disease.

Nomenclature.—The disorder is sometimes denoted as Albers-Schönberg's disease because it was he who established it as a clinical entity. The condition came to light through his finding of densely radiopaque bones in a young adult who had suffered a fracture of a femur but who was apparently otherwise in good health, his case thus representing what would now be regarded as the "benign" form of the disease. Other names which have been used for the condition include "marble bone disease" ("Marmorkrankheit") and "osteosclerosis fragilis generalisata." However, the name now favored and in common use is "osteopetrosis," which emphasizes the stonelike hardness demonstrated by the affected bones, especially of adults.

CLINICAL CONSIDERATIONS

The disease has been observed in persons of various races, and may be inherited from either parent. There is no striking sex predilection, but males seem to predominate slightly among the subjects.

In many cases, as noted, the underlying skeletal involvement is already well developed at birth ("osteopetrosis fetalis"), and the affected fetus may be born dead or survive for only a few days. In such a case, if outward manifestations of the disease are lacking (hydrocephalus, for instance) and the neonate's skeleton has not been examined roentgenographically, the presence of the condition may go undetected unless an autopsy which includes study of some of the bones is done. In other instances of osteopetrosis fetalis, the severely affected infant survives for some months or even into early childhood, but presents, in addition to radiopacity of the bones, such clinical manifestations as anemia, hepatomegaly, splenomegaly, lymphadenopathy, blindness, hydrocephalus, fractures, osteomyelitic foci, and sometimes even retardation of skeletal growth. Though varying from case to case, these clinical manifestations are all due directly or indirectly to the skeletal aberrations. (See McCune and Bradley, and Pines and Lederer.)

Cases in which the presence of the disease goes unrecognized until some time in childhood or even adult life may be regarded as belonging in the category of "osteopetrosis tarda." It seems almost certain that in these cases, too, the bones are already abnormal at birth. This may be inferred from the fact that some of these subjects give a history of having sustained a number of fractures, often from early childhood. However, in the very "benign" cases in which the presence of the disease is not uncovered until adult life is reached, it is highly probable that the skeletal changes are very slight at birth and only gradually become clearly evident roentgenographically. In a small proportion of these cases, certain of the common clinical expressions of the disease (fractures, anemia, optic atrophy, etc.) may be minimal or even absent (see Hinkel and Beiler).

A *fracture* is often the clinical manifestation that leads to the detection of a case of osteopetrosis. The first fracture may have occurred during early childhood, and other fractures are likely to occur later, if the subject continues to survive. On the other hand, some cases of so-called "benign" osteopetrosis have been reported in which no pathologic fractures have occurred. In connection with fractures, rather special interest attaches to a case which was followed for 24 years at one hospital. The patient had sustained 33 pathologic fractures, of which the first had taken place when he was 3 years of age (see Hasenhuttl).

The fractures are usually clean transverse breaks which occur upon relatively slight provocation, and are dependent mainly upon the brittleness of the petrous bones. The shafts of the long tubular bones of the limbs are the most common sites of the fractures, and a given bone may undergo several of them in the course of some years. The fractures usually heal at about the normal rate, and abundant callus is produced in the course of healing.

The development of an *anemia*, varying in degree from case to case, is intimately related to the bone changes. However, though it is essentially a myelophthisic anemia, its severity does not necessarily parallel the extent of the osteopetrosis demonstrable roentgenographically. It has also been suggested that in some cases the anemia is at least partly hemolytic in origin (see Engfeldt *et al.*). Especially if the anemia is severe, the spleen, liver, and superficial lymph nodes may be found enlarged. When such cases come to autopsy, foci of hematopoietic tissue are almost regularly found in these and other organs. Even if the anemia is not severe at first, it tends to become so as the disease progresses, though it does not necessarily do so. When it does, the number of red blood cells may become greatly reduced and include many macrocytes. Furthermore, the anemia is usually of the hypochromic variety, the color index being less than 1. The platelets, too, may become greatly reduced in number, and purpuric phenomena may appear shortly before death. In addition, especially in infants and young children, there may be a very decided terminal rise in the total leukocyte count, and large numbers of normoblasts and megaloblasts may appear in the blood.

The clinical manifestations due to *injury of intracranial structures*, ensuing from involvement of the bones of the base of the skull, are very important. More or less pronounced optic atrophy is a common finding. It seems to be due to compression of the optic nerves from narrowing of the optic foramina and/or from a pachymeningitis. The resultant defects of vision range from moderate loss of acuity to complete blindness. The visual defect is often associated with nystagmus. In occasional instances there are also manifestations (deafness, facial and ocular palsies,

Osteopetrosis

etc.) attributable to injury of other cranial nerves, apparently likewise from intraforaminal compression. Furthermore, enlargement of the head, ascribable in most instances to *hydrocephalus*, has been observed rather frequently, especially in affected neonates and in cases already diagnosed in infancy. In many of these cases the pressure of the spinal fluid has been found definitely elevated. However, there seems to be no single cause or uniform explanation for the hydrocephalus. The encroachment of the sella turcica upon the pituitary gland may lead to *hypopituitarism* (see p. 341). This helps to explain why, in some cases of osteopetrosis, the subjects are subnormal in stature and sexually underdeveloped, and why even those who reach adult life may show undue persistence of their epiphysial cartilage plates.

The appearance of an *osteomyelitic focus* is a very curious clinical manifestation rather frequently encountered in osteopetrosis. The osteomyelitis occurs most commonly in the jaw bones (especially the mandible) and may follow upon the extraction of a tooth (see Shallow *et al.*). When these bones are involved, the infection is quite likely to be a severe one, associated with fistulation and often with sequestration of bone fragments. Finally, it may be pointed out that, especially in younger subjects, the *teeth* are generally delayed in eruption and carious.

Biochemical Findings.—The serum calcium and inorganic phosphate values are ordinarily within the normal range in cases of osteopetrosis. Our own experience is in accord with these general findings. However, there are reports of some cases in which the serum calcium and inorganic phosphate values were found reduced and, on the other hand, of cases in which the serum calcium value was reported as being elevated. The serum alkaline phosphatase value is usually also within the normal range. The value was within this range in the case of an adult subject who was under treatment in our hospital, while in another of our cases (that of a youth 16 years of age) the serum alkaline phosphatase value was definitely elevated (see Bodansky and Jaffe).

In the evaluation of the mineral content of the bones in cases of osteopetrosis, it should be borne in mind that these bones are more compact (that is, of greater weight per unit volume) than normal bones. Thus it is not surprising that they have a somewhat greater mineral content than corresponding normal bones. In regard to the metabolism of calcium and phosphorus in osteopetrosis, the available data are meager. It has been suggested that there is an increased retention of absorbed calcium and phosphorus by the affected infants, but this has not been convincingly demonstrated. On the other hand, it does appear to be established that the urinary excretion of calcium is reduced in these cases, and that the propor-

Figure 38

A, Roentgenograph showing an innominate bone and some bones of the corresponding lower extremity removed at autopsy from a child 21 months of age affected with osteopetrosis. Note the striking general radiopacity of the bones, the faint, relatively radiolucent lines following the contour of the ilium, and a few similar lines extending transversely across the lower end of the femur and upper end of the tibia. (See also Fig. 40-*A*, which illustrates the gross appearance of this femur and tibia in sagittal section.)

B, Roentgenograph showing the hip area in the case of a girl 9½ years of age in whom osteopetrosis was known to have been already present in early childhood. At the age of 4, the child had incurred a pathologic fracture of the right ulna, and at the age of 6, a pathologic fracture of the left humerus. Note the lack of architectural detail (absence of cortical and spongiosa markings) and the almost uniform radiopacity of the bones. A narrow, relatively radiolucent zone following the contour of the ilium is to be observed below its upper margin.

C, Roentgenograph demonstrating the radiopacity of the bones of a knee area in the case illustrated in *B.* (See also Fig. 39-*A* and *C.*)

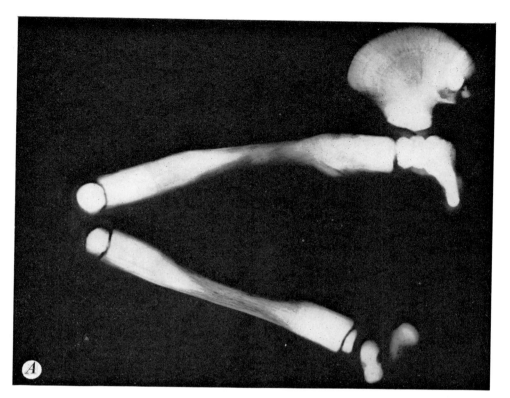

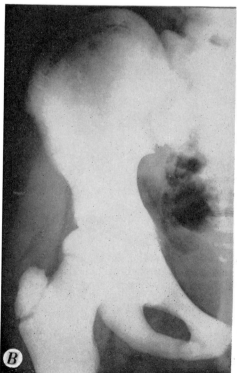

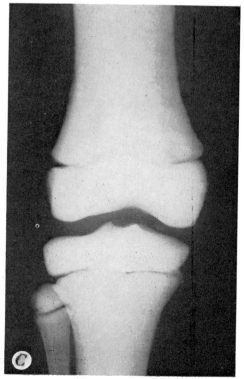

Figure 38

tion of urinary to fecal excretion is much smaller than it would normally be. (See Kramer *et al.*, Dent *et al.*, and Pincus *et al.*)

ROENTGENOGRAPHIC FINDINGS

Whether or not the clinical manifestations already suggest it, the diagnosis of osteopetrosis in the living subject is usually made on the basis of roentgenographic examination of the bones. (See Figs. 38 and 39.) The examination may have been instigated simply in the hope of clarifying a puzzling clinical picture presented by the subject. Or, instead, it may have been undertaken in connection with the routine management of a fracture (pathologic) in a patient who did not yet present any other clinical manifestations of the disease. When once a clue suggesting the disease has been obtained and the entire skeleton is roentgenographed, the diagnosis usually no longer remains in doubt. In fact, it was by its peculiar roentgenographic manifestations that the disease first attracted the attention of Albers-Schönberg in 1904. His patient, who lived to be 49 years of age, was already 26 when first studied, and even then the bones were roentgenographed merely because of a fracture of the femur, the patient being otherwise apparently in good health at that time. It was only after the report on this case had appeared in the literature that the severe (malignant) cases in infancy and childhood, presenting roentgenographic bone changes similar to those described by Albers-Schönberg in his adult case, were recognized as instances of the same disorder (see Assmann).

What is roentgenographically characteristic of the bones in this disease is the exaggerated opacity of the shadows which they cast. The more uniformly white and opaque these shadows are, the more severe is the involvement which they reflect. When the bones are extensively implicated, the architectural details in many or most of them may be so obscured that it is no longer possible to distinguish roentgenographically between corticalis and spongiosa, and in affected long tubular bones, even the major marrow cavities may no longer be clearly discernible.

In the *skull*, changes are consistently found at the base of the cranial cavity, The entire base may appear thickened, the sinuses more or less encroached upon.

Figure 39

A, Roentgenograph showing the lumbar vertebrae in the case of osteopetrosis in the 9½ year old girl about whom some clinical information has already been given in connection with Figure 38-*B*. Note, in relation to the vertebral bodies, the beginnings of a zone of relative radiolucency traversing the midsection of each body. Otherwise, these bodies are densely radiopaque.

B, Roentgenograph showing a number of the lower thoracic vertebrae in a case of "benign" osteopetrosis. Note the sandwich-like appearance of the vertebral bodies created by the presence of an upper and lower radiopaque zone separated by a clear-cut central radiolucent zone. The patient was a man 60 years of age (case II in the article by Hinkel and Beiler) who had no relevant complaints before the age of 55. At that time he began to suffer from pain and limitation of motion of the hip joints, and it was roentgenographic examination of the hips that first disclosed the presence of the disease. An arthroplasty replacement of the head of the left femur was done, and Dr. Beiler submitted to the writer for study a slice of that femoral head, along with a number of roentgenographs from this case. (See also *D* and Figure 41-*A*, *B*, and *C*.)

C, Roentgenograph of a hand from the case illustrated in *A*. Note the striking and almost uniform radiopacity presented by many of the bones.

D, Roentgenograph of a hand from the case illustrated in *B*. It is in the carpal bones that the radiopacity is most striking. Note that at the periphery of these bones there is a narrow zone of relative radiolucency creating a "bone-in-bone" effect.

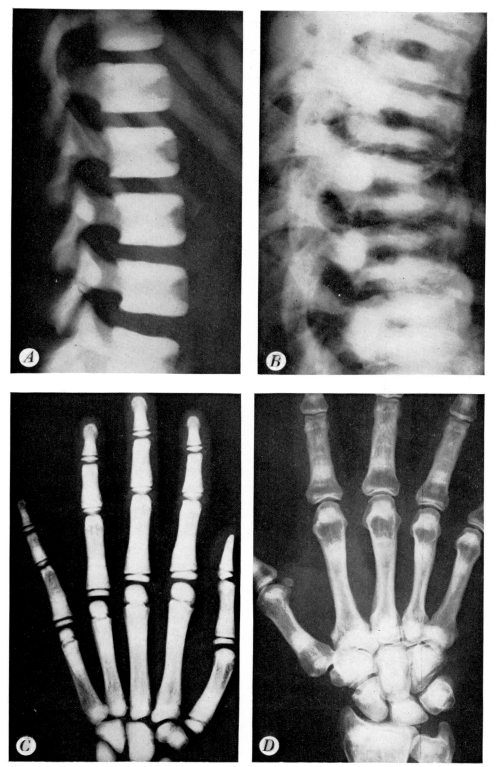

Figure 39

and the various cranial foramina also narrowed.   The sella turcica in particular usually shows pronounced thickening of its floor and also of its posterior clinoids. The resultant narrowing of the pituitary fossa and consequent compression of the pituitary gland may induce some degree of hypopituitarism (see p. 341), which may already be manifest in surviving affected infants.   Extensive alterations are often also observed in the jaw bones (especially the maxillae).

The *vertebral column*, even of an affected neonate, may already show roentgenographic deviations from the normal.   In subjects of all ages, it is in the vertebral bodies that the changes are most pronounced.   In a neonate or young infant, the vertebral bodies, though radiopaque on the whole, already show a somewhat more radiolucent zone extending horizontally across each body along the path of the main branches of the central veins.   In older children this zone of relative radiolucency is wider and stands out more clearly.   In adults the transverse zones of radiolucency traversing the vertebral bodies and separating their upper and lower zones of radiopacity are often so clear-cut as to impart a "sandwich-like" appearance to the individual bodies.   Of the *other trunk bones*, the innominate bones are likely to show the most striking changes roentgenographically.

In the *bones of the extremities*, the changes tend strongly to be bilateral and symmetrical.   However, the extent and severity of involvement of these bones may vary from case to case, though, on the whole, those of the lower limbs are the ones most heavily affected.   In any event, the metacarpals and metatarsals are often less strikingly radiopaque than the long bones of the respective extremities, and under these circumstances the phalanges are generally the least affected of the tubular bones.   The carpal and tarsal bones may be uniformly radiopaque.   On the other hand, they may present large central cores of radiopacity surrounded by rather narrow peripheral zones of relative radiolucency.

Especially in subjects who have survived at least for some years and in whom the bone changes are milder, roentgenography may reveal alternating lighter and darker bands in some of the bones, despite their generally increased opacity.   In long bones these bands run transversely and are found mainly in the metaphyses. In flat bones and small roundish ones, the bandlike shadows tend to follow the bone outlines.   Furthermore, certain of the long bones may show expansion at one end and thus present a clublike appearance.   In addition, the long bones of the lower extremities may be somewhat curved.   In some cases this curvature may be sufficient to account for the shortness of stature or may contribute to it along with the hypopituitarism.

PATHOLOGIC FINDINGS

Most of the reports relating to the pathologic changes in the bones in cases of osteopetrosis pertain to the findings in stillborn neonates and in young infants who

Figure 40

A, Photograph of the sagittally sectioned bones of a lower extremity from the case of an affected child 21 months of age. (Fig. 38-*A* illustrates the roentgenographic appearance of these bones.) Neither the femur nor the tibia shows a clear-cut major marrow cavity.   The interior of the shafts of both of these bones is almost entirely occupied by rather closely compacted osseous tissue.   It is only in the midshaft of the tibia that this tissue is still somewhat loose-meshed, and in that area the shaft cortex is still clearly delimited.

B, Photomicrograph ($\times$ 65) illustrating the histologic architecture of the compacted osseous tissue in the interior of the shaft of the femur.   There is relatively little myeloid tissue in the marrow spaces.   The clearly distinguishable cartilage matrix appears light gray. Within the cartilage matrix and bordering upon it, one can note small, dark, agglomerating blobs representing primitive osseous tissue.

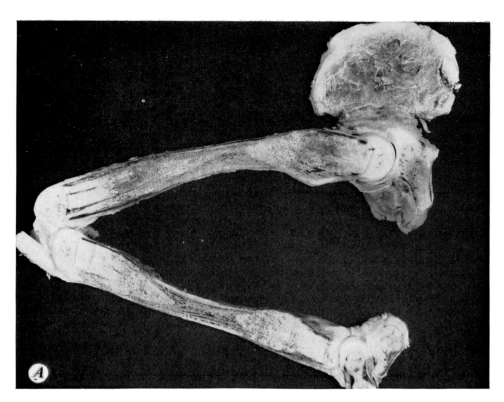

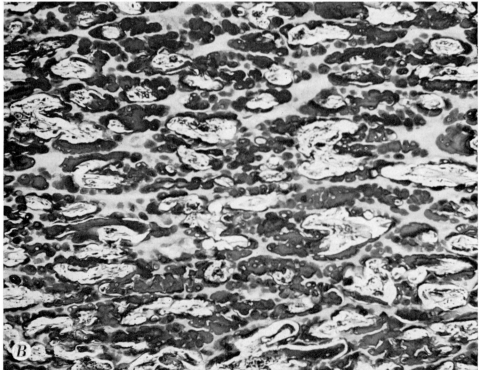

Figure 40

have succumbed to the disease. Anatomic studies relating to the bones of older children affected with osteopetrosis are less numerous, and those dealing with the status of the bones in subjects who have survived into adult life are few indeed. (See Dijkstra, Büchner, Laubmann, Gerstel, Zawisch, and Pines and Lederer.) The present writer's own experience with the pathologic anatomy of the skeletal aberrations observed in the disease is based on examination of bones removed at autopsy from four stillborn neonates and bone specimens removed surgically (for one reason or another) from one older child and three adults. In regard to the three adults, one of the specimens came from a case in the series reported by Hinkel and Beiler, another represented material removed in the case reported by Hasen-huttl, and the third came from a case treated at our own hospital. The following presentation of the pathologic findings in osteopetrosis deals only with the skeletal abnormalities.

Neonates and Young Infants.—On *gross examination* it will be found first of all that, though not much altered in shape or size, the bones removed from such affected subjects are excessively heavy. When the bones are cut open, one is struck by the large amount of more or less compacted osseous tissue which is present in the interior of the bones. (See Fig. 40.) This tissue may be so densified and may have crowded out the myeloid marrow so extensively that the cut bone surface has a grayish color only mottled with red. In certain bones the cortex may appear definitely thickened by periosteal bone apposition. In others, much or all of it may have merged so completely with the osseous tissue occupying the interior of the bone that it is no longer recognizable as a distinct cortex. The periosteum in general is easily detachable, though where periosteal bone apposition is in progress it may be somewhat thickened.

On sectioning various bones of the trunk, it appears that in these bones, too, compacted osseous tissue (rather than loose-meshed spongy bone) is present in the interior of the bones. In fact, in certain of these bones—notably, the vertebrae—the changes may be even more striking than in the long tubular bones. In infant subjects the ribs frequently show beading at the costochondral junctions. The calvarium and the base of the cranium are usually distinctly thickened and somewhat more compact than they would normally be. Finally, if centers of postnatal ossification are examined, it appears that, in addition to being perhaps somewhat retarded in their development, they are also composed of rather compacted osseous tissue and not of normal loose-meshed spongiosa.

On *microscopic examination*, too, the appearance presented by the bones of the neonate and infant subjects is striking. At sites of very active endochondral ossification (costochondral junctions of ribs and epiphysial-diaphysial junctions of long tubular bones), the zone of proliferating cartilage is abnormally wide. However, this finding is not to be taken as an indication of the presence of actual rickets superimposed upon the osteopetrosis. Instead, the cartilage cells accumulate to constitute the wide proliferating zone, because the tongues of calcified cartilage matrix formed at the sites of endochondral ossification persist instead of being resorbed in the normal way. However, what is even more conspicuous is that the compacted intramedullary osseous tissue contains cores of calcified cartilage matrix even at considerable distances from the sites of endochondral bone formation. In fact, calcified cartilage matrix cores are to be observed in the intramedullary osseous tissue even in the midshaft region of the long tubular bones, for instance. The cores of calcified cartilage matrix persist in all the bones formed by endochondral ossification, even if the affected infant survives to reach childhood or adult life.

The osseous tissue present in relation to these cartilage cores is peculiar in several ways. It is present on the surfaces of the cores and within them as small confluent blobs of primitive (nonlamellar) osseous tissue. In the writer's opinion, these frag-

ments of osseous tissue, and especially those which form in the interior of the cartilage cores, develop as a result of osseous metaplasia of the cartilage rather than
through the activity of osteoblasts. Whether in the interior of the cartilage cores or
on their surfaces, the osseous tissue is rather poor in cells. As they grow larger,
the bloblike fragments of osseous tissue tend to fuse into larger masses. What is
also remarkable in the course of the intramedullary bone formation in osteopetrosis is the sparsity of active osteoblasts and the almost complete absence of
osteoclasts. Indeed, there is hardly any evidence of osteoclastic resorption, so
prominent in connection with the continuous remodeling process under normal
conditions of endochondral bone formation. Finally, it should be noted that, though
the marrow spaces in the intramedullary osseous tissue are minute, they usually
still contain small amounts of hematopoietic elements and but little connective
tissue. That is, in affected neonates and young infants, while the myeloid marrow
is strikingly reduced in amount, it is not extensively scarred by fibrous tissue
replacement.

In bone formed through intramembranous ossification, one does not, of course,
find calcified cartilage matrix. Also, the osseous tissue formed in this way is
histologically less atypical than the endochondrally formed bone. In an affected
neonate or young infant, the calvarium, for instance, will be found to be composed
of broad, compacted trabeculae of osseous tissue. Furthermore, it will already
show a good deal of mature (lamellar) osseous tissue outlining the diploic spaces.
In relation to the tubular bones, for instance, the cortical osseous tissue laid down
beneath the periosteum will be found to be largely nonlamellar, though some
lamellar osseous tissue, also, will be present about the haversian spaces.

Older Children and Adults.—The skeletal abnormalities underlying osteopetrosis
in older children and adults are of the same order as those presented by the neonates
and young infants. (See Figs. 41 and 42.) Thus, in these older subjects, too, the
interior of the bones is found, on gross examination, to be substantially occupied by
grayish yellow, closely compacted bony tissue. On microscopic examination the
compacted bony tissue in the interior of an affected tubular bone, for instance,
will be found to present a striking histologic similarity to the corresponding tissue
in an analogous bone of a neonate. On the basis of histologic examination of a
femoral head from an adult affected with the benign form of osteopetrosis, the
writer estimates that definitely more than half of the tissue occupying the interior
of the femoral head consisted of sheets and trabeculae of calcified cartilage matrix.
Within the cartilage matrix and on the surface of its trabeculae, osseous tissue was
present.

In this adult subject (as in the neonate and infant subjects), the osseous tissue
consisted largely of confluent blobs of nonlamellar bone. Again, it was clearly
evident that much of this bone had developed as a result of bony metaplasia of the
cartilage matrix rather than through the activity of osteoblasts. In fact, although
many tissue blocks from the femoral head in question were embedded and sectioned,
the tissue slides prepared from these blocks again showed practically no osteoblasts
and also a striking lack of osteoclasts. Furthermore, because the tissue fluids
apparently could not reach the compacted osseous tissue to nourish it adequately,
many of the bone cell lacunae were empty, and undoubtedly much of the osseous
tissue was in a state of aseptic necrosis.

GENETIC AND PATHOGENETIC CONSIDERATIONS

Concerning the *genetic aspects* of osteopetrosis, it is well known that the subjects
are frequently the offspring of consanguineous marriages. When this is the case,

the parents have usually been recorded either as first cousins or vaguely as "cousins." Under these circumstances, the disease is rather likely to be manifest at birth and not infrequently takes the so-called "malignant" form. However, the offspring of a consanguineous marriage in which even one of the mates is affected with the disease may nevertheless show the disorder in its "benign" form (see Montgomery and Standard). The validity of consanguinity as a factor in the disease and the likelihood that several children in the same family will be affected are strikingly illustrated in the report by Kudrjawtzewa. The latter presents the record of a family in which osteopetrosis appeared in 3 out of 5 children of a consanguineous marriage, although in previous marriages with unrelated persons each of the parents had had only normal children. Furthermore, if a subject having the disease survives into adult life and becomes a parent, the disease may be transmitted to the offspring, even though the marriage is a nonconsanguineous one (see Pirie). Also, McPeak reports 8 cases occurring in three generations of one family.

Severely affected subjects do not reach maturity and hence do not transmit the disorder. However, as has been indicated, the condition is inheritable and seems to be transmitted mainly as an autosomal recessive trait. That the disease tends to be genetically recessive is strongly suggested by the fact that, in the majority of the cases in which osteopetrosis takes the clinically "benign" form, one cannot find evidence of the disorder in either the ancestors or the offspring of the affected subjects. Nevertheless, the possibility of an irregular dominant genetic factor is raised by the occurrence of some "parent-offspring" cases. Hereditary osteopetrosis has also been observed in rabbits (see Pearce and Brown, and Pearce). In these rabbits the disease was transmitted as a recessive trait, was present at birth, and was invariably fatal by the fourth or fifth week of life. The pathologic findings in the bones of the affected animals showed a remarkable resemblance to the findings in the bones of human neonates and young infants affected with the disease. Osteopetrosis has also been observed in chickens, and in them, too, the pathologic features are similar to those seen in humans (see Biltz and Pellegrino, and also Holmes).

The *pathogenesis* of the basic aberration in osteopetrosis has not yet been fully clarified. That the disease involves the bones preformed in cartilage as well as those not so preformed (the "membrane bones") is well known. However, as already

Figure 41

A, Roentgenograph showing the right hip area in the case of a man 60 years of age affected with "benign" osteopetrosis. Some clinical information relating to this patient is given in connection with Figure 39-*B*. Note the striking radiopacity of the femoral head and also the evidence of osteoarthritic changes at the hip joint. Several concentric zones of relative radiolucency can be observed at the upper end of the ilium.

B, Roentgenograph of two thin slices cut from the resection specimen of the femoral head shown in *A*.

C, Photomicrograph ($\times$ 65) illustrating the histologic appearance of the densely radiopaque femoral head slices shown in *B*. Note the large amount of persisting cartilage matrix, which appears light gray in the picture. The osseous tissue is nonlamellar and is also atypical otherwise.

D, Roentgenograph showing part of the right forearm and wrist from another case of "benign" osteopetrosis. The carpal bones are radiopaque, and in some of them there are outlining zones of relative radiolucency creating the effect of "bone-in-bone." Observe also the characteristic transverse radiolucent zones at the lower end of the radius. The patient was a man 58 years of age who had long been aware that he was affected with osteopetrosis. He had not suffered any pathologic fractures, but at the age of 10 he had been struck by an automobile and sustained a fracture at the upper end of the right femur. He did not know of any blood relationship between his parents. (See also Fig. 42.)

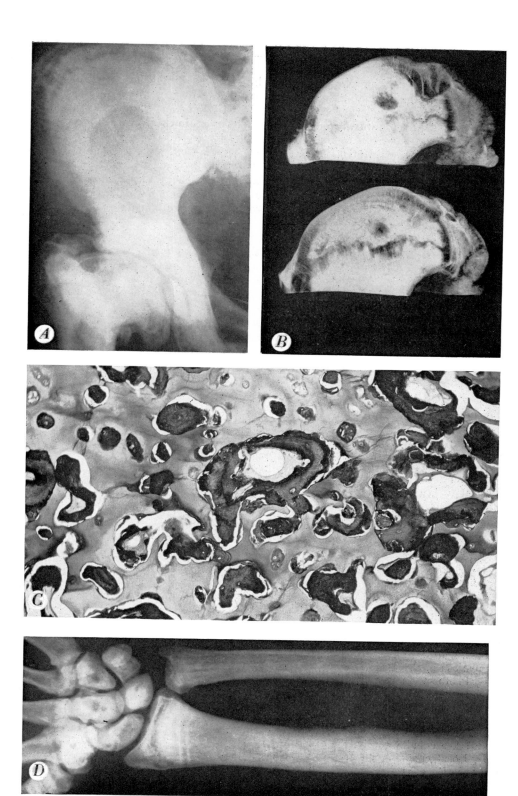

Figure 41

noted, the more striking changes are to be observed in the bones preformed in cartilage. The histologic hallmark of the disease in respect to these bones is the intramedullary accumulation and persistence of calcified cartilage matrix which, under normal circumstances, would have been resorbed in the process of growth and remodeling of the osseous tissue formed in the course of endochondral ossification. The osseous tissue deposited in and on the persisting cores of cartilage matrix is also atypical, as is the cortical osseous tissue formed through periosteal activity. Because of thickening of the bone cortices and the presence and persistence of large amounts of calcified cartilage matrix in the interior of the affected endochondrally formed bones, the latter in particular appear strikingly radiopaque on roentgenographic examination.

The general impression created by the histologic appearance of the bones in cases of osteopetrosis is that the pathogenetic mechanism underlying the aberration is primarily one of defective resorption. In the writer's opinion, too, there can be no doubt that the mechanism of resorption normally operative in relation to the pre- and postnatal growth and remodeling of the bones is profoundly disturbed in connection with the disorder. Indeed, on histologic examination of bone from affected neonates, a definite dearth of osteoclasts is to be noted, and in the bones of affected children and adults, osteoclasts may be so sparse that individual tissue sections may even fail to show any at all. It is true that the bones formed in the course of endochondral ossification show the presence of fairly large amounts of osseous tissue. However, one is struck by the fact that, to a considerable extent, the osteogenesis is not the result of osteoblastic activity. In fact, actively functioning osteoblasts are sparse, even if the affected bones come from a neonate. Much of the osseous tissue laid down in cases of osteopetrosis appears as the result of osseous metaplasia of cartilage rather than the activity of osteoblasts. When formed, this osseous tissue is nonlamellar (primitive) osseous tissue, and since it tends not to be remodeled, very little of it becomes transformed into lamellar (mature) osseous tissue. In summary, then, the writer holds that, in osteopetrosis, not only is the normal resorption mechanism disturbed, but the mechanism by which osseous tissue is normally laid down in the course of the development, growth, and maintenance of the bones is also disorganized.

Figure 42

A, Photograph illustrating the gross appearance of the cut surface of the resected right femoral head in a case of "benign" osteopetrosis. The subject was the man to whom reference was made in connection with Figure 41-D. Note that the osseous tissue is closely compacted, and that one cannot distinguish any trabecular architecture, such as is shown for comparison in B.

B, Photograph illustrating the gross appearance of the cut surface of a femoral head of an adult not affected with osteopetrosis, to illustrate the normal spongy trabecular architecture.

C, Roentgenograph of a slice about 3 mm. thick cut from the specimen shown in A. Note the striking radiopacity, and compare with D, which is a roentgenograph of a slice of about the same thickness cut from the specimen shown in B. The two roentgenographs (C and D) were taken simultaneously, the exposure time and kilovoltage used thus being the same.

D, Roentgenograph illustrating the spongy architecture of the normal femoral head shown in B.

E, Photomicrograph (× 65) demonstrating the histologic appearance of the compacted osseous tissue in the interior of the petrous femoral head shown in A. Note the presence of large fields of cartilage matrix and the atypical osseous tissue which has developed in that matrix, apparently by metaplasia.

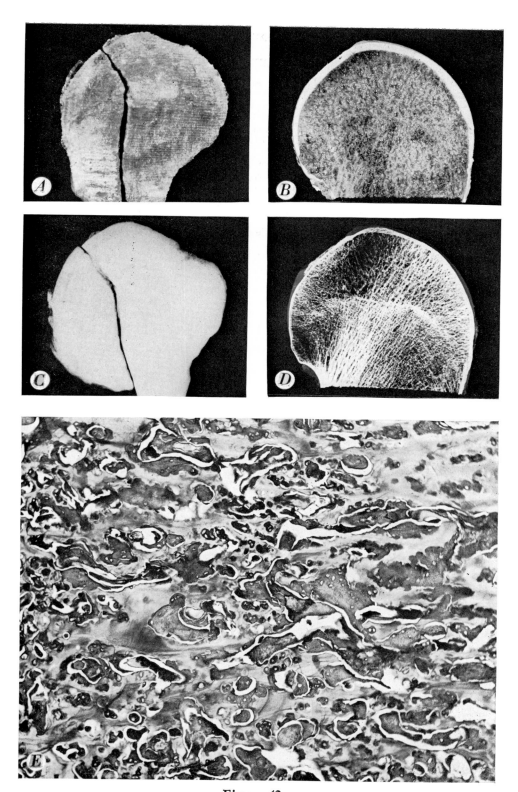

Figure 42

REFERENCES

Albers-Schönberg, H.: Röntgenbilder einer seltenen Knochenerkrankung, München. med. Wchnschr., *51*, 365, 1904.

————: Eine bisher nicht beschriebene Allgemeinerkrankung des Skelettes im Röntgenbild, Fortschr. Geb. Röntgenstrahlen, *11*, 261, 1907.

Assmann, H.: Beiträge zur osteosklerotischen Anämie, Beitr. path. Anat., *41*, 565, 1907.

Biltz, R. M., and Pellegrino, E. D.: Avian Osteopetrotic Bone, J. Bone & Joint Surg., *47-A*, 1365, 1965.

Bodansky, A., and Jaffe, H. L.: Phosphatase Studies. III. Serum Phosphatase in Diseases of the Bone: Interpretation and Significance, Arch. Int. Med., *54*, 88, 1934.

Büchner: Ueber Marmorknochenkrankheit (Nach Untersuchungen von Dr. Heidger), Zentralbl. allg. Path., *64*, 329, 1935.

Dent, C. E., Smellie, J. M., and Watson, L.: Studies in Osteopetrosis, Arch. Dis. Childhood, *40*, 7, 1965.

Dijkstra, O. H.: L'ostéogénèse dans la maladie des os marmoréens, Ann. anat. path., *12*, 131, 1935.

Engfeldt, B., Karlberg, P., and Zetterström, R.: Studies on the Skeletal Changes and on the Etiology of the Anaemia in Osteopetrosis, Acta path. et microbiol. scandinav., *36*, 10, 1955.

Gerstel, G.: Über die infantile Form der Marmorknochenkrankheit auf Grund vollständiger Untersuchung des Knochengerüstes, Frankfurt. Ztschr. Path., *51*, 23, 1937.

Hasenhuttl, K.: Osteopetrosis. Review of the Literature and Comparative Studies on a Case with a Twenty-four-Year Follow-up, J. Bone & Joint Surg., *44-A*, 359, 1962.

Hinkel, C. L., and Beiler, D. D.: Osteopetrosis in Adults, Am. J. Roentgenol., *74*, 46, 1955.

Holmes, J. R.: Radiological Changes in Avian Osteopetrosis, Brit. J. Radiol., *34*, 368, 1961.

————: Postmortem Findings in Avian Osteopetrosis, J. Comp. Path. & Therap., *71*, 20, 1961.

Kramer, B., Yuska, H., and Steiner, M. M.: Marble Bones. II. Chemical Analysis of Bone, Am. J. Dis. Child., *57*, 1044, 1939.

Kudrjawtzewa, N.: Über Marmorknochenkrankheit, Arch. klin. Chir., *159*, 658, 1930.

Laubmann, W.: Über die Knochenstruktur bei Marmorknochenkrankheit, Virchows Arch. path. Anat., *296*, 343, 1935.

McCune, D. J., and Bradley, C.: Osteopetrosis (Marble Bones) in an Infant: Review of the Literature and Report of a Case, Am. J. Dis. Child., *48*, 949, 1934.

McPeak, C. N.: Osteopetrosis: Report of Eight Cases Occurring in Three Generations of One Family, Am. J. Roentgenol., *36*, 816, 1936.

Montgomery, R. D., and Standard, K. L.: Albers-Schönberg's Disease. A Changing Concept, J. Bone & Joint Surg., *42-B*, 303, 1960.

Pearce, L.: Hereditary Osteopetrosis of the Rabbit. III. Pathologic Observations; Skeletal Abnormalities, J. Exper. Med., *92*, 591, 1950.

Pearce, L., and Brown, W. H.: Hereditary Osteopetrosis of the Rabbit. I. General Features and Course of Disease; General Aspects, J. Exper. Med., *88*, 579, 1948.

Pincus, J. B., Gittleman, I. F., and Kramer, B.: Juvenile Osteopetrosis: Metabolic Studies in Two Cases and Further Observations on the Composition of the Bones in This Disease, Am. J. Dis. Child., *73*, 458, 1947.

Pines, B., and Lederer, M.: Osteopetrosis: Albers-Schönberg Disease (Marble Bones). Report of a Case and Morphologic Study, Am. J. Path., *23*, 755, 1947.

Pirie, A. H.: The Development of Marble Bones, Am. J. Roentgenol., *24*, 147, 1930.

Shallow, T. A., Davis, W. B., and Farrell, J. T., Jr.: Osteopetrosis, Ann. Surg., *100*, 512, 1934.

Zawisch, C.: Marble Bone Disease. A Study of Osteogenesis, Arch. Path., *43*, 55, 1947.

Chapter

8

Achondroplasia

ACHONDROPLASIA is a skeletal disorder in which the subjects characteristically present: (1) a pronounced shortness of the extremities (micromelia), particularly striking in view of the fact that the trunk is only slightly stunted; and (2) some enlargement of the head, associated with a conspicuous depression at the root of the nose. Achondroplasia begins to develop very early in fetal life and appears to be dependent upon a primary disturbance of endochondral bone growth. By the seventh or eighth month of fetal life, the resultant skeletal abnormalities are already well developed. Indeed, the more severely affected fetuses usually die *in utero* near the end of gestation. However, if the fetus is born alive (and the neonate does not succumb in early infancy), the subject is quite likely to survive into adulthood or even into old age. In these milder cases of achondroplasia, the affected person is a malproportioned dwarf whose smallness and grotesqueness are associated with normal intelligence.

The condition (not a very rare one) may appear sporadically as a genetic mutation (in progeny of normal parents), and indeed, most instances of the disorder are to be accounted for in this way. However, there are also cases which occur on a hereditary basis, a surviving achondroplastic dwarf tending to transmit the disorder as a dominant character.

Nomenclature.—Achondroplastic dwarfs have played a rather strange and conspicuous role in human relations. For instance, they were modeled by the ancient Egyptians, apparently as gods. They have served as jesters in many old royal courts, and currently they often appear as circus freaks. Though such adult dwarfs have thus been familiar for many centuries, it was not until recent times that achondroplastic dwarfism in adults was brought into relation with the disorder as it appears in stillborn fetuses. Indeed, Parrot, in 1878, seems to have been the first to establish this association clearly, and it was he who gave to the condition as a whole the name "achondroplasia." Kaufmann, who studied fetal cases in particular, designated the condition in these cases as "chondrodystrophia fetalis." Both these names have their shortcomings, but "achondroplasia" seems preferable because of its broader applicability.

CLINICAL CONSIDERATIONS

The achondroplastic neonate (more often a female than a male) usually presents clear-cut manifestations calling attention to its abnormal skeleton. Specifically, the head is excessively large and the root of the nose is drawn in. The limbs, which are disfigured by rolls of fat, are, as noted, definitely short in proportion to the trunk. These manifestations are likely to be found particularly pronounced if, as is so frequently the case, the fetus has been born dead. (See Fig. 43.) Occasionally the limbs of a stillborn achondroplastic fetus are so extremely shortened as to suggest phocomelia; that is, the limbs appear like the flippers of seals (see Hughes

Jones). If the achondroplastic infant is born alive and has survived for a few days or weeks, the chances for its continued survival are already fairly good. If the subject is still alive at the end of the first year, the chances of survival into adulthood or even old age are approximately the same as those of a normal child. There is no *treatment* which is definitely known to increase the postnatal growth in those achondroplastics who continue to survive.

In the course of childhood, the disproportion between the trunk and the extremities tends to become increasingly pronounced, though the disproportionate largeness of the head does not. Except in regard to the skeleton, the achondroplastic child is likely to be fairly normal. For instance, it learns at the proper ages to walk and talk. Furthermore, the milk teeth and permanent teeth erupt at the proper time. Also, as adolescence approaches, the development of the primary and secondary sex characters shows itself to be normal.

By the time the subject reaches adulthood, his or her status as a dwarf has long been firmly established. Achondroplasia apparently underlies most cases of pathologic dwarfism encountered in adults. The adult achondroplastic is usually a little under 4 feet tall, though an individual subject may be several inches taller or shorter, in accordance with the severity of the defect. The lower extremities are likely to be of less than half the normal length, while the sitting height is ordinarily about two thirds of the normal. Thus the center of the body, which in the normal adult is at the level of the symphysis pubis, is shifted considerably upward. Muscularly, the adult achondroplastic is, as a rule, well developed and sometimes even particularly strong in view of the small size. In mental capacity, these subjects are generally average, though some are slightly below and some definitely above. However, they often suffer from emotional difficulties, probably representing affective reactions to their deformity.

In regard to the *short limbs* (micromelia) of the surviving achondroplastic, it should be pointed out first that the lower extremities are likely to be even more stunted than the upper. Indeed, the writer has observed a rather mildly affected adult subject in whom the lower extremities were so much the shorter that on casual observation the upper ones seemed almost normal in comparison. Further-

Figure 43

A, Photograph illustrating, in a neonate, the large head, depressed nasal bridge, and strikingly dwarfed extremities characteristic of achondroplasia.

B, A lateral view of the neonate shown in *A*, bringing out the pudginess of the shortened limbs. This is due to the fact that their soft tissues, relatively normal in amount, have had to accommodate themselves to limited space. (These two photographs represent material from the collection gathered by the eminent Viennese pathologist, the late Jakob Erdheim.)

C, Photograph of two stillborn neonates which have been sectioned longitudinally in the sagittal plane. The infant on the left (which is illustrated for purposes of comparison) is of normal length and proportions, while the one on the right is an achondroplastic. In regard to the length of their upper and lower extremities, the differences between the two neonates are obvious. In respect to length of the vertebral column, there is no obvious difference, but actual measurement revealed that the vertebral column of the "normal" neonate was 26.5 cm. in length, and that of the achondroplastic neonate 23 cm. Note that in the achondroplastic infant the foramen magnum is abnormally narrow, the centers of ossification for the vertebral bodies (as they appear in the longitudinal axis) are underdeveloped, and the sacrum is directed sharply backward.

D, Photograph of the macerated bones of one lower extremity of each of the two infants shown in *C*. The bones of the achondroplastic subject are easily identifiable by their small size and, in the case of the long tubular bones, also by their abnormal shape. (*C* and *D* are reproduced from the article by Knötzke, cited among the references.)

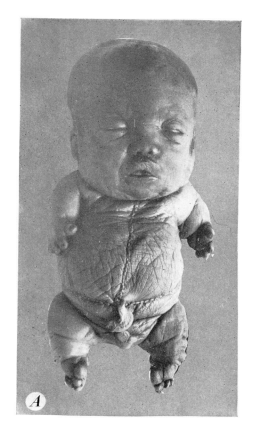
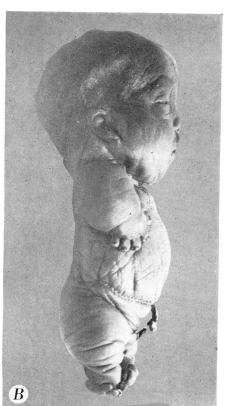
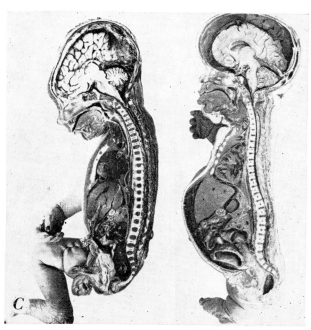
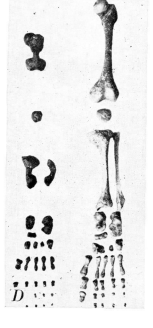

Figure 43

more, in each extremity it is the proximal segment that is more severely affected. Thus the arm is usually shorter than the forearm, and the thigh than the leg, while the normal ratio is the reverse. The hands and feet are also shortened, though relatively less so than the other portions of the extremities. The shortened fingers (except for the thumb) tend to approximate each other in length—that is, the normal differences between them in length may be obscured. Also, when the broad hand is stretched out, slight ulnar deviation is often revealed and the fingers tend to diverge in such a way that the impression of a trident (three-pronged effect) is created (see Marie). Finally, there is nearly always some limitation of extension at the elbow joints, and usually also some bowleggedness.

The large *head* of the subject has a greater transverse than anteroposterior diameter (that is, it is brachycephalic). The nose is usually of the "pug" variety, characterized by a conspicuous depression, or indentation, at the root. However, this depression may be absent in mild cases, as it was, for example, in the subject mentioned above, in whom the upper extremities appeared almost normal. (Such a case would seem to be well described as one of "attenuated achondroplasia.") When flattening of the face is pronounced, the alveolar process of the upper jaw is pushed forward, in consequence of the growth which has continued at the alveolar border to accommodate the teeth. Protrusion of the upper alveolar processes and the prominence of the lower jaw result in prognathism.

The *trunk* seems quite normal in comparison with the shortened limbs, although it, too, is really somewhat stunted. There is often a lower lumbar lordosis, which is sometimes associated with a low dorsal kyphosis. Because of the smallness of the pelvis and contraction of the pelvic inlet, pregnancy going to term in an achondroplastic woman necessitates cesarean section if the mother is to be saved. (See Fig. 44.)

Differential Diagnosis.—Clinical cases of achondroplasia rarely present any problems of differential diagnosis. In no type of pathologic dwarfism except achondroplasia does one find the peculiar disproportionate shortness of the extremities in relation to the trunk, and the depression at the root of the nose, in association

Figure 44

A, Frontal and lateral views of an achondroplastic girl 9 years of age. Note the depression of the root of the nose, the sharp lordotic angulation in the region of the lumbosacral junction, the shortness and pudginess of the limbs, and the bowing deformity of the lower extremities. The center of the body, instead of being at the level of the symphysis pubis, is actually somewhat above the umbilicus. The girl's parents showed no evidence of achondroplasia and there was no familial history of the disorder. (See Fig. 46-*A.*)

B, Lateral and frontal views of an achondroplastic man 28 years of age. All the external features of the disorder as shown in *A* are also represented here. In this case, too, the midpoint between the crown of the head and the soles of the feet was slightly above the umbilicus.

C, Photograph of a hand of an achondroplastic adult showing the typical three-pronged position ("main en trident") assumed by the fingers when these are held in extension.

D, Photograph illustrating the external conformation of three different types of dwarfs contrasted with a man of normal build. The normal man (on the extreme right) is 5 ft. 6½ in. tall. The two subjects immediately to the left are achondroplastic adults, the nearer one being 47 years of age and 4 ft. tall and the other 27 years of age and 3 ft. 9 in. tall. Next in line toward the left are two normally proportioned dwarfs. These ateleiotic dwarfs are 28 and 20 years of age respectively and measure respectively 3 ft. 4½ in. and 3 ft. 3 in. in height. The dwarfed subject on the extreme left is a female cretin 30 years of age. (This photograph is reproduced from the article on dwarfism by Rischbieth and Barrington in the *Eugenics Laboratory Memoirs,* No. 15, 1912, and the pertinent clinical information comes from the article by C. H. James which appeared in the Indian M. Gaz., **45,** 443, 1910.)

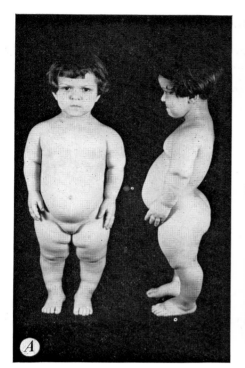

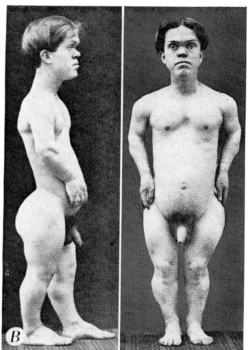

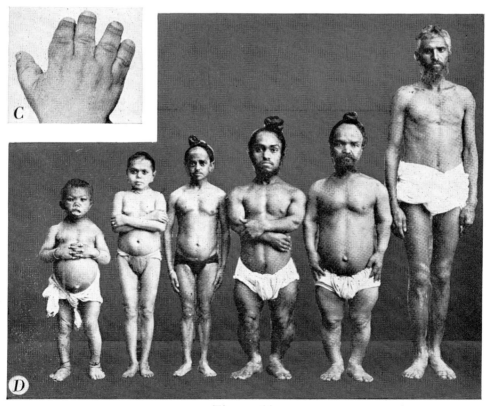

Figure 44

with good intelligence, normal sexual development, and normal health, if early infancy has been survived. Even in cases in which the disorder is present in attenuated form, roentgenographic examination almost always yields ample data for establishing the correct diagnosis. In such cases the punched-in appearance of the nose may be absent, but there is always some shortness of the limbs (especially of the lower) in comparison with the trunk. However, care must be exercised to distinguish attenuated achondroplasia from shortness of the limbs due to severe rickets in infancy and childhood.

On the basis of one or more of the characteristics listed above, achondroplasia is easily distinguishable from the pathologic dwarfism in children suffering from hypopituitarism (p. 341) or hypothyroidism (p. 346). Although a victim of mongolism exhibits dwarfism and brachycephaly as does the achondroplastic, the mongoloid subject is mentally retarded and sluggish (see Ingalls). There is also no likelihood of confusing achondroplastic subjects with those suffering from *ateleiosis* or *progeria*. In neither of the two latter conditions, and especially not in ateleiosis, is there any gross skeletal disproportion. Instead, the skeleton is merely rather uniformly, though severely, dwarfed. Furthermore, the ateleiotic dwarf remains infantile in appearance, and the progeric dwarf, even during youth, appears like a shriveled old person. The clinical and skeletal peculiarities of ateleiosis and progeria and the distinctions between these conditions and achondroplasia have been given by Keith, among others.

PATHOLOGIC FINDINGS

Gross Findings in the Achondroplastic Neonate.—The first detailed study of a series of skeletons of achondroplastic neonates was reported by Kaufmann in 1892. He showed conclusively what others before him had indicated—that the skeletal abnormalities presented by these subjects develop on the basis of an apparently primary inadequacy of cartilage cell proliferation at sites of endochondral ossification. This inadequacy results in deficient preparation of the cartilage for its replacement by bone, and hence in retardation or inhibition of endochondral bone growth. (See also Knaggs, and Knötzke.)

The *long bones* of achondroplastic neonates may be of less than half the normal length. Furthermore, in most cases the epiphyses are strikingly large and more or less misshapen. Notably in the femur or humerus, they may constitute nearly one half of the total length of the bone. The excessive size of the epiphyses accentuates the shortness of the intervening shaft. The latter is not only short, but thick, and flares at its ends to adapt itself to the enlarged epiphyses. Altogether, such long bones may have almost the shape of dumbbells. In a longitudinal section of one of these bones, it will be found that the cartilage constituting the epiphyses contains an unduly large number of cartilage vessel canals, and that the cartilaginous tissue is ordinarily quite firm. Each epiphysis is rather sharply marked off from the diaphysis, and the shaft cortex usually appears thickened.

In the *skull* the important deviations appear in that part of the base which is developed in cartilage, and especially in the body of the sphenoid and in that portion of the occipital bone which surrounds the foramen magnum. It will be observed in particular that the axial dimensions of the body of the sphenoid and the basilar portion of the occipital bone are much shorter than in the normal. In the achondroplastic neonate the sphenoid may already present as a single mass of bone, in consequence of premature fusion, or synostosis, of its ossific centers. On the other hand, in a normal neonate the sphenoid contains three separate ossific centers, which ordinarily do not fuse until months after birth. Furthermore, in the achondroplastic neonate the foramen magnum is narrowed and the size of the cerebellar fossa reduced because of premature ossification of those cartilaginously preformed portions of the occipital bone lateral to and behind the foramen magnum. The shortening of the axial diameter of the base of the skull as a whole accounts for the large round head of the achondroplastic fetus, since the calvarium is forced to expand at its sutures and fontanelles if the brain is to have adequate room. The changes in front of the foramen magnum in particular explain the deep depression at the root of the nose and also the flattening of the face. The narrowing of the foramen magnum may have led to death of the fetus through pressure upon the medulla oblongata. The bones of the calvarium, not being preformed in cartilage, tend to show a regular and adequate development of their osseous tissue.

In relation to the bones of the *trunk*, it may be stated first that the clavicles, too, since they are largely not preformed in cartilage, are likely to be only slightly stunted. The vertebral column, on the other hand, often shows abnormal curves, even in the newborn subject. In particular, there may be a kyphotic curvature of the dorsolumbar region and excessive lordotic curvature of the lumbosacral region. When the column is sectioned vertically, it will be observed that, though the vertebral bodies are of practically normal dimensions, they still consist largely of cartilage. The centers of ossification for the bodies are so much below normal size as to be strikingly peculiar. It will also be observed that the spinal canal is abnormally narrow. This narrowness may be caused by the bulkiness of the cartilage surrounding the canal, but more often, apparently, it is due to a premature synostosis of the vertebral bodies with their arches. The costal cartilages are increased in length, and, since the bony portions of the ribs are shortened, the costochondral junctions become shifted even as far as the axillary line. These junctions often show more or less pronounced beading. Most commonly, the latter is due to a cuplike encirclement of the bone by the cartilage. Sometimes, however, it arises from an overlapping of the cartilage by the bone at the junction. In the ribs, as in the tubular bones, the cortex is excessively thick. The innominate bones are smaller than they should be and are sometimes rather grotesquely distorted. Their iliac portions may be less well developed than their ischial and pubic portions, and the acetabular fossae tend to be rather small. The sacral promontory is conspicuous by its forward extension. In some neonates there may already be sacroiliac synostosis. (Many of the gross anatomic features presented by the skeleton of the achondroplastic neonate and discussed in this section are to be observed in Figures 43-C and D.)

The *other abnormalities* are few and relatively unimportant. The thick folds of skin and subcutaneous tissue so frequently observed seem to be due merely to the fact that the amount of these tissues formed is normal and hence too great for the size of the skeletal parts. The subcutaneous tissue is sometimes edematous. The muscular development may seem excessive but probably is so, again merely in proportion to the stunting of the skeleton. The viscera usually show no pathologic features. Sometimes, however, the brain presents a hydrocephalus interna, with or without hydrocephalus externa. The *glands* of *internal secretion*, like the viscera, are ordinarily spared. Occasionally, however, certain of them are found altered, and notably enlargement or atrophy of the thyroid and even atrophy of the pituitary have been reported. The latter condition may be related to the abnormal smallness of the sella turcica. Finally, it is interesting that the viscera or skeleton of the achondroplastic neonate may also present certain *incidental developmental malformations*, such as cleft palate, polydactyly, syndactyly, and/or polycystic kidneys.

Microscopic Findings in the Achondroplastic Neonate.—The histologic features characteristic of achondroplasia can be observed at all sites of endochondral ossification but stand out particularly well at the epiphysial-diaphysial junctions of long tubular bones and at the costochondral junctions. At these sites, as already noted, there is *deficiency in cartilage cell proliferation,* in contrast to what one would find at such a junction in a normal control. In particular, it will be observed that the zone of proliferating cartilage cells is rather meager and that furthermore the hypertrophic cartilage cells present have formed only short columns, if any. In addition, there is no evidence of an active advance of calcified cores of cartilage matrix into the diaphysis for the deposition of bone upon them. Nevertheless, it is clear that before birth a certain amount of endochondral bone growth must have taken place at the epiphysial-diaphysial junctions which have been modified in the manner described. This growth apparently occurs mainly, and sometimes entirely, through a feeble and distorted process (akin to the normal one) in which bits of calcified cartilage advance into the diaphysis and form a nidus upon which a small amount of bone is deposited.

At the epiphysial-diaphysial junctions of the long bones (and also at the costo-chondral junctions), a so-called *"periosteal strip"* consisting of fibrous connective tissue (in which bone may have formed) may be seen. This strip, which has received much emphasis in histopathologic descriptions of achondroplasia, seems to be able to block the endochondral bone growth which would otherwise be taking place. According to most observers, the interfering fibrous tissue of the strip arises through inward migration of connective tissue from the periosteum or perichondrium at the bone-cartilage junctions. The bone which often forms in the periosteal strip develops through direct osseous metaplasia of its constituent connective tissue. At sites of endochondral ossification where there is no direct contact with the periosteum or perichondrium (for instance, around the ossification center of a vertebral body), connective tissue tending to form a strip is brought in through the cartilage vessel canals which converge from the periosteum or perichondrium toward the ossification center.

Finally, it may be stated that, in the diaphysial cortices of the long bones, periosteal bone formation is not hindered. In fact, the cortices of such bones in the neonate subjects are often abnormally thick, although there are also cases in which these bones have been found abnormally thin and even liable to fractures. The hematopoietic tissue of the affected bones presents nothing abnormal. (See Fig. 45.)

Figure 45

A, Photomicrograph ($\times$ 3) showing the general histologic architecture of an entire femur from a somewhat premature achondroplastic stillborn fetus. Note that the shaft of the bone is abnormally short in relation to the combined size of its cartilaginous epiphyses. Note also the numerous cartilage vessel canals in the epiphyses.

B, Photomicrograph ($\times$ 12) of part of a rib from an achondroplastic female infant $7\frac{1}{2}$ months of age. Even under this low magnification, one can observe some trabeculae of bone (see arrows) apposed against the proliferating cartilage at the costochondral junction. Note also that there is a lack of calcified cartilage matrix cores extending from the costal cartilage into the rib shaft, such as would normally be present at a site of active endochondral bone growth. (See also *D.*)

C, Photomicrograph ($\times$ 5) of part of the epiphysial-diaphysial junction at the lower end of a femur from the infant whose rib is shown in *B.* Note that, as at the costochondral junction of the rib, trabeculae of bone (see arrows) are apposed against the cartilage, and that evidence of active endochondral ossification in the juxta-epiphysial region is lacking.

D, Photomicrograph ($\times$ 75) showing in greater detail the histologic appearance of part of the costochondral junction of a rib from the same achondroplastic infant in question in *B* and *C.* Though the cartilage cells in the junctional area are hypertrophic, they fail to show the normal alignment into more or less straight columns, and there are again no long cores of calcified cartilage matrix extending into the shaft of the rib. Note furthermore that the surface of the costal cartilage abutting on the shaft of the rib is being covered or "blocked" by trabeculae of osseous tissue.

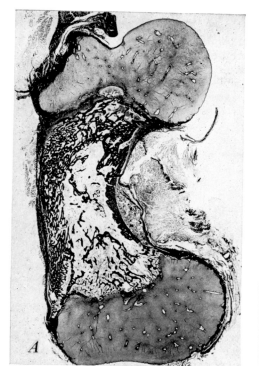

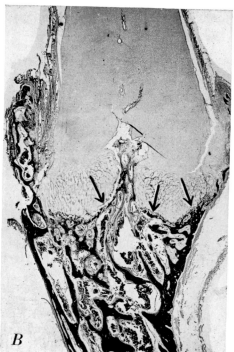

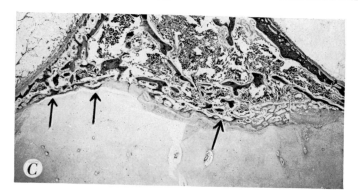

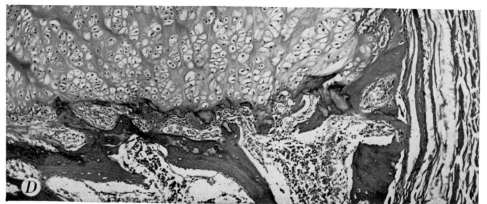

Figure 45

Findings in Achondroplastic Children and Adults.—In general, it should be borne in mind that the surviving subjects represent the milder cases of achondroplasia. Relatively few anatomic studies have been made on such cases. However, the anatomic findings (see Marum, Donath and Vogl, and Breus and Kolisko) have been well supplemented by roentgenographic studies, which have yielded additional details both on the evolution of the skeletal abnormalities in individual cases and on the variations in these abnormalities from case to case (see Fairbank, and Caffey). Thus it is known that in the affected children the centers of postnatal ossification do develop in the various cartilaginous epiphyses and in the cartilaginous precursors of the tarsal and carpal bones. Also, the time and order of appearance of these centers seem to be approximately normal. Furthermore, these children grow in height, although slowly and inadequately. The stunting of their long bones is due mainly to the feebleness of the growth at the epiphysial cartilage plates. However, a contributing factor may be premature fusion, partial or complete, of many of the epiphyses of these bones with their diaphyses.

In the adult subjects (as in the children) the *long bones* have short and stocky shafts with thick cortices. The bone ends are usually enlarged—often only slightly but sometimes quite prominently. The muscular insertions are strongly marked. In some cases, certain of the long bones may be somewhat curved. There may also be deformities at their ends. The most frequent are a coxa vara deformity of the upper end of the femur, disproportionate enlargement of the inner femoral condyle as compared with the outer, and a humerus varus deformity. Because of the changes in the ends of the femur, the subject may have a peculiar waddling gait and a genu varum. Another curious feature of achondroplasia is the high position of the head of the fibula, which may reach to the level of the upper surface of the

Figure 46

A, Roentgenograph of part of the right lower limb of an achondroplastic girl 9 years of age (see Fig. 44-*A*) showing the general contour of the illustrated parts of the affected femur, tibia, and fibula.

B, Roentgenograph of a macerated femur from a middle-aged achondroplastic dwarf illustrating the typical shortness of the bone shaft and the stubbiness of the ends of the bone.

C, Frontal view of the skeleton of an adult achondroplastic dwarf. Note the pronounced shortening of all four extremities relative to the trunk and head. The midpoint of the skeleton is at the level of the middle of the first lumbar vertebra instead of at the upper border of the symphysis pubis, as it would normally be. Note that the bones of the hands and feet are much less affected than the other bones of the corresponding extremities and thus appear relatively large. The skull is large, particularly in relation to total height, and it is brachycephalic. The vertebral bodies are broad, the ribs are thick, and the ends of the long tubular bones flare strikingly. (This photograph is reproduced from the article by Rischbieth and Barrington in the *Eugenics Laboratory Memoirs*, No. 15, 1912.)

D, Photograph showing the lower three thoracic and upper three lumbar vertebrae from an achondroplastic adult dwarf who presented a sharply angulated kyphotic gibbus having its crest at the first lumbar vertebra. The subject was 57 years of age at the time of death and had presented a dorsolumbar kyphosis since childhood. During the five years before his death, he developed progressive pain in the lower limbs and difficulty in locomotion, and eventually a spastic paraplegia appeared, due to a transverse myelitis. Anatomic examination of the vertebral column showed pronounced narrowing of the spinal canal and compression of the spinal cord from marginal exostoses which had developed in the area of the kyphosis. The autopsy was performed by Professor Jakob Erdheim of Vienna, and the findings in this case were reported by Donath and Vogl (see references). This photograph and the corresponding roentgenograph (see *E*) represent original material from the Erdheim Collection.

E, Roentgenograph of the specimen shown in *D*.

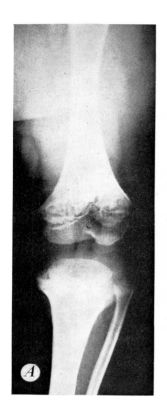

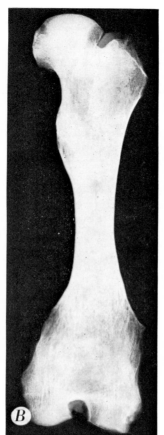

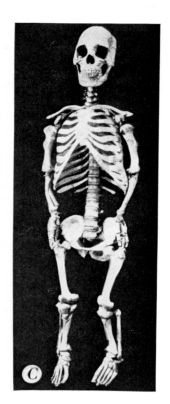

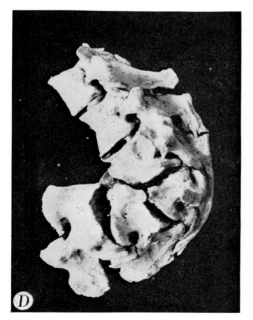

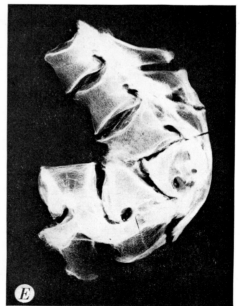

Figure 46

tibia and interfere with complete extension of the knee joint. Analogous conditions around the elbow joint cause the common lack of complete extension in this joint also.

In regard to the *skull* it is usually observed that, though the bones of the calvarium are not much thickened, the calvarial circumference is much larger than it should be, and this largeness is often accentuated by the largeness of the frontal protuberances. The abnormal shortness of the base of the cranium and the consequent drawn-in appearance of the root of the nose, which have been discussed in relation to the fetal cases, are observed in the adult subjects as well. Prognathism, too, is common in the latter.

In relation to the *trunk* it has been found that the form of the thoracic cage varies widely, being influenced by the presence of dorsolumbar kyphosis on the one hand and by the involvement of the ribs in the growth disturbance on the other. The sternum may be pushed forward or be depressed. The ribs are ordinarily described as being thick, broad, and deformed. There is also a pronounced increase in the lumbosacral angle, due to the frequently observed forward protrusion of the lower lumbar vertebrae and backward, more or less horizontal, extension of the sacrum. Furthermore, in practically all cases, the dorsolumbar region shows a more or less pronounced deviation from the normal lordosis. Thus the vertebral column in this region may be straight, but in the majority of cases there is a kyphosis, which sometimes amounts to actual gibbus formation. Instances of paraplegia of the lower extremities in achondroplastics in whom the kyphosis was associated with compression of the spinal cord have been described (see Donath and Vogl, Freund, and Spillane). The condition of the pelvis in adult achondroplastics has attracted wide attention. In addition to being very small, it usually shows: (1) severe anteroposterior flattening of the inlet; (2) a high promontorium with a decided forward projection; (3) almost backward slanting of the sacrum; and (4) exaggerated flaring of the ilia. In other cases the pelvis is generally narrowed and somewhat triangular in shape, but the outlet is relatively large. (See Fig. 46.)

The *internal organs* have revealed no consistent or striking abnormal manifestations in any of the cases coming to autopsy.

ACHONDROPLASIA IN ANIMALS

Achondroplasia has been encountered in numerous animal species. The Dexter is a breed of small cattle characterized by achondroplastic traits consisting of a short broad head and short extremities. When it is mated pure, about one fifth of the calves produced are of the so-called "bulldog" variety, in which the achondroplastic features of the parents are very exaggerated. Such calf fetuses, always stillborn, present: shortened limbs and base of skull, depressed nose, narrowed foramen magnum, lordosis, brachycephaly, inturned feet, and a shortened vertebral column (see Crew). These abnormal traits of the "bulldog" Dexter calves are analogous to those of achondroplastic human fetuses. Hereditary achondroplasia has also been observed in the rabbit (see Pearce and Brown). The affected rabbits were stillborn or died very shortly after birth, and their bones showed, both grossly and histologically, abnormalities analogous to those found in human achondroplastic neonates. Shortened hind limbs and deformed skulls, again suggesting achondroplasia, have been observed in chickens ("creeper fowl"), affected chicks already presenting evidence of the condition after the first few days of incubation (see Landauer and Dunn). The short and distorted limbs of the basset hound and dachshund likewise suggest achondroplasia. However, in these animals the skull is entirely normal, and, furthermore, when two of the same variety are mated the offspring are usually born alive, though they, too, show the short extremities.

Whether the short-leggedness of such dogs should really be considered as an expression of achondroplasia which has become stabilized genetically in a partial form is by no means clear yet, in the opinion of the present writer.

GENETIC CONSIDERATIONS

Inquiry into the family history of an achondroplastic human subject frequently fails to reveal other instances of the condition in the immediate family or antecedents. Furthermore, there are a number of recorded cases in which the achondroplasia appeared in only one of a set of twins of parents who were both free of the disorder (see Slungaard and Harris). Such sporadic or solitary cases of achondroplasia undoubtedly represent a genetic mutation. In this connection, it has been estimated that, in Denmark, 1 of every 10,000 to 12,000 neonates born to normal parents is an achondroplastic (see Mørch).

However, there are also cases in which inquiry reveals that one parent (and sometimes also a grandparent) was affected with the condition. In these familial cases the disease is inherited as a dominant character. In any event, achondroplasia is not likely to be found repeatedly in generation after generation of a family tree. In the first place, as already noted, most of the affected subjects die *in utero* or shortly after birth. Secondly, the marriage of an achondroplastic adult often yields no progeny, or no viable progeny. The possibility of hereditary transmission through the female line in the past was particularly slight because of the obstetrical difficulties created by the narrow pelvis in the female achondroplastic. For these various reasons, it is understandable why, in any country, the great majority of the surviving subjects affected with achondroplasia represent sporadic, not familial, cases of the disorder. Finally, a few instances have been recorded in which, though one parent of a family was affected with achondroplasia, the children (usually one or only a few) were free of the disorder, and their offspring in turn were also free of it. (For accounts of the family histories in large series of cases of achondroplasia, see Rischbieth and Barrington, and Mørch.)

REFERENCES

BREUS, C., and KOLISKO, A.: *Die Pathologischen Beckenformen*, Leipzig and Vienna, Franz Deuticke, *1*, 313 ff., 1904.

CAFFEY, J.: Achondroplasia of Pelvis and Lumbosacral Spine. Some Roentgenographic Features, Am. J. Roentgenol., *80*, 449, 1958.

CREW, F. A. E.: The Significance of an Achondroplasia-like Condition met with in Cattle, Proc. Roy. Soc. London s.B, *95*, 228, 1923–24.

DONATH, J., and VOGL, A.: Untersuchungen über den chondrodystrophischen Zwergwuchs. Das Verhalten der Wirbelsäule beim chondrodystrophischen Zwerg, Wien. Arch. inn. Med., *10*, 1, 1925.

————: Untersuchungen über den chondrodystrophischen Zwergwuchs. (II. Mitteilung.) Über die Beziehungen zwischen Wirbelsäule und Rückenmark und das Auftreten von Querschnittslähmungen bei chondrodystrophischen Zwergen, Ztschr. ges. Neurol. u. Psychiat., *111*, 333, 1927.

FAIRBANK, T.: *An Atlas of General Affections of the Skeleton*, Edinburgh & London, E. & S. Livingstone Ltd., 1951.

FREUND, E.: Spastic Paraplegia in Achondroplasia, Arch. Surg., *27*, 859, 1933.

HUGHES JONES, E. W. A.: Studies in Achondroplasia. I. Dystrophia Hormathica, an Unrecorded Form of Defective Ossification Akin to Achondroplasia, J. Anat., *66*, 565, 1931–32.

INGALLS, T. H.: Congenital Malformations: Environmental Influences that Act to Cause Them, Yale J. Biol. & Med., *32*, 51, 1959.

JAMES, C. H.: Three Varieties of Dwarfs, Indian M. Gaz., *45*, 443, 1910.

KAUFMANN, E.: *Untersuchungen ueber die sogenannte foetale Rachitis (chondrodystrophia foetalis.)*, Berlin, Georg Reimer, 1892.

KEITH, A.: Progeria and Ateleiosis, Lancet, *1*, 305, 1913.

————: Studies on the Anatomical Changes Which Accompany Certain Growth-disorders of the Human Body, J. Anat., *54*, 101, 1919–20.

KNAGGS, R. L.: Achondroplasia. (Chondrodystrophia Foetalis), Brit. J. Surg., *15*, 10, 1927–28.

KNÖTZKE, F.: Bemerkungen zur Wirbelsäule des Chondrodystrophen, Beitr. path. Anat., *81*, 547, 1928–29.

LANDAUER, W., and DUNN, L. C.: Chondrodystrophia in Chicken Embryos, Proc. Soc. Exper. Biol. & Med., *23*, 562, 1925–26.

MARIE, P.: L'achondroplasie dans l'adolescence et l'age adulte, Presse méd., 8^2, 17, 1900.

MARUM, G.: Über eine erwachsene chondrodystrophische Zwergin, Frankfurt. Ztschr. Path., *24*, 663, 1920–21.

MØRCH, E. T.: *Chondrodystrophic Dwarfs in Denmark*, Copenhagen, E. Munksgaard, 1941.

PARROT, J.: Sur les malformations achondroplasiques et le Dieu Phtah, Bull. Soc. anthrop. Paris, 3e Série, *1*, 296, 1878.

PEARCE, L., and BROWN, W. H.: Hereditary Achondroplasia in the Rabbit. II. Pathologic Aspects, J. Exper. Med., *82*, 261, 1945.

————: Hereditary Achondroplasia in the Rabbit. III. Genetic Aspects; General Considerations, J. Exper. Med., *82*, 281, 1945.

RISCHBIETH, H., and BARRINGTON, A.: Dwarfism. *Eugenics Laboratory Memoirs*, No. 15, London, Dulau and Co., Limited, 1912.

SLUNGAARD, R. K., and HARRIS, L. E.: Chondrodysplasia (Achondroplasia) in One of Dizygotic Twins, Am. J. Dis. Child., *86*, 788, 1953.

SPILLANE, J. D.: Three Cases of Achondroplasia with Neurological Complications, J. Neurol. Neurosurg. & Psychiat., *15*, 246, 1952.

Chapter

9

Certain Other Anomalies of Skeletal Development

In the three preceding chapters, the writer discussed "osteogenesis imperfecta," "osteopetrosis," and "achondroplasia." The inborn anomalies of skeletal development to be discussed in the present chapter are: *chondrodystrophia calcificans congenita, dysplasia epiphysialis multiplex, Morquio's disease, metaphysial dysostosis, osteopoikilosis, osteopathia striata,* and *cleidocranial dysostosis.*

The first three of these disorders not infrequently present certain overlapping features which suggest a possible kinship among them, beyond the fact that they all belong within the general category of the so-called *hereditary chondrodysplasias.* Furthermore, these three conditions also have characteristics which may result in misinterpretation of one case or another as an instance of achondroplasia in atypical form. Metaphysial dysostosis, on the other hand, though also included among the chondrodysplasias, is not likely to be confused with achondroplasia. The remaining conditions to be discussed, though representing well-defined entities among the large and varied and in part still-unclarified group of inborn anomalies of skeletal development, bear no relationship whatsoever to the so-called chondrodysplasias

CHONDRODYSTROPHIA CALCIFICANS CONGENITA

This rare anomaly of skeletal development (also frequently denoted as *"dysplasia epiphysialis punctata"*) is characterized by the presence of multiple small punctate foci of calcification in the still-cartilaginous portions of the skeleton of the affected neonate. In severely affected subjects, punctate calcifications may also be observed in the tracheal and bronchial cartilages and even in the synovial membrane of some of the joints. The foci of calcification stand out in the x-ray picture as discrete or agglomerated radiopacities. They are usually best visualized in the cartilaginous epiphyses of long tubular bones, though other cartilaginous skeletal areas often also show them. The focal calcifications reflected in the radiopacities are, of course, not present in those parts of the skeleton which develop through intramembranous ossification, as, for instance, the bones of the cranial vault and most of those of the face. The subjects not uncommonly also present certain localized developmental skeletal anomalies, cataracts, and/or dermal lesions.

That the disorder may affect several sibs in one family is clear. Its hereditary transmission has not been established, however, though it is possible that it is transmitted as an autosomal recessive trait (see Hobaek). In any event, nothing is known in regard to the pathogenesis of the condition.

Nomenclature.—In the first documented report on the disorder, the disease was described as representing an aberrant or peculiar form of achondroplasia (see Conradi). Fairbank, dissenting from this interpretation, established the condition as a clinical entity and evolved the name "dysplasia epiphysialis punctata" to designate it. However, the name "chondrodystrophia calcificans congenita,"

207

suggested by Hünermann, seems somewhat preferable. It is true that the inclusion of "chondrodystrophia" as part of the name does permit some confusion with achondroplasia. Still, the name as a whole has the advantage of pointing out that calcifications are characteristic of the disorder and that the condition is already manifest at birth. Furthermore, it avoids the impression that the calcifications are limited to the cartilaginous epiphyses. Another reason "chondrodystrophia calcificans congenita" seems preferable to "dysplasia epiphysialis punctata" is that it avoids possible confusion in terminology between "dysplasia epiphysialis punctata" and "dysplasia epiphysialis multiplex." Other names by which the disorder has been designated include "stippled epiphyses" and "chondroangiopathia calcarea (seu punctata)."

CLINICAL CONSIDERATIONS

The affected neonate (more often a female than a male) is likely to be born somewhat prematurely. Even if born alive, many of these infants die within a few months after birth. In most cases the infant's head is somewhat enlarged, and the nasal root tends to be broad and depressed. The limbs of the subject are usually dwarfed in relation to the trunk. However, in some cases there is a lack of symmetry in respect to the shortness of the limbs, and there are even cases in which only one of the limbs is strikingly dwarfed. If the subject is severely affected, all four limbs are usually abnormally short, their proximal segments (arms and thighs) being proportionally shorter than the forearms and legs. The ends of the affected long bones generally appear enlarged. At the hips, knees, and elbows, there may be limitation of motion and flexion deformity. As noted, some of the subjects also manifest local congenital skeletal deformities or anomalies. These include clubfoot, clawhand, dislocation at the hip joint, etc. Not infrequently, bilateral cataracts are already present at birth. Furthermore, the affected infant may show one or another of such dermal lesions as dyskeratosis, hyperkeratosis, or even ichthyosis.

In the occasional subject who does not succumb during infancy, the characteristic spotty radiopacities usually disappear progressively from the cartilaginous epiphyses and the various other cartilaginous skeletal areas (see Burckhardt, Fanconi, and also Raap).

ROENTGENOGRAPHIC FINDINGS

Roentgenographic examination of an affected neonate reveals, as noted, the presence of numerous discrete and/or confluent radiopacities distributed through the skeletal areas which are still cartilaginous. As to the general shape of the bones, it is to be noted in particular that the shafts of the long tubular bones (humerus, femur, tibia) are decidedly short and broad. In addition, the ends of these bones may flare to a marked degree. (See Fig. 47.)

Figure 47

A, Roentgenograph demonstrating the characteristic radiopacities in the cartilaginous epiphyses of the long bones of the upper limbs, in the still-cartilaginous portions of the vertebrae, and in the vertebral ends of the ribs in the case of an infant 5 days of age affected with chondrodystrophia calcificans congenita. Note that the cartilaginous vertebral margin of the scapula visible (the left) is also outlined by punctate radiopacities. The clavicles (which are formed in membrane) show no such radiopacities.

B, Roentgenograph showing the radiopacities in the cartilaginous portions of various bones of the lower extremities in the same case illustrated in *A,* the infant in question now being 2 months of age.

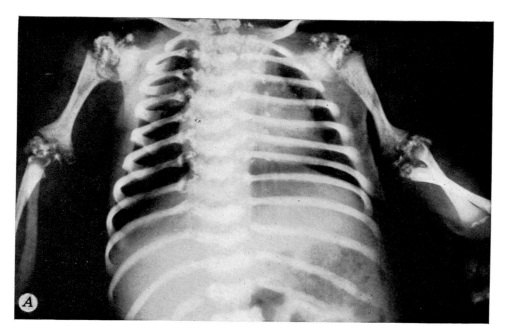

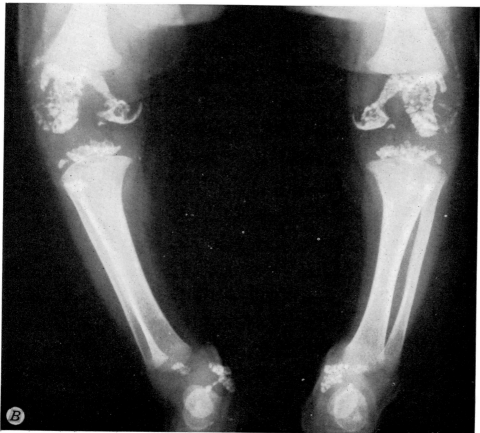

Figure 47

209

The radiopacities in question represent sites of calcification in the cartilage. Where they are small and discrete, the cartilaginous area is likely to appear stippled. On the other hand, confluence of the foci of calcification is represented by the presence of patches of radiopacity. The latter finding is most conspicuous in the cartilaginous epiphyses of certain of the long tubular bones—*viz.* upper and lower end of the femur and upper end of the tibia and humerus. When present in the cartilaginous ends of long bones, the large patches of radiopacity have, on occasion, been misinterpreted as representing multiple and often premature postnatal centers of ossification. The cartilaginous epiphyses at the lower end of the tibia, radius, and ulna are not usually heavily stippled. The cartilaginous precursors of the bones of the wrist and the epiphyses of the short tubular bones of the hands and feet are usually also not strikingly involved. The cartilage comprising the crest of the ilium, however, occasionally shows spotty radiopacities in a strandlike arrangement (see Frank and Denny). The cartilaginous posterior ends of the ribs may be stippled, and the vertebrae, too, may show stippling.

In a case studied by the writer (that of an infant 2 months of age), the bodies of the thoracic and lumbar vertebrae in particular presented an unusual appearance. Instead of standing out as a single unit, each vertebral body appeared to be divided in its longitudinal axis into two segments separated by a zone of radiolucency. This aberration seems to be the result of the development of two separate centers of ossification (one in front of the other) instead of a single center for each vertebral body. The anatomic findings relating to the case of an infant presenting a similar aberration of the vertebral column are illustrated by Harris. The subject in that case was 11 months of age, and the two centers of ossification for each vertebral body were found to be separated by a tract of cartilage extending through each body from disk to disk.

As noted, an occasional affected infant continues to survive, and in such cases there is a progressive disappearance of the characteristic radiopacities. Indeed, by the third or fourth year of life, they may no longer be demonstrable. However, the postnatal centers of ossification for the various epiphyses and the carpal and tarsal bones are nevertheless likely to be delayed in their appearance, and even the order of their emergence may deviate from the normal. In the very exceptional instance in which the course of a case of chondrodystrophia calcificans congenita (dysplasia epiphysialis punctata) has been followed from infancy through later childhood and into adolescence, it has been noted that the subject may come to present the manifestations characteristic of dysplasia epiphysialis multiplex (p. 211). A well-documented case in point is reported by Silverman. As an infant, the subject in question had presented roentgenographic findings characteristic of chondrodystrophia calcificans congenita (see Vinke and Duffy).

PATHOLOGIC FINDINGS

Comprehensive anatomic study of the skeleton has been carried out in only a few of the cases of chondrodystrophia calcificans congenita which have come to autopsy. Details on both the gross and the microscopic skeletal findings in such cases are given in the pertinent reports by Conradi and by Hässler and Schallock. In most of the other reports dealing with the pathologic anatomy of the condition, the microscopic rather than the gross anatomic findings are stressed (see Putschar, and Karlen and Cameron). In any event, it is clear from such anatomic studies as have been carried out that the bones of the calvarium and face and the shafts of the tubular bones and ribs, for instance, are of normal firmness and compactness. On the other hand, the still-cartilaginous portions of the skeleton of the affected neonate or infant show numerous scattered gray-white gritty foci of calcification.

These may be barely perceptible, of pinhead size, or even as large as lentils. In the cartilaginous epiphyses of some of the long tubular bones, such foci of calcification are usually quite prominent, and they are often also conspicuous grossly in the cartilaginous precursor of the patella. Furthermore, foci of calcification are to be observed in cartilaginous areas surrounding centers of ossification, as, for instance, in the cartilage around the ossific centers of the vertebral bodies. Occasionally they are also observed in the cartilaginous precursors of the bones of the carpus and tarsus, as well as about any centers of ossification for the tarsal bones already present in the affected infant.

On *microscopic examination* it will be noted that at sites of endochondral bone formation (costochondral and epiphysial-diaphysial junctions, for instance) the zone of proliferating cartilage cells tends to be narrower than it should be. However, it is in the cartilaginous epiphyses and the various other cartilaginous parts of the skeleton that the histologic changes characteristic of the condition are to be observed. In particular, one finds focal areas of mucoid degeneration of the cartilage. In such sites the collagen fibrils of the cartilage matrix may have been unmasked, and some microcysts may be noted. Elsewhere in the cartilage, one will observe smaller or larger tissue fields in which the cartilage matrix appears heavily calcified. In some of these areas, furthermore, the cellularity of the cartilage may be increased. Here and there, particularly where the calcification is rather heavy, the altered cartilage may also be found fragmented, and one may even note some multinuclear giant cells of the foreign-body type in the vicinity of the fragmented cartilage. In addition, fragmented calcified cartilage areas may show invasion by blood vessels and connective tissue from neighboring cartilage vessel canals. (See Fig. 48.)

DYSPLASIA EPIPHYSIALIS MULTIPLEX

Dysplasia epiphysialis multiplex (multiple epiphysial dysplasia) is a relatively rare familial and hereditary disorder of skeletal development. It is characterized by abnormalities in the evolution and growth of the centers of ossification for the epiphyses, apophyses, and epiphysioid bones. In any given case, few or many of these various centers of ossification may be found affected. The hereditary transmission of the disorder is well established, and the condition seems to be inherited as a simple dominant mendelian trait. Since the disorder is not lethal, it is not surprising that the literature includes a number of reports recording its presence in members of three or more generations of a given family tree (see Maudsley, Shephard, and also Weinberg *et al.*).

Nomenclature.—As has already been noted (see p. 210), there are indications in the literature that an infant affected with chondrodystrophia calcificans congenita (dysplasia epiphysialis punctata) who has survived into adolescence may come to present the roentgenographic picture of dysplasia epiphysialis multiplex (see Silverman). Nevertheless, in the writer's opinion, these two conditions should still be kept distinct, since the evidence at hand is not sufficient to establish them firmly as interrelated disorders. Furthermore, in regard to terminology, there can be little doubt that cases recorded in the older literature as representing "osteochondritis" in multiple sites ("familial generalized osteochondritis dissecans," for example) actually represent instances of dysplasia epiphysialis multiplex.

CLINICAL CONSIDERATIONS

In any large series of cases representing members of several generations of one family tree, the number of affected males and females is approximately the same.

Thus the disorder apparently does not predilect either sex. The stigmatized infant usually appears normal at birth, and ordinarily no aberrations in respect to growth and development become apparent clinically for at least the first 2 or 3 years of life. At some time in the course of the next few years, the subject will probably come under medical care because of shortness of stature (due primarily to shortness of the lower limbs) and/or waddling gait, genu valgum or genu varum. Nevertheless, the affected child does not usually complain of pain related to articular areas.

A subject who has reached adult life, however, may have complaints localized to joints, and especially to the hip joints. These joints in particular are prone to the development of some degree of degenerative arthritis (osteoarthritis). In relation to certain other joints, there may be laxity of ligaments and, on the other hand, some restriction of motion, unassociated with pain. In addition to shortness of stature, it is not uncommon to find that the digits of the subject's hands are short, thick, and stubby, and that their ends are blunted. However, in relation to each other, the digits usually show the normal proportions.

It is often emphasized in connection with dysplasia epiphysialis multiplex that, though the subject's stature is below normal, the vertebral column tends to be of normal length. In some cases the vertebral bodies (particularly those of the thoracic and lumbar regions) do show minor deviations in respect to shape and structure. On the whole, however, the vertebral column in dysplasia epiphysialis multiplex does not show any striking or consistent changes, and this fact is stressed as a point of differential diagnosis between that condition and Morquio's disease (see Fairbank). In Morquio's disease, one finds platyspondyly, with flattening and gross irregularity (tonguelike anterior projections) in the outline of the vertebral bodies. Otherwise, Morquio's disease and dysplasia epiphysialis multiplex have many features in common. Indeed, it may not be unreasonable to maintain that Morquio's

Figure 48

A, Roentgenograph demonstrating the appearance of bisection of the vertebral bodies which is encountered in some cases of chondrodystrophia calcificans congenita. The subject was 2 months of age, and the vertebral bodies shown (lower thoracic and lumbar) manifest a longitudinal division into two segments separated by a narrow zone of radiolucency.

B, Photograph of a drawing illustrating part of the vertebral column, sectioned longitudinally, from the case of an infant 11 months of age affected with chondrodystrophia calcificans congenita. Each of the vertebral bodies shown presents two centers of ossification (anterior and posterior) separated by a tract of cartilage.

C, Photomicrograph (low power) showing the histologic appearance of one of the vertebral bodies illustrated in B. Note the two separate centers of ossification, of which the larger one (on the left) is in the anterior position. A wide tract of cartilage separates the two centers from disk to disk. (B and C were reproduced from the monograph by H. A. Harris, Bone Growth in Health and Disease.)

D, Photomicrograph (× 120) illustrating the histologic appearance presented by an area in the cartilaginous epiphysis at the lower end of one of the femora in the case of chondrodystrophia calcificans congenita reported by Karlen and Cameron. In the upper central part of the picture, the cellularity of the cartilage is increased. In the lower right-hand portion of the illustration, the cartilage is calcified. Below and to the left, the pale-staining uncalcified cartilage shows evidences of degeneration and cystic softening.

E, Photomicrograph (× 120) from another cartilaginous epiphysis in the case referred to in D. The dark-staining area on the left is composed of rather cellular cartilage which is heavily calcified. The adjacent area on the right consists of heavily calcified cartilage which has undergone degeneration and cystic softening. The cartilage in the lower part of the field shows minute focal areas of calcification. (D and E were reproduced from the article by Karlen and Cameron in the Journal of Bone and Joint Surgery.)

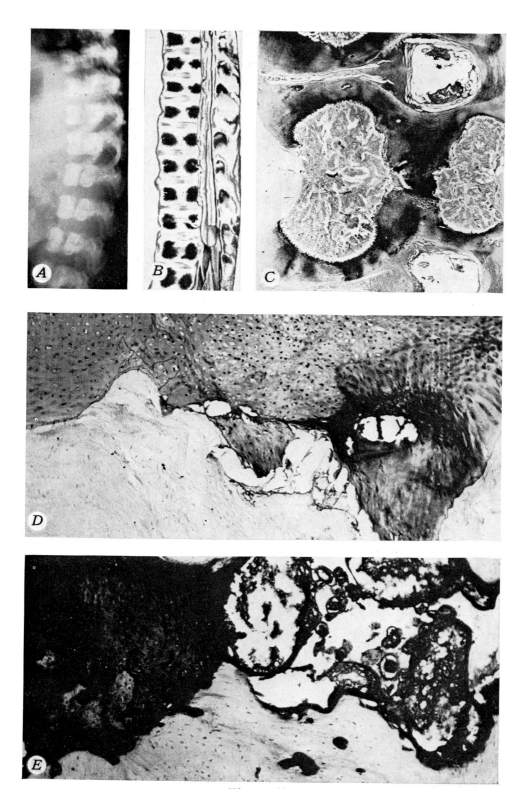

Figure 48

disease represents merely the full expression of the developmental aberration less completely manifested in dysplasia epiphysialis multiplex.

ROENTGENOGRAPHIC AND PATHOLOGIC FINDINGS

The number of ossification centers affected, as well as the distribution of the involvement over the skeleton, is by no means the same in all cases. In general, the centers of ossification most likely to show the characteristic early changes of the disorder and also to present the typical ultimate alterations in outline and structure are those in the regions of the hip, shoulder, and ankle joints. Also often affected, but usually less conspicuously, are the centers of ossification in the regions of the knees, elbows, carpus, and tarsus. The centers for the metacarpal and metatarsal heads and for the epiphyses of the phalanges, if involved at all, are usually only mildly affected. An exceptional finding in regard to the distribution of the involvement was reported by Weinberg *et al.* In their large series of cases representing six generations of one family tree, the abnormalities were consistently found limited to bones of the lower extremities. Others, too, have observed that the distribution of the lesions, whatever it may be, is somewhat similar in affected members of the same family (see Maudsley).

The centers of ossification in the various affected epiphyses, epiphysioid bones, and apophyses tend to be delayed in their appearance. The implicated ossification centers are usually found underdeveloped and irregular in outline and density, and some appear mottled or even fragmented in part or throughout. Indeed, it is not unusual to find a relatively large focus of ossification (representing the main portion of the center) with smaller ossific foci representing subsidiary centers in its

Figure 49

A, Roentgenograph illustrating the lower part of a forearm, the wrist, and part of the hand in a case of dysplasia epiphysialis multiplex in a young subject. The latter was a boy (one of a set of male twins) 12 years of age. His mother and several of his sibs (including his twin brother) were also affected with the disorder. Note the irregularity in the contour of the centers of ossification of the carpal bones. The evolving trapezium and scaphoid show two separate and adjacent centers, which appear to be fusing. The centers of ossification for the heads of the metacarpal bones present a ragged contour, as do the proximal ends of these bones. A cartilaginous epiphysis at the lower end of the radius shows punctate radiopacities in the cartilage surrounding the already evolved portion of the ossification center. Note also that the cartilaginous epiphysis at the lower end of the ulna likewise presents such punctate radiopacities. A few radiopacities of this kind are to be noted at the periphery of the distal end of the capitate and in the center of ossification at the base of the first metacarpal bone. The presence of these punctate radiopacities seems to support the idea of an interrelationship between dysplasia epiphysialis multiplex and chondrodystrophia calcificans congenita.

B and *C*, Roentgenographs showing the left elbow and right knee regions in the case to which reference was made under *A*. Note the various abnormalities presented by the evolving epiphysial centers of ossification. In particular, these centers appear irregular in contour, and some of them display small, pronglike projections. In addition, a number of small, punctate radiopacities are to be observed in the still-cartilaginous portions of some of the epiphyses.

D, Roentgenograph of a foot from the same subject. Note the striking irregularity in contour of the evolving tarsal bones. The proximal ends of the metatarsal bones are also irregular in contour, and some present short, spikelike projections, as do some of the tarsal bones. (The illustrations appearing in this figure relate to one of a number of cases of dysplasia epiphysialis multiplex reviewed by the writer with the late Dr. I. Seth Hirsch, who included the case in his published article.)

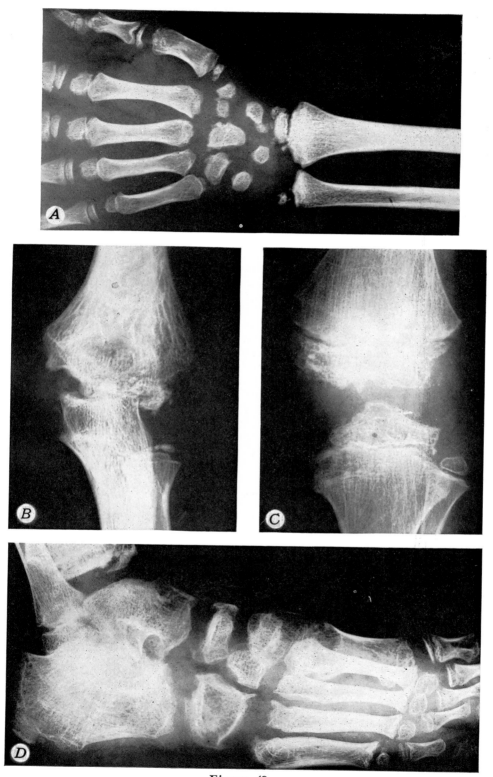

Figure 49

immediate vicinity. With the passage of time, the shadow cast by the affected ossification center may become more uniform in respect to density, the separate foci tending to coalesce, but the general contour of the center remains abnormal. Many of the centers of ossification may now present an irregular, jagged contour instead of a normal, smooth one. Subsequently they may lose their jaggedness, but the bony epiphyses or epiphysioid bones in question usually do not acquire a normal contour or full normal size. The shafts of the long bones of the lower extremities, in particular, are shorter than they would normally be, and their ends may flare somewhat. (See Fig. 49.)

In their completely evolved form, the affected femoral and humeral heads are flatter (that is, less convex) than they would normally be. The femoral condyles are also likely to be found flattened and are inclined to be rectangular, though at the same time the center for the upper epiphysial end of each tibia may still present an irregular or even jagged contour. The lower epiphysial end of each tibia is often much narrower laterally than medially, and the corresponding upper end of each astragalus may also be altered in shape, in conformity with this deformation. Thus the tibio-astragalar joint may be found to be slanted obliquely. In the joints in which the contour of the bone ends is considerably altered, osteoarthritis may evolve. Indeed, in the hip joints this complication is very common and is often already present in early adult life. (See Fig. 50.)

The occurrence of bilateral, so-called "double-layer" patellae has also been observed not infrequently in connection with dysplasia epiphysialis multiplex. Such patellae are composed of a larger anterior part and a smaller posterior part, but one or both component portions may be multipartite (see Hodkinson).

In respect to the *pathologic findings*, the literature on dysplasia epiphysialis multiplex does not seem to include any satisfactory studies in which the actual anatomic findings in the affected centers have been detailed and correlated with the well-recognized aberrations visible roentgenographically. This lack is easy to understand in view of the fact that the condition is not in itself lethal for the growing subject. Furthermore, even if an affected child does die early in life (from a

Figure 50

A, Roentgenograph of a wrist and part of the hand of a young adult affected with dysplasia epiphysialis multiplex. Note the small size and abnormal contour of the scaphoid and lunate bones and also the irregular and fragmented appearance particularly of the heads of the second and fifth metacarpal bones. The subject was a man who was 27 years of age at the time this roentgenograph was taken. Three of his brothers (including his twin brother) were also found to be affected with the disorder (see Litchman and Chirls). The other illustrations appearing in this figure relate to the same case and were also taken when the subject was 27 years of age.

B, Roentgenograph illustrating alterations in contour of the vertebral bodies in the case in question, as exemplified in the lower four lumbar vertebrae. The bodies of the second and third of these vertebrae, in particular, are distinctly shorter in height anteriorly than posteriorly.

C, Roentgenograph showing the presence of pronounced degenerative osteoarthritis in the hip joints of the subject, though he was only 27 years of age. In the hip joint on the left, a number of osteochondral bodies (joint mice) can be seen. In cases of dysplasia epiphysialis multiplex, this is a very common finding, even in young adults. Indeed, it is frequently complaints referable to the hip joint that first direct attention to the presence of the disorder.

D, Roentgenograph of one of the knee joints in this case. Note the abnormal contour of the external condyle of the femur.

E, Roentgenograph of part of one of the feet of the same subject. Note in particular that the heads of all of the metatarsal bones are flat and otherwise abnormal.

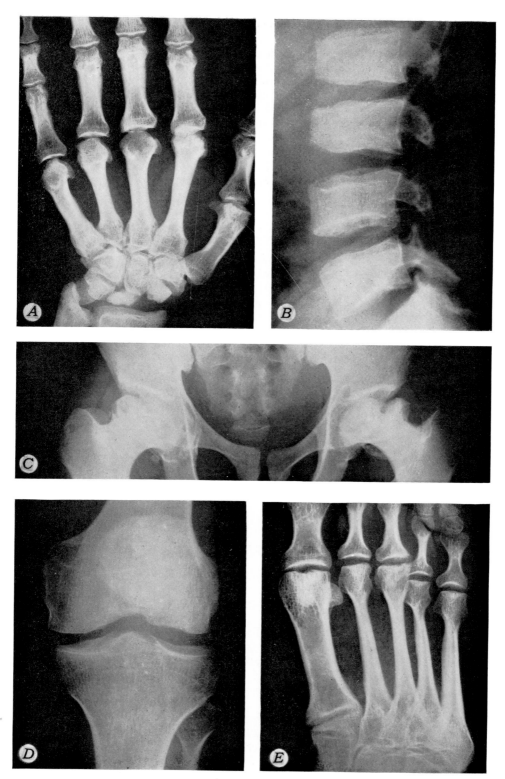

Figure 50

contagious disease or cancer, for instance), the fact that there may not yet have been any clinical manifestations referable to the skeletal disorder would make it unlikely that one or more epiphyses would be removed at autopsy for anatomic study. Anderson *et al.* did attempt to elucidate the anatomic basis for the changes in dysplasia epiphysialis multiplex and Morquio's disease through the study of biopsy material. However, their findings (chiefly inadequate chondrocyte proliferation and maturation) are not really directly pertinent, since their observations relate mainly to changes noted in the epiphysial cartilage plates and adjacent metaphysial areas and not to the epiphysial centers of ossification *per se*. On the other hand, their findings do shed some light upon the basis for retarded longitudinal bone growth in these cases.

MORQUIO'S DISEASE

The inborn anomaly of skeletal development known as Morquio's disease (or Morquio-Brailsford disease) was described independently in 1929 by the two authors in question. Both recognized that some cases representing the condition had been described in the past as instances of atypical achondroplasia. Morquio emphasized the familial character of the disorder, but, though he wished to delimit the latter as a separate clinical entity, he designated it merely as "a form of familial osseous dystrophy." Brailsford described the condition under the title of "chondro-osteo-dystrophy," and stressed the vertebral involvement in the subtitle of his paper. Indeed, it is severe and conspicuous abnormality of the vertebral column that constitutes the hallmark of Morquio-Brailsford disease. In particular, the vertebral bodies are shallow, wedged, and otherwise deformed, and the contour of the vertebral column as a whole is grossly distorted. In the latter connection, the most striking alteration is a sharply angular kyphotic deformity of the column in the dorsolumbar region. The bony components of the hip joints rank next in frequency and severity of involvement. Other skeletal areas, too, are usually affected, but the bones of the skull and face are ordinarily spared. In consequence of the skeletal changes (particularly those relating to the vertebral column), the subject is dwarfed. The intelligence is usually normal, though occasionally somewhat subnormal.

CLINICAL CONSIDERATIONS

The condition is of rare occurrence but often affects several sibs in the same family. This fact seems to point to a genetic basis for the disorder, even though the question of its hereditary transmission has not been clearly settled. Neither sex seems to be predilected.

Even subjects who come to show the disorder in severe form hardly ever present clinical manifestations of it during their infancy. When the affected child begins to try to stand or walk, such manifestations may become apparent. However, the disease often does not begin to be clearly evident clinically until the child is 4 or 5 years of age, unless, for whatever reason, the skeleton has previously been roentgenographed. By the time this age is reached, spinal deformity and difficulty in walking may be noted, and these clinical features of the disorder are usually progressive. Eventually, the crippling is likely to be so severe that the child may be unable to walk without aid. However, there are exceptions, as exemplified in the case reported by Pohl. In that case the subject, who had been under observation at the same clinic from the age of 22 months to the age of 22 years, was able not only to walk but to engage in various sports.

Typically, in a young subject severely affected with Morquio's disease, the neck is very short, and it may be so short that the head seems to be drawn in between the shoulders. Also, there is pigeon-breastedness and mid- or lower dorsal kyphosis, often associated with scoliotic deformity. The abdomen protrudes, and the lumbar lordosis is exaggerated. The gait is a waddling one, mainly because of the alterations in the hip joints. There is knock knee and flatfootedness, in association with a flexed position of the knees and hips, resulting in a crouching stance. The ends of the long bones are often though not necessarily enlarged. Some of the joints may be hypermobile, in consequence of laxity of muscles and ligaments, but others may show limitation of movement, due to the deformity of the bone ends. As indicated, the affected subjects are somewhat below the average in height, mainly because of the deformity of the vertebral column. The deformity of the vertebral column and the flexed position of the knees and hips result in the fingers reaching well below the middle of the thighs, in contrast to what is observed in achondroplasia.

ROENTGENOGRAPHIC AND PATHOLOGIC FINDINGS

The most important single *roentgenographic* finding in a child affected with Morquio's disease is flattening of the vertebral bodies. The platyspondyly is usually most striking in the dorsal region and, in itself, contributes to the shortness of the neck and trunk. Though flattened, the affected vertebral bodies show increase in their anteroposterior and transverse diameters. Their upper and lower surfaces are irregular and may be ill defined, and tend to slope toward each other anteriorly. This accounts for the wedgelike appearance of the individual vertebral bodies observed in the lateral view—an appearance which may be accentuated by the presence of a small, tonguelike anterior projection. The intervertebral disk spaces usually appear widened. In late childhood and adolescence, the abnormal contour of the vertebral bodies is frequently found to be less pronounced in the x-ray picture. This happens because the multiple secondary centers of ossification for the vertebral bodies, which appear in the cartilaginous marginal ridges ringing the upper and lower surface of each body, enlarge and eventually fuse to form an osseous marginal ridge. These bony marginal ridges, which cast a shadow, add to the apparent height of each body, especially in front, where the ridge is normally thickest.

Striking changes are also observed in relation to the hip joints. In particular, the acetabular cavities are usually large, irregularly outlined, and often abnormally deep. The various centers of ossification for the epiphyses and epiphysioid bones of the extremities tend to be delayed in their appearance and development. Furthermore, many of these centers of ossification fail to evolve normally. Some appear flattened and others fragmented. Still other centers of ossification may come to show an irregular, jagged contour instead of the normal, smooth one. Some of the epiphyses may even present a spotty or mottled appearance. The ends of the shafts of the long tubular bones frequently flare at the epiphysial-diaphysial junctional areas and show spikelike or even liplike projections curving toward the adjacent epiphysis. The metacarpal and metatarsal bones and phalanges may be stubby, and their shafts may flare at the proximal ends, which may even be somewhat lipped. (See Fig. 51.)

In regard to *differential diagnosis*, it is to be noted that, aside from the striking roentgenographic alterations in the vertebral column and acetabula in Morquio's disease, the alterations observed in the epiphyses and epiphysioid bones in that disease bear a certain resemblance to those seen in dysplasia epiphysialis multiplex (p. 211). In gargoylism (p. 542) the vertebral column may also show a sharply angulated kyphosis in the dorsolumbar region, due to backward displacement of one or more vertebral bodies. However, the vertebral column does not show general wedging of the vertebral bodies, as it does in Morquio's disease. At any rate, gargoylism represents a so-called "storage disease" which has its basis in a disturbance of endogenous metabolism. Its skeletal alterations appear to be secondary to the intracellular accumulation of a complex macromolecular glyco-protein within the bone marrow, and the accumulation of the abnormal glycoprotein in the spleen and liver results in hepatosplenomegaly (see Caffey, and Calandi and Vichi).

The differentiation between Morquio's disease and achondroplasia presents no special diagnostic problem when both conditions are present in typical form. The short trunk and relatively long extremities ordinarily found in cases of Morquio's disease contrast strikingly with the relatively long trunk and short extremities characteristic of achondroplasia. However, some highly atypical cases of Morquio's disease have been encountered and reported as instances of "spondylo-epiphysial dysplasia (pseudo-achondroplastic type)." In these cases of Morquio's disease, the skull was spared, as it usually is, and the dwarfism was very much delayed in onset. Furthermore, the epiphyses and epiphysioid bones showed the character-istic irregularities of ossification. However, the vertebral column was not so severely involved as it ordinarily is in Morquio's disease, while the extremities were more severely shortened than they usually are. Consequently the trunk appeared relatively long and the extremities relatively short, as in achondroplasia (see Maroteaux and Lamy, and Ford et al.).

There is a dearth of information in the literature relating to the *pathologic anatomy* of Morquio's disease. In fact, the writer knows of no instance in which a child affected with the disorder died and came to autopsy and in which the postmortem examination included removal and study of ample material from affected skeletal areas. The meager descriptions in the literature which relate to the pathology of Morquio's disease are based mainly on histologic findings in biopsy specimens (see Einhorn et al. and Anderson et al.). Such specimens have usually been taken from the general vicinity of epiphysial cartilage plate areas. The findings have been reported as indicating that there are degenerative changes in the cartilage matrix, and that proliferation and maturation of the cartilage cells are not progress-ing normally in the areas in question. These changes do shed light on the basis for the retarded longitudinal growth of the tubular bones. However, they do not clarify the anatomic changes underlying the spotty and fragmented roentgeno-

Figure 51

A, Roentgenograph demonstrating the striking alterations in the vertebral column which are characteristic of Morquio's disease. Note that the vertebral bodies are shallow, wedged, and otherwise deformed. Also, the contour of the vertebral column as a whole is grossly distorted, and there is an angular deformity of the column in the dorsolumbar region. The subject was a child $1\frac{1}{2}$ years of age at the time this x-ray picture and the others in this figure were taken.

B, Roentgenograph of the right ankle region in this case. The ossification centers for the astragalus and os calcis are abnormal in contour and show some pronglike (or spikelike) projections. The tibia and fibula display flaring of their shaft ends. In addition, the center of ossification for the distal epiphysis of the tibia is abnormal in contour.

C, Roentgenograph illustrating the condition of the pelvis and upper ends of the femora in this child. The abnormality in the contour of the hip joints is obvious. Both capital femoral epiphyses are very much underdeveloped. Furthermore, as is not unusual in con-nection with the various inborn anomalies of skeletal development, there are additional aberrations in this case, the upper ends of both femora showing exostotic outgrowths.

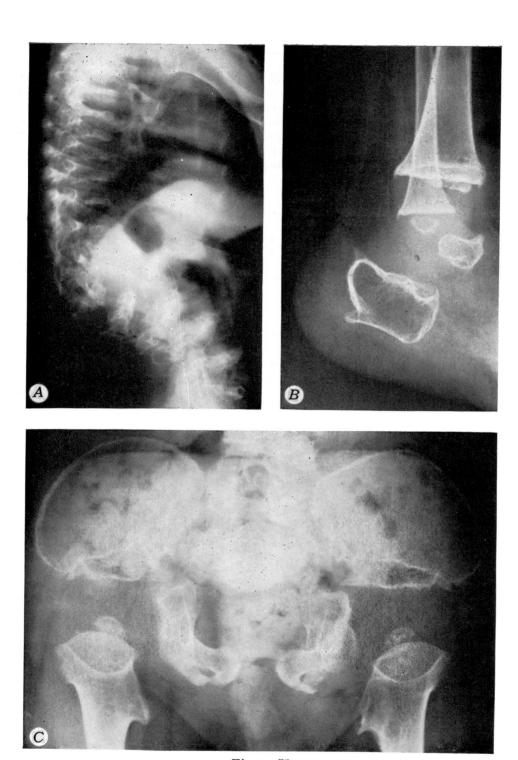

Figure 51

graphic appearance of the affected ossifying epiphyses and epiphysioid bones. The writer deduces from the roentgenographic appearances that the affected epiphyses and epiphysioid bones do not develop from a central nucleus of ossification but from multiple eccentric centers of ossification which subsequently fuse (see Hirsch). In any event, the formation of a well-rounded concept of the gross and microscopic pathology of the skeletal aberrations in Morquio's disease will have to await detailed information from study of adequate specimens removed at autopsy.

METAPHYSIAL DYSOSTOSIS

Metaphysial dysostosis is an extremely rare anomaly of skeletal development, characterized by the accumulation of cartilage in various skeletal sites—notably, in the metaphyses of the tubular bones. In the affected bone sites, the bone contour is expanded, and the area casts a variegated abnormal roentgenographic shadow reflecting different degrees of calcification of the accumulated lesional cartilage. Clinical attention was apparently first directed to the condition in 1934 by Jansen, and another unequivocal example of the disorder was reported in 1954 by Cameron *et al.* The parents and sibs of the subject in the latter case were not affected. Thus, in this instance at least, the disorder was not familial and apparently not inherited. A case of metaphysial dysostosis in a young child was also reported by Lenk. The latter records that adult members of three preceding generations in that child's family had stunted limbs, and roentgenographs of various parts of the father's skeleton suggest that his dwarfism might have had its basis in dysplasia epiphysialis multiplex.

CLINICAL CONSIDERATIONS

Metaphysial dysostosis is so rarely encountered that it is difficult to formulate a composite (generally valid) description of its clinical aspects. In the case reported by Jansen, the patient was a boy who was born with clubfeet. The ankles and lower ends of the ulnae gradually thickened. The child crawled at 6 months but was still unable to walk at 3 years, though he did manage to walk later with the help of splints. He was dwarfed, and at 10 years of age was about 12 inches below average in height. The skull and vertebral column were normal, the dwarfing being due mainly to pronounced shortening and deformity of the lower limbs. The feet were in valgus position. A follow-up of this patient was reported by de Haas *et al.* in 1969, when the subject was 44 years of age. In the course of the years, the striking feature was the development of normal bony structure associated with marked deformity and dwarfing. The joint surfaces remained intact.

In the case reported by Cameron *et al.*, deformity of both lower limbs was again the striking early clinical feature of the condition. In particular, the long bones of the lower extremities were stunted and abnormally curved in various ways. Furthermore, the ends of these long bones were enlarged and deformed, as were the ends of the long bones of the upper extremities. The costochondral junctions of the ribs were also enlarged. Except in regard to the skeleton, physical examination of the subject revealed nothing significant.

ROENTGENOGRAPHIC AND PATHOLOGIC FINDINGS

A *roentgenographic survey* of the skeleton of an affected child will show that, in addition to the striking involvement of the metaphysial areas of the tubular bones (especially the long tubular bones), there is usually also some involvement of the innominate bones and scapulae (particularly their acetabular and glenoid areas respectively) as well as the shafts of the ribs (at the costochondral junctions) and of the clavicles (at the sternal ends). A striking and contrasting feature in respect to the roentgenographic picture is the relatively normal shadow cast by such centers of ossification as may already be present for the epiphyses of the tubular bones and the epiphysioid bones of the carpus and tarsus. However, these centers of ossification are usually not so large as one would expect them to be at the age of the subject in question, and some which should have appeared by that age may not yet be present.

As to the long tubular bones, the metaphysial regions of their shafts are enlarged and expanded. Indeed, some of the affected shaft ends may be so expanded that the bone appears more or less clubbed at each end. The x-ray shadow cast by the flaring, clublike shaft ends varies with the amount of lesional cartilage present in the area and with the extent to which calcification and ossification have taken place in this cartilage. Thus there may be areas which are relatively radiolucent— that is, areas in which the lesional cartilage is not calcified or ossified. In other areas one may observe many roundish punctate and larger foci of radiopacity reflecting calcification of the cartilage matrix. In still other areas, relatively radiolucent or relatively radiopaque foci may be found which are encircled or marginated by rings of radiopacity representing calcification and/or ossification taking place around the periphery of the encircled cartilage. In the metaphysial regions of the short tubular bones of the hands and feet, changes less striking but otherwise analogous to those in the corresponding areas of the long tubular bones are to be observed.

The shadows cast by the expanded and cupped anterior ends of the ribs and sternal ends of the clavicles likewise reflect the presence of abnormal amounts of cartilage in various stages of calcification and/or ossification. This is true also for the modified acetabular areas of the innominate bones and the general region of the glenoid fossae of the scapulae. Finally, it should be noted that, like the epiphyses and epiphysioid bones, the vertebral bodies are usually spared. Furthermore, the intervertebral disks are not likely to show any abnormalities.

The problems of *differential diagnosis* raised by the roentgenographic findings in cases of metaphysial dysostosis relate to: rickets refractory to vitamin D (p. 409), rickets based on renal tubular dysfunction—so-called Fanconi rickets (p. 414), and rachitoid changes due to chronic renal insufficiency—so-called renal hyperparathyroidism (p. 321). However, any confusion that might be created on a roentgenographic basis between metaphysial dysostosis and these various other conditions is obviated by the clinical, biochemical, and/or pathologic findings (see Müller and Sissons, Evans and Caffey, and Peterson).

In regard to the *pathologic findings* in metaphysial dysostosis, the only pertinent material available for evaluation is represented by a single biopsy specimen from each of a few cases. In the case reported by Jansen, the specimen was obtained from the lower metaphysis of a tibia, and in the one reported by Cameron *et al.*, it came from the lower metaphysis of a femur. The writer has studied a biopsy specimen from the lower metaphysis of a femur in one case and from the upper metaphysis of a tibia in another.

What one observes on anatomic examination of the epiphysial-metaphysial junctional area of an affected long bone, for instance, is an extremely wide, irregular mass of cartilage protruding into the shaft. That is, one finds this mass of cartilage instead of a normal, narrow epiphysial cartilage plate. Furthermore, it is to be noted that, on the shaft side of the abnormal cartilage mass, endochondral ossification is not proceeding actively. That is, one fails to find numerous cores of calcified cartilage matrix extending into the metaphysis and forming the scaffolding on which osseous tissue normally comes to be deposited in the course of endochondral ossification. In the direction of the epiphysis, it will be noted that the abnormal mass of cartilage is rather well vascularized and, in places, quite cellular. Here and there, furthermore, one observes focal areas of degeneration of the cartilage cells, also areas in which the cartilage matrix seems to be abnormally collagenized, and other areas in which the intercellular matrix is basophilic and somewhat calcified.

Since the lesional tissue accumulating in the bones in metaphysial dysostosis is cartilage, one may be intrigued by the possible relationship of that disorder to skeletal enchondromatosis (Ollier's disease). Though skeletal enchondromatosis also represents an inborn anomaly of skeletal development, there are a number of important differences between it and metaphysial dysostosis in respect to the origin and histologic features of the lesional cartilage. The most significant difference relates to the site from which most of the cartilage issues. In metaphysial dysostosis, as noted, there can be no doubt that the cartilage takes its origin solely from certain sites of active endochondral ossification (epiphysial cartilage plates, costochondral junctions, etc.), these sites becoming abnormally altered. The epiphysial cartilage plates, for instance, no longer stand out as such, and are actually an integral part of the cartilage mass occupying and distending the metaphysial areas of affected tubular bones.

In skeletal enchondromatosis, on the other hand, the epiphysial cartilage plates contribute relatively little to the cartilage accumulating in the interior of the affected bones, and the epiphysial cartilage plates themselves do not appear abnormal on x-ray examination. Instead, most of the cartilage accumulating in the interior of the bones in skeletal enchondromatosis is derived from the cambium layer of the periosteum. Furthermore, in skeletal enchondromatosis the cartilage may be present more or less throughout the entire shaft of an affected long bone. In addition, the actual epiphysial ends of some of the tubular bones may come to

Figure 52

A, Roentgenograph illustrating the appearance of the pelvic bones and upper ends of the femora in the case of a child affected with metaphysial dysostosis. The subject in this case was a girl who was 4½ years of age at the time this x-ray picture and the others in this figure were taken. The child was born at full term, and there was a normal delivery. The chief complaint, as given by the parents, was that the child was growing very slowly and had always had difficulty in walking. The child's parents and sibs presented no skeletal aberrations. In relation to the femora, note the wide, relatively radiolucent area between their capital epiphyses and the expanded and otherwise altered proximal shaft areas. These wide zones of radiolucency are presumably occupied mainly by cartilage, as are the expanded proximal parts of the femoral shafts and also the widened iliac bones.

B and *C*, Roentgenographs demonstrating the status of one knee area and both wrist areas in this case. In the epiphysial-diaphysial junctional regions, the bone shafts are expanded, and there is a wide abnormal zone (presumably representing lobules of cartilage) interposed between the epiphyses and the corresponding shafts. These roentgenographic appearances are strikingly different from those which one observes at corresponding sites in connection with vitamin D-resistant rickets or in renal tubular rickets (of the Fanconi type, for instance).

D, Photomicrograph ($\times$ 25) illustrating the histologic architecture of a biopsy specimen obtained from an epiphysial-diaphysial junctional area in a case of metaphysial dysostosis. The tissue in the upper part of the picture is abnormally vascularized cartilage, and may be held to represent part of an extremely widened epiphysial cartilage plate. Some endochondral ossification has been proceeding on the surface where this cartilage plate is apposed to the bone shaft.

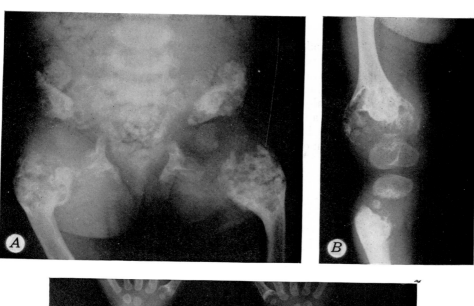

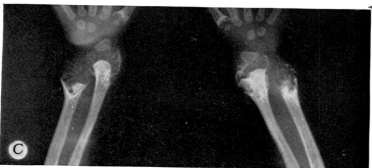

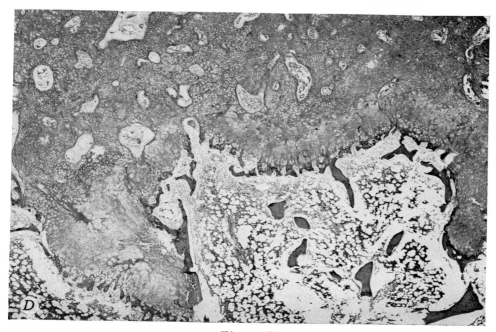

Figure 52

contain cartilage. This usually occurs after the regional epiphysial cartilage plate has disappeared and the epiphysis has fused with the shaft. That is, the cartilage present in the epiphysial ends of an affected tubular bone in enchondromatosis represents cartilage which has extended into these areas from cartilage present in the shaft (see Jaffe). Finally, the writer wishes to point out that there are also differences in histologic detail between the lesional cartilage of metaphysial dysostosis and that of skeletal enchondromatosis. In particular, the cartilage of skeletal enchondromatosis is much more cellular than that of metaphysial dysostosis. (See Fig. 52.)

OSTEOPOIKILOSIS AND OSTEOPATHIA STRIATA

Osteopoikilosis was first clearly delineated as a clinical entity by Albers-Schönberg in 1915 and independently by Ledoux-Lebard *et al.* at about the same time. In 1924, Voorhoeve described a condition, now sometimes denoted as *osteopathia striata* (or Voorhoeve's disease), which he held to represent a variant form of osteopoikilosis—an interpretation now generally favored.

In a *typical* case of *osteopoikilosis*, many of the bones of the affected subject show numerous small foci (or islands) of compact osseous tissue interspersed through the spongiosa as an integral part of its trabecular architecture. These islands of compact bone in the spongiosa appear roentgenographically as discrete or clustered, round, oval, or somewhat elongated foci of radiopacity, giving the affected bone areas a distinctive spotted or mottled appearance. The disorder is inheritable, and there are a number of reports of its occurrence in several generations of one family tree. In addition to the indicated skeletal aberration, the subject not infrequently presents skin lesions of one kind or another.

In a *typical* case of *osteopathia striata*, x-ray examination of affected bones reveals the presence of conspicuous linear striations or markings of variable thickness and extent. The striations stand out particularly well in the metaphyses of the long tubular bones, where they run parallel to the long axis. In flat bones, such as the ilium, they tend to radiate out in a fanlike arrangement. The anatomic basis for the roentgenographic picture of osteopathia striata has not been established, since appropriate studies are lacking. The striations apparently reflect the presence of abnormally thick spongy trabeculae running in a uniform direction.

As noted, it is rather generally held that "osteopoikilosis" and "osteopathia striata" are variant forms of the same basic developmental disorder. Indeed, the father of the two children with "striated" bones described by Voorhoeve, while presenting suggestive striations in a number of bones, also showed small roundish radiopacities suggestive of osteopoikilosis in the ends of some of his bones. These x-ray findings relating to the father constitute one of Voorhoeve's main reasons for holding that the two conditions were variant forms of the same disorder. The writer has seen and will illustrate a case presenting conspicuously both the prominent longitudinal striations in the long bone shafts, such as are characteristic of osteopathia striata, and the numerous spotty mottled opacities prominent in the ends of these bones, such as are characteristic of osteopoikilosis. Furthermore, some of the bones in this case showed extensive patches of diffuse intramedullary radiopacity in their shafts, and some even showed, in addition, cortical thickening due to subperiosteal new bone deposition. Thus, in this case there were additional aberrations further complicating the classification of the condition. In any event, it is still a question, in the writer's opinion, whether osteopathia striata should be regarded as representing merely a variant form of osteopoikilosis—a doubt also expressed by Fairbank. Despite these reservations, it seems appropriate, in view of the predominant opinion, to discuss osteopoikilosis and osteopathia striata in relation to each other.

Nomenclature.—The terms "mottled bones" and "spotted bones" have often been used to designate osteopoikilosis. Other names which have been assigned to the condition include "osteosclerosis disseminata," "familial disseminated osteosclerosis" and "osteopathia condensans disseminata." The latter names have often been applied when no distinctions have been made between osteopoikilosis and osteopathia striata (Voorhoeve's disease).

CLINICAL CONSIDERATIONS

Incidence.—Though osteopoikilosis and osteopathia striata are both of rather rare occurrence, by far the majority of the recorded cases (totalling somewhat over 100) represent instances of typical osteopoikilosis. As to incidence in the general population, it is of interest that a review of the x-ray films in the archives of the emergency hospital (Unfallkrankenhaus) of Vienna revealed a total of only 12 cases of typical osteopoikilosis among the 211,000 patients whose films were surveyed (see Jonasch).

In regard to *sex* incidence, the findings are not consistent, some writers stating that males are more commonly affected by osteopoikilosis, while others state the opposite. The *age* of the subjects at the time of discovery of the presence of the condition varies widely, ranging from early childhood to late adult life. Roentgenographic evidence of osteopoikilosis is usually clear-cut in affected young adults, but some indications of the presence of the disorder may already be found in early childhood if the subject was roentgenographed at that age (see Busch). The relatively few recorded cases of osteopathia striata also show a wide range of variation in respect to the age of the subject at the time the disorder was discovered.

Clinical Findings.—Since the skeletal alterations of osteopoikilosis give rise to no clinical complaints and are innocuous, these alterations are usually recognized only by chance in the course of roentgenographic examination made in connection with some other condition. In regard to osteopathia striata, there are again no complaints definitely referable to the skeletal abnormality. There are statements in the literature indicating that affected subjects are not infrequently somewhat below average in height, that some present broad hands with short fingers, and also that some of them show a predisposition to rheumatic disease. Whether these associations and the occasional presence of some additional skeletal malformation are accidental findings or causally significant remains to be ascertained.

The association of osteopoikilosis with various types of *cutaneous lesions* has already been mentioned. At least 25 to 35 per cent of the subjects show such lesions. The most common lesion of the skin is represented by patches of small (lentil- to bean-sized), roundish or oval, sharply circumscribed, yellowish white or brownish yellow nodules. These are the result of focal hyperplasia of the connective tissue of both the cutis and subcutis, and this condition is regarded as analogous to "disseminated lenticular dermatofibrosis," a hereditary cutaneous disorder (see Buschke and Ollendorff). The cutaneous nodules in question are most commonly observed on the flanks, the buttocks, and the posterior aspect of the thighs. They are not necessarily symmetrical, and it has been reported that they may come and go, especially in young subjects. Another type of skin lesion observed in some cases is represented by lentil-sized, often depressed, horny nodules (keratomas). These are located on the palms and/or soles, are present singly or in small groups, and correspond to the so-called "hereditary keratoma" (see Aigner). Scleroderma-like lesions have also been reported in an occasional case (see Windholz, and Weissmann), and the subjects of the disorder seem to show a predisposition to the formation of keloids at the sites of scars.

Genetic Aspects.—In an individual case, osteopoikilosis or osteopathia striata may appear as a *mutation* or may be *inherited*. An affected subject tends to transmit the disorder to his or her offspring, the condition being inheritable as an autosomal dominant mendelian trait. For instance, Wilcox noted the presence of osteopoikilosis in two members of the same family (father and son). Risseeuw observed a family in which osteopoikilosis was present in a father, six of his children, and a grandchild. Busch reports the finding of 14 cases of osteopoikilosis distributed over three generations in a family tree, and it seems likely that the condition extended further back in that family, since there were already three affected subjects in the first generation in which it was noted. Melnick reports on the occurrence of 17 cases of osteopoikilosis in four generations of a family, and notes that in that family tree all eight offspring of a father and mother, both of whom were affected with osteopoikilosis, were likewise affected. Voorhoeve found osteopathia striata in a father, son, and daughter. Hurt, on the other hand, records the case of a man affected with osteopathia striata whose two children were free of the disorder. Finally, in connection with inheritance, it also seems worth noting that the skeletal aberration, as reflected in the x-ray findings representing typical osteopoikilosis, is likely to become more accentuated from generation to generation of affected subjects.

ROENTGENOGRAPHIC FINDINGS

In an adolescent or young adult presenting the typical picture of *osteopoikilosis*, x-ray examination of the skeleton reveals the presence of numerous small, well-defined radiopacities, nearly always of homogeneous density. The general contour of the bones is not abnormal. The foci of radiopacity are round, oval, or somewhat elongated. While many of them are discrete, others are clustered, and still others may appear lined up in short series whose direction is that of the long axis of the bone. The radiopacities are widely distributed over the skeleton, though certain bones or skeletal regions tend to be only lightly affected or even spared. There is also variation from case to case in respect to the degree of involvement of even those bones which are predilected. Furthermore, in any particular case the distribution of the involvement is usually rather similar on the two sides of the body. That is, the involvement is more or less symmetrical. (See Fig. 53.)

Figure 53

A, Roentgenograph illustrating the spotty radiopacities characteristic of osteopoikilosis, as observed in part of the pelvis and upper ends of the femora of a young woman. The condition was discovered as an incidental finding, and a skeletal survey revealed its presence in numerous other bones also.

B, Roentgenograph of the knee area from another case of osteopoikilosis. In this case, too, the subject was a young woman, and the spotty radiopacities were also noted in practically all the other bones preformed in cartilage.

C, Roentgenograph of part of a hand of a young man who, in the course of a routine medical examination and skeletal survey, was found to be affected with osteopoikilosis. As is usual in this disorder, the bones of the hands were found less heavily spotted than those of the feet.

D, Roentgenograph of part of a foot of a young man demonstrating the mottled spotty appearance of these bones in still another case of osteopoikilosis. In this case, too, practically all the bones preformed in cartilage showed the presence of numerous roundish or oval, discrete and conglomerate radiopacities.

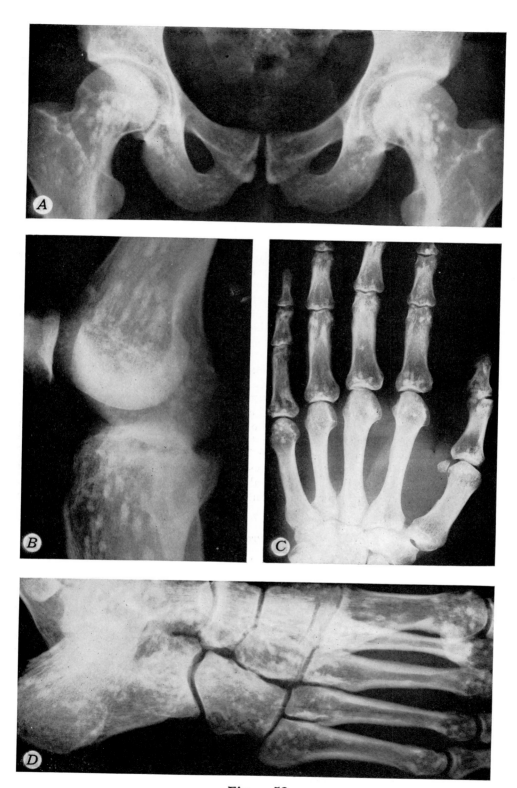

Figure 53

The long tubular bones (specifically their epiphysial ends and adjacent metaphyses) and the bones of the carpus and tarsus show the spotting in almost all cases, and it is in these regions, also, that the specially opaque areas are most numerous. In the innominate bones and scapulae, which are involved to a lesser extent, the radiopacities are likely to be most numerous in the vicinity of the acetabulum and glenoid fossa respectively. The ribs and clavicles and the bones of the vertebral column (except the sacrum) are usually only slightly affected, while the bones of the skull are not likely to be affected at all.

As implied, it is in the adolescents and young adults that the bone mottling of osteopoikilosis stands out most clearly in the roentgenographs. In families in which the disease is indigenous, affected young children already show some spotty radiopacities, particularly in the predilected bone areas. When the condition in such chidren is followed by means of serial roentgenographs, it is found that the radiopaclties become larger, more numerous, and more clear-cut. In a young child, progress .in this direction may be clearly evident even in the course of a year or two. On¹ the other hand, it has also been noted that in old adults the characteristic radiopac¹ties are likely to be less striking than they are in young adults.

In a subject presenting the typical picture of *osteopathia striata*, affected bones show linear radiopaque striations. The striations, which vary in thickness, stand out best in the long tubular bones. In them, they are observed in the metaphyses and adjacent parts of the shaft (usually sparing the epiphysial ends of the bones) and extend in the direction of the long axis of the affected bones. In the iliac portion of the innominate bones, the striations may appear fanlike, radiating toward the iliac crests. Of the bones of the feet, the calcaneus is most likely to show the striations in clear-cut form, while the bones of the hands may show them only faintly or not at all. The clavicles and the bones of the skull are usually spared.

In addition to the cases presenting the typical x-ray picture of osteopoikilosis or of osteopathia striata, there are, as noted, cases in which these two conditions appear to be present in combination or in association with some other skeletal aberration. For instance, in an otherwise typical case of osteopoikilosis observed by the writer, the frontal bones of the calvarium showed conspicuous thickening, such as one observes in hyperostosis frontalis interna, and the bones of the base

Figure 54

A, Roentgenograph showing the upper end of a femur and part of the corresponding innominate bone in the case of a boy 12 years of age presenting features of both osteopoikilosis and osteopathia striata. Note the numerous conglomerate roundish radiopacities in the capital femoral epiphysis and the faint striations in the femoral neck. The cortex of the femoral shaft is thickened in a pattern somewhat suggestive of melorheostosis, and some of the other tubular bones also showed such cortical thickening.

B, Roentgenograph illustrating the appearance of the lower end of the femur shown in *A* and also the corresponding knee joint area. The lower femoral epiphysis and the upper tibial epiphysis show numerous conglomerate radiopacities. In contrast, the lower end of the femoral shaft presents well-defined longitudinal striations, such as are characteristic of osteopathia striata (Voorhoeve's disease).

C and *D*, Roentgenographs of the lower end of the femur and the knee joint area from the case illustrated in *B* showing the appearance of these parts when the boy had attained the age of 17. In the lateral projection (*C*), the roundish radiopacities still stand out distinctly in the lower femoral and upper tibial epiphysial bone ends, while longitudinal striations have become apparent also in the upper end of the tibia. In the anteroposterior projection (*D*), the striated appearance of the lower part of the femoral shaft is striking, while the epiphysial end of the bone casts a radiopaque shadow, larger, on the whole, because of agglomeration of the spotty radiopacities.

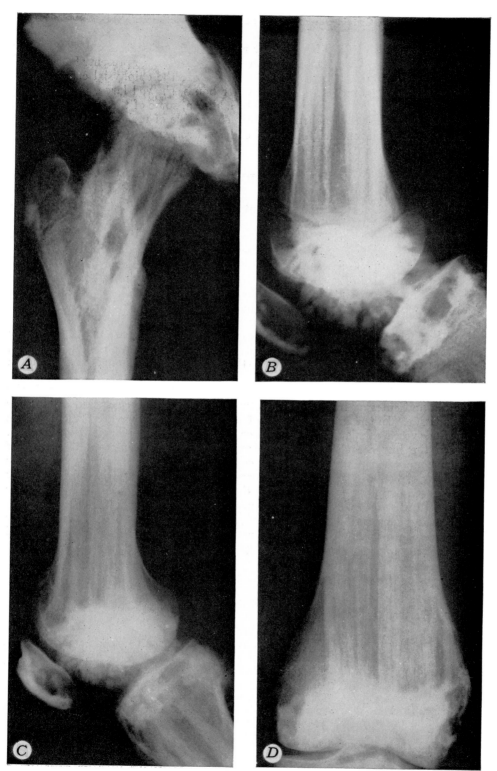

Figure 54

of the skull were also thick and diffusely radiopaque. In another case studied by the writer, the ends of the shafts of many of the long bones presented the roentgenographic appearance of osteopathia striata, while the epiphysial ends of some of these bones, along with some of the other bones, showed large, agglomerated radiopacities suggesting osteopoikilosis. In addition, some of the tubular bones in this case showed cortical thickening mildly suggestive of melorheostosis and also some extensive homogeneous patches of endosteal sclerosis. (See Fig. 54.)

PATHOLOGIC FINDINGS

As already noted, there are no pertinent anatomic studies relating to osteopathia striata, but there are a few reports on the pathologic anatomy of osteopoikilosis (see Schmorl, and Brücke). The writer, too, has had the opportunity of examining, both grossly and microscopically, a number of bones from a case of osteopoikilosis. On *gross examination* the sectioned bones in this case revealed roundish or oval foci of compact bone in the spongiosa, corresponding to the pinhead-sized or larger areas of radiopacity visible roentgenographically. These foci of compact osseous tissue were found attached to, and continuous with, spongy trabeculae presenting a normal appearance. In the epiphysial ends of the tubular bones, the roundish or oval areas of compact osseous tissue were hardly ever in contact with the bony end plate beneath the articular cartilage. In the metaphyses, on the other hand, they were usually located peripherally—that is, where the spongiosa abuts upon the bone cortex.

On *microscopic examination* the foci of compact bone dispersed through the spongiosa and entering into its architecture are found to be composed of lamellar osseous tissue. In the interior of these foci, haversian systems are present. That is, one finds vessel canals ringed by more or less concentric lamellae of osseous tissue. Between the haversian systems there are small irregular interstitial islands of lamellar bone. At the periphery of the compact islands, one notes stratified layers of lamellar osseous tissue which are separated by cement lines. We do not know how the osteopoikilotic foci arise nor is there much known about the rate of their growth. In none of the tissue sections prepared from the bones in the case studied by the writer was there any residual calcified cartilage matrix in the compact osseous foci in question. In any event, it does not seem probable that the foci are formed through endochondral ossification of cartilage rests. (See Fig. 55.)

Figure 55

A, Roentgenograph of the head of a humerus removed at autopsy in the case of a young woman in whom the presence of osteopoikilosis represented an incidental clinical finding. Note the numerous discrete and agglomerated roundish radiopacities.

B, Roentgenograph of a thin longitudinal slice cut in the sagittal plane from the humeral head shown in *A*.

C, Photomicrograph ($\times$ 4) illustrating a number of islands of compact osseous tissue interspersed through the spongiosa as an integral part of its architecture in a tissue section prepared from the humeral head illustrated in *A* and *B*. The histologic structure of the bone island indicated by the arrows is more fully presented in *D*.

D, Photomicrograph ($\times$ 25) showing in some detail the structure of the compact island of bone and its relation to the neighboring spongy trabeculae. Note that the osseous tissue is essentially of the lamellar type, and that many of the vessel canals in the focus of bone are surrounded by concentric rings of lamellar osseous tissue.

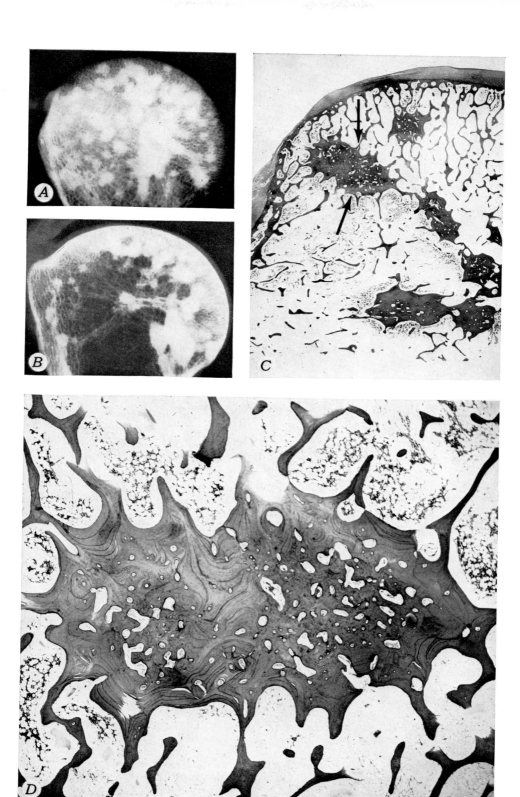

Figure 55

Finally, it seems appropriate to note that the rather frequently encountered *solitary enostosis* ("bone spot") presents anatomically the same gross and microscopic features as individual bone islands in cases of osteopoikilosis.

CLEIDOCRANIAL DYSOSTOSIS

Cleidocranial dysostosis is a skeletal disorder in which, as its name implies, the principal abnormalities are in the clavicles and the cranium. In typical cases: (1) The clavicles are incompletely formed, often being represented merely by sternal fragments, and (2) the calvarium is defective, its bones during early life being separated by abnormally large fontanelles and by wide dehiscences, especially along suture lines, although in later life these defects are usually found largely closed by irregular islands of bone. In addition to abnormalities in the clavicles and calvarium, there are usually abnormalities in other skeletal regions also, and especially in the facial skeleton. Here, many of the bones (particularly those likewise entirely or largely preformed in membrane) are small and underdeveloped, and the jaws are likely to be deformed by the presence of unerupted teeth. Marie and Sainton first gave the condition its current name, and they furthermore emphasized the hereditary factor in its occurrence.

CLINICAL CONSIDERATIONS

Though the disorder is certainly congenital, its presence not infrequently goes unrecognized until late childhood or even early adult life. It appears that the condition tends to predilect males. Typically, the most conspicuous clinical manifestation is an extraordinary mobility of the shoulders, based upon the alterations in the clavicles. In most cases the shoulders can be pulled forward, at least passively, until they almost touch in the midline. Not infrequently, too, they droop

Figure 56

A, Photograph of a woman 46 years of age affected with cleidocranial dysostosis. A short distance above the root of the nose there is an obvious depression of the forehead. It extended back to the coronal suture and was definitely wider posteriorly than anteriorly. This gutter-like depression had a yielding floor. Each clavicle was represented merely by a sternal fragment so small that the woman was able to coapt her shoulders.

B, Photograph of the calvarium from a case of cleidocranial dysostosis. The subject was a woman 60 years of age who died of a carcinoma of the body of the uterus. Note the large gutter-like defect in the frontal region. The dehiscence in the bone extends forward from the coronal suture, and the defect is filled in by fibrous tissue. Numerous wormian bones are visible along the parietal and lambdoid sutures.

C, Photograph of the macerated skull from a case of cleidocranial dysostosis in a man who was 59 years of age at the time of his death. The skull shows the characteristic calvarial defect in the frontal region.

D, Photograph displaying the lateral view of the skull illustrated in *C*. Note the numerous wormian bones composing the posterior portion of the cranium. (This illustration, and also *A* and *C*, are reproduced from the article by Hultkrantz.)

E, Roentgenograph showing the region of the left shoulder from a man 35 years of age affected with cleidocranial dysostosis. The clavicle illustrated consists of two completely separate fragments of bone.

F, Roentgenograph illustrating part of the pelvis in the case cited in *E*. Note that the superior and inferior rami of the pubic bones are not joined, and that there is a wide gap in the region of the pubic symphysis.

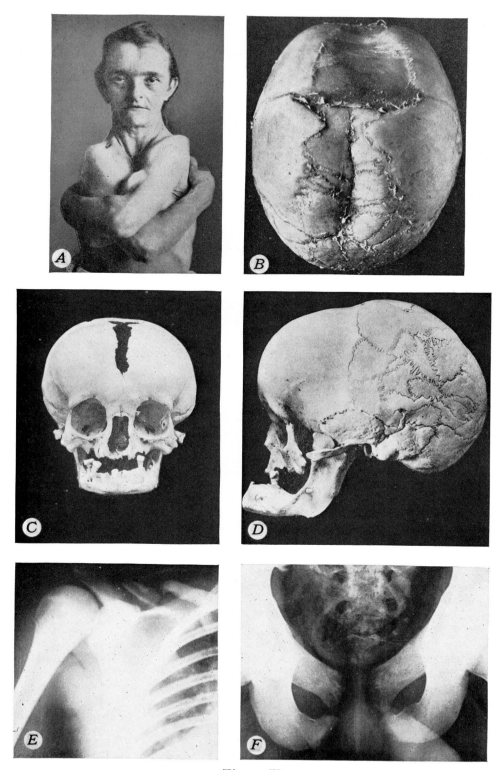

Figure 56

noticeably, but there is rarely any associated disability. Furthermore, the appearance of the subjects is striking, in that the calvarial vault seems excessively large in proportion to the face. In fact, the latter is often conspicuously small because of the receding cheeks and abnormally flat nasal root. On the other hand, the circumference of the calvarium is actually above the average, due mainly to the presence of pronounced bossing in the frontal and parietal regions. Frequently, also, an obvious furrow can be seen or felt in the frontal region between the prominent frontal bosses. Indeed, in some cases, palpation may reveal that bone is entirely lacking along the whole line of this furrow or at least in the region of the anterior fontanelle. It may even be lacking in the area of the posterior fontanelle or in the region of other sutures. The palate is very often highly arched and sometimes cleft or furrowed. Defects of the teeth (late or incomplete eruption, irregular position or development, or caries) are common, and probably arise from restriction of the tooth-forming areas by stunting of the jaws.

While it is mainly the skull and the clavicles that are involved, it should be noted that the stature of the affected subjects is usually below the average. In addition, not infrequently they show various collateral abnormalities, including, notably, deformities of the sternum, ribs, and vertebral column, subluxations of various joints, and genu valgum. These, like the shortness of stature, are difficult to explain. Apart from their skeletal abnormalities, persons affected with cleidocranial dysostosis often enjoy good health, and mentally, too, they are usually normal. (See LaChapelle and also Fitchet.)

Genetic Aspects.—Stocks and Barrington, who collected 144 cases of cleidocranial dysostosis, found that in 96 the dysostosis was known to be familial or hereditary. In the remaining 48, either there was no definite evidence of other cases in the family, or no satisfactory family history could be obtained. Others, too, have reported the high incidence of hereditary transmission of the disorder, while also indicating that in about a third of the cases it appears as a sporadic mutation (see Soule). The condition may be inherited through either parent, and if one of the parents is affected, about half of the offspring come to show the disorder. Since it is clear that the condition is a deep-rooted anomaly of skeletal development, evidently carried in the genes of the affected subject, it is to be expected that the clavicles and calvarium will present evidences of the underlying defect from the very beginning of ossification of these parts.

ROENTGENOGRAPHIC AND PATHOLOGIC FINDINGS

One of the fullest discussions of the pathology of the condition is that by Hultkrantz. The latter devoted detailed attention to the status of the skull on the basis of findings in many museum specimens, and the aberrations in this region have also been discussed by others (see Ladewig). In most reported instances, both the cranium and the clavicles have, of course, been found affected, although often to very unequal degrees. There do seem to be a few cases, however, in which the disorder was characteristic in the cranium and not manifest at all in the clavicles and, conversely (though even more rarely), cases in which the involvement seemed to be limited to the latter.

As to the *clavicles*, the most common pathologic finding is absence of part of each clavicle (outer, or acromial, end) or division of each clavicle into two sections. In the former case the clavicles are represented merely by fragments attached to the sternum, tapering off or ending abruptly at a varying distance from it. These sternal rudiments may be as little as one third or less of the length of the normal clavicle. They usually articulate normally with the sternum, but sometimes only by a lax attachment. Their nonarticulating ends may be free and very mobile. Not infrequently, however, they are bound by fibrous cords either to the coracoid process or, less commonly, to the acromion, the first rib, or the glenoid cavity of the scapula on each side. When the clavicular defect consists of division of each clavicle into two sections, the latter are nearly always separated by a fairly wide gap, which is often filled in by fibrous or ligamentous tissue. Finally, it may be noted that a few cases of cleidocranial dysostosis have been observed in which the clavicles were apparently entirely absent. Plausibly enough, the muscles normally attached to the clavicles are usually either missing, attached to substitute tissues or structures, or atrophied, in accordance with the severity of the clavicular involvement.

In regard to the *skull*, it should be recalled that the most important abnormalities are in the calvarium. Especially in young subjects, the defective ossification at the sutural borders is manifested by the presence of broad gaps bridged by connective tissue (particularly along the median suture lines), abnormally large fontanelles, and other sutures still conspicuous where normally they would already have become obliterated or nearly so. As the subject grows older, the sutural dehiscences tend to close over. However, a wide gap is likely to remain between the frontal bones. Furthermore, the calvarium usually shows a patchwork of small bones (wormian bones) representing individual unfused centers of ossification. These often replace the parietal bones or other calvarial bones to a large extent or completely. As to its general shape, the calvarium tends to present exaggerated frontal bosses, to be flattened laterally, and to be more than normally domed.

In contrast to the calvarium, the cranial base, being formed in cartilage, is not strikingly affected. However, its configuration may be somewhat distorted because of slight inhibition of growth, especially in its transverse dimension. Also, the position of the foramen magnum may have become shifted forward. The effects of the inhibition of growth of the facial skeleton have already been noted in connection with the clinical aspects of the disorder.*

Among the other skeletal abnormalities to be noted are those relating to the pubic bones. It may be found that the bodies of both pubic bones are absent, and even one or both pubic rami may be missing. The pubic rami may eventually appear, as may also the bodies of the pubic bones, but in any event the symphysis pubis tends to be unusually wide. Not infrequently one may note that there has been failure of union of one or more neural arches in the lumbar and/or dorsal region of the vertebral column. Other abnormalities occasionally encountered include the presence of epiphyses at both ends of the metacarpal and metatarsal bones. Furthermore, the terminal phalanges of the fingers and toes may be abnormally short and pointed. (See Fig. 56.)

REFERENCES

AIGNER, R.: Ueber Osteopoikilie verbunden mit Keratoma hereditarium dissipatum palmare et plantare (Brauer), Wien. klin. Wchnschr., *65*[2] (N.F.B. *8*[2]), 860, 1953.

*Under the name *"craniofacial dysostosis"* (Crouzon's disease), there has been described another hereditary anomaly of skeletal development predilecting the skull. The condition is characterized clinically by a fantastic exophthalmos, divergent strabismus, and, ultimately, often amaurosis, associated with a very short upper jaw and pronounced prognathism of the lower jaw (see Médinger and Morard). Craniofacial dysostosis results primarily from premature synostosis of the sutures of the cranium. In consequence of this process, the cranial vault becomes steep, and the appearance is that of oxycephaly (tower skull). However, the condition differs from other forms of oxycephaly in that the base of the cranial vault is very much sunken, so that the cranial cavity is more or less globular in shape. Thus the exophthalmos is due to shallowness of the ocular orbits, and the amaurosis to compression of the optic nerves in their foramina.

ALBERS-SCHÖNBERG, H.: Eine seltene, bisher nicht bekannte Strukturanomalie des Skelettes, Fortschr. Geb. Röntgenstrahlen, *23*, 174, 1915–16.

ANDERSON, C. E., CRANE, J. T., HARPER, H. A., and HUNTER, T. W.: Morquio's Disease and Dysplasia Epiphysalis Multiplex. A Study of Epiphyseal Cartilage in Seven Cases, J. Bone & Joint Surg., *44-A*, 295, 1962.

BRAILSFORD, J. F.: Chondro-Osteo-Dystrophy. Roentgenographic & Clinical Features of a Child with Dislocation of Vertebrae, Am. J. Surg., *7*, 404, 1929.

BRÜCKE, H.: Über multiple Enostosen (Osteopoikilie), Deutsche Ztschr. Chir., *239*, 554, 1933.

BURCKHARDT, E.: Ein Fall von Chondrodystrophia fetalis calcarea, Schweiz. med. Wchnschr., *68*, 330, 1938.

BUSCH, K. F. B.: Familial Disseminated Osteosclerosis, Acta radiol., *18*, 693, 1937.

BUSCHKE, A., and OLLENDORFF, H.: Ein Fall von Dermatofibrosis lenticularis disseminata und Osteopathia condensans disseminata, Dermat. Wchnschr., *86*, 257, 1928.

CAFFEY, J.: Gargoylism (Hunter-Hurler Disease, Dysostosis Multiplex, Lipochondrodystrophy); Prenatal and Neonatal Bone Lesions and Their Early Postnatal Evolution, Bull. Hosp. Joint Dis., *12*, 38, 1951.

CALANDI, C., and VICHI, G. F.: Studio clinico e radiologico su un caso di gargoilismo (malattia di Pfaundler-Hurler), Riv. clin. pediat., *62*, 9, 1958.

CAMERON, J. A. P., YOUNG, W. B., and SISSONS, H. A.: Metaphysial Dysostosis, J. Bone & Joint Surg., *36-B*, 622, 1954.

CONRADI, E.: Vorzeitiges Auftreten von Knochen- und eigenartigen Verkalkungskernen bei Chondrodystrophia fötalis hypoplastica. Histologische und Röntgenuntersuchungen, Jahrb. Kinderh., *80*, 86, 1914.

EINHORN, N. H., MOORE, J. R., OSTRUM, H. W., and ROWNTREE, L. G.: Osteochondrodystrophia Deformans (Morquio's Disease), Am. J. Dis. Child., *61*, 776, 1941.

EVANS, R., and CAFFEY, J.: Metaphyseal Dysostosis Resembling Vitamin D-Refractory Rickets, Am. J. Dis. Child., *95*, 640, 1958.

FAIRBANK, T.: *An Atlas of General Affections of the Skeleton*, Edinburgh & London, E. & S. Livingstone Ltd., 1951.

FANCONI, G.: Über einen Fall von Dysostosis enchondralis epiphysaria (Ribbingsche Krankheit) vom Typus der Mikroepiphysen im Frühstadium, Helvet. paediat. acta, *2*, 33, 1947.

FITCHET, S. M.: Cleidocranial Dysostosis: Hereditary and Familial, J. Bone & Joint Surg., *11*, 838, 1929.

FORD, N., SILVERMAN, F. N., and KOZLOWSKI, K.: Spondylo-epiphyseal Dysplasia (Pseudoachondroplastic Type), Am. J. Roentgenol., *86*, 462, 1961.

FRANK, W. W., and DENNY, M. B.: Dysplasia Epiphysialis Punctata. Report of a Case and Review of Literature, J. Bone & Joint Surg., *36-B*, 118, 1954.

DE HAAS, W. H. D., DE BOER, W., and GRIFFIOEN, F.: Metaphysial Dysostosis: A Late Follow-up of the First Reported Case, J. Bone & Joint Surg., *51-B*, 290, 1969.

HARRIS, H. A.: *Bone Growth in Health and Disease*, London, Oxford University Press, 1933, Chap. 23.

HÄSSLER, E., and SCHALLOCK, G.: Chondrodystrophia calcificans, Monatsschr. Kinderh., *82*, 133, 1940.

HIRSCH, I. S.: Generalized Osteochondrodystrophy. The Eccentrochondroplastic Form, J. Bone & Joint Surg., *19*, 297, 1937.

HOBAEK, A.: *Problems of Hereditary Chondrodysplasias*, Oslo, Oslo University Press, 1961.

HODKINSON, H. M.: Double Patellae in Multiple Epiphysial Dysplasia, J. Bone & Joint Surg., *44-B*, 569, 1962.

HULTKRANTZ, J. W.: Über Dysostosis cleidocranialis, Ztschr. Morphol. u. Anthropol., *11*, 385, 1908.

HÜNERMANN, C.: Chondrodystrophia calcificans congenita als abortive Form der Chondrodystrophie, Ztschr. Kinderh., *51*, 1, 1931.

HURT, R. L.: Osteopathia Striata—Voorhoeve's Disease. Report of a Case Presenting the Features of Osteopathia Striata and Osteopetrosis, J. Bone & Joint Surg., *35-B*, 89, 1953.

JAFFE, H. L.: *Tumors and Tumorous Conditions of the Bones and Joints*, Philadelphia, Lea & Febiger, 1958, Chap. 11.

JANSEN, M.: Über atypische Chondrodystrophie (Achondroplasie) und über eine noch nicht beschriebene angeborene Wachstumsstörung des Knochensystems: Metaphysäre Dysostosis, Ztschr. orthop. Chir., *61*, 253, 1934.

JONASCH, E.: 12 Fälle von Osteopoikilie, Fortschr. Geb. Röntgenstrahlen, *82*, 344, 1955.

KARLEN, A. G., and CAMERON, J. A. P.: Dysplasia Epiphysialis Punctata, J. Bone & Joint Surg., *39-B*, 293, 1957.

LaCHAPELLE, E. H.: *Dysostose cléido-cranienne héréditaire*, Rotterdam, Van Vleet, 1918.

LADEWIG, P.: Anatomische Untersuchung eines Falles von Dysostosis cleidocranialis, Arch. path. Anat., *291*, 540, 1933.

LEDOUX-LEBARD, R., CHABANEIX, and DESSANE: L'ostéopoecilie, forme nouvelle d'ostéite condensante généralisée sans symptomes cliniques, J. radiol. et électrol., *2*, 133, 1916–1917.

LENK, R.: Hereditary Metaphyseal Dysostosis, Am. J. Roentgenol., *76*, 569, 1956.

LITCHMAN, H. M., and CHIRLS, M.: Dysplasia Epiphysalis Multiplex, Bull. Hosp. Joint Dis., *19*, 88, 1958.

MARIE, P., and SAINTON, P.: Sur la dysostose cléido-cranienne héréditaire, Rev. neurol., *6*, 835, 1898.

MAROTEAUX, P., and LAMY, M.: Les formes pseudo-achondroplasiques des dysplasies spondylo-épiphysaires, Presse méd., *67*, 383, 1959.

MAUDSLEY, R. H.: Dysplasia Epiphysialis Multiplex. A Report of Fourteen Cases in Three Families, J. Bone & Joint Surg., *37-B*, 228, 1955.

MÉDINGER, F., and MORARD, G.: Dysostose cranio-faciale (maladie de Crouzon). Contribution a l'étude de ses manifestations oculaires, Arch. opht., *52*, 489, 1935.

MELNICK, J. C.: Osteopathia Condensans Disseminata (Osteopoikilosis). Study of a Family of 4 Generations, Am. J. Roentgenol., *82*, 229, 1959.

MORQUIO, L.: Sur une forme de dystrophie osseuse familiale, Bull. Soc. de pédiat. de Paris, *27*, 145, 1929.

MÜLLER, G. M., and SISSONS, H. A.: A Case of Renal Rickets Simulating "Metaphysial Dysostosis," J. Bone & Joint Surg., *33-B*, 231, 1951.

PETERSON, J. C.: Metaphyseal dysostosis: Questionably a form of vitamin D-resistant rickets, J. Pediat., *60*, 656, 1962.

POHL, J. F.: Chondro-Osteodystrophy (Morquio's Disease). Progressive Kyphosis from Congenital Wedge-Shaped Vertebrae, J. Bone & Joint Surg., *21*, 187, 1939.

PUTSCHAR, W. G. J.: Chondrodystrophia Calcificans Congenita (Dysplasia Epiphysialis Punctata), Bull. Hosp. Joint Dis., *12*, 514, 1951.

RAAP, G.: Chondrodystrophia Calcificans Congenita, Am. J. Roentgenol., *49*, 77, 1943.

RISSEEUW, J.: Familiaire osteopoikilie, Nederl. tijdschr. geneesk., *80*, 3827, 1936.

SCHMORL, G.: Anatomische Befunde bei einem Falle von Osteopoikilie, Fortschr. Geb. Röntgenstrahlen, *44*, 1, 1931.

SHEPHARD, E.: Multiple Epiphysial Dysplasia, J. Bone & Joint Surg., *38-B*, 458, 1956.

SILVERMAN, F. N.: Dysplasies épiphysaires: entité protéiforme, Ann. Radiol., *4*, 833, 1961.

SOULE, A. B., JR.: Mutational Dysostosis (Cleidocranial Dysostosis), J. Bone & Joint Surg., *28*, 81, 1946.

STOCKS, P., and BARRINGTON, A.: Hereditary Disorders of Bone Development. *Eugenics Laboratory Memoirs*, No. 22, London, Cambridge University Press, 1925.

VINKE, T. H., and DUFFY, F. P.: Chondrodystrophia Calcificans Congenita. Report of Two Cases, J. Bone & Joint Surg., *29*, 509, 1947.

VOORHOEVE, N.: L'image radiologique non encore décrite d'une anomalie du squelette, Acta radiol., *3*, 407, 1924.

WEINBERG, H., FRANKEL, M., MAKIN, M., and VAS, E.: Familial Epiphysial Dysplasia of the Lower Limbs, J. Bone & Joint Surg., *42-B*, 313, 1960.

WEISSMANN, G.: Scleroderma Associated with Osteopoikilosis, Arch. Int. Med., *101*, 108, 1958.

WILCOX, L. F.: Osteopoikilosis, Am. J. Roentgenol., *30*, 615, 1933.

WINDHOLZ, F.: Systemerkrankung des Skelets (Osteopoikilie), kombiniert mit einer Affektion der Haut (Dermatofibrosis lenticularis disseminata), Wien. klin. Wchnschr., *44*, 1611, 1931.

Chapter

10

Paget's Disease

In 1877, Paget described the skeletal disease which now bears his name but which he himself denoted as "osteitis deformans." His accounts of the condition related to cases in which the skeleton was extensively and severely affected—that is, to cases already showing widespread skeletal involvement and obvious deformity of individual bones. However, it has come to be recognized that cases such as Paget described, in which the disease was present in its full efflorescence, represent only a small proportion of the total cases of the disease as we now know it. Indeed, it has been made clear through roentgenographic and anatomic studies that the condition is not only fairly common but that, much more often than not, the extent of involvement of the skeleton is rather limited when the presence of Paget's disease is first recognized. In such cases the disease frequently expresses itself in alterations restricted to a few bones, and sometimes even in involvement of only one bone or bone part (see Schmorl, Jaffe, and also Goldenberg). Under these circumstances it often fails to give rise to any clinical complaints, the presence of the disease being discovered only fortuitously. This is likely to happen when, for instance, the involvement is limited to a few vertebrae or part of the pelvic girdle or calvarium.

It has also come to be recognized that, in the calvarium, Paget's disease may first be expressed roentgenographically in the form of large single or multiple areas of radiolucency unassociated with modification in calvarial thickness—the so-called "osteoporosis circumscripta cranii" (see Sosman, Schüller, and Kasabach and Dyke). The basic detailed anatomic study of calvarial osteoporosis circumscripta was made by Erdheim.* He supplied proof that it is actually an expression of Paget's disease, and that it represents, in particular, a precursor of the conventional changes of the disease in the calvarium, which may not make their appearance for some years.

The etiology of Paget's disease is still obscure, but there seem to be indications that the disease is conditioned by some genetic factor. In this connection it is of historical interest that, for a long time, "osteitis deformans" of Paget and "osteitis fibrosa cystica" of Recklinghausen were held to represent merely different forms of the same basic disorder—the "hyperostotic" and the "hypostotic" form, respectively, of so-called fibrous osteodystrophy (see Christeller). However, the discovery by Mandl in 1926 that Recklinghausen's "generalized osteitis fibrosa cystica" represented the skeletal expression of hyperparathyroidism clearly separated the two disease entities.

That the skeletal involvement in Paget's disease is more or less focal is now well established. Even when the skeleton as a whole is extensively implicated, one will usually find some areas exempted in an unsystematic way. Thus, one femur or tibia, for instance, may be spared or only slightly affected while the other is heavily involved. In general, no matter how widespread the disease may be in a given case, the bones of the hands and feet are very likely to be spared, perhaps completely.

* Many of the illustrations appearing in this chapter are reproduced from material originally collected by the eminent Viennese pathologist, Professor Jakob Erdheim.

240

In a bone part undergoing the changes of Paget's disease, the original osseous tissue becomes reconstructed through an active interplay between bone resorption and new bone apposition. The reconstructed spongy and cortical bone is peculiar not only in its gross appearance but also in its microscopic structure. In regard to the latter, the osseous tissue comes to show a histologic pattern in which innumerable osseous fragments of irregular size are faceted together and bounded by correspondingly irregular cement lines. This chaotic jigsaw (or mosaic) pattern is the histologic hallmark of the altered bone in Paget's disease.

CLINICAL CONSIDERATIONS

General Incidence.—It appears that there are geographic and racial differences in the incidence of Paget's disease. For example, the disease is reported to be exceedingly rare among the Chinese. On the other hand, it has been found to be relatively common among inhabitants of Australia of Anglo-Saxon origin who were born in that country or emigrated to it from the United Kingdom (see Barry). Furthermore, there are indications that the disease is more prevalent in Great Britain and certain parts of continental Europe than in the United States, though it is by no means a rare disorder in that country either.

At any rate, in those geographical areas where the disease is encountered frequently, it is certainly one of the more common skeletal disorders. Some idea of its actual incidence can be gained from the findings of Schmorl. In a consecutive series of 4,614 autopsies on subjects over 40 years of age, the skeleton revealed evidence of Paget's disease in 138—that is, in 3.3 per cent of the subjects. Of course, only a very small proportion of them showed it spread widely over the skeleton. The high total incidence is accounted for rather by the discovery of numerous cases in which the skeletal involvement was of rather limited extent. In many of these cases the disease was not known to have been present clinically and was found restricted anatomically—for instance, to one or a few lumbar vertebrae, part of the sacrum or of an innominate bone, or even part of the calvarium, or to several of these areas in combination.

Familial Incidence.—There are many reports of the occurrence of Paget's disease in several sibs of one family and also in various members of several generations of a given family (see Gutman and Kasabach, Rast and Weber, and Stemmermann). The writer knows of a family in which a man, one of his daughters, one of his brothers, and the son of one of his sisters all presented evidence of the disease. Furthermore, in a few instances, Paget's disease has been observed in both members of a pair of identical twins (see Martin, and Aschner *et al.*). The frequent familial occurrence of the disease points strongly to the influence of a hereditary factor. It has been suggested that the trait for Paget's disease is controlled by a simple autosomal mendelian-dominant gene (see McKusick). On the other hand, it has been proposed that it is inherited as a sex-linked recessive (see Ashley Montagu).

Sex and Age Incidence.—The relevant statistics seem to indicate that the disease is more common in males than in females. However, the difference is not great enough to suggest that the sex factor is significant in the etiology of the condition. In regard to age incidence, it is well established that in the great majority of the cases the disease does not begin to appear until about the age of 40. In a large series of cases observed by the writer, most of the patients were at least 50 years of age when the disease was first recognized. When, as occasionally happens, it is recognized in a subject between the ages of 30 and 40, it may already be well advanced but is much more likely to be of only limited extent and may even be represented only by osteoporosis circumscripta of the calvarium. Going back into the histories of some middle-aged patients, one sometimes also encounters a case in which the onset can be dated back fairly definitely to the late twenties. However, the reported occurrences of Paget's disease in any form before the age of 20 should be viewed with skepticism.

Clinical Complaints and Findings.—Many cases of Paget's disease are brought to light entirely by chance in the course of roentgenographic examination of some visceral part which has been a source of complaint. Many others are discovered when a region such as a lower limb or the lower part of the back is roentgenographed because of relatively mild pain, in the absence of external evidence of disease in the bones of the part. Sometimes osteoporosis circumscripta of the calvarium (which is asymptomatic) is discovered in the course of examination of the skull for disease of the sinuses. Occasionally, areas of circumscribed calvarial osteoporosis are present and persist for years as the sole evidence of the disease. Often, however, calvarial osteoporosis is associated with more typical changes of Paget's disease in at least one other skeletal site—usually the pelvis.

The most common and natural question arising in cases in which the skeletal involvement is still limited relates to the likelihood of progression. In this connection it should be recognized that in the great majority of cases the disease never evolves into the extreme form. Indeed, cases in which the skeletal involvement is limited often fail to show significant progression even when followed over a course of many years from the time of their initial recognition. Furthermore, even when there is progression, it is usually very slow. In fact, 10 or 15 years or perhaps more may elapse before the disorder evolves to a stage in which the skeleton is heavily implicated.

That Paget's disease may affect one bone (indeed, even a single vertebra) and remain limited to that bone is another fact now generally recognized. The question of Paget's disease limited to a long bone of a limb has elicited much discussion because of the special clinical problems it raises. It is clear that the long bone involved becomes thickened and deformed, and, if it is the tibia, the bone acquires the shape of a saber blade. Many have held that the occurrence of Paget's disease limited to a tibia can sometimes be traced back to a trauma, but this idea has been refuted by others (see Pick). When the disease is limited to a single long bone, it must be recognized that the monostotic feature of the case frequently turns out, in the course of years, to represent nothing more than the protracted localization of the disease in a single long bone before other bones become affected. In an occasional case, however, the disease evidently never comes to implicate any additional bones. In this respect the involvement of a single long bone is not different from the exclusive involvement, in one case or another, of the sacrum, one or more vertebrae, or the calvarium, for instance.

A subject who presents himself with some clinical skeletal abnormalities already suggesting Paget's disease may state, for instance, that a shin bone has become bowed, and that the skin overlying it is somewhat warm. A patient presenting more widespread involvement of the skeleton is likely to give a history of: increasing head size, increasing deafness, discomfort or vague pain in the back or lower limbs, increasing curvature of the lower limbs, or combinations of these complaints. Sometimes, even in cases showing fairly advanced skeletal changes, it is only upon the occurrence of a pathologic fracture (especially of a femur or tibia) that medical care is sought. The writer has even seen cases in which attention was first directed to the presence of the disease by the appearance of a complicating bone sarcoma in one bone or another.

The external appearance of a subject in whom the skeletal involvement is widespread is rather typical. The head is usually large and low-set and may jut forward. In males, baldness is common, and in any event the hairline is likely to have receded far back even in the women. The temporal vessels are usually very prominent and tortuous, and the ears may stand away from the head or be curved backward. The patient may be round-shouldered and show some curvature of the vertebral column in the thoracic region and possibly some deformation of the rest of the thorax. This may contribute to the cardiorespiratory difficulty so often present, but the latter is due mainly to associated cardiovascular-renal disease based on generalized arteriosclerosis.

The long bones of the lower limbs are usually much more severely affected than those of the upper, though, rarely, a case is observed in which the reverse is true. A prominent and common feature of the advanced cases is bowleggedness. In addition to lateral bowing of the femora and tibiae, there is often also anterior bowing, especially of the latter. If the tibiae are severely bowed, the skin over them is likely to be found brownishly discolored. The height of the subject is often considerably reduced because of the deformities in the trunk and lower extremities. However, the latter remain strong enough to support the body even in the most advanced stages of the disease. Altogether, in a very severe case, the sunken, protruding head, hanging arms, bent carriage, and waddling gait may even give the subject a somewhat apelike appearance.

As noted, the pain felt by subjects affected with Paget's disease is referred especially to the back and lower limbs. It tends to be exacerbated by cold and inclement weather and by muscular activity. It is very likely to be present during the first few years of the disease and is sometimes noted throughout its course. The pains in the lower limbs may be due in part to shifts in the muscle attachments. A contributory factor may be changes in the arteries of the extremities, since the larger vessels are very often found extensively calcified. However, there are cases in which the disease develops to a very advanced degree of deformity unassociated with any complaint of pain.

With the exception of the deafness (sometimes quite extreme), complaints referable to involvement of cranial nerves are rare. If they do arise, their occurrence is ascribable to compression of these nerves in their foramina. There may be retinal hemorrhages or degeneration, and choroidal changes. Mental symptoms are rare, in spite of the extensive alterations that may take place in the capacity and shape of the cranial cavity. Nevertheless, in occasional instances, altered mentality of the nature of senile dementia has been noted. It is difficult to estimate how much of the mental deterioration in such cases is related to the slow brain trauma due to compression within a reduced cranial cavity and how much is due to cerebral arteriosclerosis, but in some it is clearly due to the former (see Grünthal). Compression of the cord and/or spinal nerve roots may also occur, and a number of such cases have been reported (see Schwarz and Reback, Amyes and Vogel, Whalley, and also Melanotte). Not infrequently, this occurs in the thoracic region. The writer himself has seen several instances of paraplegia and rectal and vesical incontinence from compression of the cord (requiring laminectomy) in cases of Paget's disease. He has even seen a neuropathic fracture of a femur in a case of Paget's disease in which the cord had undergone permanent damage from compression.

BIOCHEMICAL FINDINGS

The *serum alkaline phosphatase* value is almost invariably raised in Paget's disease (see Bodansky and Jaffe, Woodard *et al.*, and Jaffe and Bodansky). In our experience, the cases presenting limited skeletal involvement yield serum alkaline phosphatase values ranging between 5 and about 25 *Bodansky units* per 100 cc. and distributing themselves rather evenly along this range, roughly in accordance with the degree and extent of the skeletal involvement. In the cases in which the latter is widespread, the values range, with few exceptions, between 50 and 150 units. The cases in which the values lie in the upper half of this range are mainly those in which the disease process is still active. The highest value observed among our patients was 258 units. In this case there was not only extensive skeletal involvement by the disease, but many of the affected bones were also the site of osteogenic sarcoma.

Ordinarily, so far as any particular case is concerned, the phosphatase value does not tend to vary much over short periods, rising only gradually in the course of some years. In the single case we studied which violated this rule, the original value of 70 units was doubled in the course of 16 months. Steady increase of the phosphatase value in a given case is an index of active progression of the disease. On the other hand, a value remaining almost unchanged over many years is usually associated with a more or less static state of the disease *per se*. However, even in such a case, a sarcoma may eventually supervene in one or another affected bone, and if the sarcoma shows osteogenic potentialities, the phosphatase level can be expected to rise again.

As is well known, the serum alkaline phosphatase value is likewise increased in cases of carcinoma associated with osteoplastic metastases to the skeleton. Carcinoma of the prostate is the outstanding example of such cases, and has, in the past, created problems of differential diagnosis from Paget's disease. However, in these cases, aside from the clue to the diagnosis which may be given by the clinical findings in regard to the prostate, the differentiation from Paget's disease is facilitated by the fact that the *serum acid phosphatase* value is nearly always found elevated (see Gutman). Thus, the information given by the acid phosphatase value usually resolves the old diagnostic problem encountered in some cases of Paget's disease with pronounced skeletal changes mainly or exclusively in the pelvic bones and/or lumbar vertebrae: Is it Paget's disease, or is it osteoplastic metastasis from a clinically occult carcinoma of the prostate? If it is a case of Paget's disease, the *acid* phosphatase value will not be found elevated, though it is frequently at the upper limit of the normal if the *alkaline* phosphatase value is very high. (For further details on this point, see p. 157.)

Ordinarily the *serum calcium* and *inorganic phosphorus* values are normal in cases of Paget's disease. In a case of Paget's disease in which a fracture has occurred (for instance, in a long bone) and a large skeletal area has been immobilized, hypercalcemia may be found. What seems to happen is that the immobilization is associated with increased resorption of calcium and phosphorus from the bones, and an increased excretion of these minerals in the urine takes place. Then, if the capacity of the kidneys to excrete them is overtaxed, one may find not only hypercalcemia but also a slight rise in the inorganic phosphorus value and even some reduction in the previously elevated alkaline phosphatase value. Indeed, in such cases, unless fluids are forced, the diet is kept low in calcium, and immobilization is kept at a minimum, so-called "chemical death" from hypercalcemia may supervene (see Reifenstein and Albright). If a patient affected with Paget's disease also develops multiple myeloma or hyperparathyroidism (and there are some recorded instances in which this has happened), the hypercalcemia present is, of course, due to the concomitant disease (see Grader and Moynihan, Kohn and Myerson, and also Hanisch).

Studies of the *mineral metabolism* have failed to yield any consistent or useful results in relation to the disease. This is understandable in view of the fact that the pathologic conditions obtaining at any one time are very complex and that, even in advanced cases, progression and healing of the bone lesions proceed side by side. Snapper reports that the calcium excretion values which he obtained in 7 cases of Paget's disease were found normal when compared with those from controls studied under the same dietary conditions. On the other hand, Rabinowitch, studying an advanced case of the disease, found a retention of calcium—that is, a positive calcium balance. The retention of calcium and phosphorus at relatively high intakes of these elements in cases of Paget's disease indicates the probability that these elements are utilized in the formation of new bone at these intakes. At low levels of intake, namely, 0.3 gm. per three-day period, the loss of calcium by a subject affected with Paget's disease may be greater than in a normal control subject (see Bodansky and Bodansky).

PATHOLOGIC AND ROENTGENOGRAPHIC FINDINGS

The pathologic changes to be found outside the skeleton in cases of Paget's disease coming to autopsy are not specific and can be briefly disposed of. In advanced cases of the disease, the aorta and larger arteries in general are found very atheromatous and sclerotic; the coronary arteries and the larger arteries of the limbs usually show extensive calcification and narrowing. The compression sometimes undergone by the brain, cranial nerves, and/or spinal cord and nerve roots has already been mentioned (p. 243). The glands of internal secretion, including the parathyroids, have not revealed anything of special interest. Minor degrees of enlargement (hyperplasia) of the parathyroids have occasionally been noted. When found, it can usually be related to the stimulatory effects upon these glands of phosphorus retention due to renal insufficiency resulting from profound nephrosclerosis. Adenomatous proliferation of one (or at most two) of the parathyroids is not observed in Paget's disease except in the rare cases in which the disease is complicated by hyperparathyroidism. In some cases, especially if the patient has been bedridden, renal calculi may be present.

Skull.—The extent of involvement of the skull may range from mere calvarial osteoporosis circumscripta to pronounced thickening of the calvarium and even extreme thickening of the base of the cranium. As already noted, *osteoporosis circumscripta* of the calvarium represents an early and peculiar stage of skull involvement. It causes no complaints and is recognized clinically through roentgenography. Where it is present, the calvarium shows increased radiolucency, unassociated with modification in thickness. When a calvarium so affected is removed and the pericranium and dura are stripped from it, the area of osteoporosis circumscripta is to be recognized by the dark (reddish violet) color presented by the inner and outer surfaces of the affected part of the calvarium. The discolored area is roundish in outline. It may be relatively small, measuring only several centimeters across, or it may be so large as to involve a substantial part of the calvarium. Instead of a single area, one may find several relatively small ones, completely separated or abutting upon each other (see Erdheim, and Collins and Winn).

In a cross-sectional slice of calvarium including both a zone of osteoporosis circumscripta and one which is still unmodified, the two zones again stand out clearly. Even with the naked eye it will be seen that, in the zone of osteoporosis, almost nothing remains of the compact inner and outer tables *per se*. That is, the diploic architecture extends practically to the outer and inner surfaces of the calvarium. It is because the marrow shines through in consequence of disappearance of the tables that the area of osteoporosis circumscripta has a violet gleam. Also mainly in consequence of this, the area appears radiolucent in comparison with the nonaffected part of the calvarium. The diploic bone in the area of osteoporosis circumscripta is loose-meshed at first. Even then, however, it already presents histologically, at least to some extent, the irregular mosaic, or jigsaw, pattern of Paget bone. As the disease progresses, the diploic bone becomes more and more close-meshed, and then it shows the mosaic pattern strikingly. The more emphati-

17

cally close-meshed the diploic bone, the fainter, of course, becomes the violet coloration of the affected area, and eventually this coloration may even disappear.
Concomitantly, because of condensation and even sclerotization of the diploic bone,
the radiolucency of the latter decreases, and densely sclerotic foci begin to stand
out as small radiopacities. (See Figs. 57 and 58.)

As the whole area becomes progressively sclerotized, thickening of the calvarium
is inaugurated by new bone deposition on both surfaces. Even in those skulls which
finally show decided thickening, the calvarium does not ordinarily become more
than 2 or 3 cm. thick at any point. However, in extreme cases it has been known to
reach a thickness of 5 cm. or more in some places. In general, the calvarium is often
thickest anteriorly, where it merges with the base. The thickening is not symmetrical, either. Thus, for instance, more posteriorly, the calvarium may be thicker
on the left than on the right. More anteriorly, the reverse may be true. On the other
hand, the entire left side may be thicker than the right side. Also, in regard to the
contour of the outer and inner surfaces of the calvarium, there is usually much more
irregularity of the inner surface than of the outer. Indeed, in consequence of considerable subdural bone apposition, the inner surface may have a good many distinct
bulges in its contour.

In a severely affected skull, the thickening involves not only the calvarium but
also the base. As a result of subdural new bone apposition on the base, one may find
that the posterior fossa has become greatly elevated. Instead of curving away from
the foramen magnum in a large, gentle concavity, the posterior fossa may be found
rising up from it in a rather abrupt slope, associated with pronounced narrowing of
the foramen. The anterior and middle fossae may also be substantially encroached
upon. Altogether, through the modifications at the base and on the inside of the
calvarium, the size of the cranial cavity may be greatly reduced and the brain may
have undergone compression. The neurological disturbances produced by com-

Figure 57

A, Roentgenograph (lateral view) of a skull showing large confluent areas of radiolucency
representing osteoporosis circumscripta cranii in still-unmodified form. Note in particular
that the bones of the calvarium are not thickened, and that no foci of radiopacity are present
within the radiolucent areas. The subject was a man 62 years of age. The x-ray pictures of his
lumbar vertebrae and pelvic bones did show the thickening and coarsened architecture characteristic of Paget's disease.

B, Roentgenograph of a calvarium removed at autopsy in the case of an elderly man. It
shows a very large focus of osteoporosis circumscripta, represented by the area of radiolucency. The latter involves the frontal and parietal bones (more on the left than on the right)
and measured 14.5 cm. in length and 13.5 cm. across. In the upper part of the picture, on the
left, a small roundish focus of radiopacity is to be noted. This would correspond to a compact
island of Paget bone which has developed within an area of calvarial osteoporosis circumscripta (see Fig. 58-*D*).

C, Photograph of the calvarium shown in *B*, made after the pericranium had been stripped
away. The site of the osteoporosis circumscripta is clearly delimited from the unaltered part
of the cranial vault by its dark border. Correspondingly, in the fresh specimen the color of
the delimiting border was a much darker red than the focus of osteoporosis as a whole. In
regard to texture and thickness, however, there was no grossly discernible difference between
the region of osteoporosis circumscripta and the rest of the calvarium.

D, Photograph of a segment of calvarium which had been macerated to demonstrate certain
differences in gross detail between an area of osteoporosis circumscripta (on the right) and a
relatively normal area (to the left). Note that, in the region of the osteoporosis circumscripta,
a clear-cut outer table is lacking, the diploic bone is exposed, but the calvarium is not thinner
in this area than in the uninvolved part. From all this, it is evident why a calvarial region affected by osteoporosis circumscripta usually appears highly radiolucent in the x-ray picture.

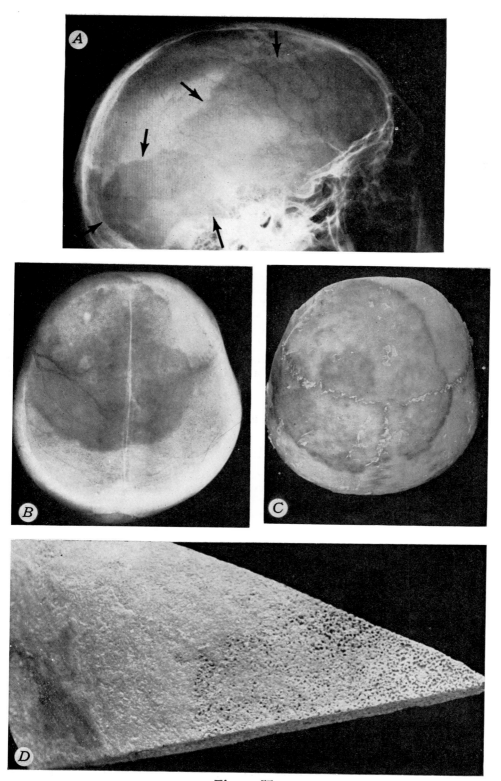

Figure 57

pression and distortion of the neuraxis which result from such advanced cranial changes are discussed by Bull *et al.*

The cut surface of an emphatically thickened calvarium usually fails to present a uniform gross appearance. In many places, practically throughout its thickness, it is composed of rather compacted but finely porous osseous tissue creating the impression of pumice stone. In other places, particularly in the thickest portions, the pumice-like osseous tissue is found oriented mainly toward the inner and outer surfaces of the calvarium. In between, one will find a zone which may present foci of wide-meshed spongiosa filled with cellular marrow, foci of cellular marrow alone, and foci of fibrous tissue which may be highly vascularized in some places. However, such variegated areas are not necessarily limited to an intermediate zone, and in some cases they are to be found near the inner or outer surfaces of the thickened calvarium. In fact, in some areas, large parts of the outer portion of the calvarium may be composed of very porous spongy bone whose marrow spaces are filled with congested myeloid marrow which may impart an intense red color to the area.

If this variegated picture of the gross pathology of a very much thickened calvarium is kept in mind, the meaning of the *roentgenographic reflections* of this pathology becomes clear. The roundish, intensely radiopaque shadows which one sees in the x-ray picture represent the sclerotized foci of osseous tissue which one sees grossly. The streaks or large areas of relative radiolucency between the tables or toward one surface of them represent the more porous osseous areas, along with the fibrous and myeloid areas mentioned. The osseous tissue which has a pumice-like appearance grossly shows moderate diffuse opacity roentgenographically. Thus, the intermingling of these shadows of various densities creates the general appearance

Figure 58

A and *B*, Roentgenographs of two thin cross-sectional slices of calvarium demonstrating the contrast between a region which is the site of osteoporosis circumscripta and one which is not yet involved or is only in an early stage of involvement. In *A*, the uninvolved part of the calvarium is on the left, and here the outer and inner tables are rather thick and compact. In the area of osteoporosis circumscripta, the tables have yielded almost completely to the diploic bone. In *B*, the changes of osteoporosis circumscripta are clearly evident on the left. Note that on the right the outer and inner tables are already thinner than they would normally be, and the diploic bone is encroaching on them. That is, in this part of the calvarium, the changes of osteoporosis circumscripta are already present, though not yet highly developed. The subject in this case was a woman 69 years of age. When the calvarium was removed at autopsy and stripped of its pericranium, the right parietal bone showed a dark red area of discoloration, measuring 4.5 cm. across, which represented the site of the osteoporosis circumscripta.

C, Photomicrograph ($\times$ 7) illustrating the histologic pattern of calvarial osteoporosis circumscripta at a site where the latter is present in its full efflorescence and is not significantly modified by secondary changes. Very little is left of either table as such. The diploic trabeculae are also thin. If examined under high magnification, the osseous tissue of the tables and diploic bone would already manifest, even at this stage, some indications of the mosaic pattern characteristic of the histologic structure of Paget bone. The subject was a man 69 years of age.

D, Photomicrograph ($\times$ 7) showing the histologic pattern presented by another area of the calvarium in the same subject. On the left, the changes of unmodified osteoporosis circumscripta are to be observed. Most of the right side of the picture is occupied by a compact focus of condensed Paget bone. If examined under higher magnification, the osseous tissue of this focus would already present clearly the so-called mosaic pattern of Paget bone.

E, Photomicrograph ($\times$ 5) showing a focus of scarring and new bone formation (in the central part of the picture) within an area of osteoporosis circumscripta cranii. The subject in this case was a woman 72 years of age.

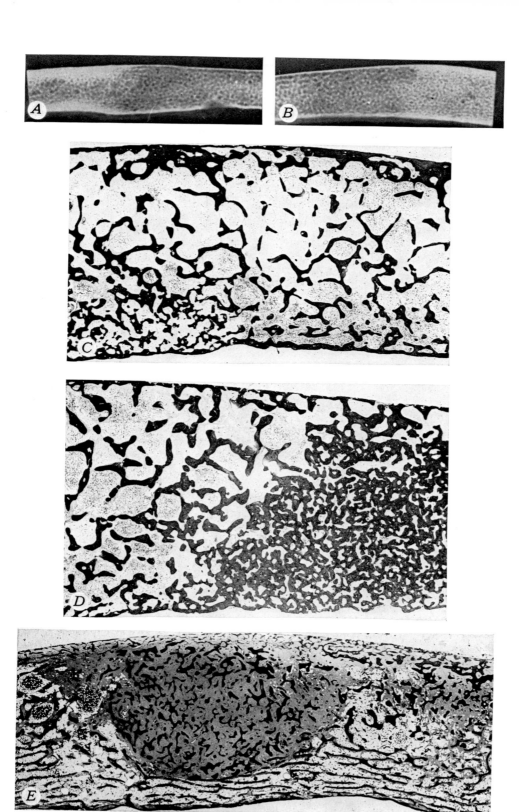

Figure 58

conventionally described as that of "cotton wool" in relation to a Paget skull so altered. (See Figs. 59 and 60.)

In regard to other parts of the skull, it is to be noted, for instance, that the diploic portion of the petrous temporal bone undergoes the modifications characteristic of Paget's disease. However, the exceedingly compact cochlear part seems to present some special resistance to the disease (see Anson and Wilson). Because of contrasts in radiopacity, the semicircular canals are likely to appear clearly in roentgenographs of an affected skull, when taken in the so-called Towne position (see Kettunen). Edema of the membranous internal ear (otitis interna serosa) has been described as sometimes occurring. Also, with heavy involvement of the floor of the cranial cavity, extensive thickening of the walls of the accessory nasal sinuses, leading even to complete obliteration of those nearest the base, has been reported (see Brunner and Grabscheid). Involvement of such facial bones as the zygomata, maxillae, and mandible does not often occur or, at least, does not often become prominent in cases of Paget's disease. When it does occur, along with profound involvement of the rest of the skull, the facial appearance may be that of leontiasis ossea. Indeed, the so-called "diffuse osteitic" form of leontiasis ossea has sometimes been interpreted as a form of Paget's disease limited to the skull. (See p. 276.)

Vertebral Column and Pelvis.—In advanced cases of Paget's disease, these bone parts are usually found involved and often extensively implicated. In fact, the disease so strongly predilects them that at least some lumbar vertebrae and/ or parts of the sacrum and innominate bones are commonly affected, even in the clinically milder cases. Indeed, it is the lumbar vertebrae and the sacrum that one would examine if a survey were being made to ascertain the incidence of nonsymptomatic Paget's disease in a general population over 40 years of age, since one could be sure that but few cases were being missed if these areas were negative.

In a given case, whatever vertebrae or sacral components are affected are usually

Figure 59

A, Roentgenograph (lateral view) of a skull illustrating pronounced changes of Paget's disease. The calvarium is strikingly thickened (particularly toward the front) and presents the "cotton wool" appearance characteristic of the advanced stage of calvarial involvement. This appearance is created by the numerous foci of radiopacity intermingled with areas of relative radiolucency. The foci of radiopacity represent areas of compact or sclerotic Paget bone, while in the radiolucent areas the Paget bone is not only less compact but often rather porous and highly vascularized. The subject was a man 48 years of age who also presented the changes of advanced Paget's disease in numerous other skeletal parts.

B, Photograph demonstrating extreme thickening of the calvarium, especially in front, and resultant compression of the brain in a case of Paget's disease. Above and to the left, the osseous tissue is rather loose-meshed and highly vascularized. Above and to the right, several foci of compact, sclerotic Paget bone stand out. Much of the rest of the thickened calvarium is composed of osseous tissue suggesting finely porous pumice stone.

C, Photograph illustrating the appearance of the base of the cranial cavity after the part of the brain shown in B had been removed. Because of the pronounced thickening of the base of the cranium, there has been considerable encroachment upon the various fossae at the base, and the foramen magnum is also somewhat narrowed. The subject was a woman 65 years of age who presented evidence of Paget's disease in various other skeletal areas and in whom a sarcoma had also developed in one of the pelvic bones.

D, Photograph showing the cut surface of a segment of greatly thickened calvarium from a case of Paget's disease. The subject was a man 68 years of age. Note that the gross architecture of the calvarium is completely different from what it would normally be. In particular, much of the osseous tissue has the appearance of finely porous pumice stone. In the midportion of the illustrated slice of calvarium, a focus of fibrous tissue is present on the left, and a focus of sclerotic bone on the right (see arrows).

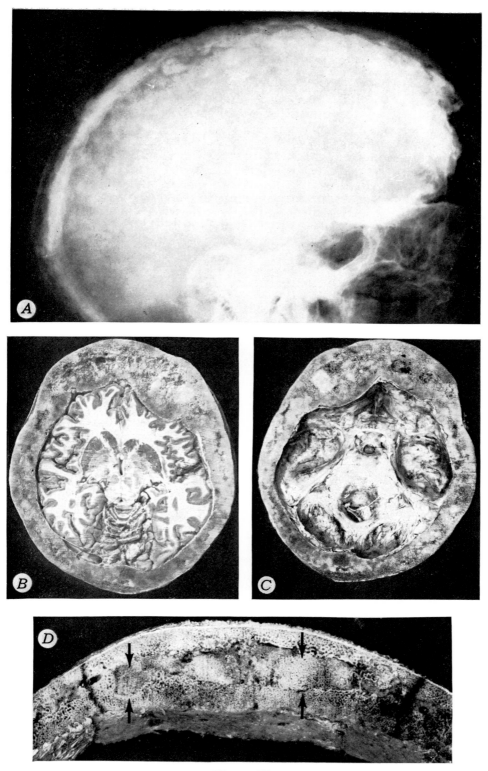

Figure 59

involved *in toto,* though the changes are more conspicuous in the bodies than in the processes. In an affected vertebral or sacral body, the reworked spongy bone at the periphery is often found closely set or compacted so as to frame the body. The more centrally placed trabeculae are ordinarily plump and thickened, and individual ones stand out as pillars with irregular surfaces. The marrow spaces between them are irregular in size and frequently large, and often still show myeloid and fatty marrow. These changes are clearly reflected in roentgenographs of the affected vertebrae, through coarsening of the trabecular markings and formation of a margin of peripheral condensation framing the bone outlines.

It is not unusual for at least some of the bodies of a severely involved vertebral column to become altered in size and shape. Some may show reduction in height, associated with expansion of the adjacent intervertebral disks which have retained their turgor, and take on, to a lesser or greater degree, the form of the so-called "fish vertebrae." These, and others which are not reduced in height, may also show increase in their transverse dimensions, through deposition of periosteal new bone The disks between adjacent bodies may be found degenerated and replaced in part or throughout. Under these circumstances, the vertebral bodies become fused, both directly and through the formation of marginal exostoses. The bone bridging the vertebrae likewise shows the modifications characteristic of the disease. These various changes may lead to kyphotic or kyphoscoliotic deformity of the column. When the latter is severely affected, the spinal canal may be found diminished in caliber (see Knaggs). The narrowing may materially reduce the perithecal space around the cord and its membrane. The presence of osseous excrescences springing from the posterior surface of the bodies and other parts of the wall of the canal sometimes creates (as already indicated in connection with the clinical findings) pressure on the cord and/or the emerging nerves (see Siegelman *et al.,* and Feldman and Seaman). (See Fig. 61.)

If the sacrum is involved, the innominate bones are usually also found affected to some degree. Implication of the entire pelvic girdle (sometimes including deformity and narrowing of its outlet) is not likely to be observed except in cases showing extensive changes in the rest of the skeleton as well. The gross changes in severely affected iliac bones resemble, in a general way, those in the calvarium, in harmony with the structural similarity between the two areas, although the iliac bones do not undergo as much thickening as one may encounter in the calvarium. Roentgenographically, such iliac bones often also cast the so-called "cotton wool"

Figure 60

A, Roentgenograph of a thin slice of a thickened and otherwise severely altered calvarium from a case of Paget's disease. As is common, the osseous tissue is generally more loose-meshed along the outer than along the inner surface of the modified calvarium. The most condensed areas of Paget bone appear as clear-cut foci of radiopacity.

B, Photomicrograph ($\times$ 5) illustrating the general histologic pattern presented by an area of thickened calvarium from a case of Paget's disease. The architectural pattern shown here corresponds approximately to what one would find if the tissue section had been prepared from the last inch or so on the right of the slice of calvarium shown in *A.* Note that, in conformity with what would be expected on the basis of that x-ray picture, the osseous tissue is rather condensed in the inner (or deepest) portion of the calvarium, and rather loose-meshed in the outer (or upper) two thirds.

C, Photomicrograph ($\times$ 5) showing the general histologic pattern presented by an area of thickened calvarium from another case of Paget's disease. Note the focus of condensed bone located to the left of the center of the picture. It is such foci that account for the radiopacities in the x-ray picture of the altered calvarium, and in particular the one shown here would correspond to one of the radiopaque foci to be seen on the left in *A.*

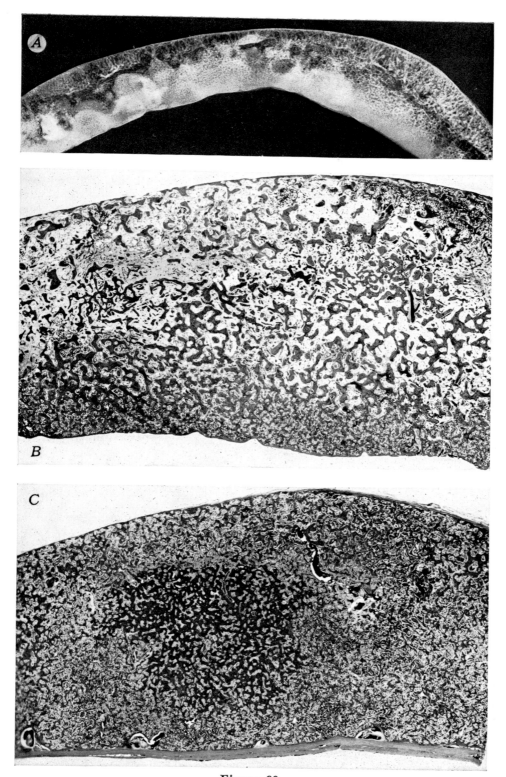

Figure 60

shadow whose anatomic basis has been described above in relation to the calvarium. The writer has even seen, in an iliac bone (as evidence of its early involvement), a large area of radiolucency resembling the so-called osteoporosis circumscripta of the calvarium in a case in which elsewhere there was clear-cut roentgenographic evidence of the disease.

Long Tubular Bones.—In a long bone the disease usually starts at one end and spreads toward the other. Though it may start at both ends and spread toward the middle of the shaft, it only rarely starts in the middle and spreads toward the ends. If one sections longitudinally a long bone which is not yet involved throughout its entire extent, the abnormal portion stands out well from the normal. The spongiosa of the affected end is found, on the whole, rather densified, and, especially just under the articular cartilage, it may be rather closely compacted and pumice-like. Any individual trabeculae which stand out are coarse, and the marrow spaces between some of these trabeculae are large and filled with red marrow. The medullary cavity in the affected area is, of course, retained (as it is even if the entire bone is diseased), but the marrow is likely to have a rust-red hue. The affected part of the cortex, too, is very different from normal cortex. Specifically, it is thickened, more or less lamellated, and of gray-red color. The line of demarcation between the modified and the still-unmodified cortex is easy to see, as the latter is still compact and yellow-white. It is also to be noted that the progress of the disease along the cortex occurs in the form of an advancing wedge of involvement. That the periosteum plays a role in the thickening of the cortex had long been suspected and was clearly proved by Freund. In general, the gross recognition of the periosteal activity is difficult, be-

Figure 61

A, Photograph of part of the vertebral column (T_8 through T_{12}), cut in the sagittal plane, showing various degrees of involvement of the vertebral bodies in a case of Paget's disease. The body of T_8 shows no grossly recognizable alterations. (See also *D*.) It is the body of T_{10} that shows the most advanced and characteristic changes of Paget's disease. Note in particular the alteration in the gross internal architecture of the vertebral body in question. The outline of this body is framed by compacted though still coarsely trabeculated Paget bone, which surrounds a central area of much looser architecture. (See also *B* and *C*.) The body of T_{12} presents only a moderate degree of involvement, but already shows the beginning of the framing of its outline. The subject was a man who was 66 years of age at the time of his death, which was due to widespread visceral metastases from a carcinoma of the ascending colon. It was a skeletal survey made in another connection about a year before his death that revealed the presence of Paget's disease, which was found to involve the calvarium, clavicles, ribs, vertebral column, pelvis, and upper parts of both femora.

B, Photograph of a thin slice cut from the body of T_{10} at a level somewhat deeper than that shown in *A*.

C, Roentgenograph of the specimen illustrated in *B* emphasizing the characteristic framing of the outline of a severely affected vertebral body.

D, Roentgenograph of a slice from T_8 showing the trabecular architecture of a vertebral body which has, as yet, been spared by the disease.

E and *F*, Roentgenograph and photograph, respectively, of part of a vertebral column cut in the sagittal plane and macerated. They show various degrees of involvement of the vertebral bodies in another case of Paget's disease. Proceeding from above downward, one notes that the third and fourth vertebrae illustrated (T_{12} and L_1) are the most severely altered. In these vertebrae there is some increase in the anteroposterior dimension, and they show particularly well the framing of their outline by condensed Paget bone. The subject was a man who was 55 years of age at the time of his death. Since the age of 45, he had had complaints (mainly of pain referred to various skeletal areas) known to be ascribable to Paget's disease. In addition to the vertebral column, many other parts of the skeleton were found severely affected by the disease.

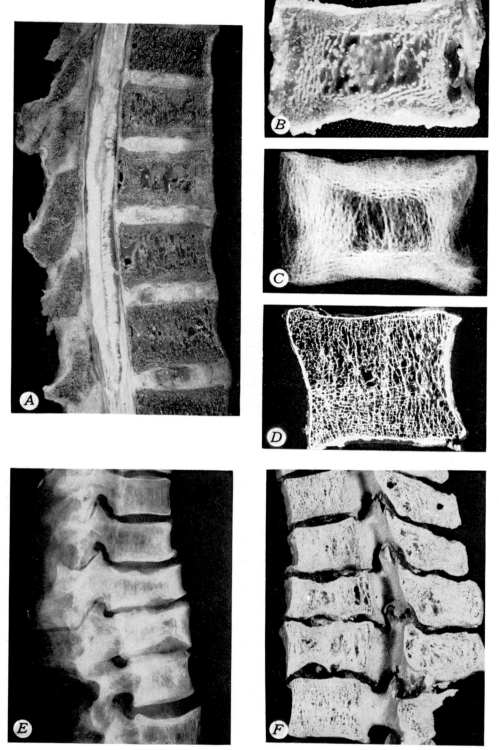

Figure 61

cause the amount of periosteal new bone formed at any one time is minute. Furthermore, it rapidly becomes transformed into Paget bone and thus ordinarily fails to stand out from the diseased cortical bone.

If the entire bone is involved, the description just given for a part applies with certain modifications to the whole. The contour of the bone is usually modified to some extent. If the affected bone is a femur, coxa vara is often present, and there may be anterior and also lateral bowing of the shaft. When it is a tibia, the latter may be considerably bowed anteriorly as well as somewhat laterally. The major marrow cavity may be found reduced in width and length because of lateral encroachment by the thickened cortex and longitudinal encroachment by the Paget bone at the ends. However, if, for any reason (such as immobilization in a cast because of fracture, or disuse associated with long confinement in bed), a bone affected by Paget's disease has become atrophic through inactivity, the major cavity may be found both lengthened and widened. Under these circumstances one can see, particularly toward the bone ends, smaller or larger foci of fatty connective tissue which, if softened, may appear as cystic spaces. It is in such a bone also that one is likely to find the clearest evidences of periosteal activity in the disease. Underneath the periosteum there may be a layer of bone of variable thickness which stands out from the deeper portion of the cortex and can be shown microscopically to be periosteal new bone. Finally, as to the articular cartilages, it is to be noted that they show nothing which is peculiar to Paget's disease. However, in an individual bone they may show the changes of senescence or alterations following upon functional degeneration attributable to malalignment of the joints. That is, the joints may come to show various degrees of degenerative arthritis.

Figure 62

A, Photograph of the upper third of a femur (sectioned in the sagittal plane) from a case of Paget's disease. The cortex of the shaft is thick. Its constituent osseous tissue is obviously not normal compact cortical bone. Instead, it is rather porous, resembling finely porous pumice stone. The greater trochanter fails to show the normal trabecular architecture and is framed for the most part by a thick layer of more porous Paget bone. Much of the neck of the femur is occupied by rather compact Paget bone resembling that of the cortex. In the femoral head the Paget bone is more loose-meshed, though individual trabeculae are thick. Note also the numerous cystlike spaces, filled with fatty marrow, in the head, neck, and greater trochanter. The subject was a woman 72 years of age in whom Paget's disease was widely distributed over the skeleton and had been known to be present for at least 10 years.

B, Photograph of the upper third of a tibia (sectioned in the sagittal plane) from another case of Paget's disease. Note again that the cortex of the shaft is thick and that its constituent osseous tissue is obviously not normal compact cortical bone. In the subchondral area the Paget bone is compact but finely porous. The subject was a man who was 76 years of age at the time of his death, which was due to chronic nephritis and uremia. The Paget's disease in this case was of very limited extent, and the tibia in question was the only bone examined at autopsy in which the changes were found to be pronounced.

C, Photograph (somewhat enlarged) of the sectioned surface of the distal quarter of a radius affected with Paget's disease. The thickened cortex is composed of rather porous Paget bone. The subchondral osseous tissue is somewhat more compact, particularly on the right. The subject was a man 65 years of age whose skeleton showed limited involvement by the disease. A roentgenographic skeletal survey showed that, in addition to the involvement of the radius, there was evidence of Paget's disease in the pelvic bones and in the upper part of a humerus. In the latter, a sarcoma had developed.

D, Photograph of the distal quarter of a femur which had been sectioned in the sagittal plane and macerated. The cortical bone is thickened, and its porous, pumice-stone-like character stands out plainly, since all the nonosseous tissue in the specimen has been cleared away. The subject was a woman 64 years of age who presented Paget's disease of only limited extent.

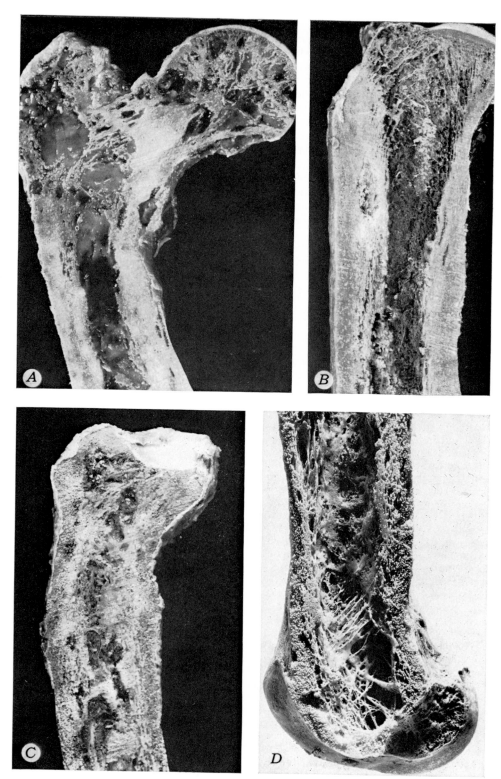

Figure 62

We come now to the roentgenographic appearance presented by a long tubular bone affected with Paget's disease. We need not dwell upon the picture revealed by such a bone when the latter is already involved along its entire extent. Under these circumstances the *x*-ray findings indicate the same pathologic changes that are shown by other heavily affected bones. However, the *x*-ray pictures presented by long bones in earlier stages of the disease do reveal some special features. In such bones the progress of the disease is characterized by radiolucency gradually spreading along the shaft. Not far behind this advancing wedge of radiolucency, and proceeding in the same direction, the conventional roentgenographic changes of the disease can usually already be noted (see Eisler). The writer has also observed a number of cases in which the radiolucency had progressed for a considerable distance along the bone shaft before the picture characteristic of Paget's disease began to appear at the bone end first affected. (See Figs. 62 and 63.)

Other Bones.—In advanced cases the ribs, too, may be heavily implicated, and when they are, the changes are usually most conspicuous in the axillary region. The clavicles are often affected, even without involvement of the ribs. Furthermore, the entire sternum may be found involved, though more often it is only its manubrium or body that is implicated. On the other hand, the carpal and tarsal and short

Figure 63

A, Roentgenograph of part of a femur demonstrating the progression of involvement by Paget's disease along the shaft in the distal direction. The portion of the femur shown represents approximately its middle half. In the lower third of the picture, the bone cortex (especially on the right) is clearly compact and of normal thickness. For some distance above this site, the cortex appears radiolucent and already somewhat thickened. The radiolucent area represents the region where the spread of the Paget's disease along the cortex is most recent and active. The microscopic appearances at a comparable site where the disease process is advancing into the still-compact cortex are shown in Fig. 64–*A*.

B, Photograph showing the cut surface of part of the shaft of a macerated femur which had been undergoing the changes of Paget's disease. In the lower third of the picture, the shaft cortex is compact and of normal thickness, and the spongiosa is fine-meshed and apparently also not altered. In the upper two thirds of the picture, the cortex is very much thickened. Note the wedgelike progression of the involvement into the still-unaltered cortical bone. Observe also that where the cortex is very much thickened the spongiosa is more wide-meshed and its constituent trabeculae are also thickened.

C, Roentgenograph showing the progress of Paget's disease downward along the shaft of a tibia. Note the thickened and radiopaque cortex in the upper portion of the picture, especially on the left. The radiolucent area below the thickened cortex represents the site where the disease process is advancing actively. Note also that the fibula is apparently not affected.

D, Photograph showing the cut surface of the lower third of a femur sectioned in the coronal plane. The subject was a man 54 years of age. In this specimen the direction of advance of the Paget's disease is from below upward. Note that, to a large extent, the osseous tissue in the condyle is rather compact, and where a trabecular architecture is present the individual trabeculae are prominent. The shaft cortex is thickest where it continues into the condylar area—that is, where it would normally be thinnest. In the fresh specimen the cortical bone appeared reddish and felt like finely porous pumice stone. The junctional area between the still-unaffected cortical bone and the thickened and altered cortex stands out even grossly near the upper end of the picture and is even more clearly apparent in *E*. The upper two thirds of this femur showed no gross evidence of Paget's disease.

E, Roentgenograph of the specimen shown in *D* demonstrating the advance of the pathologic process along the cortex. The junctional area between the altered and the still-uninvolved cortex stands out clearly. Note that the region of more recent cortical involvement is relatively radiolucent in comparison with the thickened and otherwise altered cortex below it and the still-unaffected cortex above it.

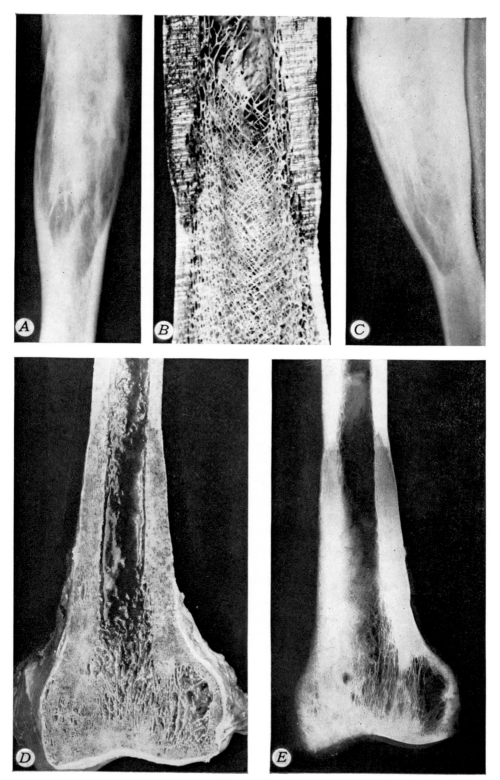

Figure 63

tubular bones are only rarely affected, even in very advanced cases, and even then only lightly.

Fractures and Infractions.—The occurrence of *fractures* is not at all uncommon in the disease. They are observed most frequently in the femur and tibia. A complete fracture may occur after a slight trauma or, apparently, even spontaneously, and the fracture line is usually transverse. Sometimes one can show, in regard to a long bone, that the fracture has occurred through an infraction (that is, an incomplete fissure fracture) which had been known to be present before (see Allen and John). The fractures in Paget's disease heal when immobilized, though slowly as a rule. The bony callus solidifying the fracture ends soon becomes transformed in the fashion characteristic of Paget's disease.

Infractions, or *fissure fractures*, are observed much more commonly than complete fractures. They, too, predilect the femur and tibia, especially the latter. They occur on the convex surface of the curved bone and extend through the cortex, penetrating to various depths. The conditions under which they occur are not known, but possibly their origin is connected with slight traumata. Ordinarily, several fissure fractures are present concurrently in a single long bone, but the writer has observed a tibia in which he was able to count 15 infractions along its shaft at one time. However, the number seen at one time may be different at a subsequent date, for some will have disappeared because they have healed by filling in, while new ones may have formed. Roentgenographically they appear as narrow, slitlike, radiolucent transverse lines. Anatomically they are genuine fissure fractures and not, as some have held, mere linear transformation zones (Umbauzonen) running across the cortex, such as one sees in connection with rickets, osteomalacia, and other porotifying skeletal conditions. The repeated occurrence and filling in of fissure fractures has been regarded as responsible, at least in part, for the increase in total length of curved long bones in the disease. (See Fig. 64.)

Evolution of the Histopathologic Pattern.—As already noted, the etiology of Paget's disease is still obscure, but there seem to be indications that the disease is conditioned by some genetic factor. It is possible that one expression of the latter is the occurrence, in the subject's later life, of aberrations in the organic matrix of the osseous tissue, resulting in an abnormal susceptibility of the bone to resorption. In a part undergoing the changes of Paget's disease, the original spongy and cortical bone is repeatedly resorbed and synchronously replaced by new bone of abnormal character. The onset of the pathologic changes does not seem to be preceded by fibrous replacement of the marrow bordering upon the osseous tissue destined for

Figure 64

A, Photomicrograph ($\times$ 5) illustrating the advance of Paget's disease along the cortex of a tibia. In the lower third of the picture, the cortex is relatively normal. In the upper two thirds of the picture, it is thickened and otherwise modified. The region of the most active progression of the disease process along the cortex (the site of the "advancing wedge" of the involvement) is in the middle third of the picture.

B, Roentgenograph of part of a femur affected with Paget's disease showing numerous incomplete transverse fissure fractures in the cortex (both anteriorly and posteriorly).

C, Photomicrograph ($\times$ 10) showing the general histologic pattern presented by one of the infraction sites in the modified cortex of the femur illustrated in *B*. Under high magnification it was apparent that the fissural defect on the left of the picture is occupied by completely disintegrated and also demineralized osseous tissue—that is, by something tantamount to a "mush" of organic bone matrix. Further to the right, in the region of the fissural infraction, the osseous tissue is in an earlier stage of disintegration. Altogether, the histologic changes at the site of a fissure fracture in Paget's disease are analogous to what one usually observes at the site of a fatigue fracture in an otherwise normal bone.

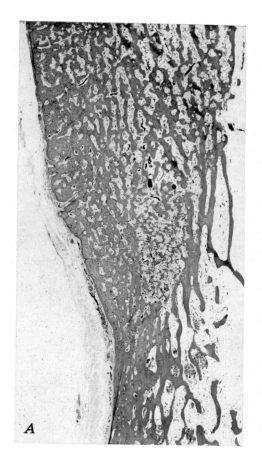

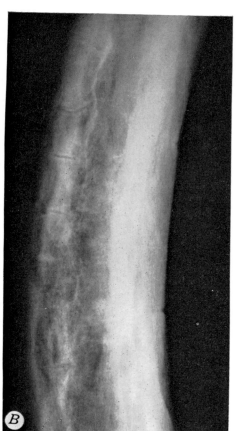

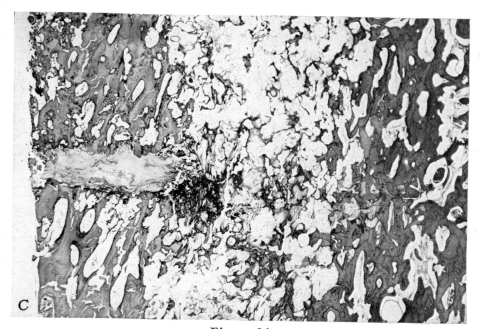

Figure 64

reworking. Instead, it seems to be associated with increased vascularity and congestion and increased cellularity of the neighboring marrow rather than with connective tissue scarring of the marrow.

However, when the transformation of the spongy trabeculae and cortical bone in an affected area has once started, the marrow in its immediate vicinity does tend to become fibrillar or distinctly fibrosed, though still manifesting a striking increase in the number of blood vessels—both arterioles and venous sinuses (see Edholm and Howarth, and also Rutishauser *et al.*). Indeed, bone blood-flow studies have indicated that, in a bone in which Paget's disease is extensive and very active, the blood flow is sometimes as much as 20 times the normal. It has been claimed that the increased blood flow may reflect what amounts to a direct communication between arterioles and venous sinuses—that is, to the existence of arteriovenous shunts in the diseased bones (see Edholm *et al.*). On the other hand, pertinent anatomic studies by Rutishauser led him to conclude that the unquestioned increase in the blood supply of the diseased bone is due to hyperplasia and hypertrophy of all the vessels (but particularly of the arterioles) in the bone rather than to direct communication between arterioles and venous sinuses.

In a bone part showing the pathologic process in an early and active stage (the *"hot phase,"* as the writer has called it), the surfaces of the individual spongy trabeculae present numerous Howship's lacunae containing osteoclasts. One also notes evidences of new bone formation at many of the sites where focal bone resorption has already occurred. The intertrabecular marrow may be merely hyperplastic and hyperemic or already rather fibrillar. In the cortex of an affected bone at this stage, osteoclasts and Howship's lacunae will also be found on the walls of haversian canals. Many of the latter are enlarged and likewise present focal deposits of new bone on their walls. Adjacent widened haversian canals may even have merged as the alterations proceed centrifugally toward the inner and outer surfaces of the cortex. The marrow in the canals is usually rather vascular and fibrillar. The thickening of the cortex results from deposition of new bone by the periosteum, but this new bone, being reworked almost as fast as it is laid down, is ordinarily indistinguishable from the rest of the cortex, at least to the naked eye.

While the Paget bone (both spongy and cortical) which comes to replace the original bone is distinctive even grossly, it is its evolving microscopic appearance that particularly characterizes it. The rapidly recurring cycles of bone resorption and bone apposition affecting both the original and any newly formed osseous tissue create the histologic picture of full-fledged Paget bone. Each new encroachment on the bone which is being resorbed leaves a resorption line, part or all of which remains as a cement line when the new bone is deposited. These lines, with the intervening fragments of bone, bestow upon the osseous tissue of Paget's disease the irregular mosaic architecture which is typical of its histologic pattern. Such osseous

Figure 65

A, Photomicrograph ($\times$ 4) of a tissue slide prepared from a block of bone representing a cross section of a tibia altered by Paget's disease. Even under this low magnification it is evident that the details of the histologic pattern, as manifested in the bone cortex, can be expected to differ from site to site. In fact, *B* of this plate and Fig. 66-*A* and *B* were prepared from different areas of the bone cortex in order to demonstrate these variations.

B, Photomicrograph ($\times$ 35) showing in greater detail the histologic pattern in one area of the cortex shown in *A*. Here the disease process is still in an active ("hot") phase. The interosseous tissue is a highly vascularized loose connective tissue. Active bone resorption by osteoclasts and new bone apposition by osteoblasts are proceeding simultaneously throughout this field, as is shown by Fig. 66-*A*, which presents a small part of it under higher magnification.

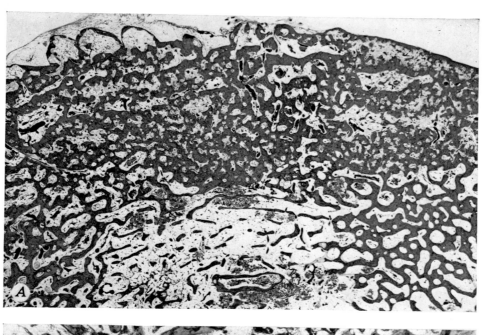

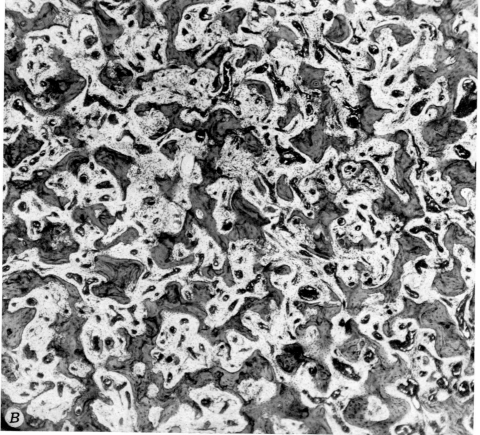

Figure 65

tissue may be briefly described as consisting of numerous irregular segments (breccie) of lamellar bone which are separated by short, irregular, and often somewhat toothed cement lines staining deeply when dyed with hematoxylin. The tiny fragments of lamellar osseous tissue are found fitted into one another in an irregular mosaic (or jigsaw) pattern and manifest but little tendency to be arranged about vessel canals to form haversian systems. Paget bone showing this histopathologic pattern in its fullest expression represents what might be called the static stage (the *"cooled-off phase"*), to contrast it with the so-called "hot phase" of the evolving histopathologic changes. Unlike the osseous tissue of the "hot phase," the osseous tissue of Paget's disease in the "cooled-off phase" does not show striking osteoclastic activity or conspicuous fibrous scarring.

It is also to be emphasized that a tissue section prepared from a bone involved by the disease may show areas in which the disease process is in the "hot phase," adjacent or close to areas in which it is in the "cooled-off phase." In addition, there may be tissue fields in which the disease process is in an intermediate or "cooling-off phase." At this stage in the evolution of the histologic changes, osteoclastic activity and fibrous scarring are less prominent than in bone areas in which the disease is in the "hot phase." However, the osseous tissue already shows the mosaic pattern, though not so characteristically as in the osseous tissue representing the "cooled-off phase." (See Figs. 65 and 66.)

TUMORS COMPLICATING PAGET'S DISEASE

In his textbook *"Tumors and Tumorous Conditions of the Bones and Joints,"* the writer has discussed and illustrated in some detail the subject of tumors complicating Paget's disease. However, for the sake of completeness, the salient facts relating to tumors complicating Paget's disease are presented here also.

Sarcoma.—It is not at all unusual for a sarcoma to become engrafted upon bones involved in Paget's disease. The writer himself has studied anatomic material from many cases in which this happened. However, one cannot state the over-all *incidence* of this complication with any degree of precision. Various appraisals of its incidence have been given, notably in relation to the cases in which the skeletal involvement is widespread. A plausible estimate is that sarcoma eventually appears in 5 to 10 per cent of the cases in which the skeleton is extensively and severely affected. However, it must be recognized that sarcomas may also appear in cases in which the skeletal involvement is relatively limited. Among those cases of Paget's disease in which the number of bones affected is not large, the incidence of sarcoma is certainly lower than 5 per cent and perhaps as low as 2 or 3 per cent. If the numerous cases of nonclinical Paget's disease of very limited extent are taken into account in the statistics on malignant transformation, the over-all incidence can safely be said to be much lower even than 2 or 3 per cent. (See Price and Goldie.)

Indeed, in these nonclinical cases of Paget's disease, it is not unusual to first dis-

Figure 66

A, Photomicrograph ($\times$ 100) showing in some detail the interplay of bone resorption by osteoclasts and new bone deposition by osteoblasts at a site where the pathologic process of Paget's disease is in an active phase.

B, Photomicrograph ($\times$ 100) showing in some detail the pattern presented by Paget bone which already manifests the characteristic mosaic architecture. Note the numerous irregular fragments of osseous tissue separated by cement lines but fitted together into a sort of jigsaw pattern.

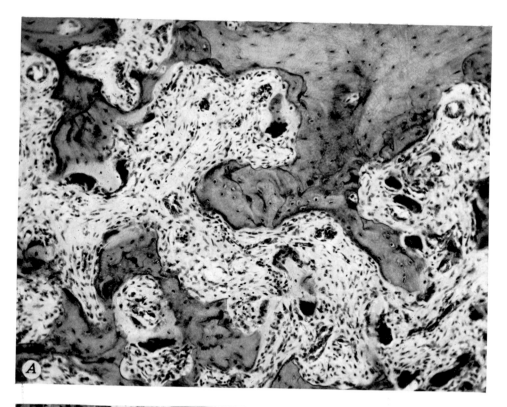

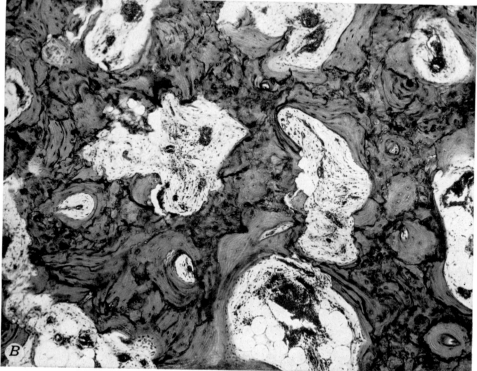

Figure 66

cover the presence of the condition because a sarcoma has become engrafted upon one or another of the affected bones. Thus the finding of a sarcoma in a bone of a middle-aged or older person may well instigate a roentgenographic examination of the rest of the skeleton for Paget's disease, since, in these age groups, sarcoma frequently has its foundation in Paget's disease (see Coley and Sharp). How limited the Paget's disease may be and still be the basis for sarcoma is illustrated by the following experiences of the writer, to which he could add others: He has observed two cases of Paget's disease limited to the cranial bones, in both of which a sarcoma appeared in the occiput; a case in which the disease appeared to be limited to the sixth thoracic vertebra, and the latter became the site of a sarcoma; a case in which the disease was limited to the pelvic bones and fifth lumbar vertebra, and a sarcoma appeared in one of the ischia; a case in which the disease was limited to the left innominate bone and the upper end of the right femur, and the latter was the site of a sarcoma; and a case of sarcoma appearing in an affected scapula, in which subsequent study also revealed Paget's disease in the pelvic bones.

In a case of widespread Paget's disease, when a sarcoma appears in one affected bone or bone part, other foci of sarcoma are usually already present or soon become apparent in other affected parts. The question naturally arises whether these other foci of sarcoma are metastatic or independent sarcomas. Autopsy findings in such cases point strongly to independent (multicentric) origin of these other sarcomas. This conception is also supported by those cases in which the Paget's disease is of limited extent but in which, some months after the appearance of the sarcoma in one bone, a focus of sarcoma appears in one or another of the few other bones affected by the disease. The idea of independent origin of the various sarcomatous foci in Paget's disease is reinforced indirectly by the fact that metastatic skeletal foci of sarcoma are not nearly so common in cases of osteogenic sarcoma appearing *de novo* as are the skeletal foci of sarcoma appearing in multiple bones in cases of Paget's disease of all degrees of severity.

Not infrequently in a case of Paget's disease complicated by sarcoma, the patient dates back the local complaints to a trauma. In connection with osteogenic sarcoma appearing *de novo* (notably, in young subjects), the writer has strong doubts about the importance of trauma in the origin of the condition. Since, in Paget's disease, the multiple foci of sarcoma seem to be independent (that is, not metastases), it also seems justifiable to question the role of trauma as an instigating factor in malignancy connected with that disease. Obviously a trauma would usually be acting only on one site and thus could not account for the development of sarcoma in Paget bones at remote sites. Thus, a trauma seems merely to attract attention to a sarcoma already present.

Clinically, it is local pain, and frequently also local swelling, that calls attention to the sarcoma or sarcomas. Roentgenographically the site of a sarcoma in a Paget bone is usually marked by a smaller or larger, irregular, mottled or uniform area (or areas) of radiolucency set against a background of bone altered by Paget's disease. On the other hand, the presence of radiopacities within the radiolucent area or in the overlying soft parts reflects ossification going on in the sarcoma. In any event, it is not very often that one sees the dense, eburnated radiopaque shadows so common in connection with osteogenic sarcoma developing *de novo*—that is, the osteogenic sarcoma predilecting adolescents and young adults.

There are indications that the sarcoma arises from the substratum of fibrous tissue in the Paget bone. For some little distance beyond the immediate site of the actual sarcoma, one can often see that the nuclei of the marrow connective tissue show plumping, fusion, and other features of atypism. These findings have been interpreted as evidences of presarcomatous transformation of the fibrous marrow (see Albertini). Be that as it may, it is certain that the sarcomas appearing in Paget's disease vary widely from case to case in respect to cellularity and other cytologic details. In the writer's experience, some of the sarcomas complicating Paget's disease are highly collagenized fibrosarcomas poor in cells. Others are highly cellular and, on the whole, anaplastic fibrosarcomas rich in sarcoma giant cells. Still others are rather cellular fibrosarcomas showing not only sarcoma giant cells but also, in some fields, numerous large multinuclear giant cells set against a background of plump spindle cells—areas which simulate malignant giant-cell tumor of bone. In other tumors, again, the sarcomatous stroma, in part or throughout, expresses osteogenic potentialities, forming considerable tumor osteoid and even osseous tissue. But even this range does not express the full variety of the cytologic possibilities. In one case studied by the writer, not only was tumor osteoid and bone being formed, but in many areas (even areas in which ossification was going on) the sarcomatous stromal tissue seemed to be composed of cells resembling malignant myeloid elements. Just as arresting as this case was one in which a chondrosarcoma as large as a child's head was present in the iliac portion of an innominate bone which, like much of the rest of the skeleton, was heavily affected with Paget's disease. It is difficult to explain this complexity of cytologic expression shown by the sarcomas appearing in relation to the disease. It would seem that the connective tissue from which they arise may reveal, even within the same tumor, manifold potentialities for differentiation and dedifferentiation along mesenchymal lines.

Thus, a biopsy specimen from one area of a particular tumor may reveal the pattern of an osteogenic sarcoma; a biopsy from another area, that of an anaplastic fibrosarcoma; and one from still another area, even a pattern suggesting a malignant giant-cell tumor. For this reason, in evaluating a pertinent biopsy specimen, the writer usually prefers to designate the tumor merely as a sarcoma complicating Paget's disease, without attempting to define more precisely the cytologic nature of the tumor as a whole.

The development of sarcoma in a case of Paget's disease is very ominous. Even if only one bone has been the site of a sarcoma, and amputation was surgically feasible and was done, the ultimate prognosis is bad, being indeed no better than for osteogenic sarcoma developing *de novo*. It is only occasionally that a patient affected with Paget's disease complicated by sarcoma survives for more than two years, though a few instances of much longer survival have been reported (see Schatzki and Dudley). The writer's own experience does not include a single case of Paget's disease complicated by sarcoma in which the patient survived as long as five years, and others report similar experience (see McKenna *et al.*). Of course, the patients developing multiple sarcomas all die soon. Most of them succumb with metastases in the lungs (and usually also elsewhere) in the course of about six months. Those who do not succumb within this time live only a little longer.

Giant-cell Tumor.—Once in a great while, a bone part affected with Paget's disease shows a tumor or even multiple tumors presenting the tissue pattern of a conventional giant-cell tumor throughout. That is, in these lesions the tumor tissue is completely devoid of ominous histologic features. With few exceptions, this occurrence has been noted only in relation to the skull. In a particularly instructive case which the writer has followed (and which he reports in some detail in his book on skeletal tumors), 12 giant-cell tumor lesions appeared successively in the course of eight years in relation to the frontal, parietal, temporal, occipital, and upper facial regions. As to the Paget's disease itself, this involved not only the skull but also the vertebral column, the innominate bones and the femora. In none of these other skeletal parts has any type of tumor developed to complicate the Paget's disease. Since this case was described, the writer has observed an instance of a giant-cell tumor of conventional pattern which developed in the humerus of a man 49 years of age who showed roentgenographic evidence of Paget's disease in many parts of the skeleton. A giant-cell tumor devoid of ominous histologic characteristics has also been noted in a tibia affected with Paget's disease (see Barry). From the experience relating to these cases, and from what one can gather from an occasional other case which has been reported in the literature, it appears that the outlook for continued survival when Paget's disease is complicated by giant-cell tumor of conventional pattern (as contrasted with sarcoma) is not bad.

TREATMENT

The treatment of Paget's disease is merely symptomatic and palliative. Fortunately, the cases in which the skeleton becomes extensively and severely affected or in which a sarcoma develops are, as indicated, definitely in the minority. Patients in whom the skeletal involvement is not extensive when they first come under medical care can be assured that the disease is not likely to progress rapidly. Even in those cases in which the skeletal involvement has already become fairly extensive, the further advance of the disease is ordinarily also slow. In an individual case, irrespective of the severity of the skeletal involvement at a given time, there may even be a remission in the progress of the skeletal changes. Under these circumstances the local complaints tend to diminish, though the roentgenographic appearance of the affected bones remains essentially the same.

Quite empirically, patients with Paget's disease are placed on well-rounded diets, special care being taken to include adequate amounts of calcium and phosphorus and vitamin D. The patient will be more comfortable if he is careful to keep warm and to wear shoes which are not too tight. The straining of a painful part, even in the course of regular work, should be avoided. If one lower limb is shorter than the other, the disparity should be corrected by a built-up shoe to relieve the strain. Postural disability due to implication of the vertebral column may call for the use of a brace.

Temporary benefits (notably, in the form of relief from pain) have been reported from drug therapy. This has included the use of aspirin in liberal doses (see Henneman), the daily ingestion of small amounts of aluminum acetate (see Helfet), and the administration of various endocrine preparations. In the latter connection, it has been claimed that if corticoids are used they should be given simultaneously with an androgen-estrogen preparation (see McGavack et al.). However, because of the well-known damaging effect of corticoid therapy even on normal bones and joints, the prolonged use of this type of endocrine therapy would seem to be ill-advised.

Roentgen therapy in small, divided doses (total dosage not more than about 500 r) has also been used in some cases against pain in an affected bone part, again with at least temporary benefit, but overradiation must be avoided with special care. When radiation is used for the relief of headache and vertigo in cases in which the skull is heavily affected, it is well to remember that this treatment may induce alopecia.

REFERENCES

VON ALBERTINI, A.: Über Sarkombildung auf dem Boden der Ostitis deformans Paget. (Kasuistischer Beitrag), Virchows Arch. path. Anat., 268, 259, 1928.

ALLEN, M. L. and JOHN, R. L.: Osteitis Deformans (Paget's Disease): Fissure Fractures—Their Etiology and Clinical Significance, Am. J. Roentgenol., 38, 109, 1937.

AMYES, E. W. and VOGEL, P. J.: Osteitis Deformans (Paget's Disease) of the Spine with Compression of the Spinal Cord. Report of Three Cases and Discussion of the Surgical Problems, Bull. Los Angeles Neurol. Soc., 19, 18, 1954.

ANSON, B. J. and WILSON, J. G.: Structural Alterations in the Petrous Portion of the Temporal Bone in Osteitis Deformans, Arch. Otolaryng., 25, 560, 1937.

ASCHNER, B. M., HURST, L. A., and ROIZIN, L.: A Genetic Study of Paget's Disease (Osteitis Deformans) in Monozygotic Twin Brothers, Acta genet. med. et gemel., *1*, 67, 1952.

ASHLEY MONTAGU, M. F.: Paget's Disease (Osteitis deformans) and Heredity, Am. J. Human Genet., *1*, 94, 1949.

BARRY, H. C.: Sarcoma in Paget's Disease of Bone in Australia, J. Bone & Joint Surg., *43-A*, 1122, 1961.

BODANSKY, A. and JAFFE, H. L.: Phosphatase Studies. III. Serum Phosphatase in Diseases of the Bone: Interpretation and Significance, Arch. Int. Med., *54*, 88, 1934.

BODANSKY, M. and BODANSKY, O.: *Biochemistry of Disease*, 2nd ed., New York, The Macmillan Co., 1952.

BRUNNER, H. and GRABSCHEID, E.: Zur Kenntnis der Ostitis deformans (Paget) der Schädelbasis. I. Das Schläfenbein, Virchows Arch. path. Anat., *298*, 195, 1936.

————: Zur Kenntnis der Ostitis deformans (Paget) der Schädelbasis. II. Die vordere Schädelgrube mit besonderer Berücksichtigung der Nebenhöhlen der Nase, Virchows Arch. path. Anat., *301*, 237, 1938.

BULL, J. W. D., NIXON, W. L. B., PRATT, R. T. C., and ROBINSON, P. K.: Paget's Disease of the Skull and Secondary Basilar Impression, Brain, *82*, 10, 1959.

CHRISTELLER, E.: Die Formen der Ostitis fibrosa und der verwandten Knochenerkrankungen der Säugetiere, zugleich ein Beitrag zur Frage der "Rachitis" der Affen, Ergebn. allg. Path. u. path. Anat., *20²*, 1, 1923.

COLEY, B. L. and SHARP, G. S.: Paget's Disease. A Predisposing Factor to Osteogenic Sarcoma, Arch. Surg., *23*, 918, 1931.

COLLINS, D. H. and WINN, J. M.: Focal Paget's Disease of the Skull (Osteoporosis Circumscripta), J. Path. & Bact., *69*, 1, 1955.

CUTHBERTSON, D. P.: Note on the Balance of Calcium, Magnesium, Phosphorus, and Sulphur in a Case of Osteitis Deformans, Glasgow M. J., *108*, 218, 1927.

EDHOLM, O. G., HOWARTH, S., and McMICHAEL, J.: Heart Failure and Bone Blood Flow in Osteitis Deformans, Clin. Sc., *5*, 249, 1945.

EDHOLM, O. G. and HOWARTH, S.: Studies on the Peripheral Circulation in Osteitis Deformans, Clin. Sc., *12*, 277, 1953.

EISLER, F.: Ein seltener Fall von Pagetscher Knochenerkrankung (Ostitis deformans), Fortschr. Geb. Röntgenstrahlen, *29*, 311, 1922.

ERDHEIM, J.: Über die Genese der Paget'schen Knochenerkrankung, Beitr. path. Anat., *96*, 1, 1935.

FELDMAN, F., and SEAMAN, W. B.: The Neurologic Complications of Paget's Disease in the Cervical Spine, Am. J. Roentgenol., *105*, 375, 1969.

FREUND, E.: Zur Frage der Ostitis deformans Paget, Virchows Arch. path. Anat., *274*, 1, 1929.

GOLDENBERG, R. R.: The Skeleton in Paget's Disease, Bull. Hosp. Joint Dis., *12*, 229, 1951.

GRADER, J. and MOYNIHAN, J. W.: Multiple Myeloma and Osteogenic Sarcoma in a Patient with Paget's Disease, J.A.M.A., *176*, 685, 1961.

GRÜNTHAL, E.: Über den Hirnbefund bei Pagetscher Krankheit des Schädels. Zugleich ein Beitrag zur Kenntnis der Entstehung systematischer Kleinhirnatrophien, Ztschr. ges. Neurol. u. Psychiat., *136*, 656, 1931.

GUTMAN, A. B.: Serum "Acid" Phosphatase in Patients with Carcinoma of the Prostate Gland, J.A.M.A., *120*, 1112, 1942.

GUTMAN, A. B. and KASABACH, H.: Paget's Disease (Osteitis Deformans). Analysis of 116 Cases, Am. J. M. Sc., *191*, 361, 1936.

GUTMAN, A. B. and PARSONS, W. B.: Hyperparathyroidism Simulating or Associated with Paget's Disease; with Three Illustrative Cases, Ann. Int. Med., *12*, 13, 1938.

HANISCH, C. M.: Paget's Disease Complicated by Multiple Myeloma, Bull. Hosp. Joint Dis., *11*, 43, 1950.

HELFET, A. J.: A New Conception of Parathyroid Function and its Clinical Application: A Preliminary Report on the Results of Treatment of Generalized Fibrocystic and Allied Bone Diseases and of Rheumatoid Arthritis by Aluminium Acetate, Brit. J. Surg., *27*, 651, 1940.

————: Paget's Disease. Considerations in its Diagnosis and Treatment, South African M. J., *26*, 703, 1952.

HENNEMAN, P. H.: Paget's Disease, J.A.M.A., *181*, 736, 1962.

JAFFE, H. L.: Paget's Disease of Bone, Arch. Path., *15*, 83, 1933.

————: *Tumors and Tumorous Conditions of the Bones and Joints*, Philadelphia, Lea & Febiger, 1958. (See p. 463.)

JAFFE, H. L. and BODANSKY, A.: Diagnostic Significance of Serum Alkaline and Acid Phosphatase Values in Relation to Bone Disease, Bull. New York Acad. Med., *19*, 831, 1943.

KASABACH, H. H. and DYKE, C. G.: Osteoporosis Circumscripta of the Skull as a Form of Osteitis Deformans, Am. J. Roentgenol., *28*, 192, 1932.

KASABACH, H. H. and GUTMAN, A. B.: Osteoporosis Circumscripta of the Skull and Paget's Disease: Fifteen New Cases and a Review of the Literature, Am. J. Roentgenol., *37*, 577, 1937.

KETTUNEN, K.: Roentgen Demonstration of the Semicircular Canals in Paget's Disease, Am. J. Roentgenol., *70*, 564, 1953.

KNAGGS, R. L.: On Osteitis Deformans (Paget's Disease) and its Relation to Osteitis Fibrosa and Osteomalacia, Brit. J. Surg., *13*, 206, 1925.

KOHN, N. N. and MYERSON, R. M.: Hyperparathyroidism Associated with Paget's Disease, Ann. Int. Med., *54*, 985, 1961.

LOOSER, E.: Ostitis deformans und Unfall, Arch. klin. Chir., *180*, 379, 1934.

MANDL, F.: Klinisches und Experimentelles zur Frage der lokalisierten und generalisierten Ostitis fibrosa, Arch. klin. Chir., *143*, 1 and 245, 1926.

MARTIN, E.: Considérations sur la maladie de Paget, Helvet. med. acta, *14*, 319, 1947.

McGAVACK, T. H., SEEGERS, W., and REIFENSTEIN, E. C., JR.: The Influence of Anabolic Steroid (Deladumone) Therapy on the Clinical and Metabolic Aspects of Paget's Disease, J. Am. Geriatrics Soc., *9*, 533, 1961.

McKENNA, R. J., SCHWINN, C. P., SOONG, K. Y., and HIGINBOTHAM, N. L.: Osteogenic Sarcoma Arising in Paget's Disease, J. Bone & Joint Surg., *44-A*, 1267, 1962.

————: Osteogenic Sarcoma Arising in Paget's Disease, Cancer, *17*, 42, 1964.

McKUSICK, V. A.: *Heritable Disorders of Connective Tissue*, St. Louis, The C. V. Mosby Co., 1956.

MELANOTTE, P. L.: Sindrome midollare transversa in corso di malattia di Paget della colonna dorsale, Clin. ortop., *12*, 631, 1960.

PAGET, J.: On a Form of Chronic Inflammation of Bones (Osteitis Deformans), Med.-Chir. Tr., *60*, 37, 1877.

————: Additional Cases of Osteitis Deformans, Med.-Chir. Tr., *65*, 225, 1882.

————: Remarks on Osteitis Deformans, Illus. Med. News, *2*, 181, 1889.

PICK, L.: Zur Frage des Zusammenhanges zwischen Unfall und Ostitis deformans (Paget), Zentralbl. allg. Path., *56*, 362, 1932–33.

PRICE, C. H. G., and GOLDIE, W.: Paget's Sarcoma of Bone, J. Bone & Joint Surg., *51-B*, 205, 1969.

RABINOWITCH, I. M.: Metabolic Studies in a Case of Osteitis Deformans, J. Nutrition, *5*, 325, 1932.

RAST, H. and WEBER, F. P.: Paget's Bone Disease in Three Sisters, Brit. M. J., *1*, 918, 1937.

REIFENSTEIN, E. C., JR. and ALBRIGHT, F.: Paget's Disease: Its Pathologic Physiology and the Importance of This in the Complications Arising from Fracture and Immobilization, New England J. Med., *231*, 343, 1944.

RUTISHAUSER, E., VEYRAT, R., and ROUILLER, C.: La vascularisation de l'os pagétique. Étude anatomo-pathologique, Presse méd., *62*, 654, 1954.

SCHATZKI, S. C. and DUDLEY, H. R.: Bone Sarcoma Complicating Paget's Disease. A Report of 3 Cases with Long Survival, Cancer, *14*, 517, 1961.

SCHEURLEN: Pagetsche Knochenkrankeit beim Kind, Kinderärztl. Praxis, *8*, 56, 1937.

SCHMORL, G.: Zur Kenntnis der Ostitis fibrosa, Verhandl. deutsch. path. Gesellsch., *21*, 71, 1926.

————: Zur Kenntnis der Ostitis deformans Paget, Verhandl. deutsch. path. Gesellsch., *25*, 205, 1930.

————: Zur Kenntnis der Ostitis deformans Paget. Aufhellungszonen in der Kortikalis und periostale Ossifikation, Fortschr. Geb. Röntgenstrahlen, *43*, 202, 1931.

————: Zur Technik der Knochenuntersuchung. Bemerkungen zur Diagnose der Ostitis deformans Paget, Ostitis fibrosa v. Recklinghausen und Osteoporose, Beitr. path. Anat., *87*, 585, 1931.

————: Über Ostitis deformans Paget, Virchows Arch. path. Anat., *283*, 694, 1932.

SCHÜLLER, A.: Über circumscripte Osteoporose des Schädels, Med. Klinik, *25*, 615, 1929.

SCHWARZ, G. A. and REBACK, S.: Compression of the Spinal Cord in Osteitis Deformans (Paget's Disease) of the Vertebrae, Am. J. Roentgenol., *42*, 345, 1939.

SIEGELMAN, S. S., LEVINE, S. A., and WALPIN, L.: Paget's Disease with Spinal Cord Compression, Clin. Radiol., *19*, 421, 1968.

SNAPPER, I.: Maladies osseuses et parathyroides, Ann. méd., *29*, 201, 1931.

SOSMAN, M. C.: Radiology as an Aid in the Diagnosis of Skull and Intracranial Lesions, Radiology, *9*, 396, 1927.

STEMMERMANN, W.: Die Ostitis deformans Paget unter Berücksichtigung ihrer Vererbung, Ergebn. inn. Med., *3*, 185, 1952.

STENHOLM, T.: *Osteodystrophia Fibrosa*, Uppsala, Almqvist and Wiksells, 1924.

SUMMEY, T. J. and PRESSLY, C. L.: Sarcoma Complicating Paget's Disease of Bone, Ann. Surg., *123*, 135, 1946.

WHALLEY, N.: Paget's Disease of Atlas and Axis, J. Neurol. Neurosurg. & Psychiat., *9*, 84, 1946.

WILSON, J. G. and ANSON, B. J.: Histologic Changes in the Temporal Bone in Osteitis Deformans (Paget's Disease), Arch. Otolaryng., *23*, 57, 1936.

WOODARD, H. Q., TWOMBLY, G. H., and COLEY, B. L.: A Study of the Serum Phosphatase in Bone Disease, J. Clin. Invest., *15*, 193, 1936.

Chapter

11

Various Hyperostoses of Obscure Origin

THE present chapter will be devoted to a number of conditions (other than Paget's disease) which are characterized by bone thickening (hyperostosis). In some of the conditions to be considered, the hyperostosis is limited to one skeletal area (or even to a part of it), while in others it is widely distributed over the skeleton. Among the disorders belonging to the former group, we shall give attention to *hyperostosis frontalis interna* and *leontiasis ossea*. Among the disorders in which the hyperostosis tends to be widely distributed over the skeleton we shall discuss: *infantile cortical hyperostosis, pulmonary hypertrophic osteoarthropathy,* and *idiopathic familial hypertrophic osteoarthropathy with pachydermia (pachydermo-periostosis).*

HYPEROSTOSIS FRONTALIS INTERNA

Hyperostosis frontalis interna is the name generally applied to skull thickening more or less restricted to the squamous portion of the frontal bone and involving in particular its subdural (or inner) surface. In the area of thickening the subdural surface of the affected squama frontalis may be rather smooth but more often presents an irregularly nodular, bumpy or warty appearance.

Attention was already directed to the type of skull thickening in question by the anatomist Morgagni more than 200 years ago. His subject was an old woman in whom the calvarial thickening was associated with virilism and obesity. This clinico-anatomic complex is often denoted as the "Morgagni syndrome," and is also referred to as the "Stewart-Morel syndrome" and as "metabolic craniopathy." Hyperostosis frontalis interna is being discussed here mainly in connection with the Morgagni syndrome, of which it is the pivotal feature. However, it should be noted that the type of skull thickening in question may be observed in elderly women in whom virilism and/or obesity are absent, and even under still other circumstances (for instance, pregnancy or acromegaly). It seems very likely that endocrine imbalance plays a crucial role in the pathogenesis of hyperostosis frontalis interna and the other manifestations of the Morgagni syndrome, though the nature of that imbalance is not yet clear.

CLINICAL CONSIDERATIONS

Hyperostosis frontalis interna is observed almost exclusively in females, irrespective of the attendant circumstances under which it is encountered. In females past the menopause who present the other manifestations of the Morgagni syndrome—obesity and virilism (as expressed by hairiness of the face and coarsening of the features)—hyperostosis frontalis interna is a common finding. Indeed, Henschen noted some degree of hyperostosis frontalis interna (ranging from slight to pronounced) in almost 40 per cent of postmenopausal females coming to autopsy. Gershon-Cohen *et al.* carried out a pertinent roentgenographic study on 128 residents (79 females, 49 males) in a home for the aged. This study revealed the presence of hyperostosis frontalis interna in 62 per cent of the females but in none of the males. Furthermore, it indicated that obesity and virilism (as expressed by hirsutism) were almost as common among those female residents of the home who presented no evidence of hyperostosis frontalis interna as among those who did present it.

The rather high incidence of hyperostosis frontalis interna reported by Henschen and by Gershon-Cohen *et al.* is ascribable to the large proportion of elderly and old women among the cases in their series. In accounts based on large series of un-selected cases covering a much wider age range, the reported incidence of the hyperostosis as observed roentgenographically is much lower. In particular, this incidence is reported as 4.8 per cent by Grollman and Rousseau, as 6.73 per cent by Moore, and as 12.2 per cent by Salmi *et al.* These various reports also point up again the rarity of hyperostosis frontalis interna among males.

The obesity commonly observed in women presenting the Morgagni syndrome is usually of the rhizomelic type. These women show striking adiposity of the lower part of the abdominal wall, the buttocks, the upper part of the thighs, the breasts, and the shoulder regions. The obese subject is quite likely to exhibit facial hirsutism, to be hypertensive, and also to have a history of menstrual irregularity, especially in the form of diminished menstrual flow or periods of amenorrhea. Headache is a common complaint and is severe in some cases. In addition, various neuropsychiatric disturbances, including depression and anxiety, may be manifested.

Stewart was impressed by the frequency with which he found hyperostosis frontalis interna in women who were insane. Morel already gave a long list of clinical phenomena likely to be observed in subjects presenting the hyperostosis under consideration. He mentioned particularly adiposity and insomnia and nocturnal restlessness. He also noted, though less often, polyphagia and polydipsia, urinary difficulties, disturbances of equilibrium, muscular asthenia, visual disturbances, headaches, and even convulsions. Indeed, Morel attempted to integrate the hyperostosis and these various clinical phenomena into a syndrome—namely, "internal frontal hyperostosis with adiposity and cerebral difficulties." To signalize the early contributions of these two investigators in regard to the clinico-anatomic complex in question, the term "Stewart-Morel syndrome," as already noted, is sometimes used as an alternative to "Morgagni syndrome." (See also Calame.)

ROENTGENOGRAPHIC AND PATHOLOGIC FINDINGS

On *roentgenographic examination* the part of the frontal bone involved in the hyperostosis is found abnormally radiopaque. The contour of the inner surface of the thickened part of the bone usually appears irregularly ridged, knobby, and/or bumpy instead of smooth. While these changes may be found limited to the squamous portion of the bone, they are not infrequently also observed on its orbital plate, and sometimes even only there. In any event, a smaller or larger area along the midline of the squamous portion of the frontal bone is usually found uninvolved. The contour of the outer surface of the affected bone is not altered anywhere.

On *anatomic examination* it will be found that the dura is even more intimately adherent to the thickened portion of the frontal bone than it would normally be. Architecturally the thickened region may show the normal proportion of diploic bone to compact tables. Usually, however, the proportion of diploic bone to tables is excessive. Either or both of the tables may even be abnormally thin. Not uncommonly, the diploic bone is dense and sclerotic. The calvarial thickening results from the deposition, by the dura, of new bone on the inner table. Concomitantly, however, this table tends to undergo spongification from the diploic side. For this reason, it is largely diploic bone that is excessive in the thickened portion of the calvarium. At autopsy in a case in which the hyperostotic squama frontalis presents one or more large knobby thickenings on its inner surface, it is not unusual to find the immediately underlying frontal part of the brain depressed. (See Figs. 67 and 68.)

There is little danger of confusing the hyperostosis frontalis interna of the Morgagni syndrome with the so-called *"pregnancy osteophytes"* which frequently develop on the inner surface of the calvarium in pregnant women. These, too, tend to appear mainly on the squamous portion of the frontal bone, but are likely to be rather flat and not particularly prominent and usually disappear after the pregnancy. In *acromegaly*, also, there may be thickening of the frontal and parietal bones from new bone depositions on their inner surface by the dura. The associated involvement of the mandible in acromegaly is so characteristic, however, that confusion with the Morgagni syndrome is again not likely to arise.

In *senile calvarial hyperostosis* the calvarial thickening is usually rather generalized. The process of its development is essentially that of new bone deposition on the inner table by the dura and progressive diploization of this table. However, the normal proportions between the tables and the diploic bone tend to be retained in senile calvarial hyperostosis, though the diploic bone may be rather densified because of thickening of its trabeculae. This diffuse form of hyperostosis is observed more often in females than in males. It probably represents an attempt at accommodation to senile brain shrinkage, but it is sometimes observed without accompanying brain shrinkage. Diffuse calvarial thickening is also commonly found in connection with general paresis and senile and epileptic dementia. In these conditions it apparently has the same cause and the same manner of development as it has in senile persons without dementia. (See Erdheim, and also Henschen.)

Figure 67

A, Roentgenograph (lateral view) of a skull presenting the changes of hyperostosis frontalis interna. The squamous portion of the frontal bone is thickened. Note that the contour of its outer surface is not altered, but that the inner surface of the thickened portion of the bone appears irregularly bumpy. The subject was a woman 50 years of age who, at the time of her first admission to our hospital ($2\frac{1}{2}$ years before her death), presented evidences of diabetes mellitus, hyperthyroidism, hypertension, and generalized arteriosclerosis. The immediate cause of her death, as revealed at autopsy, was massive hemorrhage from ruptured gastroesophageal varices secondary to portal cirrhosis of the liver.

B, Photograph showing the inner surface of the calvarium as it appeared in the autopsy specimen in the same case. Observe the bumpy excrescences in the region of the squamous portion of the temporal bone. In contrast to the bilateral and symmetrical excrescences usually observed, the thickening in this case is much more prominent on the right.

C, Photograph of two thin slices of the calvarium cut transversely in the plane perpendicular to the arc of the calvarium. Since these slices were cut below the level of the smaller excrescence (on the left in *B*), they show only the relation of the larger excrescence (on the right) to the inner surface of the calvarium. Note that the osseous tissue of the hyperostotic mass protruding from the inner surface in these slices is continuous with the diploic osseous tissue.

D, Roentgenograph of a thin slice of the calvarium cut transversely in the plane perpendicular to the arc of the calvarium. The picture demonstrates the orientation of the bumpy excrescences on the inner surface of the frontal region to the neighboring diploic osseous tissue. It also supplements the gross findings as shown in *C*.

E, Roentgenograph (anteroposterior projection) showing the altered frontal area of the calvarium illustrated in *B*. There is, of course, close correspondence between the alterations revealed by this x-ray picture and the changes observable in the gross specimen.

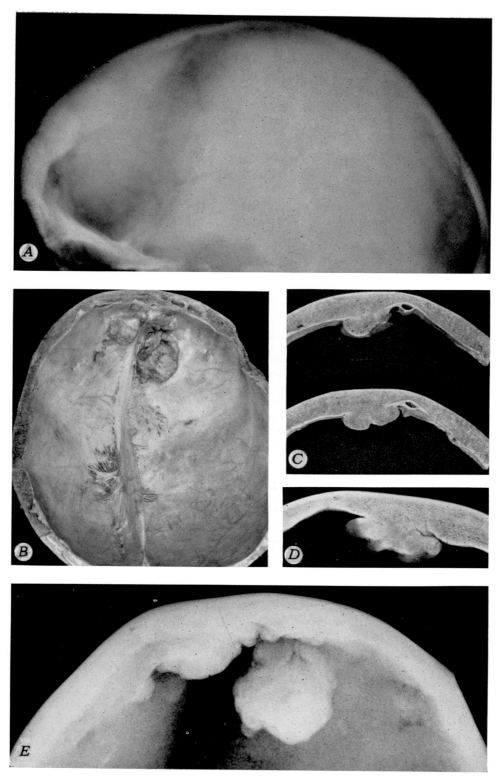

Figure 67

275

LEONTIASIS OSSEA

Disfigurement of the skull resulting from thickening of the bones of the cranio-facial skeleton is commonly denoted as *"leontiasis ossea."* In the past, this name has been used too comprehensively. In the light of later knowledge, it seems advisable to restrict the term to those cases in which the craniofacial hyperostosis is bilateral and more or less symmetrical and in which the hyperostosis is limited to the bones of the skull.

In some cases of leontiasis ossea, the thickening of the skull bones develops in consequence of a creeping periostitis manifested in the cumulative deposition of sub-periosteal new bone. In other cases the changes which lead to thickening of the skull bones start in the interior of the affected bones. In the latter cases the thickening of the bones is associated with replacement of their normal structural components by new bone. Both grossly and histologically, the altered skull bones in these cases present some of the aspects of skull bones altered by Paget's disease.

As already implied, cases in which individual skull bones undergo tumor-like expansive swelling because of an intramedullary lesion should not be included in the category of leontiasis ossea. Most often in these cases, it is a maxilla, the mandible, or one of the bones of the calvarium that is affected. If such an expanding intra-medullary lesion is composed of fibro-osseous tissue, it either represents a localized expression of fibrous (fibro-osseous) dysplasia of bone or, if the lesion is in one of the jaw bones, it may be a cementoma. Indeed, the writer believes that most of these solitary localized fibro-osseous lesions of skull bones, if not associated with analogous lesions elsewhere in the skeleton, bear the same relation to polyostotic fibrous dysplasia as a solitary osteocartilaginous exostosis or a solitary enchondroma of bone bears to multiple exostosis or skeletal enchondromatosis respectively (see Jaffe).

Cherubism ("familial fibrous swelling of the jaws") likewise does not belong in the category of leontiasis ossea (see Caffey and Williams, and Dechaume *et al.*). Obviously, one should also exclude, for instance, the symmetrical hyperostoses of the

Figure 68

A, Photograph of the inner surface of the calvarium from the case of a woman 70 years of age who presented virilism and obesity in addition to hyperostosis frontalis interna. In this specimen the changes on the inner surface of the frontal bone are bilateral and symmetrical, and the affected area presents a "warty" appearance.

B, Photograph of the inner surface of the calvarium from the case of a woman 80 years of age who likewise presented the principal manifestations of the Morgagni syndrome (virilism, obesity, and frontal hyperostosis). In this case the hyperostoses are again bilateral and symmetrical, but quite bumpy, and had caused flattening and depression of the frontal lobes of the brain. (This illustration and the one shown in *A* were kindly given to me by Professor Folke Henschen, who made important contributions to the pathologic anatomy of the Morgagni syndrome.)

C, Photomicrograph ($\times$ 2) illustrating the general histologic pattern in an area of hyperostosis frontalis interna. Note the compact outer table which has retained its normal contour. In the thickened portion of the calvarium, the osseous tissue which had been deposited under the dura had undergone spongification from the diploic side, and the regional inner table is even thinner than it would normally be.

D, Photomicrograph ($\times$ 8) showing the difference in histologic architecture between an uninvolved area of calvarium (extreme right) and an area altered by hyperostosis frontalis interna. If one projects a horizontal line to the left, starting from the inner table as indicated by the arrows, one will be following along the site of the original inner table. The osseous tissue below the hypothetical line represents the subperiosteally deposited new bone, which has been spongified and which has thus become part of the diploë of the hyperostotic area.

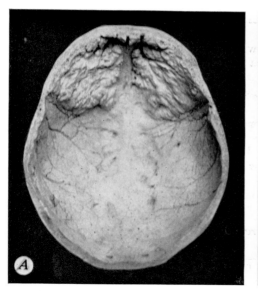

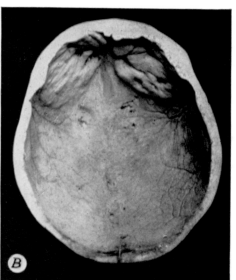

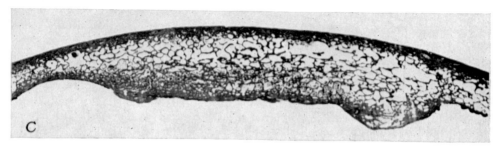

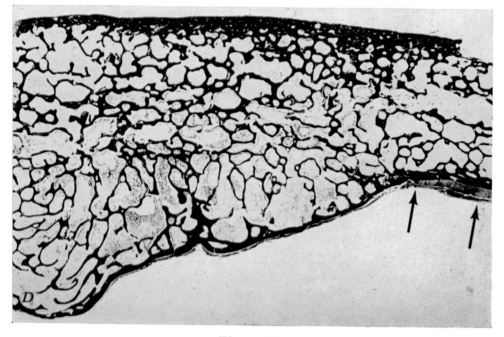

Figure 68

upper jaw which develop in connection with goundou, a tropical disease observed most commonly in natives of West Africa (see Eckert).

LEONTIASIS OSSEA RESULTING FROM CREEPING PERIOSTITIS

Leontiasis ossea developing on the basis of creeping periostitis was only occasionally encountered in the past and is very rarely encountered now. The condition evolves slowly, and, even when the disorder begins in childhood, as it usually does, it is quite likely to be compatible with survival into middle age (see Knaggs and also Lasserre). The underlying periostitis apparently represents an inflammatory response to an infectious agent. At any rate, when it has once set in, the peri-

Figure 69

A, Photograph of the skull from a case of leontiasis ossea which had developed on the basis of a creeping periostitis. Note the irregular, finely nodulated surface of the calvarium, the bony mass extending into the orbital cavity (on the left), and the thickened facial bones. (This illustration has been reproduced, with permission, from the article by Lasserre.)

B, Photograph of the skull from a case of extremely pronounced leontiasis ossea. This is the classic case of Fourcade to which both Virchow and Lebert have made reference. It is also one of those discussed by Knaggs, who has summarized the known facts in this case as follows: "Fourcade was a surgeon at Perpignan and had a son, who except for an attack of variola had enjoyed good health till he was 12 years of age (1734). At this time his father opened for him near the inner canthus of the right eye a lachrymal tumour which suppurated for a very long time. There developed at the same time on the nasal apophysis of the right superior maxilla a tumour as big as an almond, which grew till at the age of 15 it compressed the nasal cartilage in such a manner as to prevent the youth from breathing except by the mouth. The disease then extended to the inferior maxilla [mandible], which kept its normal form only at the articular extremities and alveolar borders. The superior maxillae, the walls of the orbits with the exception of the roofs, the nasal openings, the palate and malar bones were invaded and enlarged till they formed shapeless masses. At 20 years of age the face was monstrous. He had exophthalmos with myopia, difficulty in speaking, and general enfeeblement. He died, blind and phthisical, at the age of 45. The macerated head weighed 8 lb. 4 oz.; the inferior maxilla alone 3 lb. 3 oz. Great tuberous and lobulated exostoses having the density of marble protruded from the lower jaw and inferior borders of the orbits; the cranial bones were thickened, with little, smooth, and completely sclerosed excrescences. The frontal and maxillary sinuses had entirely disappeared. The rest of the skeleton was remarkable for the fragility of the bones." (This illustration has been reproduced, with permission, from the article by Knaggs.)

C and *D*, Photographs of the frontal and lateral views of the skull from the case described by Koch, which apparently represents the "osteitic form" of leontiasis ossea. The subject, a woman, was 65 years of age at the time of her death. During the last 20 years of her life, her skull had been undergoing gradual enlargement. This was associated with roaring in the ears, headaches, dizziness, and decrease in vision. At autopsy, it was found that all the bones of the skull (except some of those of the face) were thickened, and some were strikingly so. Both grossly and microscopically, the skull changes in this case resembled those observed in skulls severely altered by Paget's disease. As already indicated in the text by the present writer, Koch apparently did not establish unequivocally the absence of involvement, in this case, of bones other than those of the cranium, although he expressed his belief that they were not involved.

E, Roentgenograph of the skull from a case of leontiasis ossea of the "osteitic form." The subject, a girl, was 15 years of age when this picture was taken. Progressive enlargement of the skull had been evident for at least 8 years previously. The subject died and came to autopsy at the age of 17. The gross appearance of the calvarium, which was removed at autopsy, is shown in Figs. 70-*A* and *B*. (I am indebted to Dr. Marvin Kuschner, formerly of Bellevue Hospital, New York City, for the pertinent material in this case.)

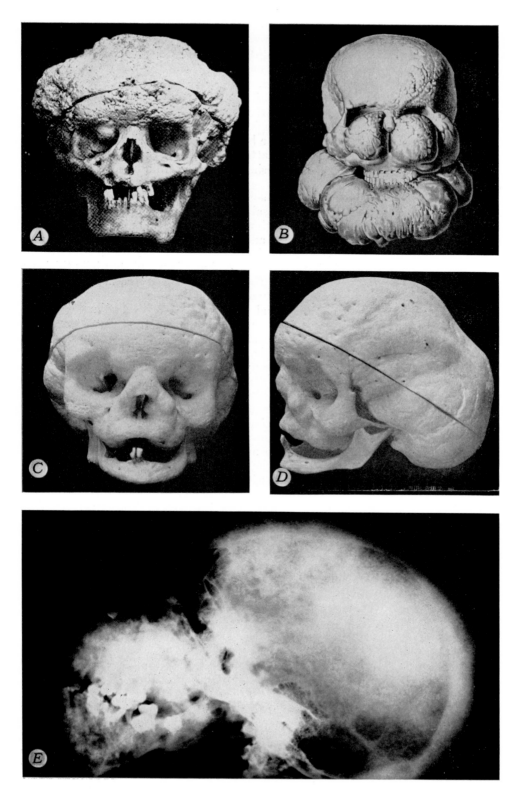

Figure 69

ostitis spreads relentlessly from one skull bone to another, causing thickening of the affected bones through subperiosteal new bone deposition. At suture lines the firm attachment of the periosteum constitutes a temporary obstacle to the spread of the periostitis. At these sites the deposit of new bone may pile up for some time before the attached periosteum is penetrated at several points and deposition on the surface of the adjacent bone begins. Though the sutures may be buried beneath the deposits when once adjoining bones have been attacked, their sites are often still indicated by sulci in the deposits. Other attached membranes, such as the temporal fascia or the palpebral ligaments, act similarly in retarding the extension and fusion of the adjacent deposits.

From study of a number of museum specimens, Knaggs deduced that the disorder usually begins in an accessory nasal sinus, the periostitis being manifested first in the deposition of new bone beneath the mucoperiosteal lining. The affection then spreads to the adjacent nasal fossa and the other sinuses opening into it, and sooner or later it extends to the lining of the nasal fossa and sinuses on the opposite side. The persistent accumulation of subperiosteal new bone substantially thickens the septum and turbinates and narrows the various accessory nasal sinuses. The disease then emerges from the nasal cavity in front and behind.

In front, it first spreads over the external surface of the maxillae, often sparing the alveolar processes. It then tends to creep upward along the frontal processes. Ultimately, because of involvement of the periosteum of the calvarial bones, osseous deposits may appear also upon the frontal and parietal bones and even the occipital bones. From the maxillae the periostitis may also spread laterally to the cheek bones or pass beneath them toward the pterygopalatine fossae. Behind, the periostitis emerges from the nasal cavity by way of the sphenopalatine foramina. On each side, the periosteal deposit may then spread in two directions. One stream moves forward to meet that passing backward along the maxilla; the other moves upward upon the great wing of the sphenoid into the temporal fossa to join the deposit covering the frontal bone. From adjacent parts the periostitis extends into the orbits and onto the arch of the palate. The extension of the disease to the mandible is difficult to explain unless one assumes with Knaggs that it takes place by way of the buccinator muscle and the pterygomandibular ligament. This assumption seems justified, since it is the outer surface, close to the insertion of these structures, that is the first part of the mandible to thicken.

Though the periosteal new bone probably remains delimited from the underlying original bone for some time, the distinction gradually becomes obliterated. Thus, eventually the thickened bones are found composed throughout of closely compacted cancellous osseous tissue. When the periosteum is stripped off, the bone surface is usually found rough, coarsely pumice-like, and studded with numerous vascular apertures. In some places the thickened skull bones may even be found eburnated. When the condition has attained full efflorescence, fantastic cauliflower-like thickening of the facial bones may give the subject's face a weirdly distorted appearance. (See Figs. 69-A and B.)

What provokes the periosteum to reactive new bone formation in these cases is not established. As already indicated, it seems likely that the instigating factor is an infectious agent, but what the responsible agent might be is not known. In this connection it should be noted that suppuration and bone sequestration do not occur as part of the disease but only as a rare complication.

During a long part of its evolution, the disease may be painless and the general health good. Eventually, however, clinical complaints develop—mainly from the mechanical effects of obstruction of the nasal and lachrymal passages and pressure upon the orbits and optic nerves from narrowing of the orbital fossae and foramina. Mental and cerebral disturbances may also appear and indeed are quite common.

In some cases, benefit has been derived from the surgical removal of hyperostoses which were compressing or otherwise injuring adjacent tissues.

LEONTIASIS OSSEA RESULTING FROM INTERNAL "FIBRO-OSSEOUS" RECONSTRUCTION

Cases of leontiasis ossea which are characterized pathologically by internal "fibro-osseous" reconstruction (commonly miscalled "fibrous osteitis") of the skull bones, and in which no analogous changes are present in skeletal parts other than the skull, are certainly very rare.

Koch reports on a case that came to autopsy which seems to be of this kind. However, close reading of his article reveals that he did not completely eliminate the possibility of involvement of other parts of the skeleton. Knaggs comments on a number of instances of the "osteitic form" of leontiasis ossea, and some of the diffusely involved skulls in question are preserved as museum specimens. In some of these cases, too, one cannot be sure that no extracranial skeletal involvement was present. In any event, however, the possibility of the existence of an "osteitic form" of leontiasis ossea unaccompanied by analogous extracranial changes cannot be denied.

The "osteitic form" of leontiasis ossea usually sets in before adulthood and sometimes causes tremendous enlargement of the head. This enlargement is likely to be much more prominent in the cranial than in the facial parts of the skull, and the lower jaw may even be entirely spared. However, there are cases in which involvement of the facial bones, and particularly of the jaw bones, is even more conspicuous than that of the calvarium. In the "osteitic form" of leontiasis ossea, as contrasted with the periostitic form, the thickened bones appear relatively smooth rather than obviously bumpy.

With an occasional exception, the impression created by skulls presenting the "osteitic form" of leontiasis ossea is similar, both clinically and anatomically, to that given by a skull heavily involved in Paget's disease. In fact, Koch regarded his case as one of Paget's disease expressing itself as leontiasis ossea. Indeed, it is probably through cases like his that the interpretation of certain cases of leontiasis ossea as Paget's disease limited to the skull came into existence (see Hamburger and Nachlas). It seems to the present writer very unlikely, however, that a skull will become affected almost in its entirety by Paget's disease while the rest of the skeleton remains entirely free of it. One hesitates, therefore, to accept "osteitic" leontiasis ossea as localized Paget's disease. Another possibility is that it represents an exuberant expression of fibrous dysplasia limited to the skull bones. However, the writer has yet to see a case in which such widespread cranial alterations were associated with extensive changes clearly representing fibrous dysplasia elsewhere in the skeleton. On the other hand, in cases of fibrous dysplasia in which many trunk and limb bones are affected, though one almost always finds one or more foci of cranial involvement, the latter does not, in the writer's experience, reach the magnitude of "leontiasis ossea" or even of "unilateral cranial hyperostosis" or "hemihypertrophy of the cranium." Altogether, one must still keep an open mind on the question of the basic nature of the "osteitic form" of leontiasis ossea. (See Figs. 69-C, D, and E, and Fig. 70.)

INFANTILE CORTICAL HYPEROSTOSIS

Infantile cortical hyperostosis is a disease of unknown cause which usually becomes manifest early in infancy, and in which the anatomic changes are centered in the bones, though not confined to them. In particular, the affected bones undergo thickening in consequence of apposition of excessive amounts of subperiosteal new bone on their cortices. The disease was first reported as a clinical entity by Caffey and Silverman in 1945, and independently by Smyth *et al.* in 1946. Dating back somewhat before that time, there are a few reports in the literature on cases in which infants showed bone lesions that would now be interpreted as manifestations of infantile cortical hyperostosis (see Roske, and de Toni). Altogether, the current impression is that the condition actually represents a relatively new disease. Though its cause is still obscure, there is increasing evidence that hereditary factors may play a role in its occurrence. The condition has been noted in several sibs of one family and/or members of several generations of one family tree. This finding supports the idea that the appearance of the disorder is determined at least in part by genetic influences, whatever its instigating cause may be (see Van Buskirk *et al.*, Gerrard *et al.*, and Clemett and Williams).

CLINICAL CONSIDERATIONS

It appears that the disease is not rare and not indigenous to any particular country or racial or cultural group. In the great majority of the cases, the subjects (apparently more often males than females) are less than 5 months of age when the disease first becomes manifest. Indeed, some of them are only a few days or a few weeks old. An occasional instance of the disease has even been discovered in a fetus late in intra-uterine life or in a fetus born prematurely (see Barba and Freriks, and Bennett and Nelson).

The manifestations of infantile cortical hyperostosis set in abruptly with hyperirritability, often associated with some fever and usually with swelling of the jaws (especially the lower jaw.) Occasionally, swelling of one or both arms or legs and/or conjunctivitis precedes the changes in the jaw regions by several days. In some cases the condition ceases to progress further, and may even be limited to involvement of the jaws. In other cases, swellings develop over additional skeletal parts, including one or both scapulae, clavicles, or various ribs on one or both sides. In these severer cases, there may be high and even prolonged fever, and the infant may be pale and anemic. An increased sedimentation rate of the red cells and a moderate degree of leukocytosis are usual under these circumstances. On palpation, the swollen parts are found hard and indurated and deeply fixed to the underlying bones. They are likely to be somewhat tender but are not discolored or abnormally warm. The swollen areas do not soften, their regression taking place by involution. Lymphadenopathy is not encountered.

In an individual case, the number of bones involved may be few or many. The involvement is likely to be migratory—that is, various bones tend to become implicated in succession. Also, in relation to a given bone, the periosteal new bone dep-

Figure 70

A, Photograph of the calvarium, removed at autopsy, in the case illustrated in Fig. 69-*E* showing the pronounced thickening of the constituent bones.

B, Photograph of the calvarium shown in *A*, after the part had been macerated.

C, Roentgenograph of a segment from a thin slice of calvarium cut from the macerated specimen shown in *B*.

D, Photomicrograph (× 10) illustrating the general histologic pattern (fibrous replacement and new bone formation) encountered in a skull affected with the "osteitic form" of leontiasis ossea.

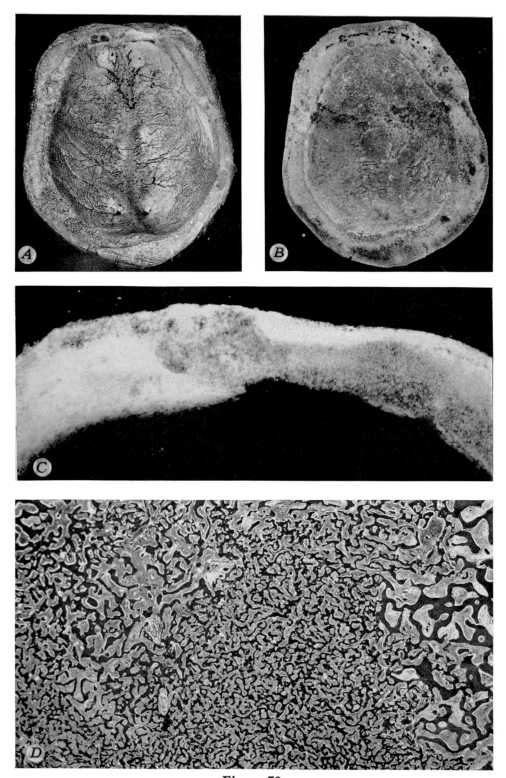

Figure 70

osition may recede and then perhaps reappear. The disease is usually self-limited, and the skeletal changes ordinarily regress completely in the course of a few months or a year or two. From all this it is clear that the *clinical course* of the condition is by no means the same in all instances. In those cases in which the skeletal involvement appears to be limited to the mandibular region (the mildest cases), the facial swelling may disappear and the disorder as a whole subside after a few weeks. Among the cases in which multiple skeletal areas are affected, some (the cases of moderate severity) run a course in which the manifestations last only for several weeks or months. In the latter cases the involvement is usually migratory, one or more new sites becoming affected while in other sites the swelling is resolving. Also, in a given area, the swelling may recrudesce after it has already subsided. In severe cases the course may be protracted or even chronic. Thus, in an individual instance, the swellings may persist and even progress for a year or two before receding. Occasionally, however, gradual regression of the various swellings is followed by repeated recrudescences of swelling in one or more parts (particularly in the jaws), and this course may continue for a number of years. Two cases of late recurrence of infantile cortical hyperostosis have been reported by Swerdloff *et al.* Furthermore, instances have been reported (and the present writer has also seen a case) in which a severely affected infant has succumbed, death usually being due to secondary infection. (See Sherman and Hellyer, Matheson and Markham, Sauterel and Rabinowicz, Caffey, and also Holman.)

ROENTGENOGRAPHIC AND PATHOLOGIC FINDINGS

As already indicated, the number of bones affected in a given case may be few or many, and in any event may vary from time to time. That is, bones not found involved at the initial *x-ray examination* may show involvement some weeks later. The characteristic deposits of new bone appearing on the cortices of the various affected bones may be present not only where the soft tissues overlying these bones are swollen, but sometimes even in areas where there is no soft-tissue swelling.

The mandible is found involved and thickened in almost all cases, and often it is the only bone affected. The clavicles, too, are rather commonly and severely implicated. Also, in some cases, one or both scapulae and numerous ribs appear clothed by thick deposits of new bone on their cortices. In relation to the long tubular bones, the amount of new bone deposited on the shaft cortex is sometimes sufficient to double or even triple the normal diameter of the bone in the midshaft area. However, the deposit tends to be uneven in thickness, and often does not extend to the ends of the shaft—that is, to its metaphysial regions. If both bones of a forearm or a leg are massively thickened, one or more bridges of bone connecting them may be seen. In contrast to the long tubular bones, the short tubular bones of the hands and feet are nearly always found free of deposits of new bone on their cortices.

The *resolution* of the bone changes as observed roentgenographically takes place along two general lines. In the course of some months, the layer of new bone deposited on the pre-existing cortex becomes increasingly compact, thinner, and less clear-cut as it undergoes amalgamation with the underlying cortex. In addition, as is common under all circumstances in which new bone is deposited on pre-existing cortical bone, the original cortical bone yields by becoming increasingly porous ("porotified"). As resorption of the original cortical bone progresses and the subperiosteally deposited new bone becomes more compact, the latter becomes the new bone cortex. The resorption or yielding of the original cortex results, in the course of a number of additional months, in widening of the marrow cavity of the affected bone. The new cortex formed from the subperiosteally deposited bone may even appear thinner than the original cortex. After another year or two, however, the altered bone may be well on the way toward a normal status in respect to the thickness of its cortex and the width and contour of its marrow cavity. (See MacLeod *et al.*)

The *histopathologic skeletal findings* in cases of infantile cortical hyperostosis naturally vary with the stage of the disease process. If a specimen obtained from a bone and its overlying soft tissues represents a very early stage of involvement, the presence of acute inflammatory changes will be noted. The periosteum will be found thickened and edematous and permeated to some degree by polymorphonuclear leukocytes. Proliferative periosteal activity is also to be observed. This is expressed by the presence of increased numbers of connective tissue cells and of osteoblasts which are lining up to form trabeculae of new bone. During this early stage in the development of the anatomic changes, the soft tissues (muscle and fascia) contiguous to the periosteum are also likely to show some edematous swelling and infiltration by polymorphonuclear leukocytes (see Eversole *et al.*).

Actually, most of the tissue specimens examined represent somewhat later stages in the evolution of the disease. Under these conditions, active inflammatory changes are no longer to be observed. However, the periosteum of the affected bone is still thickened and fibrous, as are the connective tissue septa which invest the musculature adjacent to, and even beyond, the altered periosteum. The connective tissue septa extending into the adipose tissue are also thickened. Beneath the periosteum, one now observes a layer composed of immature (coarse-fibered) trabeculae of osseous tissue of variable thickness. Between these bony trabeculae there is highly vascularized connective tissue meagerly interspersed with small lymphoid cells. If the subperiosteal layer of new bone is very thick, the underlying original cortical bone will already be found extensively rarefied (see Sherman and Hellyer).

In one of the cases studied by the writer—a case which ran a very protracted course and in which the infant died—the bones showed, roentgenographically and grossly, the characteristic thick deposits of subperiosteal new bone. On microscopic examination, however, widespread inflammatory changes were found both in the subperiosteal new bone and in the interior of the affected bones. The inflammatory changes took the form of numerous discrete foci of inflammation, the dominating cells being small round cells of the lymphoid type. There was also some connective tissue scarring within and in the immediate vicinity of these foci of inflammation, the total pattern actually suggesting granuloma formation. It is of special interest that microscopic examination of the viscera of the infant in question failed to reveal any analogous inflammatory lesions. Since the clinical and roentgenographic features in this case parallel those ordinarily observed in connection with nfantile cortical hyperostosis, the noted anatomic findings are surprising if not unique. However, it may well be that the granulomatous inflammatory changes observed in the bones represent the results of a secondary and complicating terminal infection—possibly even a virus infection. Unfortunately, no bacteriologic studies of the tissues were carried out in this case.

We do know, however, that, in various other cases of infantile cortical hyperostosis in which bacteriologic studies were made, no bacterial or viral agents were ever identified. Nevertheless, since the anatomic findings early in the disease do seem to represent inflammatory changes, the possibility of a bacterial or viral factor in the instigation or pathogenesis of the disease cannot be entirely excluded. Emphasis has been laid on the possible pathogenetic significance of thickening, through intimal proliferation, of the arterioles of the periosteum and overlying soft tissues of the affected bones. However, the writer doubts that disturbance of the blood supply to the bones plays any role in the development of the changes. (See Figs. 71 and 72.)

TREATMENT

Corticosteroids have been found to be highly effective in controlling the disorder. Their use is certainly indicated in those cases in which the infant is acutely ill and the condition appears to be progressing. For the first two or three weeks, the therapeutic dosage should be the maximum advocated for an infant, in relation to the particular corticosteroid used. After that, the dosage should be reduced gradually over the succeeding few months, since experience has shown that premature and/or abrupt cessation of the medication is likely to be followed by recrudescence of the clinical manifestations, sometimes even in exacerbated form. Under appropriate treatment, even an infant who has been very ill shows striking symptomatic improvement within a few days. This clinical improvement is associated with gradual subsidence of the swellings, though the bones may still present roentgenographic evidence of the disease for some months. (See Marquis.)

PULMONARY HYPERTROPHIC OSTEOARTHROPATHY

The principal components of the clinicopathologic complex represented by *pulmonary hypertrophic osteoarthropathy* are: (1) pulmonary disease of one type or another; (2) clubbing (drumstick enlargement) of the ends of the fingers and toes, due mainly or entirely to thickening of the subungual soft tissues; (3) periosteal new bone deposition (osteophytosis) found particularly on the tubular bones of the extremities; and (4) painful swelling of joints, apparently initiated by inflammatory changes in the synovial membrane. However, in some cases the extrapulmonary findings consist of drumstick fingers alone, or rather widespread osteoperiostitis

Figure 71

A, Roentgenograph of the jaws of a male 5 months of age affected with infantile cortical hyperostosis (Caffey's disease). At the time of admission to the hospital, the infant had a slightly elevated temperature, clear-cut swelling of the left forearm, and some swelling of the lower jaw. Along the lower margin of the mandible, a thin layer of subperiosteal new bone is apparent. Both bones of the left forearm showed thick layers of subperiosteal new bone on their shafts.

B, Roentgenograph of part of the thorax from a case of infantile cortical hyperostosis in a female 4 months of age. Note that the ribs are clothed by thick coats of subperiosteal new bone. At the time this x-ray picture was taken, the right femur and the bones of both forearms were also already affected. Within a period of about 6 months, the abnormal changes had substantially regressed.

C, Roentgenograph of the long tubular bones of the right upper extremity of a male 9 months of age affected with infantile cortical hyperostosis. The bones in question show rather well-developed subperiosteal deposits of new bone on their shafts.

D, Roentgenograph showing thick deposits of subperiosteal new bone on the long tubular bones of the lower extremities in the same case represented by C. This x-ray picture, too, was taken when the infant was 9 months old. The disease ran a chronic protracted course in this case, and the subject died and came to autopsy at the age of 15 months. (See also Figs. 72-A and B.)

E, Roentgenograph showing the left radius and ulna in a case of infantile cortical hyperostosis. The patient, 6 months of age when this picture was taken, had had swelling of the affected forearm for the preceding 2 months. There was also a brawny swelling in the region of the mandible, more prominent on the right side than on the left. A biopsy specimen was taken from the affected right fibula in this case, and the findings are illustrated in Figs. 72-D and E.

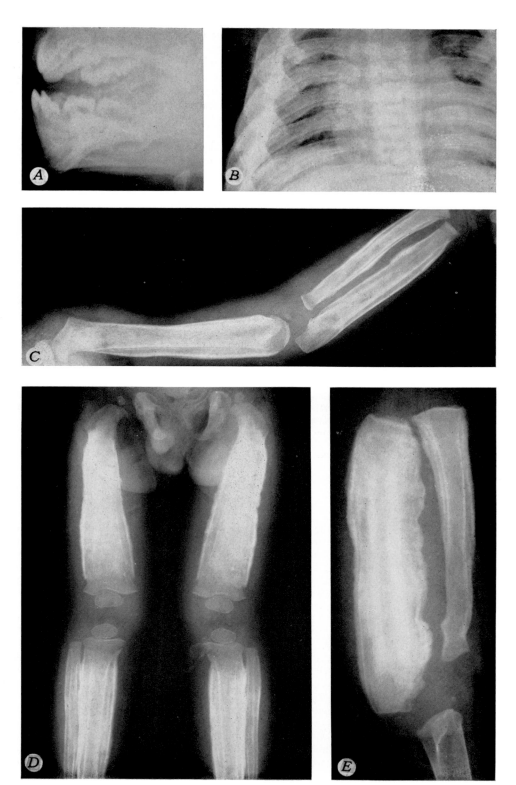

Figure 71

(osteophytosis) alone, or both of these features, with or without articular changes.

Pulmonary hypertrophic osteoarthropathy not infrequently evolves in a patient presenting pulmonary metastases from a primary bone sarcoma (most often an osteogenic sarcoma). When the underlying pulmonary lesion is not a sarcoma metastatic from a bone, it may be a sarcoma metastatic from the soft tissues, or a pulmonary carcinoma (either primary or metastatic). Furthermore, the pulmonary disease provoking a hypertrophic osteoarthropathy may even have its basis in an infection, appearing, for instance, in connection with a tuberculous or nontuberculous lung abscess or a chronic bronchiectasis.*

Dogs and various other mammals affected with primary or secondary tumors of the lung or with other intrathoracic disease have been found to show skeletal changes entirely analogous to those encountered in human cases of pulmonary hypertrophic osteoarthropathy (see Jones and Schnelle).

CLINICAL CONSIDERATIONS

In a young patient presenting pulmonary metastases from an osteogenic sarcoma of bone, manifestations of pulmonary hypertrophic osteoarthropathy may easily fail to arouse much interest because of the gravity of the subject's general condition.

* Clubbing of the fingers and toes may, of course, be observed with conditions other than pulmonary disease—notably, with cardiac disease. Osteophytosis (with or without the clubbing) is occasionally also found in connection with disease of the heart, liver (including biliary passages) and intestinal tract (see Locke). Clubbing of the fingers and toes and widespread osteophytosis have even been noted in connection with hypothyroidism developing after thyroidectomy for Graves' disease (see Thomas). Furthermore, clubbing and rather widespread periosteal new bone deposition have been reported as occurring without disease of the lungs or heart or, indeed, of any other organ. Such cases are rare and should be held apart from cases of pulmonary hypertrophic osteoarthropathy. The condition they represent is often denoted as "idiopathic hypertrophic osteoarthropathy with pachydermia." For the sake of brevity, it is also sometimes called "pachydermo-periostosis" (see p. 291).

Figure 72

A, Roentgenograph showing the status of the femur and part of the tibia and fibula from the case of infantile cortical hyperostosis illustrated in Fig. 71-*D*. This picture was taken about 6 months after the other and shows striking progression of the changes. The subject was now about 15 months of age. Death soon ensued, and an autopsy was performed.

B, Photograph of the femur shown in *A*, after the bone had been sectioned longitudinally in the frontal plane. The extreme thickening of the cortex stands out clearly. (This femur and the pertinent roentgenographs in this case were submitted to the present writer for his opinion by Dr. Asher Yaguda and Dr. Eli Rubenstein, and the writer wishes to acknowledge his indebtedness to them for permission to use this material.)

C, Roentgenograph of the right fibula and tibia from the case of infantile cortical hyperostosis already referred to in connection with Fig. 71-*E*. The upper half of the fibula shows the presence of a thick layer of subperiosteal new bone on the shaft cortex. A cross-sectional block of bone was removed from the fibula for further study. (See *D* and *E*.)

D, Roentgenograph (enlarged 2½ times) of the cross-sectional block of bone removed from the fibula shown in *C*. The remains of the original cortex are represented by the radiopaque inner circle. All the surrounding osseous tissue represents subperiosteal new bone.

E, Photomicrograph (× 6) of a tissue section prepared from the block of bone shown in *D*. Myeloid and fatty marrow are present within the marrow cavity of the fibula. The original cortical bone is rarefied and is surrounded by more or less concentric layers of new bone. Even when examined microscopically under higher power, the numerous tissue sections cut from the block of bone failed to reveal any inflammatory changes in the subperiosteal deposit of new bone or the medullary cavity of the affected fibula.

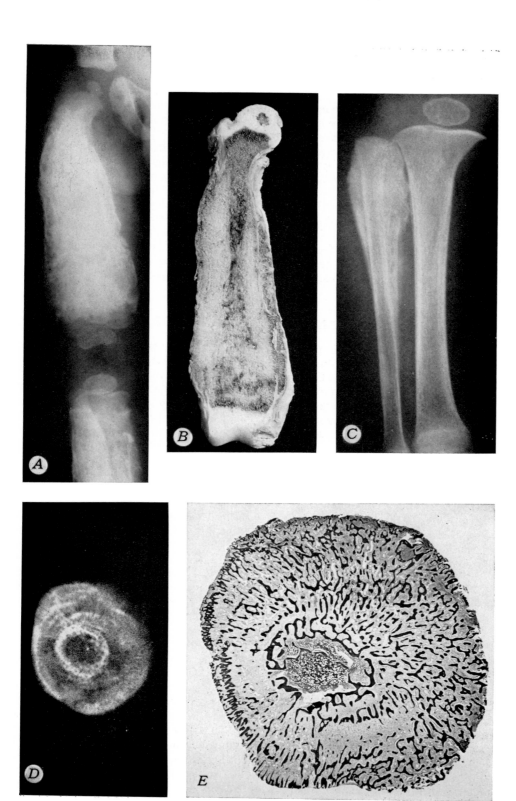

Figure 72

This may also be the case in the terminal stages of illness when an older patient is suffering from metastases to the lungs—for instance, from a soft-tissue sarcoma or from a carcinoma. In either event, it may be the casual finding of periosteal new bone deposition in the course of a roentgenographic skeletal survey that first calls attention to the presence of the condition.

On the other hand, in an occasional instance it is the manifestations of pulmonary hypertrophic osteoarthropathy that occupy the foreground of the clinical picture. This happens especially in connection with primary bronchogenic carcinoma, and sometimes the pulmonary tumor is even clinically occult. Indeed, in several pertinent cases observed by the writer, the knee joints and the small joints of the hands and feet were so painful and swollen that, if skeletal roentgenographs had not disclosed widespread osteophytosis, the presenting articular complaints and findings could have been misinterpreted as those of rheumatoid arthritis. In these cases it was only after the discovery of the osteoperiostitis that roentgenographs of the lungs were taken and the presence of a bronchogenic carcinoma was discovered.

ROENTGENOGRAPHIC AND PATHOLOGIC FINDINGS

As already indicated, it is the tubular bones of the extremities that show the periosteal new bone apposition and resultant cortical thickening most regularly and prominently (see Crump, and Gall *et al.*). Furthermore, within a given tubular bone, the involvement is usually most intense about the middle of the shaft, becoming gradually less so toward the ends of the bone. The epicondyles and the sites of insertion of ligaments and tendons usually do not become excessively prominent, but do show considerable new bone deposition nevertheless. Among the long tubular bones, the radius and ulna and the tibia and fibula are usually more severely affected than the humerus and femur. Of the short tubular bones, the metacarpals and metatarsals are more heavily involved than the phalanges. Indeed, the terminal phalanges often escape completely, though they sometimes show small osteophytic excrescences at their distal ends.

The bones of the trunk are relatively little affected and seem often to be spared altogether. However, one may find some osteophytic deposition upon the cortices of the clavicles. The cortices of the ribs are modified only slightly if at all. The same statement applies to periosteal new bone apposition on the vertebral bodies. Osteophytic thickening of the iliac crests may be observed, but new bone deposition upon the flat surfaces of the iliac bones is distinctly uncommon. The skull bones are usually completely spared. However, in rare instances, new bone deposition has been noted on the inner surface of the calvarium and on the nasal bones.

Pertinent *histologic studies* (notably by Crump) have revealed that, prior to the deposition of new bone by the periosteum, its outer, or fibrous, portion is the site of round cell infiltration. This is followed by proliferation of the inner, or cambium, layer (the osteoblastogenic layer) of the periosteum, resulting in the deposition of new bone upon the underlying original cortical bone. The osteoperiostitic deposit is laid down in layers. At first, it is sharply demarcated from the original cortex and is composed of meshy trabeculae of primitive (coarse-fibered) osseous tissue. As the deposit, which does not appear as an even cuff, becomes thicker, much of the deeper part of it undergoes lamellar reconstruction and becomes denser, though never so compact as the original cortex was. On the other hand, the latter undergoes a certain amount of porotification (as do also the deeper layers of the periosteal new bone), so that the once sharp line of demarcation between the old and new cortical bone gradually becomes less striking if the subject survives. Finally, it should be noted that there is no endosteal deposition of bone. That is, the spongy trabeculae do not become thickened or significantly reconstructed. In fact, the subcortical and subchondral spongy trabeculae tend to undergo some resorption, and where this occurs the intertrabecular marrow may even become somewhat fibrosed.

As to the status of the joints, it should be noted first that the enlargement of articular regions and the limitations of motion so often observed clinically are sometimes dependent upon thickening of the bone ends from the periosteal deposits, and are not necessarily associated with any alterations in the articular tissues themselves. Nevertheless, in some cases the latter, too, are affected. When the joints are involved, postmortem examination will reveal inflammatory changes in the synovial membrane, with thickening of the membrane and sometimes also intra-articular effusion. Under these circumstances, the synovial membrane is likely to show focal collections of round cells, evidence of hyperemia, and even connective tissue proliferation. In addition, the articular cartilages may be found modified by connective tissue pannus extending out from the inflamed membrane and by subchondral vascularization. These articular changes are especially likely to be encountered in adults whose pulmonary osteoarthropathy is of long standing. In any event, the affected joints do not become ankylosed, as they often finally do in cases of idiopathic (familial) hypertrophic osteoarthropathy with pachydermia. (See Figs. 73 and 74.)

The *pathogenetic mechanisms* underlying pulmonary hypertrophic osteoarthropathy have not yet been fully clarified. Among the explanatory concepts which have been proposed is the one which would base the condition on irritation of the periosteal and synovial membranes by circulating toxic products from the pulmonary lesion. In support of this idea, there is the finding of round cell infiltration in the outer, or fibrous, coat of the periosteum prior to the deposition of new bone by the cambium layer of the periosteum. There is also the finding of inflammatory changes in the synovial membranes of the swollen, painful joints.

However, the concept of "circulating toxic products" is yielding to the idea that the development of pulmonary hypertrophic osteoarthropathy is to be related to changes in the peripheral blood supply, induced indirectly by the underlying pulmonary disease. The presence of an increased peripheral blood flow is suggested by various clinical observations and also by direct physiological measurements. In this connection it is significant that the clinical manifestations of pulmonary hypertrophic osteoarthropathy often regress after excision of the pulmonary (or other intrathoracic) lesion or after mere interruption of the pathway of the pulmonary vagus nerve. These observations seem to indicate the existence of a reflex that passes from the diseased intrathoracic area or areas through the pulmonary vagus to produce the increased peripheral blood flow.

Apparently, though there is an increased peripheral blood flow, the excess blood (which is poorly oxygenated) passes through the arteriovenous shunts, bypassing the capillary bed. This type of blood flow tends to produce local passive congestion and poor tissue oxygenation, and in this way stimulates proliferation of the various connective tissues, including the periosteal and synovial membranes. However, the details of these various mechanisms still remain to be explored. (See Rasmussen, Hansen, Flavell, and also Huckstep and Bodkin, and Vogl and Goldfischer.)

IDIOPATHIC FAMILIAL HYPERTROPHIC OSTEOARTHROPATHY WITH PACHYDERMIA

Idiopathic hypertrophic osteoarthropathy with pachydermia represents a clinicopathologic entity to be distinguished in particular from pulmonary hypertrophic osteoarthropathy. Other names for the disorder include: *generalized hyperostosis with pachydermia, idiopathic familial generalized osteophytosis*, and *pachydermo-periostosis* (a convenient short designation). However, *pachydermo-hyperostosis* seems preferable as a short name, since it accords better with the total anatomic skeletal findings.

CLINICAL CONSIDERATIONS

The disorder is of rather rare occurrence. It is apparently not indigenous to any one country or to any racial group. The subjects are much more often males than females. That the condition is often familial is well established. It has been observed in several children of one family, in a parent and one or more of the children, and among other relatives of the affected subjects.

The manifestations of the disease generally set in during adolescence. Occasionally, however, they appear before puberty or during adult life. The disorder is insidious in its onset, but then progresses rather rapidly for a few years. During this evolutionary, or active, phase of the disease, the fingers and toes gradually thicken. Indeed, mainly because of hypertrophy of the subcutaneous tissues, the hands and feet as a whole eventually enlarge so much that they become ungainly, and they may even acquire a pawlike appearance. The distal ends of the fingers and toes are clubbed, and the convexity of the nails is strikingly accentuated. There may be complaints of excessive sweating of the hands and feet. Furthermore, because of the changes in the bones and also in the overlying subcutaneous tissues, the legs and forearms, in particular, lose their natural contours and become more or less cylindrical in shape. During the few years in which the disease is progressive, the subject may also complain of vague pains in the bones and joints. These complaints are related to the periosteal new bone deposition (osteophytosis) which extends to the articular ends of the various affected bones.

In addition to the alterations involving the limbs, there is increasing coarsening of the facial features. This results from thickening of the skin of the face and especially of the forehead. Because of hyperplasia of its sebaceous glands, the skin also appears greasy. The thickened skin of the forehead develops transverse and/or vertical folds separated by deep furrows, and the natural nasolabial folds deepen.

Figure 73

A, Photograph of a patient affected with a bronchogenic carcinoma and manifesting pulmonary hypertrophic osteoarthropathy. He was admitted to our hospital because of complaints relating to his joints, the pulmonary lesion being clinically occult. These complaints had been present for about 1 year. In particular, the finger joints, knees, ankles, shoulder joints, and wrist joints were swollen, painful, warm, and tender, and restricted in their motion. Indeed, the clinical picture at the time of admission suggested a rheumatoid polyarthritis, and the fact that the patient's complaints were to be related to a bronchogenic carcinoma was first suggested by the presence of widespread osteoperiostitis as revealed by a roentgenographic skeletal survey.

B, Photograph showing the clubbing of the ends of the fingers and the swelling of the wrist and finger joints of the left hand shown in *A*.

C, Roentgenograph of part of the hand of the patient shown in *A*. Note the periosteal new bone deposition on the proximal phalanges of the fingers and on the metacarpal bones. An osteoperiostitis was also present on the bones of the right hand, as well as on the long bones—particularly those of the legs and forearms. It was these findings that led to roentgenographic examination of the chest, which revealed the tumor in the right lung.

D, Photomicrograph ($\times$ 8) of a cross section through the midportion of the third proximal phalanx of the hand shown in *C*. The original cortical bone is undergoing resorption and is overlaid by a ring of subperiosteal new bone varying in thickness.

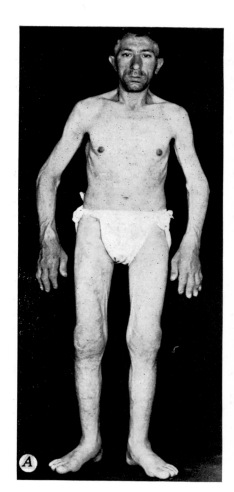

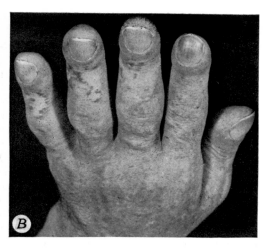

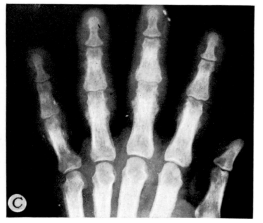

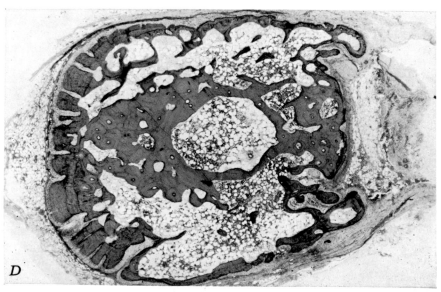

Figure 73

The scalp also thickens and likewise undergoes furrowing, its surface showing more or less coiled corrugations. In consequence of the alterations in the facial features, the subject tends to have a "worried" or "angry look" and to appear prematurely aged. (See Rimoin.)

The evolutionary (or active) phase of the disease is followed by a period, often lasting for many years, during which various chronic disabling complications set in. During this period, many of the joints become ankylosed. The small joints of the hands and feet are usually so affected because of bridging of the joints by bone which has developed in their articular capsules. Ossification of the costovertebral joints results in stiffening of the thorax, and ossification of the ligaments of the vertebral column leads to the development of a kyphosis. Concurrently the interosseous ligaments of the forearms and legs also undergo ossification. The most serious complication, which may develop late in the course of the disease, is the appearance of neurological manifestations. These are due to pressure upon the spinal cord and/or nerve roots as the result of narrowing of the spinal canal and/or the presence of vertebral osteophytes.

Although many cases of pachydermo-hyperostosis present the composite clinical picture outlined above, there are some in which one or another of the characteristic manifestations of the disorder is delayed in its appearance, never becomes pronounced, or even fails to develop at all. Thus there are cases in which the pachydermia is rather limited in extent and the alterations in the facial features are consequently inconspicuous. In other cases of the disorder, it is the periostosis (periosteal new bone deposition) that is slight, while the pachydermia is as well developed as in the classic cases.

It should also be pointed out that, particularly in these incomplete (or mild) expressions of the disorder, the external clinical appearance of the subject may resemble that of a person affected with pulmonary hypertrophic osteoarthropathy. In a classic case of pachydermo-hyperostosis, the large hands and feet may also suggest acromegaly due to hyperpituitarism. However, in pachydermo-hyperostosis, one

Figure 74

A, Roentgenograph showing periosteal new bone deposition on the *left* tibia and fibula in the case of a child presenting pulmonary metastases from an osteogenic sarcoma. The primary site of the sarcoma was the *right* tibia, and that leg had been amputated 22 months before this roentgenograph was taken. At this second admission, a skeletal survey also showed the presence of osteophytosis on both radii and ulnae and on practically all the metacarpal and metatarsal bones. The patient died $2\frac{1}{2}$ years after the amputation, and autopsy revealed not only pulmonary metastases but a number of skeletal metastases.

B, Photograph of the tibia and fibula shown in *A*, after they had been removed at autopsy and sectioned in the longitudinal plane. Note the layers of new bone on their cortices and the normal architecture of their spongiosa.

C, Photograph of a transverse slice through the shaft of the tibia shown in *B*, before that bone had been cut in the long axis. Observe that the osteophytic deposit extends around the entire circumference of the bone, but is not of uniform thickness. The original cortex stands out most clearly below and to the right. On the left, it is more obscure, because it is undergoing resorption (see *D*).

D, Roentgenograph of the slice of thickened cortex shown in *C*. Note the circumferential layering of the periosteal new bone and the small roundish radiolucencies on the left in the original cortical bone where the latter is undergoing resorption.

E, Photomicrograph ($\times$ 6) illustrating the pattern of the cortical bone and of the periosteal deposit present on the left in *C* and *D*. The subperiosteal new bone has been deposited in ringlike layers. In the central portion of the picture, the original cortex is undergoing porotification, while on the left and below, it is still compact.

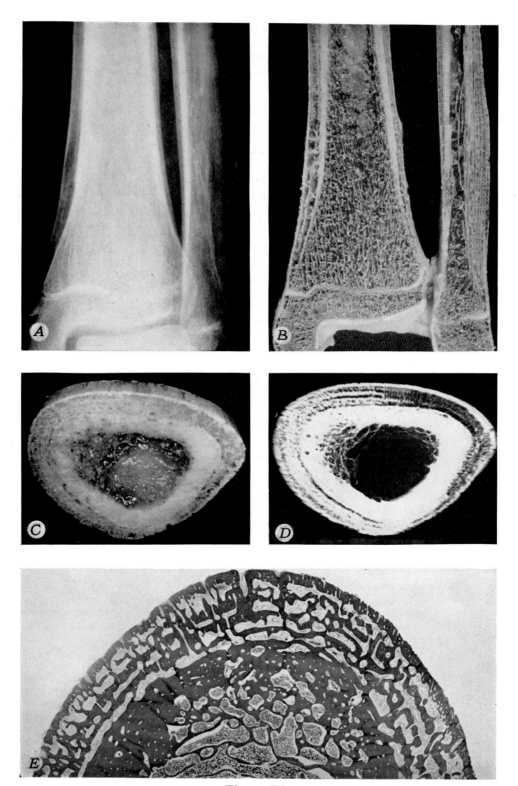

Figure 74

does not encounter (as one does in acromegaly) macroglossia, striking enlargement of the lower jaw, and the presence of abnormal visual fields. Furthermore, in pachydermo-hyperostosis, the sella turcica is normal in size and shape, and there is no "tufting" of the distal phalanges of the fingers and/or toes. (See Roy, Touraine *et al.*, Vogl and Goldfischer, Vague, and also Angel.)

PATHOLOGIC FINDINGS

The *pathologic findings* (particularly in regard to the skeletal changes) as they relate to cases of long standing have been fully described by Arnold and by Uehlinger. The latter and Freund have also given detailed descriptions of the roentgenographic skeletal findings corresponding to the anatomic findings to be noted, as given below, in cases of long standing. The changes are widespread over the skeleton and are more or less symmetrically distributed. In consequence of the periosteal new bone deposition, the various bones are found thickened. In the limbs the thickening is most striking in the long tubular bones. The shafts of these bones are definitely increased in diameter. Their articular surfaces are usually not much modified.

When stripped of its overlying soft parts, the surface of the shaft of a thickened long tubular bone appears roughened like the bark of a tree. A cross section through the shaft is very likely to reveal the absence of a clear-cut delineation between the original cortical bone (now more or less porotic or spongified) and the periosteal new bone which had been deposited on it. In contrast, a cross section through the shaft of a long tubular bone in a case of *pulmonary* hypertrophic osteoarthropathy ordinarily *does* show a sharp delimitation between the original cortex and the new bone deposited on it. This difference is accounted for by the fact that in pachydermo-

Figure 75

A, Photograph of a man 36 years of age presenting the outward clinical manifestations characteristic of pachydermo-periostosis. Note the furrowed appearance of the thickened skin of the forehead and the striking enlargement of the hands. Enlargement of the hands and feet set in when the subject was 18 years of age. The clinical details relating to this man and to his brother, who was affected with the same condition, were described by Müller.

B, Photograph of most of the bones (macerated and articulated) of the trunk and extremities from the case of pachydermo-periostosis described by Uehlinger. All the long tubular bones are strikingly thickened. The subject, a man, was 55 years of age at the time of his death. The clinical manifestations of the disorder had a late onset in this case, not appearing until he was 40 years of age.

C, Photograph of the left tibia and fibula, sectioned in the frontal plane, from the skeleton shown in *B*. The two bones are fused as a result of ossification of the interosseous ligament.

D, *E*, *F*, and *G*, Photographs illustrating various bones thickened in consequence of subperiosteal new bone deposition, from the case of pachydermo-periostosis in which the anatomic findings were described in detail by Arnold. The subject, a man, was 47 years of age at the time of his death, and his case was followed clinically for about 29 years. The clinical history was that at the age of 18 he noticed a gradual enlargement of the feet, especially around the ankles, and this was followed by enlargement of the legs and knee areas. In time, the hands also enlarged, and the fingers became so thick and the skin so tight that he had to cease working. The changes were not associated with significant pain or with alteration of the general health, and after a few years the condition ceased to progress. In addition to the bones of the extremities, the anatomic study revealed that the sternum, ribs, vertebrae, pelvis and jaw bones were also thickened by apposition of new bone. The vertebral bodies showed new bone apposition mainly along the anterior surface, and the innominate bones mainly along the crests and tubercles.

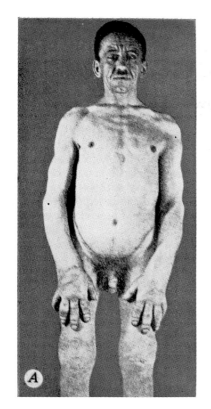
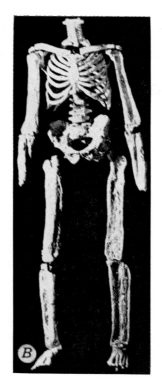
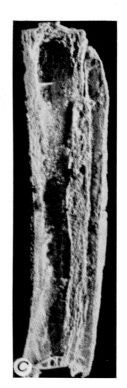
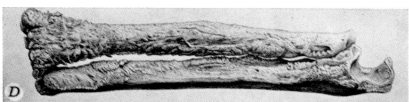
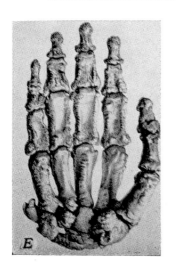
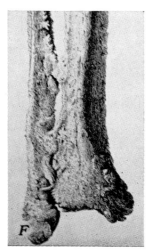
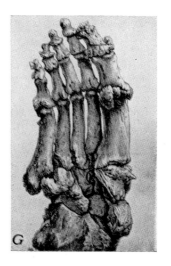

Figure 75

periostosis the subject usually survives for many years after the periosteal new bone has been laid down. Hence, enough time elapses to permit the occurrence of the various alterations in the original compact cortex and the periosteal new bone which lead to their blending.

The skull tends to be spared, except for the jaw bones which show moderate thickening, particularly of their alveolar portions. In an early stage of the disease, the vertebrae do not tend to show any modifications in contour, and the intervertebral disks are also not significantly modified. In the advanced stage, one finds the intervertebral disks very much narrowed and the various spinal ligaments ossified to a greater or lesser degree. In consequence, parts of the vertebral column become fused and the intervertebral foramina narrowed, and there may even be narrowing of the spinal canal. The interior of the vertebral bodies is also found modified, the normal spongiosa having been replaced by sparse, thick pillars of osseous tissue extending mainly in the long axis of the vertebral bodies. In regard to the various other bones of the trunk, it is to be noted that the ribs and clavicles are more or less uniformly thickened by deposits of new bone on their cortices. The innominate bones, scapulae, and sternum present irregularly bumpy osteophytic deposits at various predilected sites. On the innominate bones, these deposits are most striking at the iliac crests and about the margins of the acetabula.

The bones of the wrist and ankle are not obviously enlarged—that is, they are not significantly increased in size. Like the vertebral bodies, however, they come to show reconstruction of the spongiosa, which is replaced by small numbers of thick pillars of bone which also follow the direction of lines of tension and pressure. The ossification of the various ligaments of the vertebral column has already been mentioned. The interosseous ligaments of the forearms and legs, too, may be found extensively ossified. In subjects who have survived for many years after the onset of the disorder, bony bridging across various joints (both large and small), resulting in ankylosis, is usually also encountered. As noted, the joints of the hands and feet, in particular, are commonly found ankylosed. In fact, fusion of the bones of the wrist and midtarsus may proceed to such an extent that no lines of cleavage remain between the various bones of the parts in question, the whole area appearing as a solid block. (See Fig. 75.)

The pathologic changes in the soft (nonosseous) tissues are usually limited to the skin and subcutaneous tissues. In an individual case, the epidermis may not be particularly altered, while in another case there may be hyperkeratosis and/or parakeratosis. The connective tissue of the dermis (corium) is thickened, and the sebaceous and sweat glands are hyperplastic—often strikingly so. The hair follicles, too, may be hyperplastic. The fat of the subcutaneous tissue shows fibroblastic scarring, and the subcutaneous connective tissue in general is found thickened, collagenized, and even hyalinized in places.

The *pathogenetic mechanisms* underlying the development of idiopathic hypertrophic osteoarthropathy with pachydermia are still to be unraveled. In particular, it has still to be determined whether the altered peripheral blood flow which appears to be significant in connection with *pulmonary* hypertrophic osteoarthropathy is also operative in the idiopathic condition. Indeed, except for the genetic factor suggested by the high familial incidence of the latter disorder, nothing is known as yet about its etiology or pathogenesis.

REFERENCES

ANGEL, J. H.: Pachydermo-periostosis (Idiopathic Osteoarthropathy), Brit. M. J., *2*, 789, 1957.
ARNOLD, J.: Acromegalie, Pachyacrie oder Ostitis? Ein anatomischer Bericht über den Fall Hagner I., Beitr. path. Anat., *10*, 1, 1891.

BARBA, W. P., II, and FRERIKS, D. J.: The Familial Occurrence of Infantile Cortical Hyperostosis *in Utero*, J. Pediat., *42*, 141, 1953.

BENNETT, H. S., and NELSON, T. R.: Prenatal Cortical Hyperostosis, Brit. J. Radiol., *26*, 47, 1953.

CAFFEY, J.: Infantile Cortical Hyperostosis; A Review of the Clinical and Radiographic Features, Proc. Roy. Soc. Med., *50*, 347, 1957.

CAFFEY, J., and SILVERMAN, W. A.: Infantile Cortical Hyperostoses; Preliminary Report on a New Syndrome, Am. J. Roentgenol., *54*, 1, 1945.

CAFFEY, J., and WILLIAMS, J. L.: Familial Fibrous Swelling of the Jaws, Radiology, *56*, 1, 1951.

CALAME, A.: *Le syndrome de Morgagni-Morel. Etude anatomo-clinique*, Lausanne, H. Jaunin, 1950.

CLEMETT, A. R., and WILLIAMS, J. H.: The Familial Occurrence of Infantile Cortical Hyperostosis, Radiology, *80*, 409, 1963.

CRUMP, C.: Histologie der allgemeinen Osteophytose. (Ostéoarthropathie hypertrophiante pneumique.), Virchows Arch. path. Anat., *271*, 467, 1929.

DECHAUME, M., GRELLET, M., PAYEN, J., BONNEAU, M., GUILBERT, F., and BOCCARA, S.: Le Chérubisme, Presse méd., *70*, 2763, 1962.

ECKERT, L.: Ueber Gundu, Inaug. Dissertation, Leipzig, 1913.

ERDHEIM, J.: Über senile Hyperostose des Schädeldaches, Beitr. path. Anat., *95*, 631, 1935.

EVERSOLE, S. L., JR., HOLMAN, G. H., and ROBINSON, R. A.: Hitherto Undescribed Characteristics of the Pathology of Infantile Cortical Hyperostosis (Caffey's Disease), Bull. Johns Hopkins Hosp., *101*, 80, 1957.

FLAVELL, G.: Reversal of Pulmonary Hypertrophic Osteoarthropathy by Vagotomy, Lancet, *1*, 260, 1956.

FREUND, E.: Idiopathic Familial Generalized Osteophytosis, Am. J. Roentgenol., *39*, 216, 1938.

GALL, E. A., BENNETT, G. A., and BAUER, W.: Generalized Hypertrophic Osteoarthropathy, Am. J. Path., *27*, 349, 1951.

GERRARD, J. W., HOLMAN, G. H., GORMAN, A. A., and MORROW, I. H.: Familial Infantile Cortical Hyperostosis, J. Pediat., *59*, 543, 1961.

GERSHON-COHEN, J., SCHRAER, H., and BLUMBERG, N.: Hyperostosis Frontalis Interna Among the Aged, Am. J. Roentgenol., *73*, 396, 1955.

GROLLMAN, A. and ROUSSEAU, J. P.: Metabolic Craniopathy. A Clinical and Roentgenologic Study of So-called Hyperostosis Frontalis Interna, J.A.M.A., *126*, 213, 1944.

HAMBURGER, L. P. and NACHLAS, I. W.: Leontiasis Ossea as a Manifestation of Paget's Disease, Arch. Surg., *12*, 727, 1926.

HANSEN, J. L.: Bronchial Carcinoma Presenting as Arthralgia, Acta med. scandinav., Suppl. *266*, 467, 1952.

HENSCHEN, F.: Morgagnis Syndrom, Veröffentl. Konstitutions- und Wehrpath., *9*, 1937.

————: Über die verschiedenen Formen von Hyperostose des Schädeldachs, Acta path. et microbiol. scandinav., Suppl. *37*, 236, 1938.

HOLMAN, G. H.: Infantile Cortical Hyperostosis: A Review, Quart. Rev. Pediat., *17*, 24, 1962.

HUCKSTEP, R. L. and BODKIN, P. E.: Vagotomy in Hypertrophic Pulmonary Osteoarthropathy Associated with Bronchial Carcinoma, Lancet, *2*, 343, 1958.

JAFFE, H. L.: *Tumors and Tumorous Conditions of the Bones and Joints*, Philadelphia, Lea & Febiger, 1958. (See p. 138.)

JONES, T. C. and SCHNELLE, G. B.: Pulmonary Hypertrophic Osteoarthropathy in Dogs, Lab. Invest., *8*, 1287, 1959.

KNAGGS, R. L.: Leontiasis Ossea, Brit. J. Surg., *11*, 347, 1923–24.

KOCH, M.: Demonstration eines Schädels mit Osteitis deformans Paget (Leontiasis ossea Virchow), Verhandl. deutsch. path. Gesellsch., *13*, 107, 1909.

LASSERRE, C.: Les ostéopathies hypertrophiantes, Rev. d'orthop., *18*, 457, 1931.

LOCKE, E. A.: Secondary Hypertrophic Osteo-Arthropathy and Its Relation to Simple Club-Fingers, Arch. Int. Med., *15*, 659, 1915.

MACLEOD, W., DOUGLAS, D. M., and MAHAFFY, R. G.: Infantile Cortical Hyperostosis, Clin. Radiol., *16*, 269, 1965.

MARQUIS, J. R.: Infantile Cortical Hyperostosis, Radiology, *89*, 282, 1967.

MATHESON, W. J. and MARKHAM, M.: Infantile Cortical Hyperostosis, Brit. M. J., *1*, 742, 1952.

MOORE, S.: Hyperostosis Frontalis Interna, Surg., Gynec. & Obst., *61*, 345, 1935.

————: *Hyperostosis Cranii*, Springfield, Charles C Thomas, 1955.

MOREL, F.: *L'hyperostose frontale interne*. Syndrome de l'hyperostose frontale interne avec adipose et troubles cérébraux, Geneva, Chapalay & Mottier, 1929.

MÜLLER, W.: Über die familiäre akromegalieähnliche Skeletterkrankung, Bruns' Beitr. klin. Chir., *150*, 616, 1930.

RASMUSSEN, H.: Peripheral Vascular Disease, with Hypertrophic Osteoarthropathy, as the First Manifestation of Bronchial Carcinoma, Acta med. scandinav., Suppl. *266*, 855, 1952.

RIMOIN, D. L.: Pachydermoperiostosis (Idiopathic Clubbing and Periostosis), New England J. Med., *272*, 923, 1965.

ROSKE, G.: Eine eigenartige Knochenerkrankung im Säuglingsalter, Monatsschr. Kinderh., *47*, 385, 1930.

ROY, J. N.: Hypertrophy of the Palpebral Tarsus, the Facial Integument and the Extremities of the Limbs Associated with Widespread Osteo-periostosis: A New Syndrome, Canad. M.A.J., *34*, 615, 1936.

SALMI, A., VOUTILAINEN, A., HOLSTI, L. R., and Unnérus, C-E.: Hyperostosis Cranii in a Normal Population, Am. J. Roentgenol., *87*, 1032, 1962.

SAUTEREL, L. and RABINOWICZ, T.: Contribution a l'étude d'un nouvel aspect étiologique de l'hyperostose corticale infantile, Ann. Radiol., *4*, 211, 1961.

SHERMAN, M. S. and HELLYER, D. T.: Infantile Cortical Hyperostosis. Review of the Literature and Report of Five Cases, Am. J. Roentgenol., *63*, 212, 1950.

SMYTH, F. S., POTTER, A., and SILVERMAN, W.: Periosteal Reaction, Fever and Irritability in Young Infants. A New Syndrome? Am. J. Dis. Child., *71*, 333, 1946.

STEWART, R. M.: Localized Cranial Hyperostosis in the Insane, J. Neurol. & Psychopath., *8*, 321, 1928.

SWERDLOFF, B. A., OZONOFF, M. B., and GYEPES, M. T.: Late Recurrence of Infantile Cortical Hyperostosis (Caffey's Disease), Am. J. Roentgenol., *108*, 461, 1970.

THOMAS, H. M., JR.: Acropachy, Arch. Int. Med., *51*, 571, 1933.

DE TONI, G: Una nuova malattia dell'apparato osseo: la poliosteopatia deformante connatale regressiva, Policlin. infant., *XI*, 201, 1943.

TOURAINE, A., SOLENTE, G., and GOLÉ, L.: Un syndrome ostéo-dermopathique: La pachydermie plicaturée avec pachypériostose des extrémités, Presse méd., *43*, 1820, 1935.

UEHLINGER, E.: Hyperostosis generalisata mit Pachydermie. (Idiopathische familiäre generalisierte Osteophytose Friedreich-Erb-Arnold.), Virchows Arch. path. Anat., *308*, 396, 1941.

VAGUE, J.: La pachydermopériostose. Pachydermie plicaturée avec pachypériostose des extrémités (Syndrome de Touraine, Solente et Golé), Rev. rhum., *15*, 201, 1948.

VAN BUSKIRK, F. W., TAMPAS, J. P., and PETERSON, O. S., JR.: Infantile Cortical Hyperostosis. An Inquiry into Its Familial Aspects, Am. J. Roentgenol., *85*, 613, 1961.

VOGL, A. and GOLDFISCHER, S.: Pachydermoperiostosis. Primary or Idiopathic Hypertrophic Osteoarthropathy, Am. J. Med., *33*, 166, 1962.

Chapter

12

Primary and Secondary Hyperparathyroidism

Hyperparathyroidism represents the clinicopathologic changes produced in the course of time through the influence of excessive amounts of circulating parathyroid hormone. Instances of clinical hyperparathyroidism fall into two categories—*primary* and *secondary*. In man, *primary hyperparathyroidism* may result from: (1) parathyroid adenoma formation in one (or sometimes two) of the parathyroid glands; (2) diffuse hyperplasia of all the parathyroids (usually four); or (3) a parathyroid carcinoma. The parathyroid aberration most commonly underlying primary hyperparathyroidism is adenoma formation. The cases of *secondary hyperparathyroidism* narrow down, for practical purposes, to those in which parathyroid enlargement and hyperfunctioning has been induced by renal insufficiency of long duration. Indeed, it is well established that chronic renal insufficiency instigates diffuse hyperplasia of the parathyroids. However, under these circumstances the parathyroid enlargement is not so pronounced as it usually is in cases of *primary* hyperparathyroidism based on diffuse hyperplasia of all the parathyroids.

It is when one is dealing with *primary hyperparathyroidism* uncomplicated by renal insufficiency that one observes the characteristic biochemical and anatomical effects of an abnormal and protracted increase in the amount of circulating parathyroid hormone. The typical biochemical findings under these conditions are: an increased excretion of calcium and phosphorus (mainly by way of the urine); a hypercalcemia and hypophosphatemia; and an elevated serum alkaline phosphatase activity value. It has been clearly established that the negative calcium and phosphorus balance (excess of outgo over intake) is due to withdrawal of mineral from the bones. In consequence of a persistent drain upon the mineral stores of the skeleton, the bones undergo progressive rarefaction and fibrous transformation. The affected bones are susceptible to fractures, and so-called "brown tumors" and areas of cyst formation may also appear in them. If the hyperparathyroidism is not corrected and the condition runs its natural course for years, the bones become profoundly altered and the skeleton as a whole may come to present the classic picture of so-called generalized osteitis fibrosa cystica (Recklinghausen's disease of bone).

In *secondary (renal) hyperparathyroidism* one finds hyperphosphatemia and not infrequently hypocalcemia, along with other biochemical aberrations indicative of renal failure. The skeletal changes in these cases are not often striking, since the subjects usually succumb to the complications resulting from uremia before the alterations in the bones have had time to become pronounced. However, the skeletal changes resulting from hyperparathyroidism secondary to chronic renal insufficiency are usually more conspicuous (roentgenographically and anatomically) in children than in adults. The case of an adult in whom profound skeletal alterations of hyperparathyroidism coexist with evidence of severe renal failure may raise a problem of differential diagnosis. In particular, it may be difficult to decide in such an instance whether it was renal failure or parathyroid hyperfunctioning that was the point of departure for the pathologic condition as a whole.

In contrast to hyperparathyroidism, *hypoparathyroidism* is associated with hypo-calcemia, hyperphosphatemia, and a sharp curtailment of the urinary excretion of both calcium and phosphorus. The hypocalcemia is due specifically to a reduction of the ionized fraction of the blood calcium. Whenever, in hypoparathyroidism, the serum calcium level drops to 7.0 mg. per 100 cc. or less, hypertonia results and is manifested in muscle spasms and tetany.

Very rarely, hypoparathyroidism results from failure of the parathyroid glands to develop. In these cases of congenital absence of the parathyroids, the neonate's life is a brief and stormy one characterized by repeated convulsions and attacks of choking. Death usually ensues within a few days or some weeks after birth (see Rössle, and also Lobdell). There are also reports of newborn infants manifesting congenital *hypo*parathyroidism (in the form of tetany and/or spasmophilia) apparently attributable to the presence of *hyper*parathyroidism in the mother (see Buchs). The cause of the *hypo*parathyroidism in these neonates seems to be functional suppression of the fetal parathyroids in consequence of the excess parathyroid hormone present in the mother's blood during pregnancy. In line with this explanation is the experimental finding that, in dogs injected with parathormone over long periods of time, autopsy reveals that the parathyroids are greatly reduced in size and also show microscopic evidence of involutional atrophy (see Jaffe and Bodansky).

Occasionally, hypoparathyroidism is also encountered in older children and in adults. In some of these cases the condition represents so-called *idiopathic* hypoparathyroidism. It is likely that "idiopathic" hypoparathyroidism sometimes has its basis in degenerative changes in the parathyroids, either primary or following upon hemorrhage into them (see Danisch). In any event, the usual basis for hypoparathyroidism in adults is accidental removal or damage of the parathyroids in the course of subtotal thyroidectomy.

When the hypoparathyroidism passes from the acute into a chronic stage, attacks of muscle spasm and tetany (associated with hypocalcemia and hyperphosphatemia) may still be frequent. In addition, certain phenomena apparently due to trophic disturbances now make their appearance. More particularly, in victims of chronic hypoparathyroidism, the nails may fall off, opacities develop in the lenses, the hair fall out, and the teeth become defective. Intracranial calcification is another finding which is not unusual in hypoparathyroidism. When present, the calcification usually involves the basal ganglia of the brain and the walls of the small cerebral arteries. If well developed, the intracranial calcification is demonstrable roentgenographically. However, it should be noted that similar intracranial calcifications may be visualized on occasion in other conditions, such as encephalitis, tuberous sclerosis, toxoplasmosis, and mental deficiency (see Camp, and Levin *et al.*). The skeletal changes of hypoparathyroidism are certainly of academic interest, but they have no direct clinical or pathological significance. Experience indicates that, though the bones may become more radiopaque, the alterations which they show are not distinctive in any way (see Salvesen and Böe).

The term *pseudohypoparathyroidism* is used to denote a condition in which the subject presents various manifestations of hypoparathyroidism but fails to respond to the administration of parathyroid hormone in the manner typical of indubitable hypoparathyroidism—that is, with an elevation of the serum calcium level and an increased urinary excretion of phosphorus (phosphorus diuresis). The physical appearance of the subjects is characterized by shortness of stature, stocky build, a round face, and stubbiness of some fingers and toes (due to shortness of the fourth and/or fifth metacarpals and metatarsals). Like those affected with *true* hypoparathyroidism, the patients in cases of *pseudo*hypoparathyroidism show hypocalcemia and hyperphosphatemia, have attacks of tetany, develop cataracts, and may also come to present intracranial and/or subcutaneous calcifications. In some of the cases, mental retardation has also been observed.

Occasionally one encounters a patient presenting the physical and mental abnormalities characteristic of pseudohypoparathyroidism but *not* showing hypocalcemia, hyperphosphatemia, or tetany. Because the patients in question have a normal response to parathyroid hormone, the designation *pseudo-pseudohypoparathyroidism* has been applied to such cases. In an attempt to meet certain objections to this designation, other names for the condition, such as "*brachymetacarpal dwarfism*," have been suggested.

It is held by some that the basic defect in pseudohypoparathyroidism is a diminished responsiveness of the renal tubules (the end organ) to circulating parathyroid hormone rather than a deficiency in secretion of the hormone. However, despite the differences between pseudohypoparathyroidism and pseudo-pseudohypoparathyroidism in respect to the biochemical features, the likelihood is that the latter condition represents an abortive expression of the former. Furthermore, there are a number of reports of cases in which more than one member of a family presented the pseudohypoparathyroidism syndrome in some form. Thus it appears that both expressions of the condition may have a genetic basis. This concept is favored by the fact that a child of a mother affected with pseudo-pseudohypoparathyroidism may present the manifestations of pseudohypoparathyroidism, and vice versa. In the familial cases, the findings suggest that the disorder is transmitted as an autosomal (non-sex-linked) dominant, but this mode of transmission has not been definitely established. (See Albright *et al.*, MacGregor and Whitehead, Howat and Ashurst, Hortling *et al.*, Uhr and Bezahler, and Gibson.)

PRIMARY HYPERPARATHYROIDISM

In the older medical literature, the skeletal manifestations which are known today to be caused by primary (or idiopathic) hyperparathyroidism were usually regarded as expressions of osteomalacia. Hence an important advance was made in 1891, when Recklinghausen drew attention to the differences between the skeletal lesions of actual osteomalacia and those of the condition which came to be known as "generalized osteitis fibrosa cystica" (Recklinghausen's disease of bone). However, it was not until 1926 that the latter disease was shown to be a manifestation of parathyroid hyperfunctioning (see Mandl). It is true that, in the interim, various pathologists had become aware that there might be a relationship between certain diseases of bones and abnormalities of the parathyroid glands (see Askanazy, Erdheim, and also Maresch). (See Fig. 76.)

Yet even after it became clear that Recklinghausen's disease of bone was often associated with parathyroid enlargement, the latter was still ordinarily regarded as a response to, rather than as the cause of, the bone lesions. That is, the parathyroid enlargement in generalized osteitis fibrosa cystica was held to be secondary to the bone involvement. This view lost ground after Mandl's success in the treatment of a case of this disease by removal of a parathyroid adenoma. His finding represented a decisive advance in the determination of the true nature of that condition. It not only established the role of parathyroid hyperfunctioning in its causation, but helped to dissociate Recklinghausen's disease completely from both Paget's disease and osteomalacia. Mandl's observation was soon confirmed by many other reports of clinical improvement following upon parathyroid extirpation in Recklinghausen's disease (see Gold, Barr *et al.*, Boyd *et al.*, Hannon *et al.*, Gutman *et al.*, and also Compere).

These early clinical contributions were paralleled and extended by experimental work with potent parathyroid extracts first prepared by Hanson and by Collip. In this connection the writer and his colleagues (Bodansky and Blair) studied and reported in detail the biochemical and pathologic changes produced in animals by the injection of parathyroid extract. In particular, we were able to show that many if not all of the pathologic changes observed in the bones and various internal organs in cases of Recklinghausen's disease could be produced experimentally in susceptible animals (especially dogs) in the course of long-range studies with the hormone (see Bodansky et al., Jaffe and Bodansky, Bodansky and Jaffe, and Jaffe et al.). Additional details relating to the evolution of the concept of hyperparathyroidism, and information about the various pertinent early clinical and experimental studies carried out by us and by other investigators, are to be found summarized in the writer's comprehensive review article on hyperparathyroidism published in 1933 (see Jaffe).

Since about 1940, accumulating experience with hyperparathyroidism has given rise to an enormous body of literature on the subject. This has been largely confirmative of what was already established by that time. Notably, the more recent literature reaffirms strongly the importance of being on the alert for hyperparathyroidism in all cases presenting manifestations of renal calculi. In addition, this increasing experience with the disease has led to recognition of the importance of considering the possibility of hyperparathyroidism in patients presenting manifestations of peptic ulcer and/or pancreatitis. (See Hellström, Hellström and Ivemark, Frame and Haubrich, Fogh-Andersen, and Cope et al.)

Figure 76

A, Photograph of the severely deformed body of a woman in a case of untreated primary hyperparathyroidism of long duration. The subject was 33 years of age at the time of her death in 1925—the year in which the basis for the disease (parathyroid hyperfunctioning) and consequent appropriate treatment for it first became known. For at least 3 years before her death, there had been various complaints referable to the gastrointestinal tract which had been interpreted clinically as "gallbladder disease" and/or "chronic appendicitis." During the course of her illness, the patient had suffered from a number of fractures which occurred after slight trauma. She had also been pregnant twice. The first pregnancy had ended in abortion at $3\frac{1}{2}$ months, and the second was terminated by cesarean section several months before she died. Both pregnancies had been associated with exacerbation of her clinical complaints, including the difficulties relating to the bones.

B, Photograph showing, in posterior view, the thyroid and trachea in the case illustrated in A. Note the adenomatous left lower parathyroid. The other three parathyroids are not enlarged, and the position of each of these is also indicated by a small black bead and an arrow.

C, Photographic reproduction of a drawing of part of the bony pelvis in the same case. Note that the shape of the pelvic inlet is distorted and that the left iliac bone is greatly expanded. The cut surface of the modified ilium shows that the expanded area is occupied mainly by what appears to be a large "brown tumor." This tissue mass is intensely hemorrhagic in part (upper left) and has undergone cystic softening in the adjacent area.

D and E, Photograph and roentgenograph of the uncut right femur removed at autopsy in the case of the woman shown in A. The contour of the upper half of the femur is expanded. The angulation slightly below the middle of the shaft is the result of a fracture. The roentgenograph reveals the absence of a distinct compact cortex and of normal trabecular markings.

F and G, Photograph and roentgenograph of the right tibia in the same case. Note the cystlike distention of the contour of the midportion of the bone shaft. The roentgenograph again reveals the absence of a distinct compact cortex and of the normal trabecular markings. The bulged portion of the tibial shaft casts a "ground glass" shadow reflecting the presence of the poorly mineralized fibro-osseous tissue set in what can be assumed to be a large "brown tumor" mass which, in part, is hemorrhagic and cystic.

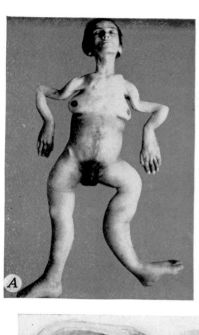

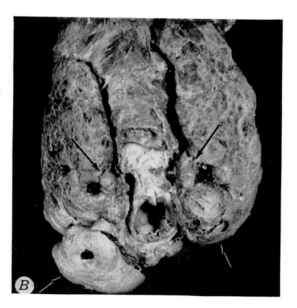

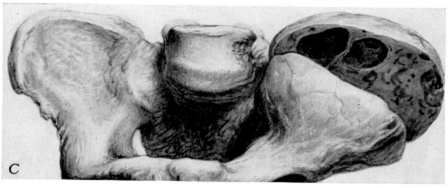

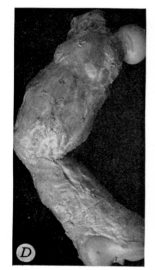

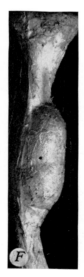

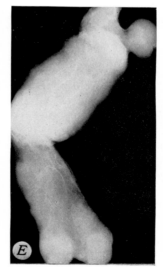

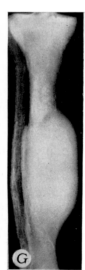

Figure 76

305

CLINICAL CONSIDERATIONS

Incidence.—While not a common disease, primary hyperparathyroidism is certainly not rare. Its incidence seems to be at least two or three times as high among females as among males. It occurs most frequently between the ages of 30 and 60 years. Though it is not unusual to observe the condition in subjects between 20 and 30 years of age, it seems to be definitely rare below 10 years. No racial, dietary, or environmental factors in the incidence of the disease have been definitely established. However, it has been noted that the disease sometimes occurs in several members of the same family, in the same or successive generations (see Jackson *et al.*, and Cassidy and Anderson).

Clinical Complaints and Findings.—The clinical complaints in primary hyperparathyroidism are referable in the main to: the hypercalcemia *per se*, renal and/or gastrointestinal disturbances, and the skeletal changes. However, it must be pointed out that not every individual patient will present, at the time the condition is diagnosed, clinical complaints arising from all these sources. Indeed, the manifestations may differ widely from case to case. Thus, rather frequently, the patient comes to the physician because of complaints from renal calculus, while roentgenographic examination of the skeleton still fails to reveal any changes or shows only slight or equivocal changes which had been causing no difficulty. Again, the patient's only complaint may be of a bone swelling (in a jaw bone, for instance) or a fracture, or vague pains referable to bones and joints, though close questioning will usually reveal other pertinent manifestations.

The increase in the calcium content of the blood plasma is due mainly to an increase in the ionized calcium fraction. This accounts for the diminished excitability of the neuromuscular junctions which is shown by many of the patients. In consequence of the hypercalcemia, some patients feel exceedingly tired, relaxed, and sluggish, and suffer from stubborn constipation. Sometimes severe gastrointestinal symptoms, such as attacks of abdominal pain, nausea and vomiting, are prominent and even the presenting phenomena. Such gastrointestinal manifestations, while usually dependent upon a pronounced hypercalcemia, occasionally have their immediate basis in a peptic ulcer (in which case, hematemesis may also have been present) or, more rarely, in a pancreatitis.

Because the kidneys are called upon to excrete excessive amounts of calcium and phosphorus, polyuria and polydipsia are common complaints. Since, as noted, urinary calculi (calcium phosphate or calcium oxalate stones) very frequently develop in connection with the disease, complaints referable to nephrolithiasis occupy a conspicuous place in the clinical picture. In some instances, considerable quantities of calcium may eventually be deposited in the kidney pyramids, resulting in nephrocalcinosis. The nephrocalcinosis by itself, or a pyelonephritis following upon an infection in the presence of calculi, may lead to severe renal insufficiency, which is thus sometimes observed as a complication of primary hyperparathyroidism when the latter is of long duration. A pronounced hypercalcemia in conjunction with hyperphosphatemia (following upon renal insufficiency) may be the basis for widespread metastatic calcifications, involving even arteries. Altogether, the extensive metastatic calcifications which one may encounter in the disease have their analogies in the manifestations presented by dogs under conditions of experimental poisoning by parathyroid hormone. (See Johnson, Morgan and Maclagan, Thomas *et al.*, and Jaffe and Bodansky.)

The complaints arising from skeletal involvement may consist at first merely of tenderness in the shins or vague aching pains, especially in the larger joints. With more advanced skeletal changes, pain in the back is common. If the vertebrae are very much softened, shortening and deformity of the column may result from compression fracture of one or more vertebral bodies. On the other hand, attention is sometimes drawn to the disease by a pathologic fracture of a long bone. The way to the diagnosis is also sometimes first opened by the discovery of a bone swelling from a solid or cystic so-called "brown tumor." As noted, such bone swellings not infrequently appear first in a jaw bone, and in such cases it may be a dentist who first suspects the presence of the disease. With pronounced involvement of the jaw bones, one may also observe malocclusion or distortion of the normal arrangement of the teeth, but the latter tend to be free of caries (see Strock).

Primary hyperparathyroidism is now commonly diagnosed before it has advanced far enough to devastate the skeleton and irreparably damage the kidneys. Indeed, the clinical picture presented by the patients has shifted from one in which severe skeletal changes occupied the foreground to one in which complaints from renal calculi are the dominant feature. In fact, a large proportion of the cases are now being diagnosed even before they present roentgenographic evidence of skeletal involvement at all, or while the latter is still limited to mild rarefaction. Indeed, it is now customary to consider the possibility of hyperparathyroidism whenever one is dealing with renal calculus and, accordingly, to examine the blood for aberrations in the serum calcium, inorganic phosphorus, and alkaline phosphatase levels. It is true that only a small minority of all patients presenting renal calculi as their principal clinical complaint are actually affected with hyperparathyroidism. However, the fact that the latter possibility is now increasingly borne in mind is leading to the discovery of hyperparathyroidism when the disease is still in an early stage of its evolution (see Albright *et al.*, and McGeown). Finally, as already indicated, an occasional instance of primary hyperparathyroidism is now brought to light through biochemical study of the blood of a patient presenting manifestations of a peptic ulcer or even of pancreatitis.

Unless the offending parathyroid tissue is removed, the disease usually progresses. The rarefied bones are susceptible to repeated fractures and deformities, and the patient may eventually become severely deformed and even hopelessly bedridden. The gravity of the condition is usually increased by renal insufficiency associated with the presence of renal calculi and pyelonephritis and even renal calcinosis. There is wide variation in the speed with which such a course is run. When the condition has reached this stage, even surgical removal of the offending parathyroid tissue may no longer save the patient's life, since the renal changes are, by now, often irreversible.

BIOCHEMICAL FINDINGS

Especially when the condition is present in an early stage and in mild form, the diagnosis of primary hyperparathyroidism must depend heavily upon the biochemical data. As already stated, the classic pertinent findings in this connection are: hypercalcemia, hypophosphatemia, elevated serum alkaline phosphatase activity, and increased urinary secretion of calcium and phosphorus (see Jaffe and Bodansky, Gutman *et al.*, and also p. 308). However, it is the presence of a hypercalcemia for which other causes can be excluded that is still the most constant and reliable finding. In particular, the likelihood that a noted hypercalcemia is actually due to hyperparathyroidism is greatly strengthened if the hypercalcemia is associated with a reduced tubular reabsorption of phosphorus, and if the hypercalcemia persists after a short series of daily cortisone injections has been given.

Hypercalcemia.—Hypercalcemia (that is, a serum calcium value above 11.0 or 11.5 mg. per 100 cc.) is, as noted, a crucially important diagnostic criterion of primary hyperparathyroidism, especially if such a value is obtained on several successive occasions. In adults showing normal values for serum inorganic phosphorus and total protein, the calcium value is normally between 9.5 and 10.5 mg.

per 100 cc. by the standard methods of analysis. The narrowness of the margin between the normal and the abnormal, and the pitfalls of the test technique make it imperative that there be no doubt as to the accuracy with which the test was performed. This is especially true if no clear-cut skeletal changes are observed roentgenographically. Under these conditions the serum calcium value may be just significantly beyond the limits of the normal, and one is compelled to rely particularly heavily upon serum calcium determination in establishing the diagnosis. In general, however, the serum calcium values in primary hyperparathyroidism range between 12 and 15 mg., and they may go even higher. In the presence of a hypercalcemic crisis, values of 18 to 20 mg. per 100 cc. are not unusual.

Hypophosphatemia.—The finding of hypophosphatemia (that is, a serum inorganic phosphorus level below 2 mg. per 100 cc.) is very helpful in the diagnosis of primary hyperparathyroidism. Indeed, a combination of hypophosphatemia with hypercalcemia is exceedingly strong evidence in favor of the diagnosis. However, it should be borne in mind that the serum inorganic phosphorus value in a case of hyperparathyroidism is often not depressed. (For purposes of comparison, one should know that in normal adults the serum inorganic phosphorus value is usually between 2.5 and 4.0 mg. per 100 cc. as determined by the methods generally used.)

Serum Alkaline Phosphatase Activity.—In cases of primary hyperparathyroidism in which definite bone changes have developed, the serum alkaline phosphatase activity value is regularly increased. In accordance with the severity of the skeletal involvement, the degree of this activity tends to range between 8 and 35 Bodansky units. When the bone changes are only incipient or not yet apparent roentgenographically, the serum alkaline phosphatase activity value may be within normal limits or is only very slightly elevated. (The normal range of serum alkaline phosphatase values for adults is 1.5 to 3.5 Bodansky units per 100 cc.)

Calcium and Phosphorus Balance Studies.—When a patient with clear-cut hyperparathyroidism is placed for a 3-day period on a diet low in calcium (and the diet is also standardized in respect to its other ingredients and its acid-base equivalents), there is a much greater loss of calcium and, usually, also of phosphorus by way of the urine and feces (especially the former) than is shown by a normal subject. However, to make an accurate calcium-phosphorus balance study requires much attention to numerous details, and for practical clinical purposes it is not often necessary in arriving at the diagnosis. Furthermore, it should be noted that in mild cases of hyperparathyroidism the negative calcium and phosphorus balance found is sometimes not sufficiently pronounced (even in a period of low calcium intake) to have diagnostic significance.

A simple clinical method of ascertaining whether a patient is excreting abnormally large amounts of calcium by way of the kidneys is to test the urine with the Sulkowitch reagent. This is a solution containing oxalate radicals buffered at such a pH that when an equal amount of the reagent is added to urine the calcium will almost immediately come down as a fine white precipitate of calcium oxalate. The patient should be on a low calcium diet (one not including milk, milk products, or nuts) for at least 3 days before collection of a 24-hour urine sample. If a test sample of this urine yields no precipitate, there is no calcium in the urine. If it yields a fine white cloud, there is a moderate amount of calcium. If it yields a precipitate which looks like milk, there is enough calcium in the urine to suggest the probability of a definite negative calcium balance (see Barney and Sulkowitch).

PATHOLOGIC AND ROENTGENOGRAPHIC SKELETAL FINDINGS

As already stated, the negative mineral balance in hyperparathyroidism is due to abstraction of mineral from the bones. The demineralization of the bones is associated with the presence of numerous osteoclasts. In consequence, there is evidence of lively osteoclastic resorption on the walls of the haversian canals of the cortical bone and on the surfaces of the spongy trabeculae. At the sites of active osteoclastic resorption, a substitutive fibrosis is to be noted. The continuation of these two processes is the foundation for the various anatomic changes which one may eventually find in the bones in one case or another of hyperparathyroidism. (For the biochemical mechanisms by which the parathyroid hormone apparently stimulates the formation of osteoclasts, and the possible mechanisms by which the osteoclasts resorb the osseous tissue at the site of their action, see p. 147.)

It must be recognized that in the very early stages of hyperparathyroidism, if mineral loss is compensated by adequate mineral intake, bone changes may be so slight as to be imperceptible on gross or roentgenographic examination, though they may be detectable on microscopic examination of an adequate biopsy specimen. In a somewhat more advanced case in which the negative mineral balance is still not pronounced, changes in the bones may be just barely perceptible on gross examination. In such cases (see, for instance, Bergstrand) the cortex of an altered long tubular bone may show only a slight porousness. Microscopically it will be found that this is due to erosive enlargement of the vessel canals of the cortex. These now contain connective tissue and have some osteoclasts on their walls. The spongy trabeculae, too, will show evidence of mild resorption, and will be found perforated and surrounded by tracts of connective tissue. The tendency toward the deposition of new bone is everywhere slight or absent. In the other bones, too, the alterations are merely those of the mild resorption and substitutive fibrosis here described. However, these bones are by no means uniformly involved. The bones of the jaws and the vertebral column, for instance, are much more likely to show the changes than those of the hands and feet.

Roentgenographically, in such cases one may find merely slight porousness of the bones. This is expressed in rarefaction (perhaps without thinning) of the bone cortices and a somewhat blurred appearance of the spongiosa. In other cases one may note, in addition, the presence of slight subperiosteal scalloping of the cortices of some of the tubular bones. The latter change is most likely to be observed in relation to the small bones of the hand, and particularly the middle phalanges. In occasional instances of hyperparathyroidism, subperiosteal erosive defects of rib cortices have also been noted. (See Steinbach *et al.*, and Noetzli and Steinbach.)

If, in a case of hyperparathyroidism, the negative mineral balance has been very pronounced and of long duration, the skeletal changes may reach their full efflorescence, as expressed in "generalized osteitis fibrosa cystica." Under such conditions the bones show severe osteofibrosis associated with the presence, here and there, of cysts and "brown tumors" and deformities. The deformities result from the effects of bone softening and fractures. It is in severely involved long tubular bones that the most striking pathologic changes are observed. The trend of the advanced changes in the other bones is similar to that in the long bones, although, of course, the changes are influenced by the shape and position of the particular bone or bones in question.

In fairly advanced cases, roentgenographic examination will reveal that the cortices of the bones are rarefied and/or thinned, and the spongy bone ends show blurring of the trabecular outlines. Also, the circumference of some bones may be expanded in places by the presence of cysts and "brown tumors." In addition, there may be infractions and fractures. If, by chance, the disease has appeared in an older child or an adolescent and progressed, the bone changes visible roentgenographically may suggest those of adolescent rickets. In these instances the long tubular bones, in particular, may show bowing, widening of the metaphyses, and slipping of certain epiphyses. (See Fig. 77.)

21

Long Tubular Bones.—A severely modified long bone may show, on gross examination, expansion of its transverse diameter in one region or in several places. It may also be distorted longitudinally, especially because of malalignments at the sites of previous infractions and fractures. If the bone is the femur, its neck is likely to be bent downward from its normal position into that of coxa vara. The periosteum of the affected bone is usually quite thin. Beneath it, there is no obvious new bone of periosteal origin, except where the integrity of the cortex has previously been threatened or actually undermined.

If a severely affected long bone is sectioned longitudinally, it will be noted that the cortex is extremely porous, much of the compact bone having been replaced by connective tissue. Indeed, in some places the cortex may even show small, discrete, gray-white or brownishly discolored gritty fibrous foci. Because of extensive resorption and substitutive fibrosis of the spongy trabeculae, the ends of the bones may present large, gray-white fibrous foci in which delicately reticulated new bone may be felt. Some softer brownish foci may also be present, these representing the so-called "giant-cell tumors" or "brown tumors" of hyperparathyroidism. The sectioned surface of the bone may also show some single and multilocular cystic spaces in its interior. The larger cysts (often multilocular) may have well-defined fibrous linings. They may be empty or contain coagula of thin, albuminous material, perhaps admixed with changed blood and cholesterol crystals. It is difficult to state

Figure 77

A, Roentgenograph of a hand of a man 50 years of age in a case of hyperparathyroidism. Note that the cortices, particularly of the phalanges, are rarefied, and that some of them show the so-called subperiosteal scalloping (see arrows). The proximal half of the fifth metacarpal bone is expanded and appears multilocular. The presence of the disease first came to light in this case when a biopsy specimen from a localized swelling of the mandible was found to present the histologic pattern of a giant-cell epulis. It was only then that a roentgenographic skeletal survey was undertaken. This revealed widespread rarefaction of the other bones, also, along with a number of discrete "cystlike" multilocular areas. Furthermore, inquiry elicited that, in the 5 years preceding the establishment of the diagnosis, the man had had several attacks of renal colic and also a surgical intervention for urolithiasis. The basis for the hyperparathyroidism in this case was diffuse hyperplasia of the four parathyroids. The patient made a slow but remarkable recovery after removal of three of the enlarged (cherry-sized) parathyroids and all but a tiny fragment of the fourth.

B, Roentgenograph of the bones in the region of the right elbow of a woman 51 years of age who had been manifesting effects of hyperparathyroidism for at least 5 years prior to the establishment of the diagnosis. Note the multilocular cystlike radiolucencies in the lower end of the humerus and the upper end of the ulna, and also the rarefaction and thinning of the cortices of these bones. Similar changes were observed in many other skeletal areas, including the tubular bones of both hands. The basis for the hyperparathyroidism in this case was found to be an adenoma of the lower left parathyroid measuring 2.5 × 2 × 1.5 cm. and consisting mainly of chief cells.

C, Roentgenograph of the bones in the region of the right hip of a woman 57 years of age who had been manifesting the effects of hyperparathyroidism for about 10 years before the diagnosis was established. Her complaints began with pain and weakness in her knees and ankles. Subsequently she manifested polyuria, polydipsia, and renal colic. Prior to removal of a parathyroid adenoma (which weighed 2.2 grams), a skeletal survey showed widespread porosity of the bones. In addition, some of them revealed large roundish foci of radiolucency which tended to be multilocular, as demonstrated in the bones of the hip area illustrated.

D, Roentgenograph of the upper ends of the left tibia and fibula from the case illustrated in *C*. The trabecular markings of the tibia are indistinct and, in places, disrupted. The cortical bone appears somewhat thinned and is certainly not so compact as it would normally be.

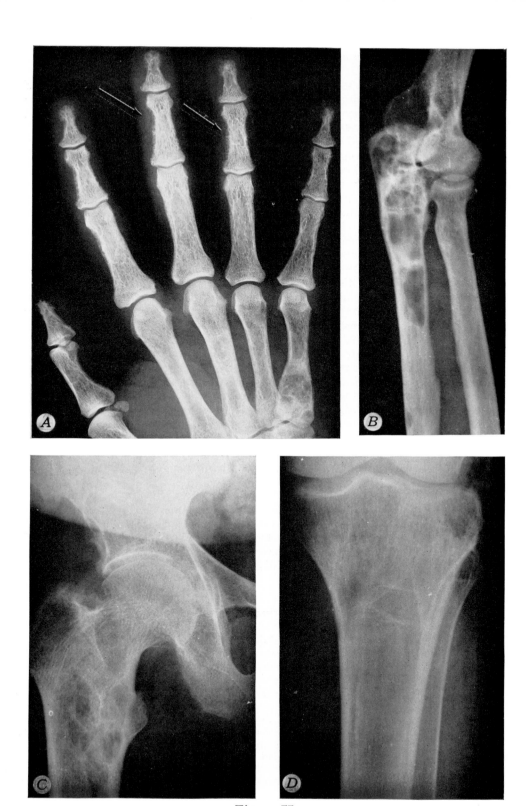

Figure 77

with certainty how these large cysts are formed, but it seems likely that some of them result from cystic degeneration developing in the whitish or brown fibrous foci. In and between the cystic spaces, there may be blood from hemorrhage, recent or old. When large, the cysts and/or fibrous foci sometimes thin the overlying cortex and expand the diameter of the bone, accounting for the bulging visible externally.

On histologic examination of various portions of such an affected long bone, it becomes apparent that where the bone (both cortical and spongy) is being resorbed and replaced by connective tissue, some rather immature new bone (fiber bone) may make its appearance in that tissue. However, new bone formation is not a striking feature in the skeletal histopathology of primary hyperparathyroidism. Also, one will note some osteoclasts wherever the original or the new bone is in the process of resorption. The abundance of osteoclasts is roughly in accordance with the liveliness of the resorptive process.

Microscopic study of the "brown tumor" areas shows that they are composed of a spindle cell connective tissue stroma and osteoclast-like giant cells. These are usually sparse and often clumped. However, it is recognized that in some places in a given "brown tumor" the multinuclear giant cells may be so numerous as to overshadow the supporting stroma. The brown color of these tumors is apparently dependent upon hemorrhage, being imparted by blood pigment which may be contained within their cellular elements. Large "brown tumors" may undergo cystic degeneration until little of the original tissue remains. On the other hand, they may heal by being converted into sclerotic connective tissue scars which may even become partly calcified. As to the mode of origin of the "brown tumors," the most plausible theory seems to be that they represent a special type of reparative reaction resulting from hemorrhage which has occurred in fibrous marrow. In the writer's opinion, the "brown tumors" of hyperparathyroidism represent giant-cell reparative granulomas and are not to be regarded as identical with solitary giant-cell tumor of bone, which represents a genuine tumor (see Jaffe). (See Figs. 78 and 79.)

Vertebral Column.—The vertebrae show the same active replacement of the original bone and marrow by fibrous tissue and new bone which characterizes the lesions in other skeletal parts. Even grossly, small cystic spaces and "brown tumors" may be apparent. Vertebral bodies thus transformed are so weakened that they may yield to the expansion of still turgid intervertebral disks. Where this occurs, the bodies undergo reduction of their vertical diameter from above and below, and mild

Figure 78

A, Photograph of the sagittally sectioned deformed left femur in another untreated case of primary hyperparathyroidism of long duration. The contour of the bone shaft is expanded, and the interior of the shaft is largely occupied by blood which clotted after the occurrence of multiple fractures which had taken place without disrupting the periosteum. In the condylar region of the femur, there is evidence of considerable fibrous tissue which has replaced the original spongy bone.

B, Photograph of a humerus, sectioned in the frontal plane, from still another case of primary hyperparathyroidism. It is apparent even grossly that the cortex of the bone shaft is rarefied. The original spongy bone of the humeral head has been replaced, and microscopic examination would show that the replacement tissue is connective tissue containing delicate trabeculae of new bone.

C, Photograph of part of the calvarium from the case of hyperparathyroidism represented by *B*. Note that a distinct inner and outer table and intervening diploë are no longer present, having been largely replaced (as microscopic examination revealed) by connective tissue and new bone (see Fig. 80-*B*).

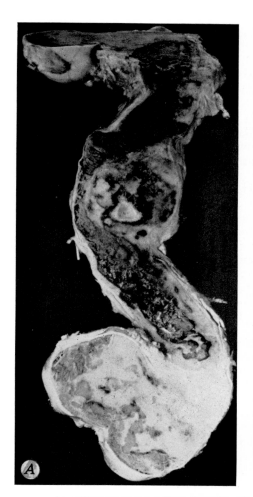
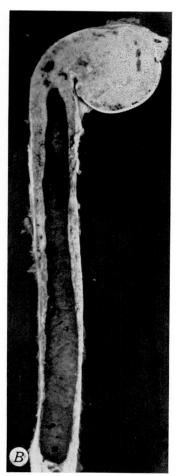
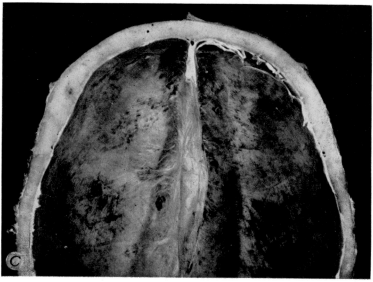

Figure 78

forms of the so-called "fish vertebrae" are created. As for the intervertebral disks themselves, their cartilage plates may show areas of focal resorption, or may even have disappeared entirely if the pathologic process in the bodies has been particularly severe. Degenerative changes may also appear in the annulus fibrosus and in the nucleus pulposus. The alterations in the vertebral column may lead to its gross deformation. In consequence of collapse of some of the thoracic vertebrae, the vertebral column not infrequently shows exaggeration of its normal dorsal kyphosis. In other instances the vertebral column may have become twisted into a pronounced kyphoscoliotic position, which, when associated with deformation of the ribs and sternum, results in a badly misshapen thoracic cage. Of course, such severe deformations of the trunk bones are now to be observed only in neglected cases in which the disease had been present for many years.

Pelvis.—In advanced cases of primary hyperparathyroidism, the pelvis, too, is likely to undergo deformation, tending to become extremely asymmetrical and also reduced in size. When replaced by pathologic new bone, the iliac bones are easily compressible and may even be flexible. They or the sacrum are sometimes expanded by cysts or "brown tumors." In the past, the pelvic deformity sometimes attained such severity as to approximate the type observed in cases of puerperal osteomalacia. In fact, this is one of the reasons that osteitis fibrosa cystica used to be confused with osteomalacia.

Calvarium.—If extensively diseased, the bones of the calvarium are usually thinned and pliable, and it may even be possible to cut them with a knife. On cross section it may appear that the structural division into inner and outer tables with intervening diploë no longer obtains. The osseous tissue of which the calvarium now consists is made up of intertwining newly formed trabeculae. In some places, gross calvarial defects may be present which are filled with fibrous tissue but nevertheless delimited by the pericranium and dura. In some instances, instead of being uniformly thinned, the calvarium may show areas of thickening. This thickening represents one of the reasons for the former occasional confusion of the skeletal lesions of Recklinghausen's disease with those of Paget's disease. A thickened region may measure as much as 2 cm. or more in depth. On cross section the surface of such an area appears injected and finely porous. It shows no evidences of the original cal-

Figure 79

A, Photomicrograph (×5) illustrating the histologic pattern presented by the articular end of an affected long bone. In the upper part of the picture, intertrabecular marrow spaces containing myeloid and/or fatty marrow are still present. In the lower part of the picture, connective tissue which has surrounded and replaced the original spongy trabeculae forms a more or less continuous mass, the marrow spaces having been substantially obliterated. The osseous tissue present in this lesional area is largely newly formed bone of the coarse-fibered variety.

B, Photograph of part of a humerus (sectioned in the frontal plane) showing a small "brown tumor" focus (see arrows) within the rarefied shaft cortex in a case of primary hyperparathyroidism.

C, Photomicrograph (×5) of a cross section showing the histologic pattern of the humerus illustrated in *B*. The section was taken to include the "brown tumor" area. The latter is visible within the cortex in the lower right part of the picture. The small dark specks which can be seen even under this low magnification represent multinuclear giant cells. The rest of the cortical bone is rarefied and shows fibrous transformation. On the endosteal surface of the cortex, fatty and myeloid marrow can be seen.

D, Photomicrograph (×6) illustrating the appearance of the cortex of a femur from a case of primary hyperparathyroidism of long duration. Practically all of the original cortical bone has been replaced by connective tissue in which delicate trabeculae of new bone (mainly coarse-fibered) are present.

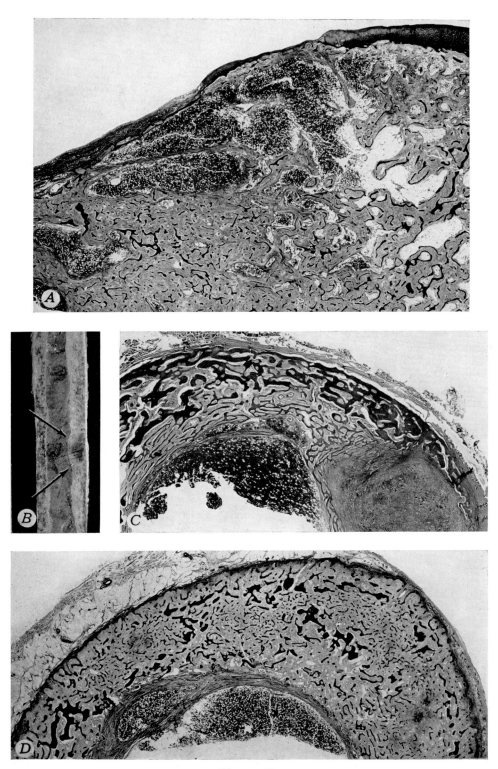

Figure 79

315

varial architecture. Roentgenographically, in advanced cases of hyperparathyroidism, the calvarium is likely to present a peculiar granular mottling (usually without thickening). The mottled shadow represents the intermingling of the new bone with connective tissue which has replaced the original bone. When the hyperparathyroidism is corrected in a case in which the calvarium had shown clear-cut granular mottling, numerous large foci of radiopacity will be observed roentgenographically as manifestations of the process of healing (see Jaffe, and Ellis and Hochstim).

Jaws.—In advanced cases the jaw bones tend to undergo pronounced fibro-osseous transformation. This is the basis for the disappearance, as observed roentgenographically, of the lamina dura (periodontal lamella) outlining the sockets of the teeth. Cysts and "brown tumors" commonly appear in the jaw bones and may distend their contour in one place or another. A "brown tumor" breaking through the attenuated and otherwise altered cortex may extend under the gum and produce a giant-cell epulis. Some teeth may fall out in consequence of involvement of the jaws, and those remaining may assume distorted positions. However, as already remarked, such teeth as remain do not seem to be very susceptible to the development of caries. (See Fig. 80.)

Articular Changes.—The articular manifestations observed in three patients with proven functioning parathyroid adenomas were described by Zvaifler et al. The roentgenographic abnormalities which they had observed in one or another of these cases consisted of articular cartilage calcification, periarticular and synovial calcification, and subperiosteal bone resorption at sites near affected joints. Moreover, they emphasized that none of these roentgenographic findings are specific for primary hyperparathyroidism but, even if present, may not give rise to clinical complaints or physical findings referable to the involved joints. (See also Dodds and Steinbach.)

PATHOLOGY OF THE HYPERFUNCTIONING PARATHYROIDS

In man, the parathyroid glands are normally four in number. They are small, flat, oval or piriform bodies, measuring, on the average, about 6 to 7 mm. in length, 2 to 3 mm. across at the widest part, and 1 to 2 mm. in thickness. Their weight in a

Figure 80

A, Roentgenograph showing the characteristic granular mottling of the calvarium observed in cases of hyperparathyroidism (primary or even secondary) in which the skeletal changes are pronounced. The case in question was one of primary hyperparathyroidism, and the relevant clinical data on this patient have been given in the legend for Fig. 77-*A.*

B, Photomicrograph (×6) illustrating the histologic pattern presented by a calvarium which would have shown granular mottling roentgenographically. Note that the architecture of the calvarium is completely altered, the inner and outer tables and diploë having been largely replaced by connective tissue containing trabeculae of new bone. The tissue section from which this illustration was prepared was taken from the calvarium shown in Fig. 78-*C.*

C, Photomicrograph (× 5) showing the fibro-osseous transformation of the lamina dura outlining the socket of a tooth. It is this process that accounts for the absence of the lamina dura (periodontal lamella) about the teeth when the jaws are examined roentgenographically in cases of hyperparathyroidism associated with advanced skeletal changes.

D, Roentgenograph of part of a jaw showing, in particular, pronounced rarefaction of the mandible and a few discrete roundish radiolucencies. The patient was a woman 28 years of age who entered the hospital with a 2-week history of epigastric distress and vomiting. Examination of the blood serum yielded the biochemical findings characteristic of hyperparathyroidism. Surgical exploration of the neck revealed a parathyroid adenoma which weighed 1.2 grams.

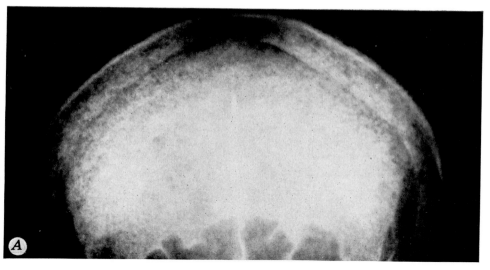

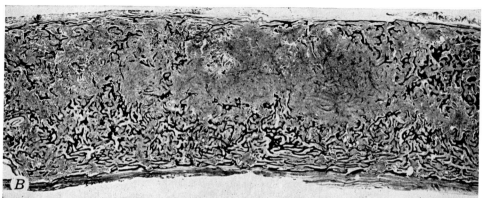

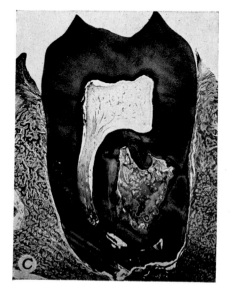

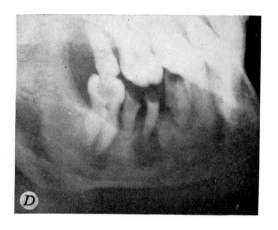

Figure 80

normal adult is likely to average about 30 mg. per gland, but an individual gland may weigh as little as 20 mg. or as much as 60 mg. The parathyroids are usually attached to the posteromedial surface of the lateral thyroid lobes—one toward the upper pole of each lobe and one toward the lower pole—but aberrations in their location are common (see Norris, and Gilmour and Martin).

The basic parenchymal cell of the parathyroid is the chief cell, and such other parenchymal cells as one may encounter in the gland are apparently derived from this cell. Before puberty, the parenchymal cells are almost all small chief cells. After puberty, more and more of them become oxyphil cells, and some become water-clear cells. Fat cells appear after puberty and increase in number until the subject is about 40 years of age.

The *parathyroid abnormality* in primary hyperparathyroidism takes several different forms (see Castleman and Mallory, Muller and Smeenk, and also Castleman). In about 85 per cent of the cases, the parathyroid hyperfunctioning is the result of the development of a benign tumorous growth—an adenoma. As a rule, the adenomatous proliferation involves only a single parathyroid gland, though in an occasional instance an adenoma develops in each of two glands. In most of the remaining 15 per cent or so of the cases in question, the hyperparathyroidism is the result of primary hyperplasia diffusely involving all four of the parathyroid glands. In addition, there are some instances in which the hyperparathyroidism is due to the presence of a functioning (hormone-producing) carcinoma which has developed in a parathyroid gland. In an occasional instance of hyperparathyroidism, the parathyroid aberration is associated with changes in various other endocrine glands. At autopsy in these cases one may find such endocrine abnormalities as pancreatic islet cell adenomas, adrenal cortical hyperplasia, and pituitary (anterior lobe) hyperplasia. (See Bergstrand, Wilton, Zollinger and Ellison, Wermer, and also Pearl *et al.*)

A parathyroid *adenoma* is more likely to develop in one of the glands of the lower pair than in one of the upper pair. In line with the fact that in its embryologic migration a parathyroid not infrequently becomes aberrantly located, it is also not unusual to find an aberrantly located adenoma. Occasionally, such an adenoma lies completely within the thyroid gland, or it may be tucked away in the neck, between the trachea and esophagus. However, the most common aberrant location is the mediastinum, either posterior or anterior.

The adenomas vary considerably in size, roughly in accordance with the severity of the skeletal changes in the cases from which they come. In individual cases the adenoma has weighed as little as 0.5 gm. or even less, and as much as 30 gm. or even more. Most commonly, the weight is somewhere between 2 and 10 gm. An adenomatously transformed parathyroid is usually soft, roundish, and yellow-brown, but this appearance may be modified by secondary changes from hemorrhage, fibrosis, and/or cystic softening. In an adenoma, one may still find a small residual focus of the original normal gland tissue. Also, as often as not, an adenoma is composed almost solely of typical chief cells. When it is not, it still contains many chief cells, though the histologic picture may be dominated in some places by fully developed water-clear cells or by transitional chief cells in the process of transformation into water-clear cells or pale oxyphil cells. (See Roth.)

When the hyperparathyroidism is induced by adenoma formation in one of the glands, the other parathyroids tend to show involutional atrophy, especially if the hyperparathyroidism is of long standing. This occurrence is in line with our findings relating to hyperparathyroidism induced experimentally in dogs. In the dogs injected with parathormone over long periods of time, the parathyroids were often found to be of only about one-half the normal size. We interpreted this observation as evidence of involutional atrophy of the parathyroid glands due to the administration of the parathormone (see Jaffe and Bodansky).

When the hyperparathyroidism has resulted from *hyperplasia* of all four glands, it will be noted that the hypertrophied glands are not all enlarged to the same degree. In a given case, an individual gland is not likely to exceed 1 gm. in weight, and some of the glands usually weigh much less. In any event, the upper two hypertrophied glands are generally larger than the lower two glands. Furthermore, the affected glands tend to be rather soft, irregular in shape, and more or less brownish in color. Histologically the glands in some cases consist of very large but fairly uniform water-clear cells which show a tendency toward acinar arrangement and toward basal orientation of their nuclei. In other cases the hypertrophied glands are found to consist mainly of chief cells, thus suggesting the histologic pattern of an adenoma, or that of an enlarged parathyroid gland observed in association with chronic renal insufficiency. It is to be noted, however, that the parathyroid enlargement (due to chief-cell hyperplasia) is ordinarily not so pronounced when it occurs in cases of chronic renal insufficiency as it is in connection with primary hyperparathyroidism due to chief-cell hyperplasia of the four glands.

As already observed, an occasional case of hyperparathyroidism develops on the basis of a *functioning parathyroid carcinoma.* A cancerous parathyroid gland usually has a firm texture and a whitish color—features which tend to distinguish it grossly from an adenoma. In some cases, furthermore, one is already alerted to the possibility that the enlarged parathyroid is cancerous by the finding of metastatic involvement of regional lymph nodes at the original surgical intervention. On histologic grounds alone, it is sometimes difficult to distinguish a carcinoma of a parathyroid from an adenoma. Removal of the cancerous parathyroid is usually followed by local recurrence and, eventually, by metastasis, especially to the liver and lungs. The metastases from parathyroid carcinomas usually likewise produce parathyroid hormone. A fully documented case of metastasizing carcinoma of a parathyroid gland in which a detailed postmortem anatomic study was carried out has been reported by Ellis and Barr. The patient in question (a young woman) died approximately 6 years after the onset of the clinical complaints of hyperparathyroidism. In addition to the presence of widespread so-called "osteitis fibrosa cystica," autopsy revealed a high degree of medial calcification of the smaller arteries, renal calcinosis without obvious nephrolithiasis, and metastatic calcification of the gastric mucosa.

Finally, it is important to note that a few cases have been observed in which a large adenoma had developed in a parathyroid gland without giving rise to skeletal lesions or other evidences of hyperparathyroidism. Obviously the adenomas in question had not been secreting parathyroid hormone. Histologically, some of these adenomas are found to consist almost entirely of oxyphil cells. These cases have come to clinical attention mainly because of the presence of a nodular mass in the neck which had given rise to dysphagia or to some discomfort from local pressure (see Maresch, Capps, and also Norris).

DIFFERENTIAL DIAGNOSIS AND TREATMENT

Differential Diagnosis.—A case of primary hyperparathyroidism in its full efflorescence rarely presents any problem of diagnosis or differential diagnosis. However, most cases seen now are less fully evolved, and some of these may be exceedingly difficult to diagnose. For instance, one may be presented with a case showing renal calculus, no clear-cut evidence of skeletal demineralization, and a serum calcium value only slightly above the upper limit of the normal—that is, somewhere between 10.5 and 11.0 mg. per 100 cc. Such a case may or may not be one of primary hyperparathyroidism, and its solution requires persistence and fine distinctions. Specifically, it requires a most thoughtful evaluation of the history, periodic serum calcium, inorganic phosphorus, and alkaline phosphatase determinations, and even also repeated measurement of the urinary calcium excretion to determine whether the patient is in negative calcium balance.

On the other hand, one must be aware that hypercalcemia does not necessarily indicate the presence of hyperparathyroidism. For instance, hypercalcemia is a relatively common finding in multiple myeloma. In some cases of cancer extensively metastatic to the skeleton, one may likewise find an associated hypercalcemia. Also, immobilization in a plaster cast of a large part of the body (especially of a young subject) may lead to hypercalcemia through disuse atrophy of the bones and a concomitant inability of the kidneys to excrete the excess calcium presented to them, the kidneys sometimes even becoming damaged in consequence. In a small but not negligible percentage of cases of sarcoidosis, hypercalcemia is also encountered. The so-called *milk-alkali syndrome* sometimes observed in patients with peptic ulcer who are consuming large quantities of milk and alkali may also raise problems of differential diagnosis. This confusion may arise from the presence of a hypercalcemia in these subjects. However, it should be noted that in some patients exhibiting the milk-alkali syndrome the presence of a peptic ulcer may actually be related to a concurrent hyperparathyroidism.

In infants and very young children, one occasionally encounters a hypercalcemia whose cause is still unknown (*idiopathic hypercalcemia of infancy*). These subjects present a variety of clinical manifestations. Some of the latter are attributable to the hypercalcemia *per se* (anorexia, vomiting, constipation, polyuria, and muscular hypotonia). In addition, the affected infants or young children usually show physical and mental retardation and a characteristic "elfin" facies (see O'Brien *et al.*). It is clear, however, that so-called "idiopathic hypercalcemia of infancy" does not have its basis in hyperparathyroidism. The serum inorganic phosphorus and alkaline phosphatase values are within normal limits unless there is concomitant renal insufficiency due to renal calcinosis. The skeletal manifestations, too, are different from those of hyperparathyroidism. Early in the course of the disease, roentgenographic examination may reveal bands of increased density in the metaphysial regions of the long bones in particular. Late in the course of the disease, the bones may show more or less increased radiopacity representing various degrees of osteosclerosis. The latter is probably related to the chronic renal insufficiency following upon the renal calcinosis manifested by those among the severely affected children who have survived for a number of years.

Apart from the possibilities suggested by the finding of a hypercalcemia, the principal problem of differential diagnosis is presented by generalized osteoporosis— senile, postmenopausal, or unexplained ("cryptogenic"). In these cases, however, one can be kept on the right track by the almost complete lack of involvement of the skull and the normality of the serum calcium, inorganic phosphorus, and alkaline phosphatase values, except sometimes under the influence of fractures and subsequent immobilization. Cases of osteomalacia and idiopathic steatorrhea in adults (rare in this country) may raise problems of differential diagnosis, but in these cases the serum calcium level is at or below the normal, and the serum inorganic phosphorus value is usually below. Paget's disease, though it may sometimes be complicated by hyperparathyroidism, is now rarely confused with it. This is true also of fibrous dysplasia of bone, even when many bones are affected by it. Finally, one must recognize that sometimes the distinction between primary and secondary hyperparathyroidism may be difficult to make, even when the presence of hyperparathyroidism is clear (see below).

Treatment.—In principle, the treatment of primary hyperparathyroidism consists of surgical removal of the offending parathyroid tissue. If the hyperparathyroidism has developed on the basis of an adenoma, the indication usually is simply to re- move the tumor. Nevertheless, it may happen that even though an adenoma has been removed, the hyperparathyroidism recurs because a second adenoma had been missed at the time of the surgical intervention or had developed subsequently. If the hyperparathyroidism has resulted from hyperplasia of all the parathyroid glands, the usual procedure is to remove three of the glands and about half (or perhaps some- what more than half) of the fourth. In these cases, consideration must be given to the danger of recurrence of the hyperparathyroidism from regrowth of the re- maining portion of the fourth gland. Concomitantly, however, the possibility of the development of chronic *hypo*parathyroidism from damage to the blood supply of the remaining parathyroid stump must also be borne in mind. (The technical problems relating to the surgical treatment of hyperparathyroidism have been discussed in detail by Cope *et al.*)

One of the principal problems connected with the surgical treatment of the hyperparathyroidism relates to postoperative hypocalcemia and tetany. During the period of convalescence, the dietary intake of calcium should be high. The presence of postoperative tetany (which is usually mild and transient) may also necessitate the intravenous administration of calcium gluconate, at least temporarily. There can be no doubt that, as a rule, the more severe the bone changes and the higher the alkaline phosphatase activity at the time of the operative intervention, the more pronounced and protracted are the postoperative hypocalcemic phenomena. The simplest and most plausible explanation for this state of affairs is that, when the condition of hyperparathyroidism is corrected, the depleted skeleton represents a sort of "vacuum" which greedily sucks in considerable circulating calcium for repair (see Bodansky and Jaffe).

Even under successful surgical management of the case, the ultimate prognosis will depend on the degree of damage already sustained by the kidneys. Indeed, if the kidneys have been severely damaged by nephrocalcinosis, death from renal insufficiency ultimately occurs, even though the offending parathyroid tissue has been removed. In the absence of permanent renal damage, successful operative intervention promptly interrupts the pathologic state as a whole. In regard to the skeleton, substantial healing of the bone lesions may be manifest within a few months, even to the point of great reduction in the size of cysts and "brown tumors." On the other hand, deformities do not become spontaneously corrected to any great extent after they have once developed.

RENAL (SECONDARY) HYPERPARATHYROIDISM

It is well known that the parathyroids tend to undergo hyperplasia in the presence of chronic renal insufficiency. Sometimes the glands show only microscopic evidence of this, but usually they also show gross enlargement. When grossly enlarged, each gland is ordinarily not more than two or three times the normal size. Exceptionally, however, the glands may be much larger. The parathyroid enlargement associated with renal disease results from hyperplasia of the chief cells, the individual cells remaining approximately of normal size (see Pappenheimer and Wilens, and Castle- man and Mallory). The parathyroid hyperplasia in these cases is usually attributed to the effects of phosphate retention, consequent lowering of the serum calcium, and the resultant disequilibrium of the calcium-phosphorus ratio of the plasma. Specifi- cally, the parathyroid hyperplasia in renal hyperparathyroidism seems to represent a functional response to the reduced level of the serum calcium—in particular, of its ionized fraction. However, it is not clear why in some cases of chronic and even protracted renal insufficiency the parathyroids are only moderately enlarged, while in occasional other cases of this nature they are tremendously enlarged. Finally, it should be noted that slight degrees of parathyroid enlargement are encountered, for instance, in some cases of multiple myeloma, Paget's disease of bone, and carcinosis extensively metastatic to the skeleton. The parathyroid enlargement appearing under these circumstances is apparently likewise the result of renal insufficiency which has developed in these cases for one reason or another.

In the presence of renal hyperparathyroidism, the inorganic phosphorus value of the serum may rise to 10 mg. or more per 100 cc. The serum calcium may drop to a level as low as 7 mg. Tetany usually fails to appear, however, since the ionized calcium fraction tends still to remain high enough to keep the neuromuscular junctions from becoming hyperirritable. On the other hand, the serum calcium may be somewhat above the normal, although the serum inorganic phosphorus is considerably increased. Such a relation indicates that the hyperparathyroidism is very pronounced. The serum alkaline phosphatase value also rises, and this rise reflects involvement of the skeleton. Taken as a whole, these biochemical findings are diagnostically significant for renal hyperparathyroidism only when it can be established that it was actually renal disease that was the point of departure for the disorder. Indeed, these findings are altogether analogous to those noted in cases of primary hyperparathyroidism in which a complicating chronic renal insufficiency from renal calculi and pyelonephritis or renal calcinosis has developed.

PATHOLOGIC FINDINGS

Renal Changes.—In childhood or adolescence the protracted renal insufficiency underlying renal hyperparathyroidism usually develops on the basis of a congenital defect (structural or functional) of the kidneys or urinary tract. This may be a congenital defect of renal development, such as polycystic kidneys. Or, instead, the kidney damage may follow some sort of functional difficulty at the urethrovesical sphincter which, from early life, has interfered with the outflow of urine. Sometimes the presence of a congenital defect cannot be established and the renal insufficiency

Figure 81

A, Photograph of the kidneys, ureters, and bladder removed at autopsy in the case of a child 3 years of age who presented evidences of secondary (renal) hyperparathyroidism. Dissection of the specimen revealed multiple ureteral strictures which were apparently congenital. The left kidney was completely atrophic and was represented only by a small saccular structure. The right kidney was hydronephrotic and also showed evidences of pyelonephritis.

B, Photograph of the neck organs from the same case. All four parathyroids are enlarged, the upper two more so than the lower (see arrows).

C, Roentgenograph of the sternal ends of the lower four right ribs (postmortem specimen) in this case. There is slight beading at the costochondral junctions. The mottled appearance (radiolucencies intermingled with radiopacities) presented by the ends of the ribs in the vicinity of the costochondral junctions is due to widening of the endochondral growth zones and also the presence of abnormal amounts of connective tissue and new bone (see Fig. 82-*A*).

D, Clinical roentgenograph, dating from about 7 months before the death of the child, illustrating the changes at the right wrist.

E and *F*, Roentgenographs of the wrist and knee areas from the case of a girl 13 years of age who came to the Outpatient Department of the hospital complaining of weakness and vague pains in the knees. That the changes apparent in the juxta-epiphysial areas of the long bones shown represented renal rickets was indicated by the biochemical findings. In particular, the serum calcium value was 5.8 mg. per 100 cc., the inorganic phosphorus 8.1, and the nonprotein nitrogen 179.

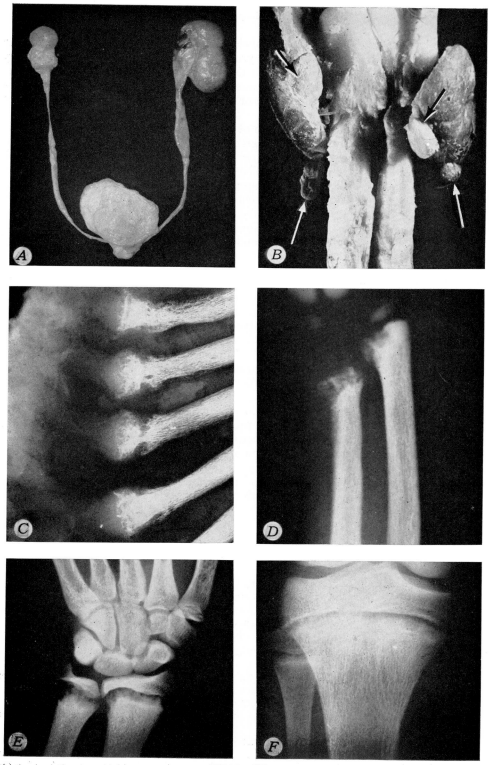

Figure 81

seems to be attributable to a primary pyelonephritis or a glomerulonephritis of long duration. In adults, renal hyperparathyroidism from protracted renal insufficiency may have its basis in a glomerulonephritis which, for some unexplained reason, is running an exceptionally protracted course. On the other hand, its basis may be bilateral renal calculi and pyelonephritis or even congenital polycystic kidneys. (See Morgan and Maclagan.) (See Fig. 81.)

Skeletal Changes.—In the usual run of cases of chronic renal insufficiency associated with slight or only moderate degrees of parathyroid hyperplasia, the alterations in the bones are relatively mild (see Ginzler and Jaffe). Our findings in such cases can be summarized as follows: The bones showing minimal changes were, of course, not altered grossly. On microscopic examination, however, they often revealed mild but clear-cut fibroporotic changes in the spongiosa. In particular, in these cases the spongy trabeculae showed scattered resorption lacunae containing osteoclasts and connective tissue, and some of them also presented, here and there, deposits of new bone. Occasionally—and specifically when the renal insufficiency had been very protracted—the bones were found even grossly altered. In these instances the spongiosa was close-meshed and the trabeculae were thickened and distorted, so that altogether the skeletal changes amounted to a mild osteosclerosis. Under these circumstances, microscopic examination reveals that the thickening of the bony trabeculae has developed through gradual accretion of new bone, despite the alternation of reparative with resorptive processes that must have been going on for a long time. The pertinent findings of Rutishauser, Mach and Rutishauser, Uehlinger, Valvassori and Pierce, and also Zimmerman are in harmony with our own.

It does not seem justifiable in these cases to inculpate hyperparathyroidism *per se* for the skeletal changes. Very likely, they are also attributable, at least in part, to the chronic acidosis of renal insufficiency. Indeed, in the cases showing osteosclerosis, a fluctuating acidosis, in which periods of bone resorption have alternated with periods of bone deposition, seems to provide a better explanation for the bone changes than do the effects of mild hyperparathyroidism alone.

However, in those relatively uncommon cases of protracted renal insufficiency in which the parathyroids have undergone pronounced enlargement, their hyperfunctioning may lead to bone changes indistinguishable from those to be seen in advanced cases of primary hyperparathyroidism. As a rule, in such instances of

Figure 82

A, Photomicrograph (× 4) illustrating the histologic architecture of one of the ribs shown in Fig. 81-*C*. Note the widening of the proliferating cartilage zone; the absence of myeloid marrow in the intertrabecular spaces beyond the proliferating cartilage; the distorted local trabecular architecture; and the focus of subperiosteal connective tissue extending into the bone, as indicated by the arrow on the left. Taken together, such histologic findings provide a plausible basis for understanding the roentgenographic appearances presented by the ribs in question.

B, Photomicrograph (× 4) illustrating the histologic architecture observed at the lower end of a femur from the same case represented by *A*. Note the widening of the proliferating cartilage zone at the epiphysial cartilage plate; the scarring of the intertrabecular marrow; and the distorted spongy trabeculae. The area indicated by the arrows is shown under higher magnification in *C*.

C, Photomicrograph (× 35) of part of the juxta-epiphysial area from *B*. The somewhat widened epiphysial cartilage plate is to be seen in the lower portion of the picture. In the juxta-epiphysial area the intertrabecular marrow is scarred, and the spongy trabeculae are distorted. Small focal areas of hemorrhage are also present.

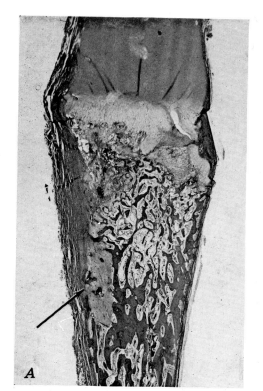

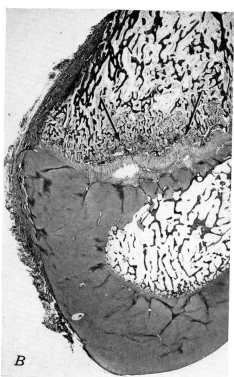

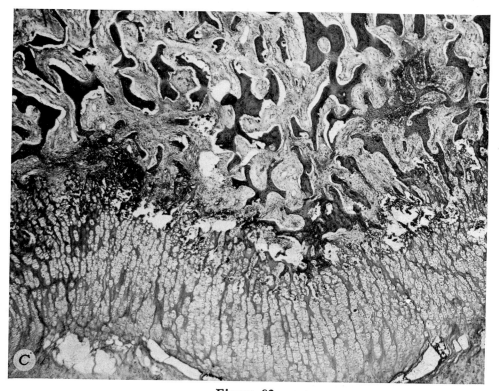

Figure 82

renal hyperparathyroidism, if the patients are children, the bones will be found stunted and will present rachitoid changes at the sites of endochondral bone growth. The calvarium may present granular mottling. Clinically, these young subjects are undersized and sometimes also manifest infantilism. Such cases have, in the past, been described under the heading of "renal rickets" or "renal dwarfism." Terminally, calcareous deposits (metastatic calcifications) are sometimes found in various soft tissues and are likely to be most prominent in the media of the small and moderate-sized arteries, in the soft tissues near joints, and in the subcutaneous tissues and skin in general.

In adults, advanced skeletal changes from renal hyperparathyroidism are encountered even more rarely. In these cases, which in general represent the adult equivalent of "renal rickets" in childhood, stunting and rachitoid changes are, of course, absent. However, the bones present essentially the same other changes as appear in the cases developing earlier in life. One may find, roentgenographically, granular mottling of the calvarium, rarefaction of the cortices of the long bones, and more or less annular areas of decreased density, representing "brown tumors" and cysts—appearances entirely like those seen in adults with primary hyperparathyroidism and severe skeletal changes. Terminally, in these cases, too, metastatic calcifications may appear (see Anderson). (See Figs. 82 and 83.)

Figure 83

A, Photograph of the lower three lumbar vertebrae and the sacrum, cut in the sagittal plane, from the case of a man 41 years of age who had died of uremia. When the subject was 20 years of age, he was hospitalized for acute nephritis, and in the interim he had suffered from the effects of chronic glomerular nephritis. The parathyroids were found enlarged, and their total weight was approximately 4 times the average for the subject's age group. It is apparent even grossly that the spongiosa of these bones is close-meshed, and the trabeculae are thickened—appearances suggesting an osteosclerosis.

B, Photomicrograph ($\times$ 2) illustrating the general histologic architecture of the first and part of the second sacral segment from the specimen shown in *A*. Note the compacted spongy trabeculae. From the details visible under higher magnification, it could be deduced that the osteosclerosis had developed through gradual accretion of new bone. Apparently, reparative processes had predominated over resorptive processes in the alternation between the two types of change which must have been going on for a long time.

C, Photograph of the three lower thoracic vertebrae, cut in the sagittal plane, from the case of a woman 60 years of age who had renal insufficiency of long duration and died of uremia. At autopsy the kidneys were found small, contracted, and heavily scarred in consequence of chronic pyelonephritis. Only three of the four parathyroids were found on dissection of the neck organs, and all three were definitely enlarged. As can be seen, the architecture of the vertebral bodies is profoundly altered. The gross changes are those which one would expect to find in a case of primary hyperparathyroidism, though actually we are dealing here with one of the rare cases in which secondary (renal) hyperparathyroidism has induced severe skeletal alterations. A roentgenographic survey of the skeleton before death demonstrated the presence of granular mottling of the calvarium and widespread porosity of the bones in general. The peripheral blood vessels showed striking ringlike calcifications, and these extended down even to the small arteries in the ends of the fingers and toes. In this connection it is to be remarked that, while the aorta was found somewhat atheromatous at autopsy, it did not show evidences of calcification.

D, Photomicrograph ($\times$ 4) showing the histologic architecture of part of a vertebral body in the case illustrated in *C*. The original trabeculae of spongy bone have been resorbed and replaced by connective tissue and new bone. In the central part of the picture, there is a large area filled with myeloid and fatty marrow.

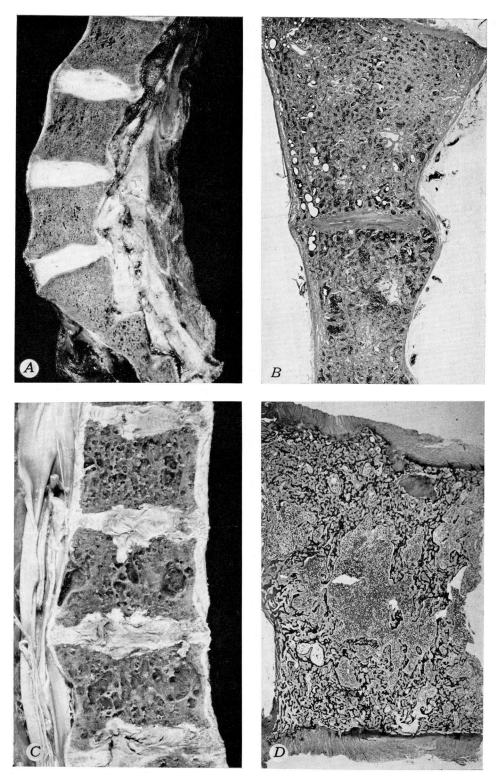

Figure 83

DIFFERENTIAL DIAGNOSIS AND TREATMENT

In a child or adolescent the presence of unexplained stunting, unexplained acidosis (non-acetone) or unexplained renal disease, separately or together, should suggest the possibility of renal hyperparathyroidism. Furthermore, in any case of so-called "late rickets," no matter how typical it seems to be, one should make sure that one is not dealing with renal hyperparathyroidism instead. Certainly if the subject is less than 10 years of age, the other possibility—that the condition is primary hyperparathyroidism—becomes remote, since the latter condition hardly ever appears at such an early age. On the other hand, in an adult the differential diagnosis between primary and secondary hyperparathyroidism is sometimes difficult. A history of renal disease (glomerulonephritis or pyelitis and pyelonephritis) in the absence of renal calculi or renal calcinosis weighs heavily in favor of the diagnosis of renal hyperparathyroidism. Nevertheless, an occasional instance of renal hyperparathyroidism may develop in an adult on the basis of bilateral renal calculi and pyelonephritis. Still, in any case of hyperparathyroidism occurring in an adult and presenting renal calculi, one must certainly consider first the idea that the renal aspect of the condition is an expression of primary hyperparathyroidism.

In cases of renal hyperparathyroidism, attention should be concentrated upon improvement of renal function, if that is possible. As to the parathyroids, it is questionable whether surgical intervention should be undertaken in any instance of renal hyperparathyroidism.

REFERENCES

ALBRIGHT, F., SULKOWITCH, H. W., and BLOOMBERG, E.: Further Experience in the Diagnosis of Hyperparathyroidism, Including a Discussion of Cases with a Minimal Degree of Hyperparathyroidism, Am. J. M. Sc., *193*, 800, 1937.

ALBRIGHT, F., BURNETT, C. H., SMITH, P. H., and PARSON, W.: Pseudo-Hypoparathyroidism—an Example of 'Seabright-Bantam Syndrome,' Endocrinology, *30*, 922, 1942.

ALBRIGHT, F., FORBES, A. P., and HENNEMAN, P. H.: Pseudo-pseudohypoparathyroidism, Tr. A. Am. Physicians, *65*, 337, 1952.

ANDERSON, W. A. D.: Hyperparathyroidism and Renal Disease, Arch. Path., *27*, 753, 1939.

ASKANAZY, M.: Beiträge zur Knochenpathologie, in *Chemische und medicinische Untersuchungen* (Festschrift für M. Jaffe), Braunschweig, F. Vieweg und Sohn, 1901.

————: Ueber Ostitis deformans ohne osteides Gewebe, Arb. Geb. path. Anat. Inst. Tübingen, *4*, 398, 1904.

BARNEY, J. D., and SULKOWITCH, H. W.: Progress in the Management of Urinary Calculi, J. Urol., *37*, 746, 1937.

BARR, D. P., BULGER, H. A., and DIXON, H. H.: Hyperparathyroidism, J.A.M.A., *92*, 951, 1929.

BERGSTRAND, H.: Ostitis fibrosa generalisata Recklinghausen mit pluriglandulärer Affektion der innersekretorischen Drüsen und röntgenologisch nachweisbarem Parathyreoideatumor, Acta med. scandinav., *76*, 128, 1931.

BODANSKY, A., BLAIR, J. E., and JAFFE, H. L.: Experimental Hyperparathyroidism in Guinea Pigs Leading to Ostitis Fibrosa, J. Biol. Chem., *88*, 629, 1930.

BODANSKY, A., and JAFFE, H. L.: Parathormone Dosage and Serum Calcium and Phosphorus in Experimental Chronic Hyperparathyroidism Leading to Ostitis Fibrosa, J. Exper. Med., *53*, 591, 1931.

————: Hypocalcemia Following Experimental Hyperparathyroidism and its Possible Significance, J. Biol. Chem., *93*, 543, 1931.

BOYD, J. D., MILGRAM, J. E., and STEARNS, G.: Clinical Hyperparathyroidism, J.A.M.A., *93*, 684, 1929.

BUCHS, S.: Angeborener Hypoparathyreoidismus von drei Brüdern infolge von Hyperparathyreoidismus der Mutter, Schweiz. med. Wchnschr., *91*, 660, 1961.

CAMP, J. D.: Symmetrical Calcification of the Cerebral Basal Ganglia. Its Roentgenologic Significance in the Diagnosis of Parathyroid Insufficiency, Radiology, *49*, 568, 1947.

CAPPS, R. B.: Multiple Parathyroid Tumors with Massive Mediastinal and Subcutaneous Hemorrhage, Am. J. M. Sc., *188*, 800, 1934.

CASSIDY, C. E., and ANDERSON, A. S.: A Familial Occurrence of Hyperparathyroidism Caused by Multiple Parathyroid Adenomas, Metabolism, *9*, 1152, 1960.

CASTLEMAN, B.: *Tumors of the Parathyroid Glands*, Atlas of Tumor Pathology, Section IV— Fascicle 15, Washington, D.C., Armed Forces Institute of Pathology, 1952.

CASTLEMAN, B., and MALLORY, T. B.: The Pathology of the Parathyroid Gland in Hyperparathyroidism. A Study of 25 Cases, Am. J. Path., *11*, 1, 1935.

————: Parathyroid Hyperplasia in Chronic Renal Insufficiency, Am. J. Path., *13*, 553, 1937.

COLLIP, J. B.: The Extraction of a Parathyroid Hormone which will Prevent or Control Parathyroid Tetany and which Regulates the Level of Blood Calcium, J. Biol. Chem., *63*, 395, 1925.

COMPERE, E. L.: Pathologic and Biochemical Changes in Skeletal Dystrophies: Analysis of Results of Treatment of Parathyroid Osteosis, Arch. Surg., *32*, 232, 1936.

COPE, O., CULVER, P. J., MIXTER, C. G., JR., and NARDI, G. L.: Pancreatitis, A Diagnostic Clue to Hyperparathyroidism, Ann. Surg., *145*, 857, 1957.

COPE, O., BARNES, B. A., CASTLEMAN, B., MUELLER, G. C. E., and ROTH, S. I.: Vicissitudes of Parathyroid Surgery: Trials of Diagnosis and Management in 51 Patients with a Variety of Disorders, Ann. Surg., *154*, 491, 1961.

DANISCH, F.: Epithelkörperchenblutungen bei Säuglingen und Kleinkindern und das Spasmophilieproblem, Frankfurt. Ztschr. Path., *33*, 380, 1926.

DODDS, W. J., and STEINBACH, H. L.: Primary Hyperparathyroidism and Articular Cartilage Calcification, Am. J. Roentgenol., *104*, 884, 1968.

ELLIS, J. T., and BARR, D. P.: Metastasizing Carcinoma of the Parathyroid Gland with Osteitis Fibrosa Cystica and Extensive Calcinosis, Am. J. Path., *27*, 383, 1951.

ELLIS, K., and HOCHSTIM, R. J.: The Skull in Hyperparathyroid Bone Disease, Am. J. Roentgenol., *83*, 732, 1960.

ERDHEIM, J.: Über Epithelkörperbefunde bei Osteomalacie, Sitzungsb. k. Akad. Wissensch., Math.-naturw. Klasse, *116*, sect. 3, 311, 1907.

FOGH-ANDERSEN, P.: Hyperparathyreoidisme, hyppighed og kirurgisk behandling, Ugesk. laeger, *116*, 796, 1954.

FRAME, B., and HAUBRICH, W. S.: Peptic Ulcer and Hyperparathyroidism: A Survey of 300 Ulcer Patients, Arch. Int. Med., *105*, 536, 1960.

GIBSON, R.: Brachymetacarpal Dwarfism or Pseudo-Pseudohypoparathyroidism with Mental Defect in Siblings, Canad. M. A. J., *85*, 70, 1961.

GILMOUR, J. R., and MARTIN, W. J.: The Weight of the Parathyroid Glands, J. Path. & Bact., *44*, 431, 1937.

GINZLER, A. M., and JAFFE, H. L.: Osseous Findings in Chronic Renal Insufficiency in Adults, Am. J. Path., *17*, 293, 1941.

GOLD, E.: Ueber die Bedeutung der Epithelkörpervergrösserung bei der Ostitis fibrosa generalisata Recklinghausen, Mitt. Grenzgeb. Med. u. Chir., *41*, 63, 1928.

GUTMAN, A. B., SWENSON, P. C., and PARSONS, W. B.: The Differential Diagnosis of Hyperparathyroidism, J.A.M.A., *103*, 87, 1934.

GUTMAN, A. B., TYSON, T. L , and GUTMAN, E. B.: Serum Calcium, Inorganic Phosphorus and Phosphatase Activity in Hyperparathyroidism, Paget's Disease, Multiple Myeloma and Neoplastic Disease of the Bones, Arch. Int. Med., *57*, 379, 1936.

HANNON, R. R., SHORR, E., McCLELLAN, W. S., and DuBOIS, E. F.: A Case of Osteitis Fibrosa Cystica (Osteomalacia ?) with Evidence of Hyperactivity of the Parathyroid Bodies. Metabolic Study I, J. Clin. Invest., *8*, 215, 1930.

HANSON, A. M.: Parathyroid Preparations, Mil. Surgeon, *54*, 554, 1924.

HELLSTRÖM, J.: Primär hyperparathyreoidism, Nord. med., *61*, 551, 1959.

HELLSTRÖM, J., and IVEMARK, B. I.: Primary Hyperparathyroidism: Clinical and Structural Findings in 138 Cases, Acta chir. scandinav., Suppl. *294*, 1962.

HORTLING, H., PUUPPONEN, E., and KOSKI, K.: Pseudo-pseudohypoparathyroidism, J. Clin Endocrinol., *20*, 466, 1960.

HOWAT, T. W., and ASHURST, G. M.: Pseudohypoparathyroidism, J. Bone & Joint Surg., *39-B*, 39, 1957.

JACKSON, C. E., TALBERT, P. C., and CAYLOR, H. D.: Hereditary Hyperparathyroidism, J. Indiana M. A., *53*, 1313, 1960.

JAFFE, H. L.: Hyperparathyroidism (Recklinghausen's Disease of Bone), Arch. Path., *16*, 63 and 236, 1933.

————: Hyperparathyroidism, Bull. New York Acad. Med., *16*, 291, 1940.

————: Primary and Secondary (Renal) Hyperparathyroidism, S. Clin. North America, *22*, 621, 1942.

————: Giant-Cell Reparative Granuloma, Traumatic Bone Cyst, and Fibrous (Fibro osseous) Dysplasia of the Jawbones, Oral Surg., *6*, 159, 1953.

JAFFE, H. L., and BODANSKY, A.: Experimental Fibrous Osteodystrophy (Ostitis Fibrosa) in Hyperparathyroid Dogs, J. Exper. Med., *52*, 669, 1930.

JAFFE, H. L., BODANSKY, A., and BLAIR, J. E.: The Influence of Age and of Duration of Treatment on the Production and Repair of Bone Lesions in Experimental Hyperparathyroidism, J. Exper. Med., *55*, 139, 1932.

JAFFE, H. L., and BODANSKY, A.: Diagnostic Significance of Serum Alkaline and Acid Phosphatase Values in Relation to Bone Disease, Bull. New York Acad. Med., *19*, 831, 1943.

————: Serum Calcium: Clinical and Biochemical Considerations, J. Mt. Sinai Hosp., *9*, 901, 1943.

JOHNSON, J. W., JR.: Primary Hyperparathyroidism with Extensive Renal Calcification and Secondary Hyperplasia of the Parathyroids, Am. J. Path., *15*, 111, 1939.

LEVIN, P., KUNIN, A. S., DONAGHY, R. M. P., HAMILTON, W. W., and MAURER, J. J.: Intracranial Calcification and Hypoparathyroidism, Neurology, *11*, 1076, 1961.

LOBDELL, D. H.: Congenital Absence of the Parathyroid Glands, Arch. Path., *67*, 412, 1959.

MACGREGOR, M. E., and WHITEHEAD, T. P.: Pseudo-hypoparathyroidism: A Description of Three Cases and a Critical Appraisal of Earlier Accounts of the Disease, Arch. Dis. Childhood, *29*, 398, 1954.

MACH, R. S., and RUTISHAUSER, E.: Les ostéodystrophies rénales. Étude expérimentale et anatomoclinique des lésions osseuses au cours des néphrites, Helvet. med. acta, *4*, 423, 1937.

MANDL, F.: Klinisches und Experimentelles zur Frage der lokalisierten und generalisierten Ostitis fibrosa, Arch. klin. Chir., *143*, 1 and 245, 1926.

MARESCH, R.: Beiträge zur Kenntnis der Hyperplasien und Tumoren der Epithelkörper, Frankfurt. Ztschr. Path., *19*, 159, 1916.

McGEOWN, M. G.: Effect of Parathyroidectomy on the Incidence of Renal Calculi, Lancet, *1*, 586, 1961.

MORGAN, A. D., and MACLAGAN, N. F.: Renal Disease in Hyperparathyroidism, Am. J. Path., *30*, 1141, 1954.

MULLER, H., and SMEENK, D.: Enkele aspecten van primaire hyperparathyreoïdie (studie van 52 waargenomen gevallen), Nederl. tijdschr. geneesk, *106*, 2314, 1962.

NOETZLI, M., and STEINBACH, H. L.: Subperiosteal Erosion of the Ribs in Hyperparathyroidism, Am. J. Roentgenol., *87*, 1058, 1962.

NORRIS, E. H.: The Parathyroid Glands and the Lateral Thyroid in Man: Their Morphogenesis, Histogenesis, Topographic Anatomy and Prenatal Growth, Contrib. Embryol., *159*, 249, 1937.

————: Primary Hyperparathyroidism. A Report of Five Cases that Exemplify Special Features of this Disease (Infarction of a Parathyroid Adenoma; Oxyphil Adenoma), Arch. Path., *42*, 261, 1946.

O'BRIEN, D., PEPPERS, T. D., and SILVER, H. K.: Idiopathic Hypercalcemia of Infancy, J.A.M.A., *173*, 1106, 1960.

PAPPENHEIMER, A. M., and WILENS, S. L.: Enlargement of the Parathyroid Glands in Renal Disease, Am. J. Path., *11*, 73, 1935.

PEARL, M. A., STERNBERG, W. H., and DINGMAN, J. F.: Unusual Cases of Hyperparathyroidism, Arch. Int. Med., *110*, 481, 1962.

VON RECKLINGHAUSEN, F.: Die fibröse oder deformirende Ostitis, die Osteomalacie und die osteoplastische Carcinose in ihren gegenseitigen Beziehungen, in *Festschrift für Rudolf Virchow*, Berlin, G. Reimer, 1891.

RÖSSLE, R.: Über gleichzeitige Missbildungen der branchiogenen Organe und über angeborenen Mangel der Epithelkörperchen, Virchows Arch. path. Anat., *283*, 41, 1932.

ROTH, S. I.: The Ultrastructure of Primary Water-Clear Cell Hyperplasia of the Parathyroid Glands, Am. J. Path., *61*, 233, 1970.

RUTISHAUSER, E.: Ostéodystrophie néphrogène, Ann. d'anat. path., *13*, 999, 1936.

SALVESEN, H. A., and BÖE, J.: Idiopathic Hypoparathyroidism. Observations on Two Cases, One Complicated by Moniliasis and Idiopathic Steatorrhea and One with an Unusual Degree of Calcium Deposition in the Bones, Acta endocrinol., *14*, 214, 1953.

STEINBACH, H. L., GORDAN, G. S., EISENBERG, E., CRANE, J. T., SILVERMAN, S., and GOLDMAN, L.: Primary Hyperparathyroidism: A Correlation of Roentgen, Clinical, and Pathologic Features, Am. J. Roentgenol., *86*, 329, 1961.

STROCK, M. S.: The Mouth in Hyperparathyroidism, New England J. Med., *224*, 1019, 1941.

THOMAS, W. C., JR., WISWELL, J. G., CONNOR, T. B., and HOWARD, J. E.: Hypercalcemic Crisis Due to Hyperparathyroidism, Am. J. Med., *24*, 229, 1958.

UEHLINGER, E.: Pathogenese des primären und sekundären Hyperparathyreoidismus und der renalen Osteomalacie, Verhandl. deutsch. Gesellsch. inn. Med., *62*, 368, 1956.

————: Die Regulation des Kalziumstoffwechsels und primärer Hyperparathyreoidismus, München. med. Wchnschr., *106*, 685, 1964.

————: Hyperkalzämie-Syndrome, München. med. Wchnschr., *106*, 692, 1964.

UHR, N., and BEZAHLER, H. B.: Pseudo-pseudohypoparathyroidism: Report of Three Cases in One Family, Ann. Int. Med., *54*, 443, 1961.

VALVASSORI, G. E., and PIERCE, R. H.: Osteosclerosis in Chronic Uremia, Radiology, *82*, 385, 1964.

WERMER, P.:   Genetic Aspects of Adenomatosis of Endocrine Glands, Am. J. Med., *16*, 363, 1954.

WILTON, A.:   On the Genesis of "Osteitis Fibrosa Generalisata" (Engel-Recklinghausen Disease), Acta path. et microbiol. scandinav., *23*, 1, 1946.

ZIMMERMAN, H. B.:   Osteosclerosis in Chronic Renal Disease; Report of 4 Cases Associated with Secondary Hyperparathyroidism, Am. J. Roentgenol., *88*, 1152, 1962.

ZOLLINGER, R. M., and ELLISON, E. H.:   Primary Peptic Ulcerations of the Jejunum Associated with Islet Cell Tumors of the Pancreas, Ann. Surg., *142*, 709, 1955.

ZVAIFLER, N. J., REEFE, W. E., and BLACK, R. L.:   Articular Manifestations in Primary Hyperparathyroidism, Arthritis Rheum., *5*, 237, 1962.

Chapter

13

Skeletal Alterations Resulting from Dysfunction of Other Endocrine Glands

IN the preceding chapter the various clinical and anatomic manifestations of hyperparathyroidism were considered in some detail. In the present chapter, attention will be centered upon the skeletal aberrations arising from dysfunction of endocrine glands other than the parathyroids. In particular, consideration will be given to the skeletal aspects of: *acromegaly* and *hyperpituitary gigantism, hypopituitary dwarfism, hypothyroid dwarfism, hyperthyroidism,* and the *Cushing syndrome.* In addition, brief mention will be made of the skeletal reflections of *eunuchism* and *gonadal dysgenesis, diabetes mellitus,* and the *adrenogenital syndrome.* Of course, the skeletal aberrations in all these conditions constitute merely one element in the endocrinological disorder as a whole. However, since we are really concerned only with the skeletal changes, details relating to the clinical, physiological, and biochemical aspects of these endocrine disorders will not be considered.

ACROMEGALY AND HYPERPITUITARY GIGANTISM

In an adult, prolonged hyperpituitarism results in *acromegaly,* and in a growing subject it is expressed in *hyperpituitary gigantism.* The basis for the hyperpituitarism is usually an adenoma (composed mainly of acidophil cells) of the anterior lobe of the pituitary gland. Sometimes, however, the hyperpituitarism has its basis in diffuse hyperplasia of the acidophil cells of the anterior lobe. The association of hyperpituitary gigantism and acromegaly with the presence of acidophil cell adenomas or diffuse hyperplasia of the acidophil cells is strong evidence that these cells are involved in the secretion of a growth-promoting hormone (somatropin). Indeed, this hormone seems to be embodied largely in the granules of the acidophil cells.

In a young subject the growth-promoting hormone of the anterior lobe of the pituitary has a direct stimulating effect on endochondral bone growth at the epiphysial cartilage plates, and hence on longitudinal growth of the bones. In an adult, long after endochondral bone growth would normally have ceased, excessive amounts of circulating pituitary growth hormone may reactivate endochondral bone growth at various existing cartilage-bone junctions (costochondral junctions, for instance).

CLINICAL CONSIDERATIONS

When hyperpituitarism sets in near or after the completion of skeletal growth (as is usually the case), the subject, without either growing fat or increasing excessively in height, comes to present a thick-set appearance, accentuated by abnormally large hands and feet and also coarse facial features—particularly a prognathous lower jaw. Marie gave the name "acromegaly" to this condition, because he recognized that enlargement of the hands, feet, and lower jaw (acral parts) appeared early in the development of the syndrome and constituted a clinically characteristic part of it. The enlargement of the hands and feet in acromegaly is created mainly by progressive hypertrophy of all their soft tissues but especially by thickening of the connective tissue of the corium and the subcutaneous connective tissue. To a small extent the enlargement may also be due to periosteal deposits upon the phalanges and metacarpal and metatarsal bones. The prognathism is the result of increase in height of the rami of the lower jaw and of deposition of bone upon its mental margin. In addition to the acral parts, the various internal organs, including the viscera and the endocrine glands other than the pituitary, also become enlarged. In fact, splanchnomegaly is a prominent feature of the pathologic anatomy of this disease. Prominent thickening of the tongue and other buccal structures is likely to create difficulty in articulation, and in consequence, speech may be difficult to understand.

A number of years may elapse between the appearance of clear-cut acral changes and the time the acromegalic seeks relief from symptoms caused by pressure of the enlarged pituitary upon the sella turcica and the neighboring tissues (see Davidoff, and Gordon et al.). In the meantime the sella has usually undergone considerable expansion, detectable roentgenographically. Headache becomes a conspicuous affliction when the enlarged pituitary begins to exert pressure against the walls of the sella. This symptom may vanish temporarily if the expanding tumor ruptures the sellar diaphragm. After bursting the latter, the adenoma may give rise to signs of compression of the optic chiasm and especially to disturbances of vision. Progression of the condition is often associated with injury to the posterior lobe of the pituitary and to the hypothalamus, leading to polyphagia, polydipsia, and polyuria. We need not dwell, however, on the manifold other clinical aspects of acromegaly which are conditioned by the controlling influence of the pituitary on other glands of internal secretion and on fat and carbohydrate metabolism.

In the more uncommon instances in which the pituitary hyperfunctioning sets in well before puberty, *exaggerated skeletal growth*, due to stimulation of endochondral ossification at the epiphysial cartilage plates (and other growth zones), usually dominates the clinical picture at first. Through the effects on the epiphysial cartilage plates of the long bones in particular, the subjects become extremely tall, reaching a height of 7 feet or more. A striking example of gigantism of this kind was described by Behrens and Barr. Their patient was a boy who was already unusually large at 6 months of age, and at 13½ years had attained a height of 7¼ feet without showing clinically any other pronounced abnormalities. At the age of 18¼ years, the subject was 8¼ feet tall. His hands, feet, and lower jaw shared in his general excessive size, but they were not disproportionately enlarged, and prognathism was as yet absent (see Humberd). Hyperpituitary giants usually die during early adult life, but if they continue to survive, they can be expected to manifest the acral changes of acromegaly in addition to their gigantism. That is, their hands and feet become enlarged out of proportion to the rest of the body, their facial features coarsen, and the lower jaw becomes prominent. Many of the circus giants are acromegalic giants. (See Fig. 84.)

Often, after the clinical manifestations of acromegaly have been present and increasing for many years, the progression of the disease ceases rather abruptly. The interruption of the clinical progress of the disease often follows upon hemorrhage into, and concomitant degeneration of, the enlarged anterior lobe of the pituitary. In fact, the damage to the gland may be so severe that manifestations of *hypopi-*

tuitarism, such as loss of libido in the male and cessation of menstruation in the female, may finally appear. If the progress of the disease does become arrested, such skeletal and visceral overgrowth as has already taken place does not regress. However, the hypertrophy of the subcutaneous tissues in the enlarged acral parts may recede to some extent.

In respect to *treatment,* large doses of estrogen have been recommended for cases showing mild degrees of acromegaly. In cases in which there are indications that the pituitary adenoma is exerting pressure effects on the local structures, a choice between surgery and irradiation may have to be made. Irradiation of the pituitary region from opposing fields (crossfire irradiation) constitutes a very hopeful therapeutic procedure in such cases. Surgical intervention in the form of partial hypophysectomy is justified only by the presence of damaging pressure upon various intracranial structures. Apart from these general therapeutic indications for advanced acromegaly, there are those dictated by other features in a given case. These features include associated deficient functioning of one or more other glands of internal secretion—for instance, the thyroid or pancreas. More recently, cryotherapy has been used in the treatment of acromegaly. References to this form of therapy have been made under such titles as "cryoablation," "cryohypophysectomy," and "hypophysial cryosurgery." (See Maddy *et al.,* Adams *et al.,* and Dashe *et al.*) The beneficial effects of the various forms of therapy used result from a fall in the plasma growth hormone. Roth *et al.* reported that all of the commonly used therapeutic procedures were equally effective.

PATHOLOGY OF THE SKELETAL ALTERATIONS

There has been little opportunity to investigate anatomically the pertinent skeletal changes as they appear in relatively young hyperpituitary giants. Still, as already

Figure 84

A, Photograph of the head of an acromegalic man 43 years of age. The manifestations of acromegaly had set in when he was about 24 years old.

B, Roentgenograph of the skull in the case illustrated in *A.* Note the exaggerated height of the rami of the mandible, and the forward and downward protrusion of the body of that bone. The frontal and maxillary sinuses are abnormally large, and the calvarium manifests definite thickening.

C, Roentgenograph showing advanced changes of osteoarthritis in the right hip joint in the same case. Because of pronounced marginal exostosis formation, the size of the femoral head is much greater than it would normally be. The contour of the head is irregular, the joint space is narrowed, and the apposing articular bone ends are sclerosed.

D, Roentgenograph of a hand in the case of another middle-aged man affected with acromegaly. Note the loose-meshed (lacelike) architecture of the distal ends of the terminal phalanges, and also the small knobby projections at these bone ends.

E, Roentgenograph showing the eleventh and twelfth thoracic vertebrae of a sagittally sectioned vertebral column from another case of acromegaly. The subject was a woman 48 years of age who had begun to manifest evidence of acromegaly when she was 28 years old. The thoracic vertebrae, in particular, showed an increase in the transverse and anteroposterior diameters of the bodies. The increased size was due to subperiosteal new bone deposition, and the extent of this in the anteroposterior plane in each of the two vertebrae illustrated is demarcated by the line toward the right of the picture.

F, Photograph of the twelfth thoracic vertebra (macerated specimen) from another case of acromegaly. The subject was a man 39 years of age who had presented manifestations of the disease since he was 21 years old. The extent of the subperiosteal new bone deposition which increased the size of the vertebral body is indicated by the arrows. (*E* and *F* were reproduced, with permission, from the article by Erdheim in Virchows Arch. path. Anat., *281,* 1931.)

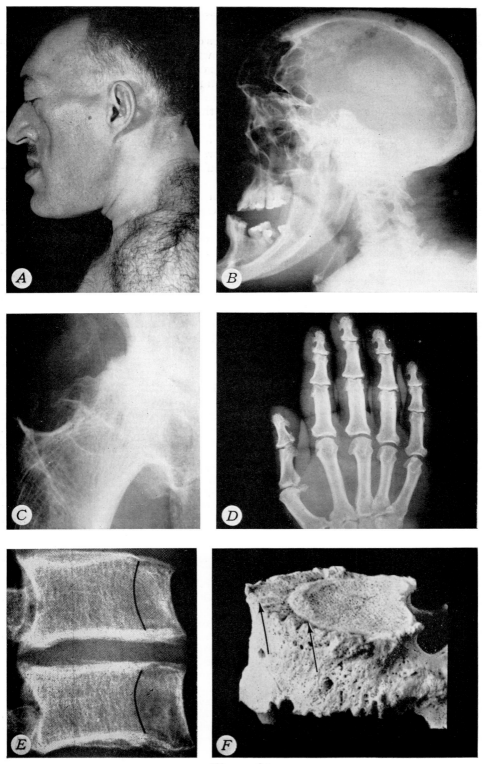

Figure 84

indicated, it has become clear that the largeness of the skeleton in these cases results from the stimulation of endochondral bone growth at the epiphysial cartilage plates or other growth zones in consequence of the excessive secretion of the growth hormone. Most of our knowledge of the skeletal alterations which arise from the dyspituitarism under discussion comes from autopsies on acromegalics whose hyperpituitarism had not set in until skeletal growth had been almost or entirely completed. Altogether, the skeletal pathology in these cases varies considerably, roughly in accordance with the age at onset and the duration of the hyperpituitarism. On the basis of this material, it appears that in these mature subjects, too, hyperpituitarism tends to bring about a stimulation and even reactivation of endochondral ossification.

In subjects in whom endochondral ossification has not yet entirely ceased, its stimulation may be expressed in somewhat exaggerated longitudinal growth, although the subjects can no longer become actual giants. If endochondral ossification has ceased at the time of onset of the hyperpituitarism, the latter will tend to reactivate endochondral ossification where it can. One place in which such reactivation is still possible even at an advanced age is at the costochondral junctions. This fact is clearly shown in a case studied by Erdheim. The subject was a woman 71 years of age in whom acromegaly was manifest only during the last 4 years of life. Despite the fact that the hyperpituitarism set in many decades after completion of skeletal growth, endochondral bone formation was nevertheless revived, though only to a very limited degree and mainly at the costochondral junctions. The

Figure 85

A, Photograph of parts of three ribs sectioned in the long axis to demonstrate the gross appearance of the costochondral junctions under normal conditions in a middle-aged adult. The subject was a well-developed man 45 years of age who had died of a fulminating streptococcal infection. The findings at the costochondral junctions of these ribs are in striking contrast to those shown in *B*, which represent analogous areas from a case of acromegaly.

B, Photograph of parts of three ribs sectioned in the long axis to demonstrate the gross appearance of the costochondral junctions in a middle-aged acromegalic. The subject was a woman who died at the age of 48 and who had presented various manifestations of acromegaly for many years. The costal cartilages are much thicker than they would normally be, and the costochondral junctions are strikingly expanded. The thickening of the costal cartilages is the result of the deposition of new cartilage upon the resting cartilage, and the enlargement of the costochondral junctions is the consequence of reactivated endochondral ossification at these sites.

C, Photomicrograph ($\times$ 7) illustrating the general histologic pattern presented by the costochondral junctional area of the *middle* rib shown in *A*. Note the tonguelike projection of the cartilage into the shaft of the rib and the smooth contour at the cartilage-shaft junction, indicating that the cartilage is in a quiescent state (see *E*).

D, Photomicrograph ($\times$ 3) illustrating the general histologic pattern presented by the costochondral junctional area of the middle rib shown in *B*. Even at this low magnification it is apparent that endochondral ossification has been reactivated (see *F*).

E, Photomicrograph ($\times$ 35) revealing in greater detail the histologic findings at the costochondral junction of the rib shown in *C* and representing the appearance which is normal for a middle-aged adult. The costal cartilage at the cartilage-bone junction is in an inactive (resting) stage, and the spongy trabeculae of the rib shaft abut upon (close off) the costal cartilage.

F, Photomicrograph ($\times$ 55) revealing in greater detail the histologic findings at the costochondral junction of the rib shown in *D* and representing the appearance which is characteristic of acromegaly of long standing. Note that the cartilage cells at the cartilage-bone junction have been proliferating and are lined up in columns, and that endochondral ossification is proceeding, though not very actively, at the costochondral junction.

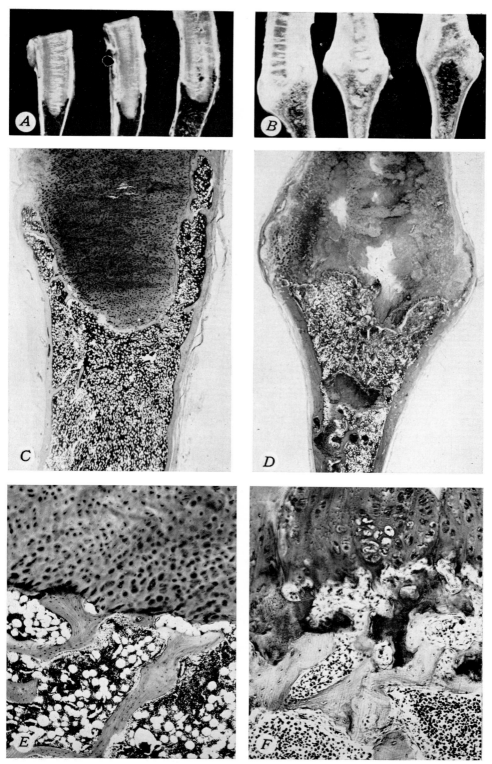

Figure 85

acromegalic state is associated furthermore with a tendency toward the gradual deposition of subperiosteal new bone, especially in certain predilected regions.

The alterations in the *skull bones* are among those most distinctive of acromegaly (see Keith). As a result of the periosteal deposition of bone upon the alveolar margins of the maxillae and mandible, the dental sockets are deepened and the teeth separated. Bone is also deposited upon the mental eminence of the mandible and along its lower margin, anterior to the grooves of the facial arteries. However, the most striking alterations in the mandible are those which take place in the rami in consequence of growth at their articular ends. The rami often become narrower and increase in height, sometimes by an inch or more. These changes result in the mandible being pushed downward and forward, and malocclusion of the teeth develops. There is also often overgrowth of the supra-orbital ridges, expansion of the frontal and maxillary sinuses, and enlargement of the malar and zygomatic bones. The modifications in the calvarium may be relatively slight. However, the calvarium is usually somewhat thicker than the normal, especially on the vault. In rare instances it may be so thick and otherwise grossly modified as to suggest the type of calvarium usually found in advanced cases of Paget's disease. As to the base of the cranium, it should be noted that the sella is enlarged in nearly all cases, although there are various other alterations which may also take place. In fact, the sellar fossa may be extremely distorted because of erosion of the sphenoid by the tumefied pituitary gland.

The *thoracic cage* often presents a striking increase in size. It is due largely to an increased length of the middle six ribs which induces a pronounced forward projection of the lower part of the sternum. In addition, the clavicles may be thicker and much longer than they would normally be. The ribs and costal cartilages are unusually wide and may even show pronounced thickening at the costochondral junctions. The rows of "beaded" costochondral junctions may also create the illusion of a rosary. The exaggerated growth of the ribs, particularly in length, is due, as already noted, to the fact that endochondral ossification has been reactivated at the costochondral junctions. Thus, if a widened costal cartilage and adjacent rib

Figure 86

A, Photomicrograph ($\times$ 3) showing parts of two thoracic vertebral bodies and the intervening intervertebral disk from a case of acromegaly. About one-third of the disk (as one goes from left to right) represents disk tissue which has been added to the pre-existing intervertebral disk in the course of the anteroposterior and lateral growth of the vertebral bodies in question. Examination under higher power would show that the cartilage on the upper and lower surfaces of the *added* disk tissue presents evidence of proliferation (see *B*). In contrast, the cartilage of the plate on the upper and lower surfaces of the *pre-existing* disk tissue would be found in a quiescent state.

B, Photomicrograph ($\times$ 25) illustrating the histologic appearance of the proliferating cartilage on the lower surface of the intervertebral disk in the area to which the arrow points in *A*. Because the photograph was prepared from a rather thick celloidin section, the histologic details relating to the proliferating cartilage cells do not stand out so clearly as they would in a thin section (see *C*).

C, Photomicrograph ($\times$ 55) from another vertebra in this case of acromegaly. Note that the cartilage on the deep surface of the intervertebral disk has been proliferating. Some of the proliferating cartilage cells are lined up in short columns, and there is some evidence of endochondral ossification. (Compare with *D*.)

D, Photomicrograph ($\times$ 35) illustrating the histologic appearance of the cartilage plate of an intervertebral disk of a middle-aged adult *not* affected with acromegaly. Note that the cartilage is in a resting (static) stage and, in particular, that there is no evidence of endochondral ossification at the cartilage-bone junction.

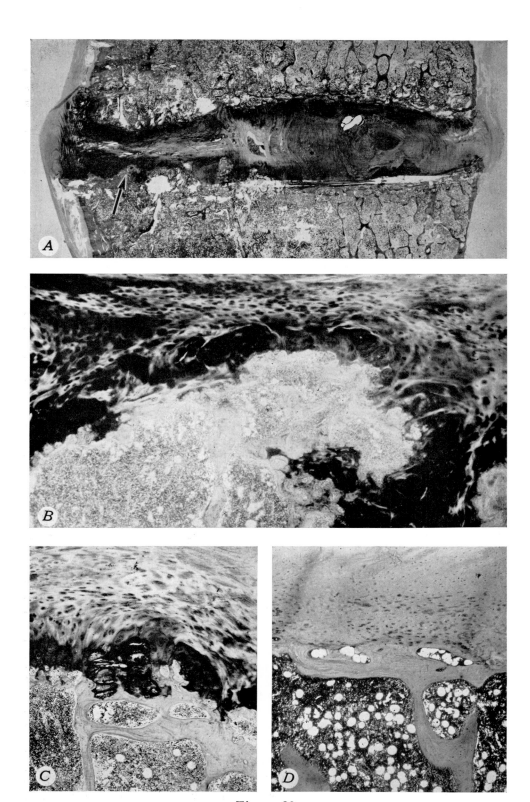

Figure 86

body are transected horizontally, the newly proliferated cartilage in the region of the costochondral junction can be recognized even grossly by its dazzling white color. On microscopic examination it appears that this cartilage proliferation is associated with the appearance, at the bone-cartilage junctions, of cartilage cells in columnar arrangement, such as one sees in regions of endochondral ossification during the growth period. (See Fig. 85.)

The changes in the *vertebral column* are also striking in acromegaly. Erdheim has described them in detail in an acromegalic woman, 48 years of age, whose disease had been clearly evident since the age of 28 and almost certainly existed before that age. In this case, especially in the thoracic region, there was an increase in the transverse and anteroposterior diameters both of the vertebral bodies and the intervertebral disks. The increase in the diameters of the vertebral bodies was the result of marginal subperiosteal new bone formation, while the increase in the size of the disks resulted from marginal subperichondrial new formation of cartilage. These processes resemble closely those by which the growth of the disks and vertebral bodies is achieved normally during the early years of life. (See Fig. 86.) Roentgenographically, the resultant squatty shape of the vertebral bodies in acromegaly has usually been interpreted as being due to a decrease in the height of the bodies, whereas actually the change in proportion is the result of widening of the bodies. Furthermore, these acromegalic changes in the vertebral column might also be misinterpreted as being merely those of spondylosis deformans (p. 762). Clinically, one is likely to find a cervicodorsal kyphosis resulting from muscular weakness.

If the acromegalic subject is not excessively tall, the *long tubular bones* usually fail to present any striking changes, though their articular ends may be less delicately modeled than those of normal bones. The cortices of the shafts are generally smooth and of normal thickness, but are sometimes pitted and marked by vascular impressions. One may even find slight periosteal new bone deposition. The various tuberosities may be more than normally prominent. The *short tubular bones* (phalanges, metacarpals, and metatarsals) may also not be much altered. They may, however, be somewhat thickened by the deposition of periosteal new bone (periosteal osteophytes). This thickening sometimes contributes to the enlargement of the hands and feet. Furthermore, the distal phalanges may show a curious terminal nodular tufting, strikingly demonstrable roentgenographically. The periosteal new bone deposition on the short and long tubular bones is not nearly so striking, however, as it is likely to be in cases of pulmonary hypertrophic osteoarthropathy (p. 286). Nor does one see, in uncomplicated acromegaly, the drumstick-like clubbed terminal phalanges characteristic of pulmonary osteoarthropathy; on the other hand, the latter does not show the conspicuously prognathous jaw of acromegaly. In the past, instances of idiopathic familial osteoarthropathy with pachydermia (p. 291) have also been confused with acromegaly.

In addition to stimulating the cartilage at costochondral junctions, hyperpituitarism may instigate proliferation in the *articular* cartilages. This is first manifest in proliferation of the cells of the radial (or columnar) zone of these cartilages, the hyperplasia and hypertrophy then spreading to the other zones. The thickened articular cartilages may finally degenerate, and ulcerations may appear on their surfaces. Furthermore, marginal exostoses may then appear. These various articular changes simulate the changes of osteoarthritis (p. 738) and may give rise to clinical manifestations, such as pain, limitation of motion, crackling on movement, and intra-articular effusion. Indeed, in cases of stabilized acromegaly, the arthritis of one joint or another may come to be the principal source of clinical complaint. This was so in a case, seen by the writer, in which a pronounced osteoarthritis of the left hip was so disabling that a major surgical intervention had to be considered, despite its special hazards for an acromegalic.

HYPOPITUITARY DWARFISM

Clinico-anatomic observations showed long ago that damage to the pituitary, and specifically to its anterior lobe, leads to stunting of the skeleton if the damage occurs during the period of skeletal growth. The pathologic skeletal findings in human cases of hypopituitary dwarfism are in accord with the observation that young animals subjected to hypophysectomy show stunting of growth. The corollary finding that pituitary extracts containing the growth hormone, or principle, at least partially counteract the stunting effects of hypophysectomy has supplied additional confirmation of the interrelationship in question. It is the skeletal reflections of hypopituitarism that will mainly concern us in the present discussion.

The underlying *pituitary lesion* responsible for hypopituitary dwarfism is not always the same. Most often the damage to the anterior lobe of the pituitary in these cases is due to destruction of the pituitary by a tumor arising from an embryonal rest of the craniopharyngeal canal. Such a tumor may develop from a rest located within the confines of the sella turcica and may remain limited to the sella, thus not injuring the midbrain. Under these conditions the subject comes to exhibit the effects of hypopituitarism alone, as expressed in the *Paltauf type* of dwarfism. More frequently, however, the tumor arises in the stalk region above the sella turcica, and there is damage both to the midbrain and the pituitary. In such cases the subject manifests the *Fröhlich type* of dwarfism. Indeed, most rests of the craniopharyngeal canal are located not in the anterior lobe proper but in the pars tuberalis of this lobe, which covers the stalk in front and behind. The tumors arising from such rests are commonly designated as craniopharyngiomas (see Cushing, and Erdheim).

Suprasellar pharyngiomas are likely to widen the mouth of the sella turcica, while the contour of the floor may remain unchanged. On the other hand, intrasellar tumors of this type tend to deform the floor of the sella while changing the mouth but little. Craniopharyngiomas are epithelial tumors. They may be solid, cystic, or partly solid and partly cystic. Their solid parts, particularly, tend to calcify and ossify, and they may become intimately adherent to the adjacent tissues. In consequence of the calcification, their presence is usually detectable on roentgenographic examination of the pituitary area.

The causes other than tumor formation which may give rise to pituitary dwarfism are less common. For instance, the dwarfism may follow upon injury to the pituitary from abnormalities in the development of the sella. Exceptionally, it ensues upon the formation of a chromophobe cell adenoma in the anterior pituitary lobe of a child. It may also result from congenital underdevelopment or cystic degeneration of the anterior lobe. It may even follow upon damage to the pituitary from an infection or from a local vascular disturbance due to an embolic thrombosis.

CLINICAL CONSIDERATIONS

The gravity of the clinical picture developing after actual damage to the pituitary in growing subjects depends upon a number of circumstances. One of these is, of course, the degree of damage to the pituitary. In this respect, however, there is a wide margin of safety. Even if the hypopituitarism has started in early childhood, the subject may not be severely stunted if a small part of the anterior lobe continues to function. The presence or absence of associated damage to the midbrain is another factor influencing the clinical picture.

In general, a lesion leading to hypopituitarism induces, in a growing subject, a pronounced immaturity and atrophy of the genital organs and a somatic underde-

23

velopment in which stunting of longitudinal growth is a conspicuous element. Furthermore, if the subject survives to an age at which the secondary sex characters and organs would normally be well differentiated, these are weakly developed. The various effects of the pituitary hypofunction are due to deficiency of the growth- and gonad-stimulating principles elaborated by the anterior lobe. In addition, because of the interrelation of this lobe with the adrenals and thyroid, these glands, too, are likely to undergo regressive anatomic changes. If pronounced hypopituitarism develops in subjects who have already completed their growth, skeletal dwarfing will be absent, although these subjects will show the other clinico-anatomic manifestations of pituitary hypofunction.

As noted, if the pituitary lesion is not associated with damage to the midbrain, the pituitary dwarfism can be said to be of the *Paltauf type*. In addition to the somatic and genital underdevelopment, dwarfs of this type present a slender and fragile build, thin skin, and very fine hair not profuse in amount. The intelligence is not affected. If the pituitary lesion is associated with damage to the midbrain, the dwarfism can be said to be of the *Fröhlich type*. Dwarfs of this type resemble the Paltauf type in genital underdevelopment and sexual immaturity but, in addition, show the plumpness and girdle-like adiposity of dystrophia adiposogenitalis. In these cases, if a suprasellar craniopharyngioma is present, there is strong likelihood that the tumor will also damage the optic chiasm, the hypothalamus, and certain cranial nerves. It may even cause hydrocephalus, through compression of the third ventricle or the foramen of Monro. In general, such patients usually come to suffer from such complaints as headaches and vomiting, visual disturbances (even amounting to blindness), hypersomnolence, and polyuria and polydipsia, in addition to manifestations due more specifically to the anterior pituitary hypofunction. It should also be pointed out that if, instead of being merely very deficient, the function of the anterior lobe becomes completely abolished, a pronounced hypophysial cachexia (the cachexia of Simmonds' disease) becomes engrafted upon the existing condition and the patient soon succumbs.

In the *treatment* of pituitary dwarfism appearing in consequence of solid or cystic craniopharyngiomas which are also producing neurological symptoms, surgical intervention is often required on the latter account. Such intervention is so serious a hazard to life, however, that it should not be undertaken unless the neurological

Figure 87

A, Photograph of part of the base of the skull (macerated specimen) from a case of hypopituitarism. Note that the cranial sutures are still wide open and that the sella turcica is considerably enlarged. The subject was a man 38 years of age and 56 inches tall who presented an infantile habitus and, in particular, underdevelopment of the masculine secondary sex characteristics. The hypopituitarism in this case had resulted from a benign cystic mixed tumor of the craniopharyngeal canal, which led to pronounced pressure atrophy of the pituitary gland.

B, Roentgenograph of the macerated specimen illustrated in A showing even more clearly that the various sutures are still wide open.

C, Photograph showing, from this case, part of the lower end of a femur sectioned in the frontal plane. Despite the fact that the subject was 38 years of age, the epiphysial cartilage plate is still clearly visible. It extends across the bone in a somewhat irregular, wavy course. (For the pertinent histologic findings, see Figs. 88-A and B.)

D and E, Photograph and roentgenograph, respectively, of the left innominate bone, still from the same case of hypopituitary dwarfism. Note that the epiphysis of the crest of the ilium has not yet fused with the body of that bone. Furthermore, fusion of the ilium, ischium, and pubis in the acetabular region has not yet occurred. Also, the inferior ramus of the pubis is not yet united with the ischium.

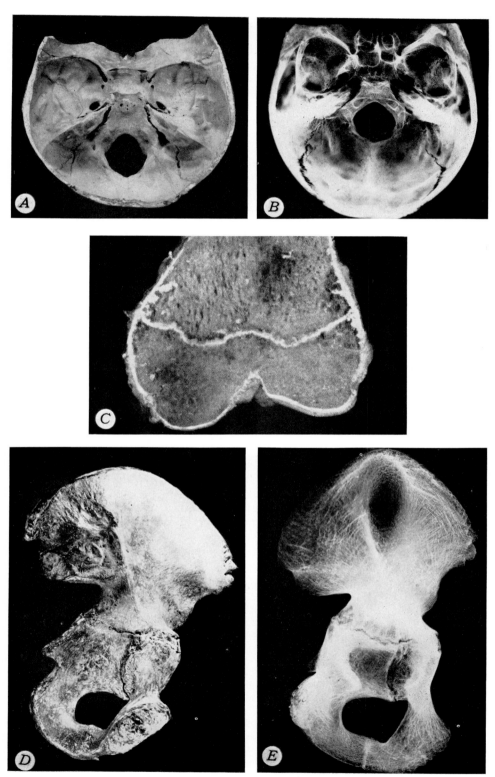

Figure 87

complaints are very severe indeed. In those cases without neurologic complaints, attempts may be made to correct the sexual and statural underdevelopment by the administration of the growth-promoting and gonadotropic hormones. However, it is in regard to growth that the best results are likely to be obtained, and it is growth hormone derived from human pituitary glands that is most effective. The use of thyroid in conjunction with the growth-promoting hormone involves the danger of instigating premature fusion of the epiphyses. Altogether, hormonal therapy in these cases, and especially for stunted children who apparently are suffering from merely "functional" hypopituitarism, should be employed with circumspection and only by one thoroughly familiar with its usage.

PATHOLOGY OF THE SKELETAL ALTERATIONS

In pituitary dwarfism the processes which underlie the condition of the skeleton are: (1) a delay in the appearance and growth of the centers of postnatal ossification; (2) a retardation and premature arrest of bone growth at epiphysial cartilage plates, sutures, and synchondroses; and (3) persistence of plates, sutures, and synchondroses far beyond the age at which they would normally have disappeared. For details on the normal chronology of postnatal ossification and epiphysial fusion, see Chapter 2.

A classic example of the skeletal changes to be observed in an adult hypopituitary dwarf was described by Erdheim. The subject was a man 56 inches tall who died at the age of 38. The bones, while small, were of fairly normal shape and proportions, although the stunting was not absolutely evenly distributed over the skeleton. In the skull the sutures (which are regions of bone growth) were found still wide open. The various components of the innominate bones had not yet fused either. Furthermore, the epiphysis for the crest of each ilium was still neither fully formed nor fused. The vertebrae, ribs, and tubular bones also showed persisting "arrested" growth zones. For instance, a sagittal section through the lower end of a femur revealed that an epiphysial cartilage plate was still present between the epiphysis and the shaft of the bone. (See Fig. 87.) The long bones of the pituitary dwarf 49 years of age described by Paltauf also showed persisting plates.

On *histologic examination* the persisting epiphysial cartilage plates of long bones in an adult pituitary dwarf show that their metaphysial surfaces are closed off by bone, and this renders endochondral ossification impossible even though the cartilage plates are still present. Thus, though they persist, the plates are functionally

Figure 88

A, Photomicrograph (× 9) illustrating the general histologic pattern of the persisting epiphysial cartilage plate at the lower end of the femur shown in Fig. 87-*C*. The plate is irregularly wavy, shows focal areas of degeneration, and is closed off by osseous tissue apposed on both its shaft surface (above) and epiphysial surface (below). The blocked-out area is represented under higher magnification in *B*. (The figures on this plate all relate to the same case, and the clinical data are in the legend pertaining to Figure 87.)

B, Photomicrograph (× 35) showing in greater detail the histologic appearance of the blocked-out area in *A*. In the central part of the picture, the cartilage of the plate still retains its hyaline intracellular matrix. There is also evidence of columnar arrangement of the cartilage cells in that portion of the plate which is closest to the epiphysis. However, evidence of endochondral ossification is lacking, and osseous tissue abuts upon the epiphysial surface of the plate.

C, Photomicrograph (× 28) of the costochondral junctional area of a rib in this case. Note that the cartilage cells in the junctional area are lined up in short columns—an arrangement which is clearly abnormal for an adult.

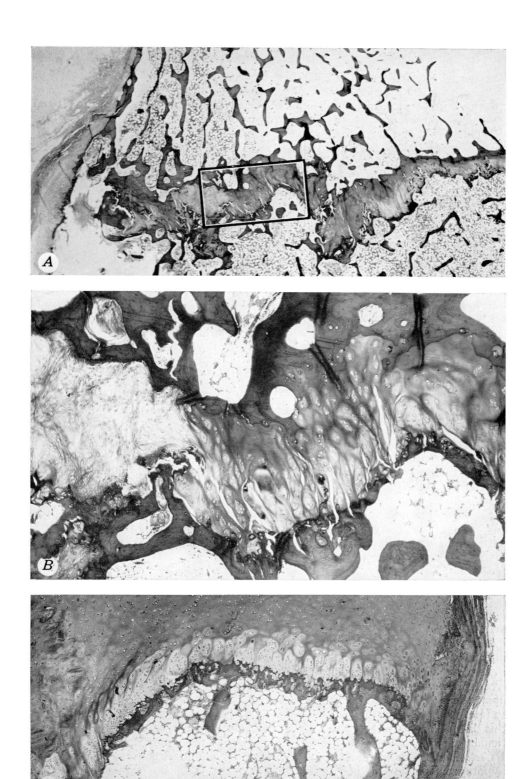

Figure 88

inactive. (See Fig. 88.) Even in subjects who have not yet reached adulthood, the plates appear more or less closed off by bone on their metaphysial surfaces, as is evident, for instance, also in the case reported by Altmann and in experimental findings on animals (see Becks *et al.*).

Some or all of the persisting plates may eventually disappear. The present writer has observed a case of pituitary dwarfism in a woman 49 years old and 47 inches tall in whom some of the epiphysial plates had vanished. Specifically, it appeared from the roentgenographs that the epiphyses of the iliac crests, the ischial tuberosities, the spinous processes of the vertebrae, and also some of the vertebral bodies were as yet unfused, while in the long bones the epiphyses had completely fused and the cartilage plates had disappeared. However, in the case reported by Priesel in which the subject lived to be 91 years of age, all the plates had finally vanished.

The skeletal changes in *thyroid dwarfism* are closely similar to those in pituitary dwarfism. It should be noted, however, that, on the whole, the skeleton of an adult pituitary dwarf is not so severely stunted as that of an adult thyroid dwarf (p. 347). The reason for this is that endemic or sporadic cretinism usually begins to be manifest shortly after birth, so that growth is stunted almost from the beginning. In contrast, hypopituitarism starting in childhood does not usually set in until the child is about 4 or 5 years of age, so that the child has had a chance to grow considerably before its growth is retarded. (It is interesting in this connection that by the end of the third year a normal child attains about half of its expected adult height.) Clinical discrimination between pituitary and thyroid dwarfism is easily possible on the basis of the grossly subnormal (idiotic or imbecilic) mentality of the cretin.

The differentiation between pituitary dwarfs and the malproportioned dwarfs of which *achondroplastics* (p. 193) are such striking examples also presents no problem. However, not every well-proportioned dwarf is a pituitary dwarf, either. Indeed, in an individual case it may be only after postmortem examination that it becomes possible to decide definitively whether one was dealing with pituitary dwarfism or dwarfism of some obscure type. As is apparent from the review of the subject of growth and maturation by Rössle, there are many poorly understood sorts of pathologically conditioned stunting and dwarfism, some of which do not fall into any clear-cut category even anatomically. The diagnostic problems relating to dwarfism in general have been discussed by McCune and by Wilkins, among others.

HYPOTHYROID DWARFISM

Cases of hypothyroidism fall into two categories—primary and secondary. In the primary cases the point of departure for the thyroid hypofunctioning is the thyroid itself. In the secondary cases the thyroid hypofunctioning results from a disordered interrelationship between the thyroid and the other glands of internal secretion. Primary hypothyroidism is the form represented notably by patients suffering from cretinism, myxedema setting in during childhood, or myxedema in adults following upon therapeutic thyroidectomy. Secondary hypothyroidism is seen in patients suffering from hypopituitarism and in some patients having Addison's disease. In this discussion we are concerned mainly with primary hypothyroidism and, in particular, with the skeletal manifestations of *cretinism* and *juvenile myxedema*.

Cretinism is the state of stunted physical, mental, and sexual development due to hypothyroidism starting in the first months of life. In some cases the underlying hypothyroidism results from an embryologic defect in thyroid development (thyroid aplasia) in a child whose parents are apparently normal. Usually, however, the hypothyroidism underlying cretinism is based on atrophy of the thyroid, conditioned by an iodine deficiency. In cretinism the thyroid is already abnormal during fetal life in consequence of this deficiency, and the continuance of the latter postnatally is associated with an early deterioration of the gland. These are the cases of so-called *endemic cretinism*. They center in regions in which simple goiter, also based on iodine deficiency, is likewise endemic in the population at large, and the cretins are often the children of goitrous mothers who themselves come from goitrous families. On the other hand, *juvenile myxedema* is a state of stunted physical and sexual and (to a lesser extent) mental development resulting from hypothyroidism starting in childhood but not in infancy. Such sporadic instances of hypothyroidism are usually due to degeneration of the thyroid. The underlying cause of the degeneration may be unknown, though sometimes it is the aftermath of inflammatory damage to the thyroid, following upon some infectious disease.

As to *hypothyroidism* setting in during *adult life*, it will suffice to say that the bone changes are negligible. In such cases the bones do tend, however, to show an increased compactness, or density, attributable to a decreased urinary excretion of calcium and phosphorus. In addition, arthritic changes of the character of osteoarthritis are common among patients developing myxedema during adult life (see Monroe). On rare occasions, *thyroid acropachy* develops in cases of hyperthyroidism following arrest of the disease by surgery or chemotherapy. The acropachy is manifested by periosteal new bone formation on the metacarpals, metatarsals and phalanges, and also by clubbing of the ends of the fingers and toes (see Thomas, King *et al.*, and Nixon and Samols).

CLINICAL CONSIDERATIONS

By the time an untreated hypothyroid infant is about a year old, its cretinism is clearly apparent in sluggishness of bodily activity, slowness of growth, and retardation of mental development. Specifically, it is soon evident that the child is late in sitting up, walking, and talking. In addition, the skin is myxedematously thickened and dry, the tongue large, and the voice hoarse. In the course of the next few years, the deficient growth becomes very conspicuous, especially in the extremities. There is usually also severe anemia and stubborn constipation associated with megacolon. The teeth show delayed eruption, and those which have erupted are imperfectly formed and manifest early decay. The mentality is now definitely subnormal, and it may even deteriorate to that of an imbecile or idiot as adult life approaches. Sexually, cretins remain immature, the gonads being atrophic and the secondary sex characters poorly developed.

In juvenile myxedema the changes tend in the same direction but are milder, especially in respect to mentality. Indeed, in these cases the stunted physical stature is often the central and dominating clinical feature. The various physical signs of thyroid deficiency in childhood, and the functional and biochemical findings helpful in arriving at a clinical diagnosis, have received considerable attention (see Wilkins and Fleischmann). In the latter connection, emphasis has been laid on the diagnostic importance of an elevated serum cholesterol value, its reduction under thyroid medication, and the tendency of the cholesterol value to rise again sharply some weeks after withdrawal of the medication.

A cretin who has reached adult age without adequate treatment may be only 3 feet or slightly more in height. However, since most cretins do receive some treatment, they usually attain a height of more than 4 feet though less than 5. The bones of the head and trunk show less stunting than those of the extremities. Hence, the adult cretin's extremities (and especially his legs) are disproportionately short in comparison with the total body length. Occasionally (notably in cases treated early and adequately), the retardation of growth is so mild that the subject is of almost average height for his sex and race.

In the *treatment* of cretinism, early diagnosis is imperative, for only through the institution of treatment during the first months of life is it still possible to avoid permanent cretinistic damage, especially to the brain. For this purpose, desiccated thyroid is used, the dosage varying with the age and needs of the individual patient. The treatment of juvenile myxedema is pursued along the same lines. Since preparations of desiccated thyroid vary greatly in strength and are not absorbed or tolerated to an equal extent by all subjects, the dosage is best controlled on the basis of the clinical effects on growth, skeletal maturation, and general well-being. The effect of thyroid upon older cretinistic imbeciles is disappointing, and, indeed, thyroid may even be contraindicated for them, since it tends to overstimulate the poorly controlled organism. In relation to prophylaxis, it appears desirable to prevent conception in myxedematous women for at least several months after their myxedema has been controlled, and to watch their offspring carefully for evidences of hypothyroidism.

PATHOLOGY OF THE SKELETAL ALTERATIONS

As already stated, the effects of hypothyroidism on the skeleton of a child are similar, in general, to those of hypopituitarism. They consist of: (1) delayed appearance and retarded growth of the various centers of postnatal ossification; (2) retarded bone growth at the epiphysial cartilage plates, synchondroses, and sutures; and (3) persistence of plates and sutures well beyond the age when they would normally have disappeared (see Langhans, de Quervain and Wegelin, and Benda). In an individual case the skeletal age, as revealed by the number and size of the postnatal centers of ossification, may be years (perhaps a decade or more) behind the chronologic age. (See Fig. 89.) For data on the normal chronology of postnatal ossification and epiphysial fusion, see Chapter 2.

Figure 89

A, Roentgenograph of a femur, tibia and fibula, and humerus removed at autopsy from a cretin 6 years of age. Centers of ossification are present only for the lower epiphysis of the femur, the upper epiphysis of the tibia, and the head of the humerus. Also, these centers are much smaller than they would be in a normal child 6 years of age. It is to be noted that ossification centers are not yet present for the head of the femur, the distal epiphysis of the tibia, and the capitulum of the humerus—centers which, in a normal child, are frequently present by the fourth month of life.

B, Roentgenograph of a hand and wrist also removed at autopsy in the case of the cretin 6 years of age. Note that no centers of ossification are present as yet in the cartilaginous epiphyses of the phalanges and metacarpal bones or in the cartilaginous precursors of any of the carpal bones. For instance, in a normal child a center of ossification for the proximal phalanx of the third finger is nearly always present by the end of the first year of life, and for the head of the third metacarpal bone by about the end of the second year of life.

C, Photomicrograph ($\times$ 12) illustrating the general histologic pattern of the epiphysial-diaphysial junctional area at the distal end of the fibula shown in *A*. It is clear even under this low magnification that active endochondral ossification is not occurring at the growth zone in question, despite the youthfulness of the subject. The juxta-epiphysial area slightly to the left of the center of this picture is shown under higher magnification in *D*.

D, Photomicrograph ($\times$ 35) demonstrating that, though the cartilage at the growth zone lines up in columns, cores of calcified cartilage matrix are not extending into the shaft, as would be normal at a site of active endochondral bone growth. Note also that the shaft surface of the cartilage growth zone has osseous tissue apposed on it. This represents an additional indication that endochondral ossification and hence longitudinal bone growth are impeded.

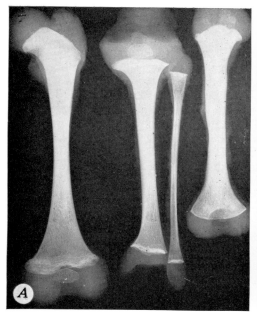

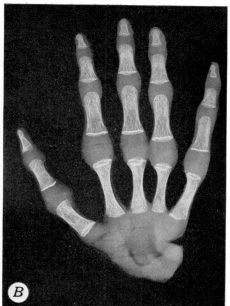

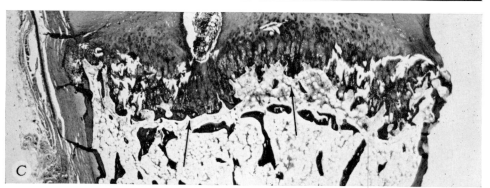

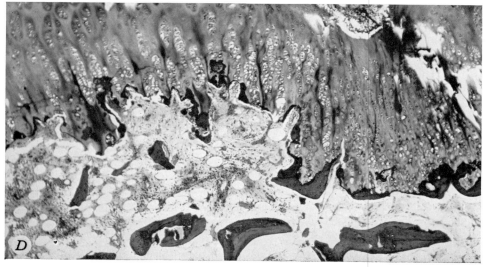

Figure 89

The dwarfism is referable mainly to the effects of the hypothyroidism on the epiphysial cartilage plates of the long bones. As noted, not only is endochondral ossification inhibited at the epiphysial cartilage plates, but the latter tend to persist, completely or in part, well beyond the normal ages for their disappearance. Thus, the plates of the long tubular bones may be found persisting even beyond the fourth decade. However, most of these plates and all the others ordinarily do disappear, albeit tardily, before this age period is reached. Histologically, the persisting epiphysial cartilage plates show little evidence of cartilage cell proliferation, and are closed off by bone which is apposed against the growth surface (that is, the surface facing the shaft of the bone). Hence, the continued presence of the plates does not create an opportunity for additional growth. It has also been observed that the synchondroses (for instance, between the individual segments of the sternum and sacrum and at the base of the skull) and the sutures of the calvarium are also usually very slow in disappearing.

In the cranium the retardation of growth is more severe in the floor than in the vault. As a result, a brachycephalic effect tends to be produced through foreshortening of the floor and a drawing in of the root of the nose in consequence of diminished growth at the spheno-occipital synchondrosis. The calvarium is occasionally thicker than it would normally be. The sella turcica is usually wide and deep. The lower jaw may become prognathous. These changes in the bones of the skull contribute greatly to the apelike countenance presented by some older cretins who have suffered from extreme hypothyroidism. Corresponding growth changes were noted in the skull bones of young thyroidectomized sheep (see Todd and Wharton).

Of interest also are certain changes observed roentgenographically in some of the postnatal centers of ossification and often referred to as "epiphysial dysgenesis." These changes are most common and most striking in the centers for the femoral heads and tarsal naviculars, though they may also be found in almost any other

Figure 90

A, Roentgenograph of part of a hand from the case of a male hypothyroid dwarf 24 years of age. Note that none of the epiphyses of the phalanges have fused as yet with the respective bone shafts. In normal subjects about 18 years of age, the epiphysial cartilage plates of these bones have usually become obliterated and the respective epiphyses fused with their shafts.

B, Roentgenograph of a knee area from the same hypothyroid dwarf as it appeared when the subject was 19 years of age. In at least 50 per cent of normal male subjects, the lower epiphysis of the femur is already fused with the shaft at about 19 years of age, and the upper epiphysis of the tibia is fused at about 18 years of age.

C, Roentgenograph showing the changes of "epiphysial dysgenesis" in the femoral heads of a male hypothyroid dwarf 29 years of age. He was born in a part of Austria in which goiter was endemic, and his mother and 2 sisters had large colloid goiters. Since his early childhood he had manifested retardation in growth and mental development. Note that the heads of both femurs are enlarged and flattened and appear fragmented. Over the years, the subject had received thyroid therapy but, for various reasons, only intermittently and in inadequate dosage. When he was 39 years of age, a resection angulation osteotomy was performed on the right hip because a severe disabling osteoarthritis had developed (see *D*).

D, Photomicrograph ($\times$ 8) of part of the right femoral head removed when the subject in the case also illustrated in *C* was 39 years of age. The inset shows the roentgenographic appearance of the femoral head just prior to its surgical resection. In the photomicrograph it is clearly apparent, even under the low magnification, that there are irregular islands of endochondral ossification in the interior of the head below the articular cartilage. The cartilage delimiting these islands of endochondral ossification has undergone degeneration in some places. The foci of endochondral ossification in the interior of the femoral head are represented in the roentgenograph by the small, roundish, radiolucent areas with clearly delimited radiopaque borders.

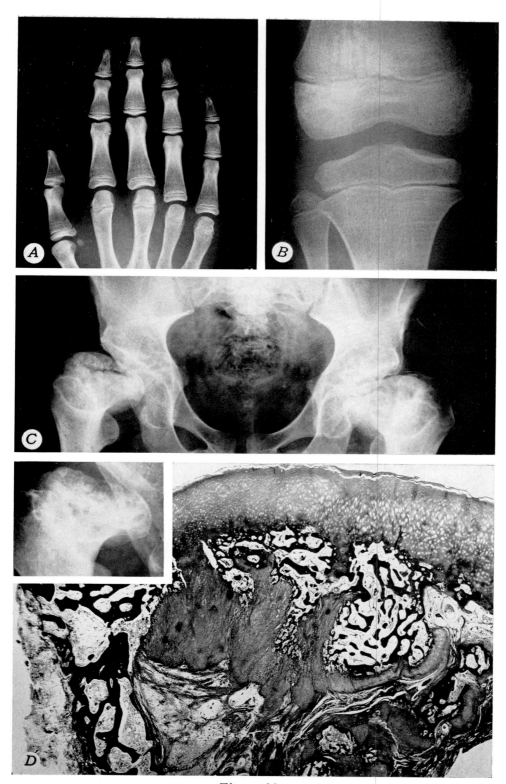

Figure 90

postnatal center. Epiphysial dysgenesis of the femoral capital epiphysis is also frequently observed in hypothyroidism of the juvenile myxedema type. In the affected centers (for instance, in the femoral heads), ossification proceeds very irregularly from multiple centers instead of from a single center. Hence, epiphysial dysgenesis in the femoral heads leads to changes which simulate roentgenographically those of Legg-Perthes disease. However, this "fragmented" appearance is the result of aberration in the endochondral ossification process in the head (see Looser). Thus it does not represent the aseptic necrosis of the head which is the basis of Legg-Perthes disease. Under treatment with thyroid, the "fragmented" appearance of the femoral head may substantially disappear within a year or two. During the course of the treatment, the abnormalities visible roentgenographically may at first be accentuated. If the hypothyroidism is not treated, however, the affected femoral head may undergo flattening and mushrooming. As a result of these changes, pronounced osteoarthritis of one or both hip joints may eventually develop. Occasionally one also finds a deformation of the upper end of the humerus (humerus varus) resulting from a sliding down of its head on the medial side. Sometimes the ossification of the lower end of the femur is so defective that bits of cartilage (with or without subchondral bone) break off and enter the knee joint, as they do in conventional osteochondritis dissecans. (See Fig. 90.)

HYPERTHYROIDISM

In adults suffering from hyperthyroidism of some years' duration, demineralization of the skeleton, often quite widespread, may be observed roentgenographically, though there may be no clinical complaints ascribable to the osteoporosis. If there are any, they are most likely to be merely vague aches and pains related to the back or limbs. However, pronounced osteoporosis of the vertebral column may result in collapse of one or more vertebrae and, thus, in definite pain and kyphosis. In some cases, fractures of ribs or even of long bones have followed upon relatively trivial trauma to the porotic bones (see Bartels and Haggart, and Bothe *et al.*). In the relatively infrequent instances in which toxic goiter appears in a young, growing subject, the latter is very likely to present, in time, clinical evidence of accelerated skeletal growth. In these cases, too, if the hyperthyroidism is of long standing, osteoporosis may become apparent.

It has been demonstrated that the osteoporosis has its basis in a negative mineral balance—that is, excess of outgo over intake of minerals (see Aub *et al.*, and Puppel *et al.*). The loss of minerals—particularly of calcium—occurs by way of both the urine and feces. The excess of calcium in the urine is usually not great enough to bring about an actual reversal of the normal ratio of urinary to fecal calcium, which is about 30:70. In this respect the negative mineral balance of hyperthyroidism contrasts with that of hyperparathyroidism (see p. 308). Furthermore, hyperthyroidism is not associated, as is hyperparathyroidism, with a strong tendency toward the formation of urinary calculi. Even in cases of hyperthyroidism in which the osteoporosis is pronounced, the serum calcium and inorganic phosphorus values are not increased above the normal. The serum alkaline phosphatase value is usually somewhat raised in such cases, perhaps to 6 or 8 Bodansky units per 100 cc.

The *treatment* of toxic goiter *per se* does not, of course, concern us here. The osteoporosis in particular can be largely or even completely forestalled by a high intake of calcium, phosphorus, and vitamin D. This regimen militates against the appearance of a negative mineral balance and the resultant skeletal demineralization. Since the feeding of a liberal and varied high caloric diet constitutes part of the medical treatment of toxic goiter, a rather high mineral intake is already assured. Nevertheless, 1 or 2 grams of supplementary calcium should be given daily to patients suffering from hyperthyroidism. This calcium should certainly be given if, for some reason, subtotal thyroidectomy has to be delayed or cannot be done.

After thyroidectomy, the osteoporosis often becomes completely corrected. However, it may be slow in clearing up, and supplementary calcium feeding is indicated then also. In older patients, if the osteoporosis does not yield to thyroidectomy, the probability is that some factor other than hyperthyroidism is also involved. Indeed, in older women the osteoporosis in a case of toxic goiter is quite likely to be related, at least in part, to the postmenopausal state.

PATHOLOGY OF THE SKELETAL ALTERATIONS

As already noted, in cases of toxic goiter appearing during childhood or adolescence, accelerated bone growth may occur. This is to be observed especially in subjects who were under 15 years of age when the hyperthyroidism set in. However, though the ultimate height of the subject often exceeds the average, he is not likely to become abnormally tall—that is, to manifest gigantism (see Holmgren). Evidently the tendency toward abnormal tallness is partly counteracted by the fact that the unduly stimulated epiphysial cartilage plates of the long bones tend to disappear earlier in these subjects than in normal persons, the epiphyses prematurely fusing with the diaphyses. In line with these clinical findings, there is the experimental finding that feeding toxic doses of thyroid to young rats leads to retardation or premature cessation of growth at the epiphysial plates of the long bones, apparently preceded by a period of stimulated growth (see Smith and McLean).

When the osteoporotic changes are advanced and grossly evident, they are rather widely distributed over the skeleton. If one strips the periosteum from a severely altered long bone, for instance, the rarefied cortex will appear strikingly hyperemic, and its outer surface will no longer be smooth. Such a bone can be cut with ease and, when opened, will show a great reduction in the quantity of the spongy trabeculae. Histologically, in a severely affected bone the osteoporosis is characterized by resorption of the cortical and spongy bone and replacement of them by connective tissue. In a femur studied by Askanazy and Rutishauser, the outer half of the bone cortex was more severely porotic than the inner. The resorptive process had led to enlargement of the vessel canals of the compacta. The enlarged canals were found filled with connective tissue containing some blood pigment and engorged blood channels, and the surfaces of the canals were indented by Howship's lacunae containing osteoclasts. Furthermore, in some places, new bone is to be found apposed upon what remains of the old. In the spongiosa, tracts of connective tissue dissecting the bony trabeculae will also be observed. Similar changes have been noted in the bones of animals receiving serial doses of thyroxin or desiccated thyroid. Indeed, in guinea pigs in whom feedings of thyroid extract had produced pronounced skeletal alterations, the bones presented resorptive and fibrotic changes simulating those of hyperparathyroidism, though of a lesser degree (see Silberberg and Silberberg).

THE CUSHING SYNDROME

In its full efflorescence, the Cushing syndrome includes: *osteoporosis* and also hirsutism, abdominal obesity, gonadal hypofunction, mild but insulin-resistant diabetes, hypertension, muscular weakness and wasting, and purplish skin striae due to disappearance of elastic fibers in the subcutaneous tissues. In addition, many of the patients manifest abnormal mental reactions, an increased susceptibility to infection, and poor healing response to surgical or accidental trauma. The condition is of rather rare occurrence. It is observed predominantly in females, and the subjects are most often in the third or fourth decade of life. A few instances of the Cushing syndrome in infants and young children have also been observed (see Darling *et al.*).

In the cases on which Cushing based his description of the disorder, he noted changes in the pituitary and in the adrenal glands. In particular, the pituitary abnormality noted was a basophil cell adenoma of the anterior lobe, and the adrenals were found enlarged in consequence of hyperplasia of their cortices. The disorder was denoted at first as "pituitary basophilism," because the hormonal aberration underlying the condition was originally held to be limited to the pituitary. However, it is now firmly established that adrenal cortical hyperfunctioning (from an adenoma, carcinoma, or merely physiological hyperactivity) plays a more direct and significant role in the production of the Cushing syndrome.

As noted, the abnormality commonly encountered in the *pituitary* is a basophil cell adenoma. This is usually located in the anterior lobe, though sometimes in the pars intermedia, and its presence is often associated with invasion of other portions of the gland by basophil cells. Be that as it may, it is held that the basophil cell adenoma formation *per se* does not have as much functional significance in relation to the Cushing syndrome as does the presence of a peculiar hyalinization and vacuolization of the basophil cells of the anterior lobe (see Crooke). However, cases have also been recorded in which all the characteristic clinical manifestations of the Cushing syndrome (including pronounced osteoporosis) have been present on the basis of an adrenocortical adenoma or carcinoma, while no adenoma or other readily discernible abnormality in the pituitary was present (see Oppenheimer *et al.*, Lescher and Robb-Smith, and Albright). It should also be noted that it is not unusual to encounter at autopsy a small pituitary adenoma composed of basophil cells, in the complete absence of the features of Cushing's syndrome (or indeed any other clinical manifestations of endocrinal dysfunction).

The cells of the *adrenal cortex* secrete gluco-corticoids (cortisol, cortisone, and corticosterones), mineralo-corticoids, androgens, estrogens, and other related compounds. Under normal conditions the secretion of these hormones is under the control of the anterior lobe of the pituitary, mediated by its secretion of the adrenocorticotropic hormone (corticotropin or ACTH). In the presence of hyperplasia of the cortex of one or both adrenal glands, or a benign or malignant tumor of the adrenal cortical tissue, the cortical cells secrete excessive amounts of the various steroid hormones in question. Under these conditions, hypersecretion of these hormones is largely independent of the stimulatory effect of ACTH (corticotropin) on the adrenal cortical cells.

In cases of the Cushing syndrome it is cortisol (hydrocortisone) and cortisone in particular that are elaborated in abnormal amounts by the adrenals. The hypercortisonism underlying the Cushing syndrome disturbs the metabolism of proteins. It seems to induce an inhibition of protein synthesis throughout the body, and this results in an excessive loss of nitrogen in the urine and feces.

The *treatment* in cases of the Cushing syndrome is necessarily directed toward reducing the output of adrenal hormones. However, it is often difficult to decide whether the treatment should first be directed toward the pituitary gland or toward the adrenal. This problem arises because of the variety of pathologic changes (often present in combination) to be observed in relation to these glands. Thus, in a particular case one may be dealing with: (1) a basophil cell adenoma (or other benign tumor) of the pituitary and hyperplasia of the adrenals; (2) hyperplasia of the adrenals and mere hyalinization (Crooke's change) of the basophil cells of the pituitary; or (3) an adenoma or carcinoma of one or both adrenals, with or without hyalinization of the basophil cells.

In the absence of roentgenographic changes in the region of the sella turcica and of clinical findings directly suggestive of a pituitary tumor, one should proceed to rule out the possibility of an adrenal tumor before undertaking treatment. Even if the presence of an adrenal tumor or other adrenal abnormality is not clearly established by x-ray examination, surgical exploration in search for an adrenal abnormality seems justifiable. In any event, surgery directed against the adrenals may well be supplemented or preceded by irradiation of the pituitary gland. However, the ultimate over-all prognosis is by no means good, irrespective of the therapeutic procedures employed (see Knowlton). Nevertheless, Glenn and Mannix maintain that the availability of replacement therapy has rendered total bilateral adrenalectomy a fairly safe procedure for hyperplasia of the adrenal cortex in cases of the Cushing syndrome.

PATHOLOGY OF THE SKELETAL ALTERATIONS

Insofar as the skeleton is concerned, the disturbance of protein synthesis in the Cushing syndrome is expressed in diminished formation of organic bone matrix (and in particular of collagen) consequent to depressed osteoblastic activity. Because wear-and-tear bone resorption (the resorption of endogenous metabolisom continues in these cases without being adequately counterbalanced by the formatin) of new bone, the total amount of osseous tissue gradually diminishes. Thus the osteoporosis of the Cushing syndrome results from a wasting away of the osseous substance. This contrasts with what is observed, for instance, in hyperparathyroidism. The latter condition is associated with active and aggressive osteoclastic bone resorption expressed in the formation of numerous Howship's lacunae and also in fibrous scarring of the bone marrow.

In brief, the osteoporosis associated with Cushing's syndrome represents what was designated by pathologists in the past as "smooth bone atrophy." In a sense, the term "bone atrophy" is more accurate anatomically than "osteoporosis" for characterizing the skeletal changes occurring not only as part of the Cushing syndrome but also in the postmenopausal and/or senescent state and under conditions of prolonged immobilization of a skeletal part. That is, we may appropriately speak of the bone atrophy associated with the Cushing syndrome, postmenopausal bone atrophy, and bone atrophy of inactivity.

In practically all cases of the Cushing syndrome, some degree of osteoporosis (bone atrophy) is apparent roentgenographically, at least in the calvarium, vertebral column, and ribs. The osteoporosis is pronounced and rather generalized in some cases, and the skeletal areas mentioned tend to be the ones most severely affected. Under these circumstances, roentgenographic examination of the vertebral column will show expansion of the intervertebral disks, and compressional collapse or wedging of some of the vertebral bodies may result in kyphotic deformity. Those vertebral bodies which have retained a relatively normal contour are likely to appear diffusely radiolucent, while those which have undergone compressional collapse appear rather radiopaque by comparison. (See Fig. 91.)

On microscopic examination of a porotic vertebral body which has largely retained its general contour (that is, has not undergone compressional collapse), one will note that the spongy trabeculae are abnormally thin and also sparse. The surfaces of such trabeculae show relatively few osteoblasts and are hardly pitted at all by Howship's lacunae. The intertrabecular marrow spaces contain myeloid and fatty marrow, and the proportion of fatty to myeloid marrow may be increased. The cortex of such a vertebral body is likewise even thinner than it would normally be. On the other hand, in a vertebral body which has undergone compressional collapse, one will note (especially in the vicinity of its superior and inferior surfaces) fragmented and aseptically necrotic spongy trabeculae, residual hemorrhage, fibrous scarring of the marrow, and new bone formation (endosteal callus).

While it is the vertebral column that ordinarily shows the most striking involvement in cases of the Cushing syndrome, the rest of the skeleton is, of course, not spared. The ribs in particular are likely to be very porotic and to show evidences of fractures, recent or healed. The long tubular bones are not found strikingly altered in shape, unless they have been fractured. In an intact long bone the periosteum is unaltered, but the cortex is thinned from the medullary side. On microscopic examination, such a cortex will show enlargement of the vessel canal spaces, but the latter contain no important amount of connective tissue. At the ends of the bone, the spongy trabeculae are also very thin. The marrow in the major marrow cavity and at the spongy ends is ordinarily very fatty. (See Mooser, Rutishauser, Follis, and also Sissons.)

Osteoporosis entirely analogous in its severity to what one may observe in cases of the Cushing syndrome may develop in a subject to whom natural or synthetic corticosteroids have been administered over long periods of time. For instance, it is not infrequently encountered as a side effect in the course of treatment of rheumatoid arthritis with corticosteroids (see Rosenberg, and Murray).

Irrespective of the occurrence of osteoporosis, patients suffering from rheumatoid arthritis (or various other diseases) and treated with corticosteroids occasionally develop destructive changes at the articular bone ends of one or another joint (see Chandler et al., and Heimann and Freiberger). The joint areas most often affected are the hip, knee, and shoulder. The joint involved may come to present changes which are occasionally so severe that they suggest those of a so-called "Charcot

Figure 91

A, Roentgenograph showing, in A-P projection, the thoracic part of the vertebral column and parts of the ribs from a case of Cushing's syndrome. The bones are strikingly porotic. The patient was a woman 30 years of age whose presenting skeletal complaints were pain in the back and weakness of the lower extremities of 6 months' duration. A few months before the onset of these complaints, amenorrhea had set in. The physical findings included truncal obesity, a rounded, moon-shaped face, and facial hirsutism. The Cushing syndrome in this case had its basis in an adenoma of the cortex of the right adrenal gland, the adenoma measuring approximately 4 × 3.5 × 1.5 cm.

B, Photograph showing, in sagittal section, part of the vertebral column, removed at autopsy, in the case of a woman 53 years of age who had presented the Cushing syndrome. The bodies of a number of the thoracic vertebrae and the first four lumbar vertebrae show evidences of compressional collapse following in the wake of pronounced osteoporosis. The patient's clinical complaints at the time of admission to the hospital had included pain in the back, facial hirsutism, weakness of the lower extremities, and truncal obesity. She had also presented the characteristic rounded "moon face," and was found to have hypertension, glycosuria, and elevated levels of urinary 17-ketosteroids and 17-hydroxycorticosteroids. The manifestations of the Cushing syndrome in her case were established as having their basis in a carcinoma of the right adrenal gland. (I am indebted to Dr. Hubert A. Sissons of the Royal National Orthopaedic Hospital of London for this photograph and the pertinent clinical data.)

C, Photomicrograph (× 4) of a tissue section prepared from the eleventh thoracic vertebral body shown in *B*. Note the general sparsity of the spongy trabeculae. Above and to the right, the dark-staining area in the vertebral body represents intervertebral disk tissue which had herniated into the body. Below and to the right, there is an area of reactive new bone formation in the vertebral body, representing internal callus.

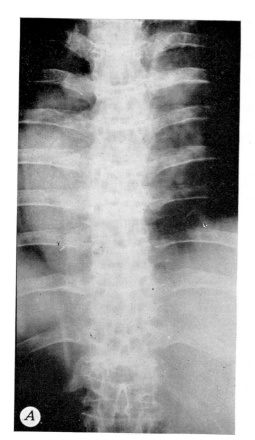

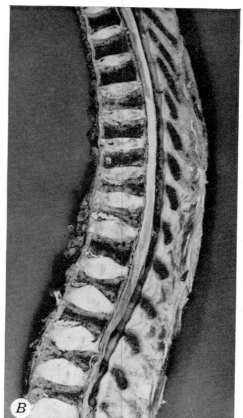

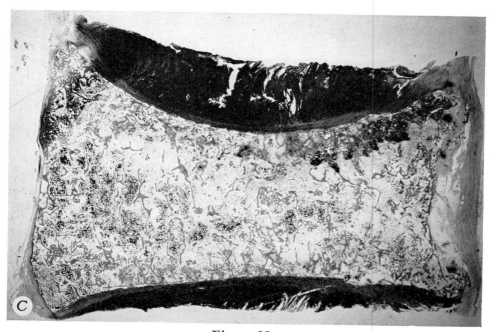

Figure 91

arthropathy." This complication has usually been observed in the wake of prolonged oral, subcutaneous, and/or intra-articular administration of cortisone and hydrocortisone, in particular. The writer has even noted the occurrence of severe destructive changes in the articular bone ends of a shoulder joint three months after the patient received only one intra-articular injection of cortisone. (See also Bentley and Goodfellow.)

The pathogenesis of *"cortisone-wrecked joints"* remains a puzzling question. In this connection it should be noted that analogous changes have *not* been reported as occurring in the large diarthrodial joints in cases of the Cushing syndrome of natural origin. It has been postulated that the articular changes sometimes observed after the administration of corticosteroids have their inception in aseptic bone necrosis. More particularly, the latter is held to result from alterations which the corticosteroids have induced in the vascular system of the affected articular bone ends. The subsequent disintegration of the joint has been thought to have its cause in reduced sensitivity of the part to accidental or undue functional trauma. (See Fig. 92.)

Whatever the pathogenesis of the "cortisone-wrecked joints," it is significant that analogous destructive articular changes were not reported during the early period of steroid hormone therapy—that is, when crude adrenocortical extracts were being administered in the course of treatment of various diseases. One explanation for

Figure 92

A, Roentgenograph of part of the vertebral column in a case of rheumatoid arthritis treated with cortisone over a period of two years. The vertebral column had become severely porotic, and a number of the vertebral bodies underwent compressional collapse. The two collapsed bodies shown in the picture are those of the eighth and ninth thoracic vertebrae. The patient was a woman 58 years of age who, in the course of her treatment with cortisone, came to manifest certain features of the Cushing syndrome, to wit: fullness of the face, facial hirsutism, and girdle obesity. For about one year before admission to the hospital, she had complained of pain in the lower part of the back. This pain increased decidedly after a fall in which she injured her back. Shortly after the fall she also complained of pain in the lower part of her left leg (see *B*).

B, Roentgenograph showing the lower part of the left tibia and fibula in this case. The bones are porotic, the cortices in particular being thin. A transverse fissure fracture (barely observable) extends across the tibia, and a small amount of callus is present on the medial surface of the tibia at the site of the infraction.

C, Roentgenograph of the right shoulder region showing pronounced alterations in the shoulder joint which had ensued upon the local injection of hydrocortisone. The patient was a man of middle age who came under medical care for pain in the right shoulder region. The x-ray pictures taken about one month after the onset of the pain showed that the latter was evidently due to the presence of calcification in the area of the supraspinatus tendon and subdeltoid bursa. At that time, however, the structure and contour of the bones entering into the formation of the shoulder joint appeared normal. After those x-ray pictures were taken, the man received 8 injections of hydrocortisone into the shoulder region over a period of about 3 weeks. The steroid-induced alterations which evolved in the articular ends of the joint in the course of the following year are revealed in this picture.

D, Roentgenograph of a knee joint (left) illustrating a steroid-induced arthropathy. The patient was a man 53 years of age who had been suffering from rheumatoid arthritis for 12 years and who had been receiving steroid hormone therapy (orally administered) for about 18 months prior to the time this x-ray picture was taken. For about one year previously the patient had been limping because the knee joint was particularly painful and swollen. The medial plateau of the tibia is depressed, and the femoral condyles show subchondral infractions. The roentgenographic appearances resemble those sometimes observed in connection with relatively mild tabetic arthropathy.

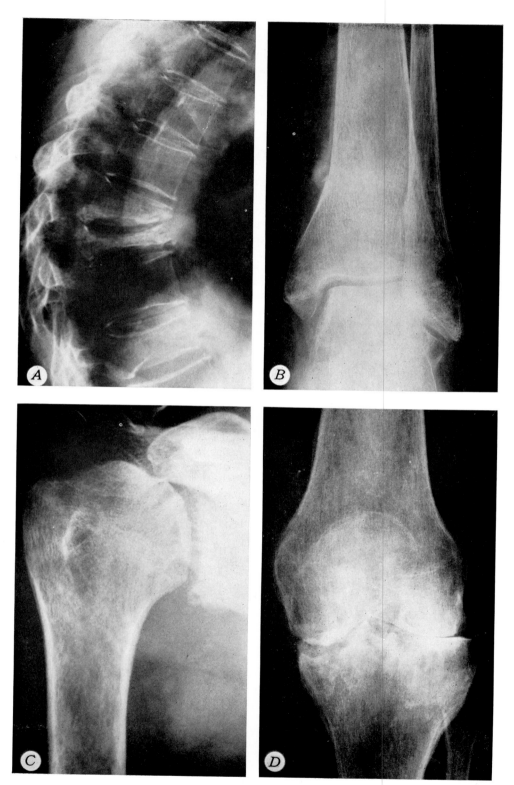

Figure 92

this may be that the crude extracts contained steroid hormones other than cortisone and hydrocortisone, and that some of these other steroid hormones (possibly androgenic in action) "antagonized" the effects of cortisone and hydrocortisone. This idea would also be in line with the fact that destructive articular changes do not occur in cases of the Cushing syndrome of natural origin (see Kream).

EUNUCHISM AND GONADAL DYSGENESIS

The fullest available studies on *eunuchs* are those which have been undertaken on male subjects castrated in childhood for various religious purposes. The members of the Skopze sect of male castrates have presented a very favorable opportunity for observing on a large scale the physical characteristics of eunuchs (see Pelikan). The effects of the testicular deficiency are much more prominent in eunuchs than in merely eunuchoid persons. In the latter the hypogonadism, though likewise originating in childhood, is a partial one, usually following upon trauma or disease.

Eunuchs who have been castrated well before puberty tend toward the feminine in their configuration. Notably, they may have narrow shoulders and broad hips. They also show a lack of hair on the face, axillae, and perineum, and a female type and distribution of the hair in the pubic and scalp regions. The skin is pale and poor in pigment. There is also a feminine tendency toward the accumulation of pads of fat in special regions—for instance, in the breasts and buttocks and over the iliac crests, the femoral trochanters, and the symphysis pubis. The voice is falsetto. The accessory sex organs, such as the penis, seminal vesicles, and prostate, are highly atrophic. The thyroid is usually small and involuted. On the other hand, the thymus is enlarged in consequence of delayed involution, and the anterior lobe of the pituitary is enlarged because of the presence of large numbers of "castration cells."

Concerning the *skeletal alterations*, it is clear that human adult males who had been castrated tend to be rather tall. Also, both their upper and their lower extremities are excessively long in proportion to the trunk (see Becker). In regard to the individual long bones of the extremities, it appears that the excess of growth tends to be greatest in the femora. Furthermore, all the long tubular bones are likely to be gracile, since their increase in diameter is not proportional to their increase in length.

It should be noted as one of the skeletal peculiarities found in castrates that the epiphysial cartilage plates (and possibly even sutures) persist beyond the age when they would normally have disappeared. In contrast to the persisting plates in hypo-

Figure 93

A, Photograph of the skeleton of a eunuchoid man 28 years of age and 6 feet in height. It is apparent that the bones of the extremities are disproportionately long in relation to the trunk. Also, it is to be noted that (because of persistence of the epiphysial cartilage plates) the iliac crests and the femoral heads have not yet fused with the rest of their respective bones. (Reproduced, with permission, from the monograph of Tandler and Grosz.)

B and *C*, Roentgenographs from the case of a eunuch 33 years of age. Note that the crest of the ilium, the lower epiphysis of the femur, and the upper epiphysis of the tibia and also the fibula have not yet fused with their corresponding bone parts, and the respective epiphysial cartilage plates have persisted.

D, Photomicrograph ($\times$ 15) showing persistence of epiphysial cartilage plate tissue between the head and shaft of a humerus in the case of a woman 32 years of age affected with hypogonadism due to congenital absence of the ovaries. Persisting cartilage plates were evident also in the innominate bones, long tubular bones, and even the phalanges. Note that the cartilage cells are lined up in columns at the surface of the plate abutting on the shaft of the bone.

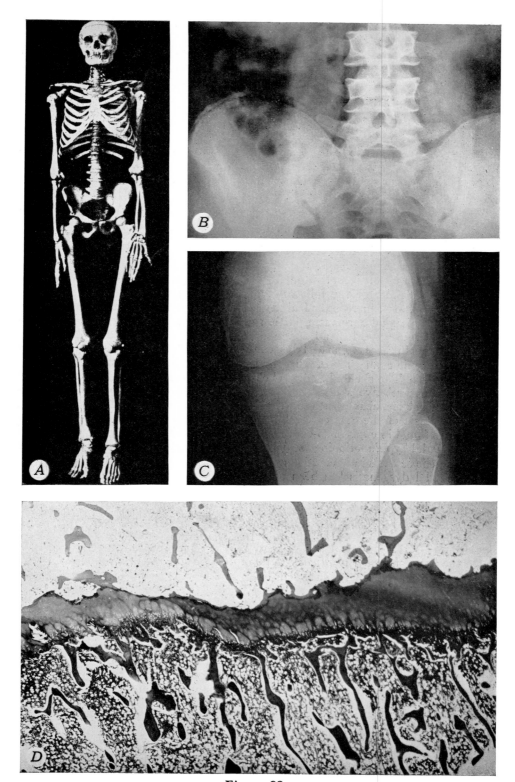

Figure 93

thyroid and hypopituitary dwarfism, the plates in cases of primary hypogonadism continue to be functionally active. This fact, of course, creates the possibility of the continuance of longitudinal growth beyond the usual growth period—a continuance which is registered notably in the long tubular bones. The skull seems to show no striking abnormalities in size or shape, though prominence of the supraorbital ridges has been recorded. Enlargement of the sella turcica, apparently resulting from hypertrophy of the anterior lobe of the pituitary, has been noted (see Tandler and Grosz). The pelvis of the castrate tends to take on the feminine configuration, though it is usually larger than the pelvis of the normal female. Thus there is often a flaring of the iliac bones and a large pelvic outlet. Finally, it may be appropriate to note that the larynx is much smaller in the castrated than in the normal man because the cartilages of the larynx fail to attain their proper size. (See Fig. 93.)

In recent years, attention has also been directed to skeletal abnormalities appearing in association with *gonadal dysgenesis* (see Finby and Archibald, Dalla Palma *et al.*, Levin and Kupperman, and also Kosowicz). The affected subjects have hypoplastic or aplastic gonads and female external genitalia. In addition, they present one or more of the following: primary amenorrhea, minimal secondary sexual development, increased pituitary secretion of follicle-stimulating hormone, and a negative sexual chromatin pattern usually characterized by a total chromosome count of 45 (XO) instead of the normal 46.

The subjects in cases of gonadal dysgenesis tend to be of short stature and to show roentgenographic changes resembling in a general way those of dysplasia epiphysialis multiplex. The skeletal findings held to be particularly suggestive of gonadal dysgenesis are: relative shortness of the fourth metacarpal bone, tibia vara deformity at the knee, changes at the wrist resembling those of Madelung's deformity, and hyperplasia of the first cervical vertebra. However, the various skeletal abnormalities found in cases of so-called gonadal dysgenesis are not really determined by the gonadal hypofunctioning as such. They can be interpreted more plausibly as having a genetic basis in aberrations of genes which are merely closely linked. Indeed, gonadal dysgenesis has been observed among females who do not present skeletal abnormalities (see Hoffenberg and Jackson).

DIABETES MELLITUS

On the basis of *roentgenographic studies* of *diabetic children* in whom the diabetes was of recent onset, it has been noted that: (1) The centers of postnatal ossification tend to show a development slightly in advance of the chronologic age, and (2) the body height is likely to be somewhat above average. However, in children with diabetes of long standing, the centers of postnatal ossification are likely to be less fully developed than in controls of the same age. Furthermore, as exemplified in the tibia, the long bones of these latter diabetics are gracile, the transverse diameter half way down the shaft being less than in the controls, and the cortex also being thinner than normal. In addition, transverse striae (Harris lines) are frequently encountered roentgenographically in the metaphyses of the long bones of these children. The earlier in childhood the diabetes has set in, the more pronounced are these various evidences of skeletal retardation likely to be. In certain children in whom the disease is of some years' duration, the long bones may also present evidences of osteoporosis and even be below average in length (see Morrison and Bogan).

The bones of an *adult diabetic* in whom the disease first appeared in middle life ordinarily present no abnormalities roentgenographically if nutrition has remained reasonably adequate. This is true even when the arteries of the extremities have become strikingly calcified, unless such factors as infection, inactivity, and tro- phoneurotic influences have had time to affect the bones (see Jaffe and Pomeranz). The occasional occurrence of neuropathic arthropathy (the so-called Charcot joint) in cases of diabetes mellitus of long standing is now a recognized complication of that disease. This complication is discussed elsewhere, since it has its immediate basis in a neural disturbance rather than in the endocrine disorder (see p. 866).

Another finding to be mentioned in connection with diabetes of adults is *dis- coloration of the bones*. This was first observed by Schmorl, who noted it, especially in the calvarium, at autopsies on adults who had suffered from diabetes mellitus. In particular, the calvarium in these cases very frequently showed a golden or muddy brown-yellow discoloration. This color change was so striking and charac- teristic that he regarded its presence, especially in the muddy brown form, as con- stituting by itself a rather reliable anatomic basis for a diagnosis of diabetes mellitus at the autopsy table. In fact, a corresponding discoloration was noted in only 3 of almost 2,000 calvaria of non-diabetic patients. Furthermore, it is rather unusual to find a calvarium of a diabetic which does not show at least some degree of yellow discoloration. In only 2 of Schmorl's 46 autopsied cases of diabetes was the yellow coloration absent entirely (the calvarium being gray or gray-white), and in these 2 cases the subjects were young.

As to the distribution of the discoloration, it was found that in the calvarium it involved both tables and the diploë. It was also observed on the floor of the cranial cavity after the dura had been stripped away. Furthermore, it was noted in the more superficial layers of the compacta of long tubular bones, but it was never so intense in these bones as in the calvarium. As yet, the substance responsible for the yellow color has not been identified either by chemical analysis of the bones or by microscopic examination. It has been proposed that it may be of the nature of the vegetable dye carotene or be in some way connected with the hypercholesterolemia so common in advanced cases of diabetes mellitus. Such suppositions still await proof.

THE ADRENOGENITAL SYNDROME

The clinical manifestations of the *adrenogenital syndrome* (adrenal virilism) are the result of excessive androgen secretion by the adrenal cortical cells in consequence of hyperplasia of the cortex of the glands or the development of a benign or malignant cortical tumor. In a female fetus, a suprarenal cortical tumor, for instance, instigates penis-like enlargement of the clitoris, associated with atrophy of the uterus and ovaries (pseudohermaphroditism), while in a male fetus it exaggerates the male sex characteristics. In a young child, such a tumor induces pubertas praecox. This has been observed mainly in male children, in whom it is manifest in premature and excessive development of the sex organs and early appearance of secondary sex characters. The subject is likely to become a so-called "little Hercules." That is, he may develop, quite prematurely, the muscular strength and primary and secondary sex characters of an adult male. If the tumor is malignant, death may ensue early from metastases. If it is not, there may be some acceleration of growth at first, but this tends to be counteracted by premature obliteration of the epiphysial cartilage plates, so that the subject ultimately fails to attain average stature for his age. In a female child the effects of a suprarenal cortical tumor are the same as in a male, so far as the skeleton is concerned. In addition, there is hypertrophy of the clitoris, obesity, and an abnormal growth of body hair with male distribution (see Glynn, Gallais, and also Jailer).

Among adults the virilizing effects of suprarenal cortical hyperplasia or tumor formation have been observed mainly in females. In adult females the virilism is manifested in hirsutism, amenorrhea, clitoral enlargement, breast atrophy, acne, voice changes, excessive muscular development, and loss of libido. When an adrenal carcinoma is present, the patient may even show some of the manifestations of the Cushing syndrome in addition to virilism. In particular, there may be hypertension, impaired glucose tolerance, and purplish skin striae, but generalized and pronounced osteoporosis, such as one sees in connection with the Cushing syndrome, is not likely to be manifest.

REFERENCES

ADAMS, J. E., SEYMOUR, R. J., EARLL, J. M., TUCK, M., SPARKS, L. L., and FORSHAM, P. H.: Transsphenoidal Cryohypophysectomy in Acromegaly, J. Neurosurg., *28*, 100, 1968.

ALBRIGHT, F.: Cushing's Syndrome, Harvey Lect., *38*, 123, 1942–43.

ALTMANN, F.: Hypophysärer Zwergwuchs bei einem weiblichen Individuum, Beitr. path. Anat., *85*, 205, 1930.

ASKANAZY, M. and RUTISHAUSER, E.: Die Knochen der Basedow-Kranken. Beitrag zur latenten Osteodystrophia fibrosa, Virchows Arch. path. Anat., *291*, 653, 1933.

AUB, J. C., BAUER, W., HEATH, C., and ROPES, M.: Studies of Calcium and Phosphorus Metabolism. III. The Effects of the Thyroid Hormone and Thyroid Disease, J. Clin. Invest., *7*, 97, 1929.

BARTELS, E. C. and HAGGART, G. E.: Osteoporosis in Hyperthyroidism, New England J. Med., *219*, 373, 1938.

BECKER, P. F.: Ueber das Knochensystem eines Castraten, Arch. Anat. u. Physiol. (Anatomische Abteilung), p. 83, 1899.

BECKS, H., SIMPSON, M. E., and EVANS, H. M.: Ossification at the Proximal Tibial Epiphysis in the Rat, Anat. Rec., *92*, 109, 1945.

BEHRENS, L. H. and BARR, D. P.: Hyperpituitarism Beginning in Infancy. The Alton Giant, Endocrinology, *16*, 120, 1932.

BENDA, C. E.: *Mongolism and Cretinism*, 2nd ed., New York, Grune & Stratton, 1949.

BENTLEY, G., and GOODFELLOW, J. W.: Disorganisation of the Knees Following Intra-articular Hydrocortisone Injections, J. Bone & Joint Surg., *51-B*, 498, 1969.

BOTHE, F. A., SIMPSON, H. M., and ROWNTREE, L. G.: Traumatic and Spontaneous Fractures in Exophthalmic Goiter, Surg., Gynec. & Obst., *75*, 357, 1942.

CHANDLER, G. N., JONES, D. T., WRIGHT, V., and HARTFALL, S. J.: Charcot's Arthropathy Following Intra-articular Hydrocortisone, Brit. M.J., *1*, 952, 1959.

CROOKE, A. C.: A Change in the Basophil Cells of the Pituitary Gland Common to Conditions Which Exhibit the Syndrome Attributed to Basophilic Adenoma, J. Path. & Bact., *41*, 339, 1935.

CUSHING, H.: *The Pituitary Body and its Disorders*, Philadelphia, J. B. Lippincott Co., 1912.

————: The Basophil Adenomas of the Pituitary Body and Their Clinical Manifestations (Pituitary Basophilism), Bull. Johns Hopkins Hosp., *50*, 137, 1932.

————: *Intracranial Tumours*, Springfield, Charles C Thomas, 1932.

————: "Dyspituitarism": Twenty Years Later, with Special Consideration of the Pituitary Adenomas, Arch. Int. Med., *51*, 487, 1933.

DALLA PALMA, L., CAVINA, C., GIUSTI, G. and BORGHI, A.: Skeletal Development in Gonadal Dysgenesis, Female in Phenotype, Am. J. Roentgenol., *101*, 876, 1967.

DARLING, D. B., LORIDAN, L., and SENIOR, B.: The Roentgenographic Manifestations of Cushing's Syndrome in Infancy, Radiology, *96*, 503, 1970.

DASHE, A. M., SOLOMON, D. H., RAND, R. W., FRASIER, S. D., BROWN, J., and SPEARS, I.: Stereotaxic Hypophyseal Cryosurgery in Acromegaly and Other Disorders, J.A.M.A., *198*, 591, 1966.

DAVIDOFF, L. M.: Studies in Acromegaly. III. The Anamnesis and Symptomatology in One Hundred Cases, Endocrinology, *10*, 461, 1926.

ERDHEIM, J.: Nanosomia pituitaria, Beitr. path. Anat., *62*, 302, 1916.

————: Über Wirbelsäulenveränderungen bei Akromegalie, Virchows Arch. path. Anat., *281*, 197, 1931.

————: *Die Lebensvorgänge im normalen Knorpel und seine Wucherung bei Akromegalie*, Berlin, Julius Springer, 1931.

FINBY, N. and ARCHIBALD, R. M.: Skeletal Abnormalities Associated with Gonadal Dysgenesis, Am. J. Roentgenol., *89*, 1222, 1963.

FOLLIS, R. H., JR.: The Pathology of the Osseous Changes in Cushing's Syndrome in an Infant and in Adults, Bull. Johns Hopkins Hosp., *88*, 440, 1951.

GALLAIS, A.:   Le Syndrome génito-surrénal, Paris Thèses, No. 225, 1912.

GLENN, F., and MANNIX, H., JR.:   Diagnosis and Prognosis of Cushing's Syndrome, Surg. Gynec. & Obst., *126*, 765, 1968.

GLYNN, E. E.:   The Adrenal Cortex, its Rests and Tumours; its Relation to other Ductless Glands, and especially to Sex, Quart. J. Med., *5*, 157, 1912.

GORDON, D. A., HILL, F. M., and EZRIN, C.:   Acromegaly: Review of 100 Cases, in *Year Book of Endocrinology*, p. 93, 1962–1963 Series.

HEIMANN, W. G. and FREIBERGER, R. H.:   Avascular Necrosis of the Femoral and Humeral Heads after High-Dosage Corticosteroid Therapy, New England J. Med., *263*, 672, 1960.

HOFFENBERG, R. and JACKSON, W. P. U.:   Gonadal Dysgenesis in Normal-looking Females: A Genetic Theory to Explain Variability of the Syndrome, Brit. M. J., *1*, 1281, 1957.

————:   Gonadal Dysgenesis: Modern Concepts, Brit. M. J., *2*, 1457, 1957.

HOLMGREN, J.:   *Uber den Einfluss der Basedow'schen Krankheit und verwandter Zustände auf das Längenwachstum*, Leipzig, Metzger & Wittig, 1909.

HUMBERD, C. D.:   Giantism. Report of a Case, J.A.M.A., *108*, 544, 1937.

JAFFE, H. L. and POMERANZ, M. M.:   Changes in the Bones of Extremities Amputated Because of Arteriovascular Disease, Arch. Surg., *29*, 566, 1934.

JAILER, J. W.:   Virilism, Chapt. 11 in *Hormones in Health and Disease*, edited by R. L. Craig, New York, The Macmillan Co., 1954.

KEITH, A.:   An Inquiry into the Nature of the Skeletal Changes in Acromegaly, Lancet, *1*, 993, 1911.

KING, L. R., BRAUNSTEIN, H., CHAMBERS, D., and GOLDSMITH, R.:   A Case Study of Peculiar Soft-Tissue and Bony Changes in Association with Thyroid Disease, J. Clin. Endocrinol., *19*, 1323, 1959.

KNOWLTON, A. I.:   Cushing's Syndrome, Chapt. 12 in *Hormones in Health and Disease*, edited by R. L. Craig, New York, The Macmillan Co., 1954.

KOSOWICZ, J.:   The Deformity of the Medial Tibial Condyle in Nineteen Cases of Gonadal Dysgenesis, J. Bone & Joint Surg., *42-A*, 600, 1960.

————:   The Roentgen Appearance of the Hand and Wrist in Gonadal Dysgenesis, Am. J. Roentgenol., *93*, 354, 1965.

KREAM, J.:   Personal communication.

LANGHANS, T.:   Anatomische Beiträge zur Kenntniss der Cretinen. (Knochen, Geschlechtsdrüsen, Muskeln und Muskelspindeln nebst Bemerkungen über die physiologische Bedeutung der letzteren.), Arch. path. Anat., *149*, 155, 1897.

LESCHER, F. G. and ROBB-SMITH, A. H. T.:   History of a Case of Carcinoma of the Adrenal Cortex with Cushing's Syndrome, Proc. Roy. Soc. Med., *27¹*, 404, 1933–34.

LEVIN, J., and KUPPERMAN, H. S.:   Skeletal Abnormalities in Gonadal Dysgenesis, Arch. Int. Med., *113*, 730, 1964.

LOOSER, E.:   Über die Ossifikationsstörungen bei Kretinismus, Verhandl. deutsch. path. Gesellsch.: *24*, 352, 1929.

MADDY, J. A., WINTERNITZ, W. W., NORREL, H., QUILLEN, D., and WILSON, C. B.:   Acromegaly, Treatment by Cryoablation, Ann. Int. Med., *71*, 497, 1969.

MARIE, P.:   Sur deux cas d'acromégalie; hypertrophie singulière noncongénitale des extrémités supérieures, inférieures et céphalique, Rev. méd., *6*, 297, 1886.

McCUNE, D. J.:   Dwarfism, Clinics, *2*, 380, 1943.

MONROE, R. T.:   Chronic Arthritis in Hyperthyroidism and Myxedema, New England J. Med., *212*, 1074, 1935.

MOOSER, H.:   Ein Fall von endogener Fettsucht mit hochgradiger Osteoporose, Virchows Arch. path. Anat., *229*, 247, 1920–21.

MORRISON, L. B. and BOGAN, I. K.:   Bone Development in Diabetic Children, Am. J. M. Sc., *174*, 313, 1927.

MURRAY, R. O.:   Steroids and the Skeleton, Radiology, *77*, 729, 1961.

NIXON, D. W., and SAMOLS, E.:   Acral Changes Associated With Thyroid Diseases, J.A.M.A., *212*, 1175, 1970.

OPPENHEIMER, B. S., GLOBUS, J. H., SILVER, S., and SHASKIN, D.:   Suprarenal Virilism and Cushing's Pituitary Basophilism, Tr. A. Am. Physicians, *1*, 371, 1935.

PALTAUF, A.:   *Uber den Zwergwuchs in anatomischer und gerichtsärztlicher Beziehung*, Vienna, A. Hölder, 1891.

PELIKAN, E.:   *Gerichtlich-medizinische Untersuchungen über das Skopzenthum in Russland*, Giessen, J. Ricker, 1876.

PRIESEL, A.:   Ein Beitrag zur Kenntnis des hypophysären Zwergwuchses, Beitr. path. Anat., *67* 220, 1920.

PUPPEL, I. D., GROSS, H. T., McKORMICK, E. K., and CURTIS, G. M.:   Calcium, Phosphorus and Vitamin D Therapy in Hyperthyroidism, J.A.M.A., *121*, 1175, 1943.

DE QUERVAIN, F., and WEGELIN, C.: *Der endemische Kretinismus*, Berlin, Julius Springer, 1936.

ROSENBERG, E. F.: Rheumatoid Arthritis, Osteoporosis and Fractures Related to Steroid Therapy, Acta med. scandinav., *162* (suppl. 341), 211, 1958.

RÖSSLE, R.: Wachstum und Altern. Zweiter (pathologischer) Teil, Ergebn. allg. Path., *20²*, 369, 1923–24.

ROTH, J., GORDEN, P., and BRACE, K.: Efficacy of Conventional Pituitary Irradiation in Acromegaly, New England J. Med., *282*, 1385, 1970.

RUTISHAUSER, E.: Osteoporotische Fettsucht. (Pituitary Basophilism), Deutsches Arch. klin. Med., *175*, 640, 1933.

SCHMORL, G.: Über abnorme Färbungen der Knochensubstanz, Virchows Arch. path. Anat., *275*, 13, 1930.

SILBERBERG, M. and SILBERBERG, R.: The Effects of Thyroid Feeding on Growth Processes and Retrogressive Changes in Bone and Cartilage of the Immature Guinea Pig, Growth, *2*, 327, 1938.

SISSONS, H. A.: The Osteoporosis of Cushing's Syndrome, J. Bone & Joint Surg., *38-B*, 418, 1956.

SMITH, E. E. and McLEAN, F. C.: Effect of Hyperthyroidism upon Growth and Chemical Composition of Bone, Endocrinology, *23*, 546, 1938.

TANDLER, J. and GROSZ, S.: *Die biologischen Grundlagen der sekundären Geschlechtscharaktere*, Berlin, Julius Springer, 1913.

THOMAS, H. M., JR.: Acropachy, Arch. Int. Med., *51*, 571, 1933.

TODD, T. W. and WHARTON, R. E.: The Effect of Thyroid Deficiency upon Skull Growth in the Sheep, Am. J. Anat., *55*, 97, 1934.

WILKINS, L.: Epiphysial Dysgenesis Associated with Hypothyroidism, Am. J. Dis. Child., *61*, 13, 1941.

WILKINS, L. and FLEISCHMANN, W.: The Diagnosis of Hypothyroidism in Childhood, J.A.M.A., *116*, 2459, 1941.

Chapter

14

Osteoporosis of the Senescent and/or Postmenopausal State

As is generally recognized, *osteoporosis* is a fairly common (though by no means inevitable) finding in connection with gonadal deficiency (especially in women) and in elderly persons in general. Though the osteoporosis may be widely distributed over the skeleton, it is the bones of the trunk (particularly those of the vertebral column) that are most consistently and most severely affected. Interestingly enough, even when the involvement of the skeleton is extensive, the calvarium usually shows little if any evidence of osteoporosis. The pathogenesis of the condition is still not entirely clear, and it seems likely that multiple factors interact to bring it about. One of these factors, emphasized by Chalmers and Ho, is diminished physical activity with advancing age.

Anatomically the osteoporosis in question (sometimes denoted as *primary osteoporosis*) is characterized by: (1) a reduction in the amount of osseous tissue per unit of bone volume; (2) conspicuous sparsity and thinning of the spongy trabeculae of the affected bones, not associated with active osteoclastic resorption and scarring of the intertrabecular marrow; and (3) usually some thinning and porosity of the cortices of the affected bones, again without evidence of significant osteoclastic resorption.

The osteoporosis showing these anatomic features was denoted by pathologists in the past as "smooth bone atrophy" (see Pommer, and Gerth). That designation was employed because the reduction in the amount of spongy and cortical osseous tissue per unit volume of bone was not the result of osteoclastic activity. On this account, the surfaces of the spongy trabeculae and of the haversian canals of the cortical bone are found relatively smooth instead of being pitted by Howship's lacunae, to which osteoclasts are oriented. On the positive side, the type of osteoporosis represented by the term "smooth bone atrophy" was originally conceived as resulting primarily from diminished osteoblastic activity. The consequence of reduced osteoblastic activity is deficient deposition of calcifiable organic bone matrix, which would compensate for the osseous tissue continually being resorbed in the course of endogenous skeletal metabolism. Currently, evidence is accumulating to the effect that changes in the chemical composition of the mucopolysaccharides of the ground substance, due to malfunctioning of the osteocytes (the bone cells), also play a part in the evolution of the osteoporosis. (See Pathogenesis.)

CLINICAL CONSIDERATIONS

The senescent and/or postmenopausal state constitutes the most common basis for the development of osteoporosis. As already noted, the latter by no means occurs in all women who have undergone the menopause (natural or artificial) or in all persons who have become elderly. Nevertheless, the *incidence* of osteoporosis is consistently higher in elderly women than in elderly men, as is to be expected in view of the fact that in women the influence of senescence is augmented by that of the menopause. The reported statistical data are in general accord on this point. The different reports do show somewhat different estimates of the over-all incidence of the osteoporosis in women and men and its occurrence in the different age groups. However, there is general agreement that the incidence of osteoporosis rises consistently from the fifth decade, and sharply after the beginning of the eighth decade.

In one report, covering 136 non-ailing men and women ranging in age from 63 to 95 years, the over-all incidence of osteoporosis involving the vertebral column, as revealed roentgenographically, is stated to be very high, though no percentage is given (see Gershon-Cohen *et al.*). In this group of cases, furthermore, 11 of the 54 men (20 per cent) and 24 of the 82 women (29 per cent) showed compression fractures of one or more vertebral bodies. These fractures were most commonly encountered in the lower thoracic vertebrae (most often the twelfth), and when a lumbar vertebral body was affected it was most often the first lumbar. The compression fractures were "asymptomatic" in the sense that they were not associated with severe pain and serious disablement, which usually appear in connection with post-traumatic fractures of vertebral bodies in adults not affected with osteoporosis.

In another report, relating to a series of 218 ambulatory women ranging in age from 45 to 79 years, the incidence of roentgenographically demonstrable osteoporosis of the spine is given as 29 per cent (see Smith *et al.*). It should be noted that only about one third of these women were 65 years of age or older. In this series of 218 cases, only 4.6 per cent of the women showed wedging or compression fractures of one or more vertebral bodies. The lower incidence of vertebral fractures among these subjects is apparently attributable to the fact that so high a proportion of them were under 65 years of age.

An elderly person whose vertebral column has been gravely altered by the osteoporosis has usually lost at least several inches in height. This loss is due mainly to the development of a rounded kyphosis in the thoracic portion of the vertebral column, whose mobility is also reduced. The rounded back shortens the trunk, the lower ribs come to lie close to the iliac crest, and the limbs hence appear disproportionately long. Despite the severity of the changes revealed on roentgenographic examination (especially in the vertebral column), the clinical complaints are often surprisingly mild. When clinical complaints are reported, they are most likely to include pain in the bones (especially the vertebral column and pelvis) and pain referred to the region of the loins and down the lower limbs. The pain is most pronounced when movement follows a period of rest—notably when the patient first

Figure 94

A, Roentgenograph of the calvarium in the case of a woman 61 years of age affected with postmenopausal osteoporosis. As is usual in these cases, the bones of the cranial vault present an essentially normal appearance in comparison with what is observed in the bones of the axial skeleton and even of the limbs in the same case.

B and *C*, Roentgenographs of part of the thoracic vertebral column and the upper two thirds of the right tibia and fibula from the same patient whose calvarium is illustrated in *A*. The vertebral bodies appear very much "washed out" because of sparsity of the spongy bone. Several of the intervertebral disks are moderately expanded, and the vertebral bodies show a slight degree of marginal lipping (spondylosis) anteriorly. The tibia and fibula manifest pronounced thinning of their cortices and also diminution of the trabecular markings at the upper ends of these bones.

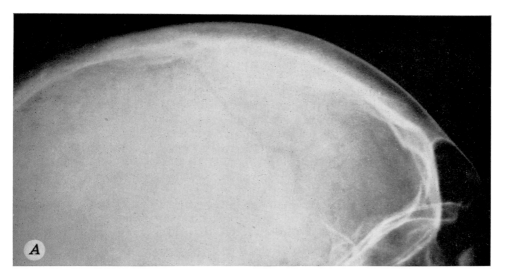

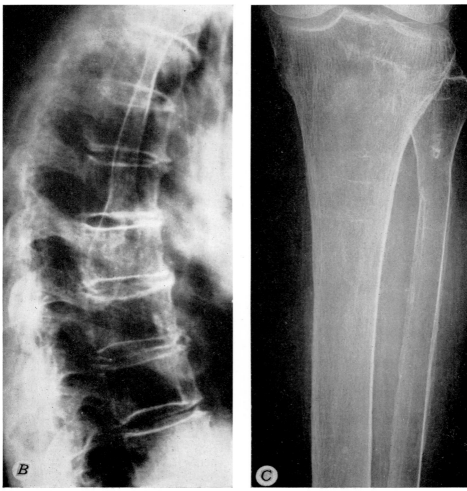

Figure 94

rises in the morning. Aggravating influences include bending movements and stair-climbing, and sometimes changes in the weather. (See Fig. 94.)

Among subjects having advanced osteoporosis of the vertebral column, there is a high incidence of transcervical and intertrochanteric femoral fractures. In a series of 100 aged women in whom such a fracture had taken place, it was found that 76 per cent showed roentgenographic evidence of osteoporosis of the vertebral column (see Urist). In another series, consisting of 124 women (in the sixth, seventh, and eighth decades of life) with femoral fractures, the incidence of osteoporosis was 84 per cent (see Stevens *et al.*). Usually in these cases the occurrence of the femoral fracture is related to some minor incident, such as stumbling or rising abruptly from a chair, and an ensuing fall. In most instances the fall is actually the consequence rather than the cause of the fracture, the latter occurring because the upper end of the femur is already porotic. Under these circumstances the femoral fracture is often to be interpreted as a "spontaneous," or "pathologic," fracture, since a trau-matic factor sufficient to account for the fracture is absent. The degree of osteo-porosis present in the fractured femur just before the occurrence of the fracture can be evaluated on the basis of the roentgenographic findings relating to the opposite (nonfractured) femur.

It has been stated by some workers that, despite attempts at fixation with metallic appliances, there is a high incidence of nonunion in connection with fractures of the femoral neck in cases of osteoporosis. Others have reported, however, that the proportion of successes in the treatment of femoral neck fractures (with metallic appliances) was not significantly different in patients with osteoporosis from what it was in patients without osteoporosis. That is, the fate of the fracture did not appear to be influenced by the presence or absence of osteoporosis or by the degree of the osteoporosis. Impacted fractures (whether or not there was osteoporosis) yielded the highest incidence of union (see Stevens and Abrami).

In regard to the *biochemical findings* in the blood in osteoporotic elderly persons otherwise not ailing, it is known that the serum calcium, inorganic phosphorus, and alkaline phosphatase values are within the normal range. However, if one or more fractures are present, the phosphatase value may be somewhat elevated. The gen-erally normal serum biochemical findings differentiate the osteoporosis in question from other conditions in which the roentgenographic findings sometimes suggest that disorder, *viz.*: osteomalacia, hyperparathyroidism (primary or secondary), and certain exceptional instances of diffuse myelomatosis. It is only rarely that tissue examination as provided by bone biopsy is needed or indicated to help establish the diagnosis.

ROENTGENOGRAPHIC AND PATHOLOGIC FINDINGS

It is in the bones of the trunk (vertebral column, sternum, ribs, and pelvis) that the osteoporosis first becomes manifest. In time, it may also become evident in the long and short tubular bones. In the skull bones, as already noted, it shows itself late and in very mild form if at all. In any event, a considerable amount of depletion of the osseous tissue of an affected skeletal part must occur before the presence of the osteoporosis is revealed in clinical roentgenographs. This depletion has been estimated at about 30 per cent. Such estimates have their foundation in data cor-relating the information to be obtained from roentgenographic and anatomic exami-nation of porotic bones with the results of chemical assays of the ash or mineral content of such bones. Since a rather large amount of the osseous tissue must be lost before the osteoporosis reveals itself in the clinical roentgenographs, various procedures, including x-ray densitometry, have been tried as means of establishing the presence of osteoporosis early in the course of its development (see Barnett and Nordin). None of these procedures has yet proved practical on a clinical basis. However, study of postmortem material and, in particular, of slabs of sagittally sectioned vertebral bodies has shown that the radiodensity of these bone slabs is statistically correlated with the calcium content of the osseous tissue of the vertebral bodies in question (see Caldwell and Collins).

It is in the *vertebral bodies* that the roentgenographic and/or anatomic aspects of the evolution and progression of the osteoporosis observed in the postmenopausal and senile states can most easily be followed. As is common knowledge, a normal vertebral body consists almost entirely of spongy osseous tissue, the delimiting cortical shell, where present, being very thin. Indeed, the upper and lower surfaces of a vertebral body, centrally to the corresponding marginal ridge, are devoid of cortex. In these regions the cartilage of the pertinent intervertebral disk is apposed upon condensed spongiosa. The spongiosa of the vertebral body as a whole forms a latticework which is rather loose-meshed in the middle portion of the body and relatively close-meshed in the upper and lower portions. (See Figs. 12-*C* and *D*.)

In the evolution of the osteoporosis in a *vertebral body*, the spongy trabeculae become thinner and sparser, but those which are transversely oriented usually show the changes earlier and to a greater degree. Consequently, many of the transversely oriented trabeculae disappear, and the longitudinally directed trabeculae, though thinned, become more conspicuous. Accordingly, the porotic vertebral bodies will tend to show faint longitudinal striations in the roentgenograph. These stand out much more clearly, of course, in an *x*-ray picture representing a specimen of vertebral column removed at autopsy than in a corresponding clinical *x*-ray picture (see Uehlinger). With further progression of the osteoporosis, the longitudinally directed trabeculae become fewer and less conspicuous, the affected vertebral bodies consequently acquiring a sort of "washed-out" appearance in the roentgenograph. (See Figs. 95 and 96.)

The stage is thus set for alterations in the contour of the vertebral bodies, the diminished trabecular framework no longer being adequate for the static load imposed upon it. The turgor of relatively intact intervertebral disks pressing against yielding vertebral bodies may make many of the latter (especially those of the lower thoracic and lumbar region) take on a biconcave shape. In the thoracic region, in particular, one or more of the vertebral bodies may become narrowed in the dorsoventrad direction, the wedge formation representing the end result of compressional collapse and fracture. It is the dorsoventrad narrowing of thoracic vertebral bodies that accentuates the normal dorsal curvature of the vertebral column, sometimes to the extent of producing a pronounced kyphotic deformity. Microscopic examination of a wedged vertebral body will show some necrotic spongy trabeculae and fibrous scarring, and also newly deposited bone and other evidences of endosteal callus formation. Roentgenographically, the shadow cast by a wedged vertebra in which a fair amount of endosteal callus is already present may be relatively radiopaque in comparison with the shadow cast by neighboring porotic vertebrae not so altered.

As already indicated, the *long* and *short tubular bones* may eventually also show definite roentgenographic evidence of osteoporosis. Anatomically, however, the spongy osseous tissue of these bones is likely to manifest osteoporosis in the form of thinning and sparsity of the trabeculae, while the bone cortex still does not present any clear-cut porotic changes roentgenographically. As the severity of the osteoporosis increases, the cortical bone, too, comes to show it. The involvement of the bone cortex advances from its inner, or medullary, surface toward the outer, or periosteal, surface. The haversian canals become enlarged, and adjacent ones may fuse, so that the compact cortical bone becomes progressively porotic. Where the porosity of the cortical bone has progressed considerably, the latter may appear stratified in the x-ray picture. At a still more advanced stage of the osteoporosis, much or all of the cortex of a severely porotic long tubular bone may have undergone resorption, so that the cortex is represented merely by a thin and rather faint radiopaque shadow. It is natural that such severely porotic long bones are subject to fractures if they undergo even slight trauma (direct or indirect). The high incidence of fractures of the neck of the femur in cases of osteoporosis of the senescent and/or postmenopausal state bears witness to this fact.

Altogether, in the course of the evolution of the osteoporosis in a tubular bone, the trabeculae of the spongy osseous tissue become thin, and many of them also disappear. The cortical bone, too, becomes rarefied and often very thin. However, in the absence of fractures, these alterations are not associated with reactive fibrosis either in the spongy marrow spaces or within the enlarged haversian canals of the cortical bone. Also, the surfaces of the spongy trabeculae and of the haversian canals are smooth. That is, they are not, as already noted, pitted by Howship's

Figure 95

A, Roentgenograph of part of the vertebral column, in lateral projection, from a case of generalized osteoporosis in a woman 60 years of age. On the day before admission to the hospital, she fell and sustained a fracture of the lower end of the tibia and fibula of the right leg, the bones of which were also porotic. The osteoporosis involving the bones of her vertebral column came to light in the course of a roentgenographic skeletal survey. Note that the intervertebral disk spaces are widened. The eleventh thoracic vertebral body shows evidence of compressional collapse and is, in part, more radiopaque than the merely porotic vertebral bodies immediately above and below it. The increased radiopacity of the eleventh thoracic vertebra is the result of reparative new bone formation (intramedullary callus formation) which has taken place in response to the compressional collapse. The contour of the body of the ninth thoracic vertebra is also altered.

B, Photograph of part of the vertebral column (sectioned longitudinally) from a case of postmenopausal osteoporosis. The subject, who was 57 years of age, entered the hospital because of back pain. She stated that 8 weeks prior to admission she had bent over to pick up an object from the floor and felt a sudden sharp pain in the back. Clinically, she presented an exaggerated dorsal kyphosis, and the ribs could be palpated below the iliac crests. A spine fusion was done, but the patient died one day after the surgical intervention. All the intervertebral disks shown are expanded, and three of the vertebral bodies illustrated are strikingly deformed in contour. The wedged vertebral body in the upper part of the picture is the ninth thoracic vertebra, and *C* is a survey photomicrograph of a histologic section prepared from that body. The biconcave vertebral body in the lower part of the picture is the first lumbar vertebra, and *D* is a survey photomicrograph of a histologic section prepared from that body. As observed at autopsy, the ovaries were very small, having undergone involution. The sectioned ovaries revealed no primary follicles.

C, Photomicrograph ($\times$ 4) showing the general histologic architecture of the ninth thoracic vertebral body illustrated in *B*. Note the general sparsity of spongy bone. The compressional collapse of this vertebral body must have occurred not long (possibly only a few days) before the subject came to autopsy. This interpretation is based on the fact that examination of the section under higher magnification failed to reveal evidence of proliferation of osteogenetic connective tissue and new bone formation, which would constitute part of the reparative reaction to the collapse of the vertebral body.

D, Photomicrograph ($\times$ 4) showing the general histologic architecture of the first lumbar vertebral body illustrated in *B*. This collapsed body presents abundant evidence of reparative new bone formation (intramedullary callus). Numerous trabeculae of new bone can be seen even at this low magnification. Under higher magnification, much of the new bone is found apposed on trabeculae of pre-existing osseous tissue. These trabeculae can be seen to be nonviable, and some are also disintegrating. These nonviable trabeculae show a lack of osteocytes (bone cells), which would normally be present.

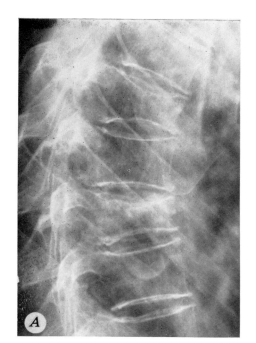

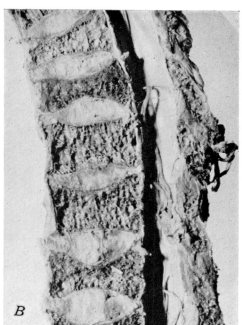

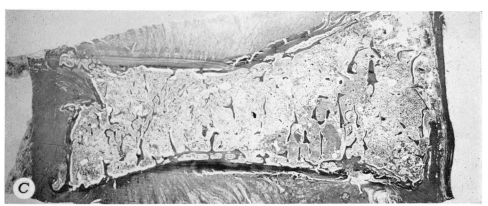

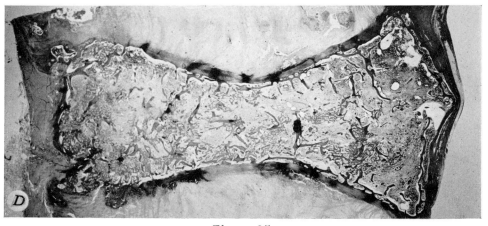

Figure 95

lacunae, to which osteoclasts are oriented. Furthermore, despite the reduction in the amount of bone substance, the microscopic architecture of the porotic osseous tissue *per se* shows no obvious deviation in histologic detail from nonporotic osseous tissue as observed in a normal age control (see Urist). In particular, it appears normal in respect to the organization of its collagen fibers (as revealed by polarization microscopy), the mineral density of the osseous tissue (as revealed by microradiography), and the appearance of its osteocytes (as revealed by conventional light microscopy).

The fact that in postmenopausal osteoporosis (often presenile) and senile osteoporosis the loss of bone substance is not conditioned by osteoclastic activity distinguishes this type of osteoporosis from the porosity of the bones which is encountered in connection with hyperparathyroidism, for instance (see p. 309). In cases of the Cushing syndrome, the underlying hypercortisonism disturbs the metabolism of proteins and induces inhibition of protein synthesis. Insofar as the skeleton is concerned, this inhibition is expressed in diminished formation of organic bone matrix (and in particular of collagen) by the osteoblasts (see p. 355). Thus there is a definite anatomic kinship between the osteoporosis associated with the Cushing syndrome and that observed in the postmenopausal and/or senescent state. (See Fig. 97.)

PATHOGENESIS

It is generally recognized that the porotic osseous tissue encountered in the postmenopausal and/or senescent state shows no aberration from normal osseous

Figure 96

A, Roentgenograph of part of the vertebral column in the case of a woman 71 years of age who manifested generalized osteoporosis. Note the compressional collapse of the first lumbar vertebra. The "washed-out" appearance of the other vertebral bodies is the result of reduction of the trabecular markings. The patient was admitted to the hospital because she had fallen and suffered a comminuted fracture at the lower end of the left radius. She had apparently had no complaints referable to the skeleton prior to her fall. At some time in the past, she had had a panhysterectomy, and for a number of years she had been under treatment for hypertension and attacks of angina pectoris. About $2\frac{1}{2}$ weeks after admission, she died suddenly, and autopsy revealed that the immediate cause of death was coronary thrombosis.

B, Photograph showing in longitudinal sagittal section the collapsed first lumbar vertebra illustrated in *A,* the porotic but not collapsed vertebral bodies immediately above and below it, and also the expanded corresponding intervertebral disks. In the two vertebral bodies which have not undergone compressional collapse, there is a pronounced sparsity of the spongy trabeculae. The relatively few trabeculae which are clearly distinguishable are directed mainly in the vertical plane, the horizontally directed trabeculae being even sparser (see *C*). The vertebral body which has collapsed presents evidence of intramedullary callus formation (see *D*).

C, Photomicrograph ($\times$ 4.5) showing the general histologic architecture of part of a vertebral body from this case which has retained a relatively normal contour. There is a striking sparsity of spongy trabeculae, and the few trabeculae present are directed mainly in the vertical plane. The bone marrow is heavily interspersed with fat cells. (For histologic details, see Fig. 97–*A*.)

D, Photomicrograph ($\times$ 4) showing the general histologic architecture of the posterior half of the collapsed first lumbar vertebra. In contrast to what one observes in *C,* the interior of this vertebral body reveals evidence of considerable new bone formation taking place in a substratum of highly vascularized osteogenetic connective tissue. (For histologic details, see Fig. 97-*B*.)

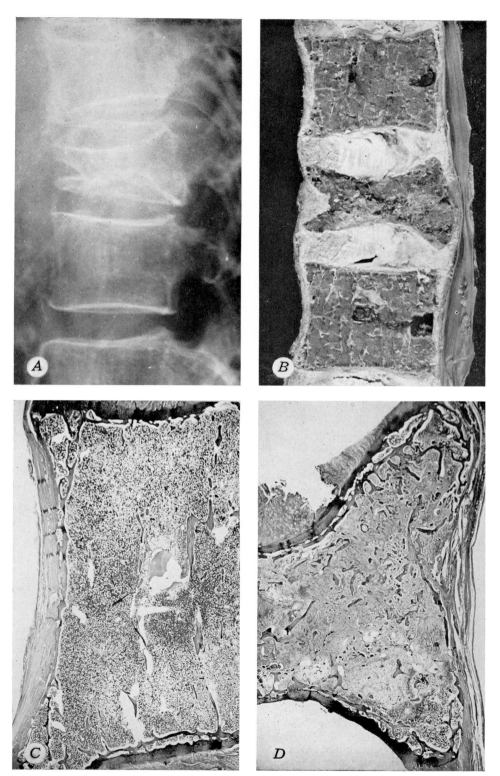

Figure 96

tissue in the proportions of mineral matter to organic matter. Also, the composition of the apatite representing the bone mineral is not different in osteoporotic bone from what it is in normal bone. However, the organic matter of the osseous tissue does show quantitative and qualitative aberrations in respect to the proportions of the various mucopolysaccharides in the ground substance of the organic matrix in comparison with these proportions in youthful subjects (see Casuccio). There are also indications that, in osteoporotic bone, the collagen of the organic matrix (which is laid down by the osteoblasts) is defective in its ultrastructure (see Little *et al.*). Nevertheless, it should be pointed out that somewhat analogous changes in the composition of the mucopolysaccharides of the organic matrix are to be noted in the osseous tissue of elderly persons free of osteoporosis.

Various concepts have been proposed to account for the pathogenesis of the osteoporosis. One of these concepts (see Albright, and Reifenstein) is the idea that the osteoporosis is instigated by a hormonal imbalance and, in particular, by a relative increase in the proportion of circulating adrenal gluco-corticoids (which are antianabolic hormones) in relation to circulating sex hormones (which are anabolic hormones). On the other hand, a single hormonal factor is stressed by Urist *et al.* That factor is held to be 17-hydroxycorticosteroids acting in persons possibly predisposed to osteoporosis by the lack of an "antiosteoporotic factor" which would normally protect the bones from the antianabolic effects of 17-hydroxycorticosteroids. It has also been proposed that the osteoporosis results from a prolonged though mild negative calcium balance arising in predisposed subjects in consequence of a chronic calcium deficiency due to a low mineral content of the diet and/or diminished absorption and reabsorption of calcium from the intestinal tract (see Nordin).

The interesting and varied pathogenetic mechanisms just outlined should be considered in the light of the possibility that the osteoporosis represents merely one facet of a general involutional process which occurs in all aging and senile persons and which in some of them becomes particularly conspicuous in the skeleton. As is well known, it is through the activity of the osteoblasts that the organic matrix of osseous tissue is formed. Therefore, there is much to suggest the possibility that in some subjects the process of aging is associated with progressive involution of the

Figure 97

A, Photomicrograph ($\times$ 40) illustrating the condition of the trabeculae and intertrabecular marrow of the vertebral body shown in Figure 96-*C*. Note the absence of osteoclasts along the surface of the trabeculae and also the absence of fibrous scarring of the marrow. The myeloid marrow is heavily interspersed with fat cells, as is usually the case in the porotic vertebral bodies in the condition in question.

B, Photomicrograph ($\times$ 40) illustrating in higher detail the histologic appearance presented by the collapsed first lumbar vertebra shown in Figure 96-*D*. The substratum of osteogenetic connective tissue is highly vascularized. New bone formation is in evidence. Furthermore, in some places the newly formed osseous tissue (coarse-fibered bone) can be observed apposed upon pre-existing nonviable lamellar osseous tissue. The pre-existing osseous tissue has largely undergone aseptic necrosis in the wake of compressional collapse of the vertebral body, which has led to comminution of the spongy trabeculae and interference with the local blood supply.

C, Photomicrograph ($\times$ 9) illustrating the general histologic architecture of part of a rib in a case of advanced generalized osteoporosis. The subject was a man 70 years of age. The cortex of the rib is extremely thin, and the spongy bone very sparse. Rib fractures just beyond the costochondral junction are not uncommon in cases of osteoporosis of the senescent state, and the anatomic basis for their occurrence is evident from this illustration.

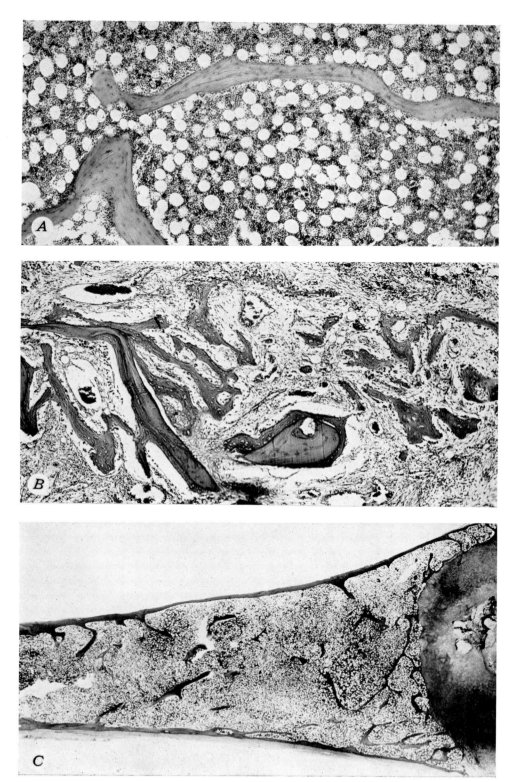

Figure 97

osteogenetic connective tissue and in particular of the osteoblasts. It is also known that the osteocytes (which arise from osteoblasts that have become entrapped in mineralized bone matrix) help to maintain the vitality (structural and metabolic) of the organic bone matrix. Therefore the decadence of these cells in the course of advancing age undoubtedly influences the quantitative and qualitative composition of the mucopolysaccharides (and possibly also of the collagen) of the organic bone matrix. Hence, depressed activity of the osteoblasts and the alteration of the bone matrix through malfunction of the osteocytes would result in a disturbance in the metabolism of the osseous tissue and thus lay the foundation for the osteoporosis (see Jaffe and Pomeranz, and Rutishauser and Majno). However, it is quite possible that the progressive alteration in the metabolic activity of the osteoblasts and osteocytes which occurs concomitantly with the aging process is nevertheless conditioned to some extent by a hormonal imbalance—probably a deranged ratio of circulating antianabolic hormones to circulating anabolic hormones. It appears that in all aging subjects there is a *slight* decrease (about 10 per cent) in the amount of circulating antianabolic steroids, but a *marked* decrease (50 to 80 per cent) in the amount of circulating anabolic steroids (see Reifenstein). The decrease in the anabolic hormones is much greater in the aging female than in the aging male, and thus there is a greater imbalance between the anabolic and the antianabolic hormones in the female. This difference is believed to account for the higher incidence of the osteoporosis in the aging female.

The development of the osteoporosis of the postmenopausal and/or senescent state clearly involves the interaction of multiple factors, some of which are still obscure. In accordance with the progressive reduction in the amount of osseous tissue in the skeleton, the evolution of the osteoporosis is inevitably associated with a prolonged, however mild, negative calcium balance. Naturally, one assumes in this connection that the dietary calcium intake of the subject is within reasonably normal limits, and that there is no interference with absorption of the mineral from the gastrointestinal tract, such as obtains, for example, in relation to steatorrhea. Under these conditions, aberrations from the normal in respect to the composition and proportions of the mucopolysaccharides of the organic matrix, and diminished deposition of collagen by the osteoblasts, are to be inculpated in the negative calcium balance. That is, though adequate bone mineral (as represented by calcium) may be available, it may fail to be retained in the bone matrix in sufficient amounts and hence be excreted in correspondingly increased amounts, so that a negative calcium balance results.

If one assumes that the negative calcium balance in a given case of osteoporosis is as much as 100 mg. per day, it would take about 9 years for the osteoporosis to develop to such a degree that it is clearly apparent roentgenographically. This calculation rests on the estimate that about 30 per cent of the 1,100 gm. of calcium contained in the skeleton of a normal, well-developed adult has to be lost before the osteoporosis becomes clearly apparent in clinical roentgenographs. It also presupposes that the dietary intake of calcium by the subject is not grossly inadequate, for on a very low calcium intake the negative calcium balance would be much more pronounced, and the osteoporosis would become evident sooner. Since the osteoporosis may develop even in a person whose calcium intake is adequate in terms of the standard minimal requirement, it is to be assumed that those in whom the condition develops are persons whose natural requirement for calcium is abnormally high. Furthermore, they apparently cannot adapt to a minimal daily calcium intake in the manner characteristic of older persons who remain free of osteoporosis. In any event, on an adequate calcium intake, a subject in whom the osteoporosis is already very pronounced may no longer show the negative calcium balance evident during the long period when the osteoporosis was evolving. On the other hand, it has been found that osteoporotic subjects whose daily calcium intake is very high (amounting to as much as 2 gm.) may come to show a strongly positive calcium balance (see Fraser).

TREATMENT

The treatment of osteoporosis of the senescent and/or postmenopausal state has remained a problem. *General measures* commonly employed include a well-rounded diet (high in protein and adequate in calcium), encouragement of activity, and the use of analgesics for the relief of pain. In addition, *hormonal therapy* is widely employed.

Though subjective improvement in general well-being is often achieved, roentgenographic changes indicating significant improvement in the condition of the bones have not been observed. Nevertheless, hormonal therapy is still generally used, on the principle that one of the basic factors underlying the development of the osteoporosis is a hormonal imbalance between the circulating anabolic steroids (androgen and estrogen) and the antianabolic steroids (gluco-corticoids).

Treatment of the osteoporotic subjects with anabolic hormones, especially over long periods of time, seems to arrest the progress of the osteoporosis but fails to restore the bones to their normal density (see Henneman and Wallach). This fact strongly suggests that the hormonal imbalance in question may be only a predisposing factor rather than the determining factor in the osteoporosis of the senescent state. As already pointed out in the discussion of the pathogenesis of the osteoporosis, the actual determining factor may well reside in various chemical and structural changes occurring in the organic matrix of the osseous tissue. These changes would represent only one aspect of the involutionary changes taking place, to a greater or lesser extent, in the body as a whole. On this basis, it is understandable that the osteoporosis of the senescent and/or postmenopausal state has sometimes been viewed as an irreversible (though arrestable) involutional atrophy of the bones (see Jaffe, and Casuccio).

REFERENCES

ALBRIGHT, F.: Osteoporosis, Ann. Int. Med., *27*, 861, 1947.
BARNETT, E. and NORDIN, B. E. C.: Radiological Assessment of Bone Density. I. The Clinical and Radiological Problem of Thin Bones, Brit. J. Radiol., *34*, 683, 1961.
CALDWELL, R. A. and COLLINS, D. H.: Assessment of Vertebral Osteoporosis by Radiographic and Chemical Methods Post-Mortem, J. Bone & Joint Surg., *43-B*, 346, 1961.
CASUCCIO, C.: An Introduction to the Study of Osteoporosis (Biochemical and Biophysical Research in Bone Ageing), Proc. Roy. Soc. Med., *55*, 663, 1962.
————: Concerning Osteoporosis, J. Bone & Joint Surg., *44-B*, 453, 1962.
CHALMERS, J., and HO, K. C.: Geographical Variations in Senile Osteoporosis: The Association with Physical Activity, J. Bone & Joint Surg., *52-B*, 667, 1970.
FRASER, R.: The Problem of Osteoporosis, J. Bone & Joint Surg., *44-B*, 485, 1962.
GERSHON-COHEN, J., RECHTMAN, A. M., SCHRAER, H., and BLUMBERG, N.: Asymptomatic Fractures in Osteoporotic Spines of the Aged, J.A.M.A., *153*, 625, 1953.
GERTH: Zur Frage der Osteoporose, Virchows Arch. path. Anat., *277*, 311, 1930.
HENNEMAN, P. H. and WALLACH, S.: A Review of the Prolonged Use of Estrogens and Androgens in Postmenopausal and Senile Osteoporosis, Arch. Int. Med., *100*, 715, 1957.
JAFFE, H. L.: Hyperparathyroidism (Recklinghausen's Disease of Bone), Arch. Path., *16*, 63 and 236, 1933 (see p. 247).
JAFFE, H. L. and POMERANZ, M. M.: Changes in the Bones of Extremities Amputated Because of Arteriovascular Disease, Arch. Surg., *29*, 566, 1934.
LITTLE, K., KELLY, M., and COURTS, A.: Studies on Bone Matrix in Normal and Osteoporotic Bone, J. Bone & Joint Surg., *44-B*, 503, 1962.
NORDIN, E. C.: Osteoporosis, in *Bone Metabolism*, edited by H. A. Sissons, London, Pitman Medical Publishing Co. Ltd., 1962, p. 113.

Pommer, G.: Über Osteoporose, ihren Ursprung und ihre differentialdiagnostische Bedeutung, Arch. klin. Chir., *136*, 1, 1925.

Reifenstein, E. C., Jr.: The Relationships of Steroid Hormones to the Development and the Management of Osteoporosis in Aging People, Clinical Orthopaedics, *10*, 206, 1957.

——: Osteoporosis, in *Bone as a Tissue*, edited by K. Rodahl, J. T. Nicholson, and E. M. Brown, Jr., New York, McGraw-Hill Book Company, Inc., 1960, p. 83.

Rutishauser, E. and Majno, G.: Physiopathology of Bone Tissue: The Osteocytes and Fundamental Substance, Bull. Hosp. Joint Dis., *12*, 468, 1951.

Smith, R. W., Jr., Eyler, W. R., and Mellinger, R. C.: On the Incidence of Senile Osteoporosis, Ann. Int. Med., *52*, 773, 1960.

Stevens, J., Freeman, P. A., Nordin, B. E. C., and Barnett, E.: The Incidence of Osteoporosis in Patients with Femoral Neck Fracture, J. Bone & Joint Surg., *44-B*, 520, 1962.

Stevens, J. and Abrami, G.: Osteoporosis in Patients with Femoral Neck Fractures. A Follow-up Study, J. Bone & Joint Surg., *46-B*, 24, 1964.

Uehlinger, E.: Zur Diagnose und Differentialdiagnose der Osteoporose, Schweiz. med. Jahrb., 1958, p. 39.

Urist, M. R.: Observations Bearing on the Problem of Osteoporosis, in *Bone as a Tissue*, edited by K. Rodahl, J. T. Nicholson, and E. M. Brown, Jr., New York, McGraw-Hill Book Company, Inc., 1960, p. 18.

Urist, M. R., Zaccalini, P. S., MacDonald, N. S., and Skoog, W. A.: New Approaches to the Problem of Osteoporosis, J. Bone & Joint Surg., *44-B*, 464, 1962.

Chapter

15

Rickets and Osteomalacia

THE two main causes of rickets and its adult counterpart, osteomalacia, are: (1) lack of vitamin D and (2) disordered functioning of the renal tubules without disease of the renal glomeruli.* The *lack of vitamin D* may be due to: a simple inadequacy of the supply of vitamin D; or loss of ingested vitamin D—for instance, in conditions associated with chronic steatorrhea. In the cases of rickets or osteomalacia due to *disordered functioning of the renal tubules*, the dysfunction may consist of: defective tubular resorption, or defective tubular excretion. The so-called *vitamin D-resistant rickets* (or *refractory rickets*) was formerly considered to be the result of the development by the body of refractoriness (unresponsiveness) to vitamin D. Current experience indicates that refractory rickets actually belongs in the category of rickets due to disordered functioning of the renal tubules, and represents one clinical expression of such malfunctioning.

Though the substantial part of our knowledge of rickets and, to a lesser extent, of osteomalacia has been derived from cases developing through simple inadequacy of the supply of vitamin D, it is rather the cases developing as a result of renal tubular dysfunction that are in the foreground of our current interest concerning these conditions. Anatomically, irrespective of the underlying cause, rickets and osteomalacia are characterized by the presence of abnormal quantities of osteoid (that is, organic bone matrix deficient in bone mineral) wherever osseous tissue is being laid down. Thus, in both conditions, broad osteoid borders are to be found along the margins of the spongy trabeculae and along the walls of the haversian canals. In addition, in rickets the sites of endochondral bone formation show: (1) deficient calcification of the matrix of the proliferating cartilage; (2) an abnormal accumulation of cartilage; and (3) considerable deposition of osteoid. Along with these anatomic criteria of rickets and osteomalacia, there are clinical *biochemical criteria*, viz.: a tendency toward a somewhat lowered serum calcium value, a definitely lowered serum phosphate value, and a definitely raised serum alkaline phosphatase value. Also, there is evidence of chronic acidosis in the cases of rickets due to renal tubular malfunction, except in those cases belonging in the category of so-called refractory, or vitamin D-resistant, rickets.

As an addendum to this chapter, it seems appropriate to consider the syndrome of *hypophosphatasia* (p. 437). That condition, which is often already clinically manifest at birth, is not, of course, the result of vitamin D deficiency nor of malfunctioning of the renal tubules. As the name hypophosphatasia implies, the disorder is characterized by diminished formation and activity of the enzyme

---

* The so-called renal rickets and renal osteomalacia (also denoted as renal hyperparathyroidism and renal osteodystrophy) are conditioned by actual pathologic changes in the nephron units of the kidneys. The disordered homeostasis resulting from the consequent chronic renal insufficiency leads to parathyroid hyperplasia and hyperfunctioning. The latter in turn is one of the influences contributing to the development of the skeletal alterations observed in cases of protracted renal insufficiency (see p. 321).

phosphatase (specifically alkaline phosphatase). In consequence of the low alkaline phosphatase content of the various body fluids and tissues, the metabolism of calcium and phosphorus is disordered, and in relation to the bones, there is diminished mineralization of the organic matrix which is laid down in the course of pre- and postnatal skeletogenesis.

It is the excessive amounts of osteoid at sites of endochondral bone growth that result in roentgenographic pictures suggestive of those encountered in cases of rickets due to vitamin D deficiency or renal tubular malfunctioning. It is because of these anatomic and roentgenographic findings that hypophosphatasia is being discussed in this chapter. However, the serum biochemical findings in this condition are not at all in accord with those to be noted in the other forms of rickets. Indeed, in hypophosphatasia the serum calcium value is at the high normal level, or there may be an actual hypercalcemia; the serum phosphate value is at the high normal level (and is, of course, abnormally high if there is a complicating renal insufficiency); and the low serum alkaline phosphatase value (and occasional absence of serum alkaline phosphatase activity) is also in contrast to what one finds in rickets due to vitamin D deficiency or renal tubular malfunction.

RICKETS DUE TO SIMPLE LACK OF VITAMIN D

Rickets due entirely or mainly to simple lack of vitamin D (ordinary nutritional rickets) was formerly a very common disease in those parts of the temperate zone which have cold winters, and especially in large crowded cities of these parts. Its victims were older infants and very young children, and the disease only rarely developed after the third or fourth year. Those affected had lacked sufficient exposure to the antirachitic (ultraviolet) rays of the sun, while concomitantly their vitamin D intake had been too small to compensate for this lack. Furthermore, if, in addition to the vitamin D deficiency, there was a dietary deficiency of calcium and/or phosphorus, the development of rickets was strongly favored. Two instances of congenital rickets based on maternal malabsorption have been recorded by Begum *et al.*

Wherever the prophylactic use of vitamin D is systematically practiced, full-fledged cases of infantile rickets of the simple nutritional type have become rare. The decade 1918–1927 saw the achievement of practical mastery over the disease. In the United States, the main contributors toward this achievement included the New York group (Hess, Sherman, and Pappenheimer), the Baltimore group (Park, Shipley, and McCollum), and the Wisconsin group (Steenbock and Hart). In England, Mellanby and Korenchevsky were among the leading contributors. Goldblatt made a comprehensive and systematic survey to 1931 of the vast amount of work by these and the great numbers of other investigators who together have laid the foundation for our present understanding of rickets. The monograph by Hess also includes a scholarly summary of the historical aspects of the disease. The one by Mellanby traces particularly the background of experimental rickets.

Experimental Rickets and Rachitoid States.—The development of the technique for producing rickets experimentally was the entering wedge in the conquest of the disease. Actively growing young rats constituted the principal subjects in the experimental production of rickets. In these animals the vitamin D deficiency had to be combined with a disturbance of the calcium-phosphorus ratio in the diet if rickets was to develop. The optimal ratio of calcium to phosphorus in the diet is between 2:1 and 1:1 for humans and rats alike, but, even with an optimal ratio, certain minimal amounts of both of these elements are necessary for normal skeletal development.

In rapidly growing rats, a distortion of the calcium-phosphorus ratio to 4:1

(or more), in the absence of vitamin D, promptly produces rickets. If the proportion is reversed by increasing the phosphorus until the calcium-phosphorus ratio is 1:4 (or more), a condition somewhat like rickets develops, although this condition resembles osteoporosis more closely than it does typical rickets. Distortion of the calcium-phosphorus ratio produces these ill effects because a great excess of one of these elements tends to interfere with the absorption of the other. In rats, this interference can be abolished to a great extent by an increase in the vitamin D intake.

The question has often been raised whether such experimental rickets actually corresponds to human rickets. So far as the pathology of the changes and the methods by which they can be achieved are concerned, the low-phosphorus rickets of rats does seem to be the exact counterpart of human rickets. This is true despite the fact that in infants developing rickets there need be no previous distortion of the calcium-phosphorus ratio in the diet, and even the phosphorus intake is usually adequate.

Rachitoid bone lesions—that is, bone lesions which resemble those of experimental nutritional rickets, though not identical with them—can also be produced when more or less soluble salts of strontium, magnesium, beryllium, aluminum, or iron are added to the diet in great excess. Specifically, such salts tend to render the phosphorus in the diet unabsorbable by combining with it to form poorly soluble or insoluble phosphates. In consequence, bone lesions akin to those of low-phosphorus rickets are likely to appear. Thus, the addition of excesses of one or another metallic salt has an effect similar to that of a high-calcium low-phosphorus rachitogenic diet, the element added acting in the same way as an excess of calcium (see above). It is interesting to note, however, that vitamin D (which can correct or ameliorate the effects of distortion of the calcium-phosphorus ratio through excess of calcium) is futile against rachitoid lesions resulting from the feeding of excesses of the minerals here being considered. It should also be pointed out that, if the bones presenting these rachitoid lesions are ashed, they show traces or larger amounts of the particular metal used in the experiment. (See Lehnerdt, Shipley *et al.*, Jacobson, and Storey.)

CLINICAL CONSIDERATIONS

It is possible for a neonate to be born with rickets (*congenital rickets*) if its mother, during the pregnancy, had osteomalacia in severe form (see Maxwell *et al.*). However, in infants of non-osteomalacic mothers, even if vitamin D deficiency is present from birth, the bones do not usually begin to develop rachitic changes much before the fourth month of age, and the period of clinically flagrant rickets is that between 8 and 18 months. In the case of *premature* infants, both the onset and the period of floridity of the disease occur earlier.

The clinical picture of rickets to be given will trace the course which a case would take (though such cases are now rarely seen) if the disease began early in infancy and continued without treatment or spontaneous remission for about two years. The disease sets in so insidiously that it is usually not until characteristic skeletal changes are already detectable clinically that one discovers that the child is suffering from rickets (see Eliot and Park). In a rachitic infant 3 or 4 months of age, the only manifestation of the disease may be some widening of the calvarial sutures and the anterior fontanel. However, there may also be some slight beading at the costochondral junctions, and a suggestion of enlargement of the wrist ends of the radius and ulna and of the malleoli at the ankle. Such infants may still seem fairly healthy and lively and may still be gaining normally in weight.

At 6 to 9 months of age (or earlier, especially in premature infants), craniotabes may already be so extensive as to involve a large part of the back of the calvarium,

Figure 98

A, Photograph of a female rachitic child 14 months of age. Note the two highlighted areas on the forehead (representing bossing of the frontal bones) and the forward protrusion of the front of the chest (representing the so-called chicken breast). The clinical history obtained on the child's admission to the hospital was that she was born at full term, was never breast fed, and could not as yet stand up without support. Physical examination revealed the presence of craniotabes and a widely open anterior fontanel. There was also: marked beading at the costochondral junctions of the ribs; enlargement of the ends of the long bones at the wrists and ankles; knock knee; and bowing of the lower portion of the shaft of each tibia. The serum calcium, phosphate, and alkaline phosphatase values on admission were, respectively: 10.0 mg. and 2.8 mg. per cent, and 93 Bodansky units per 100 cc. The child was now placed on therapeutic doses of vitamin D, and 6 weeks later the serum phosphate value had risen to 4.8 mg. and the alkaline phosphatase value had dropped to 25 Bodansky units. Concomitantly, there was striking clinical improvement in the child's condition.

B, Photograph of the calvarium removed at autopsy and freed of adjacent soft tissues in a case of rickets. The slight but definite elevation on each of the still-unfused frontal bones corresponds to the bilateral bossing of the frontal region which had been noted clinically. The child died of pneumonia when he was about 2 years of age.

C, Roentgenograph of ribs removed at autopsy in a case of rickets showing the characteristic rachitic changes at the costochondral junctions. The subject was a boy 16 months of age whose death was due to a bronchopneumonia complicating diphtheria. Note the irregularity of the chondral ends of the rib shafts and their more or less cuplike appearance. Each cupped area represents a rachitic intermediate zone, which is a region substantially occupied by osteoid. Note also that in some of these ribs the cortex lacks clear demarcation, apparently in consequence of the presence of non-mineralized bone matrix (osteoid) beneath the periosteum.

D, Roentgenograph illustrating, for the sake of contrast with *C*, some ribs removed at autopsy from a nonrachitic control subject who died of acute glomerulonephritis which developed as a complication of scarlet fever. Note that the chondral end of each rib shaft is sharply delimited by a linear radiopaque shadow representing the zone of provisional calcification. Furthermore, in comparison with *C*, the cortices of these control ribs are clearly set off.

E, Photograph of the cut surface of the right femur (sectioned in the frontal plane) from a case of active rickets in a female child who died at the age of 8 months. The child was born at full term and had never received prophylactic vitamin D. She was brought to the hospital because she had fallen out of bed 2 days before admission and had suffered a fracture of the *left* femur. Actually, the child was *in extremis* when she was brought in, manifesting cyanosis, convulsions, and high fever, and she died 2 days after admission. Though it had already been recognized clinically that rickets was present, the physical state of the child had precluded the drawing of blood for the determination of serum calcium, phosphorus, and alkaline phosphatase values. The autopsy revealed that the immediate cause of death was a bronchopneumonia, and confirmed the presence of advanced rachitic changes in the bones. Note the widening of the epiphysial cartilage plate area at the lower end of the femur. The histologic details relating to this area are illustrated in Figure 99-*C*.

F, Roentgenograph of a femur from another case of rickets illustrating the x-ray picture which the femur shown in *E* could be expected to present. Note the somewhat radiolucent area in the neck of the femur at its junction with the head. This area represents a rachitic intermediate zone presumably containing osteoid and also some cartilage projecting from the cartilage plate. At the lower end of the femoral shaft, there is a corresponding radiolucent area representing the widened epiphysial cartilage plate and the accumulated cartilage and osteoid in the juxta-epiphysial region of the lower metaphysis. The shaft cortex is thin, and somewhat above the middle of the shaft there is evidence of callus formation at the site of an infraction of the cortex.

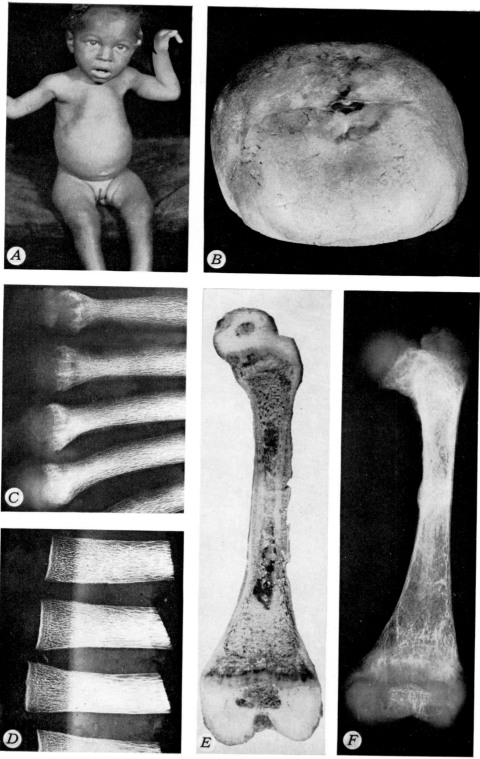

Figure 98

385

while the frontal region or its eminences may show some bossing. The anterior fontanel will be found strikingly large, and the posterior fontanel may still be palpable. (Normally the anterior fontanel closes during the second year of postnatal life, but the posterior fontanel is already closed at about 2 months after birth.) The head of the rachitic infant is likely to show some deformation from flattening on one or the other side or in the back, and the hair may be sparse over the latter region. Dentition will be found delayed. Beading of the costochondral junctions may already be so prominent that these junctions stand out on each side as a rosary. The thoracic cage may appear further deformed from exaggerated forward protrusion of the sternum and from a flaring of the costal margins along the attachment of the diaphragm, creating the so-called Harrison grooves. In addition, especially in relatively active infants, the enlargement at the wrists and ankles may now be considerable, and there may even be the beginnings of curvature of the long bones, especially those of the lower extremities. Furthermore, the infant may have a "potbelly" and may also be unable to sit up without support.

By the time the untreated rachitic child has reached the age of 15 to 24 months, all the skeletal manifestations are found exaggerated, except the craniotabes (which has usually disappeared) and the patency of the anterior fontanel (which has usually at least diminished). Thus, because of increase in the prominence of parietal bossing, together with depression of the anterior fontanel and coronal and sagittal sutures, the top of the head may be flat and squarish. Delay in dentition is still quite apparent; furthermore, in those few teeth which have erupted, the enamel may be defective near the gums, so that the teeth are subject to caries. In the thoracic cage, exaggeration of the skeletal changes is shown by increased protrusion of the sternum (chicken-breastedness) and indentation of the chest wall along the lines of the costochondral junctions, so that the rosary is no longer easily palpable. The Harrison grooves are now well developed, and, along the attachment of the diaphragm, retraction of the sides of the chest is prominent with each inspiration. Furthermore, there may be some dorsal curvature of the spine; if present, it usually affects the entire thoracic column and is rarely associated with any sharp angulation. The enlargement of the ends of the long bones at the wrists and ankles has increased in prominence, and enlargement is now shown also by the bone ends at the knees and elbows. The proximal and middle phalanges of the fingers may be thickened, and the joints between them may appear constricted. Thus, the fingers may present sausage-like enlargements.

The poor muscular development also becomes more clearly apparent. Thus, in order to maintain a sitting posture, the young child with advanced rickets may have to hold itself up by its hands or balance itself by crossing its legs. Furthermore, the child may be unable to pull itself to a standing position or to stand even with support, and walking is correspondingly delayed, or these acts may be executed very clumsily. When such a rachitic child does sit up or walk, the associated functional stresses and strains upon the shafts of the long bones increase the likelihood of their becoming deformed. In such subjects the lower extremities are usually definitely bowed, and there may be knock knee. The gait may be waddling and coxa vara deformity present. The lumbar region may show exaggerated lordosis. If the rachitic state continues into later childhood, the patient is likely to present truly striking deformities and stunting of height sufficiently severe to amount to actual dwarfism. (See Fig. 98.)

BIOCHEMICAL FINDINGS

Mineral Balance Studies.—*Normal infants* and *young children* ingesting an adequate amount of calcium and phosphorus are in positive balance in regard to these minerals. That is, their day-to-day total combined urinary and fecal loss of these minerals is less than the intake. On an adequate (or optimal) calcium and phosphorus intake, healthy young and pre-adolescent children are in positive calcium balance to the amount of about 20 per cent of the intake, and in positive phosphorus balance to the amount of about 14 per cent of the intake. In such subjects, about 90 per cent of the excreted calcium appears in the feces and 10 per cent in the urine, while about 65 per cent of the excreted phosphorus appears in the urine and about 35 per cent in the feces (see Macy). Of the calcium retained, about 99 per cent is utilized in the mineralization of the osseous tissue that is being formed. Of the phosphorus retained, 70 to 75 per cent is utilized in this way, and the rest of the retained phosphorus contributes to the formation of the proteins of the soft tissues.

In the *rachitic infant* or *child*, less calcium and phosphorus are available to the skeleton because the combined urinary and fecal excretion of these minerals is greater than in the normal child on an adequate calcium and phosphorus intake. However, the amount of these minerals excreted in the rachitic child rarely exceeds the intake, so that the calcium and phosphorus balance tends to remain positive, though on a level much below the normal. Furthermore, the proportion of the fecal to the urinary excretion of calcium becomes even higher than in the normal subject, the urinary excretion of calcium dropping sharply below 10 per cent. Also, the proportion of fecal to urinary excretion of phosphorus rises and may even be the reverse of the normal. As a result of all this, wherever organic bone matrix is being formed during the rachitic state, the deposition of bone mineral—a form of hydroxyapatite (p. 125)— is diminished or greatly deficient. As already noted, poorly mineralized organic bone matrix is designated as osteoid, and it is the presence of abundant osteoid that characterizes the histologic picture of both rickets and osteomalacia.

The reason for the increased fecal excretion of calcium and phosphorus in the rachitic state resides in the fact that, in the absence of adequate amounts of vitamin D, there is a reduction in the absorption of calcium and apparently also of phosphorus from the intestinal tract. However, the underlying mechanism by which vitamin D acts to promote the absorption of calcium and phosphorus is not fully understood. Nevertheless, it appears that vitamin D, when available in adequate and physiologic amounts, tends to raise the citrate content of the blood plasma and tissue fluids. In consequence, an increase in the amount of citrate tends to occur in the lumen of the gastrointestinal tract, and on this account the absorption of calcium (and secondarily of phosphate) may be increased. The manner in which this increase might be mediated by the citrate seems to be related to its ability to preferentially complex calcium and thus bring into solution at least some of the poorly soluble calcium phosphate salts present in the gastrointestinal tract. The calcium citrate is readily absorbed as such, and the phosphate ions which were freed from the poorly soluble calcium phosphate then also become available for absorption. Support for the idea of this mechanism may be deduced, for example, from: the ameliorating effects of orally administered sodium citrate on experimentally induced rickets in rats; the reduced concentration of citric acid in the bones of rachitic rats as compared with normal controls; and also the observation that rachitic children show reduced levels of plasma citrate, the levels rising in the course of treatment with vitamin D (see pp. 138, 140, and 143).

Serum Biochemical Findings.—The serum *calcium* value in most cases of rickets is at the low limit of normal (that is, about 10.0 mg. per 100 cc.) or only slightly below this. The serum *inorganic phosphorus* value is almost regularly below 4.0 mg. per 100 cc. and often below 3.0 mg. (normal 4.5 to 5.5 mg. per 100 cc.). On the other hand, in those cases of rickets in which there has also been a deficiency in calcium intake, the serum calcium value may be even under 7.0 mg. per 100 cc.

(these subjects usually manifesting tetany), while the serum inorganic phosphorus is likely not to be strikingly reduced. One may also use the product of the calcium and inorganic phosphorus values as an indication of the presence of rickets, though it is not an absolute one. It has been stated that in infants a product under 30 is definitely indicative of rickets in almost all cases. However, our own experience shows that it may be as high as 40 or even a little higher without eliminating the possibility of rickets, especially in an infant who has been born prematurely. As to the *alkaline phosphatase* activity value in rickets, it has been found that this may rise to 20 to 30 Bodansky units in mild cases, to 60 in pronounced cases, and above 60 (to as high as 190 units) in very severe cases. Normal alkaline phosphatase values for young children lie between 5 and 14 units and average about 7.7 units. (See Howland and Kramer, Bodansky and Jaffe, and Jaffe and Bodansky.)

GROSS PATHOLOGY

A case of florid rickets ascribable merely to the lack of vitamin D (well-developed nutritional rickets) is now, of course, rarely seen where the administration of vitamin D to infants and young children is common practice. However, a sketch of the full pathologic picture of the disease can still serve to clarify the understanding of rickets on whatever basis and of whatever degree of severity. Very detailed descriptions of the pathology of the disease as it was seen before the vitamin D era are to be found in the monographs by Pommer, by Schmorl, and also by Recklinghausen.

As noted, the essential pathologic feature of rickets is deficient deposition of bone mineral in the organic bone matrix being laid down throughout the skeleton during the rachitic state. Such bone matrix is commonly designated as osteoid, since it more or less completely lacks the inorganic matter of full-fledged osseous tissue. Resorption of the calcified osseous tissue already present before the onset of the rickets is ordinarily not accelerated, but sometimes it is strikingly so.

In the cases showing accelerated resorption, there may also be meagerness of osteoid formation. Under these circumstances there results a combination of rickets and osteoporosis in which the bones have thin and porous cortices and wide marrow spaces interspersed with relatively few and thin spongy trabeculae. This is the picture of the so-called "atrophic" or "porotic" form of rickets, in which the bones are fragile and highly susceptible to fracture. It was observed in generally undernourished rachitic subjects. On the other hand, if the vitamin D deficiency was not absolute and the patients were otherwise well nourished, the disease was likely to show itself in the so-called "hypertrophic" or "hyperplastic" form. In such cases the bone cortices, though porous, were thick because of exuberant deposition of osteoid by the periosteum, and the marrow spaces were narrowed because of the presence of abundant spongy osteoid trabeculae. Fractures were less common in these "hypertrophic" than in the "atrophic" cases, and the condition was altogether less ominous, but the bones became considerably misshapen when the disease had continued for any length of time.

Skull.—Craniotabes (that is, the presence of areas of thinning and softening in the calvarium) is one of the most constant findings in rickets. In the affected calvarial regions, the original calcified osseous tissue has been substantially resorbed, and any new osseous tissue deposited is lacking or highly deficient in bone mineral. In the development of areas of craniotabes, there is more extensive resorption from the dural surface than from the pericranial surface of the calvarium. A severely affected region may even present gaps filled in only by connective tissue. The softened area of the calvarium can be depressed by the finger, but it snaps back again with a crackle when released.

It is rare in rickets to find craniotabes elsewhere than in the posterior parts of the parietal bones and the upper part of the occipital bone, well away from the lambdoid and sagittal sutures. The areas are rarely symmetrically distributed and are more likely to be found, and usually better developed, on the side of the head on which the infant habitually lies. An individual area is commonly about 2.5 cm. in diameter, but it may be considerably smaller or, on the other hand, involve a large part of the back of the calvarium. Rachitic craniotabes is generally not found before the third or fourth month and usually disappears by the eighth or ninth month—that is, when growth of the skull has slowed.

Softening of the calvarium may be observed at birth in otherwise normal infants born prematurely. If present, the softening is ordinarily found along the margins of the sutures, though it sometimes involves large portions of the occipital or parietal bones. Normal full term fetuses, too, may show ossification defects in the calvarium at birth. All such congenital (nonrachitic) craniotabetic areas disappear spontaneously by the third or fourth month of life. However, if an infant with areas of congenital calvarial softening develops rickets, those areas may remain unossified and constitute additional areas of rachitic craniotabes (see Abels).

Normally, the anterior fontanel begins to diminish in size soon after birth and is completely closed not later than the eighteenth to twenty-fourth month. In rare instances in otherwise normal subjects, it shows a tendency (apparently hereditary) to remain slightly open throughout life. In the rachitic infant, this fontanel is abnormally large, its margins are usually found soft, and the sutures as they approach it are quite wide. Indeed, as late as the third or fourth year in protracted cases of rickets, the anterior fontanel may still be found somewhat patent, though its base has become firm.

Thickening of the vault is also observed in rickets, though not in every case. When present, it is not found evenly distributed over the vault. It usually affects the frontal and parietal bones (and is most pronounced in the region of their eminences), while the occipital bone is either entirely spared or at least much less severely involved than the others. If the disease has persisted into the second or third year of life, the thickening of the predilected parts may be very pronounced. Wherever it appears, the thickening of the vault is almost entirely a manifestation of excessive deposition of new bone on its outer surface by the pericranium, but, to a small extent, deposition of new bone on its inner surface by the dura may have contributed to the calvarial thickening.

Altogether, though the size of the cranial cavity tends to remain unchanged, the circumference of the vault may be increased, and its shape will certainly be altered if the thickening of the calvarium is pronounced. As to shape, the top of the head in advanced rickets most commonly presents the so-called "caput quadratum" because of the four mounds produced by the prominent frontal and parietal bosses. However, if only the frontal region is prominent and projects forward beyond the plane of the face, the so-called "Olympic brow" is created, while if only the parietal bosses are prominent and the occiput is flattened, the head may have a triangular shape.

Thoracic Cage.—The first changes are reflected in the costochondral junctions. In the normal infant the latter appear as spindle-shaped swellings more pronounced on the inner surface of the thoracic cage than on the outer. In the rachitic infant these junctions are enlarged and rounded, while still remaining more prominent on the inside. Though their size varies more or less in accordance with the severity of the disease, the costochondral junctions form two series of beady enlargements, commonly referred to as the *rachitic rosary*. The "beadiness" results from marked widening of the zone of proliferative cartilage at the costochondral junction and the presence of a wide rachitic intermediate zone at the shaft end of the junction.

26

Thus the beading of the ribs has the same pathologic foundation as the enlargement that takes place at the epiphysial-diaphysial junctions of certain long bones, but the alterations are grossly demonstrable much earlier in the ribs.

Though the rib shafts of a rachitic infant are porous and yielding, it is the changes at the costochondral junctions that initiate the deformation of the thoracic cage which regularly occurs if the modifications at the junctions are severe. The deformity may consist merely of a furrow on each side, caused by sinking in of the ribs (especially the middle six) in the region of the costochondral junctions. If the body of the sternum has been pushed forward, as it often has, the front of the chest resembles more or less closely a pigeon breast, especially if, at the same time, the manubrium has been elevated and the xyphoid points inward. Occasionally, instead of chicken-breastedness, one finds funnel-breastedness, which results from forward arching of the costal cartilages so pronounced that the sternum forms the floor of a groove. Furthermore, the front of the chest may present grooves (Harrison grooves) extending from the lower end of the sternum toward the mid-axillary lines and resulting from depression of the ribs along the attachment of the diaphragm.

The clavicles may show increased anterior bowing, and if the rickets is severe, they, like the ribs, may be the site of fractures. As the rachitic subject grows older, muscle weakness favors the development of dorsal kyphosis, apparent particularly in the sitting posture. If the bones of the pelvis and those of the lower extremities also become distorted, the resultant altered statics may aggravate the deformity of the thorax through the development of a scoliosis and a lumbar lordosis.

Pelvis.—Mild rickets in infancy usually leaves no deep or significant imprint upon the ultimate form and shape of the pelvis. On the other hand, if the rickets is severe and protracted into childhood, the effect on the pelvis may come to be very pronounced. In such cases one may find an exaggerated anterior projection of the sacral promontory and sickle-like curvature of the sacrum and coccyx. These changes are associated with general flattening of the pelvis and severe lumbar lordosis. This is likely to be very grave for the female, since the resultant narrowness of the external conjugate may seriously interfere with childbirth later on.

Long Bones.—In the "atrophic" form of rickets the long bones of the extremities usually present little or no gross enlargement at their epiphysial-diaphysial junctions. When sectioned, however, these bones reveal wide rachitic intermediate zones at these junctions. Furthermore, the shaft cortex is found thin and porous, while the spongy trabeculae are sparse and slender, and this condition of the shaft explains the frequency of fractures and infractions in these cases. If such subjects survive and the disease continues, the changes presented by the bones gradually come to be those of the so-called "hypertrophic" form, which is the form that rickets more often assumes from the beginning.

In the "hypertrophic" cases the epiphysial-diaphysial junctions of the long bones may be obviously enlarged. In some of these bones the epiphysis and the rachitic intermediate zone may be found tilted or actually displaced upon the diaphysis, and periosteal new bone will be found filling in the angles created by the malposition and thus smoothing the transition between the epiphysis and the shaft. The shafts themselves, instead of being thin, as in the "atrophic" form, are very likely to show cortical thickening from the deposition of wide concentric layers of poorly mineralized osseous tissue by the periosteum. In such bones, excessive amounts of endosteal osseous tissue, also poorly mineralized, may likewise have been formed, so that the major marrow cavity is encroached upon and the spongy trabeculae at the bone ends are thick and set close together. Analogous cortical thickening may be presented by the *short tubular bones*, and when the proximal and middle phalanges are so affected, they appear sausage-like in shape.

Fractures, Curvatures, and Stunting of Growth.—Though there may be bending or twisting at the rachitic intermediate zones of the bones, fractures seem never to occur through these zones. Any fractures present are located in the shafts, often of the long tubular bones though more often of the ribs. As noted, fractures occur much more commonly in the "atrophic" than in the "hypertrophic" form of rickets, and are seldom associated with tearing of the periosteum and displacement of the fracture ends. Roentgenographically, they present as transverse or slanting, slit- or bandlike zones of radiolucency. When present, they are usually multiple and often bilateral and symmetrical. They may or may not traverse the bone completely. The bone ends on either side of the zone of radiolucency are ordinarily not sharply delimited and, as also noted, not displaced. The apparent loss of continuity of the shaft at such a site is often referred to as a pseudofracture, to contrast it with a conventional fracture. E. Looser was among the first to stress the occurrence of these zones of rarefaction ("*Aufhellungszonen*") in cases of rickets and osteomalacia. He believed that they develop as a result of local microinfractions engendered by mechanical stress, and that, in the course of healing, the area is reconstructed and filled in with an osteoid callus, the area becoming what he designated as an "*Umbauzone*." Since this internal callus is deficient in bone mineral, its roentgenographic shadow is more radiolucent than that of the neighboring rachitic bone.

Curvature of the bone shafts results most often from misdirection of growth following upon tilting of the epiphysis, but may arise from fractures or infractions of the shaft, from mere yielding of it, or through several or all of these influences together. On the whole, the long bones of the upper extremities are much less likely to show severe curvatures than those of the lower. However, the shaft of the humerus may be found bowed outward, or outward and forward, slightly above the insertion of the deltoid, while the radius and ulna may show exaggeration of their normal curvatures.

In the lower extremities the most typical deformities encountered are *bowlegs* (genu varum) and *knock knees* (genu valgum). The O-type of bowleg is presented when all the long bones bend outward in a lateral plane from the hips to the ankles. However, the curvature, because of limitation of it to either the thigh or the leg bones, may be less nearly circular. The knock knee position, in which the knees approximate or overlap one another, is usually complicated by a bowing outward of the femora and also sometimes of the tibiae and fibulae. With lateral bowing of the long bones, there is frequently some forward bowing in addition. Also, *coxa vara* may be present in a form so pronounced that the neck of the femur may form a right angle or even an acute angle with the shaft. Following posterior tilting of the lower epiphyses of the tibia and fibula and subsequent misdirection of growth, one may find the so-called "*saber shin*" deformity of the lower third of the leg.

If the rickets is severe and has continued for several years, the height of the subject is usually considerably below the normal and is very likely to remain so. In fact, many of the older textbooks describe adults so stunted as a result of protracted rickets in childhood that they fall into the category of dwarfs. The dwarfing in cases of rickets is related in part to the disturbance in endochondral bone growth. Mainly, however, it is brought about by curvatures of the long bones of the lower limbs and by pronounced lordotic and kyphoscoliotic deformity of the vertebral column. Rachitic dwarfs may have to be differentiated from achondroplastic dwarfs (p. 198), but the distinction is usually not difficult.

Teeth.—Rickets, especially if severe, retards the eruption of the deciduous teeth. The retardation may be very pronounced, and when the teeth in question do erupt they usually fail to appear in the normal sequence. Furthermore, the deciduous teeth may present defects of the enamel (found especially in the upper incisors and close to the gums) and caries (found especially in the molars). The permanent teeth, too, may have been disturbed in their development if the rickets has been severe. In certain of these, the enamel may show areas of hypoplasia, the extent and severity of which will depend upon the gravity and duration of the rickets. It is to be doubted, however, that rickets in infancy and early childhood is a factor increasing the susceptibility of the permanent teeth to caries.

MICROSCOPIC PATHOLOGY

Changes at Cartilage-Shaft Junctions.—*Normally*, the course of endochondral ossification as manifested at cartilage-shaft junctions is essentially as follows: (1) Cartilage cells in the proliferative zone advance in orderly columns toward the shaft, enlarging as they proceed; (2) as they approach the shaft, the hypertrophied cartilage cells are penetrated and destroyed by blood vessels advancing against them from the marrow; (3) coincidentally, the cartilage matrix between these cells becomes calcified; and (4) osteoblasts around the penetrating vessels lay down organic bone matrix (which quickly becomes mineralized) upon spicules of calcified cartilage matrix.

As had been shown by various early investigators, the *rachitic disorder* induces changes at cartilage-shaft junctions reflecting a disorganization of this whole process of endochondral ossification (see Park). Specifically, the advance of the cartilage cells toward the shaft no longer proceeds in orderly columns. In addition, there is delayed maturation and inadequate destruction of the advancing cartilage cells by the marrow capillaries, so that these cells accumulate and the zone of proliferative cartilage becomes abnormally wide. Indeed, relatively few marrow vessels will be found penetrating the cartilage, and those which do penetrate extend into it at various angles and to various levels, instead of running in channels parallel to the long axis of the shaft and keeping abreast of each other. One also finds in rickets that the widened proliferative zone is being vascularized to some extent by vessels extending in from the perichondrium, while still others come from the adjacent resting cartilage. These junctional changes are most pronounced where growth is normally most rapid. Hence the sites where they stand out most clearly are the costochondral junctions of the middle six ribs and the epiphysial-diaphysial junctions at the lower end of the femur and the upper end of the tibia.

Histologic examination of one of these rachitic junctions reveals, between the penetrating marrow vessels, irregular tongues and strands of cartilage extending into the shaft from the main body of the proliferative cartilage. It will also be noted that the deposition of bone mineral in the cartilage matrix along the line of destructive advance of the marrow vessels has been fragmentary or has failed to take place at all. Where the cartilage is being eroded and has marrow vessels abutting upon it, some osteoid (osseous tissue deficient in bone mineral) will be found to have been deposited. The cartilage on which the osteoid abuts is usually found to have undergone certain modifications. Specifically, in some places, both its matrix and its cells have taken on the appearance of osteoid. The cartilage so transformed has been called "cartilaginous osteoid." In other places the cartilage will be found in various stages of degeneration or in a state of regressive transformation into what seems to be connective tissue. Furthermore, the metaphysial marrow is often rather fibrous, especially around the blood vessels, which may be fairly numerous. In this fibrous marrow there are many thick and irregular osseous trabeculae covered with broad seams of osteoid and constituting a finely porous and vascularized spongioid tissue.

Altogether, then, at cartilage-shaft junctions there gradually forms a zone of disorganized and intermingled cartilage and shaft elements which may be described as the "rachitic metaphysis" or "rachitic intermediate zone." At the lower end of the femur this zone may be as much as 1 or 2 cm. wide in a case of active rickets of some duration. Furthermore, because of lack of rigidity of the rachitic intermediate zone (ascribable to the osteoid nature of its osseous tissue), deformities are likely to develop at the cartilage-shaft junctions as a result of functional stresses and strains. Their occurrence is associated with displacements (sometimes quite pronounced) of the epiphyses and chondral cartilages out of their normal positions. However, fractures seem never to develop through the rachitic intermediate zone, apparently because the very plasticity which permits its bending tends to prevent breaks. (See Fig. 99.)

In more recent studies of the rachitic changes at sites of endochondral ossification, various histochemical techniques and biophysical methods (electron microscopy, microradiography, and interference microscopy) have been used. These investigations have confirmed in general the findings given above (which were obtained on the basis of stained tissue sections studied with the light microscope), and have added certain supportive details. Furthermore, it was demonstrated that the osteoid of rickets shows atypical orientation of its collagen fibers, though structurally the collagen fibers of osteoid appear to be identical with those of mineralized bone matrix. (See Robinson and Sheldon, Hjertquist, Engfeldt and Zetterström, Rohr, and also Thomas.)

Changes in the Bone Shafts.—In the rachitic state the newly formed cortical and spongy osseous tissue of the shafts is also deficient in bone mineral. The original cortex tends to become porous, and borders of osteoid will be found lining its enlarged haversian canals and spaces. In well-nourished and relatively active rachitic infants, the cortices may, in addition, be found somewhat thickened by poorly mineralized new bone (osteoid) laid down by the periosteum. This thickening apparently develops in response to mechanical irritation of the periosteum by pull from muscles, tendons, and fasciae. On the shafts of some of the long bones, this periosteal deposit of osteoid may measure several millimeters in thickness. In such cases the osteoid seams on the trabeculae of the cancellous bone are also wide, and the marrow spaces of the spongiosa, as well as the major marrow cavity, may be narrow. Beneath the osteoid borders lining the haversian canals of the cortex and the spongy trabeculae, there usually is some osseous tissue whose matrix is moderately well mineralized. The amount of this mineralized osseous tissue becomes reduced by resorption during the progress of the disease.

Bowing may appear in the shafts because of weakening of the cortex. Fractures and infractions may also play a part in the bone deformities. Aside from deformities on these accounts, the shafts frequently show some which have their origin in the displacements that have occurred at the cartilage-shaft junctions. When an epiphysis or chondral cartilage is displaced out of the line of the shaft, continuation of growth at the cartilage-shaft junction is associated with the development, in this region, of an angulation which shifts further along the shaft during subsequent growth of the bone.

The Repair of the Rachitic Process.—As revealed microscopically, this repair sets in very promptly upon the institution of antirachitic treatment. In the rachitic intermediate zone the process of healing is inaugurated by the deposition of bone mineral in the distal border of the proliferative cartilage. This is followed by the appearance of foci of calcification at various points in the rest of the intermediate zone. Soon, by means of extension and enlargement of the bushes of blood vessels, which bear osteoblasts upon them, the widened proliferative cartilage around and between these bushes is converted into bony trabeculae.

By now the original zone of delimitation between the cartilage and shaft has been re-established as the proliferative cartilage zone. The cartilage cells in this region now mature in normal fashion, the intercellular cartilage matrix calcifies, and well-mineralized osseous tissue comes to replace the proliferating cartilage. Furthermore, any new osseous tissue forming elsewhere than at sites of endochondral bone growth is also normally calcified. Similarly, the osteoid borders of the cancellous trabeculae, the osteoid linings of the haversian spaces, and the osteoid lamellae under the periosteum and in the interior of the bone become permeated with bone mineral. Remodeling, as compared with mere recalcification, of the osseous tissue may take months or even years.

ROENTGENOGRAPHIC FINDINGS

Normally, the line of demarcation at cartilage-shaft junctions as seen roentgenographically is slightly concave at some junctions, slightly convex at others, and straight at still others. The appearance of a distinct cupping concavity where it is not normally present constitutes an important though not infallible sign of rickets. This sign appears most promptly where the juncture ordinarily has a slight natural concavity or is at least flat and not convex. For practical purposes, the findings in the lower end of the ulna and radius probably represent the best roentgenographic guide to the status of the subject in respect to rickets (see Eliot and Park).

Cupping of the lower end of the ulna is a valuable cue in the early diagnosis of the disease, cupping of the lower end of the radius coming much later. (It should be remembered, however, that, in infants with severe rickets, cupping present anatomically may fail to stand out roentgenographically because of a particularly pronounced lack of bone mineral in the junctional regions.) With the cupping, or

Figure 99

A, Photograph (somewhat enlarged) showing the cut surface of part of a rib from a case of severe rickets. The upper end of the picture shows a small portion of costal cartilage. The irregularly mottled area immediately beyond the latter consists of a widened zone of proliferating costal cartilage. The more uniformly whitish area beyond the proliferating cartilage consists of an accumulation of osteoid and cartilage representing the rachitic intermediate zone—an area which would appear relatively radiolucent in the x-ray picture.

B, Photomicrograph ($\times$ 6) of part of a rib illustrating the general architecture of a costochondral junctional area in a case of rickets. The upper end of the picture shows costal cartilage in a resting stage. Beyond that cartilage there is the proliferating cartilage zone, which is abnormally wide and irregular and shows tonguelike extensions into the adjacent portion of the rib shaft. In that part of the shaft, numerous trabeculae of non-mineralized bone matrix are present and intermingle with cartilage which has separated off and come down from the zone of proliferating cartilage. The cortex of the rib is thin, and on the left side of the picture, trabeculae of inadequately mineralized bone matrix are observed beneath the periosteum. Under higher magnification the spongy trabeculae in the interior of the rib shaft would be found to have narrow osteoid borders.

C, Photomicrograph ($\times$ 4) illustrating the general histologic architecture of the lower end of the rachitic femur shown in Figure 98-E. In this picture the secondary center of ossification in the epiphysis is much smaller than it is in Figure 98-E, because the plane of the section extends through the periphery of the ossification center rather than through its middle. Above the epiphysis (which is largely cartilaginous), one notes the dark-staining, widened, irregular, proliferating cartilage zone, from which tongues of cartilage are extending into the metaphysis. The lighter-staining tissue in the metaphysis is osteoid—that is, non-mineralized organic bone matrix. The spongy trabeculae in the interior of the femur, beyond the osteoid zone, would be found to have narrowed osteoid borders if photographed under higher magnification.

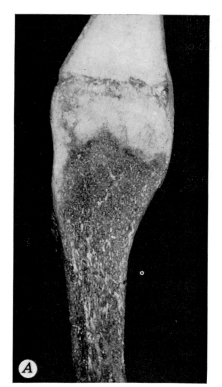

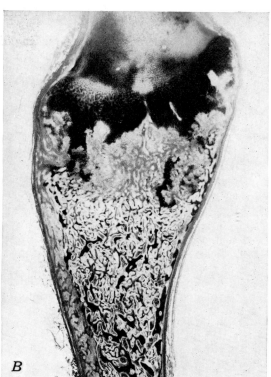

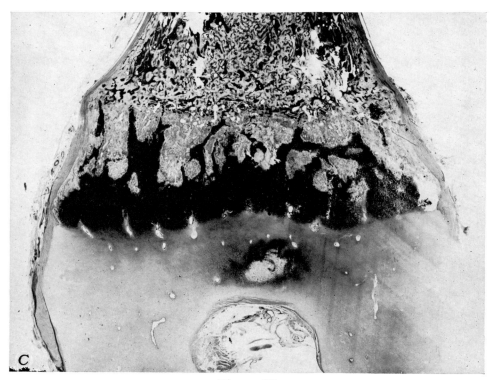

Figure 99

even without it, there may be some flaring of the end of the shaft. One may also see, extending along the margin of the shaft and even on to that of the cartilage, straight or somewhat arched linear spurs representing areas of calcification in the fibrous cuff at the junction. The end of the shaft may be fuzzy or may present a more definitely frayed appearance due to the presence of irregular threadlike shadows extending from the shaft toward the cartilage. Or, instead, the end of the shaft may appear stippled because of the presence of irregular deposits of bone mineral in the proliferative zone in the immediate vicinity of the junction. Furthermore, in clear-cut cases, one usually finds widening of the zone between the end of the shaft and the center of ossification in the epiphysis.

The shaft cortex shows more or less decreased radiodensity. At the same time, if the rickets is of the hypertrophic type, the cortex may show more or less thickening, due to the deposition of layers of new bone by the periosteum, and the marrow cavity may appear somewhat narrowed by endosteal bone formation.

The first *roentgenographic sign of repair* in response to treatment is the appearance of a transverse linear shadow beyond and parallel to the end of the shaft. This shadow indicates that, with the resumption of normal endochondral bone formation, calcification has begun again in the cartilage matrix of the proliferative zone. Soon one also notes splotchy longitudinal shadows representing mineralization occurring in the rachitic intermediate zone. Concomitantly, mineralization of the osseous tissue deposited by the periosteum becomes apparent roentgenographically. Altogether, slowly but surely, the texture of the bones returns toward the normal. Years may pass, however, before all roentgenographic evidences of the pre-existing rickets are completely obliterated, and indeed, if the rickets has been present for a considerable time, some permanent deformities may remain. (See Fig. 100 and also Fig. 98-*C*, *D*, and *F*.)

TREATMENT

The problem of rickets is now largely one of prevention, by securing to infants (from about the third week of life) adequate amounts of vitamin D as a supplement

Figure 100

A, Roentgenograph showing the bones in the region of the wrist in a case of active rickets. The patient was a male child $1\frac{1}{2}$ years of age. Note the cupping at the lower end of the radius and ulna, representing pronounced rachitic intermediate zones in the metaphyses of the bones in question. The cortices of the metacarpal bones in particular, though rarefied, are thicker than they would normally be. This is an indication that the child was well nourished on the whole, even though it lacked vitamin D.

B, Roentgenograph of the same wrist area as in *A* taken 4 weeks after administration of therapeutic doses of vitamin D had been started. Note that there is now clear-cut evidence of mineralization in the rachitic intermediate zones—a manifestation of healing.

C, Roentgenograph of the wrist area taken 10 weeks after *B*. The rachitic intermediate zones are now almost completely filled in, so that there is no longer any local evidence of clear-cut rickets.

D, Roentgenograph of the lower extremities of a female child 2 years of age who was admitted to our hospital because of severe knock knee deformity due to rickets. This deformity had been present for about 1 year and was increasing in severity. There was also anterior bowing of both tibiae and evidence of coxa vara deformity at the upper ends of the femora. Inquiry revealed that the child had not previously received any prophylactic vitamin D. She was now placed on an antirachitic regimen.

E, Roentgenograph of the lower extremities of this child taken about 15 months after antirachitic therapy had been started. The rickets has healed, but the rachitic deformities persist. The child was readmitted to the hospital for the surgical correction of the deformities.

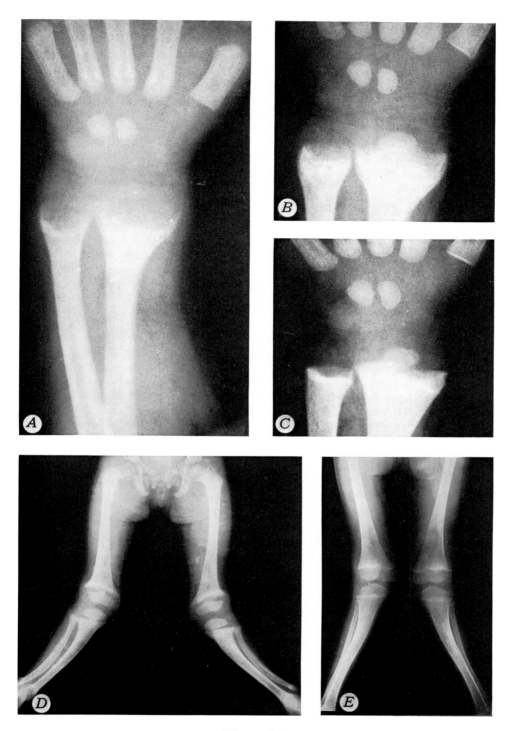

Figure 100

to an otherwise proper diet. The prophylactic use of one or another of the antirachitic substances should be continued until the child is at least 3 years of age and, in large cities with cold winters, perhaps even into late childhood. The advisability of continuing vitamin D into late childhood and particularly during periods of illness seems to be suggested by the findings of Follis *et al.* It was noted by them that ribs removed at autopsy from children of various ages, dead of various causes (but obviously not affected with clinical rickets), rather often showed osteoid borders on the spongy trabeculae at the costochondral junctions. This finding was interpreted as an indication of nonclinical rickets and was often observed even in children who had received known amounts of vitamin D for varying periods before death.

The rare case of vitamin D-deficiency rickets encountered now, while it may be active, usually manifests only mild skeletal changes. Such a case of rickets can rapidly be brought under control and cured by daily doses of vitamin D as small as 5,000 to 10,000 units continued for 2 or 3 months, after which the daily administration of prophylactic doses of 500 to 1,000 units will keep the condition from recurring.

As already indicated, the administration of vitamin D increases the absorption of calcium and phosphorus from the gastrointestinal tract, and one consequence of this is the improvement of the mineral balance in regard to calcium and phosphorus. The mechanism by which this is accomplished is mentioned on p. 144. Because of the improvement of the mineral balance resulting from the administration of vitamin D, the serum calcium value tends to rise to the normal level, as does the serum inorganic phosphorus value.

In the course of correction of the rachitic state, the elevated alkaline phosphatase value recedes toward the normal. Altogether, the alkaline phosphatase value is not only a good index of the severity of the rickets, but usually also a better guide to the adequacy of the antirachitic treatment and a more accurate indication of the complete abolition of the rachitic state than the calcium value or even the inorganic phosphorus value. It is to be noted that the inorganic phosphorus value is likely to rise promptly even under somewhat inadequate treatment. The phosphatase value drops decidedly only when the antirachitic treatment is adequate, and does not reach the normal level in its fall until the healing of the rickets is really complete (see Bodansky and Jaffe).

The treatment so far as rachitic deformities are concerned depends upon a number of factors. If the disease has been cured before severe deformities have had a chance to develop, one may expect any slight aberrations present to disappear, substantially or entirely, in the course of time. Their disappearance can be facilitated by the use of braces. If the deformities are severe and disfiguring (especially in the lower extremities) and have not subsided to any great extent by the time the child is 3 or 4 years old, the curved bones should be straightened by orthopaedic procedures. The treatment of rachitic scoliosis may range from exercise and support in mild cases to fusion of the deformed part of the column in very severe cases.

NUTRITIONAL OSTEOMALACIA

Osteomalacia due to a lack of vitamin D in association with undernutrition never found in this country the unfortunate combination of circumstances necessary for its development. Formerly, such cases of osteomalacia were rather common in India and in certain parts of China (see Wilson, and Maxwell). The writer has been informed that it is not unusual to encounter them in those countries even now. In the past, osteomalacia of the type in question was also common even in many countries of continental Europe and in Great Britain, but under ordinary conditions one rarely observes such a case in these countries now (see Dent and Smith).

In the vast majority of the cases, the subjects were females. The disease usually set in during young adulthood (or adolescence)—at any rate, well before middle age. Persons in whom the disease had begun early in adolescence ordinarily showed a combination of osteomalacic and rachitic changes (late rickets). When occurring in a female, the condition had, in its etiologic background, not only a lack of vitamin D from prolonged confinement indoors, but also a dietary deficiency in regard to fats, proteins, and calcium, and the exhausting demands made on the calcium supply by repeated pregnancies or pregnancy during adolescence.

CLINICAL CONSIDERATIONS

If the subject is a female and pregnant (as is commonly the case), she may be in her first pregnancy or may have gone through a number of pregnancies. If she is a multipara, inquiry may reveal that in previous pregnancies there had already been some difficulties suggesting osteomalacia. As to her present complaint, though this may have been ushered in abruptly by sharp bone pains and fever, it is much more likely to have been ushered in merely by bone pains, which have only gradually become severe. Ordinarily, these pains are localized at first in the lower part of the back and in the groin, but gradually they spread. They also come to be associated with muscular difficulties, connected particularly with rising from a squatting or sitting position and with walking, which is done with a waddling gait. As the pregnancy progresses, both the bone pains and the muscular weakness grow worse and the patient may become bedridden and almost helpless.

By this time, pronounced skeletal deformities have usually developed, especially in the vertebral column, ribs, sternum, and pelvis. It is the changes in the pelvis that make the subsequent delivery so dangerous for both the mother and her infant, and that account for the necessity of cesarean section or craniotomy in so many of these cases. Though the teeth may loosen and fall out, their susceptibility to caries seems not to be increased in osteomalacia.

The osteomalacic subject is also very likely to suffer from attacks of tetany or from such less obvious indications of neuromuscular hyperirritability as numbness of the limbs and muscular cramps and spasms. These manifestations are attributable to reduction in the serum calcium value (particularly the ionized calcium fraction), which almost regularly occurs in the disease. Serum calcium values of about 7.5 mg. per 100 cc. are common, and values as low as 5.0 mg. have been reported in chronic cases. The serum inorganic phosphorus is frequently also below normal, values around 2.0 mg. being common. A number of metabolic studies have been made on Chinese subjects suffering from the type of osteomalacia under consideration. These show, in relation to calcium and phosphorus metabolism, that in the control periods before the administration of vitamin D there is excessive loss of calcium and phosphorus in the feces. They also show that urinary excretion of calcium drops almost to zero. In other words, the disorder of calcium and phosphorus metabolism is essentially similar to that observed in nutritional rickets (vitamin D-deficiency rickets). The administration of vitamin D corrects the disordered calcium and phosphorus metabolism of these osteomalacic subjects in the same manner as it does in rachitic children (see Hannon et al., and Liu et al.).

Because of the pains and hyperirritability, the subject may shrink from being touched or even approached. Altogether, she may become completely incapacitated. The disease sometimes progresses steadily, the subject dying of some intercurrent disorder. More often, however, its course is characterized by progressions and remissions. It is common for the disease to flare up in the course of lactation or shortly after its termination. If, during a subsequent pregnancy, conditions are still favorable to the development of osteomalacia, all its manifestations are more severe than they were before. It is of interest that at birth the bones in offspring of osteomalacic women only very rarely show frank rickets, though it is not unusual to find them porotic.

"War Osteopathy" or "Hunger Osteomalacia."—In central Europe during and shortly after the war of 1914–1918, there occurred numerous cases of a condition variously designated as "war osteopathy," "hunger osteomalacia," or simply "osteomalacia." This appeared particularly in parts of Austria (especially in and around Vienna) and parts of Germany and Poland. Though the condition did resemble mild genuine osteomalacia, it also differed from the latter in various respects. Thus, only a relatively small proportion of cases occurred during adolescence (14 to 20 years), and in addition there was a pronounced predominance of males in this group. Also, there were practically no cases between the ages of 20 and 40 years. Finally, the incidence of the disease rose rapidly after the age of 40, though the large majority of the older subjects were females. The condition was characterized by pains in the lower back, thighs, and legs, and difficulty in climbing stairs and in walking, which was executed with a waddling gait. Often there was also bone tenderness, especially in the vertebral column. In addition, the subjects frequently manifested tetany. (See Edelmann, Beninde, and also Dalyell and Chick.) During the war of 1939–1945, instances of "hunger osteomalacia" also appeared in various countries of central Europe (see Maratka). These reports bring out, furthermore, that the patients' deficiencies were by no means limited to vitamin D, and that they were suffering from general under-nutrition and lacked specifically an adequate intake of calcium, phosphorus, fat, and animal protein. In addition, the reports stress the idea that the condition was quickly reversible by the institution of a proper dietary regimen, supplemented by vitamin D. In subjects succumbing to "hunger osteomalacia," anatomic examination of the bones revealed that the latter were rather porotic—a finding which was in harmony with the general marasmic state of the subjects (see Partsch).

PATHOLOGIC FINDINGS

Gross Pathology.—The various skeletal regions are by no means evenly affected in osteomalacia, though the skeletal involvement is generalized. On the whole, it is the vertebral column, pelvis, ribs, and sternum that usually show the severest gross changes. So far as these trunk bones are concerned, the only difference which is likely to be found between the puerperal and the nonpuerperal cases of osteomalacia pertains to the involvement of the pelvis. In the former cases this part is often gravely altered, while in the latter cases it only infrequently shows any obvious change. Of the long bones, it is the femora that in general most often show severe gross changes. Indeed, except for the humeri (upper ends), these are the only long bones that may appear much altered. In the skull, strikingly enough, gross changes seem to be infrequent and slight in osteomalacia. However, even in bones showing but little obvious alteration, the histologic evidences of the disease are ordinarily clear-cut. Furthermore, in bones which superficially seem practically normal, microscopic examination will probably reveal at least osteoid seams on the trabeculae and on the surfaces of the haversian canals.

In osteomalacia, resorption of the firm osseous tissue, together with replacement of the latter by yielding osteoid, makes the bones both pliable and fragile and hence susceptible to distortions, curvatures, and fractures. Typically, in a subject with advanced skeletal changes, the *thorax* will be found shortened in the vertical plane, narrowed and flattened from side to side, and deepened from front to back. In the creation of this status, a large part is played by the presence of sharp dorsal kyphosis, which is most severe at D_8 or D_9 and which may be associated with a dorsal scoliosis. The ribs may be found badly bent and overlapping each other. The sternum may present a number of angulations. There may also be an exaggerated lumbar lordosis, with forward protrusion of the promontory of the sacrum and even more pronounced forward protrusion of the fourth and fifth lumbar vertebrae.

The deformity of the lower part of the vertebral column contributes considerably to the evolution of the *pelvic deformity*, which is one of the most characteristic features of the disease. In connection with the forward protrusion of the sacral promontory, the iliac bones may have been dragged forward also. Below the sacral promontory the inward curve of the sacrum and coccyx may be sharply accentuated, the latter being directed transversely toward the pubis. In addition, because of upward protrusion of the femora, the acetabular fossae may be found very much deepened, so that the pelvic hollow is reduced in this way too. The pubic arch may show beaking, and the ischial tuberosities are often abnormally close together.

As noted, the shafts of the *long bones* are not very likely to appear deformed, even when they have become highly porotic. If the subject is an adolescent, however, they may be considerably deformed, especially in the lower extremities, which may show coxa vara in association with knock knees or bowlegs. Furthermore, in such subjects there may be broadening at certain cartilage-shaft junctions (those of the ribs and long bones particularly), and widened metaphysial zones, such as one sees in rickets, may be demonstrable.

Fractures may be encountered, notably in the ribs and in the shafts of the long bones, and it is not uncommon to find two or three fractures in each rib, in various stages of healing. The ribbon-like zones of rarefaction observed roentgenographically and representing local infractions filled with osteoid callus, as was discussed in connection with rickets (p. 391), are also seen in cases of osteomalacia. In osteomalacia, too, these infractions may be multiple and often bilateral and symmetrical. Common sites, in addition to the ribs, are the femoral necks, the ischia, the rami of the pubic bones, and the axillary margins of the scapulae.

Where a bone has been subjected to undue loading or mechanical bending, its interior is likely to be occupied by excessive amounts of compacted osteoid trabeculae. These areas of densified spongiosa appear gray-white and have a finely porous and firm rubbery consistency. If the vertebral column is distorted, vertebral bodies are particularly likely to show compacted spongiosa. It either extends rather uniformly through the body or appears in bands adjacent to the intervertebral disks, the compacted spongiosa being separated by a central zone of more or less porotic spongiosa. Areas of densified spongiosa are also frequently observed in the upper ends of the femora or humeri and in the ribs where the latter have undergone physiologic or pathologic curvature. Occasionally the calvarium is seen to have been rather elaborately reconstructed, the original osseous tissue having been replaced throughout by closely compacted diploic bone. Where fractures and infractions have occurred in the shafts of the long bones or ribs, rather extensive areas of compacted endosteal callus may also be found.

Microscopic Pathology.—Large sections of the monographs by Pommer and by Recklinghausen are devoted to describing and explaining the histology of the bone changes in osteomalacia. The pathologic foundation for these various skeletal changes is created by: (1) thinning of the original spongiosa and porotification of the original cortical bone, and (2) the substitution, for the resorbed tissue, of osteoid which (especially in the interior of the bone) may be formed in excessive amounts and condensed where it has been subjected to undue loading or mechanical bending. Furthermore, it is to be noted that the osteoid seams and borders show a lamellar arrangement of the collagen fibers and thus represent lamellar osteoid. On the other hand, osteoid developing in connection with endosteal callus may be coarse-fibered, but sooner or later this primitive osteoid becomes transformed into lamellar osteoid. It is also significant histologically that, in osteomalacia, osteoclasts are conspicuous by their scarcity, being found only at sites of callus formation and, even here, only in small numbers. At these sites, also, the marrow is likely to show fibrous scarring. Elsewhere, the marrow tends to remain myeloid and/or fatty, in accordance with its original nature.

RICKETS AND OSTEOMALACIA DUE TO LOSS OF INGESTED VITAMIN D

With steatorrhea from whatever cause, ingested vitamin D fails, for the most part, to be absorbed from the gut, being largely lost through the fatty stools, since vitamin D is fat-soluble. The body is also likely to suffer from calcium deprivation, since much of the ingested calcium undergoes combination with fatty acids in the intestinal contents and is excreted in the stool in the form of insoluble calcium soaps. It is this loss to the body of ingested vitamin D and of calcium that underlies the development of the rachitic or (in adults) osteomalacic skeletal changes which develop in neglected cases of chronic steatorrhea. Furthermore, in the light of our modern knowledge of nutrition, it is clear that a person (or an experimental animal) affected with chronic steatorrhea also suffers from impaired absorption of many other essential dietary components, including other vitamins. All this explains the complexity of the general clinical picture presented in cases of protracted steatorrhea

THE CELIAC SYNDROME

The term "celiac syndrome" is now often used in a rather general sense to characterize the clinical complex resulting from intestinal malabsorption in older infants and young children. The principal disease entities giving rise to mal-absorption in children and resulting in steatorrhea, along with various other manifestations, are: "gluten-induced enteropathy"; "idiopathic celiac disease"; "cystic fibrosis of the pancreas"; and "exudative enteropathy" (see di Sant'Agnese and Jones).

In *gluten-induced enteropathy* there is a sensitivity to ingested wheat, and the basis for the celiac syndrome in these cases is apparently a disorder in metabolism relating in particular to the gluten of the wheat. It is believed that the disordered metabolism is the result of a deficiency of certain intestinal mucosal proteolytic enzymes required for the proper hydrolysis of the gliadin fraction of the wheat gluten. This enzyme deficiency is to be regarded as an inborn error of metabolism. It leads in turn to the impaired absorption of fat from the intestines. In the cases interpreted as representing *idiopathic celiac disease* (or *idiopathic steatorrhea*), the absorption of fat from the intestines is greatly reduced (for some unknown reason), but there is ordinarily no sensitivity to ingested wheat gluten. When the under-lying condition is *cystic fibrosis of the pancreas*, it is pancreatic achylia (perhaps along with other factors) that is the basis for the malabsorption syndrome. The cases of *exudative enteropathy* are those in which the malabsorption syndrome, as expressed in steatorrhea, apparently results from an excessive exudation of serum proteins into the intestinal tract. In some cases, exudative enteropathy seems to be due to abnormalities relating to the intestinal lymphatics. (See Andersen, van de Kamer *et al.*, Gordon, and also Weijers and van de Kamer.)

The classical clinical picture of the celiac syndrome (irrespective of its underlying cause) is to be interpreted as the result of a multiple nutritional deficiency state with primary and secondary components. The affected children are ordinarily 6 months to 18 months of age when clear-cut manifestations of the disease appear. The disease sets in with the occurrence of repeated bouts of diarrhea. The stools are large, foul-smelling, pale, fatty, and foamy, and the abdomen becomes enlarged. The bouts of diarrhea are usually initiated by an upper respiratory infection. As the disease state continues, growth becomes retarded, and malnutrition develops. The latter is due to the defective absorption of fats, the loss of carbohydrate through fermentation, and the inadequate absorption of proteins.

Defective absorption of vitamin D and calcium results in *hypocalcemia*, tetany, porosity of the bones, and eventually even rachitoid bone changes. As noted, vitamin D is lost to the body because it is fat-soluble and hence passes out in the abnormally fatty stools. There is inadequate absorption of calcium because the calcium becomes combined with the excessive fatty acids in the intestinal contents to form insoluble (nonabsorbable) calcium soaps. The poor absorption of vitamin A renders the patient susceptible to infections, particularly of the respiratory tract. Defective absorption of vitamin K is followed by a prolonged prothombin time and by hemorrhages. Defective absorption of iron and other blood-forming components is followed by hypochromic anemia, and occasionally even a pernicious type of anemia develops. Clinical manifestations attributable to deficiencies of vitamins B and C and even E may also appear.

The *anatomic changes* which are found in the *duodenum* and *proximal part* of the *jejunum* in cases of celiac disease in children are the same as those observed in subjects suffering from nontropical sprue, and are discussed on p. 406. These changes are apparently not reversible even if the disease becomes clinically latent and the subject reaches adulthood. The changes in question may underlie the recrudescences of the disease. As to the *skeleton*, it used to be observed that, in those patients in whom the disease set in during infancy or early childhood and who survived beyond the age of 7 or 8, the bones were not only porotic but also presented rachitoid changes. Thus, these children often showed genu valgum (or genu varum), some enlargement of the epiphyses at the wrists, knees, and ankles, beading at the costochondral junctions, chicken-breastedness or a funnel-shaped chest, curvature of the vertebral column, some curvature of the long bones (especially in the lower extremities), and bossing of frontal eminences (see Parsons). *Roentgenographically* the bones showed cupping and other rachitoid phenomena at the epiphysial-diaphysial and costochondral junctions. The presence of pathologic fractures, favored by the general porosity of the bones, was also noted (see McCrudden and Fales). In particularly severe cases, dentition was delayed and the teeth were likely to be underdeveloped and subject to caries.

In general, the *anatomic* condition of the affected bones in an advanced case in a child suffering from celiac disease was clearly that of low-calcium rickets (atrophic rickets). The *serum biochemical* findings in these cases also confirmed the presence of a low-calcium vitamin D-deficiency rickets. After puberty, victims of celiac disease in a still-active form were likely to present some degree of infantilism, expressed in underdevelopment of the gonads and secondary sex characters and delay in fusion of epiphyses with their shafts. If the disease continued without control into adulthood, the skeletal deformities became even more pronounced, the victims becoming skeletal cripples.

This description of the celiac syndrome of children is pertinent to the condition as it formerly existed, but it should be borne in mind that the entire clinical outlook on celiac disease has undergone a great change in recent years. Previously, the mortality rate for celiac disease (also known as "Gee's disease") was somewhere between 15 and 25 per cent, the majority of the deaths occurring during the second or third year of life. Now, under appropriate treatment (a diet high in protein and simple carbohydrates, low in fat and starch, rich in various vitamins, and minimal in respect to gluten), the distressing manifestations of the disease can be brought under control. However, the malabsorption of fat may still be present, as demonstrable by chemical analysis of the stools (see Andersen and di Sant'Agnese, and also di Sant'Agnese). Under these circumstances, if the disease still reflects itself in the skeleton, the changes tend to be merely those of a mild osteoporosis rather than those of flagrant rickets. In any event, the disease may become latent in some affected children and then flare up again during early adult life as nontropical sprue—i.e., adult celiac disease (see Thaysen). In particular, its recrudescence may be triggered by a persisting infection in the intestinal tract or elsewhere.

NONTROPICAL SPRUE

Nontropical sprue is a name commonly applied to those rare cases of *idiopathic steatorrhea* which become manifest in adult (usually early adult) life. It seems clear that there is a genetic factor in the occurrence of the disease. The inherited metabolic defect apparently relates to a deficiency in certain proteolytic enzymes

Figure 101

A, Photograph of the cut surface of the upper half of a femur (sectioned in the fronta plane) from a case of nontropical sprue. Note that the cortex of the femur is rarefied (especially at the left of the picture), and that at the right it is thinner than it would normally be. In the neck of the femur (particularly in its central portion), the spongy trabeculae are thin and sparse. The subject (a man who had never left the United States) was 38 years of age at the time of his death. He entered our hospital about 3 months before his death from pneumonia. When he was 21 years of age (that is, 17 years before his death), he suffered an attack of what he described as "severe dysentery." This involved not only diarrhea but also the presence of blood in the stools, and he was aware that he was losing weight. Under medical care, the acute aspects of the disorder abated, and he was free of the pertinent complaints for some years. However, there were several recurrences of his difficulties— 8 years, 3 years, 2 years, and 1 year before his admission to our hospital. During the last recurrence he was having 6 or 7 loose, fatty stools each day, and he also came to have bleeding gums, as well as ecchymoses on various parts of the body. Repeated biochemical analyses of the blood showed that the total serum protein content was low, as was the serum calcium and phosphate content. For example, on one occasion the following representative values were obtained: total protein 5.1 gm. per 100 cc., the albumin fraction being 1.2 and the globulin 3.9; serum calcium 8.9 mg. per cent, phosphate 2.9 mg., and urea nitrogen 10.2 mg.

B, Photomicrograph ($\times$ 8) showing, in cross section, the general architecture of the rarefied cortical bone to be seen on the left in *A*. Note that the cortex is almost completely spongified except for a thin layer of relatively compact bone at the periphery. The spaces between the bony trabeculae in the rarefied cortex are occupied by fatty marrow.

C, Photograph showing the lower part of the vertebral column (sectioned in the sagittal plane) from this case of nontropical sprue. Note that the trabecular architecture of the vertebral bodies is well preserved and that the spongiosa seems to be even more close-meshed than it would normally be. Such an appearance of the vertebral bodies is not infrequent in connection with osteomalacia of moderate severity.

D, Photomicrograph ($\times$ 100) showing osteoid borders on the spongy trabeculae of a tissue section prepared from one of the vertebral bodies shown in *C*.

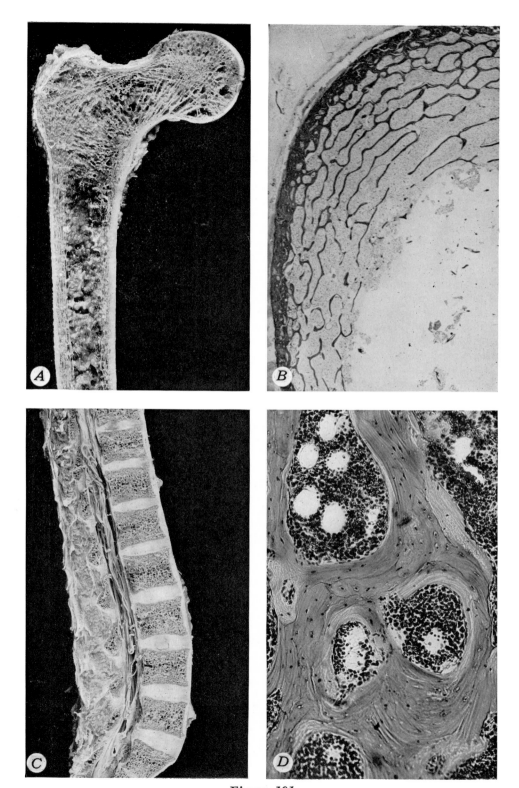

Figure 101

27

in the mucosa of the intestines, with resultant disturbances in the absorption of various substances from the intestinal tract. Indeed, as already noted, a case of nontropical sprue may actually represent the expression of celiac disease which has been latent during childhood and which has been activated or triggered during adult life by some infection.

In arriving at the *diagnosis* of nontropical sprue, one relies heavily on the clinical history, the laboratory findings, and the roentgenographic skeletal findings (see Bennett *et al.*). Considerable diagnostic significance also attaches to the histologic appearance of tissue (mucous membrane) obtained from the duodenum and/or upper portion of the jejunum by means of a peroral biopsy. However, there is a good deal of variability in the clinical manifestations of the disease among the different affected subjects. Furthermore, even when the disease appears in siblings, its clinical manifestations may be sufficiently different in these subjects to obscure the fact that one is dealing with the same disease (see Rally *et al.*).

Characteristically, there is a history of diarrhea and abdominal distention, along with crampy abdominal distress. Sometimes, however, though the stools are large, they are firm, and there is a history of constipation or a history of constipation alternating with diarrhea. Under these conditions the true nature of the disease may go unrecognized for a long time. Also, the finding of a fecal fat value above 10 per cent of the intake or above 25 per cent of the dried fecal weight is strongly suggestive of steatorrhea.

The *serum biochemical* values correspond to those of osteomalacia (see p. 399). Sometimes the serum calcium, instead of being only slightly lowered, drops even below 7 mg. per 100 cc., and in such cases tetany may appear. Furthermore, in a case of idiopathic steatorrhea in an adult, there is a decrease in the serum carotene content and also in the vitamin A. The prothrombin time is increased. One may find a severe anemia, which is usually of the hypochromic type. The finding of hypochromia in association with macrocytosis is helpful by itself in arriving at the diagnosis of nontropical sprue. Hypochlorhydria and achlorhydria are common though not regular findings.

In a case of nontropical sprue with protracted steatorrhea, there are usually also complaints relating to the skeleton. These include pains in the bones and joints, and tenderness of the bones to palpation. *Roentgenographic examination* of the bones will then show that they are rarefied, though not necessarily thinned. In cases of nontropical sprue of long standing, one may also find radiolucent zones (the so-called pseudofractures of Milkman or "Aufhellungszonen" of Looser). If a number of these radiolucent zones are present, they may be found symmetrically distributed in relation to ribs and long bones. As already noted earlier in connection with rickets and osteomalacia in general, such radiolucent zones reflect the presence of areas filled in with osteoid callus which is poorly mineralized in comparison with the bordering osseous tissue. *Microscopic examination* of bones from a case of nontropical sprue with advanced bone changes will also show the presence of osteoid borders on the spongy trabeculae and on the walls of the haversian spaces of the cortical bone. Thus the writer found such histologic evidence of osteomalacia in the various rarefied bones removed at autopsy in the case of a man dying at 38 who had suffered from idiopathic steatorrhea for 17 years. (See Fig. 101.)

In children and adults affected with celiac disease and nontropical sprue respectively, the *mucous membrane* of the *duodenum* and *proximal portion* of the *jejunum* shows anatomic changes which are held to be of diagnostic significance. Specimens of mucous membrane in pertinent cases have been obtained for study by means of suction biopsy, and the findings have been compared with those from control specimens obtained by the same means. In cases of celiac disease and nontropical sprue, the biopsy specimen is found devoid of normal villi, the surface being barren and knobby and the subsurface vasculature sparse and disorganized. These findings are in sharp contrast to the appearance of the mucous membrane obtained from normal control specimens, which presented a delicate villous surface and numerous subsurface capillaries (see Rubin *et al.*). Microscopic examination of stained tissue sections prepared from the grossly abnormal biopsy specimens confirmed the reduction in the extent of the epithelial surface, which results from the diminution in the number of villi and the blunting of those still present. In addition, it was sometimes noted that the epithelial cells at the luminal surface were flattened and that the lamina propria of the mucous membrane was infiltrated with plasma cells.

There is increasing evidence that the changes observed in the mucous membrane of the duodenum and jejunum in cases of *celiac disease* and *nontropical sprue* are irreversible. That is, they tend to persist throughout life, even though the patient does not present obvious clinical manifestations of the disease. The similarity of the anatomic changes in the mucous membrane of the duodenum and proximal portion of the jejunum in cases of celiac disease of childhood and nontropical sprue appearing in adult life is held to support the idea that these two conditions represent merely different phases of the same basic disease. Somewhat analogous anatomic changes are observed in the mucous membrane of the small intestine in cases of *tropical sprue*. However, such changes are not observed in various other conditions leading to intestinal malabsorption (see Rubin *et al.*, Shiner and Doniach, and Swanson and Thomassen).

The *treatment* of patients with nontropical sprue involves many problems and is often merely palliative. The condition is a chronic illness characterized by multiple nutritional deficiencies, and the remissions which are often achieved through therapy are very likely to be interrupted by recurrences of the manifestations, sometimes in very severe form (see Green and Wollaeger). The calcium intake may well be increased by the administration of calcium lactate. The diet should be one which is low in fat and residue, as low as possible in gluten, and high in protein and simple carbohydrates. This diet should be supplemented by a high multiple vitamin intake, but in particular by large amounts of vitamin D, vitamin K, and the vitamins of the B complex. Large doses of liver extract, alone or in combination with vitamin B_{12} and/or folic acid, should also be given. A patient who has become seriously ill may require, in addition, intravenous infusions of whole blood, human serum albumin, and/or various supportive aqueous solutions.

RICKETS AND OSTEOMALACIA DUE TO DEFECTIVE RENAL TUBULAR REABSORPTION OR EXCRETION

The cases which concern us here are those instances of rickets or of osteomalacia which are generally regarded as having their point of departure in *disordered functioning* of the renal tubules, not associated with actual pathologic changes in the kidneys. The malfunctioning of the renal tubules is held to manifest itself in defective tubular reabsorption and/or defective tubular excretion. Thus we are *not* concerned here with those cases in which skeletal alterations are associated with pathologic changes in the renal nephrons as a whole, and the consequent retention of catabolites (urea, creatinine, phosphate, etc.) in the body fluids which is due to diminished glomerular filtration in particular. The skeletal changes developing as a result of actual disease of the kidneys are of the nature of so-called "osteitis fibrosa" and are secondary, at least in part, to parathyroid hyperplasia and hyperfunctioning which has developed because of the renal (and notably glomerular) insufficiency. The skeletal changes occurring on this basis are thus ascribable to some extent to the effects of hyperparathyroidism secondary to renal disease. In such cases, if the victim is a child whose renal insufficiency is of some years' duration, the skeletal changes which develop are found associated with abnormalities at the sites of endochondral bone growth. Histologically, the changes at those sites do not correspond closely to the changes observed in simple vitamin D-deficiency rickets (nutritional rickets). However, they do simulate the latter changes clinically and roentgenographically, thus accounting for the names of "renal rickets" or "renal dwarfism" used in the past to denote the condition. The skeletal changes associated with renal disease involving dysfunction of the nephrons as a whole are discussed under "renal (secondary) hyperparathyroidism" (p. 324).

The cases of rickets and osteomalacia regarded as being due to defective renal tubular functioning *per se* seem to have in common a decrease in the renal tubular reabsorption of phosphate. However, there are differences among the cases in respect to additional aberrations in the functioning of the renal tubules, and in some cases there may be still other metabolic abnormalities. Accordingly, a number of classifications have been proposed to distinguish subgroups of cases presenting different combinations of the metabolic aberrations in question. Dent, in 1952, sorted cases of functional renal tubular rickets and osteomalacia into 6 subgroups. Others, too, have shown that the various cases can be subgrouped in one way or another (see Fanconi and Girardet, Jackson and Linder, Fraser and Salter, and also Stanbury).

It was emphasized by Dent himself that the classification he proposed in 1952 represented merely an attempt to bring some order into the diversity of those syndromes already generally regarded by that time as resulting from renal tubular malfunctioning. The classification which he suggested still has value. The 6 subgroups (or types) of functional aberration of the renal tubules resulting in rickets or osteomalacia were distinguished by him as follows: In Type I the sole defect is one relating to the reabsorption of phosphate. (As noted above, a defect in the renal tubular reabsorption of phosphate—a high renal clearance of phosphate—is usually likewise present in the cases falling into the other subgroups or types.) In Type II there is a defect in the reabsorption of glucose in addition to phosphate. In Type III the distinguishing aberration relates to the reabsorption of glucose and amino acids. In Type IV the special features are deficient reabsorption of glucose, amino acids, and potassium, and also an inability on the part of the renal tubules to acidify the urine. In Types V and VI, in addition to diminished tubular reabsorption of phosphate, there is a renal loss of potassium, together with an inability to acidify the urine and also a deficiency of ammonia formation (particularly in Type VI).

In 1964, Dent and Friedman called attention to two cases of renal tubular rickets not fitting into any of the 6 types mentioned above. The rickets in those cases was based on a renal tubular defect in the reabsorption of phosphate, calcium, amino acids, and protein. Two apparently similar cases have been reported by Gentil *et al.* A case of hypophosphatemic rickets in which the subject presented hyperglycinuria, glucosuria, and glycil-prolinuria was reported by Scriver *et al.* A case of acquired vitamin D-resistant osteomalacia characterized by hypercalcemia, low serum bicarbonate, and hyperglycinuria was reported by Henneman *et al.* There can be no doubt that, in time, cases of rickets and osteomalacia resulting from still other aberrations in renal tubular functioning and associated metabolic defects will come to be distinguished. This is understandable when one considers the possible defects in the renal tubular reabsorption of the amino acids alone. The blood plasma contains at least 20 distinct amino acids which are filtered into the tubules by the renal glomeruli. At least in theory, the renal tubular defect in regard to the reabsorption of the amino acids may relate to one, a few, or all of these acids. Furthermore, the aberration in reabsorption may also vary quantitatively from case to case in respect to individual amino acids.

Be that as it may, the writer will limit his discussion of renal tubular malfunctioning to several of the more common and relatively well-delineated rachitic (and/or osteomalacic) entities representing the condition. The entities he will consider are: "refractory rickets"; "Fanconi rickets"; and the rickets and osteomalacia of the so-called Butler-Albright syndrome. Refractory rickets corresponds to Types I and II of Dent's classification. Fanconi rickets corresponds to his Types III and IV. The third entity to be discussed—rickets and osteomalacia of the so-called Butler-Albright syndrome—results from defective renal tubular *excretion* and has its basis in renal tubular acidosis. It corresponds to Types V and VI of Dent's classification.

REFRACTORY RICKETS

In the past, so-called vitamin D-resistant rickets (better denoted as refractory rickets) was held to evolve because the body had become unresponsive to vitamin D in doses which would be entirely adequate for the cure of simple vitamin D-deficiency rickets of young children. As already noted, current experience indicates that "refractory rickets" actually belongs in the category of rickets due to disordered functioning of the renal tubules. Other names which have been applied to the condition are: "familial hypophosphatemia," "familial vitamin D-resistant rickets," and "phosphate diabetes."

CLINICAL CONSIDERATIONS

Though of relatively infrequent occurrence, so-called refractory rickets is the most common form of rickets resulting from malfunctioning of the renal tubules in the absence of obvious pathologic changes in them. It is recognized that the condition is often a familial and inherited disorder, though its occurrence may also be sporadic or at least apparently sporadic (see Tobler *et al.*, Winters *et al.*, Dancaster and Jackson, and Dent and Harris). The patient is usually a child 3 or 4 years of age, but may be an older child, perhaps 8 years of age, when first coming under medical care for the condition. Indeed, in one of the several cases studied by the writer, the patient was almost 12 years old when her rickets set in. Occasionally a case of the disease is recognized and diagnosed when the subject is still a young infant (see Schoen, and also Schoen and Reynolds).

In a typical case of refractory rickets, the clinical history is likely to reveal that the patient had received prophylactic vitamin D in infancy and had not manifested rickets during that period or perhaps even during the second year of life. It may also reveal that for some months there has been increasing muscular weakness and that deformity of the lower limbs (usually knock knee) has been developing. Physical examination shows rachitic swelling at the wrists, ankles, and costochondral junctions identical with that seen in the simple vitamin D-deficiency rickets of young children. Roentgenographic examination of the bones confirms the presence of rachitic changes. (See Fig. 102.)

The *serum biochemical values* are likewise those of nutritional rickets—that is, rickets due to simple lack of vitamin D—*viz.*: an average normal or low normal calcium, a low inorganic phosphorus, and an elevated alkaline phosphatase. The *urinary excretion* of calcium is extremely low, in accordance with the recognized diminished absorption of calcium (and also phosphorus) from the intestinal tract in rickets in general. Calcium balance studies made in this connection show that practically all the calcium being lost by the body is excreted in the feces—a finding which is also to be noted in the ordinary vitamin D-deficiency rickets of infancy and childhood.

Since the serum urea nitrogen and/or nonprotein nitrogen values are within the normal range in cases of refractory rickets, the possibility of a rachitoid state based on a renal (glomerular) insufficiency—that is, renal hyperparathyroidism—is ruled out. However, cases of so-called refractory rickets (vitamin D-resistant rickets) have to be differentiated from cases of Fanconi rickets and cases in which skeletal aberrations arise from other defects of renal tubular reabsorption. As already indicated, vitamin D-refractory rickets differs biochemically from the other forms of rickets due to renal tubular malfunctioning, in that the malfunctioning seems to relate mainly if not solely to deficient reabsorption of phosphate by the renal tubules. Thus a protracted hypophosphatemia and a striking increase in the urinary excretion of phosphorus are important guidelines for the diagnosis of the condition. However, in these cases, even greater differential diagnostic importance attaches to: the absence of acidosis; the fact that the urinary excretion of ions other than phosphorus is not abnormal; and the fact that there is also no abnormality relating to the urinary excretion of amino acids and proteins, and usually none in regard to the renal tubular reabsorption of glucose. The roentgenographic appearance of the bones in cases of metaphysial dysostosis is likely to resemble that of refractory

Figure 102

A, Roentgenograph of a knee area in the case of a boy 4 years of age affected with refractory rickets. This picture was taken at the time of his initial admission to the hospital, at which time the serum calcium value was 9.4 mg. per cent, the phosphate value 3.3 mg., and the alkaline phosphatase value 24.7 Bodansky units per 100 cc. Note that there are rachitic changes at the epiphysial-metaphysial junctional areas at the lower end of the femur, and also that as yet there are practically no indications of rickets in the corresponding region of the upper end of the tibia. The clinical record states that the boy was born at full term, and that he was given cod liver oil from the age of 6 months on. He started to walk at the age of 14 months, but walking became more difficult as he grew older because of the progressive development of knock knee. Physical examination revealed not only pronounced genu valgum but also frontal bossing, flattening of the skull posteriorly, slight beading at the costochondral junctions, and a mild degree of pigeon-breastedness. On the assumption that the child's condition represented merely an instance of simple vitamin D-deficiency rickets, bilateral tibial osteotomies were carried out to correct the genu valgum, and only therapeutic (not massive) doses of vitamin D were administered.

B, Roentgenograph illustrating the appearance of a knee area in this case $2\frac{3}{4}$ years after the roentgenograph shown in *A* was taken. The boy had been readmitted to the hospital because of a recurrence of the knock knee deformity. On this admission the serum calcium value was 8.7 mg., the phosphate value 2.3 mg., and the alkaline phosphatase value 53 Bodansky units. Note that in this picture the rachitic changes are greatly advanced in comparison with those shown in *A*.

C, Roentgenograph showing the rachitic changes at the lower end of a radius and ulna in this case. This picture was taken at the same time as the picture of the knee area shown in *B*. The boy was now started on massive doses of vitamin D (about 100,000 units daily). After some months, the amount of vitamin D administered was reduced to 50,000 units per day. The therapeutic effect of the large doses of the vitamin is reflected in *D*.

D, Roentgenograph of both knee areas in this case of refractory rickets taken 11 months after treatment with massive doses of vitamin D was begun. Note that the rachitic intermediate zones at the epiphysial-diaphysial junctional areas are substantially filled in, in accordance with healing of the rickets. At this stage, the serum calcium value was 10.3 mg., the phosphate value 4.7 mg., and the alkaline phosphatase value 10.1 Bodansky units— findings which are within normal limits for a child of the patient's age. (Compare with *B*, which represents the status of the knee areas before intensive vitamin D therapy was begun.)

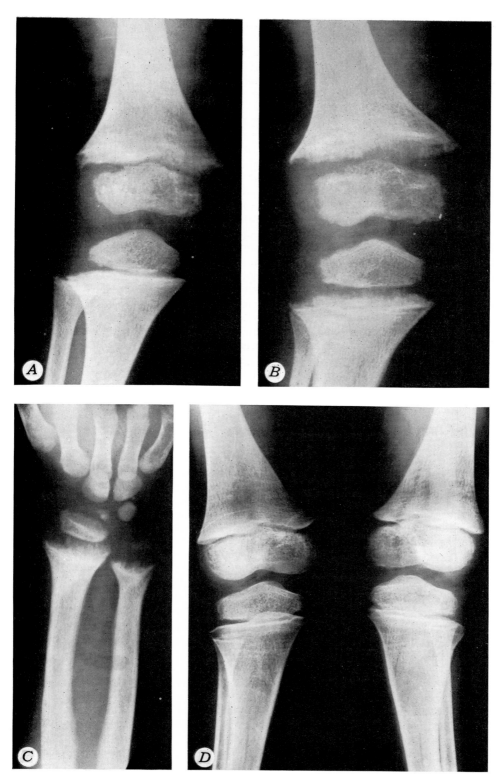

Figure 102

rickets, and this resemblance may raise a problem of differential diagnosis. However, in cases of metaphysial dysostosis, hypophosphatemia is not encountered and the histologic findings at sites of endochondral ossification are also not those of rickets (see p. 223).

TREATMENT

The treatment of refractory rickets (so-called vitamin D-resistant rickets) is directed toward the prevention of stunted growth and skeletal deformities, which would ensue if the rachitic state persisted. Since the condition represents a chronic metabolic disorder, its management should be started as early in life as possible and continued through the years. The basic principles underlying the treatment are: an ample and well-rounded diet rich in calcium; a particularly high daily intake of vitamin D; and clinical control of the patient in respect to avoidance of *hypervitaminosis D*. The high daily intake of vitamin D which is necessary for the healing of the rickets and the prevention of its recurrence (maintenance of the nonrachitic state) lies very close to an amount which might induce the toxic manifestations of hypervitaminosis D. Even under adequate and sustained vitamin D therapy, skeletal deformities present before the treatment was begun usually require surgical correction (by osteotomy), since they often fail to respond completely to the medical treatment. In any event, lapses in the regulated medical care of the subjects will result in recurrence of the rickets and/or the skeletal deformities.

However, it should be pointed out that in some cases of refractory rickets the underlying defect in the renal tubular reabsorption of phosphate is relatively mild. In these cases, of course, the control and even cure of the condition under regulated medical care is much more easily accomplished. Furthermore, smaller doses of vitamin D are required, and hence the danger of toxic effects due to hypervitaminosis D is reduced.

The regimen for treatment recommended by Stearns and also by Tapia *et al.* is essentially the following: Vitamin D is administered in daily doses ranging from 50,000 units for young children to 100,000 units for children above 6 years of age. The effectiveness of the vitamin D in increasing the absorption of calcium and phosphorus from the intestinal tract is registered in an increased urinary excretion of calcium. For this reason, before the vitamin D therapy is instituted, a 24-hour urine specimen is collected, and the urinary calcium excretion of the rachitic subject is compared with the expected 24-hour urinary calcium excretion of a corresponding normal subject on a similar daily calcium intake.

The aim of the vitamin D therapy in respect to urinary calcium excretion is to raise the latter toward the mean normal value and maintain it at least at that value. To that end, the calcium excreted in the urine by the rachitic subject on the high daily intake of vitamin D is determined at intervals of 3 to 5 days. If a rise in urinary calcium excretion does not occur promptly, the vitamin D dosage is increased, the dose being doubled at intervals of a week or less until the desired rise has been obtained. As the vitamin D dosage is stepped up, the urinary calcium excretion can be expected to rise steadily and to reach the normal mean value in the course of about 4 weeks.

To forestall the development of the toxic manifestations of hypervitaminosis D, consideration must be given to a reduction in the vitamin D dosage as the urinary calcium excretion value nears the mean normal level. To this end, the vitamin D dosage is adjusted downward, usually by 25,000 units at a time, so that the 24-hour urinary calcium excretion remains approximately at a mean value normal for children of corresponding weight and calcium intake.

As Stearns points out, it is often not until weeks after the *urinary* calcium excretion has begun to exceed the normal range that the *serum* calcium value rises above the normal level. Urinary calcium values 3 standard deviations or more above the normal mean already constitute evidence of *hypervitaminosis D,* whether the serum calcium is elevated or not. Under such circumstances, the dosage of vitamin D should be reduced promptly. If overdosage with vitamin D is continued, anorexia, nausea, vomiting, occasional hematuria, and polyuria with hyposthenuria are signs that the hypervitaminosis D has become acute. Under these conditions, the hypervitaminosis may even aggravate the skeletal changes. The aggravation occurs because hypervitaminosis D has a demineralizing effect upon the bones like that produced by excessive amounts of circulating parathyroid hormone.

Roentgenographic changes indicating amelioration of the rachitic state do not appear early in the course of treatment. Indeed, after a month of adequate treatment, no roentgenographic evidence of healing may yet be observed. In a child who is receiving large doses of vitamin D and is not manifesting evidences of overdosage, the surgical correction of a deformity by osteotomy may precipitate the appearance of vitamin D intoxication. Hence, if surgery is contemplated, the administration of vitamin D should be discontinued some time before the intervention.

THE OSTEOMALACIC COUNTERPART OF REFRACTORY RICKETS

In an occasional instance, the metabolic defect underlying refractory rickets has been noted as setting in during adolescence or even during adult life (see McCance). Under these circumstances, the condition comes to express itself as *osteomalacia.* The biochemical findings in these cases of osteomalacia are, of course, like those to be observed in cases of refractory rickets. The *treatment* outlined above for the latter condition is likewise appropriate for these cases of osteomalacia.

Jackson *et al.* report the case of a woman in whom clinical complaints referable to the skeleton set in at the age of 24. By the time she was 32 years of age, she showed pronounced changes indicative of osteomalacia, including, of course, the so-called Looser zones (pseudofractures) in various bones. Mineral balance studies revealed diminished absorption of calcium and phosphorus from the intestinal tract, and there was also evidence of greatly diminished reabsorption of phosphorus from the renal tubules.

Yoshikawa *et al.* also reported a case apparently belonging in the category of vitamin D-resistant osteomalacia in which profoundly severe skeletal changes were present before treatment was instituted. The patient was a woman who had appeared to be in good health up to the age of 48, when she began to complain of general weakness and of pain in the lower extremities. The pronounced skeletal changes evolved in the course of the following 6 years. She, too, manifested a striking decrease in the renal tubular reabsorption of phosphorus, and also showed evidence of impaired absorption of calcium and phosphorus from the intestinal tract. Biochemical study showed furthermore that there was no amino-aciduria or glucosuria, and these findings eliminated the possibility that the osteomalacia in this case represented the adult counterpart of Fanconi rickets (p. 431).

In a pertinent case of osteomalacia studied by the writer, the patient (a woman) was 57 years of age at the time of her death. For about 2 years before she died, she had been aware of increasing muscular weakness. She also complained of pains relating to various bones and joints. Biochemical studies revealed the presence of a pronounced *hyper*phosphaturia, a *hypo*phosphatemia, a low normal serum calcium value, and an elevated serum alkaline phosphatase value. Roentgenographic examination of the skeleton revealed a linear radiolucency (Looser-Milkman zone) in the neck of each femur and fractures in many of the ribs on each side of the chest. Various bones were removed at autopsy, and gross and microscopic examination of these bones confirmed the presence of osteomalacia. (See Figs. 103 and 104.)

FANCONI RICKETS

In 1936, Fanconi proposed the concept of defective renal tubular reabsorption on a functional basis as the foundation for cases of severe rickets and dwarfism associated with renal glucosuria, chronic acidosis, and a *normal* serum nonprotein nitrogen value. Thus he clearly set this form of rickets apart from the already well-recognized skeletal aberrations known to result from pathologic changes in the kidneys associated with an *elevated* serum nonprotein nitrogen value. That is, he delimited the form of rickets now classed under his name from those cases of rickets now commonly referred to as instances of "renal (glomerular) rickets" and/or "renal hyperparathyroidism." In conformity with the serum biochemical pattern usual for nutritional or vitamin D-deficiency rickets, the cases of uncomplicated *renal glycosuric rickets* of Fanconi present a hypophosphatemia, an elevated serum alkaline phosphatase value, and a low normal calcium value. Furthermore, in the cases of Fanconi rickets, the serum CO_2 value is generally reduced—often markedly.

In the cases of the Fanconi group (Fanconi rickets and the osteomalacia of adults which corresponds to it), the underlying *metabolic disorder* centers around a disturbance in amino acid metabolism. This is expressed in amino-aciduria, the urine showing fairly large amounts of 10 to 20 of the various amino acids. Indeed, Fanconi had already noted that the urine of his patients contained abnormally

Figure 103

A, Photograph of the upper end of a femur sectioned in the frontal plane in a case of osteomalacia representing the adult counterpart of refractory rickets. Note the narrow bandlike area at the junction of the head and neck of the bone. This band of osteoid would have presented in an x-ray picture as a narrow zone of radiolucency—a so-called "Aufhellungszone" of Looser. The subject, a woman, was 57 years of age at the time of her death, which was due primarily to pneumonia. About $1\frac{1}{2}$ years before her death, she began to experience pains in various bones and joints (especially the knees) and increasing general weakness. At this time, roentgenographic examination of the skeleton disclosed the presence of numerous "fracture lines," especially in the ribs. The serum calcium value was 9.5 mg. per cent, the phosphate value 1.5 mg., and the alkaline phosphatase value 11.1 Bodansky units per 100 cc. The patient was found to have an exceedingly high urinary clearance of phosphorus. However, there was no evidence of amino-aciduria or acidosis.

B, Photomicrograph ($\times$ 2) illustrating the general histologic pattern of the Looser line, which represents the band of osteoid extending across the femur at the head-neck junction. The presence of this Looser line does not signify that, at this site, there had been an actual discontinuity (that is, a complete fracture) between the head and neck of the femur. Instead, it represents a zone of reconstruction ("Umbauzone") developing perhaps in consequence of mechanical stress which has induced microfractures of individual spongy trabeculae and provoked the deposition of osteoid.

C, Photograph of one of the ribs in this case removed at autopsy and sectioned in its long axis. Note the angulation at the costochondral junction and also the one in the shaft of the rib several inches beyond that junction. At both these sites the interior of the rib contains callus which is mainly still poorly mineralized organic bone matrix. At autopsy, practically all the other ribs were found to present at least several fractures.

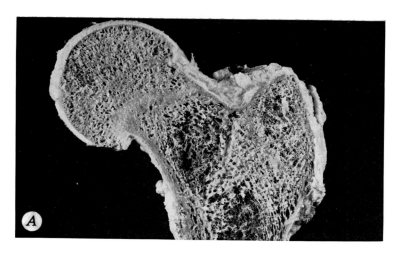

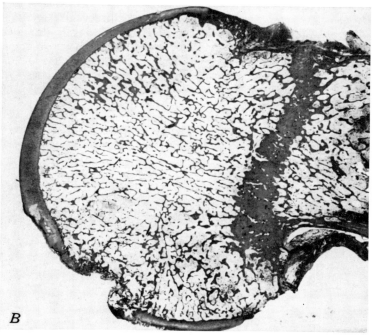

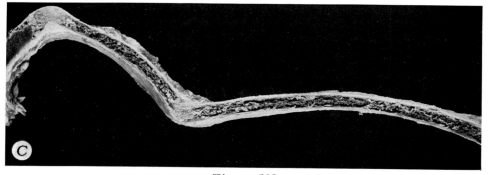

Figure 103

large amounts of organic acids and suggested that these acids consisted, at least in part, of amino acids. In 1943, McCune *et al.* confirmed Fanconi's hypothesis and demonstrated that in their case the organic acids present in the urine in abnormal amounts were: amino acids, 82 per cent; lactic acid, 11 per cent; and beta-hydroxy-butyric acid, 7 per cent. In addition to the amino-aciduria there is glucosuria, as is recognized in the term *"renal glycosuric rickets"* of Fanconi, sometimes used for the condition. Despite the glucosuria, the blood sugar value is within normal limits. A large increase in the phosphorus content of the urine (phosphaturia) has often been reported, but there are also some reports to the contrary.

These biochemical aberrations (amino-aciduria, glucosuria, and also the phosphaturia, if present) have usually been ascribed, in the past, to defective reabsorption of these substances from the renal tubules on a functional basis. However, in relation to the amino-aciduria in particular, it has been postulated more recently that, since it is accompanied by amino-acidemia, it may well be the result of an overflow from the blood because of a *pre*renal disturbance in protein and/or amino acid metabolism rather than of malfunctioning of the renal tubules in respect to the reabsorption of amino acids (see Bickel *et al.*). However, the likelihood is that both of these mechanisms are implicated in the amino-aciduria. Another common finding in the disease—a feature which is likewise an expression of the disordered amino acid metabolism—is cystinosis (the storage of cystine in various tissues and organs of the rachitic subject). Even when considerable, the amount of cystine in the urine in cases of Fanconi rickets does not exceed the total amount of the other amino acids in the urine.

In respect to *nomenclature*, the name "Lignac-Fanconi disease" is commonly used for those cases of Fanconi rickets in which cystinosis is already present. The cases of Fanconi rickets not yet manifesting the damaging effects of cystinosis are often denoted as instances of de Toni-Fanconi disease or Debré-de Toni-Fanconi disease. Lignac's finding (reported in 1926) of cystine storage in 3 children showing glucosuria along with rachitic deformities and dwarfism led to the joint appellation of Lignac-Fanconi disease. At autopsy in these cases, many of the tissues, including the liver, spleen, lymph nodes, and kidneys, revealed a crystalline substance which

Figure 104

A, Photograph of most of the vertebral column, removed at autopsy and sectioned in the sagittal plane, from the case of osteomalacia considered in connection with Figure 103. Note the very marked kyphosis. The apex of its curve is at the eighth thoracic vertebra, whose body is sharply wedged (see arrow). On sectioning the vertebral column, it was apparent that the bone could be cut with abnormal ease. The cut surface appeared grayish, and the trabeculae, though close-set, yielded to pressure from the fingers, indicating that the osseous tissue was not fully mineralized.

B, Photomicrograph ($\times$ 1.5) showing the wedged eighth thoracic vertebral body and also the seventh and ninth thoracic vertebral bodies. The body of the seventh thoracic vertebra is somewhat narrowed in its vertical dimension. Though close-set and compressible, the spongy trabeculae are actually thicker than they would normally be, and the spongy marrow spaces are consequently less prominent than they should be. The intervertebral disks are somewhat expanded, though not so much as those in the lumbar region (see *A*).

C, Photomicrograph ($\times$ 75) establishing the presence of wide osteoid borders on the relatively thick spongy trabeculae of these vertebral bodies. At the upper end of the picture, one can see part of the cartilage plate of an intervertebral disk. The mineralized bone matrix of the spongy trabeculae stains darkly, while the non-mineralized bone matrix, representing the osteoid borders, appears almost white in comparison. Note that the intertrabecular marrow spaces contain myeloid and fatty marrow, that there is no evidence of a scarring reaction, and that osteoclasts are not in evidence either.

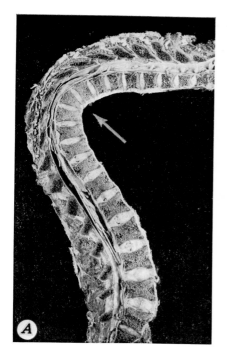

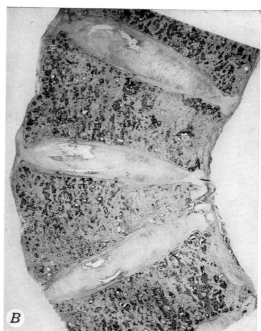

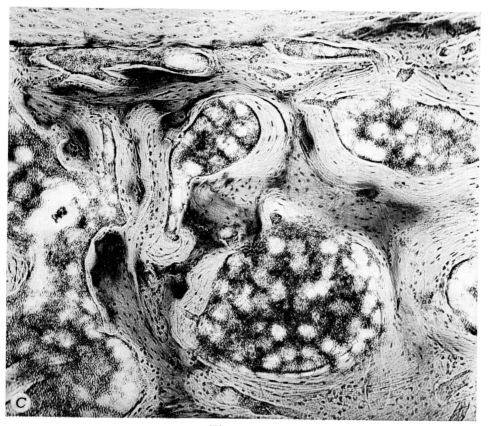

Figure 104

417

was identified as cystine. The names of Debré and de Toni are linked to that of Fanconi because, before 1936, the former workers described cases which conformed to those described by Fanconi as cases of "nephrotic glycosuric dwarfing with hypophosphatemic rickets." However, it was Fanconi who first clearly delimited these cases from cases of "rickets" due to pathologic changes in the renal nephrons as a whole and the consequent chronic renal insufficiency.

CLINICAL CONSIDERATIONS

The disease is encountered only infrequently and seems to be genetically determined. It is apparently inherited as a simple mendelian recessive trait. In a given family, siblings are not uncommonly affected. The disease tends to present itself clinically either in a form which runs an *acute* and severe course or in a form which runs a *chronic* course (see Bickel *et al.*).

In the cases pursuing an *acute course*, the clinical manifestations generally set in during the first year of life, and onset before the age of 6 months has occasionally been noted. In the case of an infant in whom the disease has set in early, inquiry is likely to reveal that the infant has manifested refusal of food, vomiting, polydipsia, polyuria, and constipation. In consequence, the infant has failed to grow or gain weight or may even have been losing weight. When first coming under medical care, the undersized, more or less marasmic subject may not as yet present clear-cut skeletal evidence of rickets. Continuance of the vomiting and refusal of food aggravate the dehydration and acidosis and also the hypokalemia, if the latter is present. The hypokalemia also contributes to the occurrence of circulatory collapse, which often results in prompt death of the acutely sick young child. It is also to be noted that, during the entire clinical course of the disease in its acute form, intermittent bouts of fever (often quite high) are not uncommon.

In the cases pursuing a *chronic course*, the clinical manifestations are mild, at least at first, and the course of the disease is relatively slow, though still progressive. In this expression of the disease, its manifestations usually do not become evident before the second or third year of the child's life and often not until several years later. In some cases representing this so-called chronic form of the disease, the presenting complaints may, it is true, be loss of appetite, polyuria, polydipsia, vomiting, constipation, etc. However, these complaints are by no means so severe as they are in the acute form of the condition. In other cases representing the chronic form of the disorder, it is the rachitic changes in the bones that call attention to its presence, and the general indications of poor health do not appear until later.

In addition to the skeletal changes (rickets and the associated porosity of the bones, rachitic deformities, and dwarfing), there is usually photophobia. The latter may or may not be associated with the presence of cystine deposits in the cornea and/or conjunctiva. It is, of course, in the older children, in whom the chronic form of the disease has been present for some years, that one observes the severest skeletal changes, and the osteoporosis also makes the bones of these children liable to fractures. The various skeletal abnormalities are understandable in the light of the protracted negative calcium and phosphorus balance resulting from excessive loss of these minerals by way of the stool.

In a pertinent case studied by the writer, the patient was 8 years of age on admission to the hospital, but had muscular weakness dating back for 1 year. Examination on admission showed that the patient, a girl, was rather undersized. She had a fairly marked degree of bilateral knock knee and other evidences of rickets, including rachitic rosary and rachitic enlargements at the wrists. Roentgenographic examination of the bones showed pronounced rachitic changes. The patient was under our observation for $3\frac{1}{2}$ years and died at the age of 12 with extremely severe skeletal alterations. Her death occurred in the course of a hypokalemic crisis.

During the years in which this child was hospitalized, she manifested glucosuria (which, on occasion, exceeded 1.0 per cent), while her blood sugar was always found to be at a normal or low normal level. It was also repeatedly demonstrated that the urine contained excessive amounts of phosphate and of organic acids—mainly various amino acids. Furthermore, the urine showed an increased ammonia content and an increased titratable acidity. The serum phosphate value was always low, and on many occasions in the last year or so of her life it was even less than 1.0 mg. per cent, representing a striking hypophosphatemia. The serum alkaline phosphatase value was always elevated, and at times was found to be as high as 64 Bodansky units per 100 cc. Except terminally, the nonprotein nitrogen value was within normal limits.

In cases running a protracted course, the liver and spleen may be found somewhat enlarged on palpation. This finding reflects the deposition of cystine in crystalline form in these organs, and cystine deposition also occurs in the kidneys, bone marrow, and lymph nodes, as well as in still other tissues. Direct renal damage from the deposition of cystine crystals may lead to severe interstitial scarring and glomerular and tubular alterations, and chronic renal insufficiency and uremia may consequently develop. On this account, the original clinical complex of rickets with *hypo*phosphatemia and normal values for the serum nonprotein nitrogen may change to that of rachitoid skeletal changes with evidences of "osteitis fibrosa" associated with *hyper*phosphatemia and elevated serum nonprotein nitrogen values. That is, a case starting out with a typical picture of Fanconi rickets sometimes evolves, in consequence of severe renal cystinosis, into the clinical and anatomic picture of renal (glomerular) rickets or renal (secondary) hyperparathyroidism, as it did in the well-documented case reported by R. Looser. Indeed, the detailed autopsy findings reported by Looser related to one of the cases on which Fanconi, in 1936, based his clinical concept of the condition. The affected child (a girl) began to show evidence of so-called Fanconi rickets at about 15 months of age and died when she was about 8 years of age.

ROENTGENOGRAPHIC AND PATHOLOGIC FINDINGS

The *roentgenographic* appearance of the bones in cases of Fanconi rickets is naturally in conformity with the severity of the basic disorder and with its duration in the individual case. When skeletal changes first become apparent roentgenographically, they are entirely analogous to those of ordinary nutritional vitamin D-deficiency rickets. As in the latter cases, the ends of the rib bodies show cupping and flaring at the costochondral junctions, and the local beadlike swellings create a rachitic rosary along each side of the chest wall. Changes of the same nature are to be observed at the ends of the shafts of long bones. The cupping at the lower end of the shaft of the ulna and also of the radius is readily demonstrable, and the rachitic intermediate zones are likely to be conspicuous in these areas. (See Fig. 105.)

The progress of the rachitic changes leads to various skeletal deformities, including coxa vara, knock knee, and bowlegs, which in themselves contribute to the dwarfing of the subject. In time, the bones may also become strikingly porous. The porosity of the bones results from thinning and rarefaction of the cortical bone, sparsity of the spongy trabeculae, and thinning of those which are still present. The added effect of the osteoporosis increases the deformities and also renders the bones readily susceptible to fractures as well as to so-called pseudofractures.

In regard to the *pathologic findings* in Lignac-Fanconi disease, we are, of course, mainly concerned here with those relating to the bones. However, some attention will also be given to the cystine present in the tissues and to the status of the kidneys in the disease—matters which are considered in detail by R. Looser, and also by Baar and Bickel.

Cystine crystals can be found, at least in small amounts, in all or most of the organs. They are to be found in the cells of the so-called reticuloendothelial system, and are not encountered in the parenchymal cells of the various organs. For instance, they can be demonstrated in the Kupffer cells of the liver, the reticulum cells of the spleen, lymph nodes, and bone marrow, and also in the histiocytes of the supporting connective tissues of the body. If cystine crystals are present in only small amounts in a given tissue, sections prepared for microscopic study may fail to reveal them unless the tissue has been fixed in alcohol and stained with basic fuchsin. When a given tissue contains the crystals in large amounts, they may be observed even if the tissue has been fixed in neutral formalin and the prepared tissue sections are stained with hematoxylin and eosin—conditions which tend strongly to favor solution of the crystals. Examination of properly prepared tissue

Figure 105

A, Roentgenograph (taken at the time of admission to the hospital) of the upper end of a humerus of a female child 8 years of age affected with renal tubular rickets of the Fanconi type. Note the wide rachitic intermediate zone. The mother indicated that the child was delivered normally and walked at 1 year, and that dentition had progressed normally during infancy. Furthermore, the mother stated that at the age of 3 years the child was well nourished and had straight legs and good posture. Clinical details relating to the subsequent 4 years (that is, the period between 3 and 7 years) are not available, since the child was then living with a relative far away from the mother. At 7 years of age, the child came to live with the mother again. At this time, the latter noticed that the child's knees were deformed, that she walked with a limp, and that these difficulties were becoming worse. On admission to the hospital it was noted that the child was undersized for her age, had fairly pronounced "knock knee," walked with a "scissors-like" gait, could get around only with assistance, and demonstrated striking muscular weakness. There was also slight lateral compression of the chest, a suggestion of Harrison's grooves, and enlargement of the ends of the long bones at the wrists. Biochemical examination of the blood on admission yielded the following values: serum calcium 10.9 mg. per cent, phosphate 1.3 mg., and alkaline phosphatase 29.5 Bodansky units per 100 cc. The blood sugar value was 89 mg. and the nonprotein nitrogen 22 mg. In the course of the succeeding 3 months, many repeat examinations of the blood were done, and the values obtained were not significantly different from those obtained at the time of the initial studies. Furthermore, 11 examinations of the urine were carried out during the period of the child's first admission to the hospital. In 9 of these 11 examinations, glucose was found in the urine, the values ranging from 0.5 per cent to 2.0 per cent. The presence of amino-aciduria was also established, as was a high urinary clearance of phosphate.

B, *C*, *D*, *E*, and *F* represent reproductions of roentgenographs of various other skeletal parts in this case, also taken at the time of the child's first admission to the hospital. The changes of rickets are, of course, most severe at the sites where longitudinal growth by endochondral ossification is normally most rapid. That is, the rachitic changes are very pronounced at the lower end of the radius and ulna, at the lower end of the femur and upper end of the tibia and fibula, and at the lower end of the tibia and fibula. The changes at the upper ends of the femora are not so striking as those in the other skeletal areas shown, since longitudinal growth is less active at the upper end of the femur than it is at these other sites. It is also to be noted, however, that a mild degree of coxa vara is present at the upper ends of the femora. Despite all the therapeutic efforts directed toward the correction of the rickets, the disease process advanced. At the age of 12, the child died during a hypokalemic crisis, and an autopsy was performed. (See Figs. 106, 107, 108, and 109 for some of the skeletal changes.)

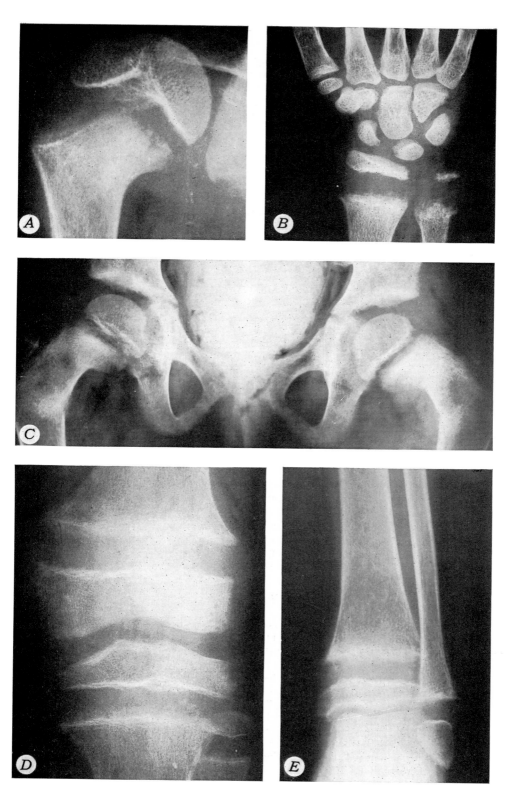

Figure 105

sections under polarized light will usually show the presence of the crystals, since the latter are doubly refractile. It seems fairly well established that the cystine crystals are not incorporated into the cells of the reticuloendothelial system through phagocytosis, but are formed within the cells. It is also to be noted that the presence of the cystine crystals in the cells does not tend to provoke a foreign-body reaction.

In respect to the *kidneys*, Clay *et al.* state that the renal tubular dysfunction underlying Fanconi rickets is to be related to a congenital structural anomaly of the tubules. On the basis of microdissection of the nephrons and histologic examination of stained tissue sections, they report finding that the proximal convoluted tubules were abnormally short, and that where the tubules joined the glomeruli (and for some little distance beyond the junctional area) the proximal convoluted tubules were constricted. Nevertheless, in an occasional case, routine anatomic examination of the kidneys reveals very little if any deviation from the normal. However, in cases which have run a protracted course, the renal changes are often very pronounced. The earliest changes are represented by granular degeneration of the epithelial cells of the proximal convoluted tubules, which may be associated with thickening of the basement membranes of the glomeruli. With further advance of the pathologic alterations, one finds evidence of interstitial round cell infiltrations, and still further progression of the condition results in an anatomic picture corresponding to that of interstitial nephritis. Finally, diffuse interstitial fibrosis makes its appearance. Under these circumstances, one finds that many of the renal tubules are atrophic and/or dilated, and that many of the glomeruli are necrotic, fibrosed, or even completely hyalinized. When such advanced changes are present, the kidneys will be found contracted, and such kidneys have been denoted by R. Looser as "glomerulosclerotic contracted kidneys."

As already noted, in cases in which the kidneys develop such severe pathologic changes, renal insufficiency becomes manifest. Under these circumstances, the normal serum nonprotein nitrogen value and the striking *hypo*phosphatemia of uncomplicated Fanconi rickets are, of course, replaced by an elevated nonprotein nitrogen value and a *hyper*phosphatemia. The renal insufficiency leads to parathyroid hyperplasia and hyperfunctioning. The resultant hyperparathyroidism in turn becomes a factor in modifying the pathologic changes in the bones. In particular, the original pathologic changes, which were analogous to those of simple nutritional vitamin D-deficiency rickets, come to have engrafted upon them the scarring effects of chronic renal insufficiency and hyperparathyroidism. Thus, to

Figure 106

A, Roentgenograph of a number of ribs removed at autopsy in the case of Fanconi rickets on which some information on the clinical history is given in connection with Figure 105-*A*. Note the general porosity of the ribs, and the numerous bands of radiolucency (Looser lines) extending across the long axis of the ribs. The broadening and deformity of the rib shafts at the costochondral junctions account for the distorted shadows at the left of the picture.

B, Photograph showing the cut surface of parts of 3 of the ribs illustrated in *A*. The arrows point to an area which cast the radiolucent shadow of a Looser line.

C, Photomicrograph ($\times$ 2) of a rib in this case. Proceeding from left to right, one can observe: a portion of resting chondral cartilage; the widened proliferating cartilage zone; the rachitic intermediate zone, containing osteoid; and a clearly defined area (see arrows) which would have appeared as a Looser line of radiolucency in the x-ray picture.

D, Photomicrograph ($\times$ 12) illustrating the general histologic architecture of the area indicated by the arrows in *C*. Most of the tissue occupying the midportion of the picture is bone matrix which appears mineralized only in spots.

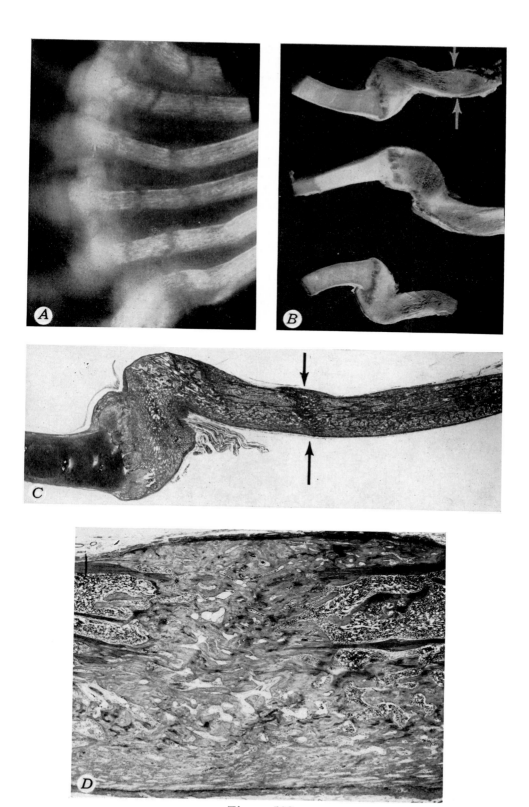

Figure 106

a greater or lesser extent, the pathologic picture is now that of rachitoid changes and "osteitis fibrosa"—the anatomic picture of so-called "renal (glomerular) rickets" or "renal (secondary) hyperparathyroidism."

However, in the case of Fanconi rickets which the writer had followed for about 4 years and which came to autopsy, there was only a minimal deposition of cystine in the kidneys, and the latter had therefore not undergone sclerotic changes. Furthermore, since chronic renal insufficiency did not develop, the rachitoid bone changes did not have engrafted upon them the scarring effects of chronic renal insufficiency. Various *skeletal parts* and *individual bones* were removed at the autopsy for roentgenographic, gross, and microscopic examination. In particular, we removed for study the calvarium, the dorsolumbar portion of the vertebral column, a number of ribs, and all the long tubular bones of the left lower extremity. The most pronounced changes were observed in the ribs and long bones.

The *ribs* showed enlargement at the costochondral junctions and also striking angulation deformity in the junctional areas. On roentgenographic examination the ribs were found to be porotic, and the body of each rib presented a number of slitlike radiolucent zones directed more or less at right angles to the long axis of the rib. As microscopic examination revealed, these radiolucent zones represented areas of microinfraction which had become filled in by osteoid callus. Because of its lack of bone mineral, this callus was more radiolucent than the somewhat better mineralized osseous tissue neighboring upon it. (See Fig. 106.)

The *femur* was also grossly misshapen. The head and neck of the bone presented a pronounced coxa vara deformity. When sectioned in the frontal plane, the upper half of the femur showed conspicuous widening of the epiphysial cartilage plate between the head and neck, and a considerable amount of osteoid in the femoral neck beyond that plate. Distal to the intertrochanteric area, the cortex of the upper part of the femoral shaft was extremely thin. Roentgenographic examination

Figure 107

A, Photograph of the upper third of the left femur removed at autopsy and sectioned in the frontal plane. (For the pertinent clinical data, see Fig. 105-A.) Note the striking coxa vara deformity which had developed in the course of the 4 years since the child's first admission. (Compare with Fig. 105-C.) The dark area at the junction of the head and neck of the bone represents the irregular and extremely wide epiphysial cartilage plate. The whitish, rather homogeneous tissue area beyond the cartilage plate is composed of fairly closely compacted trabeculae of bone matrix which, in part, is poorly mineralized. What one can see of the shaft cortex is thin.

B, Roentgenograph of the gross specimen shown in A. The center of ossification for the femoral head appears on the extreme right. The rather wide, fairly homogeneous shadow between that ossification center and the neck of the bone represents the broadened epiphysial cartilage plate area. Note, beyond the plate area, the wedge-shaped radiolucent zone in the femoral neck (see arrows). This is a so-called "Aufhellungszone" or "Umbauzone" of Looser, also denoted as a "Milkman line." It is clear from comparison with the corresponding area in A that there is no discontinuity (fracture line) in the femoral neck at the site of the radiolucency in question. The latter reflects merely the presence in the femoral neck of an area of bone matrix, which is poorly mineralized in comparison with the bone matrix on each side of the area of radiolucency. The x-ray picture also shows the thinness and rarefaction of the femoral cortex, as well as the general porosity of the bone.

C, Photomicrograph ($\times$ 2) showing the head, neck, and intertrochanteric portion of the femur illustrated in A and B. It reinforces the information conveyed by those illustrations. Note in particular that there is indeed no fracture line in the femoral neck. The latter is filled with trabeculae of bone, though at this low magnification one can only faintly see that the matrix of the osseous tissue in the area of radiolucency (shown in B) is less mineralized than the adjacent osseous tissue.

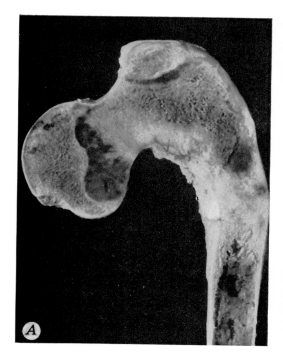

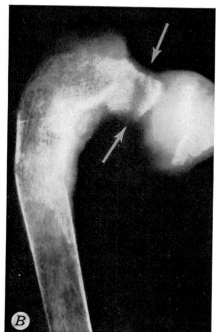

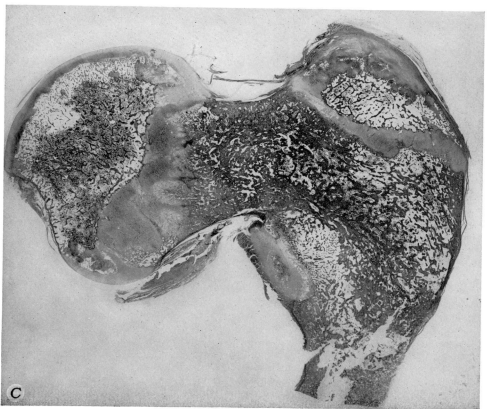

Figure 107

425

of the sectioned specimen revealed, in the femoral neck, a bandlike radiolucency, commonly denoted as a pseudofracture or Looser-Milkman line. However, as the gross and microscopic findings made clear, there was no actual discontinuity or fracture line in the femoral neck, the area represented by the radiolucent zone being completely occupied by osteoid callus. (See Fig. 107.) As one could deduce from the microscopic findings in regard to the epiphysial cartilage plates at other juxta-epiphysial areas, the osteoid callus in the femoral neck was not laid down through skeletogenic activity at the regional epiphysial cartilage plate. Instead, it must have developed as a response to microfractures occurring in the femoral neck as a result of mechanical stress.

The lower part of the left femur and the upper part of the left tibia were sectioned in the long axis and also roentgenographed. In the x-ray pictures the shaft cortices of these bones were found thin and the trabecular markings were sparse and blurred. At the epiphysial-diaphysial junctional area of the lower part of the femur and upper part of the tibia, there was a broad, relatively radiolucent area whose roentgenographic appearance suggested that of a very prominent rachitic inter-mediate zone. However, on gross examination of the sectioned bone parts, these broad radiolucent zones were found to represent mainly very wide epiphysial cartilage plates. What was even more striking and significant was the practical absence of osteoid along the surface of these plates abutting on the corresponding bone shaft. This finding is in sharp contrast to what one would expect to observe in the epiphysial-diaphysial junctional areas in a case of simple vitamin D-deficiency rickets or in a case of so-called refractory rickets.

Microscopic examination of the epiphysial-diaphysial junctional areas in question revealed that, though the epiphysial cartilage plates were wide, the cartilage cells toward the shaft surface of these plates were, in many places, not lined up in columns. Furthermore, the matrix of this cartilage, whether its cells were arranged

Figure 108

A, Photograph showing the cut surface of the lower half of the femur removed at autopsy in the same case illustrated in Figure 107. The cortex of the femoral shaft is extremely thin and porotic, and the angulation in the midportion of the picture represents the site of an infraction of the shaft. In the lower part of the picture, one can see the greatly widened epiphysial cartilage plate.

B, Roentgenograph of the specimen shown in A. This brings out the porosity of the bone in general and the thinness and porosity of the cortical bone in particular. It also demon-strates that, beyond the widened epiphysial cartilage plate, there is no distinct cuplike concavity in the metaphysial portion of the shaft (resulting from the accumulation of osteoid there), such as one would find in a case of ordinary nutritional (vitamin D-deficiency) rickets.

C, Photomicrograph ($\times$ 1) of a section prepared from the specimen shown in A. Proceeding from above downward, one can note that the shaft cortex above the site of angulation is extremely porotic. In the region of the angulation, the interior of the bone is occupied by new bone (callus) which is apparently not mineralized, since otherwise it would have cast a relatively radiopaque shadow (see B). Note also that, on the shaft side of the epiphysial cartilage plate, osteogenesis (expressed in the formation of osteoid and/or mineralized bone matrix) is practically in abeyance. As mentioned in the text, this lack of osteogenesis is apparently due, at least in part, to the protracted loss, from the body, of amino acids, which enter into the formation of the collagen of the organic bone matrix.

D, Photomicrograph ($\times$ 30) demonstrating in greater detail the histologic appearances in one area of the plate-shaft junction shown in C. From below upward, one sees some of the cartilage cells of the plate. Note that there is no evidence of mineralization of the cartilage matrix, that the cartilage cells near the shaft are not being penetrated by capillary blood vessels, and that there are no tongues of mineralized cartilage matrix extending into the shaft, as there would normally be.

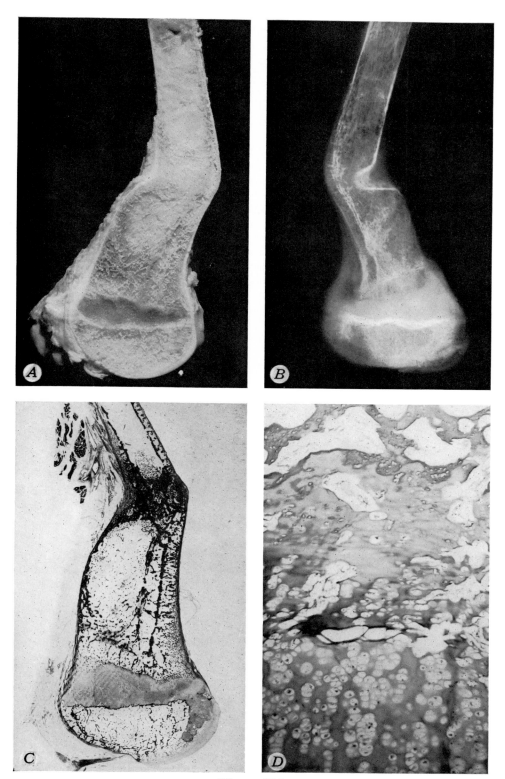

Figure 108

in columns or not, showed no evidence of calcification. In addition, only a few tongues of cartilage and/or cartilage matrix were projecting from the widened plates into the adjacent diaphysis. Another surprising finding was the abutment of spongy bone against the shaft surface of the plates and the heavy collagenization of the cartilage matrix in the immediate vicinity of contact between the cartilage and bone. All these histologic findings were clear evidence that endochondral bone formation was not occurring at the epiphysial-diaphysial junctions and, in addition, was actually being blocked. In a general way, the histologic appearances at these junctions were reminiscent of those encountered at epiphysial-diaphysial junctions in youthful subjects affected with achondroplasia and, to a lesser degree, in subjects affected with hypopituitarism. The practical cessation and "blocking" of endochondral bone formation found at the epiphysial cartilage plates was also observed about the periphery of the epiphysial centers of ossification at the lower end of the femur and upper end of the tibia.

On the basis of these findings, one may infer that, in this child affected with Fanconi rickets, the almost complete lack of endochondral bone formation found terminally at the epiphysial cartilage plates could be attributed to the protracted amino-aciduria. Because of the urinary loss of the amino acids, osteoid was not being laid down at the epiphysial cartilage plates, since these acids are essential for the formation of collagen. Furthermore, the protracted negative protein balance was possibly also reflected in an inadequate synthesis of growth hormone by the anterior lobe of the pituitary. Normally, this hormone stimulates cartilage proliferation along the shaft surface of the epiphysial cartilage plates and is thus a dynamic factor in endochondral bone formation.

Altogether, one may conclude from these roentgenographic, gross, and microscopic findings that, in cases of Fanconi disease running a chronic course and not complicated by renal insufficiency, the anatomic picture presented by the affected bones gradually shifts from that of clear-cut rickets to a picture in which the dominant changes are those of osteoporosis. In summary, then, one may say that it is the protracted lack of amino acids necessary for collagen formation and for the synthesis of growth hormone that constitutes the basis for the shift in question—that is, for the eventual emergence of "rickets that is no longer typical rickets histologically." (See Figs. 108 and 109.)

Figure 109

A, Photograph showing the cut surface of the upper half of the tibia removed at autopsy in the same case illustrated in Figures 107 and 108. The epiphysial cartilage plate is very much widened, and the cortex of the bone is extremely thin.

B, Roentgenograph of the specimen shown in A. This, too, brings out the porosity of the bone in general and the thinness of the cortical bone in particular. Beyond the widened epiphysial cartilage plate, there is again no cuplike rachitic intermediate zone resulting from the local accumulation of osteoid.

C, Photomicrograph ($\times$ 1) likewise demonstrating the general porosity of the bone and particularly of the cortex, and the absence of osteoid on the shaft side of the epiphysial cartilage plate.

D, Photomicrograph ($\times$ 30) showing in greater detail the histologic appearances in one area of the plate-shaft junction illustrated in C. Proceeding from above downward, one sees some of the cartilage cells of the plate. Note that there is a lack of organized arrangement of these cells, that there is evidence of focal degeneration of the cartilage, and that there is no evidence of columns of calcified cartilage matrix extending into the shaft. In fact, one may interpret the histologic appearances presented as indicating not only that the formation of osteoid at the plate-shaft junction has ceased, but that the shaft surface of the plate is blocked off.

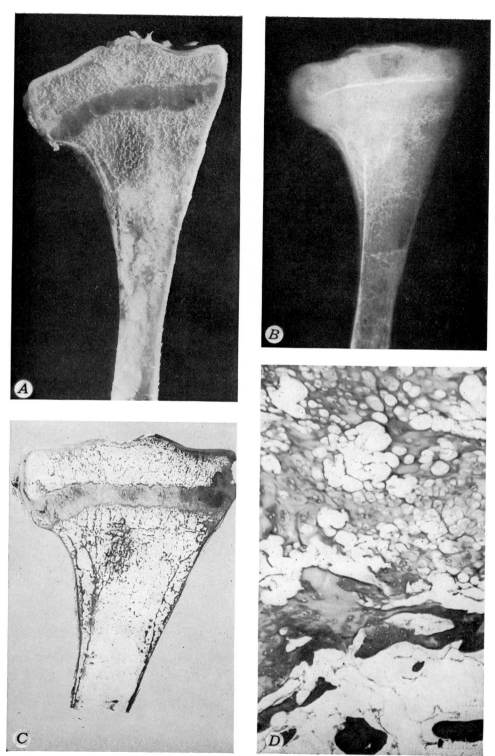

Figure 109

PROGNOSIS AND TREATMENT

At present, it appears that the ultimate prognosis in cases of Fanconi rickets (Lignac-Fanconi rickets) is unfavorable. Indeed, it is rather unusual for the affected child to survive into adolescence. The prognosis is doleful, because no way has yet been found for controlling the basic metabolic defect—that is, the disordered amino acid metabolism. The latter accounts both for the loss of large quantities of various amino acids by way of the urine (amino-aciduria) and for the storage of cystine in the various tissues of the body (cystinosis). There can be no doubt that the advanced pathologic changes very frequently present in the kidneys in the later stages of the disease are attributable at least in part to the accumulation of cystine in the kidneys. The consequent renal insufficiency (and the accompanying azotemia and *hyper*phosphatemia) in itself dooms the child to an early death.

In a case of Fanconi rickets not yet manifesting renal (glomerular) insufficiency, vitamin D in large doses is commonly administered. This increases the absorption of calcium and phosphorus from the gastrointestinal tract and may improve, at least temporarily, the condition of the bones. In addition, therapeutic efforts are directed toward counteracting the acidosis and also the hypokalemia. The latter, if pronounced, may induce a hypokalemic crisis resulting in death of the child.

However, despite all therapeutic efforts directed toward improving the condition of the affected child who came under our care at the age of 8, the child died at the age of 12 years. The immediate cause of death was a hypokalemic crisis, and the skeleton showed profound alterations. For many months before the child died, she received massive daily doses of vitamin D (often as much as 250,000 units). Over certain periods, the vitamin D was even supplemented by the daily administration of alkali, but it still failed to prevent the progress of the disease.

THE OSTEOMALACIC COUNTERPART
OF FANCONI RICKETS

The existence, in adults, of an osteomalacic state developing on a basis analogous to that of Fanconi rickets has become evident. Hunter seems to have been the first to direct attention to cases of pronounced bone rarefaction and osteomalacia associated with renal glucosuria. Cooke *et al.* reviewed the 6 cases which had accumulated in the literature to 1947 and added a case of their own. Among these collected cases is the one reported by Milkman. That one has been the basis for the term "Milkman's disease" as the name for a skeletal disorder. Specifically, he described the case of a woman who was 43 years of age at death and who had been ill for 9 years, mainly because of a generalized skeletal disability but who had also presented renal glucosuria. Roentgenographically, the skeleton appeared rarefied. Milkman observed what he described as multiple, spontaneous, symmetrical pseudo-fractures of idiopathic nature. As noted in several places in this chapter, such pseudofractures represent, in anatomic terms, bone sites filled with osteoid which casts the shadow of an unhealed fracture line because the osseous tissue neighboring on the osteoid is relatively more radiopaque. As also noted, they correspond to what E. Looser had described in 1920 as the "Umbauzonen" (zones of reconstruction) to be observed in cases of ordinary rickets and osteomalacia due to malnutrition and vitamin D deficiency. That they may occur in cases of rickets and osteomalacia having their basis in disordered functioning of renal tubules is not at all remarkable, and the roentgenographic picture corresponding to so-called Milkman's disease thus requires no special explanation. The case of the woman presenting multiple pseudofractures which was reported by Aufranc *et al.* is also clearly an instance of the osteomalacic counterpart of Fanconi rickets.

The patients affected with the type of osteomalacia in question are usually middle-aged. There is evidence that the disorder is inherited as a mendelian recessive character. The establishment of the presence of the disease in a given family may facilitate recognition of the condition in an individual case before the appearance of roentgenographic changes in the bones (see Dent and Harris). Indeed, for some time before this, the principal complaints may be muscular weakness and vague "rheumatic" pains in the lower part of the back, the hips, or even the feet.

The earliest roentgenographic skeletal findings may be "Looser zones" of radiolucency (the so-called pseudofractures), which are often bilateral and symmetrical. Such zones are most likely to be observed in the ribs, scapulae, pubic bones, and/or femoral necks. At the time such radiolucent zones are first noted roentgenographically, the bones in general may still appear fairly normal in respect to radiopacity and gross architecture. However, as the disease progresses, the bones become demineralized, the cortices appear thin and rarefied, and the trabecular markings become blurred and even obliterated in places. Fractures and deformities are the inevitable consequences of the advanced osteomalacic state. Eventually the fractures, deformities, and generalized porosity of the bones may become so severely incapacitating that the patient is confined to bed as a skeletal cripple. This was the course pursued in the case of a woman who was 35 years of age when she first presented herself at our hospital with complaints of pain in various bones and joints. The pains increased, and 3 years later the patient was admitted to Montefiore Hospital, where it was noted that each femoral neck had a transverse zone of radiolucency ("Looser zone"). Progressive demineralization of the bones and multiple fractures continued during the next 10 years, and the patient became severely deformed and died when she was 48 years of age. (See Figs. 110 and 111.)

As in rickets and osteomalacia in general, the *serum* calcium is within normal limits or only slightly lowered. However, the serum inorganic phosphorus value is consistently below normal; indeed, the hypophosphatemia may even be striking. The serum alkaline phosphatase value is, of course, elevated. In addition, biochemical study of the serum usually reveals some reduction in the potassium content and a lowered CO_2 combining power. In the cases in question, the *urine*, in addition to containing glucose, is found to contain large amounts of amino acids. However, in contrast to what one finds in cases of Fanconi rickets, the various organs and tissues in cases of osteomalacia representing its adult counterpart fail to reveal cystine storage as an expression of disordered amino acid metabolism. Also in contrast to Fanconi rickets, the urinary excretion of calcium in these cases is extremely high. The disordered functioning of the renal tubules also presents as a defect in acidification of the urine, an inability to concentrate or dilute it adequately, and the presence of protein in it.

The proper *treatment* is the administration of large doses of sodium or potassium bicarbonate and large quantities of vitamin D. Naturally, the serum calcium value must be watched to forestall the toxic manifestations of hypervitaminosis D. The dietary intake of calcium and phosphorus can be supplemented by the oral administration of calcium phosphate. The administration of a citric acid—sodium citrate mixture daily is useful in combatting the acidosis. Despite intensive therapy, the amino-aciduria tends to persist. Temporary clinical improvement is obtained in some cases, but the ultimate prognosis remains poor (see Andersen, and also Astrup and Kjerulf-Jensen).

RICKETS AND OSTEOMALACIA OF THE BUTLER-ALBRIGHT SYNDROME

Butler *et al.* and Albright *et al.* have described cases of rickets and osteomalacia whose basis seems to lie in an aberration of the excretory capacity of the renal tubules, again in the absence of defective glomerular functioning. It is believed that in these cases the renal defect resides specifically in a decreased ability of the renal tubules to make ammonia and excrete an acid urine. A chronic acidosis is present, as evidenced by a low serum CO_2 and an increase of the serum chloride content. The urinary ammonia and titratable acidity are low. One also obtains the usual rachitic or osteomalacic serum values in regard to calcium, inorganic phosphorus, and alkaline phosphatase. The nephrocalcinosis and nephrolithiasis sometimes also found are attributable to hypercalciuria. The latter occurs since the calcium, being a base, is in overdemand because of the chronic acidosis.

The bones may come to show an advanced degree of rarefaction. Multiple and even symmetrical bands of radiolucency (the so-called pseudofractures or "Aufhellungszonen") may be found in some of the bones if a complete skeletal survey is made. In an occasional case, these may be present even in the absence of pronounced generalized rarefaction of the bones. Furthermore, if the patient is still growing, rachitoid changes may be observed roentgenographically in the juxta-epiphysial zones. In the occasional case which has come to autopsy, the histologic examination of the bones shows the presence of osteoid margins on the trabeculae, substantiating the diagnosis of rickets or osteomalacia.

Albright *et al.* found that the condition responds remarkably to combined treatment with fairly large doses of vitamin D and alkalinizing salt. The alkalinizing salt mixture used for treatment consists of 140 gm. of citric acid and 98 gm. of sodium citrate dissolved in 1 liter of water. The patient takes 50 to 100 cc. of this mixture daily, in accordance with the amount needed to overcome the acidosis. The amount of supplementary vitamin D usually necessary in these cases ranges between 50,000 and 100,000 units daily. It appears that, after the skeletal aberration is corrected by this treatment, the alkalinizing salt alone suffices to prevent

Figure 110

A, Roentgenograph of the pelvis and upper ends of the femora as they appeared early in the clinical course of a case of osteomalacia presumably due to renal tubular malfunction and representing the adult counterpart of Fanconi rickets. Note the presence of a so-called Looser line (see arrows) in the neck of each femur. The patient, a woman, was 35 years of age when she was admitted to our hospital with a history of pain in the lower part of the back. The pain had been present for about 3 months, had been gradually increasing, and had become so disabling that it was difficult for her to walk any distance. In the course of the next few months, the patient began to complain of pains in various joints, and the initial clinical impression was that she was suffering from some form of arthritis. However, examination of the urine showed the presence of amino acids, though no detailed determinations were made in respect to them. Three years later (at the age of 38), the woman was admitted to Montefiore Hospital, where this x-ray picture was taken and where the fact that she was suffering from osteomalacia was first definitely established. A biopsy specimen from a fibula was submitted to the writer for histologic examination, and at the same time a specimen of blood was sent to Dr. Aaron Bodansky for biochemical analysis. The serum calcium and phosphate values were 9.5 and 1.5 mg. per cent respectively, and the serum alkaline phosphatase value was 10 Bodansky units per 100 cc. The blood sugar and urea nitrogen values were respectively 86 and 9.5 mg. Nevertheless, the urine showed a small amount of glucose. The biopsy specimen was reported by the writer as indicating the presence of osteomalacia, and ruling out the presence of hyperparathyroidism.

B, Roentgenograph illustrating the appearance of the lower two thirds of the femora 10 years after the roentgenograph shown in *A* was taken—that is, when the patient was 48 years of age. The shaft of the left femur is the site of a pathologic fracture. Furthermore, in comparison with *A*, the cortices of the femora now appear as mere "pencil lines" of radiopacity. (See also Figs. 111-*A* and *B*, showing the roentgenographic picture presented by various other bones examined at the same time.)

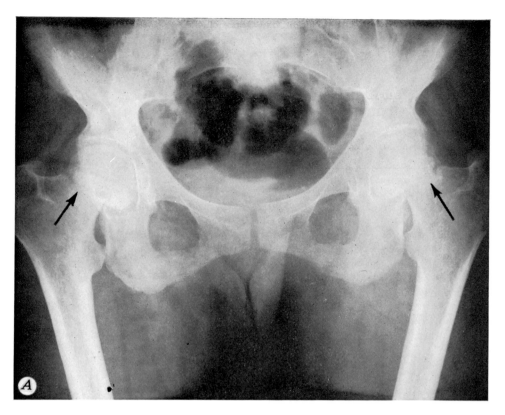

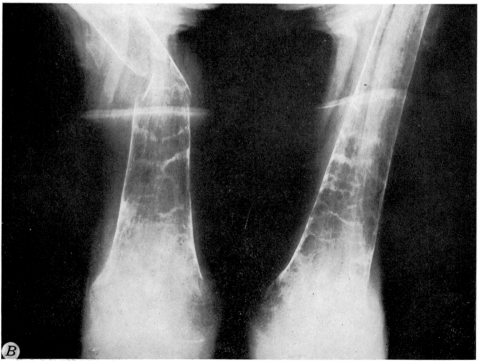

Figure 110

433

the recurrence of the rickets or osteomalacia. Furthermore, under this treatment, the severity of the nephrolithiasis tends to diminish.

SKELETAL EFFECTS OF DISORDERS OF OTHER INTERNAL ORGANS

Chronic Obstructive Jaundice.—In the presence of long-standing complete obstruction of the bile passages, changes may appear in the bones. For example, in infants with congenital atresia of these passages, the bones may become rather porotic, and rachitoid changes may even appear at costochondral and epiphysial-diaphysial junctions. Reports on such cases are to be found in the literature under the heading of "hepatic rickets" (see Gerstenberger and also Thoenes and Gruson).

In an old woman who had suffered for 5 years from biliary obstruction and cholangitic cirrhosis, Šikl noted osteomalacic alterations in the bones removed at autopsy. Such a finding in cases of chronic biliary obstruction in adults is rare. Indeed, under these circumstances the bones rarely present more than mild resorptive changes, visible only microscopically. These are manifested by the presence of Howship's lacunae and osteoclasts, subperiosteally and on the surfaces of the haversian canals and spongy trabeculae. In addition, in such adult subjects the inner table of the calvarium may present thin sheets of newly deposited bone laid down by the dura. On inspection of the calvarium, this new deposit of bone may show a greenish tint from bile staining, but if it does not, fixation of the calvarium in 10 per cent formalin for some days will make the discoloration stand out. Indeed, it is only bone deposited during the cholemic state and not yet fully calcified that is found discolored by bile in a case of cholemia.

Biliary Fistula.—If bile is excluded from the intestinal tract through the agency of a biliary fistula, severe and generalized porosity of the bones may develop. This fact was first noted early in the present century by Pavlov in dogs with experimental biliary fistulae. Such dogs, of course, also manifest steatorrhea. The changes in

Figure 111

A, Roentgenograph illustrating the pronounced porosity of the bones of both legs and both feet in the case of osteomalacia represented in Figure 110. This x-ray picture was taken when the patient was 48 years of age—that is, about 13 years after she began to complain of pains relating to the bones and joints. Both fibulae show an infraction line at the junction of the middle and lower thirds of the shaft.

B, Roentgenograph illustrating the status of the long bones of one of the upper extremities, taken at the same time as the x-ray picture shown in *A*. The humerus is the site of a pathologic fracture, and the lower third of the radius shows a transverse zone of radiolucency likewise representing an infraction line.

C, Photomicrograph ($\times$ 55) representing the histologic appearance of a tissue section prepared from a part of the ilium removed at the autopsy in this case, which was performed at Montefiore Hospital. The woman had died 6 months after the x-ray pictures shown in *A* and *B* were taken, and the autopsy was performed by Dr. Samuel H. Rosen, the hospital pathologist at that time, who removed many of the bones for study. Note the wide borders of non-mineralized bone matrix (osteoid) about the marrow spaces, and the absence of osteoclasts and fibrous scarring of the marrow—histologic findings which establish the diagnosis of osteomalacia. (I am indebted to Dr. Rosen for having made tissue available to me for study so that I might complete my records on this case. I am also indebted to Dr. Louis Leiter, formerly Chief of the Medical Division of Montefiore Hospital, for granting me permission to review the recorded clinical data on this patient, who was under the care of his department.)

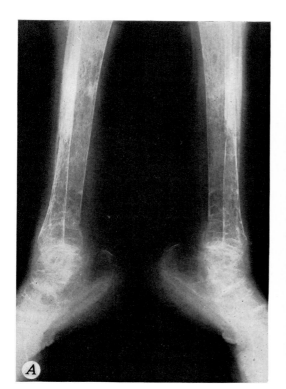

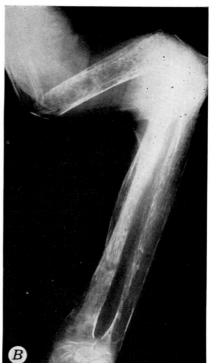

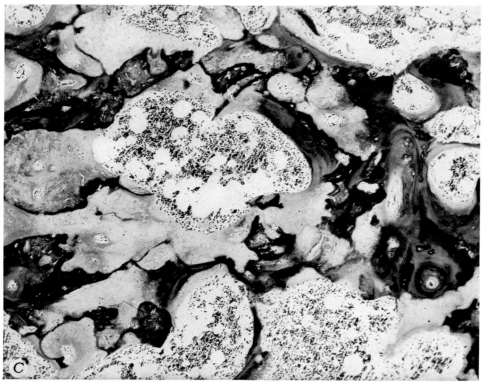

Figure 111

435

their bones begin to appear within a few months after the fistula is created. By the end of a year, in the surviving animals, the bones have usually become so extremely porotic that they are abnormally fragile and pliable. Though all the bones are affected, those of the trunk are likely to be the ones most severely involved. Indeed, eventually the vertebral column may be found twisted, the rib cage deformed into a chicken breast shape, and various bones (especially ribs) fractured, though held together by callus. On microscopic examination it will be noted that the cortical bone is rarefied, the haversian canals are enlarged, and the spongy trabeculae are thinned. The surfaces of the haversian canals and trabeculae show narrow osteoid borders.

Pathogenetically the most important factor in the development of the bone changes seems to be that, when bile is absent from the intestinal tract, the absorption of vitamin D (the calcifying vitamin) is impaired (see Seifert, and Heymann). In this connection it was demonstrated that in a dog with a biliary fistula the porosity of the bones could be influenced in the direction of healing by the subcutaneous administration of vitamin D (see Tammann). Furthermore, such treatment can change a negative calcium-phosphorus balance to a positive one in a dog with a biliary fistula (see Greaves and Schmidt). Pertinent human material on the question of the bone changes in cases of biliary fistula is very meager. However, in the case, described by Seidel, of biliary fistula of long standing (complicated by obstructive jaundice), the porotic bones, on microscopic examination, showed numerous osteoclasts and Howship's lacunae but no osteoid borders.

Pancreatic Fistula.—As a result of experimental pancreatic fistula, the exclusion of pancreatic juice from the intestinal tract leads to porotic bone changes similar to, though generally milder than, those resulting from biliary fistula. The bone changes do not have time to become very severe, since the animals require special care (including the administration of adequate doses of bicarbonate of soda) if they are to be kept alive for any length of time. The porosity of the bones has its basis in steatorrhea. Specifically, impairment of fat absorption from the intestinal tract in the presence of a pancreatic fistula tends to make the ingested calcium unavailable to the bones, since it becomes bound to the fats in the form of insoluble calcium soaps.

Gastrectomy.—It has been demonstrated by Bussabarger *et al.* that gastrectomy in dogs leads to porosis of the bones, but whether this osteoporosis actually represents osteomalacia is not clear. If the gastrectomy has been performed at a very early age, profound skeletal changes may appear and be expressed in severe bone deformities and even spontaneous fractures. The bone changes develop in the surviving dogs despite the fact that they are maintained on a diet well balanced in every respect, including calcium, phosphorus, and vitamin D content, and fed in the large amounts required by gastrectomized animals. Without losing sight of possible additional underlying factors, these workers emphasized the importance of the absence of hydrochloric acid from the intestinal contents, the absence of the reservoir function of the stomach, and the presence of a postcibal acidosis ("acid tide") in the production of postgastrectomy osteoporosis.

Severe demineralization of the bones, thought to represent osteomalacia, has also been described as a sequel to gastrectomy in man (see Pyrah and Smith, and Du Berger *et al.*). In the case described by Pyrah and Smith, the patient was a woman on whom gastrectomy was performed when she was 38 years of age. Fourteen years later, clinical and roentgenographic manifestations of osteomalacia were clearly evident. In that case the osteomalacia was attributed to the steatorrhea which developed after the gastrectomy. The patients in the 5 cases reported by Du Berger *et al.* were also rather young adults at the time the gastrectomy was performed. The time interval between the gastrectomy and the recognition of the presence of osteomalacia was usually only a few years. In none of the clinical summaries of these 5 cases is there mention of postgastrectomy steatorrhea.

HYPOPHOSPHATASIA

The concept of hypophosphatasia as a disease entity had its foundation in a case study reported by Rathbun in 1948. The subject was a male infant who was born at full term, showed manifestations of the disease at birth, and died when he was about 9 weeks of age. *Clinically* the affected infant presented a rather globular head, beading at the costochondral junctions, rachitoid deformities at the wrists, and bowing of the legs. *Roentgenographically,* all the bones appeared very deficient in mineral matter. In the cranial vault there were only a few small patches of radiopacity representing areas of mineralized osseous tissue. The rest of the vault cast a faint "ground glass" shadow, since it was composed of non-mineralized bone matrix. Rachitoid changes were evident at the costochondral junctions and at the epiphysial-diaphysial junctions of the long tubular bones. *Biochemical studies* made during the life of the infant revealed, in the course of repeated examinations, that the serum alkaline phosphatase value was extremely low, and on some occasions, no serum alkaline phosphatase activity whatever was detected. The serum calcium value was at the high normal level or slightly above this, as was the serum phosphate value. Bones removed at *autopsy* of the infant confirmed the presence of rachitoid changes at sites of endochondral bone formation. Bone samples were also extracted for phosphatase and showed an abnormally low alkaline phosphatase content. Samples of the kidneys, lungs, and mucous membrane of the small intestine likewise showed strikingly low alkaline phosphatase activity.

Rathbun's well-documented case report opened up a new area of inquiry in the general field of skeletal disease relating particularly to infants and young children. The earlier medical literature was searched for cases which seemed to belong in the category of hypophosphatasia. In consequence, several cases came to light which had been reported as instances of atypical osteogenesis imperfecta or of achondroplasia. Furthermore, additional examples of hypophosphatasia soon came to be recognized and recorded (see Sobel *et al.*, Neuhauser and Currarino, and Schlesinger *et al.*). The case reported by Engfeldt and Zetterström was described under the name of "osteodysmetamorphosis fetalis." In 1957, two rather comprehensive reviews of the literature, with added personal observations on their own cases, were published by Fraser and by Currarino *et al.* The various studies following upon the one by Rathbun furnished the additional information: (1) that the disorder is genetically conditioned; (2) that at least one parent of an affected infant or young child usually has an abnormally low serum alkaline phosphatase value even in the absence of clear-cut skeletal aberrations; (3) that an affected child and its stigmatized parent show an increased urinary excretion of phosphoethanolamine (amino ethyl phosphoric ester) in addition to the reduced serum alkaline phosphatase value; and (4) that hypophosphatasia should be regarded as representing one of the inheritable (or inborn) disorders of endogenous metabolism.

CLINICAL CONSIDERATIONS

Hypophosphatasia is of rare occurrence. Fraser estimated its *incidence* in the Toronto area of Canada at approximately 1 case per 100,000 live births. As already noted, the disorder is *genetically conditioned*, and the preponderant evidence is that it is inherited through the action of an autosomal recessive gene. However,

29

it has also been maintained that in some instances the inheritance is apparently due to the action of an autosomal dominant gene (see Silverman). Furthermore, since hypophosphatasia is genetically conditioned, affects sibs, and usually shows a recessive autosomal inheritance, it is to be expected that one or another parent will be heterozygotic for the condition. Such a parent may be expected to show diminished serum alkaline phosphatase activity and/or phosphoethanolaminuria without manifesting any skeletal abnormalities.

Clinical expressions of the disorder as represented by skeletal changes: (1) are often already present at birth; (2) not infrequently appear in the course of the first few weeks or months of life or, at any rate, during infancy; and (3) occasionally are not noted until early or later childhood. These differences in the time of appearance of the clinical manifestations seem to indicate merely that the severity of the inborn metabolic defect is greater in some cases than in others.

An affected neonate whose skeleton is already extensively involved at birth usually does not survive for more than a few hours or days. In those infants in whom the skeletal changes do not become apparent for several weeks or a few months after birth, indications of general illness (anorexia, vomiting, fever, convulsions, etc.) ordinarily first occupy the foreground of the clinical picture. If such an infant continues to survive, craniosynostosis and retardation of growth have time to become evident. Nevertheless, many of these infants die before reaching the age of one year. In a case of hypophosphatasia in which the presence of the disease does not reveal itself until some time during early childhood, it is often retarded skeletal growth, skeletal deformities (genu valgum, for instance), and premature loss of deciduous teeth that direct attention to the condition (see Sobel *et al.*, Ritchie, James and Moule, Pimstone *et al.*, and also McCormick and Ripa). Those subjects in whom the disease does not become apparent until childhood eventually come to show gradual clinical improvement. Furthermore, the prognosis insofar as continued survival is concerned takes a definite turn for the better.

Finally, it is believed that an occasional instance of osteoporosis and bone fragility in an adult has its basis in the same disorder of endogenous metabolism that is responsible for the skeletal manifestations of hypophosphatasia in infants and young children. Support for the idea that the bone fragility and osteoporosis in such a case may represent the adult counterpart of hypophosphatasia of children comes from the finding that such an adult may have had so-called "rickets" in childhood, has an abnormally low serum alkaline phosphatase value, and shows the presence of phosphoethanolamine in the urine.

Biochemical Findings.—The significant biochemical aberrations recorded so far in connection with the disease are: (1) a striking reduction in the *alkaline phosphatase* activity value of the serum, the bones (especially at sites of endochondral bone formation), and various other tissues (kidneys, liver, intestinal mucosa, etc.); and (2) the almost regular presence in the urine of *phosphoethanolamine*—a substance which is ordinarily not detectable in random samples of the urine of normal persons (see McCance *et al.* and Fraser *et al.*). It has not yet become clear why phospho-ethanolamine accumulates in the blood and is excreted in the urine in cases of hypophosphatasia. One of the explanatory possibilities suggested by Fraser is the idea that phosphoethanolamine represents the natural substrate, present in the tissues, which the enzyme phosphatase hydrolyzes to liberate phosphate ions. Since there is a great deficiency of alkaline phosphatase in these cases, the phospho-ethanolamine is not adequately hydrolyzed, accumulates in the blood, and is excreted in the urine. However, as noted, this concept has not yet been validated.

The *serum calcium* value is almost regularly increased, and in severely affected neonates and very young infants the *hypercalcemia* is often pronounced. In affected older infants and young children, hypercalcemia may not be present and is not likely to be striking if found. The absorption of calcium from the intestinal tract does occur in hypophosphatasia (though at a level somewhat below the normal). A possible explanation for the hypercalcemia may be that the absorbed calcium, not being utilized toward the mineralization of the organic bone matrix which is being laid down, accumulates in the blood. In the absence of renal insufficiency, the *serum phosphate* value is within the normal range, though frequently at the upper limit of the normal. If renal insufficiency has developed, hyperphosphatemia is, of course, present. The renal insufficiency is commonly the result of nephrocalcinosis following in the wake of hypercalcemia.

ROENTGENOGRAPHIC AND PATHOLOGIC FINDINGS

Neonates and Young Infants.—As noted, an affected neonate whose skeleton is already extensively involved at birth usually does not survive for more than a few hours or a few days. Such an infant presents a globular head and soft calvarium, obvious shortening and gross bowing deformities of the limbs, and beading at the costochondral junctions. On the basis of the neonate's external appearance alone, one might mistakenly suppose, in one case or another, that one was dealing with an instance of achondroplasia. However, *roentgenographic examination* of the skeleton promptly corrects that impression. Indeed, in the most severely affected neonates, many of the bones and/or component parts of bones may not be apparent in the roentgenographs because they are so poorly mineralized. In other cases, though most of the bones can be seen, their shadows indicate that they are under-developed and still poorly mineralized, and some of the long tubular bones may present infractions, fractures, and angulation deformities. Furthermore, the metaphysial ends of the shafts of these bones may show very wide radiolucent zones. The latter may present some faint, streaky radiopacities—an indication of disordered endochondral bone formation at the shaft surfaces of the epiphysial cartilage plates. (See Fig. 112.)

Anatomically the epiphysial cartilage plates are found widened, and their proliferating cartilage zones show a disordered arrangement of their cartilage cells and absence of mineralization of the matrix of the proliferating cartilage. Beyond these abnormal cartilage plates, the wide, relatively radiolucent metaphysial areas contain abundant amounts of non-mineralized bone matrix. Analogous changes are observed at the costochondral junctions, the enlarged (beadlike) end of each rib shaft also being occupied by a wide zone of osteoid. These findings are similar to those observed at the wide rachitic intermediate zones in cases of vitamin D-deficiency rickets, for instance. Furthermore, in hypophosphatasia, as in such cases of rickets, osteoid seams can be observed on the spongy trabeculae and on the walls of the haversian canals, and trabeculae of osteoid are likely to be found under the periosteum of various bones.

The softness and pliability of the *calvarium* which is almost consistently observed in affected neonates is likewise the result of defective ossification. Indeed, a substantial part of the organic bone matrix laid down in the membranous precursor of the calvarium may fail to be mineralized. Thus, roentgenographic examination of the calvarium may show some islands of radiopacity which are separated by narrow or wide, relatively radiolucent areas. Naturally the radiopaque areas in the calvarium are the sites where the organic bone matrix has been mineralized. The relatively radiolucent areas represent the sites where the organic bone matrix is poorly mineralized or completely lacking in mineral.

At autopsy, despite the fact that the calvarium may show only a few small plaques of osseous tissue as representatives of component bones, the usual suture lines can be observed and present an approximately normal appearance. In the ordinary course of events, the calvarium grows and expands along the suture lines. Since, in hypophosphatasia, the intramembranous deposition of bone matrix along these lines proceeds only slowly, one can understand why affected neonates present bulging of the anterior fontanelle and why the surviving children not infrequently come to manifest indications of craniosynostosis.

The *kidneys* of affected infants who succumb shortly after birth almost regularly show pathologic changes. These are the consequence of calcium deposition, the nephrocalcinosis being attributable to the hypercalcemia present in affected neonates and very young children. The calcium is found both in the renal cortex and in the medulla, but is likely to be most concentrated in the junctional area between the cortex and the medulla. Furthermore, the calcium granules are observed mainly in the interstitial connective tissue around the renal tubules, though some of the tubules may show calcium within their lumina. Mild inflammatory changes representing a reaction to the calcium deposition may also be found. In the presence of nephrocalcinosis, the kidneys may also come to show evidences of scarring if the affected infant survives for more than a few months.

Older Infants and Young Children.—In some cases, as noted, the underlying defect is less severe and the skeletal changes do not become evident until several weeks or months after birth (though still within the period of infancy). Further-

Figure 112

A, Roentgenograph showing part of the calvarium from a case of hypophosphatasia in a female infant 6 months of age. The calvarium is neither of normal thickness nor uniformly mineralized. In the upper part of the picture, there is a large, irregular area of radiolucency reflecting the almost total absence of mineralized bone matrix in the region in question. The infant was 6 months of age when she was admitted to The Children's Hospital Medical Center of Boston, where this x-ray picture and the others on this plate were taken. Previously, she had been admitted to another hospital because of fever and a bulging fontanel. On x-ray examination at that hospital, it was discovered that the infant had skeletal abnormalities, and she was then transferred to The Children's Hospital Medical Center. On admission there, it was observed that the anterior fontanel bulged, but there was no papilledema. The child was small and underweight for her age, and her extremities were flabby and hypotonic. During the infant's hospitalization, for a period of about 1 month, repeated serum calcium, phosphate, and alkaline phosphatase determinations were carried out. The serum calcium values were all within the normal range. The serum phosphate value was found to be at the lower limit of the normal. However, the serum alkaline phosphatase value was greatly depressed. It was found to be as low as 1 Bodansky unit per 100 cc. and, on occasion, less than 1 Bodansky unit.

B, Roentgenograph showing the bones of an upper extremity in this case of hypophosphatasia. Note the relative radiolucency of the lower metaphysis of the radius and ulna. This is the result of deficient mineralization of the organic bone matrix laid down in the course of endochondral bone formation at the corresponding epiphysial cartilage plates. Also worthy of note is the curious fact that the secondary centers of ossification pertaining to the phalanges and metacarpal bones shown in this picture are relatively radiopaque.

C, Roentgenograph demonstrating the appearance of bones of both lower extremities in this case. The extensive areas of radiolucency in the metaphyses of the bones shown are striking. They are clearly due to the lack of mineralization of the organic bone matrix which has been laid down. The stippled appearance of the secondary centers of ossification about the knee area stands out in contrast to the radiolucency of the neighboring metaphyses. (I am indebted to Dr. Edward B. D. Neuhauser, Radiologist-in-Chief of The Children's Hospital Medical Center, for the opportunity of studying and reproducing the roentgenographs on this plate, and also for the clinical data relating to the infant in question.)

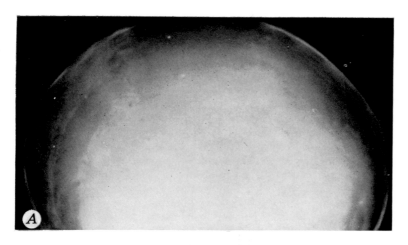

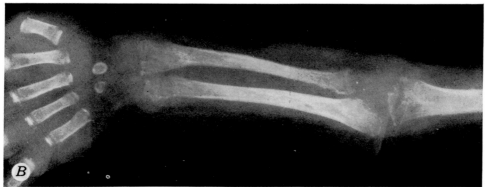

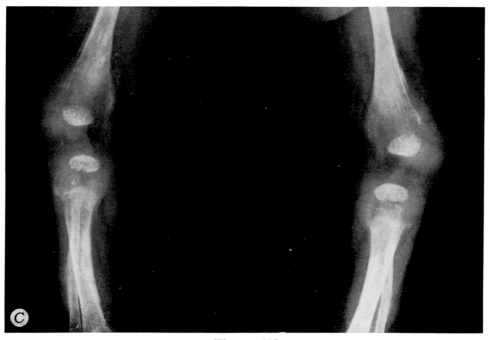

Figure 112

441

more, in an occasional instance, they may not become apparent until very early childhood. In all these cases, including those in which the subjects are still infants, the roentgenographic manifestations of the disorder are usually of lesser magnitude than in the severely affected neonates. In fact, the older the child at the time the presence of the disease becomes apparent, the less conspicuous are the skeletal changes likely to be. For example, the shadow cast by the calvarium may indicate that the component bones are fairly well mineralized. In relation to the long tubular bones, the juxta-epiphysial regions of the shafts may show relatively little widening of the epiphysial cartilage plates; nor do the metaphyses ordinarily present wide bandlike areas of radiolucency (wide rachitic intermediate zones) adjacent to the epiphysial cartilage plates. Nevertheless, the metaphyses of some of the bones may show larger or smaller, single or confluent areas of radiolucency abutting upon the epiphysial cartilage plates and possibly representing foci of osteoid and/or cartilage. While the size and contour of the epiphyses (the secondary centers of ossification) are within normal limits, the epiphyses are somewhat more radiolucent than one would expect them to be. Also, the cortices of the bone shafts may appear porotic and thinner than they normally are. In relation to the cases in this group, there is a dearth of anatomic material obtained at autopsy. However, biopsy examinations have been carried out on a few children, and these have revealed that the histologic changes (for instance, at sites of endochondral bone formation) are still those of rickets.

PROGNOSIS AND TREATMENT

If the child continues to survive, serial roentgenographic examinations will reveal that there is a tendency toward gradual improvement in the skeletal picture. The life expectancy also improves, provided that nephrocalcinosis and renal insufficiency are not present. The improved clinical and roentgenographic status of these subjects is not associated with a significant rise in the serum alkaline phosphatase value or a significant reduction in the urinary excretion of phosphoethanolamine. Any skeletal deformities which have developed are not likely to recede, and the retarded skeletal growth (shortness of stature) is not overcome as the child grows older.

Despite the fact that the roentgenographic skeletal findings mimic those of vitamin D-deficiency rickets, the administration of vitamin D in amounts exceeding the ordinary prophylactic dose is contraindicated in view of the frequent presence of hypercalcemia. Bongiovanni et al. report that a high phosphate intake may be beneficial in the treatment of the disorder. Through the use of cortisone, Fraser obtained, in one of his cases, clinical and roentgenographic improvement, and also an increase in the serum alkaline phosphatase value and a reduction in the serum calcium value. Withdrawal of the cortisone led to reversal of the improvement, and resumption of the cortisone to renewed improvement. Those children who develop clinical indications of craniosynostosis may require early craniectomy.

REFERENCES

ABELS, H.: Über die Natur der angeborenen Schädelerweichungen und der Früherweichungen im Säuglingsalter, Ztschr. Kinderh., *50*, 381, 1930.

ALBRIGHT, F., BURNETT, C. H., PARSON, W., REIFENSTEIN, E. C., JR. and Roos, A.: Osteomalacia and Late Rickets, Medicine, *25*, 399, 1940.

ANDERSEN, B. F.: Fanconis syndrom, Nord. med., *55*, 469, 1956.

ANDERSEN, D. H.: Celiac Syndrome. III. Dietary Therapy for Congenital Pancreatic Deficiency, Am. J. Dis. Child., *70*, 100, 1945.

—————: Celiac Syndrome. VI. The Relationship of Celiac Disease, Starch Intolerance, and Steatorrhea, J. Pediat., *30*, 564, 1947.

ANDERSEN, D. H. and DI SANT'AGNESE, P. A.: Idiopathic Celiac Disease. I. Mode of Onset and Diagnosis, Pediatrics, *11*, 207, 1953.

ASTRUP, P. and KJERULF-JENSEN, K.: Fanconi's Syndrome. Renal Tubular Resorption Anomaly with Aminoaciduria and Osteomalacia, Ugesk. laeger, *119*, 482, 1957.

AUFRANC, O. E., JONES, W. N. and HARRIS, W. H.: Multiple Pseudofractures, J.A.M.A., *190*, 842, 1964.

BAAR, H. S. and BICKEL, H.: Morbid Anatomy, Histology and Pathogenesis of Lignac-Fanconi Disease, Acta paediat., *42*, Suppl. 90, 171, 1952.

BAKWIN, H., BODANSKY, O. and SCHORR, R.: Refractory Rickets, Am. J. Dis. Child., *59*, 560, 1940.

BEGUM, R., COUTINHO, M. DE L., DORMANDY, T. L., and YUDKIN, S.: Maternal Malabsorption Presenting as Congenital Rickets, Lancet, *1*, 1048, 1968.

BENINDE, —: Die Verbreitung der durch die Hungerblockade hervorgerufenen Knochenerkrankungen unter der Bevölkerung Preussens (Rachitis, Spätrachitis, Osteomalacie), Veröffentl. Geb. Med.-Verwalt., *10*, 121, 1920.

BENNETT, I., HUNTER, D. and VAUGHAN, J. M.: Idiopathic Steatorrhoea (Gee's Disease). A Nutritional Disturbance Associated with Tetany, Osteomalacia and Anaemia, Quart. J. Med., *1*, 603, 1932.

BICKEL, H., BAAR, H. S., ASTLEY, R., DOUGLAS, A. A., FINCH, E., HARRIS, H., HARVEY, C. C., HICKMANS, E. M., PHILPOTT, M. G., SMALLWOOD, W. C., SMELLIE, J. M. and TEALL, C. G.: Cystine Storage Disease with Aminoaciduria and Dwarfism, Acta paediat., *42*, Suppl. 90, 1952.

BICKEL, H., SMALLWOOD, W. C., SMELLIE, J. M. and HICKMANS, E. M.: Clinical Description, Factual Analysis, Prognosis and Treatment of Lignac-Fanconi Disease, Acta paediat., *42*, Suppl. 90, 27, 1952.

BODANSKY, A. and JAFFE, H. L.: Phosphatase Studies. III. Serum Phosphatase in Diseases of the Bone: Interpretation and Significance, Arch. Int. Med., *54*, 88, 1934.

—————: Phosphatase Studies. V. Serum Phosphatase as a Criterion of the Severity and Rate of Healing of Rickets, Am. J. Dis. Child., *48*, 1268, 1934.

BONGIOVANNI, A. M., ALBUM, M. M., ROOT, A. W., HOPE, J. W., MARINO, J., and SPENCER, D. M.: Studies in Hypophosphatasia and Response to High Phosphate Intake, Am. J. M. Sc., *255*, 163, 1968.

BUSSABARGER, R. A., FREEMAN, S. and IVY, A. C.: The Experimental Production of Severe Homogeneous Osteoporosis by Gastrectomy in Puppies, Am. J. Physiol., *121*, 137, 1938.

BUTLER, A. M., WILSON, J. L. and FARBER, S.: Dehydration and Acidosis with Calcification at Renal Tubules, J. Pediat., *8*, 489, 1936.

CLAY, R. D., DARMADY, E. M. and HAWKINS, M.: The Nature of the Renal Lesion in the Fanconi Syndrome, J. Path. & Bact., *65*, 551, 1953.

COOKE, W. T., BARCLAY, J. A., GOVAN, A. D. T. and NAGLEY, L.: Osteoporosis Associated with Low Serum Phosphorus and Renal Glycosuria, Arch. Int. Med., *80*, 147, 1947.

CURRARINO, G., NEUHAUSER, E. B. D., REYERSBACH, G. C. and SOBEL, E. H.: Hypophosphatasia, Am. J. Roentgenol., *78*, 392, 1957.

DALYELL, E. J. and CHICK, H.: Hunger-osteomalacia in Vienna, 1920. I. Its Relation to Diet, Lancet, *2*, 842, 1921.

DANCASTER, C. P. and JACKSON, W. P. U.: Familial Vitamin D-Resistant Rickets, Arch. Dis. Childhood, *34*, 383, 1959.

DEBRÉ, R., MARIE, J., CLÉRET, F. and MESSIMY, R.: Rachitisme tardif coexistant avec une néphrite chronique et une glycosurie, Arch. méd. enf., *37*, 597, 1934.

DENT, C. E.: Rickets and Osteomalacia from Renal Tubule Defects, J. Bone & Joint Surg., *34-B*, 266, 1952.

DENT, C. E. and HARRIS, H.: Hereditary Forms of Rickets and Osteomalacia, J. Bone & Joint Surg., *38-B*, 204, 1956.

DENT, C. E. and FRIEDMAN, M.: Hypercalcuric Rickets Associated with Renal Tubular Damage, Arch. Dis. Childhood, *39*, 240, 1964.

DENT, C. E., and SMITH, R.: Nutritional Osteomalacia, Quart. J. Med., *38*, 195, 1969.

DI SANT'AGNESE, P. A.: Idiopathic Celiac Disease. II. Course and Prognosis, Pediatrics, *11*, 224, 1953.

DI SANT'AGNESE, P. E. A. and ANDERSEN, D. H.: Celiac Syndrome. IV. Chemotherapy in Infections of the Respiratory Tract Associated with Cystic Fibrosis of the Pancreas, Am. J. Dis. Child., *72*, 17, 1946.

DI SANT'AGNESE, P. A. and JONES, W. O.: The Celiac Syndrome (Malabsorption) in Pediatrics, J.A.M.A., *180*, 308, 1962.

DU BERGER, R. L., MASSON, G. and SYLVESTRE, J.: Milkman's Syndrome—Five Cases of Severe Osteomalacia Following Gastric Surgery, J. Canad. A. Radiologists, *11*, 57, 1960.

EDELMANN, A.: Ueber gehäuftes Auftreten von Osteomalazie und eines osteomalazieähnlichen Symptomenkomplexes, Wien. klin. Wchnschr., *32*, 82, 1919.

ELIOT, M. M. and PARK, E. A.: Rickets. Chapt. 36 in *Practice of Pediatrics*, Vol. 1, edited by J. Brennemann, Hagerstown, Md., W. F. Prior Co., 1937.

ENGFELDT, B. and ZETTERSTRÖM, R.: Osteodysmetamorphosis Fetalis, J. Pediat., *45*, 125, 1954.

————: Biophysical Studies of the Bone Tissue of Dogs with Experimental Rickets, Arch. Path., *59*, 321, 1955.

FANCONI, G.: Der frühinfantile nephrotisch-glykosurische Zwergwuchs mit hypophosphatämischer Rachitis, Jahrb. Kinderh., *147*, 299, 1936.

FANCONI, G. and GIRARDET, P.: Familiärer persistierender Phosphatdiabetes mit D-vitamin-resistenter Rachitis, Helvet. paediat. acta, *7*, 14, 1952.

FOLLIS, R. H., JR., JACKSON, D. A. and PARK, E. A.: The Problem of the Association of Rickets and Scurvy, Am. J. Dis. Child., *60*, 745, 1940.

FOLLIS, R. H., JR., PARK, E. A. and JACKSON, D.: The Relationship of Vitamin D Administration to the Prevalence of Rickets Observed at Autopsy During the First Two Years of Life, Bull. Johns Hopkins Hosp., *92*, 426, 1953.

FRASER, D.: Hypophosphatasia, Am. J. Med., *22*, 731, 1957.

————: Clinical Manifestations of Genetic Aberrations of Calcium and Phosphorus Metabolism, J.A.M.A., *176*, 281, 1961.

FRASER, D., YENDT, E. R. and CHRISTIE, F. H. E.: Metabolic Abnormalities in Hypophosphatasia, Lancet, *1*, 286, 1955.

FRASER, D. and SALTER, R. B.: The Diagnosis and Management of the Various Types of Rickets, Pediat. Clin. North America, May, 417, 1958.

FRENCH, J. M., HAWKINS, C. F. and COOKE, W. T.: Clinical Experience with the Gluten-free Diet in Idiopathic Steatorrhea, Gastroenterology, *38*, 592, 1960.

GENTIL, C., HABIB, R., LeTAN VINH, COLIN, J., GABILAN, J. C., COURTECUISSE, V., ALAGILLE, D., and LELONG, M.: Nanisme avec rachitisme, hypercalciurie et protéinurie, Semaine hôp. Paris, *38*, 784, 1962.

GERSTENBERGER, H. J.: Rachitis hepatica, Monatsschr. Kinderh., *56*, 217, 1933.

GOLDBLATT, H.: Die neuere Richtung der experimentellen Rachitisforschung, Ergebn. allg. Path. u. path. Anat., *25*, 58, 1931.

GORDON, R. S., JR.: Exudative Enteropathy, Lancet, *1*, 325, 1959.

GREAVES, J. D. and SCHMIDT, C. L. A.: Studies on Calcium and Phosphorus in Bile-fistula Dogs, Proc. Soc. Exper. Biol. & Med., *29*, 373, 1931–32.

GREEN, P. A. and WOLLAEGER, E. E.: The Clinical Behavior of Sprue in the United States, Gastroenterology, *38*, 399, 1960.

HANNON, R. R., LIU, S. H., CHU, H. I., WANG, S. H., CHEN, K. C. and CHOU, S. K.: Calcium and Phosphorus Metabolism in Osteomalacia. I. The Effect of Vitamin D and its Apparent Duration, Chinese M. J., *48*, 623, 1934.

HENNEMAN, P. H., DEMPSEY, E. F., CARROLL, E. L. and HENNEMAN, D. H.: Acquired Vitamin D-Resistant Osteomalacia: A New Variety Characterized by Hypercalcemia, Low Serum Bicarbonate and Hyperglycinuria, Metabolism, *11*, 103, 1962.

HESS, A. F.: *Rickets Including Osteomalacia and Tetany*, Philadelphia, Lea & Febiger, 1929.

HEYMANN, W.: Metabolism and Mode of Action of Vitamin D; Importance of Bile in the Absorption and Excretion of Vitamin D, J. Biol. Chem., *122*, 249, 1937.

HJERTQUIST, S.-O.: Biophysical Studies of Epiphyseal Growth Zones and Adjacent Compact Bone Tissue in Normal and Rachitic Dogs and Rats, Acta Soc. med. upsalien., *66*, 202, 1961.

HOWLAND, J. and KRAMER, B.: Calcium and Phosphorus in the Serum in Relation to Rickets, Am. J. Dis. Child., *22*, 105, 1921.

HUNTER, D.: Studies in Calcium and Phosphorus Metabolism in Generalized Diseases of Bones, Proc. Roy. Soc. Med., *28*, 1619, 1935 (see p. 1634).

JACKSON, W. P. U. and LINDER, G. C.: Innate Functional Defects of the Renal Tubules, with Particular Reference to the Fanconi Syndrome, Quart. J. Med., *22*, 133, 1953.

JACKSON, W. P. U., DOWDLE, E. and LINDER, G. C.: Vitamin-D-Resistant Osteomalacia, Brit. M. J., *1*, 1269, 1958.

JACOBSON, S. A.: Bone Lesions in Rats Produced by the Substitution of Beryllium for Calcium in the Diet, Arch. Path., *15*, 18, 1933.

JAFFE, H. L. and BODANSKY, A.: Serum Calcium: Clinical and Biochemical Considerations, J. Mt. Sinai Hosp., *9*, 901, 1943.

————: Diagnostic Significance of Serum Alkaline and Acid Phosphatase Values in Relation to Bone Disease, Bull. New York Acad. Med., *19*, 831, 1943.

JAMES, W. and MOULE, B.: Hypophosphatasia, Clin. Radiol., *17*, 368, 1966.

KORENCHEVSKY, V.: *The Aetiology and Pathology of Rickets from an Experimental Point of View*, Medical Research Council, Special Report Series, No. 71, London, His Majesty's Stationery Office, 1922.

Lehnerdt, F.: Zur Frage der Substitution des Calciums im Knochensystem durch Strontium, Beitr. path. Anat., *47*, 215, 1910.

Lignac, G. O. E.: Über Erkrankungen (u. a. Nephrose und Nephritis) mit und durch Zystinablagerungen in verschiedene Organe, Krankh. Forsch., *2*, 43, 1925–26.

———: Zystinbefunde bei einer bestimmten Kinderkrankheit, Verhandl. deutsch. path. Gesellsch., *21*, 303, 1926.

Liu, S. H., Hannon, R. R., Chu, H. I., Chen, K. C., Chou, S. K. and Wang, S. H.: Calcium and Phosphorus Metabolism in Osteomalacia. II. Further Studies on the Response to Vitamin D of Patients with Osteomalacia, Chinese M. J., *49*, 1, 1935.

Looser, E.: Über pathologische Formen von Infraktionen und Callusbildungen bei Rachitis und Osteomalakie und anderen Knochenerkrankungen, Zentralbl. Chir., *47*, 1470, 1920.

Looser, R.: Ein Fall von Cystinspeicherung mit renalem Zwergwuchs und Rachitis, Ann. paediat., *163*, 251, 1944.

Macy, I. G.: *Nutrition and Chemical Growth in Childhood*, Vol. 1, Springfield, Charles C Thomas, 1942.

Maratka, Z.: Contribution a l'étude clinique et histopathologique des ostéopathies de carence, Arch. mal. app. digest., *35*, 318, 1946.

Maxwell, J. P.: The Modern Conception of Osteomalacia and its Importance to China, Chinese M. J., *49*, 47, 1935.

———: Osteomalacia, Proc. Roy. Soc. Med., *40*, 738, 1947.

Maxwell, J. P., Hu, C. H. and Turnbull, H. M.: Foetal Rickets, J. Path. & Bact., *35*, 419, 1932.

McCance, R. A.: Osteomalacia with Looser's Nodes (Milkman's Syndrome) Due to a Raised Resistance to Vitamin D Acquired about the Age of 15 Years, Quart. J. Med., *16*, 33, 1947.

McCance, R. A., Fairweather, D. V. I., Barrett, A. M. and Morrison, A. B.: Genetic, Clinical, Biochemical, and Pathological Features of Hypophosphatasia, Quart. J. Med., *25*, 523, 1956.

McCormick, J. and Ripa, L. W.: Hypophosphatasia, J. Am. Dent. A., *77*, 618, 1968.

McCrudden, F. H. and Fales, H. L.: Complete Balance Studies of Nitrogen, Sulphur, Phosphorus, Calcium, and Magnesium in Intestinal Infantilism, J. Exper. Med., *15*, 450, 1912.

McCune, D. J., Mason, H. H. and Clarke, H. T.: Intractable Hypophosphatemic Rickets with Renal Glycosuria and Acidosis (the Fanconi Syndrome), Am. J. Dis. Child., *65*, 81, 1943.

Mellanby, E.: *Experimental Rickets*, Medical Research Council, Special Report Series, No. 61, London, His Majesty's Stationery Office, 1921.

Milkman, L. A.: Pseudofractures (Hunger Osteopathy, Late Rickets, Osteomalacia), Am. J. Roentgenol., *24*, 29, 1930.

———: Multiple Spontaneous Idiopathic Symmetrical Fractures, Am. J. Roentgenol., *32*, 622, 1934.

Neuhauser, E. B. D. and Currarino, G.: Hypophosphatasia, Am. J. Roentgenol., *72*, 875, 1954.

Park, E. A.: Observations on the Pathology of Rickets with Particular Reference to the Changes at the Cartilage-shaft Junctions of the Growing Bones, Bull. New York Acad. Med., *15*, 495, 1939.

Parsons, L. G.: Case of Intestinal Infantilism, Birmingham M. Rev., *74*, 33, 1913.

———: The Bone Changes Occurring in Renal and Coeliac Infantilism, and their Relationship to Rickets. I. Renal Rickets, Arch. Dis. Childhood, *2*, 1, 1927.

———: The Bone Changes Occurring in Renal and Coeliac Infantilism, and their Relationship to Rickets. II. Coeliac Rickets, Arch. Dis. Childhood, *2*, 198, 1927.

Partsch, F.: Ueber gehäuftes Auftreten von Osteomalazie, Deutsche med. Wchnschr., *45*, 1130, 1919.

Pimstone, B., Eisenberg, E. and Silverman, S.: Hypophosphatasia: Genetic and Dental Studies, Ann. Int. Med., *65*, 722, 1966.

Pommer, G.: *Untersuchungen über Osteomalacie und Rachitis*, Leipzig, F. C. W. Vogel, 1885.

Pyrah, L. N. and Smith, I. B.: Osteomalacia Following Gastrectomy, Lancet, *1-B*, 935, 1956.

Rally, C. R., Munroe, D. S. and Bogoch, A.: Idiopathic Steatorrhea Presenting with Different Manifestations in Sisters, Canad. M. A. J., *90*, 345, 1964.

Rathbun, J. C.: Hypophosphatasia, Am. J. Dis. Child., *75*, 822, 1948.

von Recklinghausen, F.: *Untersuchungen über Rachitis und Osteomalacie*, Jena, Gustav Fischer, 1910.

Ritchie, G. MacL.: Hypophosphatasia: A Metabolic Disease with Important Dental Manifestations, Arch. Dis. Childhood, *39*, 584, 1964.

Robinson, R. A. and Sheldon, H.: Crystal-Collagen Relationships in Healing Rickets. In *Calcification in Biological Systems*, edited by R. F. Sognnaes, Washington, D. C., American Association for the Advancement of Science, p. 261, 1960.

Rohr, H.: Autoradiographische Untersuchungen über das Knorpel/Knochen-Längenwachstum bei der experimentellen Rattenrachitis, Ztschr. ges. exper. Med., *137*, 248, 1963.

————————: Reifung der Knorpelzellen der Epiphysenfuge bei der experimentellen Ratten-rachitis, Ztschr. ges. exper. Med., *137*, 532, 1963.

RUBIN, C. E., BRANDBORG, L. L., PHELPS, P. C. and TAYLOR, H. C., JR.: Studies of Celiac Disease. I. The Apparent Identical and Specific Nature of the Duodenal and Proximal Jejunal Lesion in Celiac Disease and Idiopathic Sprue, Gastroenterology, *38*, 28, 1960.

RUBIN, C. E., BRANDBORG, L. L., PHELPS, P. C., TAYLOR, H. C., JR., MURRAY, C. V., STEMLER, R., HOWRY, C. and VOLWILER, W.: Studies of Celiac Disease. II. The Apparent Irreversibility of the Proximal Intestinal Pathology in Celiac Disease, Gastroenterology, *38*, 517, 1960.

SCHLESINGER, B., LUDER, J. and BODIAN, M.: Rickets with Alkaline Phosphatase Deficiency: An Osteoblastic Dysplasia, Arch. Dis. Childhood, *30*, 265, 1955.

SCHMORL, G.: Die pathologische Anatomie der rachitischen Knochenerkrankung mit besonderer Berücksichtigung ihrer Histologie und Pathogenese, Ergebn. inn. Med. u. Kinderh., *4*, 403, 1909.

SCHOEN, E. J.: The Question of Normal Height in Patients With Vitamin D-Resistant Rickets, J.A.M.A., *195*, 524, 1966.

SCHOEN, E. J. and REYNOLDS, J. B.: Severe Familial Hypophosphatemic Rickets, Am. J. Dis. Child., *120*, 58, 1970.

SCRIVER, C. R., GOLDBLOOM, R. B. and ROY, C. C.: Hypophosphatemic Rickets with Renal Hyperglycinuria, Renal Glucosuria, and Glycyl-Prolinuria, Pediatrics, *34*, 357, 1964.

SEIDEL, H.: Permanente Gallenfistel und Osteoporose beim Menschen, München. med. Wchnschr., *57*, 2034, 1910.

SEIFERT, E.: Zur Frage der porotischen Malazie nach Gallenfisteln, Bruns' Beitr. klin. Chir., *136*, 496, 1926.

SHINER, M.: Duodenal Biopsy, Lancet, *1*, 17, 1956.

SHINER, M. and DONIACH, I.: Histopathologic Studies in Steatorrhea, Gastroenterology, *38*, 419, 1960.

SHIPLEY, P. G., PARK, E. A., McCOLLUM, E. V., SIMMONDS, N. and KINNEY, E. M.: Studies on Experimental Rickets. XX. The Effects of Strontium Administration on the Histological Structure of the Growing Bones, Bull. Johns Hopkins Hosp., *33*, 216, 1922.

ŠIKL, H.: Osteomalacie bei langdauernder Erkrankung der Gallenwege, Frankfurt. Ztschr. Path., *55*, 120, 1941.

SILVERMAN, J. L.: Apparent Dominant Inheritance of Hypophosphatasia, Arch. Int. Med., *110*, 191, 1962.

SOBEL, E. H., CLARK, L. C., JR., FOX, R. P. and ROBINOW, M.: Rickets, Deficiency of "Alkaline" Phosphatase Activity and Premature Loss of Teeth in Childhood, Pediatrics, *11*, 309, 1953.

STANBURY, S. W.: Some Aspects of Disordered Renal Tubular Function, Advances Int. Med., *9*, 231, 1958.

STEARNS, G.: A Guide to the Adequacy of Therapy in Resistant Rickets due to Familial or Essential Hypophosphatemia, J. Bone & Joint Surg., *46-A*, 959, 1964.

STOREY, E.: Strontium "Rickets": Bone, Calcium and Strontium Changes, Australasian Ann. Med., *10*, 213, 1961.

————————: Intermittent Bone Changes and Multiple Cartilage Defects in Chronic Strontium Rickets in Rats, J. Bone & Joint Surg., *44-B*, 194, 1962.

SWANSON, V. L. and THOMASSEN, R. W.: Pathology of the Jejunal Mucosa in Tropical Sprue, Am. J. Path., *46*, 511, 1965.

TAMMANN, H.: Über die Beeinflussung der porotischen Osteomalazie nach Gallenfistel durch das D-Vitamin, Bruns' Beitr. klin. Chir., *142*, 83, 1928.

TAPIA, J., STEARNS, G. and PONSETI, I. V.: Vitamin-D Resistant Rickets, J. Bone & Joint Surg., *46-A*, 935, 1964.

THAYSEN, T. E. H.: *Non-Tropical Sprue. A Study in Idiopathic Steatorrhoea*, London, Oxford University Press, 1932.

THOENES, F. and GRUSON, W.: Zur Frage der "Rachitis hepatica," Monatsschr. Kinderh., *67*, 134, 1936.

THOMAS, W. C., JR.: Comparative Studies on Bone Matrix and Osteoid by Histochemical Techniques, J. Bone & Joint Surg., *43-A*, 419, 1961.

TOBLER, R., PRADER, A. and TAILLARD, W.: Die familiäre primäre vitamin-D-resistente Rachitis (Phosphatdiabetes), Helvet. paediat. acta, *11*, 209, 1956.

DE TONI, G.: Remarks on the Relations between Renal Rickets (Renal Dwarfism) and Renal Diabetes, Acta paediat., *16*, 479, 1933.

VAN DE KAMER, J. H., WEIJERS, H. A. and DICKE, W. K.: Coeliac Disease. IV. An Investigation into the Injurious Constituents of Wheat in Connection with their Action on Patients with Coeliac Disease, Acta paediat., *42*, 223, 1953.

WEIJERS, H. A. and VAN DE KAMER, J. H.: Celiac Disease and Wheat Sensitivity, Pediatrics, *25*, 127, 1960.

WILSON, D. C.: Osteomalacia (Late Rickets) Studies, Indian J. M. Res., *18*, 951, 963, 969, 975, 1931.

WINTERS, R. W., GRAHAM, J. B., WILLIAMS, T. F., McFALLS, V. W. and BURNETT, C. H.: A Genetic Study of Familial Hypophosphatemia and Vitamin D Resistant Rickets with a Review of the Literature, Medicine, *37*, 97, 1958.

YOSHIKAWA, S., KAWABATA, M., HATSUYAMA, Y., HOSOKAWA, O. and FUJITA, T.: Atypical Vitamin-D Resistant Osteomalacia, J. Bone & Joint Surg., *46-A*, 998, 1964.

Chapter

16

Scurvy and Certain Other Vitamin-Conditioned Disorders

THE preceding chapter was devoted to rickets and osteomalacia—conditions which, when encountered now, are much more often found to be the result of malfunctioning of the kidneys than to be of nutritional origin on the basis of vitamin D deficiency. On the other hand, the underlying factor in scurvy in man continues to be a deficient intake of vitamin C. Since the skeletal manifestations of scurvy are rather specific, the present chapter will be devoted mainly to these. However, some attention will also be given to skeletal alterations resulting from metabolic imbalance conditioned by various other vitamins. These alterations will be only briefly considered, in view of the fact that they do not represent changes which can be regarded as specific for the particular vitamin imbalance in question.

SCURVY

Scurvy results from a protracted deficiency of vitamin C in the diet. Although the disease may appear at any age, the cases are customarily subgrouped and discussed under the headings of *infantile scurvy* (scurvy of infancy and childhood) and *adult scurvy*.

Infantile scurvy was apparently first referred to by Glisson, in 1650, in his monograph "The Rickets." Indeed, he distinguished "the rickets" from "the scurvy" and understood that the two diseases may occur together. However, infantile scurvy as a disease entity was not generally recognized until Barlow very clearly differentiated it clinically and pathologically from rickets and showed its essential unity with adult scurvy. Prior to this, Möller did give a clinical description of infantile scurvy, though he misinterpreted the syndrome as "acute rickets." *Scurvy in adults* was already mentioned in the medical writings of about the middle of the sixteenth century. It became familiar because it was a scourge among sailors on protracted voyages. It is interesting that the earliest writings on scurvy in sailors already mentioned the fact that it could be cured through the use of citrus fruit juices. Long before the discovery of vitamin C and its pathogenetic relation to scurvy, the provision of citrus fruit juices to sailors on long voyages led to a marked decrease in the incidence of scurvy among them (see Vogel).

The current era of our understanding of scurvy began with the work of Hopkins and of Holst and Frölich which directed attention to the concept that scurvy is a deficiency disease. Subsequently, Harden and Zilva demonstrated that it was due specifically to deficiency of a vitamin which they designated as vitamin C. Then came the well-controlled animal experiments of Wolbach and Howe which did so much to relate the anatomic changes produced by vitamin C deficiency in animals to those of human scurvy. With the firm establishment of scurvy as the vitamin C deficiency disease came the isolation of this vitamin in crystalline form by Szent-Györgyi and by Waugh and King, and then its synthetization. Much of the background material dealing with vitamin C deficiency and its relation to scurvy is to be found summarized to about 1920 in the monograph by Hess and to about 1954 in the monograph by van Wersch.

CLINICAL CONSIDERATIONS

In general, scurvy is characterized by a hemorrhagic tendency, manifested in small or large hemorrhages in the skin, in the gums, at muscle attachments, under the periosteum, etc. Particularly in cases involving children up to $1\frac{1}{2}$ years of age, one notes not only subperiosteal hemorrhage but also changes at various sites of endochondral bone formation. The latter changes are most striking at the costochondral junctions of the ribs and at the epiphysial-diaphysial junctions of the long tubular bones—that is, at sites where endochondral bone formation is normally most active. When advanced, the alterations induced by scurvy at these various sites usually include the occurrence of infractions and fractures on the shaft side of the junctions in question. The disease also gives rise to dental changes, but these have been studied mainly in experimental scurvy of growing guinea pigs.

Infantile Scurvy.—The basis of infantile scurvy in a simple vitamin C deficiency is so generally recognized, and the prophylactic use of vitamin C is so widely practiced, that full-fledged cases of infantile scurvy are no longer commonly encountered. In such instances of the disease as are still being observed, inquiry usually reveals that the children in question have been bottle-fed (their milk thus containing very little vitamin C), and that furthermore they have not received an adequate prophylactic amount of vitamin C in the form of ascorbic acid as a medicinal preparation or in the form of orange juice (see Woodruff and also Whelen *et al.*).

As a rule, scurvy develops only after the infant has lacked the vitamin more or less completely for 6 to 10 months. However, the prodromal period may be shorter, especially if the mother's intake of vitamin C during pregnancy was insufficient to permit much storage of it by the fetus. On the average, the age of the infant when scurvy becomes clinically manifest is 8 to 13 months, although, under conditions tending to shorten the prodromal period, the subject may be several months younger (see Burns). In fact, Jackson and Park reported a case of apparently congenital scurvy in a 20 day old infant.

Latent, or subclinical, scurvy may be present for some weeks or months before there is manifest scurvy. The term "latent scurvy" is used to denote a stage of the disease in which the nature of the ailment is not clearly evident clinically. In an infant, this stage of the disease may be, and apparently often is, expressed merely in digestive disturbances and general debility. However, though there are as yet no hemorrhagic manifestations in the skin or gums, there may already be increased capillary fragility testifying to the true nature of the disease. Of course, the finding of a lowered plasma and especially white cell-platelet ascorbic acid value will help to establish the presence of vitamin C deficiency. Furthermore, roentgenographic examination of the bones may already reveal some early changes suggestive of the disease (see p. 458).

The transition from latent to manifest scurvy is ordinarily made in the course of a few days. Now, indications of hemorrhage (of varying intensity and extensiveness) are added to the more general clinical features of the latent period. In an instance of florid infantile scurvy (such as one hardly ever encounters at present), the skin is pallid, but usually presents scattered petechial hemorrhages, a few larger ecchymotic areas, and, not infrequently, a fine macular eruption. In such cases, ecchymosis of the eyelids is rather common, and unilateral ocular proptosis is sometimes observed. The gums are usually swollen and purplish red and, sometimes, even friable and ulcerated. These conditions obtain particularly at the sites of the central incisors, especially if these teeth have already erupted. Petechiae may also be present in the mucous membrane of the palate. In many cases, occult blood can be found in the urine. In the severest expressions of the disease, the hemorrhagic phenomena frequently included frank hematuria and sometimes also hematemesis and melena. In addition (because of the high susceptibility of such scorbutic subjects to intercurrent infections), complications, such as otitis media, pneumonia, diphtheria, bacillary dysentery, etc., used often to develop, becoming the immediate cause of death (see Jaffe).

An infant severely affected with scurvy is inactive and tends to lie on its back, holding its extremities in whatever position will bring least pain because of the presence of subperiosteal hemorrhages and the infractions and fractures. In consequence of the severity of involvement of the femur, tibia, and fibula, it is quite common to find the lower extremities semiflexed at the knees and hips, and the thighs externally rotated. Slight bulging of the lateral aspects of the legs may be observed. In addition, though by no means frequently, the infant may hold its

Figure 113

A, Roentgenograph of the upper portion of the anterior part of the rib cage from a case of moderately severe scurvy. The subject was a female child who was 20 months of age at the time of her death. At autopsy it was found that the bodies of the ribs were somewhat enlarged at the sternal ends. Note in particular that at the costochondral junction the sternal end of each rib shows a narrow, transverse zone of increased radiopacity, beyond which many of the ribs present a transverse, slitlike zone of radiolucency. The zones of radiopacity represent the local accumulation of calcified cartilage matrix. This is the result of suppressed and disordered endochondral bone formation at the junctions. If the process of bone formation at these sites had not been disordered (in consequence of protracted vitamin C deficiency) and had run its normal course, the calcified cartilage matrix producing the zones of radiopacity would have been largely resorbed. The slitlike radiolucencies represent infractions of the local cortex of the rib shafts on either the pleural or pectoral surfaces.

B, Photograph showing the upper part of the body of a severely scorbutic female infant who had died of pneumonia at the age of 9 months. Note the rosary-like effect produced by the prominent enlargement of the costochondral junctions, and also that the costal cartilages (especially the lower ones) are depressed and appear concave. These alterations have their basis in: subperiosteal hemorrhage at the sternal ends of the rib bodies; disruption of continuity at the costochondral junctions (due to infractions and fractures in the region of these junctions); forward displacement of the sternal ends of the rib shafts; and backward displacement of the corresponding costal cartilages.

C, Photomicrograph ($\times$ 12) illustrating the general histologic pattern in the region of the costochondral junction of a rib from another case of advanced scurvy. In that case the scurvy was equivalent in severity to the scurvy which had produced the rosary-like swellings at the costochondral junctions shown in *B*. Note, beginning at the left, that endochondral bone formation is not apparent, and that there is a slitlike space marking the separation between the costal cartilage and the shaft of the rib. On the shaft side of the junctional area, the interior of the rib shows a narrow zone of detritus ("Trümmerfeldzone"). The rib cortex is extremely thin and presents fractures in the vicinity of the costal cartilage. Spongy bone is very sparse in the interior of the rib shaft. On the pleural side of the shaft, there is evidence of rather recent subperiosteal hemorrhage. On the pectoral side, the subperiosteal hemorrhage is being organized, and there is some subperiosteal new bone formation.

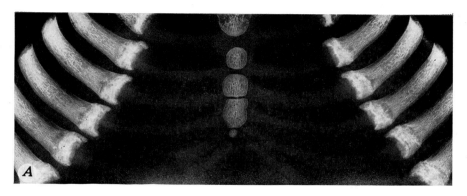

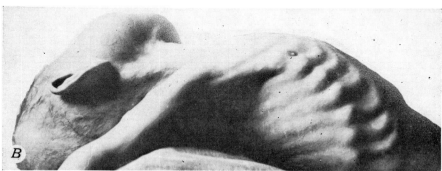

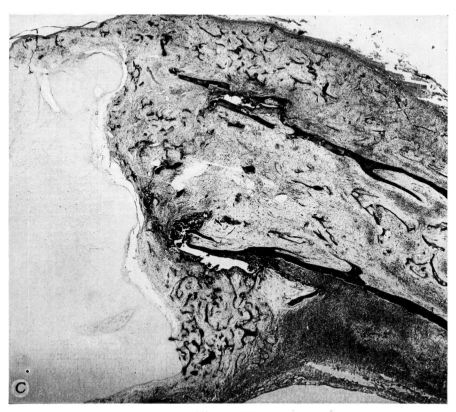

Figure 113

arms at right angles to the chest, with the elbows either extended or flexed. Palpation will reveal brawny induration, especially of the lower limbs. The latter are so painful to the touch that the infant may cry out even when it is merely approached. On the other hand, palpation of the upper extremities is ordinarily much less painful. The costochondral junctions are frequently very tender to touch and are prominent, the eminences being firm and sharply angulated. There may also be moderate enlargement of the cartilage-shaft junctions of long bones, especially at the wrists and ankles. The joints are not swollen or immobile, although, as is already apparent, the infant is very reluctant to move them. (See Fig. 113.)

Adult Scurvy.—Among adults (as among infants and young children), scurvy is now relatively uncommon, since the ordinary diet in most countries now easily meets the minimal vitamin C requirement for adults. The occasional instances of scurvy still encountered in adults in this country are usually ascribable to general undernutrition and/or dietary fads, perversions of appetite, or the presence of some other disease (especially chronic diarrhea). It should be noted also that long-standing infections, debilitating diseases, and postsurgical stress, for instance, increase the body's vitamin C requirement (see Harris et al.).

The gradualness with which scurvy develops in an adult is shown in the vitamin C deficiency experiment of Crandon on himself. In his case, morphologic evidence of scurvy in the form of nonhealing of an incision wound was not observed until he had been on the deficiency diet for 6 months, although the plasma ascorbic acid level had dropped to zero after about 6 weeks and the white cell-platelet (buffy coat) ascorbic acid concentration after about 12 weeks. It is also interesting that gingivitis and bleeding of the gums failed to develop in the course of the experiment, and that their appearance can thus evidently be prevented by careful oral hygiene (see Crandon et al., and also Hodges et al.).

In the instances of adult scurvy now encountered among civilians, the subjects are likely to be elderly people and are much more often males than females (see Vilter et al., and Chazan and Mistilis). Inquiry reveals that their food consumption has been meager, poorly balanced, and notably lacking for many months in fresh fruits and vegetables. The clinical manifestations of the disease as presented by such subjects include nonspecific complaints of weakness and excessive fatigue, poor appetite, and loss of weight. The specific clinical indications of manifest scurvy in adults all relate to hemorrhagic phenomena. The latter include: petechiae in the skin (commonly in the form of perifollicular hemorrhages); ecchymoses due to bleeding into the subcutaneous tissues, especially of the thighs; and hemorrhages into the gums. Furthermore, hyperkeratosis of the hair follicles, associated with the presence of so-called "corkscrew hairs," is commonly observed, as are edema and hypertrophy of the gums—especially of the interdental papillae. (See also Mitra.)

CLINICAL LABORATORY FINDINGS

In regard to *clinical laboratory findings*, it is to be noted that, in infants and young children with manifest scurvy, *anemia* is very likely to be present. The hemoglobin level tends to be below 10 gm. per 100 ml. of blood. The specific type of anemia encountered varies. For instance, it may be a hypochromic anemia of iron deficiency, a megaloblastic anemia, or even a hemolytic anemia due to increased fragility of the erythrocytes (see Vilter et al., and Goldberg). In the absence of an acute bacterial infection, the leukocyte and platelet counts tend to remain within normal limits, but when such an infection is present, the white cell count is naturally elevated. The bleeding and coagulation times also tend to be within normal limits, but in severe cases, one or both of these may be found increased.

The *serum calcium* and *phosphorus* values are not abnormal in scurvy unless the latter is associated with rickets. The *serum alkaline phosphatase* value is depressed in the presence of manifest scurvy. As reflected in balance studies, calcium and phosphorus metabolism seems likewise not to be disordered in scurvy except in advanced stages in which metabolism as a whole is disordered. Humphreys and Zilva demonstrated this experimentally in guinea pigs, but investigations along this line on human subjects have necessarily been unsatisfactory.

As already noted, vitamin C deficiency *per se* is reflected in reduction of the *plasma ascorbic acid* level, but more significantly in the *white cell-platelet* (buffy coat) *ascorbic acid concentration*, which is the last fraction to be depleted before the onset of clinical scurvy (see Ralli and Sherry). Indeed, the ascorbic acid concentration of the buffy coat is a better gauge of the status of the tissues in general in respect to ascorbic acid than is the ascorbic acid value of the blood plasma. As a matter of fact, a nonscorbutic subject who has not ingested any vitamin C for a few days may have a plasma ascorbic acid value below 0.1 mg. per 100 cc. and still have normal stores of vitamin C in the tissues. Persons affected with scurvy nearly always have plasma ascorbic acid concentrations below 0.1 mg. per 100 cc. (that is, concentrations too low to be estimated by current methods) unless they had received vitamin C within a day or so before the determination was made. Furthermore, in cases of scurvy the ascorbic acid concentration of the buffy coat is nearly always less than 4 mg. per 100 gm. (see Crandon *et al.*).

PATHOGENESIS AND PATHOLOGY

Pathogenesis.—The skeletal (including dental) aberrations developing as a result of vitamin C deficiency represent only one aspect of the fundamental specific effect of the deficiency. This is a depressing effect upon the formation and maintenance of intercellular material in the supportive tissues throughout the body. As already suggested by Aschoff and Koch on the basis of human autopsy material, and proved experimentally by Wolbach, this depressing effect is registered in the collagen of the purely fibrous structures, of the skeletal tissues, and of the cement material (especially that binding the endothelium of blood vessels). This concept of the pathogenesis of the disease harmonizes the pathologic findings of infantile scurvy with those of adult scurvy, and also reconciles the changes of human with those of experimental scurvy.

Specifically, the deficient formation of intercellular cementing material (ground substance) in blood vessels favors the occurrence, at any age and in any susceptible subject, of hemorrhage in the gums, in the skin, under the periosteum, etc. The osteogenic activity of the osteoblasts is depressed, and as a result, the deposition of new organic bone matrix (which consists of collagen fibrils and ground substance) is greatly reduced or fails to take place at all. In rapidly growing subjects the lack of formation of new organic bone matrix is most conspicuous at those cartilage-shaft junctions where endochondral bone growth would normally be most active. Indeed, at these junctions the arrest of osteogenesis, the presence of large numbers of modified osteoblasts, and the disorganization of the local cartilaginous and osseous tissue together create a histologic picture characteristic of scurvy. The odontoblasts stop forming new dentin, so that the growth of teeth is arrested. In scorbutic guinea pigs the dental changes are most pronounced in the incisors, since these teeth grow faster than the others. Furthermore, since guinea pig incisors continue to grow

30

throughout life, they can develop scorbutic changes even if the vitamin C deficiency is first imposed when the animals are full-grown. Immediately upon the institution of antiscorbutic treatment, the whole pathologic process begins to be reversed, and within 24 to 48 hours the reactivation of osteoblasts and odontoblasts has led to the formation of much new bone matrix and dentin.

It may well be that the basic aberration caused by protracted vitamin C deficiency leading to scurvy resides in some phase of protein metabolism. As was already pointed out elsewhere (see p. 118), collagen constitutes the major extracellular fibrous protein of all vertebrates and most invertebrates. The collagen of bone is secreted by the osteoblasts as soluble unaggregated macromolecules. These then aggregate to form the insoluble collagen fibrils. Chemically, the collagens of the various species are very similar in composition but may differ in the proportions of their amino acids and in the distribution of protein-bound carbohydrate.

Collagen contains high concentrations of glycine, proline, and hydroxyproline. It also contains lysine and hydroxylysine, but in lower concentrations. Hydroxyproline and hydroxylysine are not found in proteins other than collagen. It is suspected, though not yet established, that the biochemical defect in collagen formation resulting from ascorbic acid deficiency may be related to an inability on the part of the animal to hydroxylate proline to hydroxyproline and lysine to hydroxylysine (see Gould and also p. 120).

Gross Pathology.—A number of detailed discussions of the pathologic anatomy of scurvy are available which are based on autopsy findings during the era when cases of florid scurvy were still common (see Schmorl, Fraenkel, and also Aschoff and Koch). Among the comprehensive studies which date from a later period and which include instances of clinically latent scurvy are the ones by Park *et al.*, and Follis *et al.*

At autopsy the gross findings in a human case of advanced scurvy include pallor of the skin as a whole and the presence of contrasting petechiae and larger areas of hemorrhagic discoloration in the skin. The gums, too, almost regularly present hemorrhages (in the infants, especially at sites of newly erupted teeth), and hemorrhages may likewise be found in the mucosa of the tongue, palate, and cheeks. On incision of the skin, the hemorrhages are usually encountered also in the subcutaneous tissues. The muscles in cases of infantile scurvy are very likely to be found free of hemorrhage. In adult cases, however, the muscles often show patchy discoloration, especially at their attachments, and some muscle bellies may even be saturated with blood. The subperiosteal hemorrhages will be discussed in connection with the skeletal findings.

The mucosae of the digestive and urinary tracts, too, may present areas of hemorrhagic discoloration, as may the parenchyma of the kidneys. Such discoloration is sometimes also noted in the pericardium, pleura, and peritoneum. The cavities lined by these structures may contain blood or serohemorrhagic effusions, especially if these linings have been inflamed. In infantile scurvy the central and peripheral nervous systems ordinarily show no deviations from the norm, but a pachymeningitis hemorrhagica interna has occasionally been observed. In adult cases, hemorrhages in the sheaths of the peripheral nerves are rather common. No changes strictly referable to scurvy are to be found in the heart. The cardiac hypertrophy and dilatation of the left ventricle which have been noted in some cases of infantile scurvy are probably more accurately ascribable to an associated vitamin B_1 deficiency.

The *ribs,* in affected infants and young children, present rather sharp and firm ridgelike enlargements at their cartilage-shaft junctions and subperiosteal hemorrhage for some distance along the shafts. Palpation usually reveals a depression on the cartilage side of each enlarged costochondral junctional area and sometimes also on the bony side. The junctional beading results from subperiosteal hemorrhage and from depression and displacement of the cartilage backward and inward in consequence of infraction or fracture of the rib shaft near the junction. In adolescents and young adults, the ribs are still likely to show junctional changes to some extent in addition to subperiosteal hemorrhage.

In advanced scurvy the *long bones* show hemorrhagic effusion under the periosteum. This is commonly observed and is most pronounced in the infantile cases, and is found especially in relation to the long bones of the lower limbs. In an affected bone the effusion may have elevated the periosteum at one or both ends of the shaft or even over its entire length. The subperiosteal hemorrhage observable in these bones or elsewhere is attributable in part to bleeding and in part to tissue trauma associated with the infractions and fractures. (See Fig. 114.) In infantile cases, no matter how severe the subperiosteal hemorrhage has been, blood is rarely found in any of the articular cavities. In scorbutic adults, however, it is quite likely to be present in some of the joints, and under these circumstances the synovial membranes are usually hemorrhagically infiltrated, as are the joint capsules near their attachments. Furthermore, in adults there may be evidence of bleeding at synchondroses.

The other bones do not usually show much gross modification. However, in some cases there is subperiosteal hemorrhage on the ophthalmic surface of the orbital plate of the frontal bone. Indeed, there may have been so much distention here as to produce an exophthalmos. Little is known about involvement of the other cranial bones. In regard to the jaw bones, subperiosteal hemorrhages have occasionally been observed. In relation to the scapulae and innominate bones, they do not seem to have been noted.

Especially in infantile cases, the epiphysial-diaphysial regions of the long bones and the costochondral junctions of ribs often show some hemorrhagic discoloration of the marrow. The latter, where it is not discolored by hemorrhage, appears as a gelatinous or mucoid tissue. Throughout the junctional regions in question, bone trabeculae are particularly few and thin, and the shaft cortex, too, is abnormally thin. Fissures, infractions, and fractures are usually to be noted just shaftward of the junction. Though the cortex may also be quite thin further along the shaft, fractures and infractions are only rarely found elsewhere than in the area mentioned. Hemorrhage in the major marrow cavities of long bones is rare in scorbutic infants though not uncommon in scorbutic adults. In the ossification centers of the epiphyses and of the carpal and tarsal bones, the gross changes are much less severe than in the junctional areas, and specifically do not include fractures.

Microscopic Pathology.—Here we shall discuss only those changes involving the *bones* and *teeth* of the growing subject. In respect to these structures, the microscopic findings in the human cases are richly supplemented by those obtained in experimental scurvy of guinea pigs. Some of the better known experimental studies of scurvy are those of Holst and Frölich, Höjer, and Wolbach and Howe.

The sequences involved in normal osteogenesis at the epiphysial-diaphysial regions of long bones and at the costochondral junctions of the ribs have been summarized elsewhere (see p. 14) and need not be repeated here. In an advanced case of scurvy, microscopic examination of a costochondral junction, for instance, will show that the cartilage cells at the proliferation zone are not as regularly arranged as they would normally be. Also, extending shaftward for some little distance from the proliferation zone, one finds a sort of latticework of trabeculae of calcified cartilage matrix strikingly free of borders of osseous tissue. Throughout the junctional region and its vicinity, there is likewise a sparsity of newly formed osseous trabeculae. In addition, there is evidence of extensive resorption of whatever cortical and spongy bone was present in the junctional area before the onset of the scurvy. The local marrow is composed of spindle and stellate cells, is poor in blood vessels, and shows traces of fresh and older hemorrhages. This framework marrow ("Gerüstmark") extends in irregular strands for a greater or lesser distance shaftward in accordance with the severity of the scorbutic process. The spindle and stellate cells are mainly dormant osteoblasts, and between them there may be a considerable amount of a peculiar homogeneous material (fibrinogen and collagen) which eosin stains pink. Because of the thinness and general inadequacy of the shaft cortex in the immediate vicinity of the costal cartilage, the cortex is likely to show microscopic infractions and fractures. Even the lattice in the interior of the shaft may be extensively fractured. In fact, the whole area may be so broken up that it appears as a zone of detritus ("Trümmerfeldzone"), and one may find the costal cartilage completely separated from the shaft or even collapsed down upon the shaft like a mushroom.

In the main, this picture is produced in scurvy because, as noted, osteoblastic activity is depressed, and in consequence, wherever osseous tissue would normally be forming, the deposition of collagenous bone matrix by the osteoblasts is reduced or arrested. The striking picture presented in young scorbutic subjects at costochondral junctions and at epiphysial-diaphysial junctions of long bones thus reflects the fact that bone formation fails to occur at sites of endochondral bone growth, because the prerequisite organic matrix is not being laid down there. The microfractures, hemorrhages, detritus, and connective tissue scarring also found at such sites seem to be largely secondary, as Follis pointed out, to the basic structural weakness engendered by the lack of bone formation. Furthermore, although in scurvy the alkaline phosphatase activity values of the serum and bone are reduced, this, too, reflects the depression of osteoblastic activity rather than any inherent disturbance in the physiology of calcification in this disease. (See Figs. 115 and 116.)

In regard to the changes in the teeth of scorbutic infants, few studies have been made. Boyle, who examined the tooth germs of two scorbutic infants, found no abnormalities in the ameloblasts and odontoblasts or their intercellular substances (enamel and dentin, respectively). In one of the infants he found hemorrhages and cyst formations in the enamel organ. In a case of self-imposed scurvy of a human adult, interruptions developed in the lamina dura around the teeth (see Crandon *et al.*).

Figure 114

A, Photograph (somewhat enlarged) showing the distal end of the left tibia, sectioned in the long axis, from a case of very severe scurvy. The subject was a female child who died of an intercurrent infection when she was 16 months of age. Massive subperiosteal hemorrhage was present, as is clearly demonstrated by the blood clot between the periosteum and cortex on the right side of the picture. On the left side, the periosteum is separated from the cortex and only a small amount of blood clot still remains, the rest of it having become detached and lost in the course of preparation of the specimen. In the juxta-epiphysial region, there is a fracture line extending transversely across the shaft of the bone.

B, Roentgenograph (also somewhat enlarged but in reversed position) of the gross specimen shown in *A*. It, too, demonstrates the elevation of the periosteum, the subperiosteal hemorrhage, and the fracture line across the shaft of the bone in the juxta-epiphysial region. The increased radiopacity along the surface of the fracture line reflects the fact that the fracture has occurred through the accumulated trabeculae of calcified cartilage matrix which were extending shaftward from the epiphysial cartilage plate.

C, Photomicrograph ($\times$ 8) demonstrating the general histologic pattern of a tissue section prepared from the lower end of the tibia illustrated in *A* and *B*. The transverse fracture line is clearly evident. (See also Fig. 116.)

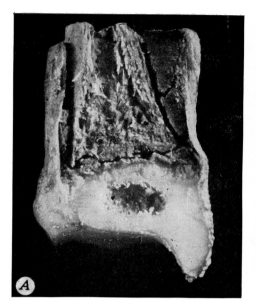

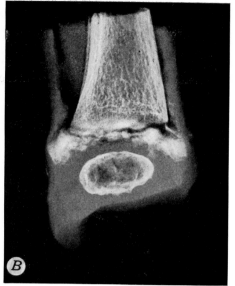

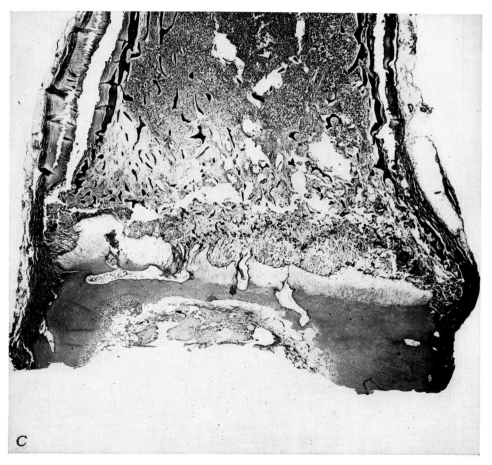

Figure 114

457

All this contrasts with the striking dental changes developing in experimental scurvy of guinea pigs. The dental changes in these animals are most prominent in the incisor teeth. These teeth show arrest of growth, and their pulp, which is hyperemic, becomes separated from the dentin by liquid. The deposition of new dentin has clearly not been going on, and there are evidences that some of the previously existing dentin has been resorbed. When the scurvy is more advanced, hemorrhages can often be noted in the dental pulp, and the latter may also show phleboliths and irregular patches of osteoid ("denticles"). Signs of damage to the teeth are likely to persist in guinea pigs for some time after all residua of the disease have disappeared elsewhere after the administration of adequate amounts of vitamin C.

ROENTGENOGRAPHIC FINDINGS

The roentgenographic skeletal findings presented by *children* affected with scurvy are easy to understand if the pathology of infantile scurvy is borne in mind. The roentgenographic findings relating to advanced cases of infantile scurvy have been described in detail by Wimberger and also by McLean and McIntosh, among others. The correlation of the earliest changes of infantile scurvy detectable roentgenographically with the coexisting pathologic findings has been studied and discussed by Park *et al*. Their study shows that one must still rely upon clinical rather than upon roentgenographic findings for the diagnosis of scurvy when the latter is still in a very early stage. By the time the affected child presents clinical indications of scurvy, roentgenographic skeletal changes are sufficiently clear-cut to aid in the diagnosis (see McCann).

In clinical cases of *infantile* scurvy, it is in the long bones of the lower extremities that the roentgenographic manifestations of scurvy can most readily be followed. At the time of transition of the disease from the latent to the manifest form, the soft tissues about these bones will be found distended, mainly because of subperiosteal hemorrhage. The bones themselves show thinning of the cortices and blurring and disappearance of the trabeculae in the metaphyses ("ground-glass" atrophy)— alterations which reflect the long-standing suppression of osteoblastic activity and resorption of existing bone. There is often also widening and densification of the provisional calcification zone at the epiphysial-diaphysial junctions, constituting evidence of retarded resorption of the spicules of calcified cartilage matrix extending from the cartilage plate. If the disease is more advanced, one may find, instead of the metaphysial "ground-glass" atrophy, a wide area of striking rarefaction (corresponding to the zone of detritus) in the region immediately shaftward of the zone of provisional calcification. It is across this area of rarefaction that the sub-

Figure 115

A, Photomicrograph ($\times$ 10) of a tissue section prepared from the lower end of a fibula in a case of scurvy which was still of only moderate severity at the time of death of the affected child. The cortex of the bone is thin and is defective at its lower end on the left. The cartilage cells of the growth zone are lined up in columns, but endochondral bone formation is depressed though not entirely abolished (see *B*).

B, Photomicrograph ($\times$ 50) showing, under higher magnification, the area blocked out in *A*. The intertrabecular marrow shows numerous small and somewhat flattened cells, many of which represent dormant osteoblasts. Such intertrabecular marrow constitutes the so-called "Gerüstmark," or framework marrow.

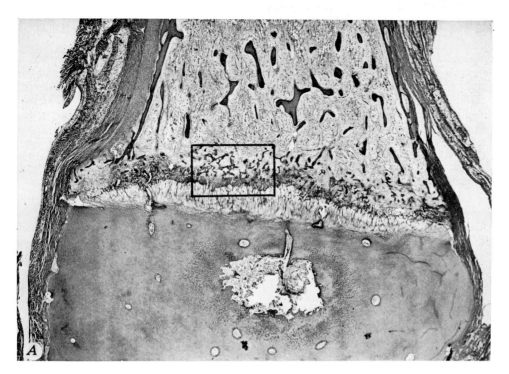

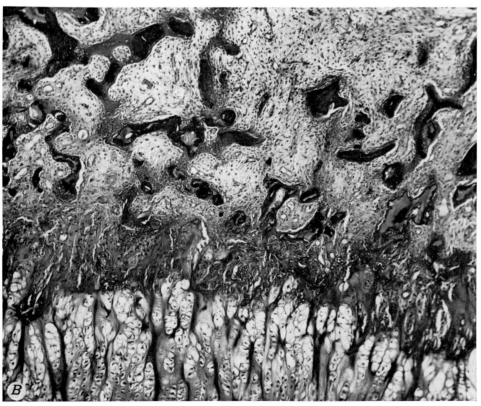

Figure 115

epiphysial infractions (sometimes leading to epiphysial displacements) occur in scurvy. In the presence of infractions there may be collapse or mushrooming of the epiphysis onto the shaft, so that the area of rarefaction has become wholly or partially obliterated. Now one may be able to note calcified spurs projecting laterally in the vicinity of the epiphysial-diaphysial junctions, indicating the formation there of callus or subperiosteal new bone. (See Fig. 117.)

Sooner or later, one can also observe widening and densification of the provisional calcification zone at the periphery of the epiphysial centers of ossification, and these centers, too, come to show striking rarefaction.

The earliest and most conspicuous roentgenographic manifestation of healing is the extensive deposition of new bone under the elevated periosteum and the progressive settling down of the latter as the hemorrhage under it is resorbed. Furthermore, with healing, the outline of the original cortex becomes more prominent and the trabecular markings reappear rather promptly in the metaphyses, though their reappearance in the centers of ossification may be very slow.

In *adults* the roentgenographic findings which may be encountered in cases of scurvy include: osteoporosis due to deficiency in the formation of collagen, the basic constituent of organic bone matrix; subperiosteal new bone formation occurring in the wake of subperiosteal and/or parosteal hemorrhage; and intra-articular effusions resulting from intra-articular hemorrhages (see Joffe). Naturally, the longer the subject has suffered from vitamin C deficiency and the severer the clinical manifestations of the disease in the case in question, the greater is the likelihood that one will find skeletal changes roentgenographically.

In a case of protracted and well-developed scurvy in an adult, a high degree of osteoporosis of the *vertebral column* and compressional collapse of one or several vertebral bodies represent a common finding. Roentgenographically, a severely affected vertebral column in a case of adult scurvy presents essentially the same appearance that a severely affected vertebral column presents in a case of Cushing's syndrome, therapeutically induced hypercortisonism, or the postmenopausal state (see Figs. 91, 92, and 95). It is particularly in relation to the *long bones* of the lower limbs that roentgenographic changes are likely to be present in scorbutic adults. These bones may manifest osteoporosis, as expressed in slight thinning of their cortices. In some cases of severe and protracted scurvy in adults, there may also be a slight amount of subperiosteal new bone deposition on the thinned cortices of these long bones.

Figure 116

A, Photomicrograph ($\times$ 6) of a tissue section prepared from the lower end of a femur in the same case of florid scurvy as that in which the lower end of a tibia was shown in Figure 114. The center of ossification for the epiphysis shows practically no osseous trabeculae. This deficiency is in accord with the fact that the epiphysial centers of ossification in cases of florid scurvy are usually found very porotic on roentgenographic examination. In the juxta-epiphysial area just beyond the epiphysial cartilage plate, a fracture line extends all the way across the width of the bone. In the general region of the fracture, there is evidence of hemorrhage and splintering of columns of cartilage matrix and also of such osseous trabeculae as are present. Altogether, the area through which the fracture line extends represents a so-called zone of detritus ("Trümmerfeldzone"). The area delimited by the arrows is shown in B.

B, Photomicrograph ($\times$ 50) showing in greater detail the area delimited by the arrows in A. It shows the histologic appearance of the zone of detritus where it abuts on the epiphysial cartilage plate. (See also Fig. 117–E.)

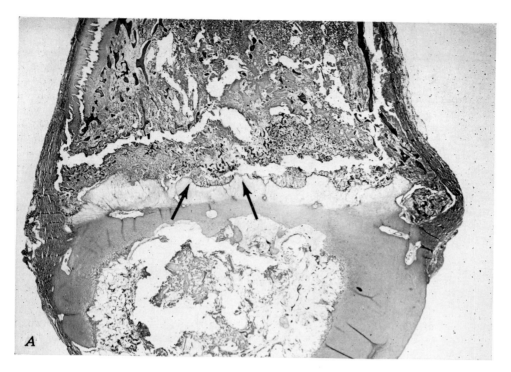

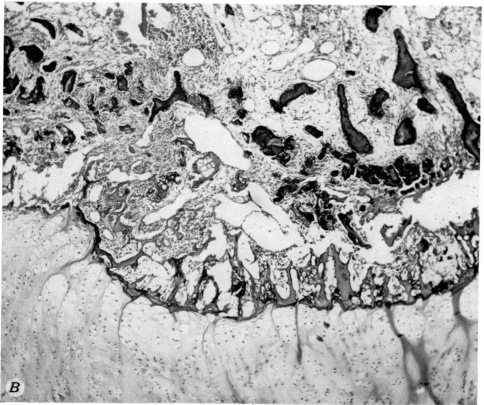

Figure 116

The striking elevation of the periosteum of long bones which is observed in cases of *infantile scurvy* and which is due to subperiosteal hemorrhage is ordinarily not observed in cases of scurvy in adults. As is well known, the periosteum covering the femur, for instance, of an infant or very young child is easily detachable from the cortex, while in an adult the periosteum is firmly adherent to the cortex. It is for this reason that, in cases of infantile scurvy, one may note striking elevation of the periosteum, due to subperiosteal hemorrhage, while in adult scorbutics such elevation is apparently prevented by the closer adherence of the periosteum to the bone. There can be no doubt, however, that, in an adult scorbutic, some subperiosteal hemorrhage does occur, and whatever subperiosteal bone formation takes place in such subjects is attributable at least in part to the hemorrhage. To some extent, also, the subperiosteal bone apposition may be the result of irritation of the periosteum by hemorrhages into the soft tissues neighboring upon the bones.

Intra-articular hemorrhages in cases of scurvy in adults have been noted mainly

Figure 117

A, Roentgenograph of the right knee area in a case of scurvy in a male child who was 14 months of age at the time of his admission to the hospital. The history given by the mother was that the child's lower limbs were extremely tender and that he made no effort to crawl or walk. A number of petechial hemorrhages in the skin were also evident, and the presence of scurvy was suspected. Note the "ground-glass" appearance of the lower end of the femur, due to absence of the normal trabecular markings. In the upper left-hand part of the picture, there is elevation of the periosteum, apparently as a result of subperiosteal hemorrhage.

B, Roentgenograph of the right knee area in a case of scurvy in a male child who was 18 months of age at the time of his admission to the hospital. The mother stated that the child was breast-fed for the first 4 months of life, and that thereafter he was fed cow's milk. However, the child had never received any orange juice or vegetables. Physical examination revealed hemorrhagic bluish gums and marked swelling and tenderness of the right thigh. Note the striking elevation of the periosteum at the lower end of the femur, due to massive subperiosteal hemorrhage. Within a few days after the child was placed on an adequate diet, including a large supplement of tomato and orange juice, there was remarkable improvement in his general physical status, and the various specific manifestations of scurvy began to recede.

C, Roentgenographs (from left to right) of the lower parts of the left fibula and tibia, right tibia and fibula, and the lower part of the left femur. They were removed at autopsy in a case of florid scurvy. The subject was a male child who was 20 months of age at the time of his death. In the juxta-epiphysial regions of all of these bones, there are narrow zones of increased radiopacity reflecting the accumulation there of calcified cartilage matrix. One can also note, in these x-ray pictures, suggestive indications of transverse infraction lines extending across the bone shafts in the juxta-epiphysial areas (see arrows). The resultant severance of continuity between the shafts and the epiphyses was also manifested by the presence of crepitation at these sites in the cadaver even before the bones were removed at autopsy.

D, Roentgenograph of both knee areas from a case of florid scurvy in a young child. In the femur on the left, there is a wide zone of detritus ("Trümmerfeldzone") in the juxta-epiphysial area, and the epiphysis has become separated from the shaft. In the femur on the right, there is as yet no clear-cut separation of the lower femoral epiphysis from the shaft, although there are spurs of new bone formation on the cortex of the femoral shaft in the juxta-epiphysial region.

E, Photograph (inset) of the cut surface of the lower end of a femur from the case of florid scurvy to which reference was made in Figure 116. This photograph is intended to illustrate what the lower end of the femur shown on the left in *D* might have been expected to reveal if it had been removed at autopsy, sectioned in the long axis, and photographed.

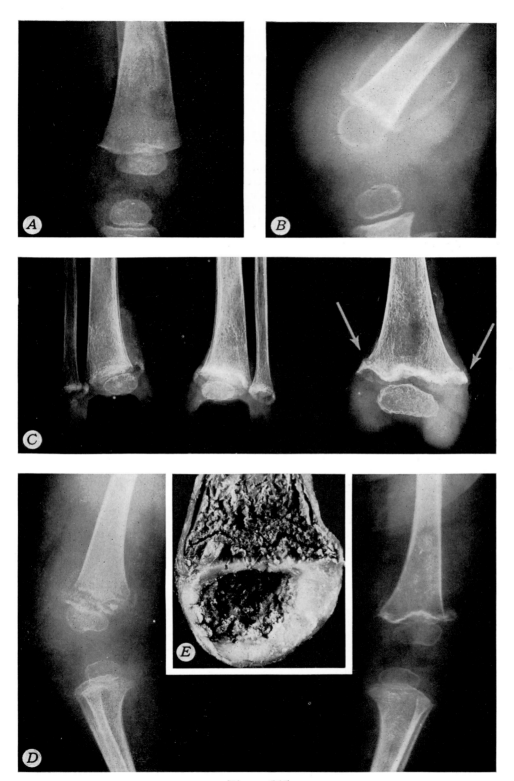

Figure 117

in relation to the lower limbs and, with rare exceptions, only in the knees and ankles. The manifestations of the intra-articular hemorrhages are not specific. That is, they are ordinarily the same as those encountered with intra-articular effusion or hemorrhage occurring on any other basis.

TREATMENT

Improvement in well-being in a case of scurvy usually begins to be noticeable within 48 hours after the institution of treatment with vitamin C. The vitamin may be given in the form of foods (notably citrus fruit juices or tomato juice) or in the form of synthetic ascorbic acid. The latter may be administered orally, intramuscularly, or intravenously. Orange juice contains about 50 mg. of ascorbic acid per 100 gm., and tomato juice about 30 mg. The minimal daily requirement of ascorbic acid as a prophylactic against scurvy is about 25 mg., while about 100 mg. of vitamin C daily will maintain the blood plasma and white cell-platelet ascorbic acid levels at optimal values—about 0.7 mg. per 100 cc. and 25 mg. per 100 gm. respectively. In a case of scurvy, 500 to 600 mg. of vitamin C administered daily should suffice to bring the ascorbic acid content of the plasma and the white cell-platelet fraction of the blood to the optimal, or saturation, values within a few weeks.

Figure 118

A, Roentgenograph of a forearm in the case of a male child 24 months of age who had been receiving about 100,000 units of vitamin A daily during the preceding 7 months. Note the subperiosteal new bone deposition on the ulna illustrated. The other ulna also came to show cortical thickening due to subperiosteal new bone deposition, as did the cortex of the left fifth metatarsal bone. For additional clinical information relating to this case, see Case 6 in Caffey's article, "Chronic Poisoning Due to Excess of Vitamin A," Am. J. Roentgenol., *65*, 12, 1951. (I am indebted to Dr. David H. Baker, Director of Radiology at the Babies Hospital, New York City, for making this illustration available to me from the files of his department.)

B, Roentgenograph showing periosteal new bone deposition on the shaft cortex of the left femur in another case of hypervitaminosis A. The child, a girl 18 months of age, also presented periosteal new bone deposition on the shaft cortex of the right femur, the left tibia, the second metatarsal bone of the left foot, and the fourth metatarsal bone of the right foot. In addition, the epiphysial cartilage plates of the bones in the region of the knees and ankle joints appeared somewhat narrower than they would normally be, reflecting the depressing effect exerted by hypervitaminosis A on the proliferation of cartilage cells.

C, Roentgenograph of part of the left foot in the same case to which reference is made in *B*. Note the thickening of the cortex of the second metatarsal bone, due to subperiosteal new bone deposition. (The child in question was a patient of Dr. Donald R. Reed of Irvington-on-Hudson, New York, and the roentgenographs from which *B* and *C* were reproduced came from the files of the Department of Radiology of the Babies Hospital, New York City. They were kindly placed at my disposal by Dr. Baker, to whom, as well as to Dr. Reed, I wish to express my thanks.)

D, Diagrammatic representation illustrating the distribution of the hyperostoses in the 7 cases of hypervitaminosis A reported by Caffey. The bones represented in black showed hyperostosis. The numbers opposite each bone shown in black indicate the number of times that particular bone was found affected out of the total possible number of these bones on both sides of the body in all 7 patients. For instance, in these 7 patients, hyperostosis was present in 5 of the 14 clavicles, 5 of the 168 ribs, 1 of the 14 radii, all 14 of the 14 ulnae, etc. (I am indebted to Dr. John Caffey and to PEDIATRICS [the journal of the American Academy of Pediatrics] and to its publisher, Charles C Thomas, for permission to reproduce this illustration.)

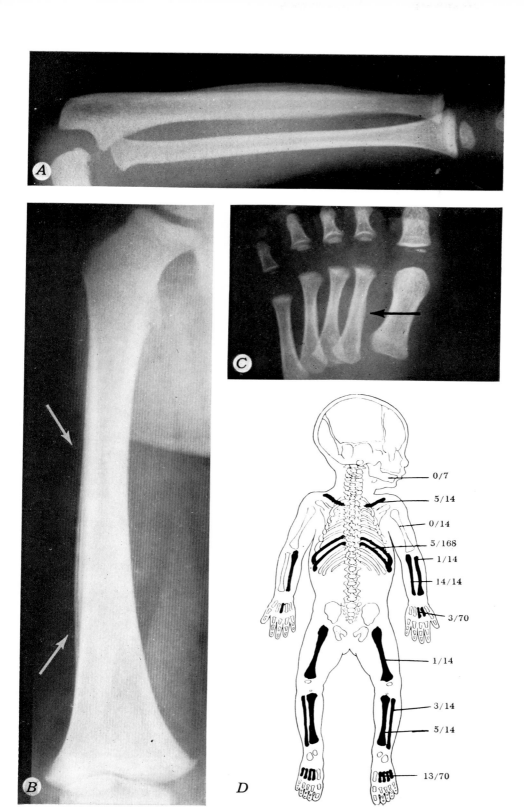

Figure 118

Under treatment, the pain, hemorrhages, and swellings rapidly recede, and the subject is usually clinically well in 3 or 4 weeks. The disappearance of the anemia can be accelerated by the oral administration of iron. A scorbutic infant should be handled as little and as gently as possible while under treatment. Even in very severe cases of infantile scurvy, such as are now hardly ever seen, it can confidently be expected that the skeletal changes will completely disappear. The time required for the restoration of the skeleton to a normal status varies and could conceivably be as long as several years. Great care should be taken to prevent cross infection, which was responsible for most of the deaths in the cases of advanced scurvy reported in the older literature. After the extremities are no longer tender and clinical cure has been achieved, the vitamin C intake can be reduced to the optimal vitamin C requirement and then to the prophylactic antiscorbutic requirement.

HYPOVITAMINOSIS A

Vitamin A and its precursors represent a dietary factor essential for the developing fetus, the growing child, and also for the adult. In the pregnant female, a pronounced deficiency in the supply of vitamin A may result in early death of the fetus and subsequent abortion. If the deficiency is less pronounced and the fetus continues to develop, it may be stillborn, in which case it is nevertheless likely to present abnormalities of skeletal development. When the vitamin A deficiency is relatively mild during the course of pregnancy, the neonate may be free of obvious skeletal abnormalities but is likely to show ophthalmic defects. In the infant and growing child, the most conspicuous manifestations of vitamin A deficiency emerge from the effects of the deficiency upon the epithelial cells and structures. In the adult, too, the most obvious clinical evidences of vitamin A deficiency have their basis in the effects of the deficiency on epithelium. In such adults the principal manifestations of the deficiency, more or less in descending order of frequency, are: night blindness, photophobia, dry and scaly skin, atrophic and dry conjunctivae (xerophthalmia), blepharitis, and follicular hyperkeratosis (see Jeghers, and also Krupp).

Experimental studies of the effects of vitamin A deficiency on animals have emphasized the finding that normal epithelium (wherever epithelium is present) undergoes atrophy and that the original epithelium is replaced by a stratified keratinizing epithelium. The keratinizing metaplasia follows upon focal proliferation of the basal epithelial cells—cells normally involved in maintaining the integrity of the epithelium. The newly proliferated epithelial cells replace the original epithelial cells and develop into a stratified keratinizing epithelium (comparable in all its layers to the epidermis). In cases of protracted vitamin A deficiency in human infants, keratinizing epithelial metaplasia appears first in the trachea and bronchi. It is only late in the course of the deficiency that keratinization develops in the epithelium of the cornea and conjunctival sac, resulting in xerophthalmia. (See Goldblatt and Benischek, Gudjónsson, and also Moore, Wolbach, and Wolbach and Howe.)

Skeletal Findings.—In relation to vitamin A deficiency, we have *not* come to recognize, in clinical medicine, a specific skeletal picture in analogy with the skeletal pictures appearing in connection with deficiency of vitamins C and D. *Experimentally*, however, it has been shown that vitamin A deficiency in very young animals of various species affects the skeleton in such a way that dramatic damage to the nervous system is likely to ensue. As to the precise mechanism by which the neural damage is induced, there are two divergent opinions.

Mellanby attributed the neural damage to direct pressure from locally thickened bone. He ascribed this bone thickening to accelerated and excessive appositional (periosteal and endosteal) bone formation, which he studied particularly in relation to the skull bones and cervical vertebrae of his experimental animals. Wolbach, on the other hand, denies the primary importance of the mechanism just described in the causation of the neural damage. He ascribes it instead to overcrowding of the central nervous system by an underdeveloped bony casing, resulting from retarded endochondral bone growth. More particularly, he and his co-workers found that, in vitamin A deficiency, endochondral bone growth ceases before the rate of growth of the animal as a whole is seriously affected. As a result, the bony framework encasing the still-growing nervous system becomes too small to contain the latter properly, and the foundation for the damage to the nervous system is laid. The overcrowding of the nervous system leads to multiple herniations of the cerebrum and cerebellum into arachnoidal villi, dislocation of the brain as a whole toward the foramen magnum, and buckling and herniation of nerve roots into intervertebral foramina and even into the bodies of vertebrae.

Of course, the retarded endochondral bone growth in susceptible vitamin A-deficient animals was not found limited to the bones encasing the nervous system. Indeed, vitamin A deficiency was found to produce a prompt cessation of cartilage cell proliferation and hence of endochondral bone growth. Also, though endochondral bone growth was retarded, appositional (that is, periosteal and endosteal) bone formation was found to continue along strictly normal lines until inanition supervened in the animal. The long bones were found shorter and thicker than they would normally be. Their shortness was ascribed to failure of endochondral bone growth, and their increased thickness to the fact that appositional bone growth continued but remodeling was retarded.

In this way, the effects of vitamin A deficiency differ from those of deficiencies in certain individual vitamins of the B complex or of the entire B complex. These deficiencies, though they eventually retard skeletal growth, do so evenly, because they act on general nutrition and retard growth in general (see Silberberg et al.). Furthermore, there is a close parallelism between the cytologic changes resulting from retarded skeletal growth due to vitamin B complex deficiency and those resulting from a quantitatively restricted but adequately balanced diet. Also, it has been shown that in young rats, in whom body growth as a whole was retarded by caloric restriction, skeletal growth was retarded in roughly the same proportion (see Handler et al.).

Teeth.—The effects of vitamin A deficiency have been intensively studied in relation to the continuously growing incisor teeth of rats and guinea pigs. In such teeth this deficiency has been found to cause atrophy and metaplasia of the ameloblasts and atrophy of the odontoblasts. Changes similar to those observed in the enamel organ of rats, though milder, have been described by Boyle as occurring in the tooth germs of a human infant with vitamin A deficiency. It has also been found that the incisor teeth of rodents, early in the deficiency, already show inadequacy and irregularity of dentin formation, due to inadequate differentiation of the odontoblasts and their failure to arrange themselves in normal fashion. Along with this change, there is evidence of lack of differentiation of the ameloblasts. This results in a great reduction in the deposition of enamel, and consequently hypoplasia of the enamel is a prominent manifestation of advanced vitamin A deficiency. Nevertheless, the odontogenic epithelium (the enamel organ) continues its proliferative activity, and cords of undifferentiated ameloblasts invade the pulpal tissues, where they form nests of cells. These cells are able to stimulate the neighboring odontoblasts to abortive efforts at dentin formation, leading to the development of numerous concretions. This mechanism is in line with the fact that the cells of the enamel organ are normally organizers of the mesenchymal pulp cells into functional odontoblasts. Indeed, rats subjected to long periods of incomplete intermittent vitamin A deficiency show tumor-like formations and tooth duplications at the formative end of the incisor teeth (see Schour *et al.*, Orten *et al.*, and Burn *et al.*).

HYPERVITAMINOSIS A

It has been shown that congenital malformations, both skeletal and nonskeletal, appear in the offspring of animals (notably rats and mice) if vitamin A in large amounts is given to the pregnant female, especially if the administration is begun early in the course of the pregnancy. The skeletal anomalies which have been noted in such offspring have been found to include: cleft palate, underdevelopment of the mandible, spina bifida, and maldevelopment of the cranium (see Cohlan, Giroud and Martinet, Inaba, and Kalter and Warkany). Experimental studies on weanling rats and guinea pigs, young dogs, and chicks who have been given massive doses of vitamin A over a period of weeks have centered mainly upon the effects of the hypervitaminosis upon the skeletal tissues (see Wolbach, Maddock *et al.*, and Wolbach and Hegsted).

Clinical instances of hypervitaminosis A have been observed in man (both in children and adults). In these cases the skeletal manifestations of vitamin A intoxication have been noted only in older infants and very young children, though these subjects also present various nonskeletal abnormalities. In adults the effects of the intoxication were registered mainly elsewhere than in the bones. In cases involving adults, there is anorexia and weight loss, but it is dermatological aberrations that occupy the forefront of the clinical picture. These include widespread loss of hair, fissures of the lips, and dry and itchy scaling skin (see Sulzberger and Lazar, Hillman, Di Benedetto, and Raaschou-Nielsen).

The nonskeletal abnormalities presented in cases involving infants and young children are reported as including dry, scaly skin, sparsity and coarseness of hair, hepatomegaly, splenomegaly, anemia, and clubbing of the fingers (see Josephs). Hyperirritability, tender and deep swellings of the limbs (especially the forearms), and limitation of motion of the limbs are regularly encountered in children suffering from hypervitaminosis A. Cortical hyperostosis is also a common feature in these cases, and is discussed below.

Skeletal Findings.—In weanling *rats* and *guinea pigs*, hypervitaminosis A has been found to produce striking skeletal changes very rapidly. It causes premature maturation and vascularization of the epiphysial cartilage plates. In the course of a few weeks, these reach the adult stage of exhaustion in the rat, and even disappear completely in the guinea pig. However, the amount of linear growth of the long bones during this time is at most only that corresponding to the age of the animal. Indeed, particularly large overdoses of vitamin A may even retard the longitudinal growth of these bones. Also, in hypervitaminosis A, there is an acceleration of the remodeling of the transverse diameter of the bones. In the rat, for instance, at sites of the most active remodeling (the juxta-epiphysial areas), fractures may appear in a week as the result of the resorption of the pre-existing cortical bone from the periosteal side and its replacement by as yet incompletely ossified new cortex from the endosteal side. (See also Wolke and Nielsen.)

In *infants* and *young children* the ingestion of large amounts of vitamin A (usually much more than 75,000 units daily) over a period of about 6 months or more is almost certain to induce hypervitaminosis A, and quite likely to lead to the development of cortical hyperostosis (see Toomey and Morissette, Dickey and Bradley,

Rothman and Leon, and Caffey). Occasionally, also, the hypervitaminosis A may be found to have had an injurious influence upon various epiphysial cartilage plates in affected children (see Pease). Through questioning of the parent or guardian, it may be brought to light that for many months the child had been ingesting large amounts of halibut or percomorph liver oil, the latter containing about 60,000 units of vitamin A per gram.

The sites at which the cortical hyperostoses become manifest roentgenographically are usually the areas where deep and firm tender swellings have already been noted clinically. In each of the 7 cases of hypervitaminosis A reported by Caffey, roentgenographic evidence of cortical hyperostosis was found to be present in both ulnae and one or more metatarsal bones (exclusive of the first metatarsal). Though both ulnae were involved in all 7 cases, there was only 1 case in which a radius was affected. In regard to the other long tubular bones in this series, it is significant that in only 1 case was a femur involved, and the humerus was not implicated in any instance. Involvement of a metacarpal bone was exceptional. (See Fig. 118.)

Special diagnostic significance attaches to the fact that in no case was there evidence of hyperostosis affecting the mandible. The lack of swelling of the face, particularly of the lower jaw, and the absence of involvement of the mandible are important in themselves in differentiating the cortical hyperostosis of hypervitaminosis A from that of infantile cortical hyperostosis (p. 282). In addition, there are the following differential diagnostic criteria: (1) Infantile cortical hyperostosis usually sets in by the fourth month of life, while the cortical hyperostosis of hypervitaminosis A ordinarily becomes manifest only after the twelfth month of life; (2) the high incidence of hyperostosis of the metatarsal bones contrasts with the rarity of involvement of these bones in Caffey's disease; (3) biochemical analysis of the blood will reveal striking elevation of the vitamin A concentration level in cases of hypervitaminosis A.

The discontinuance of the ingestion of excessive amounts of vitamin A usually brings prompt relief from the irritability, anorexia, and other nonskeletal manifestations of the condition. The cortical hyperostoses may be expected to disappear in the course of time. However, it is still a question whether the skeleton remains free of permanent damage in all children who have suffered from protracted hypervitaminosis A.

In *experimental* hypervitaminosis A, as noted above, the epiphysial cartilage plates undergo various changes which result in their premature maturation, and for this reason the animals in question come to manifest retarded longitudinal growth. In this connection it has been shown, furthermore, that toxic doses of vitamin A bring about considerable disorganization of the epiphysial cartilage plates, both in respect to the preformed matrix of the cartilage and in respect to the ability of the chondrocytes of the plates to synthesize chondroitin sulfate. In consequence, there is a depletion of cartilage matrix, due to accelerated degradation of its chondroitin sulfate and also to depressed synthesis of this protein polysaccharide complex—the essential chemical constituent of cartilage matrix (see Fell and Thomas, and McElligott). There are also experimental findings favoring the idea that the damaging effects of hypervitaminosis A on epiphysial cartilage plates of animals (and incidentally also on articular cartilages) can be largely prevented by the simultaneous administration of cortisone (see Thomas *et al.*).

In some of the *clinical* cases of hypervitaminosis A, retardation of the longitudinal growth of bones, due to damaging effects upon their epiphysial cartilage plates, has also been noted. In the cases of hypervitaminosis A in children reported by Pease, x-ray pictures of the forearms and knees revealed cortical hyperostoses, most frequent in the ulnae. However, the pertinent roentgenographs also showed irregularity and narrowing of the epiphysial cartilage plates (especially in the knee

31

regions) and broadening of the shafts of the lower ends of the femora and upper ends of the tibiae. This broadening of the metaphyses in question is apparently due to disordered local remodeling. In conformity with the experimental findings, the damage to the epiphysial cartilage plates in these children may be irreversible if the hypervitaminosis A has been protracted. In particular, the plates may become disrupted and tend to disappear prematurely. In 3 of the 7 cases followed by Pease, growth of the lower extremities was seriously impaired because of the damage to the cartilage cells at the sites of endochondral bone growth, which, in the lower extremities, is most active at the epiphysial cartilage plates of the lower end of the femur and upper end of the tibia.

HYPERVITAMINOSIS D

Not long after the introduction of irradiated ergosterol as an antirachitic agent, it was established that the administration of excessive amounts of vitamin D (in the form of irradiated ergosterol) could produce pathologic changes both in experimental animals and in human beings (children as well as adults). The amount of vitamin D (irrespective of its derivation) which will have such an effect is not the same for all animal species. For instance, it is known that the toxic dose is much smaller, proportionally, for dogs than for rats. In his sensitiveness to massive doses of vitamin D, man apparently stands much closer to the dog than to the rat. Nevertheless, in man, the spread between the therapeutic and the toxic dose is certainly considerable.

The early *experimental findings* of Pfannenstiel and of Kreitmair and Moll on the effects of excessive doses of vitamin D upon animals were soon confirmed and extended by others. Thus Shohl *et al.* gave huge doses of irradiated ergosterol to very young rats on a normal diet and found that the animals developed anorexia, lost weight and strength, and died within 2 weeks. During life, the rats showed hypercalcemia, and at autopsy many of the soft tissues presented degeneration, necrosis, inflammatory infiltrations, and metastatic calcifications. The latter were particularly conspicuous in the muscularis mucosae of the stomach, the muscle and vessels of the heart, the renal tubules and vessels, the aorta, and the lungs. The arterial calcifications were mainly in the medial coat. In the bones of these animals there was evidence of demineralization.

Soeur (working under the present writer) observed similar changes in guinea pigs and rats given toxic doses of vitamin D. Terminally, the blood of these animals showed hyperphosphatemia, and the bones were so extensively rarefied in some places that they had fractured. It has also been demonstrated that animals in which hypervitaminosis D has been induced show a pronounced increase in the urinary excretion of calcium and phosphorus, unless there is a severe renal insufficiency. Upon analysis of the bones of such animals, the calcium and phosphorus in the ash are found to be decreased.

The degenerative and necrotizing changes noted in the soft tissues by Shohl *et al.* were as severe in the rats fed diets deficient in either calcium or phosphorus as in those receiving normal diets. However, the metastatic calcifications were less severe and were also delayed in their appearance in the animals receiving the deficient diets. Conversely, it has been demonstrated that, in rats given toxic doses of vitamin D, a diet abnormally high in calcium or in phosphorus is more toxic than a diet in which these minerals are present in optimal amounts (see Duguid *et al.*, and Shelling and Asher).

Considerable attention has also been centered upon the hypercalcemia and the metastatic calcifications produced in the experimental animals by toxic doses of vitamin D. The calcium and phosphorus at sites of metastatic calcifications represent, in large measure, minerals mobilized from the bones. The question of whether the metastatic calcifications are limited to sites of previous degenerative tissue damage from the excess of vitamin D has been answered in the negative by Ham. In regard to the hypercalcemia and hyperphosphatemia, it is difficult to account for the fact that the blood can carry these high concentrations of calcium and phosphate. One of the explanations which has been given is that they are present in the blood and tissue fluids as a colloidal calcium phosphate complex. These calcium phosphate complexes do not diffuse easily and therefore tend to become deposited in the various tissues. Also, the places where acids are formed (namely, the lungs, the kidneys, and the mucosa of the fundus of the stomach) are tissue sites which are rendered alkaline when these acids are elaborated—a fact which particularly favors the deposition of calcium phosphate in these tissues.

In regard to *man*, the first reports of vitamin D intoxication related mainly to infants and young children who had been given inordinately large doses of the vitamin for the treatment of rickets and other skeletal disorders (see Putschar, and also Thatcher). Not long thereafter, instances of vitamin D intoxication in adults began to be recorded. In the latter cases the condition developed mainly as a result of the administration of large doses of vitamin D preparations for the treatment of rheumatoid arthritis (see Danowski *et al.*) and also other conditions, such as Paget's disease (see Wells and Holley). In some subjects the intoxication was caused by self-overdosing with vitamin D and mineral salts (see Bauer and Freyberg, and also Mulligan). These reports made it very clear that the indiscriminate and protracted consumption of large doses of vitamin D by adults not only lacked therapeutic value in most cases but involved dangers when not controlled. Even in rickets and osteomalacia due to renal tubular malfunction, in which the protracted use of large doses of vitamin D is indicated (see p. 412), periodic determinations of serum calcium for evidence of hypercalcemia and frequent examination of the urine for albumin are mandatory, so that any ominous findings along these lines may be noted and the vitamin D therapy either reduced or temporarily discontinued.

CLINICAL CONSIDERATIONS

There is a wide variation in individual susceptibility to vitamin D intoxication. Occasionally a patient displays indications of it on as little as 50,000 units of vitamin D per day, taken for only a few weeks. On the other hand, some patients have tolerated even as much as 500,000 units of vitamin D for many months before manifesting toxic effects. However, in the presence of renal insufficiency, doses only a few times the therapeutic dose may already prove toxic. Also, it has been observed that gastrointestinal dysfunction (especially constipation and diarrhea) increases the susceptibility to toxic effects. In addition, it is clear from the experimental studies that a high mineral intake (notably of calcium) increases the susceptibility.

In both children and adults, intoxication from hypervitaminosis D produces a variety of acute symptoms and signs (see Paul, Chaplin *et al.*, and Swoboda). The general manifestations include nausea, vomiting, diarrhea, abdominal cramps, and polyuria and polydipsia. These lead to loss of weight, weakness, and general impairment of health. Additional indications of the intoxication are the presence of albumin and/or red blood cells and casts in the urine, and progressive impairment of ability to concentrate the urine. The serum calcium value is elevated—sometimes strikingly. The occurrence of so-called "band keratitis" has been noted in several accounts and has been ascribed to the hypercalcemia. The latter is undoubtedly also the basis for many of the general manifestations of hypervitaminosis which have been noted above. (Entirely analogous clinical evidences of hypercalcemia may be observed in cases of hyperparathyroidism.)

If renal insufficiency develops as a result of nephrocalcinosis, the serum inorganic phosphorus value and the serum nonprotein nitrogen value will be found increased. Other baleful effects of protracted hypervitaminosis D and the concomitant renal insufficiency are the deposition of calcium in the arteries and arterioles, and sometimes also the appearance of massive deposits of calcium in various para-articular sites. The soft-tissue calcifications are particularly likely to occur in cases in which the hypervitaminosis D has been associated with a high daily intake of calcium. The bones, too, come to show changes, in accordance with the severity and chronicity of the hypervitaminosis D. These changes become apparent roentgenographically, but are not likely to give rise to clinical complaints unless the alterations are very pronounced. Finally, it is to be noted that hypervitaminosis D, particularly when associated with renal damage and pronounced hypercalcemia, has been known to result in the patient's death.

ROENTGENOGRAPHIC AND PATHOLOGIC FINDINGS

On *roentgenographic examination* the bones of *young children* who have received large doses of vitamin D reveal the presence of narrow bandlike zones of radiopacity at sites of endochondral bone growth. The zones of radiopacity stand out particularly well at the epiphysial ends of the shafts of the long tubular bones. This finding is in accord with the fact that endochondral bone growth is normally very active at these sites. The radiopacities in question reflect the heavy calcification of the matrix of the proliferating cartilage at these sites of bone formation and growth. Further along the bone shafts, the metaphyses may appear more or less radiolucent because of the presence of focal osteoporosis. It has also been observed that the original cortex of the shafts of various bones may become rarefied, while at the same time the cortex as a whole undergoes thickening as a result of periosteal new bone apposition on the pre-existing cortex (see Swoboda). That protracted overdosage with vitamin D in children may be the basis for metastatic calcification involving blood vessels, various organs (particularly the kidneys), and para-articular

Figure 119

A, B, C, and D, Roentgenographs showing striking soft-tissue and para-articular calcifications as manifestations of vitamin D intoxication. The patient was a woman 79 years of age who was affected with rheumatoid arthritis. She had ingested large amounts of vitamin D for several years. The actual daily intake of the vitamin D could not be ascertained. She entered the hospital primarily because she had fallen and sustained a fracture of the upper part of the shaft of the left femur (not shown in this figure). For some days before she was admitted, she had suffered from nausea and vomiting—manifestations of the vitamin D intoxication. Biochemical examination of the blood revealed that the serum calcium value was 14 mg. per cent and the nonprotein nitrogen value 63 mg. per cent. Note the tremendous distention of the acromial and deltoid bursae, which cast radiopaque shadows because they are filled with calcareous material. Note also the roentgenographic evidence of rheumatoid arthritis in the hand, and the porosity of the various other bones shown in this figure. The patient died of uremia 10 days after admission to the hospital, but no autopsy was performed.

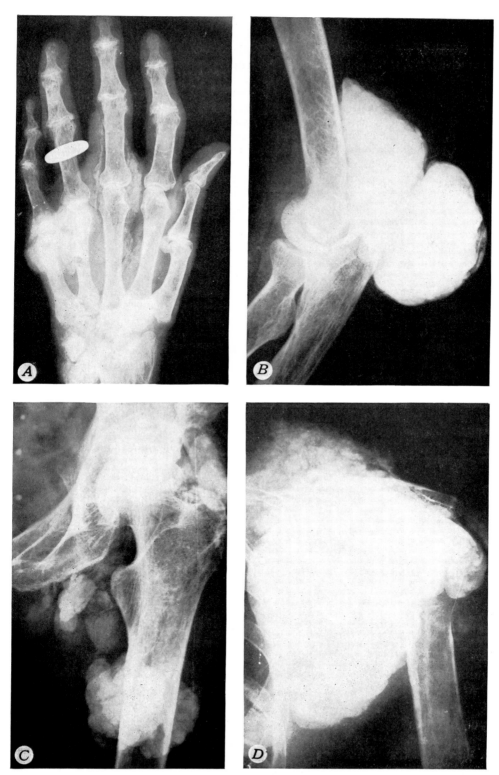

Figure 119

soft tissues is well known. In affected children, metastatic calcifications have also been observed in such intracranial structures as the falx cerebri and the tentorium cerebelli.

The bones of *adults* who have ingested massive doses of vitamin D over long periods of time frequently show roentgenographic evidence of osteoporosis, which may be of limited extent or generalized over the skeleton (see Christensen *et al.*, and Holman). The extent and severity of the osteoporosis are naturally related to the degree and duration of the hypervitaminosis. However, in a particular case the osteoporosis may be attributable in part to some other condition (such as the post-menopausal state) or to the disease (most often rheumatoid arthritis) for which the massive doses of vitamin D had been administered for therapeutic purposes.

The literature includes records on adults who presented roentgenographic evidence of osteoporosis and whose death was related to vitamin D intoxication. A number of these adults came to autopsy, but no detailed studies seem to have been made of the actual pathologic status (gross and/or microscopic) of the porotic bones. Attention in these cases had been centered mainly upon the metastatic calcifications and in particular on the findings in regard to the nephrocalcinosis. In any event, it has been established on the basis of experiments on animals that vitamin D in toxic doses mobilizes the mineral from the bones and causes widespread osteoclastic bone resorption. In fact, the demineralization and porosity of the bones induced by toxic doses of vitamin D in animals resemble the skeletal changes found in connection with experimental hyperparathyroidism (see Jaffe). Indeed, in a clinical case of hypervitaminosis D involving a woman affected with rheumatoid arthritis who had been taking massive doses of vitamin D for years, the skeletal changes observed roentgenographically by the writer were so pronounced that they even resembled those which have been encountered in some clinical cases of hyperparathyroidism. In that case, roentgenographs of the skull also revealed the so-called "granular mottling" of the calvarium, which is a striking feature in cases of hyperparathyroidism of long standing. The woman in question also developed massive para-articular calcifications. (See Fig. 119.)

When massive *para-articular calcifications* are encountered in cases of hypervitaminosis D, the subjects nearly always present, in addition, some evidences of renal insufficiency. The calcifications in question vary widely in size. Roentgenographically they appear as lobulated masses, not necessarily uniform in radiopacity. They are formed through the deposition of calcific material in bursae neighboring upon joints or overlying bony prominences, in tendon sheaths, and sometimes even within articular capsules. If the subject affected with hypervitaminosis D has rheumatoid arthritis or gout, heavy calcific incrustations may also appear in various rheumatoid nodules or gouty tophi, respectively. An affected bursa, for instance, will be found filled with thick, white, granular, calcareous material. On microscopic examination the wall of the bursa will show granules of calcium, particularly near its inner surface. There will also be evidence of an inflammatory reaction, associated with the presence of foreign-body giant cells in response to the incrustation of the bursal walls with the calcareous material.

TREATMENT

The treatment of cases of vitamin D intoxication is necessarily directed toward the restoration of the serum calcium value to the normal level and the counteraction of the dehydration and serum electrolyte imbalance. These aims can be achieved by: stopping the intake of vitamin D; placing the patient on a diet which is very low in calcium; forcing fluids to an extent which will raise the output of urine to about

2,000 cc. per day; and also combatting the electrolyte imbalance by the administration of supplements of potassium.

As a means of quickly reducing the hypercalcemia, cortisone has proved to be of value. In doses of 150 to 200 mg. per day, cortisone can be expected to restore the serum calcium value to the normal level within about 2 weeks, whereas without the use of cortisone, 2 or 3 months may be required to abolish the hypercalcemia (see Connor *et al.*, and Verner *et al.*). If the nephrocalcinosis and the resultant renal damage are still relatively mild, the treatment outlined above can also be expected to check or even reverse any manifestations of renal insufficiency. In the absence of irreversible renal damage, the various para-articular soft-tissue calcifications are also likely to recede, at least in part. Finally, it is to be noted that the effectiveness of cortisone against the hypercalcemia of hypervitaminosis D makes it useful as a criterion for differential diagnosis between the hypercalcemia of hypervitaminosis D and that of hyperparathyroidism. In the latter condition, the hypercalcemia is not reduced by cortisone (see Adams, Dent, and Anderson *et al.*).

REFERENCES

ADAMS, F. D.: Reversible Uremia with Hypercalcemia Due to Vitamin-D Intoxication, New England J. Med., *244*, 590, 1951.

ANDERSON, J., HARPER, C., DENT, C. E., and PHILPOT, G. R.: Effect of Cortisone on Calcium Metabolism in Sarcoidosis with Hypercalcaemia, Lancet, *2*, 720, 1954.

ASCHOFF, L., and KOCH, W.: *Skorbut: Eine pathologisch-anatomische Studie*, Jena, G. Fischer, 1919.

BARLOW, T.: On Cases Described as "Acute Rickets" which Are Probably a Combination of Scurvy and Rickets, the Scurvy Being an Essential, and the Rickets a Variable, Element, Med.-Chir. Tr., *66*, 159, 1883.

BAUER, J. M., and FREYBERG, R. H.: Vitamin D Intoxication with Metastatic Calcification, J.A.M.A., *130*, 1208, 1946.

BOYLE, P. E.: Manifestations of Vitamin-A Deficiency in a Human Tooth-germ, J. Dent. Res., *13*, 39, 1933.

————: The Tooth Germ in Acute Scurvy, J. Dent. Res., *14*, 172, 1934.

BURN, C. G., ORTEN, A. U., and SMITH, A. H.: Changes in the Structure of the Developing Tooth in Rats Maintained on a Diet Deficient in Vitamin A, Yale J. Biol. & Med., *13*, 817, 1941.

BURNS, R. R.: The Unusual Occurrence of Scurvy in an Eight Week Old Infant, Am. J. Roentgenol., *89*, 923, 1963.

CAFFEY, J.: Chronic Poisoning Due to Excess of Vitamin A, Pediatrics, *5*, 672, 1950.

————: Chronic Poisoning Due to Excess of Vitamin A, Am. J. Roentgenol., *65*, 12, 1951.

CHAPLIN, H., JR., CLARK, L. D., and ROPES, M. W.: Vitamin D Intoxication, Am. J. M. Sc., *221*, 369, 1951.

CHAZAN, J. A., and MISTILIS, S. P.: The Pathophysiology of Scurvy, Am. J. Med., *34*, 350, 1963.

CHRISTENSEN, W. R., LIEBMAN, C., and SOSMAN, M. C.: Skeletal and Periarticular Manifestations of Hypervitaminosis D, Am. J. Roentgenol., *65*, 27, 1951.

COHLAN, S. Q.: Congenital Anomalies in the Rat Produced by Excessive Intake of Vitamin A During Pregnancy, Pediatrics, *13*, 556, 1954.

CONNOR, T. B., HOPKINS, T. R., THOMAS, W. C., JR., CAREY, R. A., and HOWARD, J. E.: The Use of Cortisone and ACTH in Hypercalcemic States, J. Clin. Endocrinol., *16*, 945, 1956.

CRANDON, J. H., LUND, C. C., and DILL, D. B.: Experimental Human Scurvy, New England J. Med., *223*, 353, 1940.

CRANDON, J. H., LANDAU, B., MIKAL, S., BALMANNO, J., JEFFERSON, M., and MAHONEY, N.: Ascorbic Acid Economy in Surgical Patients as Indicated by Blood Ascorbic Acid Levels, New England J. Med., *258*, 105, 1958.

DANOWSKI, T. S., WINKLER, A. W., and PETERS, J. P.: Tissue Calcification and Renal Failure Produced by Massive Dose Vitamin D Therapy of Arthritis, Ann. Int. Med., *23*, 22, 1945.

DENT, C. E.: Cortisone Test for Hyperparathyroidism, Brit. M. J., *1*, 230, 1956.

DI BENEDETTO, R. J.: Chronic Hypervitaminosis A in an Adult, J.A.M.A., *201*, 700, 1967.

DICKEY, L. B., and BRADLEY, E. J.: Hypervitaminosis A, Stanford M. Bull., *6*, 345, 1948.

DUGUID, J. B., DUGGAN, M. M., and GOUGH, J.: The Toxicity of Irradiated Ergosterol, J. Path. & Bact., *33*, 353, 1930.

————: The Toxicity of Irradiated Ergosterol. II. J. Path. & Bact., *35*, 209, 1932.

FELL, H. B., and THOMAS, L.: Comparison of the Effects of Papain and Vitamin A on Cartilage, J. Exper. Med., *111*, 719, 1960.

FOLLIS, R. H., JR: Effect of Mechanical Force on the Skeletal Lesions in Acute Scurvy in Guinea Pigs, Arch. Path., *35*, 579, 1943.

FOLLIS, R. H., JR., PARK, E. A., and JACKSON, D.: The Prevalence of Scurvy at Autopsy during the First Two Years of Age, Bull. Johns Hopkins Hosp., *87*, 569, 1950.

FRAENKEL, E.: Die Möller-Barlowsche Krankheit, Fortschr. Geb. Röntgenstrahlen, *12*, 207, 1908.

GIROUD, A., and MARTINET, M.: Malformations embryonnaires par hypervitaminose A, Arch. franç. pédiat., *12*, 292, 1955.

GOLDBERG, A.: The Anaemia of Scurvy, Quart. J. Med., n.s.*32*, 51, 1963.

GOLDBLATT, H., and BENISCHEK, M.: Vitamin A Deficiency and Metaplasia, J. Exper. Med., *46*, 699, 1927.

GOULD, B. S.: Ascorbic Acid and Collagen Fiber Formation, Vitamins & Hormones, *18*, 89, 1960.

GUDJÓNSSON, S. V.: *Experiments on Vitamin A Deficiency in Rats and the Quantitative Determination of Vitamin A*, Copenhagen, Levin & Munksgaard, 1930.

HAM, A. W.: Mechanism of Calcification in the Heart and Aorta in Hypervitaminosis D, Arch. Path., *14*, 613, 1932.

HANDLER, P., BAYLIN, G. J., and FOLLIS, R. H., JR.: The Effects of Caloric Restriction on Skeletal Growth, J. Nutrition, *34*, 677, 1947.

HARDEN, A., and ZILVA, S. S.: Experimental Scurvy in Monkeys, J. Path. & Bact., *22*, 246, 1919.

————: The Antiscorbutic Requirements of the Monkey, Biochem J., *14*, 131, 1920.

HARRIS, L. J., PASSMORE, R., and PAGEL, W.: Vitamin C and Infection: Influence of Infection on the Vitamin-C Content of the Tissues of Animals, Lancet, *2*, 183, 1937.

HESS, A. F.: *Scurvy: Past and Present*, Philadelphia, J. B. Lippincott Company, 1920.

HILLMAN, R. W.: Hypervitaminosis A. Experimental Induction in the Human Subject, Am. J. Clin. Nutrition, *4*, 603, 1956.

HODGES, R. E., BAKER, E. M., HOOD, J., SAUBERLICH, H. E., and MARCH, S. C.: Experimental Scurvy in Man, Am. J. Clin. Nutrition, *22*, 535, 1969.

HÖJER, J. A.: Studies in Scurvy, Acta paediat., suppl. *3*, 1, 1924.

HOLMAN, C. B.: Roentgenologic Manifestations of Vitamin D Intoxication, Radiology, *59*, 805, 1952.

HOLST, A.: Experimental Studies Relating to "Ship-beri-beri" and Scurvy. I. Introduction, J. Hyg., *7*, 619, 1907.

HOLST, A., and FRÖLICH, T.: Experimental Studies Relating to "Ship-beri-beri" and Scurvy. II. On the Etiology of Scurvy, J. Hyg., *7*, 634, 1907.

————: Über experimentellen Skorbut, Ztschr. Hyg., *72*, 1, 1912.

HOPKINS, F. G.: Feeding Experiments Illustrating the Importance of Accessory Factors in Normal Dietaries, J. Physiol., *44*, 425, 1912.

HUMPHREYS, F. E., and ZILVA, S. S.: Metabolism in Scurvy. III. The Absorption and Retention of Calcium and Phosphorus by Guinea-Pigs, Biochem. J., *25*, 579, 1931.

INABA, T.: Experimentally Reproduced Congenital Malformations of Rats by Excessive Vitamin A Diet, J. Osaka City Med. Center, *7(7)*, 60, 1958.

JACKSON, D., and PARK, E. A.: Congenital Scurvy, J. Pediat., *7*, 741, 1935.

JAFFE, H. L.: The Influence of Purulent Infection on the Development of Experimental Scurvy, J. Infect. Dis., *40*, 502, 1927.

————: Hyperparathyroidism (Recklinghausen's Disease of Bone), Arch. Path., *16*, 63 and 236, 1933.

JEGHERS, H.: The Degree and Prevalence of Vitamin A Deficiency in Adults with a Note on Its Experimental Production in Human Beings, J.A.M.A., *109*, 756, 1937.

JOFFE, N.: Some Radiological Aspects of Scurvy in the Adult, Brit. J. Radiol., *34*, 429, 1961.

JOSEPHS, H. W.: Hypervitaminosis A and Carotenemia, Am. J. Dis. Child., *67*, 33, 1944.

KALTER, H., and WARKANY, J.: Experimental Production of Congenital Malformations in Strains of Inbred Mice by Maternal Treatment with Hypervitaminosis A, Am. J. Path., *38*, 1, 1961.

KREITMAIR, H., and MOLL, T.: Hypervitaminose durch grosse Dosen Vitamin D, München. med. Wchnschr., *75*, 637, 1928.

————: Hypervitaminose nach grossen Dosen Vitamin D, München. med. Wchnschr., *75*, 1113, 1928.

KRUPP, M. A.: The Incidence of Nutritional and Vitamin Deficiency, J.A.M.A., *119*, 1475, 1942.

MADDOCK, C. L., WOLBACH, S. B., and MADDOCK, S.: Hypervitaminosis A in the Dog, J. Nutrition, *39*, 117, 1949.

McCANN, P.: The Incidence and Value of Radiological Signs in Scurvy, Brit. J. Radiol., *35*, 683, 1962.

McElligott, T. F.: Decreased Fixation of Sulphate by Chondrocytes in Hypervitaminosis A, J. Path. & Bact., 83, 347, 1962.

McLean, S., and McIntosh, R.: Healing in Infantile Scurvy as Shown by X-Ray, Am. J. Dis. Child., 36, 875, 1928.

Mellanby, E.: Skeletal Changes Affecting the Nervous System Produced in Young Dogs by Diets Deficient in Vitamin A, J. Physiol., 99, 467, 1941.

————: Nutrition in Relation to Bone Growth and the Nervous System, Proc. Roy. Soc. London, s.B.132, 28, 1944.

————: Vitamin A and Bone Growth: The Reversibility of Vitamin A-Deficiency Changes, J. Physiol., 105, 382, 1947.

Mitra, M. L.: Vitamin-C Deficiency in the Elderly and Its Manifestations, J. Am. Geriatrics Soc., 18, 67, 1970.

Möller: Zwei Fälle von akuter Rachitis, Königsberg. med. Jahrb., 3, 135, 1862.

Moore, T.: The Pathology of Vitamin A Deficiency, Vitamins & Hormones, 18, 499, 1960.

Mulligan, R. M.: Metastatic Calcification Associated with Hypervitaminosis D and Haliphagia, Am. J. Path., 22, 1293, 1946.

Orten, A. U., Burn, C. G., and Smith, A. H.: Effects of Prolonged Chronic Vitamin A Deficiency in the Rat with Special Reference to Odontomas, Proc. Soc. Exper. Biol. & Med., 36, 82, 1937.

Park, E. A., Guild, H. G., Jackson, D., and Bond, M.: The Recognition of Scurvy with Especial Reference to the Early X-Ray Changes, Arch. Dis. Childhood, 10, 265, 1935.

Paul, W. D.: Toxic Manifestations of Large Doses of Vitamin D as Used in the Treatment of Arthritis, J. Iowa M. Soc., 36, 141, 1946.

Pease, C. N.: Focal Retardation and Arrestment of Growth of Bones Due to Vitamin A Intoxication, J.A.M.A., 182, 980, 1962.

Pfannenstiel, W.: A Summary of Recent Work on Vigantol (Irradiated Ergosterol), Lancet, 2, 845, 1928.

Putschar, W.: Über Vigantolschädigung der Niere bei einem Kinde, Ztschr. Kinderh., 48, 269, 1929.

Raaschou-Nielsen, W.: Chronic Intoxication with Vitamin A in Adults, Dermatologica, 123, 293, 1961.

Ralli, E. P., and Sherry, S.: Adult Scurvy and the Metabolism of Vitamin C, Medicine, 20, 251, 1941.

Rothman, P. E., and Leon, E. E.: Hypervitaminosis A, Radiology, 51, 368, 1948.

Schmorl, G.: Zur pathologischen Anatomie der Barlow'schen Krankheit, Beitr. path. Anat., 30, 215, 1901.

Schour, I., Hoffman, M. M., and Smith, M. C.: Changes in the Incisor Teeth of Albino Rats with Vitamin A Deficiency and the Effects of Replacement Therapy, Am. J. Path., 17, 529, 1941.

Shelling, D. H., and Asher, D. E.: Calcium and Phosphorus Studies: IV. The Relation of Calcium and Phosphorus of the Diet to the Toxicity of Viosterol, Bull. Johns Hopkins Hosp., 50, 318, 1932.

Shohl, A. T., Goldblatt, H., and Brown, H. B.: The Pathological Effects upon Rats of Excess Irradiated Ergosterol, J. Clin. Invest., 8, 505, 1930.

Silberberg, M., Levy, B. M., and Younger, F.: Skeletal Changes in Growing Vitamin B Complex Depleted Rats and the Course of Repair, Proc. Soc. Exper. Biol. & Med., 67, 185, 1948.

Soeur, R.: De l'effet de l'ergostérol irradié sur l'os, Arch. internat. méd. expér., 6, 365, 1931.

————: Étude expérimentale de l'os dans l'intoxication par l'ergostérol irradié, Presse méd., 39, 1003, 1931.

Sulzberger, M. B., and Lazar, M. P.: Hypervitaminosis A, J.A.M.A., 146, 788, 1951.

Swoboda, W.: Die Röntgensymptomatik der Vitamin-D-Intoxikation im Kindesalter, Fortschr. Geb. Röntgenstrahlen, 77, 534, 1952.

Szent-Györgyi, A.: Identification of Vitamin C, Nature, 131, 225, 1933.

Thatcher, L.: Hypervitaminosis-D, with Report of a Fatal Case in a Child, Edinburgh M. J., 38, 457, 1931.

Thomas, L., McCluskey, R. T., Li, J., and Weissmann, G.: Prevention by Cortisone of the Changes in Cartilage Induced by an Excess of Vitamin A in Rabbits, Am. J. Path., 42, 271, 1963.

Toomey, J. A., and Morissette, R. A.: Hypervitaminosis A, Am. J. Dis. Child., 73, 473, 1947.

Verner, J. V., Jr., Engel, F. L., and McPherson, H. T.: Vitamin D Intoxication: Report of Two Cases Treated with Cortisone, Ann. Int. Med., 48, 765, 1958.

Vilter, R. W., Woolford, R. M., and Spies, T. D.: Severe Scurvy: A Clinical and Hematologic Study, J. Lab. & Clin. Med., 31, 609, 1946.

Vogel, K.: Scurvy—"The Plague of the Sea and the Spoyle of Mariners," Bull. New York Acad. Med., 9, 459, 1933.

WAUGH, W. A., and KING, C. G.: Isolation and Identification of Vitamin C, J. Biol. Chem., 97, 325, 1932.

WELLS, H. G., and HOLLEY, S. W.: Metastatic Calcification in Osteitis Deformans (Paget's Disease of Bone), Arch. Path., 34, 435, 1942.

VAN WERSCH, H. J.: Scurvy as a Skeletal Disease, Utrecht, Dekker & van de Vegt N.V., 1954.

WHELEN, W. S., FRASER, D., ROBERTSON, E. C., and TOMCZAK, H.: The Rising Incidence of Scurvy in Infants, Canad. M. A. J., 78, 177, 1958.

WIMBERGER, H.: Klinisch-radiologische Diagnostik von Rachitis, Skorbut und Lues congenita im Kindesalter, Ergebn. inn. Med. u. Kinderh., 28, 264, 1925.

WOLBACH, S. B.: Controlled Formation of Collagen and Reticulum. A Study of the Source of Intercellular Substance in Recovery from Experimental Scorbutus, Am. J. Path., 9, 689, 1933.

————: Vitamin-A Deficiency and Excess in Relation to Skeletal Growth, J. Bone & Joint Surg., 29, 171, 1947.

WOLBACH, S. B., and BESSEY, O. A.: Vitamin A Deficiency and the Nervous System, Arch. Path., 32, 689, 1941.

WOLBACH, S. B., and HEGSTED, D. M.: Hypervitaminosis A and the Skeleton of Growing Chicks, Arch. Path., 54, 30, 1952.

WOLBACH, S. B., and HOWE, P. R.: Intercellular Substances in Experimental Scorbutus, Arch. Path., 1, 1, 1926.

WOLKE, R. E., and NIELSEN, S. W.: Pathogenesis of Hypervitaminosis A in Growing Porcine Bone, Lab. Invest., 16, 639, 1967.

WOODRUFF, C.: Infantile Scurvy, J.A.M.A., 161, 448, 1956.

Chapter

17

Gout

As AN independent disorder, gout (*primary gout*) is a metabolic disease which has its basis in an inborn error in the intermediary metabolism of purines and related compounds, the result of which is an abnormally high production of uric acid. The term "*secondary gout*" relates mainly to cases in which some of the clinical manifestations of gout appear in persons affected with various hematologic diseases, and particularly with leukemia. Secondary gout occurring in association with a blood dyscrasia does *not*, of course, have its foundation in an inborn error of purine metabolism. Instead, the increased formation of uric acid in secondary gout is the result of accelerated degradation of endogenous nucleic acids and nucleoproteins liberated from blood cells which are undergoing destruction in the natural course of the disease itself, and especially in consequence of treatment. In an occasional instance of chronic renal insufficiency in man, the retention in the blood and tissue fluids of nonprotein nitrogen constituents (including uric acid) may likewise be associated with bouts of articular complaints. Because of the hyperuricemia and the articular complaints, these nephritic patients, too, may be held to be affected with secondary gout. In fowl, secondary gout appearing in the course of chronic renal insufficiency is by no means a rare occurrence (p. 487). In this chapter, except where specific reference is made to secondary gout, the discussion relates only to primary gout.

As a result of the underlying metabolic derangement in primary gout, the amount of uric acid formed within the body is increased, as already noted, and the uric acid content of the various body fluids is raised. The metabolic uric acid pool remains high despite the fact that the urinary excretion of uric acid is ordinarily also increased. However, in the presence of renal insufficiency in a gouty subject, the urinary excretion of uric acid will be decreased, and concomitantly the uric acid content of the various body fluids will be further increased.

The essential pathology of gout centers about the deposition of urates in various tissues and especially in the articular and periarticular tissues, which indeed are sites of predilection for the lesions specific for the disease. The most common initial clinical indication of the presence of gout is an attack of *acute articular inflammation*. Usually, the joint first affected is the metatarsophalangeal joint of a great toe. However, in certain cases the presenting acute articular inflammation centers in some other joint—most often a knee or ankle or some foot joint other than a metatarsophalangeal joint. Occasionally the acute articular manifestations of gout appear in a number of joints simultaneously or in rapid succession, the articular involvement taking the form of an acute polyarthritis.

After repeated acute attacks of gouty arthritis, sometimes recurring over many years in one or several joints, *chronic gouty arthritis* tends to set in unless appropriate prophylactic treatment, including particularly the use of uricosuric drugs, is carried out. If chronic arthritis does develop (as it so often did in the past), it is characterized by permanent and destructive alterations in many joints and in the articular ends of the bones entering into the formation of these joints. In these cases of gout, it was the joints of the hands and feet that showed the most striking alterations. The changes presented by a more or less severely affected joint area result from the deposition of urates in the articular cartilages, synovial membrane, and articular bone ends, and the presence of tophi (masses of urates) in the para-articular soft tissues, including bursae and tendons. Chondrocalcinosis (pseudo-gout) is discussed in Chapter 4 (p. 101).

CLINICAL CONSIDERATIONS

Incidence.—The characteristic manifestation of gout—acute attacks of arthritis in the great toe (podagra)—has made the disease familiar as a clinical entity for several thousand years. In accounts of the history of gout, the idea is always stressed that it used to be very common. For instance, it is reputed to have been rather prevalent in Italy and other Mediterranean countries in the days of the Roman Empire. The impression is also given that it was common in England in the time of Sydenham. He suffered from the disease himself and, about 1683, gave a vivid description of its clinical manifestations. To judge from the account of the disease given by Garrod, it seems to have been quite prevalent in England and in other parts of the world about 150 years ago. These impressions of the high incidence of the disease in the past should, however, be evaluated in the light of the fact that they reflect mainly its presence in persons of religious, social, scientific, or political prominence rather than among the population at large. The eminence of these persons in the history of their times and countries lent emphasis to their affliction by the disease and helped to make it familiar, while perhaps exaggerating its actual incidence. (See Rodnan and Benedek.)

The *current incidence* of gout is somewhat difficult to establish. It has been estimated, however, that, in countries having a high standard of living, gout accounts for 0.1 to 0.5 per cent of all morbidity, and that 2 to 5 per cent of the cases of so-called "rheumatic diseases" in those countries really represent manifestations of gout (see Mellinghoff and Gross). It is illuminating in this connection that, although gout is common in Southern Rhodesia among its inhabitants of European origin, it seems to be rarely encountered among the native Africans (see Shepherd-Wilson and Gelfand). In regard to its incidence in the United States, estimates indicate that the disorder is present in about 5 per cent of patients seen in clinics devoted to the diagnosis and treatment of arthritic conditions (see Robinson). Indeed, the more consistently the possibility of gout is borne in mind in connection with sufferers from arthritis, the greater is the likelihood that cases of gout will be revealed among them (see Steindler). It may well be that the reported higher incidence of the disease in some countries than in others reflects merely a greater awareness of the possibility of its presence among arthritic patients in those countries.

The factors of *age* and *sex* in relation to the incidence of gout have long been recognized. In respect to *age*, it is well established that in the large majority of the cases the patients are middle-aged or elderly adults at the time they suffer the initial attack of acute articular inflammation which signalizes that they are affected with the metabolic dyscrasia underlying the disease. Nevertheless, exceptional instances have been reported in which the initial articular inflammation set in during childhood (see Bernstein and also Berk) or, at the other extreme, during advanced old age (see Talbott). In a case of gout in a young subject which was followed by the writer, the patient was 9 years of age when first seen at the hospital. However, inquiry revealed that the manifestations of the disorder (progressive swelling of the right foot and the presence of an ulcerated tophus in the region of the big toe) were already of 2 years' duration at that time (see Vorhaus). In the cases in which the presence of gout becomes apparent during childhood or early youth, the disorder is likely to take a severe form, and the subject may die of renal failure or the complications of hypertension before reaching middle age. The special severity of the gout in these young subjects can often be traced to the fact that there is a background of the disease in the families of both parents (see Emmerson).

In respect to *sex*, it is well known that the vast majority of the affected subjects are males, only about 5 per cent being females. (See statistical data cited by Kaegi.) There is as yet no generally accepted explanation for the infrequency of gout among females. Gout ordinarily sets in later in life in females than in males. Indeed, a female only rarely manifests the disease before reaching the menopause. An instance of chronic deforming gouty arthritis in a female 27 years of age was reported by Recht. In that case the episodes of acute articular inflammation began when the subject was 5 years of age, and the joints first affected were those of the fingers. In the case of gout in a young person which was seen by the writer and which is mentioned above, the subject was likewise a female.

Hereditary Factor.—Inquiry into the family background in a case of gout frequently reveals that the disease is indigenous in the family. In at least 50 per cent of the cases, one can elicit evidence of inheritance of the disease. In the presence of a positive family history, it is usually the father of the subject who was also afflicted with gout. An affected female from a family in which gout is present may likewise transmit the trait to her offspring.

In relation to the hereditary nature of the underlying metabolic disorder, it has been established that, in families in which there are cases of gouty arthritis, the relatives who do not manifest the arthritis or other clinical features of gout: (1) commonly reveal serum uric acid values which are slightly higher than the average for normal control subjects, and (2) not infrequently even reveal serum uric acid values within the lower part of the range for subjects affected with gouty arthritis. A serum uric acid value of more than 6 mg. per cent (and definitely a value above 7 mg. in males) is ordinarily regarded as indicative of hyperuricemia (p. 490). As is to be expected from the fact that gout is of rather infrequent occurrence among females, the finding of a definite hyperuricemia among the asymptomatic female relatives of gouty arthritic subjects is less common than it is among the corresponding males. Altogether, in families in which gout is present, many of the subjects (about 25 per cent or more) who are not afflicted with gouty arthritis present serum uric acid values which approach or actually represent those of hyperuricemia. That the *essential hyperuricemia* in these families has a genetic basis is also generally recognized. It has been maintained that the essential hyperuricemia is inherited as a single dominant trait with incomplete penetrance, the transmitting link being autosomal and not sex-linked. However, agreement is still lacking about the precise genetic pattern for the transmission of the trait in question. (See Talbott and Coombs, Stecher *et al.*, Smyth *et al.*, Hauge and Harvald, and also Gutman.)

Contributory Factors.—In families in which hyperuricemia has been shown to be present among the relatives of subjects affected with gouty arthritis, it is only a small percentage of the relatives having hyperuricemia that come to manifest articular complaints. Furthermore, the hyperuricemia may be present for decades in those who do ultimately develop gouty arthritis. In fact, it is only rarely that the acute articular involvement sets in before the third decade of life, and the large majority of victims first experience the acute articular complaints characteristic of gout during middle age or even later. In a hyperuricemic subject who has not as yet experienced articular complaints, these may be brought on by dietary indiscretions. In particular, persistent *overeating* (especially of foods which are rich in nucleoproteins and hence yield high amounts of purines) and the *drinking* of much wine and malt liquor may precipitate the onset of gouty arthritis in these predisposed subjects. The idea of overindulgence in food and alcohol as an instigating agent in the causation of an acute attack of gouty arthritis is a traditional one.

Figure 120

A, Roentgenograph of the metatarsophalangeal joint area of a big toe showing characteristic changes of gout. The soft-tissue shadow on the left represents a tophus. The head and neck of the metatarsal bone reveal erosion, which, in the lowest part of the affected area, appears as a U-shaped defect. The patient, a 64-year-old man, had had symptoms of gout for about 8 years. Two hemispherical tophi, each measuring about $3 \times 2 \times 2$ cm., were removed from the metatarsophalangeal area shown. The joint space was opened, revealing whitish streaking of the articular cartilages caused by urates in them. The joint capsule was thickened, and the minute whitish specks in the synovial membrane also represented urates. (See Fig. 123.)

B, Roentgenograph of the metatarsophalangeal joint area of a left big toe showing changes of gout more pronounced than those seen in *A*. The roundish area of radiolucency in the shaft of the proximal phalanx represents a large deposit of urates (compare with Fig. 124-*B*), as do the radiolucencies in the head of the metatarsal bone. The articular surfaces of the lateral halves of the phalanx and metatarsal bone are fuzzily irregular, undoubtedly because of heavy incrustation of the cartilages with urates, and penetration of urates from the altered cartilages into the subchondral bone areas. The patient was 67 years of age when this x-ray picture was taken, and his serum uric acid value was 8.2 mg. per cent. The man had had attacks of gouty arthritis for 15 years. The first acute attack was in the right big toe (see *C*), and he subsequently had repeated attacks of acute painful arthritis involving the metatarsophalangeal joints of the big toes, one or both knees, wrists, shoulders, and ankles (see *F*).

C, Roentgenograph of the metatarsophalangeal joint of the right big toe of the patient referred to in *B*. This was the joint first involved, and as a result of progressive destruction of the articular cartilages, partial ankylosis developed.

D, Roentgenograph of both feet, in which the changes of gout in both big toes are very marked. In the left foot, advanced destructive alterations in the proximal phalanx and the head of the metatarsal bone of the big toe are evident; a large soft-tissue mass (tophus) can be seen in the space between the first and second metatarsal bones; the end of the fourth toe is enlarged, and the outline of the middle phalanx is no longer visible, that phalanx apparently having been substantially replaced by uratic material. In the right foot, clear-cut changes are evident only in the bones of the big toe. The patient was 42 years old when he was admitted to the hospital because of chronic deforming tophaceous gouty arthritis involving both feet and both hands. He had had gout for approximately 10 years. At the time of admission, his serum uric acid value was 9.4 mg. per cent and the urea nitrogen was 14 mg. To correct the difficulties in walking, appropriate surgery was undertaken, and a photograph of one of the resected tophaceous masses is shown in Figure 126-*A*.

E, Roentgenograph of a knee area (from another case of gout) presenting alterations in the femur, patella, and tibia. The areas of relative radiolucency, clearest in the tibia, are undoubtedly the result of urate deposition. The patient, a 42-year-old man, had suffered from gout fror 20 years. The first acute attack of the arthritis was localized in the left big toe. During the subsequent years, he had manifestations of gouty arthritis not only in the big toes but also in the joints of the hands, wrists, ankles, knees, and elbows. At the time of his first admission to the hospital, the serum uric acid value was 7.3 mg. per cent; on later admissions it was sometimes as high as 13 or even 15 mg. per cent. However, his nonprotein nitrogen values remained within the normal range, indicating that no renal damage had yet taken place. (Also see Fig. 125).

F, Roentgenograph depicting an oval area of radiolucency in the region of the articulation between the lower end of the *right* tibia and fibula in the case of the man referred to in *B* and *C*. Analogous roentgenographic changes were also observed at the articulation between the *left* tibia and fibula.

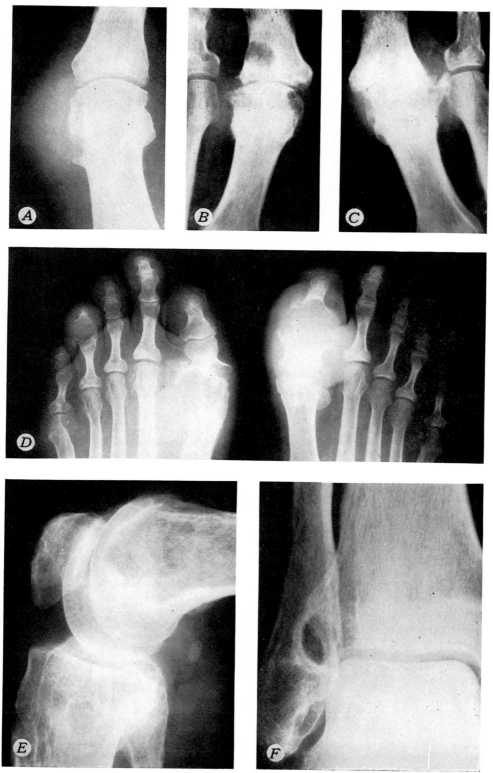

Figure 120

However, current opinion tends to minimize the importance of such overindulgence and to stress instead the precipitating influence of other factors, such as drugs (penicillin, for example), physical and/or emotional trauma, acute infections, blood loss, etc.

Clinical Complaints and Findings.—As already noted, gout usually sets in clinically as an *acute attack of arthritis* in the metatarsophalangeal joint of a great toe. Characteristically, the attack begins abruptly at night with local pain which wakes the patient from sleep. The pain is moderate at first, may become almost intolerable in the course of an hour or two, and usually abates considerably toward morning. In the absence of appropriate treatment, the pain is likely to recur for a few nights, though generally in milder form. The arthritis is regularly accompanied by fever, ordinarily not exceeding 2° or 3° F. The affected toe is exquisitely tender and quickly becomes swollen. The overlying skin is purplish red and shiny, and its veins are strikingly distended. Within 3 or 4 days, the pain and tenderness disappear, but the joint region remains doughily swollen and the epidermis scales off. (The condition may also appear in the other big toe, following there a similar though generally milder course.) Within a few weeks, all visible evidence of the acute local disturbance has usually vanished, though some pain may persist in the affected toe for months. There may be deviations from this typical course and severity of the podagra. Thus it is sometimes only after a series of acute attacks in rapid succession that a long period of remission occurs. Again, the initial attack relating to the great toe may be so mild that the patient hardly notices it at all and only remembers it years later, when subsequent, more severe attacks have shed light upon its nature.

Instead of a great toe, some other articular region may, as previously noted, be the site of the first attack. Thus the initial acute articular involvement may occur elsewhere in the foot or, more rarely, in a finger or fingers, wrist, knee, jaw, or even the cervical region. In these instances (unless it is established early that the patient has a hyperuricemia), the diagnosis of gouty arthritis may be delayed for a long time. The writer has observed a case in point. The patient was a woman 37 years of age who gave a history of three successive attacks of pain and swelling in the right knee, with only partial subsidence of the swelling after each acute epi-

Figure 121

A, Photograph of the hands and wrists in a case of chronic deforming tophaceous gouty arthritis. The picture dates from a time before the introduction of the uricosuric drugs in the treatment of gout, when such pronounced changes were still the rule in protracted cases. The patient was a man who was 58 years of age at the time this picture was taken. He reported that 13 years earlier (that is, at the age of 45) he had suffered his first attack of gouty arthritis, which involved the right big toe. In the intervening years, both hands and both feet came to present knobby enlargements, due to deposits of large masses of urates in and about the bones and joints of the hands and feet. At the time this picture was taken, the serum uric acid value was 6.2 mg. per cent. While the patient was in the hospital, he began to present evidences of renal insufficiency, and concomitantly the serum uric acid value rose to 11.4 mg. per cent.

B and *C*, Roentgenographs of both hands and wrists in this case. The swellings at the wrists and those present in relation to the fingers (as shown in *A*) are tophi which stand out in these x-ray pictures as soft-tissue masses of more or less uniform density. Note the extensive destruction which has been induced in many of the bones by the urate deposition in and about their articular ends. The tophaceous material present between the second and third metacarpal bones of the left hand reveals a number of faint punctate radiopacities. These represent small foci of calcium deposition in the masses of urates.

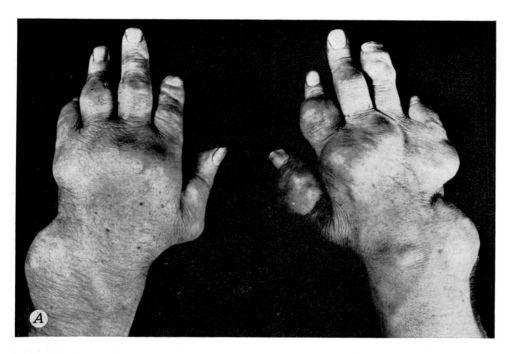

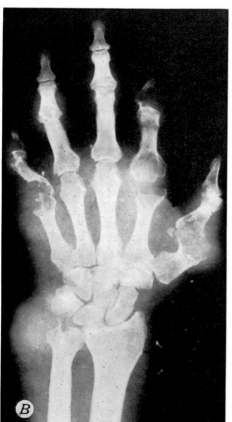

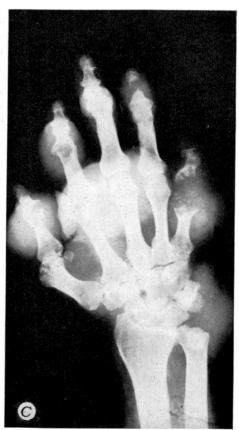

Figure 121

sode. Gradually the affected region became chronically enlarged. Because of its nontypical location, the gouty nature of the arthritis was not suspected, and synovectomy was performed. On the articular cartilage of the femur and tibia, the surgeon found whitish patches which he considered to be urate incrustations. Microscopic examination of the synovial membrane showed the presence of numerous small collections of urates within the synovium. However, it was not until about 3 years after the onset of gouty arthritis in the right knee joint that the patient first experienced an attack of pain in a great toe. As already indicated, it is only rarely that gouty arthritis sets in as an acute polyarthritis. When it does, many joints may become inflamed in rapid succession and the fever is likely to be high, so that altogether the condition may simulate an acute rheumatic polyarthritis (rheumatoid arthritis).

It is well known that a patient may suffer from acute articular attacks of gout for many years, one or more joints becoming acutely inflamed again and again, before the changes of *chronic gouty arthritis* evolve. It should be noted at once, however, that the return to a clinically normal condition between the acute attacks in any particular joint does not imply the complete absence of pathologic changes in the articular tissues of the joint in question. Thus, if one opens a joint that has been the site of repeated acute attacks without persisting clinically obvious changes, deposits of urates may be clearly perceptible even grossly, especially in the articular cartilages. Nevertheless, not all patients who have suffered from repeated attacks of acute articular gout come to show chronic deforming gouty arthritis. In those who do, sooner or later one or more joints may fail to return even clinically to a normal state. Slowly, each successive acute attack now contributes to the development of permanent, externally visible changes. In addition, alterations of a slowly progressive character may begin to evolve in joints which have not suffered directly from the acute attack or attacks. Thus, in a patient seen by the writer, tremendous gouty deformations of the finger joints and wrist joints of both hands evolved (quite painlessly) in the course of years, although the only acute attacks of gouty arthritis from which this patient had ever suffered had been limited to one great toe.

The older the patient at the time the articular manifestations of gout set in, the less likely is it that the articular changes will become pronounced. In those cases in which they do, it is in the joints of the fingers and toes that the alterations are most common and most advanced. Eventually, the digits may show the bumpy projections and distortions which characterized the typical gout hand or gout foot encountered so often in the past. In some cases, severe changes also develop in larger joints—especially the knee, elbow, ankle, and wrist joints. The shoulder and hip joints only infrequently show destructive changes, and the joints of the vertebral column present them only rarely. Ultimately, many affected articular regions may become strikingly modified, but it is the pronounced involvement and distortion of the joints of the hands and feet that cause the greatest inconvenience, since it may be difficult for the patient to walk or to feed himself. (See Figs. 120 and 121.)

Locally, in such cases one can observe or palpate knobby swellings (*tophi*) resulting from the deposition of urates in and around joint capsules, in bursae mucosae, and in tendon sheaths. They thicken the affected joints and periarticular tissues and weaken the muscles, either directly or indirectly, through limitation of motion. The skin over the tophi frequently becomes so thinned as to disclose the underlying chalky uratic material. Especially about the joints of the fingers and toes and in the olecranon and prepatellar bursae, the tophi may show periodic spurts of reactive inflammation and softening, and may even develop local ulcerations through which uratic material is discharged. Gradually, in chronic gout, urate deposits may also accumulate in other sites, such as the eyelids and the alae of the nose. However, their most common extra-articular site is the pinna of the ear. In the absence of tophi elsewhere, those in this location are of great diagnostic value.

As the disease progresses, the general health is likely to suffer eventually through visceral disturbances expressed especially in cardiovascular and renal disease. In some cases the clinical picture is dominated by these disturbances, although, concomitantly, chronic articular changes may also develop. In fact, it is the visceral complications of gout that ultimately cause death, which ensues from cerebral hemorrhage, thrombosis of cerebral arteries, occlusion of a coronary artery, or uremia.

BIOCHEMICAL CONSIDERATIONS

The inculpation of uric acid in the pathogenesis of gout dates back to the discovery by Scheele in 1776 of uric acid as an organic substance, and the demonstration by Wollaston in 1797 that tophi from gouty patients contain sodium urate crystals. Garrod, in 1848, using the crude techniques then available, contributed the highly significant finding that the amount of uric acid in the blood is greater in patients affected with gout than in non-gouty persons. The work of Fischer, published in 1907, relating to the derivation of the purine substances and the chemical structure of uric acid, constitutes a foundation for much of the knowledge we now possess in regard to the chemistry of uric acid. Also extremely important in the understanding of the metabolic defect underlying gout are the contributions of Stetten. He demonstrated that nucleic acid purines are not the only source for the formation of uric acid in the human body. In particular, he showed that purines which ultimately give rise to uric acid may be synthesized in the body from certain amino acids (glycine, for instance) and other substances of low molecular weight, such as carbon dioxide, ammonia, and formic acid.

Intermediary Metabolism of Uric Acid.—In man, uric acid (trioxypurine) is predominantly the end product of the metabolism of purine substances, while urea is the end product of the metabolism of amino acids. In birds and reptiles, uric acid is formed as an end product of the metabolism both of purines and of amino acids. Normally, man is thus a *ureotelic* animal—that is, he ordinarily eliminates most of his ingested nonpurine nitrogen in the form of urea. By contrast, birds and reptiles, for instance, are *uricotelic* animals, since they form and eliminate mainly uric acid and not urea in the course of metabolism of substances containing nitrogen.* In the gouty human subject, the uric acid metabolism tends more or less in the direction of what is characteristic of the uricotelic species. That is, in a person affected with gout (as compared with a normal person), there is an accentuation of

---

* It is thus not surprising that gout has been observed in various members of the avian species. In fowl, a condition designated as "visceral gout" has been familiar for a long time. It is characterized by the deposition of urates in various internal organs (particularly the kidneys) and on the various serous membranes, instead of in the articular cartilages, synovial membranes, and periarticular tissues. In rare instances, some of the articular cartilages may also show small deposits of urates. Since so-called visceral gout of fowl is held to be secondary to renal damage (usually of the nature of a pyelonephritis), the condition is also frequently denoted as "renal gout." The deposition of urates in the viscera and serous membranes in the affected fowl seems to be dependent upon a profound hyperuricemia resulting from the renal failure, and not upon disordered intermediary metabolism of uric acid. Only very rarely is full-fledged *articular gout* observed in fowl, and in these instances, urate deposits are not encountered in the various internal organs and/or serous membranes (see Siller). In parakeets as contrasted with fowl, articular (or synovial) gout occurs almost as frequently as does visceral gout. However, in parakeets, as in fowl, if articular gout is present, the serous membranes also fail to show deposits of urates (see Schlumberger). Still, unlike visceral gout, articular gout of fowl and other birds probably does have its basis, at least partly, in disordered metabolism of purine substances, as does human gout.

the formation of uric acid from purines which are derived from certain amino acid precursors and the substances of low molecular weight which were mentioned above.

In summary, so far as the formation of uric acid in the body is concerned, we know that in *normal persons* the purine substances from which it is derived may originate: (1) from the nucleic acids and nucleoproteins of body cells; (2) from the nucleic acids and nucleoproteins contained in the cells of ingested foods; (3) through degradation of chemical substances formed in the course of endogenous synthesis of nucleic acids and other purine substances, such as free nucleotides; and (4) from various nonpurine precursors, as mentioned above (see Seegmiller and Laster). In *persons affected with gout*, the uric acid formed in the body has these same four origins, but, as already noted, the formation of uric acid from purines derived from various nonpurine precursors (route 4) is greatly accentuated.

Figure 122

A, Photograph showing the gross changes observed in a knee joint opened at autopsy in a case of gout. The patient was a man 51 years of age who died of renal insufficiency 5 weeks after admission to the hospital, and in whom the presence of gout was discovered fortuitously in the course of the autopsy. The articular cartilage of the femoral condyles appears almost glaringly white, on the whole, because of the presence of urates in it. On the left, part of the articular surface of the tibia and one of the menisci can also be seen, and these, too, show whitish streaks and patches representing urate deposits (see *C*). The whitish specks in the synovial membrane and in the patellar ligament also represent urate deposits, and the articular cartilage of the patella is likewise heavily incrusted with urates. The clinical record in this case indicates that, for approximately 2 or 3 years before admission to the hospital, the patient had various articular complaints which had prompted a diagnosis of "rheumatoid arthritis" by his physician. One week before admission, both knee joints and the left second toe became swollen. On admission the serum urea nitrogen value was 69 mg. per cent, and it rose to 172 mg. per cent shortly before the patient's death. At that time the serum creatinine value was 15.6 mg. per cent. Unfortunately, despite the fact that numerous serum biochemical evaluations were made, the patient's physician did not request a serum uric acid determination. That the anatomic changes presented by this knee joint are those of gout is indubitable. The only question remaining unanswered is whether this is a case of clinically atypical "primary gout" or a case of "secondary gout." In the latter event, the urate deposition in the articular tissues would have its basis in the loading of the various body fluids with urates in consequence of the chronic renal insufficiency. The amount of urate deposition observed in the articular tissues in this case is exceptional in gout secondary to renal insufficiency. However, histologic examination of the kidneys lent support to the possibility that these articular changes might nevertheless represent an expression of secondary (renal) gout. Indeed, though the kidneys showed very advanced scarring and glomerular and tubular alterations, microscopic examination failed to reveal urate deposits either in the renal tubules or in the renal interstitial tissues. In all probability, if the articular changes in this case were an expression of "primary gout," the kidneys would have shown deposits of urates.

B, Photograph of the fifth lumbar vertebra from the same subject to whom reference is made in *A*. The articular cartilages of the vertebral facets show whitish discoloration, which is due to the presence of urates. The whitish specks in the nucleus pulposus of the intervertebral disk likewise represent urate deposits, and considerable amounts of urates were also present in the anterior ligament of the vertebral column.

C, Photograph of the complete tibial component of the knee joint illustrated in *A*. The urate deposits in the articular cartilage of both tibial condyles, both menisci, and the capsule of the knee joint are clearly evident.

D, Photomicrograph ($\times$ 125) showing smaller and larger deposits of urates in the synovial membrane of the capsule of the knee joint illustrated in *A*. Since the tissue was not fixed in absolute alcohol, the crystalline structure of the urates has been obliterated. (See Fig. 126.)

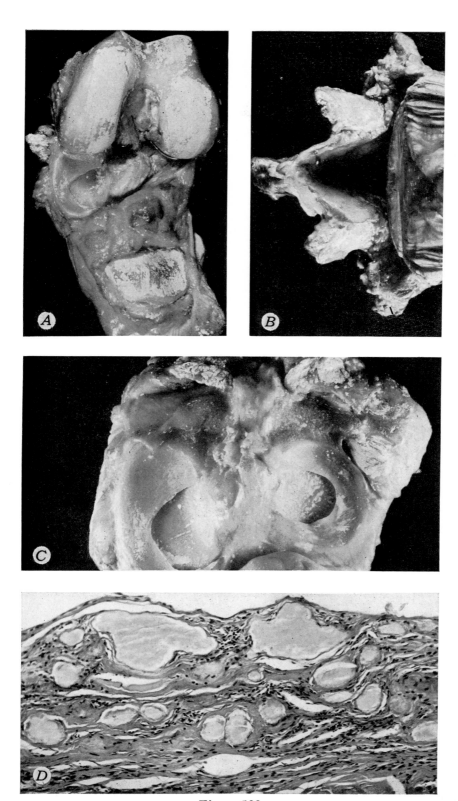

Figure 122

Chemically, the nucleic acids are complex polynucleotides of high molecular weight in which the individual nucleotides contain a purine or pyrimidine base. In part, the various individual nucleotides are differentiated in accordance with the type of purine or pyrimidine base of which they are composed. In the nucleic acids, groups of these nucleotides are arranged in repeating units. The arrangement of these units, as well as the arrangement of the different nucleotides in relation to one another, appears to be characteristic of the nucleic acid itself. It is the purine bases of the nucleotides that are the main source of uric acid, the latter resulting from the degradation of the nucleic acids and their nucleotides.

Excretion of Uric Acid.—In a person *not* affected with gout, such uric acid as is formed daily (a relatively small amount) is excreted mainly in the urine, but some is also eliminated by way of sweat and tears, and in the feces. Nearly all the uric acid formed in the body is eliminated as such, because, unlike most other mammals, man lacks the enzyme uricase, which, by uricolysis, would degrade most of this uric acid to allantoin, which would then be excreted. On a diet low in purines, a normal subject excretes between 300 and 500 mg. of uric acid in the urine per 24 hours. The amount of uric acid excreted daily in the urine consists largely of the uric acid in the glomerular filtrate which is *not reabsorbed* by the renal tubules, and to a small extent of uric acid which is *secreted* by the renal tubules. It is generally agreed that, in a normal adult, only about 5 per cent of the uric acid in the glomerular filtrate fails to be reabsorbed. Because the formation of uric acid in the body is so much greater in the gouty than in the normal subject, the urinary excretion of uric acid is much higher in the gouty subject, provided there is no renal insufficiency. Indeed, it may even be 2 or 3 times as great as the average for normal persons. Since the amount of uric acid in the daily glomerular filtrate is much greater in the gouty than in the normal subject (because of the hyperuricemia), the daily urinary excretion of uric acid is naturally likewise greater, even though the proportion of uric acid reabsorbed by the renal tubules may be the same in the two subjects.

Rieselbach *et al.* have pointed out that "diminished urate secretion per nephron observed in some patients serves as the basis for their hyperuricemia and gout and represents an entity distinct from gout which occurs on a renal basis due to a markedly diminished nephron population. If it could be established that this were on the basis of an intrinsic tubular defect, it would be reasonable to use the term 'primary renal gout' for such cases."

The high urinary excretion of uric acid ordinarily observed in a gouty subject is related to the fact that the metabolic pool of uric acid is much greater in the gouty than in the normal person. In a normal adult the uric acid pool, as expressed in the "miscible" uric acid, has been found by Stetten to be about 1.2 gm. He defines the miscible pool of uric acid in man as the uric acid in the various body fluids which is free to mix with intravenously injected, isotopically labeled uric acid—that is, metabolically active uric acid. It is estimated that, in the normal subject, somewhat less than half of the uric acid in the metabolic pool is eliminated in the course of a day and synchronously replaced, the size of the pool thus remaining constant. In some gouty subjects the miscible pool may be as large as 20 or 30 times the normal, because of a pronounced imbalance between the formation of uric acid and its elimination, in favor of the former. Since the metabolic pool of uric acid is high in the gouty person, and since uric acid and many of its salts have a very low solubility, the gouty subjects accumulate excesses of uric acid in the various tissues. However, the role played by the accumulation of uric acid in the articular tissues in the instigation of the acute attacks of articular pain and swelling is not clear.

Serum Uric Acid Values.—For normal adults, the serum uric acid values ordinarily range between 3 and 6 mg. per cent and average about 4 mg. Within this range, normal adult males tend to have slightly higher serum uric acid values than normal adult females. For normal infants and children, the average serum uric acid value is lower than for normal adults. A serum uric acid value of more than 6 mg. per cent (and definitely a value above 7 mg. in males) represents a hyperuricemia. In cases of gout in which the patients are not undergoing treatment with uricosuric drugs, serum uric acid values of 8 to 10 mg. per cent are not unusual. In the presence of a complicating renal insufficiency, the serum uric acid values are often much higher.

There are many conditions in addition to primary gout which may be associated with the presence of hyperuricemia. These include: (1) renal insufficiency (based on nephritis of one kind or another); (2) hematologic diseases (such as leukemia, myeloid metaplasia, multiple myeloma, polycythemia vera, and hemolytic anemia); and (3) so-called idiopathic hyperuricemia—that is, hyperuricemia found in persons who are in good health and who present no family history of gout. (See Fig. 122.)

As already noted, it has been established that some patients affected with hematologic disorders (especially myeloid leukemia) and showing a hyperuricemia will come to suffer from attacks of arthritis indistinguishable clinically from the acute articular manifestations of gout. The articular manifestations encountered in subjects with blood dyscrasias have been designated as "secondary gout." The development of "secondary gout" in persons with leukemia, for instance, is apparently related to: (1) the liberation of excessive amounts of nucleic acid from the leukemic cells in the course of their disintegration; and (2) the consequent appearance, in the blood, of abnormally large amounts of purines and their metabolic end product, uric acid (see Gutman, and Whitaker *et al.*). There is little information as yet in regard to the emergence of clinical gout among persons known to have "idiopathic hyperuricemia." On the other hand, it has been established that persons who have a family history of gout and are known to have hyperuricemia, but who have been free of symptoms of gout, not infrequently do come to develop clinical gout.

PATHOLOGIC FINDINGS

Our knowledge of the pathologic changes insofar as they relate to an initial attack of acute gouty arthritis is based upon the occasional instances in which involved metatarsophalangeal joints were subjected to surgical exploration on the mistaken assumption that these joints were the site of pyogenic infection (see Gudzent). However, most of the descriptions of the pathologic anatomy of gout have been derived from autopsy findings in cases of gout of long standing in which severe chronic deforming articular and para-articular changes had evolved. As is well known, the current therapeutic management of gout can be counted upon to delay or forestall the development of such pronounced skeletal changes. Therefore it is in the older literature that one finds most of the detailed descriptions of the disease as it presents itself when it has had a chance to attain its full efflorescence (see Garrod, Moore, Pommer, Lang, and also Brogsitter). In the more recent literature it is only occasionally that one still encounters reports which deal with the anatomic changes characterizing gout in its florid form (see Lichtenstein *et al.*, and Rosenquist *et al.*).

In the few cases in which a metatarsophalangeal joint involved in an *initial attack* of acute gouty arthritis has been explored surgically, it was found that there was pronounced swelling and redness of the synovial membrane and more or less serous effusion into the articular cavity. It is reported that, in the cases in question, urate deposits were not visible to the naked eye in the articular cartilages and periarticular tissues. However, it seems very likely that, if specimens of these tissues had been taken for histologic study and examined microscopically, some urate crystals could already have been detected, at least in the synovial membrane. In this connection it should be borne in mind that it is advisable to use absolute alcohol as a fixative (and not a watery fixative) for the tissue being prepared for microscopic examination. Otherwise the crystalline structure of the urate deposits may be blurred through partial dissolution. In any event, if some synovial fluid is withdrawn from an acutely inflamed joint in a case of gout and this fluid is examined microscopically with the aid of polarized light, urate crystals (either free or within polymorphonuclear leukocytes or monocytes) can usually be demonstrated (see McCarty).

The question of the role played by urates in the initiation of an acute attack of gouty arthritis has received a good deal of attention. That such an attack represented an inflammatory response to the presence of urate crystals in the involved joint was already postulated by Garrod. This idea seemed to be refuted when it was later found that if sodium urate *in solution* was injected into joints it did not induce an inflammatory response. Support for Garrod's hypothesis came from subsequent experimental studies on man and lower animals (dogs in particular) which demonstrated that the intra-articular injection of microcrystals of sodium urate *did* induce inflammatory reactions which often closely simulated the "spontaneous" attacks of acute gouty arthritis (see Malawista and Seegmiller, and also Faires and McCarty).

In relation to the provocative action of crystalline sodium urate in the causation of acute attacks of gouty arthritis, we know that the synovial fluid, being a dialysate of the blood plasma, *normally* contains small quantities of uric acid, though, of course, in solution. It therefore seems reasonable to ask why the uric acid which, even in gouty subjects, had entered the joint in solution as a dialysate from the plasma acquires crystalline form and perhaps thus provokes an attack of acute gouty arthritis. Undoubtedly the low solubility of uric acid and its salts, and its relatively high concentration in the synovial fluid of the gouty subject are factors in this change. It may well be that crystallization of the soluble uric acid may be induced by microcrystal "seeds" of urate, by localized inflammatory changes in the synovial membrane, or by still other factors. However, it seems highly probable that, in addition to the presence of uric acid in crystalline form in the synovial fluid, there are also other influences (still unknown) determining the occurrence of an attack of gouty arthritis. Dried smears of synovial fluid examined microscopically with polarized light will show birefringent needle-shaped intra- and extracellular urate crystals (see Good and Frishette).

In the course of further *evolution of the gouty changes* in a joint, various amounts of the urate salts which have entered its articular cavity as a dialysate from the

Figure 123

A, Photomicrograph ($\times$ 30) depicting collections of urates within the articular cartilage of the proximal end of the proximal phalanx of a big toe shown in Figure 120-*A*. At the extreme left and right, there is evidence that the urates are extending through the calcified zone of the articular cartilage and penetrating to a slight extent into the subchondral bone cortex. In the central portion of the articular cartilage, there is a larger focus of urates which is still confined to the cartilage. Note also that there are no urate deposits as yet in the marrow spaces of the spongiosa.

B, Photomicrograph ($\times$ 150) illustrating small collections of urates in the somewhat thickened and proliferated synovial membrane of the affected metatarsophalangeal joint to which reference was made in *A*. The individual uratic foci stand out clearly because they are ringed by cells, some of which are foreign-body giant cells. In this instance, too, the tissue was not fixed in absolute alcohol, and the crystalline structure of the urates has thus again been obliterated.

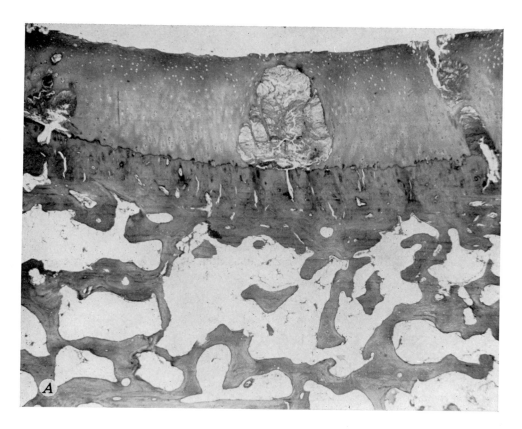

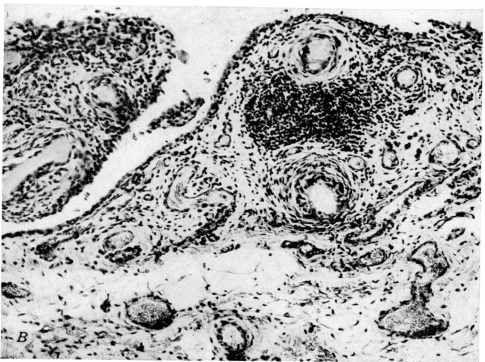

Figure 123

plasma are taken up by the articular cartilages and by the synovial membrane. The special susceptibility of *articular cartilage* to urate deposition is due, in the opinion of Pommer: (1) to the succulence of this tissue, (2) to the torpidity of its fluid exchange, and (3) to its particular chemical constitution (chondroitin sulfuric acid content, high sodium content, etc.). As already noted, it is the synovial fluid that is the source from which the cartilage imbibes the urates. Whether the urates are taken first into the cartilage cells proper or into the intercellular cartilage matrix is not yet clear. Another question is that of whether the cartilage is necrotic before the urates are deposited. The weight of evidence is against this idea, but certainly articular cartilage in which large amounts of urates have accumulated does present evidence of necrosis.

In the cartilages of an affected joint, the earliest urate deposits are observed on and just within the articulating surfaces (that is, close to the joint space) in the form of microscopic foci of urate crystals or granules (see Sherman). Through the development of additional foci of urate deposition, and through the spread and

Figure 124

A, Photograph of part of a fifth toe, sectioned in the sagittal plane, showing deposits of urates in the terminal and middle phalanges and, to a slight extent, in the soft tissues neighboring upon these bones. The patient was an elderly man who had had manifestations of gout for many years and who died of renal insufficiency.

B, Photograph illustrating the appearance of the cut surface of part of the proximal phalanx of the big toe from the same patient mentioned in *A*. A roundish focus of uratic material extending to the articular surface of the bone is clearly apparent within the spongiosa. In the immediate vicinity of the focus, the articular cartilage of the phalanx is no longer clearly discernible. However, on each side of the uratic focus, some articular cartilage is still present, although apparently modified. On the right, in the spongiosa immediately above the persisting articular cartilage, uratic material is also evident.

C, Photograph of part of a proximal phalanx and head of a metatarsal bone from the same case, again showing uratic foci in both bones in the vicinity of the metatarsophalangeal joint. It is evident that the uratic material has also distended the capsule of the joint, and that, in the immediate vicinity of the urate deposit, the articular cartilage of both the bones in question has been destroyed (see *E*).

D, Photograph of the cut surface of part of two midtarsal bones. Note the two roundish foci of uratic material in the tarsal bone shown in the lower half of the picture.

E, Photomicrograph ($\times$ 5) illustrating the general histologic pattern of the pathologic changes of gout as revealed in an affected metatarsophalangeal joint. A heavy deposit of urates is present in the synovial membrane, and the fibrous coat of the joint capsule is distended. Part of the articular cartilage of the two apposed bones has been destroyed, and it can be seen that urates have penetrated for a short distance into the spongiosa of each of these bones. Note that, beyond these urate deposits, the intertrabecular marrow spaces of the bones are free of urates. (Compare with *F*.)

F, Photomicrograph ($\times$ 30) illustrating the histologic pattern of the pathologic changes of gout as revealed in a phalanx in which the intertrabecular marrow spaces beyond the articular cartilage contain accumulations of urates which had apparently been deposited there directly. The articular cartilage at the extreme right of the picture shows small surface defects which have resulted from the deposition of urates. The surface of the rest of the articular cartilage lacks the normal smoothness, presumably because it, too, has been the site of urate deposition, and the altered superficial cartilage has consequently sloughed off. On the left of the picture, beyond the articular cartilage, a large deposit of urates is apparent. This seems to have developed in the region of attachment of the articular capsule to the bone cortex. Immediately beneath the articular cartilage, one can observe a narrow zone of spongiosa which is essentially free of urates. Beyond this zone, however, the marrow spaces of the spongiosa do show urate deposits, the dark dots in these deposits representing multinuclear foreign-body giant cells.

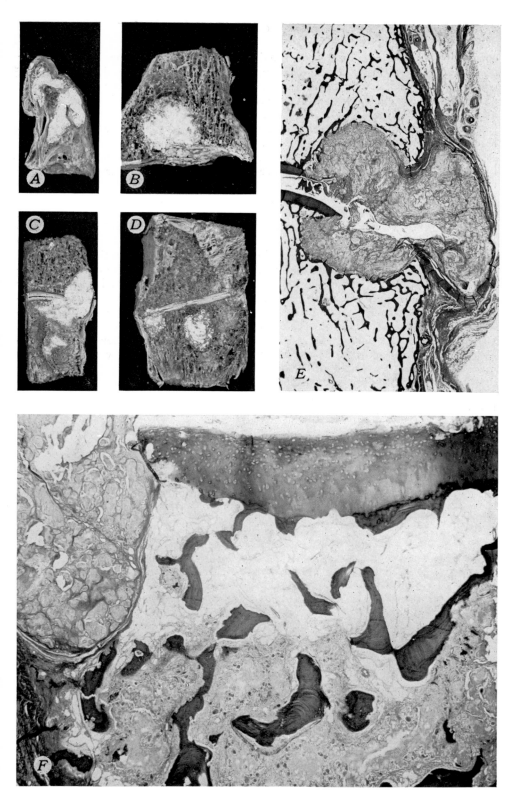

Figure 124

confluence of those already present, the deposits come to be distinguishable grossly as whitish incrustations. These may appear as smaller or larger discrete patches, or one or both of the articular cartilages of an individual joint may even be found almost uniformly chalky white. As the articular cartilages of a joint become more and more heavily incrusted with urates, defects due to sloughing off of superficial fragments of damaged cartilage may be observed. Eventually, the affected cartilages may show large areas of ulceration. (See Figs. 123 and also 122.)

As noted, the *synovial membrane* shares in the articular changes of gout. It becomes inflamed and proliferates as a result of the deposition of urates in it. The urates may appear as white foci (punctiform or larger) which are likely to be especially obvious in the thickened villi. On histologic examination the urate agglomerations within these foci are usually found to be surrounded by a narrow, ringlike border of connective tissue containing multinuclear giant cells (foreign-body giant cells) and other inflammatory cells—mainly macrophages. If the synovial membrane has not been fixed in absolute alcohol, the uratic material will appear granular rather than in the form of rodlike crystals. The changes in the synovial membrane will be found to be particularly pronounced if the articular cartilages are severely affected. In such cases, sequestrated fragments of urate-incrusted cartilage may be an additional source of irritation of the synovial membrane, acting mechanically or through the chemicotoxic effect of the urates. In consequence, the synovial membrane (especially of larger joints) becomes considerably thickened. Furthermore, some connective tissue pannus may grow out from its edges and creep over the articular cartilages, thus playing a part in the future development of ankylosis of the joint. Urate deposits may also be found in the fibrous coat of the joint capsule. In advanced cases of gout, these deposits may be large and numerous, and the fibrous coat of the capsule will show inflammatory thickening.

Figure 125

A, Photograph of the right hand and part of the forearm in the case of the man affected with chronic deforming tophaceous gouty arthritis to whom reference was already made in connection with Figure 120-E. At the time this picture was taken, the patient was 47 years of age, and had already been a victim of gout for 25 years. The fingers show knobby swellings and are otherwise obviously deformed. The position and sausage-like enlargement of the fourth finger interfered seriously with the functioning of the hand, and was subsequently ablated on this account (see B). The swelling on the ulnar aspect of the wrist represents an exceedingly large tophus, and the small swelling proximal to it on the forearm is also a tophus.

B, Photograph showing both halves of the cut surface of the swollen and deformed fourth finger of the hand illustrated in A, the finger having been disarticulated through the metacarpophalangeal joint. The tophaceous deposits which had caused the enlargement of the finger, particularly in the region of the middle and proximal phalanges, stand out clearly. The proximal interphalangeal joint still shows articular cartilage on both of the bones entering into the formation of that joint. The distal interphalangeal joint is no longer clearly delineated, having been disrupted by the accumulation of uratic material in the articular cavity and in the proximal end of the terminal phalanx and the distal end of the middle phalanx (see C).

C, Photomicrograph ($\times$ 1) of a celloidin section prepared from one of the halves of the finger illustrated in B. It shows the general architecture of the pathologic changes. The uratic material of the tophus appears grayish, and the focal collections of urates are more or less delineated by darker-staining areas which represent inflammatory cells. Many of these, as higher magnification would show, are multinuclear foreign-body giant cells. Note also that uratic material is discernible in the distal interphalangeal joint and in both of the phalanges entering into the formation of that joint.

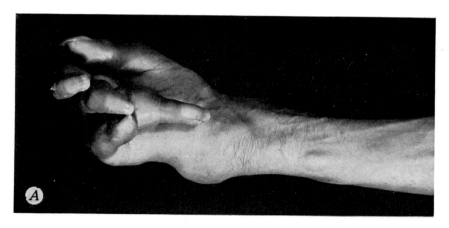

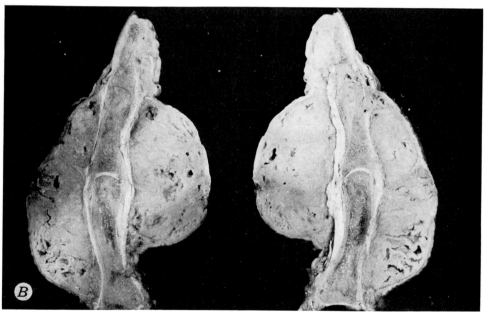

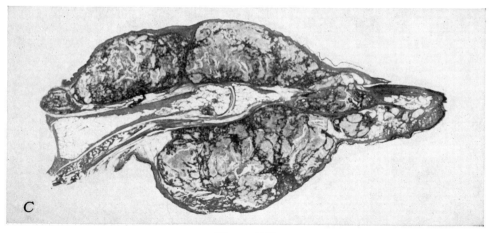

Figure 125

497

In addition to the articular cartilages and synovial membrane (and even the fibrous coat of the joint capsule), the *bones* entering into the formation of the joint may come to present smaller or larger deposits of urates. Because of penetration of the entire thickness of the articular cartilages by urates, adjacent portions of the bony end plate are likely to be perforated through vascularization. This is one of the ways in which urates present in the joint cavity enter the subchondral area to form uratic deposits in the bone. Especially when the articular changes are very florid, some uratic foci located in the immediate subchondral bone and even those present deeper in the spongiosa undoubtedly form there as independent deposits resulting from the direct deposition of urates in the bone marrow. However, some of the largest foci of urate deposits encountered in the articular ends of bones are the result of erosion or penetration of the bones by urate deposits present as tophi in the local periosteum or ligaments and tendons. Indeed, in relation to the para-articular tissues, the heaviest deposits of urates occur at the sites of attachment of ligaments and tendons. Also, any bursae in the vicinity of affected joints (for instance, prepatellar or olecranon bursae) may come to show urate deposits in their walls. Large para-articular tophi sometimes become impregnated with smaller or larger amounts of calcium salts. Deposits of calcium salts may occasionally also be observed in uratic deposits in the synovial membrane and/or within tophi in the articular bone ends of a gouty joint. (See Figs. 124, 125, and 126.)

Finally, it should be pointed out that, in a case of gout coming to autopsy, one may also find some evidence of involvement of the *axial skeleton*. The changes in the axial skeleton are, of course, never so severe as those in the appendicular skeleton. In an advanced case of gout, one or more vertebral bodies may show small intramedullary urate deposits. These are usually oriented to the contiguous intervertebral disks, which are themselves the site of some urate deposits even though the articulations between the vertebral bodies represent amphiarthroses

Figure 126

A, Photograph showing the cut surface of a large tophus removed from the region of one of the big toes illustrated in Figure 120-*D*. The legend pertaining to that figure includes clinical data relating to the patient in question. The cut surface of the tophus portrays the characteristic whitish appearance created by the presence of the urates. If a tiny fragment of such a tophus were smeared on a slide and examined microscopically (under direct or polarized light), the urates would appear as needle-like rods. Sometimes the cut surface of a tophus is so strikingly white that one might be misled into thinking that the whitish appearance had resulted from the presence of calcium. It is true that tophi occasionally come to contain calcium salts. However, such tophi are usually heavily radiopaque in the x-ray picture, while those which do not contain calcium are not.

B, Photomicrograph ($\times$ 30) showing the histologic pattern of a tissue section prepared from the tophus shown in *A*. The specimen was fixed in formalin, and the paraffin section was stained with hematoxylin and eosin. Many of the individual agglomerations of urates are roundish in contour and show variable numbers of large, dark-staining cells about the periphery of each agglomeration. These represent multinuclear giant cells (foreign-body giant cells). The details of their architecture cannot, of course, be discerned under this low magnification.

C, Photomicrograph ($\times$ 125) illustrating the appearance, under the light microscope, of the filamentous urate crystals observable in a tissue section prepared from a tophus when the tissue specimen has been fixed in absolute alcohol, embedded in paraffin, and stained with hematoxylin and eosin. (Compare with *D*.)

D, Photomicrograph ($\times$ 125) illustrating, under polarized light, the same tissue field shown in *C*. The urate crystals now stand out much more distinctly, and it is apparent that large groups of the crystals intersect each other.

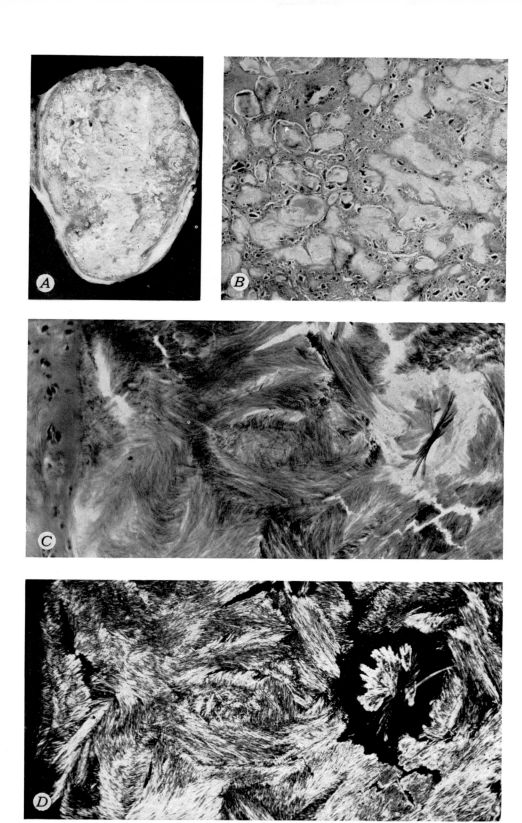

Figure 126

and not synovial joints. When the intervertebral disks and/or vertebral bodies are the sites of urate deposits, small deposits are likely to be encountered also in the paravertebral ligaments. In a case studied by the writer, the articular cartilages of some of the vertebral joints (facet joints) were also found incrusted with urates (see Hall and Selin). Involvement of one or both sacroiliac joints may be encountered in some cases with advanced peripheral gout (see Malawista *et al.*).

Extraskeletal accumulations of urates in the form of tophi may also be found elsewhere than in relation to joints. These tophi are probably best exemplified by those so often appearing in the *pinna of the ear*. There they are manifest as small knobs consisting of a central chalky core surrounded by a fairly thick capsule of connective tissue. Microscopically, the core shows dense agglomerations of urate crystals in partly or completely necrotic connective tissue. When appropriately stained, the core may also show considerable calcium. In the inner portion of the capsule, which is the looser and more cellular, there may be multinuclear giant cells. These phagocytic cells are usually in intimate contact with the urate crystals and may even enclose some of them. In the immediate vicinity of such a tophus, inflammatory infiltrations along the vascular channels can also be observed.

Of the various viscera, it is the *kidneys* that are most likely to show involvement in cases of gout. It has been known clinically for a long time that patients affected with gout frequently suffer from *renal calculi* and often pass gravel in the urine. These calculi are composed of urates, and the passage of such calculi often precedes the onset of the initial acute attack of gouty arthritis. It should be pointed out, however, that persons not affected with gout may also pass urate stones. Nevertheless, in any subject who does pass them, the possible presence of the gouty diathesis should be suspected and further investigated. (See Yü and Gutman.)

The actual structural changes occurring in the kidneys in cases of gout are very likely to lead to progressive renal failure, and this is often the cause of death. The renal blood vessels (like those elsewhere in the body) commonly exhibit advanced *atherosclerosis*. In consequence, the kidneys are likely to become contracted, and cardiovascular-renal difficulties may ensue. In addition, *urate deposits* frequently accumulate. These deposits tend to center in the medullary portion of the kidney where they assume a fan-shaped, or striated, distribution, especially when the urates are in the collecting tubules. The epithelium of the tubules undergoes necrosis, and there may be scarring and foreign-body reactions about them. On the other hand, in some cases the urates may be found deposited particularly in the interstitial tissues of the renal medulla rather than in the tubules. In such instances, too, a good deal of interstitial inflammatory scarring is to be observed. In brief, the advanced renal changes appearing in gout include, notably, glomerular and arterial hyalinization, tubular atrophy, interstitial fibrosis and inflammation, and also tophus formation (see Greenbaum *et al.*, and Gonick *et al.*). Finally, there are indications that, within families in which one or more members manifest articular gout and others merely show essential hyperuricemia, some of the latter members may develop hypertension and other complications of renal disease ("hyperuricemic nephropathy") even in the absence of articular gout (see Duncan and Dixon). (See also Munck.)

Aside from the more common nonskeletal sites of urate deposition (the kidneys and the pinna of the ear), one or more urate deposits (usually small) have been found in individual cases in various other sites, including particularly the cartilages of the upper and lower air passages. A very exceptional but unequivocal instance of a tophus present within the posterior mitral leaflet of the heart has been recorded (see Bunim and McEwen). A case in which a tophus within the heart had affected the conduction bundle and caused a complete heart block is mentioned by Hench and Darnall. A few cases have also been reported in which the gouty subject developed so-called benign pericarditis, and it has been suggested that the pericarditis appearing terminally in cases of uremia may likewise have its basis in a pronounced hyperuricemia (see Paulley *et al.*).

DIAGNOSIS AND TREATMENT

Diagnosis.—The importance of diagnosing gout early in its clinical course—that is, in its pretophaceous stage—is crucial. Indeed, in the current therapeutic management of the condition in its pretophaceous stage, it is now possible to forestall or at least largely minimize both the destructive articular changes and the para-articular alterations (resulting from the formation of large tophi in the bones and neighboring soft parts) which characterize the disease in its full efflorescence. Once the possibility of gout in its pretophaceous stage is borne in mind, the diagnosis of the condition becomes a relatively simple matter. In arriving at the diagnosis, the important criteria are: (1) a history of one previous attack or recurrent attacks of acute articular inflammation (usually in the region of a great toe) setting in abruptly and subsiding after a few days or weeks without residual impairment of function; (2) the finding of hyperuricemia, represented by a serum uric acid level of 6 mg. per cent or more; and (3) the prompt relief of the acute articular pain through the administration of colchicine if the patient is seen during an acute attack.

Roentgenographic examination of a joint area which is the site of an initial acute attack of articular gout will not as yet demonstrate any bone changes of diagnostic significance. After repeated acute attacks involving one or more joints and sometimes extending over a period of years, smaller or larger defects in the articular bone ends of such joints are likely to be visible roentgenographically. As already indicated, such defects are due to the accumulation of urates in the bones at the sites in question, and the larger bone defects are usually associated with the presence of soft-tissue shadows representing masses of urates (tophi) in the articular capsule of the joint and/or in the para-articular soft tissues. If one is dealing with an instance of tophaceous gout, the demonstration of urate crystals in material obtained from one of the soft-tissue swellings is an unequivocal criterion of the presence of gout.

Treatment.—Only the principal guides for treatment will be given here, since it is recognized that, in an individual case, the management of the patient may have to be modified to meet existing medical circumstances (see Talbott and also Gutman). In general, the treatment of gout involves: (1) the management of the gouty person as a whole; (2) the immediate and adequate treatment of an acute attack of gouty arthritis; (3) measures directed toward mitigating or forestalling future acute attacks whose cumulative effect is likely to be the appearance of tophaceous gout and destructive articular changes; and (4) the management of the patient in cases in which, for one reason or another, the disease has progressed to the stage in which severe crippling gouty arthritis has developed.

The most important items in the *general management* of the patient are: (1) a well-balanced diet, moderate in respect to the total amount of food consumed; (2) in regard to the protein substances in the diet, the avoidance of foods rich in purines (notably liver, sweetbreads, kidney, tongue, and meat extracts); (3) avoidance of, or at least great moderation in, the use of alcoholic beverages; (4) the intake of large quantities of water; (5) maintenance of regularity of bowel movements; and (6) moderate but regular exercise.

In the treatment of an acute attack of gouty arthritis, *colchicine* remains the most useful drug for allaying the pain and reducing the local inflammatory changes. The onset of prodromal symptoms or an actual acute attack of gouty arthritis

33

(whether or not this has been preceded by other acute attacks) calls for the immediate institution of a *therapeutic course of colchicine.* This course usually consists of the oral administration of 0.5 mg. of colchicine every hour (or 1 mg. every 2 hours) without interruption until: There is relief of pain, or gastrointestinal disturbances in the form of nausea and/or diarrhea develop, or a total of 7.5 to 10 mg. of colchicine has been administered (see Robinson). The onset of gastrointestinal disturbances is an indication for the immediate discontinuance of the colchicine in therapeutic dosage, at least for a few days. The gastrointestinal distress can usually be relieved by paregoric. If the pain continues to be severe, salicylates and/or codeine will contribute to the patient's comfort. Moreover, bed rest and the sparing of the acutely inflamed joint from functional use and even from pressure are indicated until the inflammatory manifestations of the acute attack have subsided. After the acute attack has abated, the administration of colchicine in maintenance dosage totaling about 1.5 mg. daily (in divided doses) is often effective in forestalling the occurrence of subsequent acute attacks or at least reducing their frequency, and thus diminishing the likelihood of the development of chronic tophaceous gout (see Yü and Gutman). The administration of colchicine is indicated before any surgical procedure is carried out on a person affected with gout, and also before the patient is likely to be confronted with a stressful situation. Other drugs effective against acute attacks of gouty arthritis include phenylbutazone (Butazolidin) and corticotropin (ACTH).

For the prevention and/or amelioration of chronic deforming gouty arthritis, drugs which induce a negative urate balance and increase the elimination of urates by way of the urine ("uricosuric" drugs) are administered. A potent eliminant of urates by way of the urine is probenecid (Benemid). Probenecid, a drug of low toxicity, is usually administered in doses of 0.5 to 1 gm. daily, and is given in conjunction with maintenance doses of colchicine. Colchicine itself has no urate eliminant properties, while, on the other hand, the uricosuric drugs have no ameliorating effect upon the pain and inflammatory aspects of the acute attack. The uricosuric effect of Benemid or other urate eliminants results from the blocking action of these drugs upon the reabsorption of urates from the renal tubules through their selective action upon the lining cells of the tubules. Concomitantly, the urate eliminants can be expected to reduce the serum urate level, often to normal, and thus to minimize the deposition of urates in various tissues. For patients receiving Benemid, an ample fluid intake is important, as are measures directed toward keeping the urine alkaline (through the administration of sodium bicarbonate, for instance). When probenecid and drugs with similar action are given over a period of several years or at least of many months, they frequently also reduce the size of the already established tophaceous deposits, provided, of course, the subject is not suffering from chronic renal insufficiency (see Smyth, Gutman and Yü, Bartels, de Sèze *et al.,* and also Svendsen).

Though probenecid was among the first urate eliminants to be widely employed in the treatment of gout, a number of additional and apparently more potent uricosuric agents have now come into use. They include, notably, sulfinpyrazone (Anturane) and zoxazolamine (Flexin) and are particularly indicated for patients who have failed to respond adequately to probenecid. These more potent urate eliminants are useful mainly during the periods between acute attacks of the gouty arthritis—that is, during the intercritical or quiescent phases of the disease. When administering these newer uricosuric drugs, a large fluid intake and alkalinization of the urine will aid in the prevention of urate deposition in the urinary tract. This aim is also furthered by keeping the dosage of these drugs as low at first as possible while still maintaining its therapeutic effectiveness (see Seegmiller and Grayzel, and Lucey). Patients who are being given these newer uricosuric drugs should also receive maintenance doses of colchicine, especially if the dosage of these uricosuric drugs is being gradually increased (see Leng-Lévy *et al.*).

Additional progress in the therapy of gout is represented by the concept of employing drugs which inhibit or reduce the synthesis of uric acid in the course of endogenous purine metabolism. One of these drugs (Allopurinol) is hydroxy-pyrazolo (3,4-d) pyrimidine. This is an isomer of hypoxanthine which acts by inhibiting the enzyme xanthinoxidase, thereby reducing the conversion of the oxypurines xanthine and hypoxanthine into uric acid. In consequence, the plasma uric acid level falls and the amount of uric acid excreted in the urine is decreased, while the urinary excretion of xanthine is increased (see Hall *et al.*, and Delbarre *et al.*). Allopurinol (HPP) is usually administered in daily doses of about 300 mg. If the patient develops an acute attack of gouty arthritis in the course of its use, colchicine should be given in addition. In cases in which gout is associated with renal impairment, Allopurinol seems preferable to the uricosuric drugs, which may aggravate the renal damage by loading the renal tubules with uric acid.

Although, as indicated, modern drug therapy is of definite value in ameliorating or preventing the development of destructive chronic tophaceous lesions, there are still cases in which the *surgical removal of tophaceous deposits* is appropriate. This is true especially when one or both hands or feet are distorted by tophaceous masses in the soft tissues and there is concomitant involvement of underlying bone, so that function of the parts is grossly impeded. Other indications for surgery include pain from pressure upon nerves and/or the presence of draining sinuses (with or without infection) extending from the surface of the tophus into underlying bone. The appropriate surgical procedures, the postoperative care of the patient, and the cosmetic effects which may be achieved through surgery are discussed in the various articles on the surgical management of chronic tophaceous gout (see Woughter, Straub *et al.*, and Larmon and Kurtz).

REFERENCES

BARTELS, E. C.: Gout—Now Amenable to Control, Ann. Int. Med., *42*, 1, 1955.

BERK, M. E.: Gout: Report of an Unusual Case in a Young Man, Am. J. M. Sc., *215*, 290, 1948.

BERNSTEIN, S. S.: Gout in Early Life, J. Mt. Sinai Hosp., *14*, 747, 1947.

BROGSITTER, A. M.: Histopathologie der Gelenkgicht, Deutsches Arch. klin. Med., *153*, 257, 1926.

————: Histopathologie der Gelenkgicht, Deutsches Arch. klin. Med., *154*, 1, 1926–27.

BUNIM, J. J., and McEWEN, C.: Tophus of the Mitral Valve in Gout, Arch. Path., *29*, 700, 1940.

DELBARRE, F., AUSCHER, C., LABROUSSE, C., and DE GERY, A.: Le traitement de la dyspurinie goutteuse par les paramétabolites et, notamment, par un inhibiteur de la xanthine-oxydase, Presse méd., *73*, 1275, 1965.

DE SÈZE, S., RYCKEWAERT, A., and D'ANGLEJAN, G.: Le traitement de la goutte par le probénécide, Rev. rhumat., *30*, 93, 1963.

DUNCAN, H., and DIXON, A. ST. J.: Gout, Familial Hyperuricaemia, and Renal Disease, Quart. J. Med., *29*, 127, 1960.

EMMERSON, B. T.: Heredity in Primary Gout, Australasian Ann. Med., *9*, 168, 1960.

FAIRES, J. S., and McCARTY, D. J., JR.: Acute Arthritis in Man and Dog after Intrasynovial Injection of Sodium Urate Crystals, Lancet, *2*, 682, 1962.

FISCHER, E.: *Untersuchungen in der Puringruppe*, Berlin, Julius Springer, 1907.

GARROD, A. B.: Observations on Certain Pathological Conditions of the Blood and Urine in Gout, Rheumatism and Bright's Disease, Med.-Chir. Tr. London, *31*, 83, 1848.

————: *A Treatise on Gout and Rheumatic Gout. (Rheumatoid Arthritis.)* 3rd ed., London, Longmans, Green, & Co., 1876.

GONICK, H. C., RUBINI, M. E., GLEASON, I. O., and SOMMERS, S. C.: The Renal Lesion in Gout, Ann. Int. Med., *62*, 667, 1965.

GOOD, A. E., and FRISHETTE, W. A.: Crystals in Dried Smears of Synovial Fluid, J.A.M.A., *198*, 80, 1966.

GREENBAUM, D., ROSS, J. H., and STEINBERG, V. L.: Renal Biopsy in Gout, Brit. M. J., *1*, 1502, 1961.

GUDZENT, F.: *Gicht und Rheumatismus*, Berlin, Julius Springer, 1928.

GUTMAN, A. B.: Primary and Secondary Gout, Ann. Int. Med., *39*, 1062, 1953.

GUTMAN, A. B., and YÜ, T. F.: Prevention and Treatment of Chronic Gouty Arthritis, J.A.M.A., *157*, 1096, 1955.

HALL, A. P., HOLLOWAY, V. P., and SCOTT, J. T.: 4-Hydroxypyrazolo (3,4-d) Pyrimidine (HPP) in the Treatment of Gout: Preliminary Observations, Ann. Rheumat. Dis., *23*, 439, 1964.

HALL, M. C., and SELIN, G.: Spinal Involvement in Gout, J. Bone & Joint Surg., *42-A*, 341, 1960.

HAUGE, M., and HARVALD, B.: Heredity in Gout and Hyperuricemia, Acta med. scandinav., *152*, 247, 1955.

HENCH, P. S., and DARNALL, C. M.: A Clinic on Acute, Old-fashioned Gout; with Special Reference to Its Inciting Factors, M. Clin. North America, *16*, 1371, 1933 (see p. 1376).

KAEGI, P.: Echte Gicht bei der Frau, Schweiz. med. Wchnschr., *85*, 698, 1955.

LANG, F. J.: Gelenkgicht (Arthritis urica), Handb. spez. path. Anat. u. Histol. Knochen u. Gelenke, *9(3)*, 309, 1937.

LARMON, W. A., and KURTZ, J. F.: The Surgical Management of Chronic Tophaceous Gout, J. Bone & Joint Surg., *40-A*, 743, 1958.

LENG-LÉVY, J., DAVID-CHAUSSÉ, J., AUBERTIN, J., and LASSERRE, M.: L'Anturan dans le traitement de la goutte, J. méd. Bordeaux, *139*, 57, 1962.

LICHTENSTEIN, L., SCOTT, H. W., and LEVIN, M. H.: Pathologic Changes in Gout, Am. J. Path., *32*, 871, 1956.

LUCEY, C.: Anturan in the Treatment of Gout, Irish J. M. Sc., *6*, 113, 1961.

MALAWISTA, S. E., and SEEGMILLER, J. E.: The Effect of Pretreatment with Colchicine on the Inflammatory Response to Microcrystalline Urate, Ann. Int. Med., *62*, 648, 1965.

MALAWISTA, S. E., SEEGMILLER, J. E., HATHAWAY, B. E., and SOKOLOFF, L.: Sacroiliac Gout, J.A.M.A., *194*, 954, 1965.

McCARTY, D. J., JR.: Phagocytosis of Urate Crystals in Gouty Synovial Fluid, Am. J. M. Sc., *243*, 288, 1962.

MELLINGHOFF, C. H., and GROSS, R. H.: Erfahrungen über die Gicht, insbesondere über die uricosurische Therapie mit Anturan, Ztschr. Rheumaforsch., *21*, 42, 1962.

MOORE, N.: Some Observations on the Morbid Anatomy of Gout, St. Bartholomew's Hosp. Rep., *23*, 289, 1887.

MUNCK, A.: Die Niere bei der Gicht, Beitr. path. Anat., *133*, 409, 1966.

PAULLEY, J. W., BARLOW, K. E., CUTTING, P. E. J., and STEVENS, J.: Acute Gouty Pericarditis, Lancet, *1*, 21, 1963.

POMMER, G.: *Mikroskopische Untersuchungen über Gelenkgicht*, Jena, Gustav Fischer, 1929.

RECHT, L.: A Case of Severe Gout in a Woman Aged 27, Acta med. scandinav., *150*, 189, 1954.

RIESELBACH, R. E., SORENSEN, L. B., SHELP, W. D., and STEELE, T. H.: Diminished Renal Urate Secretion Per Nephron As a Basis for Primary Gout, Ann. Int. Med., *73*, 359, 1970.

ROBINSON, W. D.: Current Status of the Treatment of Gout, J.A.M.A., *164*, 1670, 1957.

RODNAN, G. P., and BENEDEK, T. G.: Ancient Therapeutic Arts in the Gout, Arthritis Rheum., *6*, 317, 1963.

ROSENQUIST, R. C., SMALL, C. S., and DEEB, P. H.: Unusual Manifestations of Gout, Arch. Path., *68*, 1, 1959.

SCHEELE, K. W.: Examen chemicum Calculi urinarii, Opuscula, *2*, 73, 1776.

SCHLUMBERGER, H. G.: Synovial Gout in the Parakeet, Lab. Invest., *8*, 1304, 1959.

SEEGMILLER, J. E., and LASTER, L.: The Metabolic Origin of Uric Acid, in *Progress in Arthritis*, edited by J. H. Talbott and L. M. Lockie, New York, Grune & Stratton, 1958 (p. 341).

SEEGMILLER, J. E., and GRAYZEL, A. I.: Use of the Newer Uricosuric Agents in the Management of Gout, J.A.M.A., *173*, 1076, 1960.

SHEPHERD-WILSON, W., and GELFAND, M.: Gout in the African, Central African J. Med., *8*, 181, 1962.

SHERMAN, M. S.: Pathologic Changes in Gouty Arthritis, Arch. Path., *42*, 557, 1946.

SILLER, W. G.: Avian Nephritis and Visceral Gout, Lab. Invest., *8*, 1319, 1959.

SMYTH, C. J.: Current Therapy of Gout, J.A.M.A., *152*, 1106, 1953.

SMYTH, C. J., COTTERMAN, C. W., and FREYBERG, R. H.: The Genetics of Gout and Hyperuricemia—An Analysis of Nineteen Families, J. Clin. Invest., *27*, 749, 1948.

STECHER, R. M., HERSH, A. H., and SOLOMON, W. M.: The Heredity of Gout and Its Relationship to Familial Hyperuricemia, Ann. Int. Med., *31*, 595, 1949.

STEINDLER, A.: On Atypical Gout, Bull. Hosp. Joint Dis., *12*, 404, 1951.

STETTEN, D., JR.: On the Metabolic Defect in Gout, Bull. New York Acad. Med., *28*, 664, 1952.

————: Gout, Perspectives in Biol. & Med., *2*, 185, 1959.

STRAUB, L. R., SMITH, J. W., CARPENTER, G. K., JR., and DIETZ, G. H.: The Surgery of Gout in the Upper Extremity, J. Bone & Joint Surg., *43-A*, 731, 1961.

SVENDSEN, H. M.: Probenecidbehandling av arthritis urica, Tidsskr. norske laegefor., *77*, 1049, 1957.

SYDENHAM, T.: *Selected Works. With a Short Biography and Explanatory Notes*, by J. D. Comrie, London, John Bale, Sons & Danielsson, Ltd., 1922. (P. 57: A Treatise on the Gout.)

TALBOTT, J. H.: The Diversity of Gouty Arthritis and Its Complications, Ann. Int. Med., *31*, 555, 1949.

———: *Gout*, New York, Grune & Stratton, 1957.

TALBOTT, J. H., and COOMBS, F. S.: The Concentration of Serum Uric Acid in Non-affected Members of Gouty Families, J. Clin. Invest., *17*, 508, 1938.

VORHAUS, M. G.: Gout in Woman, Bull. Hosp. Joint Dis., *10*, 202, 1949.

WHITAKER, J. A., SHAHEEDY, M., BAUM, J., JAMES, J., and FLUME, J. B.: Gout in Childhood Leukemia, J. Pediat., *63*, 961, 1963.

WOLLASTON, W. H.: On Gouty and Urinary Concretions, Philosoph. Tr. Roy. Soc. London, *87*, 386, 1797.

WOUGHTER, H. W.: Surgery of Tophaceous Gout, J. Bone & Joint Surg., *41-A*, 116, 1959.

YÜ, T. F., and GUTMAN, A. B.: Efficacy of Colchicine Prophylaxis in Gout: Prevention of Recurrent Gouty Arthritis Over a Mean Period of Five Years in 208 Gouty Subjects, Ann. Int. Med., *55*, 179, 1961.

———: Uric Acid Nephrolithiasis in Gout: Predisposing Factors, Ann. Int. Med., *67*, 1133, 1967.

Chapter

18

Gaucher's Disease and Certain Other Inborn Metabolic Disorders

The diseases based upon inborn errors of metabolism are numerous. Gout, which is one of these diseases, was given detailed consideration in the preceding chapter, since gout is a relatively common disorder and conspicuously involves the joints and para-articular tissues. In the chapter devoted to rickets and osteomalacia, attention was given to several disease entities which also have their basis in inborn errors of metabolism, but which were discussed in that chapter because the skeletal manifestations of the diseases in question take the form of rickets or osteomalacia. Thus that chapter contains a discussion of hypophosphatasia, which develops because of an inborn deficiency in the formation of the enzyme alkaline phosphatase (p. 437). It also gave consideration to rickets and osteomalacia based on defects (apparently inborn) in the capacity of the renal tubules to reabsorb various substances filtered out by the glomeruli (p. 407). The conditions discussed under the heading of "the celiac syndrome" in that chapter include gluten-induced enteropathy (p. 402), which is likewise the result of an inborn enzyme defect.

In the present chapter we shall devote attention to a few of the many *lipidoses* and, in particular, to *Gaucher's disease* and *Niemann-Pick disease*, making some reference in the latter connection to *amaurotic family idiocy*. These three lipidoses all have a hereditary basis, and each of them may pursue either an acute fulminating course or a less rapidly progressive course, which, in the case of Gaucher's disease, is not infrequently mild and chronic. The other conditions to be discussed include *essential familial hypercholesterolemia* (a hereditary disorder of cholesterol metabolism), *gargoylism*, or *Hurler's syndrome* (a hereditary disorder of mucopolysaccharide metabolism), and *ochronosis* (a hereditary disorder based upon an inborn error of intermediary metabolism involving the amino acids tyrosine and phenylalanine). Another condition which will be considered is *lipid (cholesterol) granulomatosis*—a very rare condition whose basis in an inborn error of metabolism has not yet been clearly established but which may well represent an expression of so-called familial or idiopathic hyperlipemia.

GAUCHER'S DISEASE

Gaucher's disease is characterized by the presence, in various tissues, of cells laden with cerebrosides—mainly glucocerebroside, which is an analogue of the lipid kerasin, a galactocerebroside. The cells in question (commonly designated as Gaucher cells) are modified reticulum cells and histiocytes. They are most abundant in the spleen, liver, bone marrow, and lymph nodes.

Formerly it had been held that the reticulum cells and histiocytes imbibed the cerebrosides present in their cytoplasm from the circulating tissue fluids. The current conception is that the glucocerebroside found in the cytoplasm of the modified reticulum cells and histiocytes (the Gaucher cells) is actually synthesized by them. Furthermore, it is maintained that the glycolipids of the stroma of the red blood cells are the precursor substances of the cerebrosides found in the Gaucher cells. The following possibilities have been entertained to explain the accumulation of glucocerebroside in the reticulum cells and histiocytes: (1) an excessive formation of glucocerebroside from the glycolipids; (2) an intracellular enzymatic defect characterized by an inability of the cells to hydrolyze or degrade the accumulating glucocerebroside; and (3) the intracellular degradation of the glucocerebroside to a highly insoluble compound, even though the actual amount of glucocerebroside formed is not excessive (see Statter and Shapiro, Svennerholm and Svennerholm, Kennaway and Woolf, and also Patrick).

It is the accumulation of the Gaucher cells in the spleen, liver, bone marrow, and lymph nodes that gives rise to the characteristic clinical and anatomic features of the disease. In sufficiently protracted cases, these features consist notably of splenomegaly, hepatomegaly, and skeletal alterations, but also include hematologic abnormalities and lymphadenopathy.

Of historical interest is the fact that, though Gaucher seems to have been the first to describe the disease, his interpretation of its pathologic basis was incorrect. He believed that the disease which bears his name was "a primary epithelioma of the spleen," and in particular that it represented an "idiopathic hypertrophy of the spleen without leukemia." The modern conception of the condition was formulated by Mandlebaum and Downey, who associated the formation of the Gaucher cell with a disorder of endogenous metabolism. Subsequently, Epstein and also Lieb reported that the distinctive substance in the cytoplasm of the Gaucher cell consists mainly of kerasin (galactocerebroside). More precise chemical studies made later by others demonstrated that the lipid present in the Gaucher cells was mainly glucocerebroside—an analogue of kerasin (see Rosenberg and Chargaff). The modern conception of the pathologic anatomy of Gaucher's disease (and particularly of its skeletal aspects) dates from the work of Pick. He not only described in detail the changes to be observed in the liver, spleen, and lymph nodes, but gave special attention to those occurring in the bones.

CLINICAL CONSIDERATIONS

It seems likely that in most if not all of the cases of Gaucher's disease the underlying metabolic disorder is already present at birth. However, there are wide variations in the clinical course of the disease, apparently conditioned by differences among the affected subjects in regard to the severity of the basic metabolic imbalance. As a rule, the disease progresses slowly and insidiously and its presence is not discovered until some time during childhood and occasionally even not until adulthood. In these cases, which ordinarily pursue a protracted (or chronic) course, it is usually enlargement of the spleen that first directs attention to the disease. Occasionally the disease progresses so rapidly after birth that the subject succumbs during infancy. In these cases (representing the so-called acute, or malignant, form of the condition), the clinical manifestations are those of a rapidly advancing cachexia associated not only with enlargement of the spleen and liver but also with neurological disturbances. However, increasing consideration is being given to the possibility that in the acute, or malignant, form of the disease one is dealing with a more complex metabolic disorder than that present in the cases in which the clinical course is protracted.

Incidence and Genetic Aspects.—Gaucher's disease is a rather uncommon disorder. It exhibits a *racial incidence*, indicated by the striking preponderance of persons of Hebrew descent among the subjects. Moreover, it has been found that within the Hebrew group the disease is much more prevalent among Jews whose ancestors had lived for centuries in central and northern Europe (Ashkenazic Jews) than among Jews whose ancestors had lived for centuries in Spain, Turkey (European part) and other countries bordering upon the Mediterranean (Sephardic Jews). Indeed, it is held that Gaucher's disease is about 30 times as common among Ashkenazic Jews as among all other ethnic groups together, including Sephardic and Oriental Jews (see Fried and also Groen).

In regard to *sex incidence*, the statistical indications are that about as many males as females are affected. In relation to *age*, the presence of the disease is usually not apparent clinically until the subject has passed infancy. Many of the cases come to light during early or later childhood, and most of the rest during puberty or early adult life. However, there are some cases in which the disorder runs a very mild and torpid course, so that its presence may not be discovered until the subject is middle-aged or even elderly.

The *familial incidence* of Gaucher's disease is well established. Statistical evaluations have shown that, in groups of families in which the condition is known to exist, about one third of the members of the collected families are likely to be affected. Among the affected members there will be some (including adults) in whom the disease is still asymptomatic, its presence being established through the finding of Gaucher cells in stained smears of bone marrow obtained from the sternum or ilium (see Brill *et al.*, Hoffman and Makler, and Atkinson).

The *genetic aspects* of the disorder have not yet been fully clarified. When the metabolic defect underlying the disease appears for the first time in a family, it represents a mutation. Subsequently the genetic defect seems usually to be transmitted as an autosomal recessive trait, but there are some instances in which it seems to be transmitted as a somewhat aberrant autosomal dominant trait. In any event, in a family in which an ancestor had the disease, the likelihood that the latter will be present among the children and grandchildren of that ancestor is less than 50 per cent (see Hsia *et al.*, and Matoth and Fried).

Clinical Course and Findings.—As already noted, there are wide variations in the clinical course of the disease. Thus there are cases in which the clinical course is rather rapidly progressive. In some of these cases (representing the so-called *acute form* of the disorder), there are already clinical indications of the disease during the first few months of life, and the affected child usually dies before reaching the end of its first year. In other cases (representing what might be called the *subacute form* of the disease), the affected infant first shows evidence of the disorder during the second 6 months of life but survives for only a few years.

An infant who presents the acute, or malignant, form of Gaucher's disease has usually been born at full term of parents not affected with the disease. The infant ordinarily appears to be developing normally during the first month or two of life. After this, the child manifests gastrointestinal disturbances, fails to gain in weight, and presents other evidences of malnutrition. At this stage of the disease, the spleen and liver are already enlarging, although they may not yet be palpable. Soon thereafter, various neurological disturbances set in. These may take the form of a general hypertonia, expressed in an opisthotonos position of the head, exaggerated reflexes, and also tonic or clonic spasms of various voluntary muscles. In addition, the infant may exhibit strabismus, laryngospasm, and/or dysphagia. On the other hand, instead of showing hypertonia, the affected subject may be apathetic and hypotonic (see Frisell). The possible anatomic basis for the neurologic abnormalities in the malignant form of the disease is considered in the section dealing with the pathologic findings (p. 518).

Finally, it should be noted that the cases in which the presence of Gaucher's disease becomes apparent in infancy and in which the clinical course is rapid may represent a form of the disease based upon a more complex disturbance of lipid metabolism than the cases in which the disease runs a chronic course (see de Lange).

A *chronic course* is the one pursued by Gaucher's disease in most instances. In this form of the disorder the disease progresses slowly, and its presence may first be revealed clinically during later childhood or even during adult life. In these cases the disease, if properly treated, is not incompatible with survival into middle adult life and even into old age.

It is nearly always enlargement of the spleen that first directs attention to the disease, but some authentic cases have been reported in which there was no splenomegaly (see Morgans). The liver may already be found enlarged when the splenomegaly is discovered. Like the spleen (though less rapidly, and not in the same proportion), the liver becomes still larger as the disease progresses. The superficial lymph nodes, as a rule, are not enlarged. Even early in the disease, there may already be diffuse or spotty yellow-brown pigmentation of the skin largely confined to the face, neck, and hands. In addition, one or both eyes may show, especially on the nasal side, a yellow-brown wedge-shaped thickening of the bulbar conjunctiva (pinguecula), the base of the wedge lying toward the sclerocorneal junction. The hematologic findings at this stage of the disease usually reveal anemia (generally of the hypochromic type and ordinarily not severe), leukopenia (not associated with significant changes in the differential count), and also a thrombocytopenia of mild to moderate degree. (See Pick, Reich *et al.*, and Medoff and Bayrd.)

Though ordinarily the clinical picture is dominated by enlargement of the spleen and liver, it is not unusual to find, in addition, skeletal alterations, at least on roentgenographic examination of the bones. It may even be pain caused by a skeletal lesion that first directs attention to the presence of the disease. One of the most common sources of pain referable to the skeleton is partial collapse of one or both femoral heads and resultant deformity of the femoral head and neck. Extensive necrosis of Gaucher cells in the shaft of a long bone may follow upon thrombosis of intra-osseous blood vessels. This may give rise to an episode of acute and severe bone pain, and be associated with local heat, local swelling, and some fever. Concomitantly the leukocyte count may be elevated, and the total clinical picture may suggest acute hematogenous pyogenic osteomyelitis. The clinical complex in question has been designated as "aseptic osteomyelitis in Gaucher's disease" (see Yossipovitch *et al.*). However, it has sometimes led to an unnecessary surgical intervention because of misinterpretation of the clinical findings as those of pyogenic osteomyelitis.

Clinical difficulties relating to the skeleton may arise in other ways also. Occasionally a fracture of the shaft of an involved long bone or rib, for instance, may take place. When vertebral bodies are severely affected, there may be kyphosis resulting from collapse of one or more vertebral bodies. Those rare cases in which the skeletal involvement is extensive and complaints ascribable to it come to dominate the clinical picture have sometimes been held to represent the "osseous form" of the disease, and it has been pointed out that in some families all the affected members manifest the disease in this form (see Pick).

As already noted, the chronic cases often pursue a course extending over several decades. Instances have been reported in which subjects have survived beyond middle life. Late in the course of the disease, there may be a pronounced thrombocytopenia, associated with bleeding from various mucous membranes and with hemorrhage, following even slight trauma, into the skin, subcutaneous tissues, and deeper tissues. In the past (that is, before the era of antibiotics), death was usually due to an intercurrent disease, only rarely resulting directly from cachexia or anemia.

In the clinical *diagnosis* of Gaucher's disease, the most helpful guide is the presence of splenomegaly, although, as noted, there are rare cases in which splenomegaly is not evident. The demonstration of Gaucher cells in stained *smears of bone marrow* (ordinarily obtained from the sternum) is incontrovertible evidence of the presence of the disease. Moreover, it is only exceptionally that one cannot demonstrate the Gaucher cells in sternal marrow smears when the disease is actually present. Failure to find them under these circumstances should lead one to suspect faulty technique rather than absence of the cells in question. Such failure can often be avoided if one examines particularly the thicker parts of the smear, which are usually located along its periphery. In the stained marrow smears, the cells stand out because of their large size, often measuring as much as 40 micra in diameter. Each cell has one or two nuclei. These tend to be small in proportion to the size of the cell as a whole and are usually eccentrically located. The cell cytoplasm presents a coarse, meshy, wrinkled, fibrillar texture.

A biochemical finding of diagnostic significance in relation to Gaucher's disease is an *elevated serum acid phosphatase* value. In 8 cases of Gaucher's disease reported by Tuchman *et al.*, the serum acid phosphatase values (as determined by the Carr modification of the King-Armstrong method) ranged from 4.8 to 11.7 units. Furthermore, in only one of these 8 patients was the value below 7.0 units. The normal values obtained by the method used range only up to 4.0 units. Significance attaches also to the fact that 3 of the 8 patients were females, and that 3 of the 5 males were less than $9\frac{1}{2}$ years of age. In a case of Gaucher's disease reported by Tuchman and Swick, a number of serum acid phosphatase determinations were

Figure 127

A, Roentgenograph showing changes in the upper end of the right femur in the case of a boy 7 years of age affected with Gaucher's disease. The femoral head is flattened, and the shadow it casts shows intermingled areas of radiopacity and radiolucency reflecting the results of the aseptic necrosis which has taken place in the capital femoral epiphysis. The normal trabecular markings in the femoral neck have been largely obliterated, undoubtedly because of crowding of the intertrabecular marrow spaces with Gaucher cells and consequent pressure atrophy of the local osseous trabeculae.

B, Roentgenograph showing striking changes in the head and neck of the left femur in the case of a boy 9 years of age affected with Gaucher's disease. One year before this picture was taken, he had undergone splenectomy. Six months after that surgical intervention, he began to experience pain in the hip. The pain increased and was associated with a limp. Physical examination revealed diminished internal and external rotation at the hip joint, limitation of abduction, and evidence of some atrophy of the left lower extremity. Note the pronounced flattening of the head, its "fragmented" appearance, the increased radiopacity of the femoral neck, and the subperiosteal new bone deposition on its cortex.

C, Roentgenograph illustrating the status of the hip joints and the proximal halves of both femora in a woman 28 years of age affected with Gaucher's disease who had undergone splenectomy about 20 years before this x-ray picture was taken. She had bouts of pain referable to the hip joints, and mobility of the latter was restricted. The head of each femur is enlarged and presents extensive alterations in contour, and the acetabulum on each side slopes. In the head and neck of the femur on the left, numerous small roundish radiolucencies intermingled with areas of radiopacity are to be noted. The shaft cortex of that femur is much thinner than the cortex of the opposite femur and is also mottled with small focal radiolucencies. (I am indebted to Dr. Raphael R. Goldenberg, formerly Director of Orthopaedic Surgery at St. Joseph's Hospital, Paterson, New Jersey, for placing at my disposal the x-ray pictures from which this illustration and Figure 128-*C* and *D* were reproduced.)

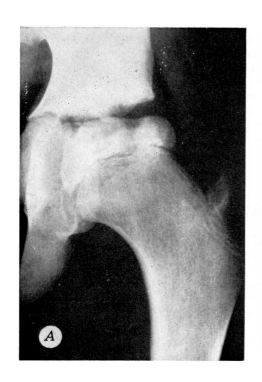

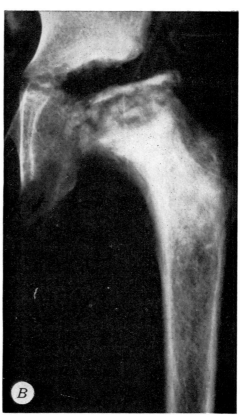

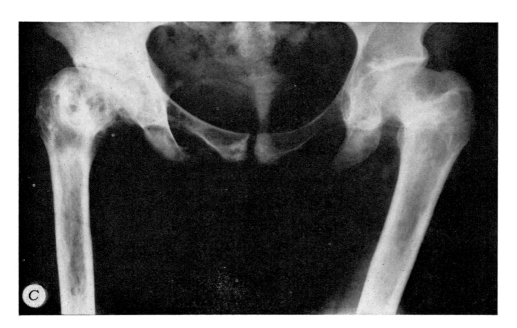

Figure 127

carried out, and all the values were found to be above 7.0 units as determined by the Gutman modification of the King-Armstrong method (normal values obtained by that technique being 0.5 to 3.0 units). In that case the patient was a man 68 years of age who showed evidences of "prostatism." The associated high acid phosphatase value naturally suggested the possibility of a carcinoma of the prostate. When this possibility was eliminated by biopsy of the prostate, it was realized and established that the case was one of asymptomatic Gaucher's disease. That the serum acid phosphatase value is elevated in Gaucher's disease is now a firmly established fact. Since the increased serum acid phosphatase is of nonprostatic origin, it is to be considered a reflection of the underlying metabolic abnormality (see Crocker and Landing).

ROENTGENOGRAPHIC FINDINGS

It has long been recognized that there is wide variation in the roentgenographic skeletal changes to be observed among the different cases of Gaucher's disease. Whether and to what extent bone changes will be found depends mainly upon the age of the subject and on whether, in the case in question, there has been sufficient infiltration of the bone marrow by Gaucher cells to affect the osseous tissue directly. As a rule, those subjects manifesting the disease in its chronic form (that is, older children, adolescents, or adults) show at least some roentgenographic skeletal alterations, but occasionally an affected young child already shows very pronounced changes. (See Figs. 127 and 128.) Infants manifesting the disease in its acute, or

Figure 128

A, Roentgenograph illustrating the so-called "clubbing" of the distal part of the femoral shafts in a case of Gaucher's disease. The medial surface of the femur on the left is slightly convex in contour instead of being concave, as it would normally be. The medial surface of the femur on the right shows alterations tending in the same direction, but to a lesser degree. Note also that in both femora the cortex, especially on the medial side of the shaft, is thinned. The reduced radiodensity of the shafts of both bones indicates the presence of osteoporosis, which is also due in part to thinning of the spongy bone. The patient was a man who was 27 years of age at the time of his first admission to the hospital. His spleen was enlarged, but his difficulties related mainly to the hip joints (see B), which had been more or less painful since he was 10 years of age.

B, Roentgenograph showing the flattening deformity of the femoral heads of the patient mentioned in A.

C and D, Roentgenographs of the distal thirds of the right femur (C) and left femur (D) in the case of the woman 28 years of age to whom reference was made in connection with Figure 127-C. The large oval radiolucent defect apparent in the right femur had evolved spontaneously—that is, it does not represent the result of a surgical intervention. It may be inferred from our knowledge relating to the pathologic anatomy of Gaucher's disease that the lesional tissue at the site of the defect had undergone necrosis and partial fibrous replacement, and that the local spongy and cortical bone had also become necrotic and had been extensively resorbed. The trabecular markings below the well-delineated defect in the shaft of the right femur show thinning and disorganization. This reflects the crowding of the intertrabecular marrow spaces with Gaucher cells, resorption of spongy trabeculae in consequence of pressure from the compacted cells and/or necrosis of masses of these cells. In the left femur the roundish area delineated by the arrows apparently represents an earlier stage in the evolution of the clear-cut radiolucent defect shown by the right femur. The mottled radiolucencies in the rest of the shaft and in the condylar region of the left femur reflect the resorption of spongy and cortical bone ensuing upon secondary changes (necrosis and scarring) in the Gaucher material.

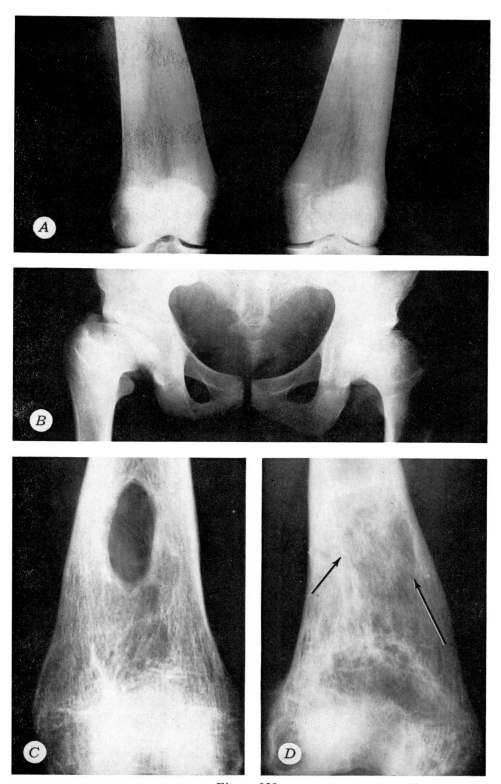

Figure 128

malignant, form ordinarily do not have skeletal changes observable roentgeno-graphically, since they usually die before the end of the first year of life. (See Strickland, Rourke and Heslin, Tennent, Jackson and Simon, and also Levin.)

In cases of chronic Gaucher's disease, one of the most common findings is some degree of expansion of the contour of various long tubular bones and thinning of their cortices. This is most frequently observed in the lower part of the shaft of each femur. The expansion of the lower end of the femoral shaft is characterized by thinning of the cortex and by loss of the normal concave outline of its medial wall. Thus, instead of being concave, the medial wall of the femoral shaft may be straight or somewhat convex, and this change may be associated with some localized thinning and bulging of the lateral wall also, thus producing the so-called "Erlen-meyer flask" appearance. In addition, the somewhat bulged lower portion of the femoral shaft is likely to show partial obliteration of the normal trabecular mark-ings in consequence of pressure atrophy of spongy trabeculae.

In some cases one may find not only diffuse rarefaction of the lower ends of the femora but discrete patchy or loculated areas of radiolucency resulting from destruc-tion of the local spongy bone and even resorption of the neighboring cortex. Inter-mingled with the radiolucent areas, there may also be irregular areas of radiopacity representing sclerotic changes occurring in reaction to necrosis of intramedullary masses of Gaucher's cells. Occasionally, also, there may be evidence of a slight degree of subperiosteal new bone deposition. These various changes are not, of course, necessarily limited to the femora, but have also been observed in other long tubular bones. The undermining of the integrity of long tubular bones may result in pathologic fractures, and severely affected vertebral bodies have been known to undergo collapse. (See Greenfield.)

The *head* of one *femur* (or more commonly of both femora) frequently presents rather striking roentgenographic changes. The latter commonly set in during childhood, ordinarily between the ages of 5 and 10 years, and the changes are likely to become advanced in the course of about a year (see Arkin and Schein, Todd and Keidan, Amstutz and Carey, and also Wood). Under these circum-stances, the femoral head appears flattened and fragmented, the picture suggesting conventional Legg-Perthes-Calvé disease, which is, of course, the result of so-called idiopathic necrosis of the capital femoral epiphysis (p. 566). Actually, the altera-tions in the femoral head in Gaucher's disease have their basis in crowding of the marrow spaces of the spongiosa in the capital femoral epiphysis and in the femoral

Figure 129

A, Photomicrograph ($\times$ 125) of a tissue section prepared from the spleen which had been removed from the boy referred to in Figure 127-*B*, which illustrates the roentgenographic changes in the head of the left femur in that case. The splenectomy had been done when the boy was 8 years of age. The pulp of the spleen is crowded with the clearly delineated large cells representing Gaucher cells.

B, Photomicrograph ($\times$ 1,100) showing several Gaucher cells in a thin (1 μ) section prepared from a Vestopal-embedded block and stained by the PAS technique. The striations visible in the cytoplasm are held to contain the glucocerebroside which accumulates in the Gaucher cells. (This illustration from the article by Fisher and Reidbord was reproduced with the kind permission of the authors and the editor of the American Journal of Pathology.)

C, Photomicrograph ($\times$ 125) illustrating the histologic pattern presented by the Gaucher cells in an intertrabecular marrow space of a rib removed at autopsy in a case of Gaucher's disease. On the left, most of the Gaucher cells are roundish or polyhedral. Toward the right, it can be seen that many of the Gaucher cells are spindle-shaped rather than polyhedral. The subject in this case was a man 46 years of age who died of cardiac failure following myocardial infarction.

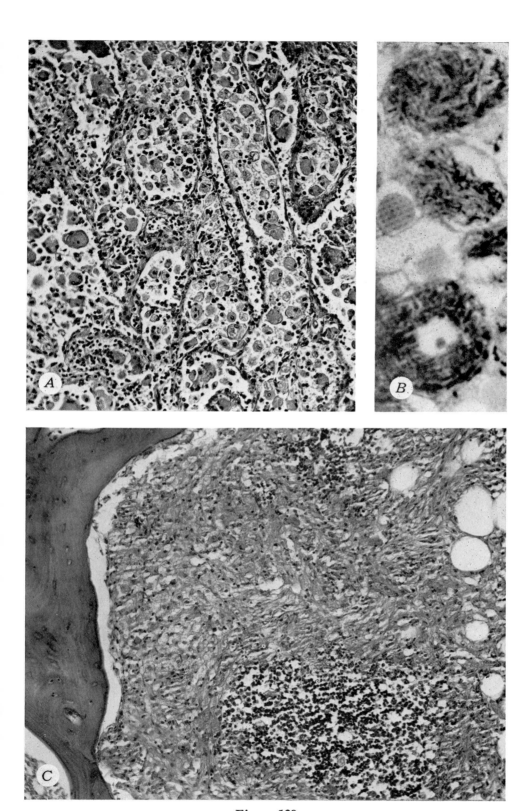

Figure 129

neck by masses of Gaucher cells. The resultant compression of the intra-osseous blood vessels, and/or infiltration of the walls of these vessels, by the Gaucher cells interferes with the local blood supply, and thus leads to aseptic necrosis of part or even most of the femoral head. Partial restitution of the altered capital femoral epiphysis can often be obtained by prolonged treatment of the child with non-weight-bearing in abduction. In any event, residual deformity of the femoral head is usually the basis for the development of osteoarthritis of the hip joint if the subject survives into middle age. Finally, it should be noted that, in an occasional case, roentgenographic changes analogous to those appearing in the femoral heads have also been noted in the humeral heads (see Rourke and Heslin).

PATHOLOGIC FINDINGS

Histology of the Gaucher Cell.—In its typical form, as observed notably in the spleen, the Gaucher cell is a large polyhedral cell. In the bone marrow the Gaucher cells may present the same general appearance, but it is more likely that many of them will be found elongated and even spindle-shaped rather than polyhedral. Sections prepared from splenic tissue which has been fixed in formalin or Zenker-acetic acid and stained with hematoxylin and eosin show that the cytoplasm of the Gaucher cells is faintly eosinophilic and that it contains barely visible eosinophilic striations. The nucleus (of which an individual cell may have more than one) is often eccentrically located.

Electron microscopy has revealed that the cytoplasmic striations observed in sections viewed with the light microscope correspond to ultramicroscopic bodies of various shapes (see Fisher and Reidbord). Furthermore, the localization of the PAS-reactive material and protein to these bodies suggests that the latter contain the glucocerebroside which is the product of the metabolic aberration underlying Gaucher's disease (see DeMarsh and Kautz). These studies add support to the current belief that the accumulation of the cerebroside in question in the Gaucher cells (mainly modified reticulum cells) is the result of an intracellular enzymatic defect—possibly a deficiency of *glucocerebrosidase* (see Patrick). The presence of hydrolytic enzymes (particularly acid phosphatase) in the Gaucher cells seems to give additional weight to this concept (see Crocker and Landing). (See Fig. 129.)

Figure 130

A, Photograph of the cut surface of the upper half of a femur removed at autopsy in a case of Gaucher's disease. The patient, a woman, was 29 years of age at the time of her death. That she was affected with Gaucher's disease was already recognized when she was 12 years of age, and she had undergone splenectomy when she was 20 years of age. The enlarged spleen weighed 1,332 gm. Because the marrow spaces of the spongiosa are substantially filled with Gaucher cells, the spongiosa appears grayish. The part of the major marrow cavity shown in the picture is filled with Gaucher material which is grayish white in its proximal portion and hemorrhagically discolored in the distal portion of the area shown. In this case the femoral head has retained a more or less normal contour, apparently because there had been no substantial necrosis of the Gaucher cells.

B, Photograph showing the cut surface of four thoracic vertebral bodies representing part of the vertebral column removed at autopsy in a case of Gaucher's disease. The patient was a man 42 years of age whose spleen had been enlarging since he was 15 years old. He died the day following splenectomy, the spleen weighing 5,000 gm. The marrow spaces of the spongiosa of the vertebral bodies are substantially filled with Gaucher cells, which give the cut surface of the vertebrae a grayish color.

C, Photograph showing in somewhat greater detail the gross appearance of the vertebral body which is second from the top in *B*.

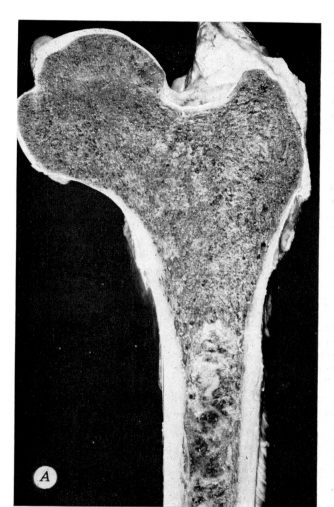

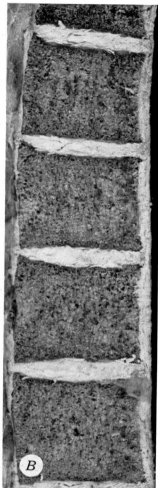

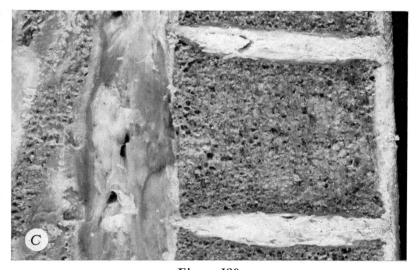

Figure 130

Nonskeletal Tissues.—The *spleen* is of a firm consistency and is usually very much enlarged and sometimes tremendously enlarged. In any group of collected cases, the weight of the spleen will be found to average about ten times the normal. When the spleen is sectioned, the reddish background of its cut surface appears mottled with gray-white or gray-yellow areas of many different sizes, representing accumulations of the Gaucher cells. Scattered over the surface, one will also find some larger or smaller cavernous foci filled with blood. In addition, there are usually some fibrous nodules representing areas in which masses of Gaucher cells, cavernous foci, or anemic or hemorrhagic infarcts have become scarified. While the *liver*, too, is enlarged, its weight on the average is only about twice the normal. Like that of the spleen, the cut surface of the liver presents numerous pale areas of various sizes. In some cases, furthermore, the liver may be rather cirrhotic. The intra-abdominal and intrathoracic *lymph nodes* will be found enlarged and otherwise involved, while the superficial ones tend to remain unaffected.

As evidences of the pronounced blood destruction which goes on in the disease, and of the *accumulation of blood pigments* (especially hemosiderin) in the spleen, liver, and lymph nodes, these tissues often show a chocolate-brown discoloration. In addition, some *iron-free pigment* may be found, for instance, in the smooth muscles of the stomach and intestines or uterus, or in the voluntary musculature. Autogenous pigment also causes the brown discoloration of the skin.

Various histologic changes have been reported as being present in the *central nervous system* of infants succumbing to the disease in its malignant form. Unfortunately, however, the number of pertinent studies is meager and there is a lack of agreement in regard to details. In the account by Oberling and Woringer, it was reported that the large and medium-sized pyramidal cells of the parietal and occipital region of the cerebral cortex showed vacuolation of the cytoplasmic matrix of

Figure 131

A, Photograph of a drawing showing the cut surface of the upper half of the right tibia, femur, and humerus removed at autopsy in the case of a man 56 years of age affected with Gaucher's disease. Since the age of 15 years, the subject had complaints relating to the right hip. These consisted of pain associated with a limp, and eventually the pain was so severe that walking had become extremely difficult. There is deformation of the femoral head, which has collapsed in consequence of necrosis of the Gaucher cells filling the intertrabecular marrow spaces. The femoral neck and the medullary cavity of the shaft show masses of scar tissue which has formed in response to necrosis of accumulated Gaucher cells. The involvement of the cortical bone has resulted in very extensive rarefaction of the latter. The changes presented by the tibia and humerus were similar to those in the femur. (This illustration was reproduced from Pick's monograph on Gaucher's disease, with the kind permission of the publishers.)

B, Photomicrograph ($\times$ 5) illustrating the histologic changes in the head of a femur in a case of Gaucher's disease. On the left side of the picture the marrow spaces of the spongiosa are filled with Gaucher cells, most of which, if visualized under higher magnification, would be found still viable. As one moves from the left toward the right of the picture, it becomes apparent that the Gaucher cells in many of the intertrabecular marrow spaces have undergone necrosis, and in some areas all of them are necrotic. Higher magnification would show that, in those areas where the Gaucher cells in these marrow spaces are necrotic, the spongy osseous tissue has also undergone aseptic necrosis. As a consequence of the necrosis, an osteochondral fragment (an osteochondritis dissecans-like body) has become delimited, though it is still attached on the right. If it had become completely detached, as it often does, and remained free in the joint cavity, this osteochondral body would have undergone enlargement by accretion and formed the core of a so-called "joint mouse." The subject in this case was a woman 38 years of age who showed similar changes in the opposite femur and also extensive changes of Gaucher's disease in many other bones.

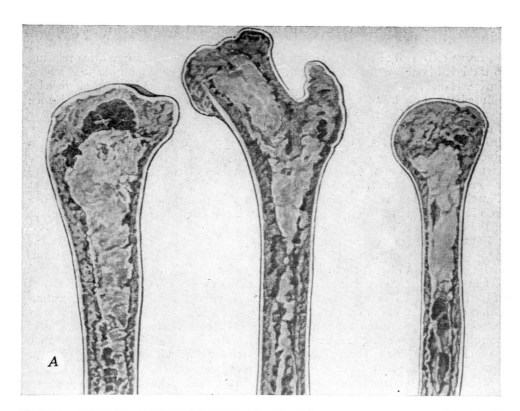

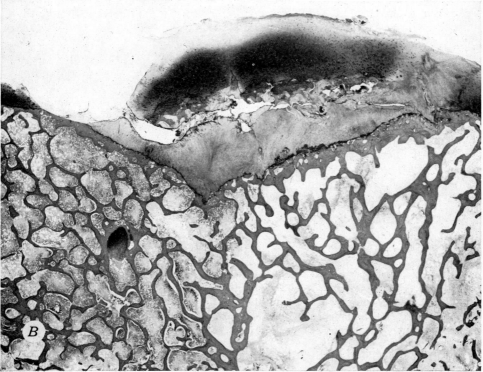

Figure 131

the nerve cells, and also degenerative changes and/or other abnormalities relating
to the Nissl bodies within the matrix.   In regard to the neuropathologic changes,
Banker *et al.* reported that in the 3 cases they studied the cerebral cortex showed a
diffuse but patchy loss of nerve cells in layers 3 and 5 of the cortex and a prominence
of microglia and Gaucher cells in the same location.   The salient findings in the
thalamus, basal ganglia, brain stem, spinal cord, and cerebellum in these cases were
profound nerve cell loss and a mild degree of intracytoplasmic accumulation of a
glycolipid.   Various microscopic changes in the ganglion cells of the brain have also
been recorded by others (see Lindau, Köhne, and also Geddes and Moore), but still
others have failed to find them (see Hamperl).   At any rate, there can be no doubt
that the central nervous system is affected in infants succumbing to Gaucher's disease in its malignant form, although certain inconsistencies relating to the details
of the changes have still to be clarified.

Bones.—The roentgenographic findings described above naturally express the
gross anatomic changes which have taken place in the bones.   The contributions
of Pick relating to the pathologic anatomy (and especially to the skeletal changes)
of Gaucher's disease have supplied a firm foundation of knowledge on this aspect
of the disorder.   The various anatomic studies have revealed that the mere accumulation of Gaucher cells in the marrow spaces of an affected bone is not necessarily
associated with obvious roentgenographic changes.   However, atrophy and/or
necrosis of Gaucher cell masses may occur, and this, with the resultant reactive
proliferation of dense fibrous tissue, is often the foundation for bone changes
observable roentgenographically.   Specifically, where such calloused tissue accumulates, the spongy trabeculae are usually resorbed and the adjacent cortex may even
become thinned from the medullary side.   Thinning of the cortex sometimes leads
to expansion of the diameter of the affected bone, but there is no tendency toward
perforation of the cortex in these cases.   Furthermore, it is important to note that,
no matter how severely the osseous tissue of a bone is affected, there is little tendency toward periosteal new bone formation or toward the infiltration of the periosteum or the periosteal surface of the bone with Gaucher cells.   (See Figs. 130
and 131.)

As to individual skeletal parts, it may be noted first that in a heavily involved
calvarium the marrow of the diploic spaces will be found replaced, largely or completely, by yellowish or grayish deposits representing agglomerations of Gaucher
cells.   The intervening trabeculae may be markedly thinned, but the tables of the
calvarium, though thinned, are not likely to be perforated.

If severely affected *long bones* are sectioned in the long axis and examined grossly,
in some, the marrow cavity will be found to contain conspicuous walnut-sized
nodules which stand out strikingly from such myeloid tissue as still remains relatively
intact.   These nodules may be soft or firm, are partly encapsulated by fibrous tissue,

Figure 132

A, Photomicrograph ($\times$ 7) illustrating alterations induced by Gaucher's disease in the
cortex and spongiosa at the lower metaphysis of the femur in the case of the woman on whom
clinical data were given in the legend of Figure 131-*B*. The cortical bone shown in the upper
part of the picture is extensively rarefied. The marrow spaces of the rarefied cortex and of
the spongiosa below it are largely occupied by compacted Gaucher cells. In many places
these cell masses have undergone necrosis, and the necrotic Gaucher cells are in the process
of being replaced by connective tissue. (See *B*.)

B, Photomicrograph ($\times$ 125) showing a field from *A*. In the lower part of the picture, a
mass of necrotic and disintegrating Gaucher cells can be seen. The upper part of the picture
shows connective tissue which is surrounding and replacing the necrotic Gaucher cells and
which represents part of the scarring reaction.

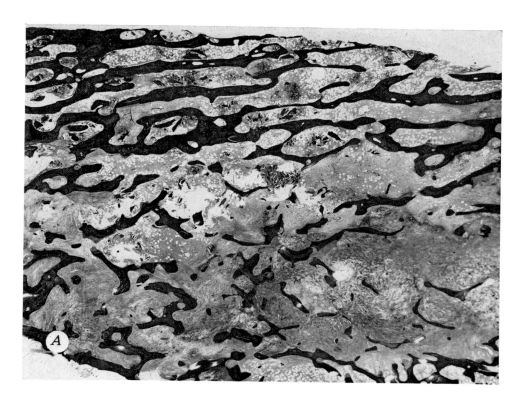

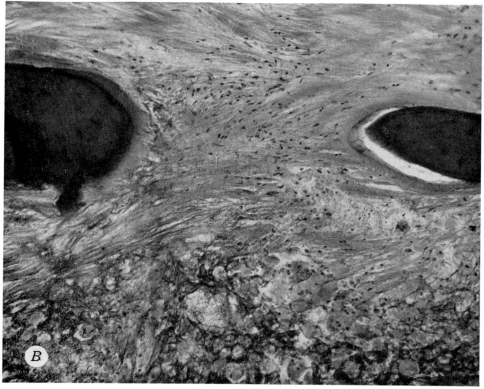

Figure 132

and are usually gray-white or more or less greenishly pigmented, though sometimes hemorrhagically discolored. Other sectioned long bones may show, instead of discrete nodules, tissue of similar appearance and consistency substantially filling the marrow cavity. Much of this abnormal tissue in the interior of the bone represents masses of necrotic Gaucher cells, modified to some extent by reactive secondary changes. (See Fig. 132.)

As already noted, substantial necrosis of the Gaucher cells in the head of a severely affected femur commonly results in collapse of the femoral head, and if the subject is a child, the roentgenographic picture of the upper end of the femur may simulate that of idiopathic Legg-Perthes-Calvé disease. The shaft of a severely affected long tubular bone may show rarefaction and thinning of the cortex, especially near the ends of the shaft. Where the cortex has been thinned, the shaft may appear somewhat expanded. Such expansion is particularly likely to occur in the neck and lower end of the femur and the upper end of the tibia. As has already been pointed out in connection with the roentgenographic findings, it is quite common for the expansion of the lower half of the femur to take a form which tends to resemble an Erlenmeyer flask.

Occasionally, especially in the lower dorsal or upper lumbar region, *vertebral bodies* are found so severely involved that they have collapsed and instigated the formation of a gibbus. Such a body becomes converted into a yellowish brown mass containing bone detritus. The mass tends gradually to disappear, and fusion may take place between the intervertebral disks formerly adjoining the collapsed and destroyed vertebra. When, in such a case, the Gaucher material develops subdurally, it may lead to compression of the spinal cord.

TREATMENT

Only palliative measures are known. No special dietary regimen seems to be of any particular benefit. In principle, however, the diet should be kept low in animal fat. If the spleen is not enlarged to a degree that it creates great discomfort, splenectomy should not be done. Indeed, this procedure may hasten the early appearance of skeletal lesions as the bone marrow begins to store more of the Gaucher material. In the presence of a severe anemia, a tendency toward hemorrhage, and a spleen so large as to create discomfort, splenectomy seems on the whole advisable. After splenectomy (although the procedure is somewhat hazardous in these cases) there is frequently improvement for some time in regard to the anemia and the hemorrhagic diathesis. Roentgen therapy directed against the enlarged spleen may contract it considerably, although this treatment, too, seems to have little influence upon the general course of the disease. Roentgen therapy seems indicated also for painful bone lesions, but the dosage should be kept low to avoid the danger of further necrosis of bone. In connection with surgical procedures (local or palliative) for the treatment of skeletal lesions, it must be borne in mind that such procedures carry with them the danger of local infection.

NIEMANN-PICK DISEASE

In *Niemann-Pick disease* the basic metabolic disorder expresses itself in the intracellular accumulation of abnormal amounts of lipids (notably phospholipids) in the various tissues, and particularly in the spleen, lymph nodes, liver, and bone marrow. The lipid-laden cells (reticulum cells and histiocytes) appear swollen and present a pale, foamy cytoplasm. It is the accumulation of the phospholipid sphingomyelin in these cells that especially characterizes the disorder. However, the tissue content in respect to other phospholipids (such as lecithin and cephalin) is also definitely increased, though not nearly to the same degree as sphingomyelin. In addition to a strikingly elevated phospholipid content, the various affected organs and tissues also show a definitely high cholesterol content. The biochemical mechanism underlying the disordered lipid metabolism still requires clarification, though there are indications that it is based on intracellular enzymatic aberrations.

Niemann recognized that the anatomic findings in his case (that of an infant who died when she was about $1\frac{1}{2}$ years of age) bore some similarity to those of Gaucher's disease, but felt that he was dealing with a condition distinct from Gaucher's disease and entitled his article "Ein unbekanntes Krankheitsbild." Pick's description of the pertinent gross and anatomic findings made clear that it was indeed a condition distinct from Gaucher's disease, and his contribution justifies the designation "Niemann-Pick disease." The early clinical and anatomic findings relating to the disease were soon supplemented by chemical and histochemical studies. Through these it was established (as noted above) that the characteristic swollen cells with pale, foamy cytoplasm observed in the affected organs and tissues harbored the phospholipids and particularly sphingomyelin (see Klenk, Menten and Welton, and also Thannhauser). Many reviews relating to Niemann-Pick disease and founded on personal cases and also collected cases culled from the literature have appeared (see Videbaek). A detailed study covering the various aspects of the disease and based on 18 cases from the records of the Children's Medical Center in Boston appeared in 1958 (see Crocker and Farber).

Niemann-Pick disease was originally regarded as a condition which became clinically manifest early in infancy and usually resulted in the death of the child within the first few years of life. However, accumulating experience has revealed cases which pursued a slower clinical course, some subjects surviving into early adult life. A problem which has not yet been completely resolved is the question of the relation between Niemann-Pick disease and Tay-Sachs disease (the infantile form of amaurotic family idiocy). Pick maintained that the two diseases have their basis in the same metabolic disturbance, even though, in Tay-Sachs disease, the pathologic alterations strongly predilect the nervous system, while in Niemann-Pick disease they involve it only slightly and incidentally, if at all.

CLINICAL CONSIDERATIONS

In respect to *incidence* it is clear that Niemann-Pick disease is of rare occurrence and shows no predilection for either sex. As to race, the accumulating data still indicate that a large proportion (possibly 50 per cent) of the subjects are of Jewish ancestry. Thus, it is no longer held that Jews are almost the sole victims of the disease. That the condition has a *genetic basis* has been well established, and the available data point to a recessive mode of transmission. In particular, in a family in which the condition is present in one of the offspring, there is considerable likelihood that one or more siblings of the subject will also be found affected. However, there is no direct evidence, as yet, of transmission of the disorder from one generation to another.

A *fulminating clinical course* is pursued by many of the cases in which the condition becomes manifest during early infancy. In such cases, jaundice may already be present at birth and is likely to persist for many months. Expansion of the abdomen, due to early and progressive enlargement of the liver and spleen, also becomes apparent in early infancy. In addition, the superficial lymph nodes may be found enlarged. There may be loss of visual acuity and even blindness, associated with a red patch in the macular area of each fundus. The affected infant usually becomes severely emaciated and deteriorates rapidly, both physically and mentally. In such cases the children often die during the first year of life, and a large majority are dead by the end of the second year of life.

On the other hand, there are cases which run a *less rapidly progressive clinical course*, despite the fact that the manifestations of the disease can already be observed during infancy. In these cases, jaundice may likewise have been present during infancy, but has ordinarily subsided after some months. Enlargement of the liver and spleen takes place more gradually, and expansion of the abdomen consequently tends to be less conspicuous. Nevertheless, most of the patients in whom the disease becomes manifest in infancy but pursues this milder course also die during childhood—usually by the time they are 6 years of age. For variable periods of time prior to their death, these subjects, too, show progressive mental and physical deterioration. Moreover, a few cases have been reported in which the disease pursued an even *more chronic* and relatively benign clinical course. In these cases the presence of the disease is, as a rule, not recognized until early childhood, when it is revealed through the finding of splenomegaly and hepatomegaly.

In connection with the general question of *survival*, Videbaek in 1949 reviewed the literature relating to 72 recorded cases, to which he added 1 of his own. In 47 of these cases there was information about the time elapsing between the finding of an enlarged spleen and liver (which led to the diagnosis of Niemann-Pick disease) and the death of the patient. In these 47 cases the average elapsed time between the establishment of the diagnosis (usually at some time during infancy) and the death of the patient was 9 months. More particularly, Videbaek's "survival diagram" relating to these 47 cases shows that 50 per cent of the affected children were dead by about 9 months after the disease had been diagnosed, 75 per cent were dead by about 12 months, and only 2 of the 47 patients (that is, about 5 per cent) survived as long as 18 months after the disease had been diagnosed. Of the 18 patients affected with Niemann-Pick disease whose cases were reported in 1958 by Crocker and Farber, 15 had already died when the review was made. Of these patients, 7 died between the ages of 4 months and 2 years, 5 between 3 and 6 years, and 3 between 12 and 20 years. Forsythe *et al.* in 1959 reported 3 cases of Niemann-Pick disease in which the presence of the condition was recognized at the ages of 3, 4, and 5 years, respectively, and in which the patients were reported as being still alive and in good general health at the ages of 19, 10, and 9 years, respectively.

PATHOLOGIC FINDINGS

The gross and microscopic pathologic findings as described by Pick still represent a firm foundation for our knowledge of this aspect of the disease and have been well supplemented by the studies of others, including notably Crocker and Farber. At autopsy in a case of Niemann-Pick disease, the normal fat depots will be found greatly depleted. The enlarged spleen, liver, and lymph nodes and also the bone marrow, as well as many other organs and tissues, show yellowish discoloration. This is due to the fact that these tissues contain great numbers of cells whose cytoplasm is rich in lipids and, as already noted, particularly in sphingomyelin.

The cells in question (so-called "foam cells") are modified reticulum cells and histiocytes (fixed macrophages) and are also often denoted as Niemann-Pick cells. In an advanced case of Niemann-Pick disease, these cells are indeed widely distributed throughout the organs and tissues of the body, including the supporting connective tissues. The Niemann-Pick cells are large, rounded cells. Each cell usually has a single nucleus, though it may be polynuclear, and the nuclei are relatively small in proportion to the cytoplasm, which is abundant. The cytoplasm of an individual cell may appear faintly granular, or granular and finely vacuolated. Less often, the cytoplasm is entirely vacuolated, and sometimes it appears completely occupied by a few large vacuoles. Because of its high phospholipid content, the cytoplasm of the Niemann-Pick cells reacts positively (showing black droplets and granules) when stained by the Smith-Dietrich method. Since the cytoplasm also contains cholesterol, it is found to be sudanophilic and also to contain doubly refractile droplets and needles when stained by appropriate methods.

Nonskeletal Tissues.—The enlarged *spleen* may weigh at least 3 or 4 times as much as it normally would, and is also abnormally firm. The cut surface of a spleen in which the Niemann-Pick cells have substantially replaced the cells of the splenic pulp may appear yellowish brown instead of presenting the normal deep red color. The *liver*, too, is firmer in consistency and lighter in color than it would normally be, but is relatively much less enlarged than the spleen. On microscopic examination the liver, if still only mildly affected, may present merely small numbers of Niemann-Pick cells in the sinusoids between the cords of liver cells. A liver in which the involvement is very pronounced will show crowding of its sinusoids with Niemann-Pick cells, and the parenchymal cells of the liver may even present striking vacuolation of their cytoplasm. In regard to the *lymph nodes*, those oriented to the viscera are the ones most likely to show considerable enlargement. There may be packets of enlarged nodes, yellowish in color, about the head of the pancreas, in the mesentery, and at the hilus of the liver and of the spleen. Much of the parenchyma of such lymph nodes will be found replaced by the characteristic foam cells. Collections of lymphoid tissue elsewhere than in the lymph nodes proper (in the thymus and in the gastrointestinal tract, for instance) also show, to a greater or lesser degree, the presence of such cells. The *lungs* often show the foam cells within the pleura and the alveolar spaces, and some foam cells may even be present in the alveolar septa. The characteristic Niemann-Pick cells are also to be found in the trachea and bronchi and especially in their mucous glands.

The pathologic changes relating to the *nervous system*, and particularly to the *brain*, have been the object of special attention because of the question of the relation of Niemann-Pick disease to Tay-Sachs disease (the infantile form of amaurotic family idiocy). In both these conditions there is storage of lipid in the cortex of the brain, in the spinal cord, and in the spinal ganglia. In association with Bielschowsky, Pick made a detailed examination of the central nervous system in a case of Niemann-Pick disease and reported that, microscopically, sections of the central nervous system revealed storage of a lipid substance in the ganglia and glia cells. In regard to morphology and staining qualities, this substance was interpreted as being identical not only with the lipid substances in the other organs and tissues of the subject in question, but also with the lipids which are usually found in the nerve and glia cells in infantile amaurotic family idiocy.

The apparent identity of the histologic findings in the two conditions led Pick and Bielschowsky to the conclusion that Tay-Sachs disease has its basis in the same metabolic disturbance as Niemann-Pick disease, except that in Tay-Sachs disease the pathologic changes center mainly in the brain, spinal cord, and spinal ganglia. Furthermore, it is stressed (1) that the changes consistently observed in the nervous system in cases of Tay-Sachs disease are not consistently observed there in cases of Niemann-Pick disease, and (2) that in Tay-Sachs disease the spleen and possibly other internal organs sometimes show the presence of foam cells resembling those observed in these organs in Niemann-Pick disease. In a classic case of amaurotic family idiocy which came to autopsy under the writer's supervision and was reported by Davison and Jacobson, the subject showed not only the pathologic changes typical of Tay-Sachs disease in the central nervous system, but also the presence in the visceral organs of foam cells resembling those observed in Niemann-Pick disease. (See Fig. 133.)

However, more recent detailed chemical and histochemical studies are indicating that, though Tay-Sachs disease and Niemann-Pick disease are both lipidoses, the metabolic disorder underlying Tay-Sachs disease is more complex than that underlying Niemann-Pick disease (see Norman *et al.*). In Tay-Sachs disease it is the lipid ganglioside (a glycolipid containing neuraminic acid) that accumulates both in the cortex and in the white matter of the brain rather than the lipid sphingomyelin, which is abundantly present in the brain in cases of Niemann-Pick disease. Furthermore, in Tay-Sachs disease the vacuolated cells (foam cells) present in the liver and spleen contain a large excess of hexosamine (a polysaccharide), while in Niemann-Pick disease the foam cells are rich in sphingomyelin.

Skeletal Tissues.—Although the changes in the bone marrow have been given considerable attention, there is a dearth of information about the actual anatomic changes observable in relation to the osseous tissue of the bones *per se*. To some extent, however, the anatomic changes relating to the bones can be deduced from the roentgenographic findings.

Since the *bone marrow* is a site of predilection for the accumulation of the lipid-bearing foam cells, the bone marrow may appear strikingly yellow if it is heavily infiltrated with these cells. Even if the color of the bone marrow does not show any significant deviation from the normal, microscopic examination will still reveal the presence of large numbers of foam cells in it.

From those few instances in which one or more long tubular bones of an affected infant have been removed at autopsy and sectioned in the long axis, it is evident that one may find some alterations in the gross architecture of the osseous tissue proper, in addition to the changes, already noted, relating to the bone marrow (see Baumann *et al.*). Under such circumstances the cortex of the bone will be abnormally thin and the spongy trabeculae also thin and reduced in number. Altogether, since the amount of osseous tissue per unit volume is reduced, and since the osseous tissue present appears adequately mineralized, the bone in question may be regarded as presenting the features of a nonspecific osteoporosis. In the absence of superimposed deficiency in the subject's intake of vitamins C and D, the junctional areas between the shaft of the long bone and its epiphyses are likely to be sharply delimited. Furthermore, in an infant or young child affected with Niemann-Pick disease, the emergence of the various secondary centers of ossification tends to be delayed, in accordance with the general poor health of the subject. Thus, in harmony with the anatomic findings (crowding of the marrow spaces with Niemann-Pick cells, thinning and sparsity of the spongy trabeculae, and thinning of the

Figure 133

A, Photomicrograph ($\times$ 125) of a tissue section prepared from a vertebral body removed at autopsy in the case of a child 2 years of age affected with Niemann-Pick disease. The marrow spaces of the spongiosa are substantially filled with lipid-laden cells which have largely replaced the myeloid cells. (I am indebted to Dr. Sydney S. Lazarus of the Isaac Albert Research Institute, Brooklyn, New York, for the tissue section.)

B, Photomicrograph ($\times$ 960) prepared from a section of the cerebral cortex of a child who died at the age of 19 months and who had presented the classic clinical manifestations of amaurotic family idiocy. The section was stained with Bielschowsky stain. The ganglion cells of the cerebral cortex are swollen, and the cytoplasm of these cells shows coarse silver granules representing the abnormal lipid. (This illustration was reproduced from the article by Davison and Jacobson dealing with a case which came to autopsy under the present writer's supervision.)

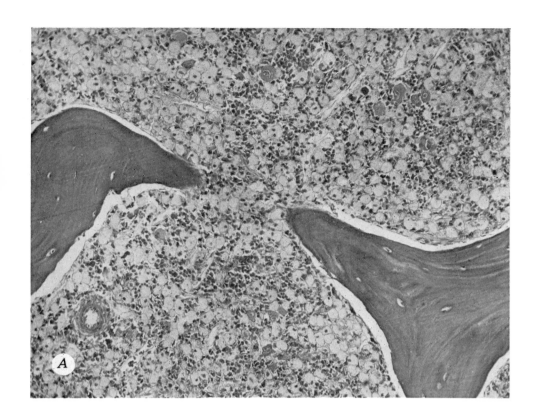

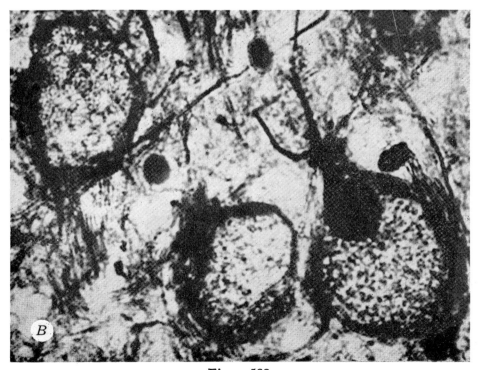

Figure 133

cortical bone), roentgenographic examination of the femora, for instance, may show some expansion of the lower part of their shafts, in addition to a more or less uniformly increased radiolucency of the bone areas, including the secondary ossification center of the lower end of each femur (see Gildenhorn and Amromin).

Finally, it should be noted that, in Niemann-Pick disease, collapse of the capital femoral epiphyses, such as commonly occurs in Gaucher's disease, has *not* been observed. Nor is one apt to find small or large definitely circumscribed areas of increased radiolucency, such as are likewise observed in Gaucher's disease. This seems to be the case even in those instances of Niemann-Pick disease in which the subject has survived into later childhood or into adult life.

TREATMENT

No medical means have yet been found by which it is possible to correct the enzymatic defect underlying Niemann-Pick disease. The treatment of the affected child has to be directed toward management of the practical problems relating notably to general hygiene, feeding, and efforts to combat any infections that may develop. If the spleen is very large, its removal not only militates against its possible rupture but may give relief from hypersplenism (especially anemia) and the effects of local pressure. However, splenectomy apparently does not influence, either for better or for worse, the general course and prognosis of the disease. Repeated transfusions (of whole blood and/or plasma) have proved to be of benefit to the patient's general well-being.

ESSENTIAL FAMILIAL HYPERCHOLESTEROLEMIA

Essential familial hypercholesterolemia is a hereditary disorder of cholesterol metabolism in which the primary effect is an increase in the body pool of cholesterol. This increase is apparently determined largely by enhanced intracellular enzymatic synthesis of cholesterol, though it is probably also determined to some extent by an increased absorption of exogenous cholesterol. Other factors which have not yet been fully elucidated probably also play some part in augmenting the body pool of cholesterol in the condition.

Though the subjects show abnormally high total serum cholesterol values, the proportion of the free cholesterol to cholesterol esters tends to remain within the normal range (about 30 per cent of the total being free cholesterol and 70 per cent in the form of esters). Serum cholesterol values of 400 to 500 mg. per cent are a common finding, but in an individual case (in accordance with the age of the subject and the severity of the metabolic defect) the value may be as high as 700 or 800 mg. or as low as 350 mg. If the metabolic defect is very severe, the serum cholesterol value will be high even during childhood, but in general the cholesterol value tends to rise as the subject grows older. However, in any large series of cases, the peak values are found in the 30- to 60-year age group. Among subjects older than 60 years, the average values are generally below the peak values. It should also be noted that, in essential familial hypercholesterolemia, the serum values for total fatty acids (that is, non-esterified fatty acids and a much larger fraction in the esterified form present as triglycerides) and phospholipids are increased above the normal, and it is lecithin that accounts for the rise in the phospholipids. (Normal serum cholesterol values are 120 to 290 mg. per cent at 30 years of age, 135 to 315 at 40 years, and 150 to 340 at 50 years.)

CLINICAL CONSIDERATIONS

Essential familial hypercholesterolemia shows no sex predilection. As a hereditary disorder the condition has been held by some to be transmitted as an incompletely dominant trait (see Wilkinson *et al.*, and Adlersberg). However, the interpretation now more generally accepted is that the condition is transmitted as a simple mendelian dominant trait (see Wheeler and Sprague, Piper and Orrild, and Harris-Jones *et al.*). In the assessment of the manner of inheritance of the disease, one source of confusion in evaluating individual cases has been the presence or absence of cholesterol deposits (*xanthomas*) in various soft tissues of the subject, in association with the hypercholesterolemia. In some cases the deposits of cholesterol in the soft tissues seem to be limited to the eyelids (*palpebral xanthelasma*), while in other cases one may find, in addition, xanthomatous involvement of tendons (*xanthoma tendinosum*) and also large, more or less nodular, tumor-like xanthomatous masses in the subcutaneous and periarticular tissues at sites of pressure (*xanthoma tuberosum*).

In a family in which one parent has essential familial hypercholesterolemia and the other does not have it, hypercholesterolemia can be expected to be present in about half of their offspring. While some of the hypercholesterolemic offspring do not develop xanthomas, a very large proportion do develop them in one form or another. In those subjects in whom the serum cholesterol value is greatly increased above the normal, the eventual appearance of xanthomas is almost the rule. However, even in these subjects, it is ordinarily not until adult life (usually about middle adult life) that xanthomas become manifest. With advancing age, the xanthomas tend to increase in size. In elderly subjects with pronounced hypercholesterolemia, the presence of xanthomas in one form or another is the rule; however, if the xanthomas do not appear before middle life, they are not likely to be widely distributed or very prominent.

The over-all incidence of arcus senilis and of coronary atherosclerosis and angina pectoris is higher in subjects affected with essential familial hypercholesterolemia than in the general population. The incidence of angina pectoris and death from coronary occlusion is certainly abnormally high in subjects under the age of 50, and coronary occlusion has been found to be a cause of death in subjects as young as 30 or 40 years of age. However, in those surviving beyond the age of 55 or 60, the incidence of death from coronary occlusion is practically within the normal range.

Against this background of essential familial hypercholesterolemia as a disease complex, we can now center our attention upon the question of skeletal involvement and, in particular, upon the large xanthomas which may develop in the skin and subcutis, in tendons, and in other soft tissues in the general vicinity of joints. (See Fig. 134.) It should be pointed out, however, that soft-tissue xanthomas analogous to those developing in connection with essential familial hypercholesterolemia may also appear in other conditions, such as idiopathic hyperlipemia, biliary cirrhosis, and hypothyroidism (see Fleischmajer).

PATHOLOGIC AND ROENTGENOGRAPHIC FINDINGS

Xanthoma Tuberosum and/or Tendinosum.—A focus of *xanthoma tuberosum* may be defined as a smooth or nodular protuberance which has resulted from the massive local accumulation of cholesterol-bearing foam cells in the skin and subcutis. The tuberous xanthomas tend to develop bilaterally in multiple sites, and some attain considerable size. Nevertheless they are, as a rule, painless. Their sites of predilection are: the heel, the dorsum of the foot, the back of the elbow, and the back of the hand—sites where the skin and underlying soft tissues are commonly subjected to pressure. When the xanthomas are present in multiple sites, the condition is often denoted as *"xanthoma tuberosum multiplex."*

A large focus of xanthoma tuberosum usually evolves through the confluence of a number of small neighboring xanthomas, and the fused mass continues to grow, sometimes attaining a size of several inches in its largest dimension. On palpation, the xanthomatous mass may yield somewhat to pressure, but if it contains a good deal of fibrous tissue it will be found firm and indurated. The epidermis covering the xanthoma may appear thin but otherwise normal, or instead it may show evidences of hyperkeratosis. The color of the actual lesional tissue may be yellow throughout or may range from yellow through orange and even to brown if the lesion is large and is of long standing. The cut surface of the xanthoma will present, in addition, some scattered whitish strands representing fibrous connective tissue.

The term *"xanthoma tendinosum"* refers to swelling of a tendon area due to massive infiltration of the region with cholesterol-bearing foam cells. The sites of predilection for xanthomatous involvement of tendons are the same as those for xanthoma tuberosum, and these two expressions of xanthoma formation may be present in the same anatomic area. Aside from appearing in tendons, xanthomas may develop in other connective tissue structures, such as a ligament or a sheet of fascia, or even in the periosteal covering of a bone.

On *microscopic examination* of these xanthomas, it is apparent that, while some of the cholesterol-bearing foam cells are fixed or wandering macrophages which have taken up the lipid, the bulk of the lesion has resulted from the imbibition of cholesterol by the local connective tissue cells to form these foam cells. In the course of the latter process, the intercellular collagen fibers are crowded out. Where the lesional tissue has been traumatized in some way and cholesterol has consequently been liberated from the cells, one finds focal areas of necrosis, foreign-body giant cells, and also so-called cholesterol slits. (See Fig. 135.)

Skeletal Involvement.—The literature relating to essential familial hypercholesterolemia yields only very meager information bearing upon changes in the bones. Most of the references to such changes have been recorded in articles dealing with the roentgenographic findings in cases presenting xanthoma tuberosum and/or tendinosum. The bone changes noted in these cases are alterations occurring mainly in the phalanges of the hands and feet and induced by pressure erosion of

Figure 134

A, Photograph showing swelling of both thumbs due to xanthoma formation in the soft tissues overlying the interphalangeal joints. This illustration and the others on this plate pertain to the same patient and were taken at the time of his first admission to the hospital. The subject was a man 28 years of age who entered the hospital because of the presence of "lumps" (para-articular soft-tissue masses) of which he had been aware for 3 years. The "lumps" were neither painful nor tender, and they had not induced any limitation of function. The serum cholesterol value was 482 mg. per cent, the uric acid 5.1 mg., and the nonprotein nitrogen 16.8 mg. (See also Fig. 135.)

B, Photograph of the anterior aspect of both knee regions showing small bilateral protuberances representing xanthomas in the region of the patellar ligaments.

C, Photograph illustrating massive xanthomas oriented to, and involving, the Achilles tendon at the back of each foot. In addition to the large protruding xanthomas, one can also note that the Achilles tendon above each mass is swollen as a result of involvement.

D and *E,* Roentgenographs showing, in lateral projection, the posterior part of the left and right foot shown in *C.* Note that the xanthomatous mass oriented to the back of each calcaneus has induced only a slight degree, at most, of pressure erosion of each of these bones.

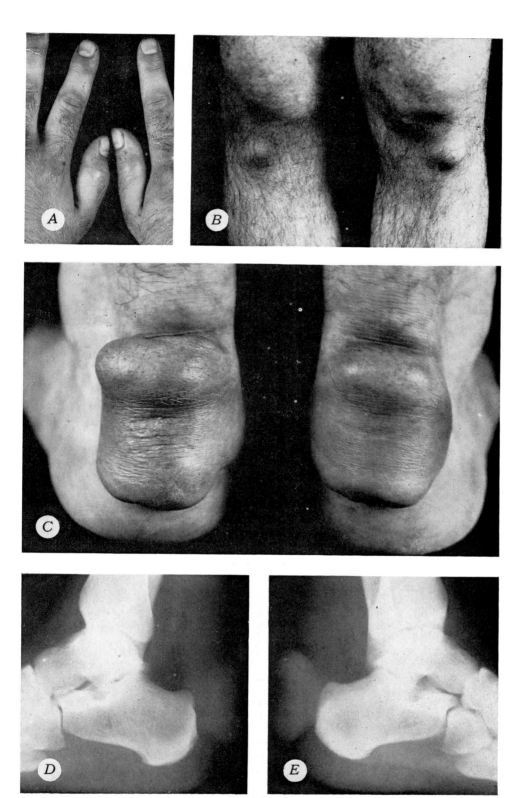

Figure 134

one or another of these bones by xanthomas located in the overlying soft tissues (see Merrill, Gaál, and also March *et al.*).

The radiolucent defects appearing in consequence of the pressure erosions are roundish or oval in shape, and are usually limited to the cortex of the affected bone. However, in regard to those phalanges in which the erosion defects are very large, the roentgenographic findings suggest that the xanthomatous tissue has probably also penetrated into the interior of the bone. On the whole, these roentgenographic changes in the phalanges are rather similar to those which may be encountered in cases of gout in which large tophi developing in the fingers and/or toes have caused pressure erosion of phalanges and even penetrated into the interior of some of them. In an occasional instance, one or more metacarpal or metatarsal bones may also present evidence of pressure erosion of the cortex near the head of the bone, especially if the proximal phalanx of the corresponding finger or toe also shows involvement. Thus the bone erosions induced by the xanthomas tend to be limited to short tubular bones of the hands and feet. In contrast, even when very large xanthomas develop in tendons (such as the Achilles tendon) and in the tissues around the elbow, their presence is ordinarily not associated with erosion of the regional long tubular bones. However, occasionally one may encounter an erosion on the posterior surface of one or both calcaneal bones if the corresponding Achilles tendon is very much thickened by xanthoma formation. Small focal erosions in the calvarium were noted in the case reported by Gaál. These had apparently resulted from the presence of a number of small palpable xanthomas which had developed in the pericranium and/or galea aponeurotica.

Rather surprisingly, the literature pertaining to essential familial hypercholesterolemia seems to contain no direct pathologico-anatomic observations relating to the question of whether cholesterol-bearing foam cells accumulate in the bone marrow in this disease, and whether such intramedullary deposits might constitute a point of departure for bone changes. Many cases of idiopathic familial hypercholesterolemia have come to autopsy, and the presence or absence of such changes could, of course, have been ascertained by examination of various bones (such as ribs, parts of vertebrae, or iliac bones) removed at autopsy. The writer himself has never performed or supervised an autopsy in one of these cases, so that he lacks personal experience on this question. It does not seem likely to him, however, that

Figure 135

A, Photograph of the back of the left elbow from the same patient on whom clinical data were given in connection with Figure 134. The area is the site of a large, protruding xanthoma, and a large xanthoma was also present on the back of the right elbow. The mass was excised. The lesional tissue was yellowish in color, of rubbery consistency, and adherent to the skin. It was infiltrating the triceps tendon, which was very much thickened.

B, Roentgenograph of the elbow region shown in *A*. Despite the massiveness of the xanthoma, there is little if any evidence of pressure erosion of the underlying bones.

C, Photomicrograph ($\times$ 55) prepared from a tissue section of the xanthoma shown in *A* and *B*. The tissue field illustrated shows numerous so-called cholesterol slits, many of which have foreign-body giant cells bordering upon them. Interspersed between the cholesterol slits are foam cells and also some thick collagenous fibers. The lighter portion of the illustrated field (upper right) is composed of compacted cholesterol-bearing foam cells which, as is shown by *D*, are intact and thus have not provoked the secondary reactive changes which are present in the rest of the tissue field and which are due to the liberation of cholesterol from degenerating foam cells.

D, Photomicrograph ($\times$ 250) showing the intact cholesterol-bearing foam cells in greater detail.

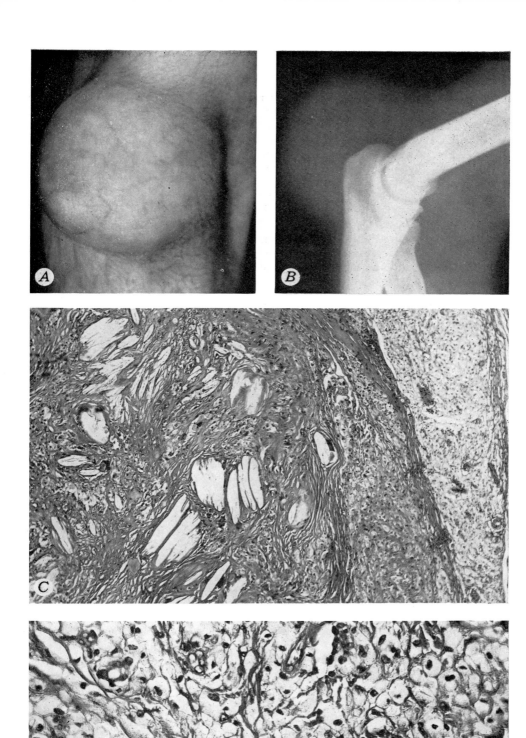

Figure 135

masses of cholesterol-bearing foam cells resulting in xanthoma formation in the marrow cavity of one bone or another frequently occur in this disease. Indeed, if intramedullary xanthoma formation does occur, the resultant scarring reaction may lead to resorption and/or destruction of spongy trabeculae and even focal resorption of cortical bone, which will certainly be reflected in the x-ray pictures of involved bones. Pertinent cases were described by Koch and Lewis, and also by Brusco *et al.*

In the following section of this chapter, the skeletal changes of lipid (cholesterol) granulomatosis will be discussed on the basis of 2 cases reported by Chester and 1 case from the files of the present writer. In the case from the writer's files, 2 serum cholesterol determinations were done, and the values obtained were within the normal range. Furthermore, in that case there was no palpebral xanthelasma, nor were there any xanthomatous deposits in tendons or any massive tuberous xanthomatous deposits in the vicinity of joints. It was noted that in Chester's 2 cases palpebral xanthelasma was present, but this is a finding which by itself does not suffice to indicate the presence of essential familial hypercholesterolemia. Furthermore, in 1 of his 2 cases (the one showing the more widespread lipid granulomatosis), a postmortem blood specimen yielded a serum cholesterol value of only 102 mg. per cent—a value much below normal and one which would seem to indicate at least that the antemortem value was not within the range of hypercholesterolemia. Thus, on the basis of the clinical and anatomical findings in these cases of lipid (cholesterol) granulomatosis, the skeletal changes described in connection with them should not be regarded as representing part of the anatomic picture of essential familial hypercholesterolemia.

TREATMENT

Since the basic metabolic disorder in essential familial hypercholesterolemia is at an endogenous cellular level (specifically, an enhanced intracellular enzymatic synthesis of cholesterol), it is not to be expected that the mere dietary restriction of cholesterol can completely counteract the resulting hypercholesterolemia. Nevertheless, it is definitely useful to reduce the daily total caloric intake, and it may be of value to restrict the intake of foods such as eggs, cream, butter, and fatty meat, since all these foods are rich in cholesterol and/or saturated fatty acids. Such a regimen serves at least to reduce the body's exogenous supply of cholesterol and, more importantly, neutral fats from animal sources. The consumption of a diet composed largely of various vegetables, fruits, and certain vegetable oils has a double advantage. The nutritive value of vegetable fats is equal to that of animal fats, but the sterols present in vegetables are absorbed to only a limited extent, so that there is a desirable reduction in the exogenous source of cholesterol. When fat is needed and used in the preparation of foods, or wanted for the enhancement of some food item being consumed (such as bread), it is advantageous to have the vegetable fat take the form of corn oil or margarine prepared from corn oil. The value of corn oil is attributable to its high content of unsaturated fatty acids. Furthermore, when corn oil is made to constitute a substantial part of the food intake for some time, the serum cholesterol value is lowered. Though the mechanism by which this reduction takes place is not yet clear, it seems to be related to the unsaturated fatty acid content of the corn oil (producing an enhanced synthesis of cholesterol esters containing unsaturated fatty acid moieties). However, if the corn oil regimen is discontinued, the serum cholesterol value rises again.

LIPID (CHOLESTEROL) GRANULOMATOSIS

In a paper entitled "Lipoid Granulomatosis," Chester (who worked under the Viennese pathologist Erdheim) included in his presentation of the lipidoses in general a pathologic condition which he regarded as distinctive and, in particular, as clearly different from both Niemann-Pick disease and so-called Schüller-Christian disease. It was on the basis of the anatomic findings in 2 cases that he described the condition thus delineated. In both of the subjects in question (a woman of 44 and a man of 69), the pathologic findings indicated that the granulomatous changes found in the viscera in one case and in the bones in both cases were provoked by the presence of foam cells containing cholesterol. The cholesterol accumulating in the marrow of the various bones led to fibrous scarring, associated, in one of the cases, with extensive intramedullary new bone formation, resulting in patches of osteosclerosis. The writer's experience includes 1 case similar to the 2 cases singled out by Chester. It seems to the writer that the case described by Sørensen also falls into this category. The roentgenographic changes in the bones and the biopsy findings relating to the bone specimen in that case seem to support this impression. In Sørensen's case there was a pronounced hyperlipemia, the values for neutral fat and fatty acid being strikingly elevated, and the values for phospholipids and cholesterol somewhat elevated. These chemical findings indicate the presence of so-called idiopathic hyperlipemia in that case, and it may well be that the bone changes observed are to be correlated with that hyperlipemia. In Chester's cases and in the case seen by the writer, determinations of the total lipid in the serum were not carried out. Nevertheless, to keep all such cases distinct from other conditions (such as Schüller-Christian disease and essential familial hypercholesterolemia) in which cholesterol likewise accumulates at various sites, it might not be inappropriate to designate the condition in question here as Erdheim-Chester disease, if one did not wish to avoid the use of still another eponym.

Schüller-Christian disease (p. 897) affects older children and adults. It runs a chronic and progressive course and represents, in a sense, a florid expression of eosinophilic granuloma—a peculiar histiocytic inflammatory reaction (inflammatory histiocytosis) in response to some as yet unknown agent. In the course of progression of Schüller-Christian disease, more and more bones come to show destructive lesions (though the latter respond to radiation therapy), and visceral involvement is also part of the disease complex. The complete Christian triad (calvarial defects, diabetes insipidus, and exophthalmos) may or may not be manifest, but the destructive lesions in the bones are a source of clinical complaints. In any event, the lesions of Schüller-Christian disease, if not treated, eventually become lipidized, collagenized, and even heavily scarified—in short, largely converted into xanthogranulomata. However, there can be no doubt that the cholesterol deposition found in the end stages of Schüller-Christian disease represents a secondary phenomenon and that, for this reason, Schüller-Christian disease does not fall into the category of the primary lipidoses, of which the classic examples are Gaucher's disease, Niemann-Pick disease, and Tay-Sachs disease. Thus, in Schüller-Christian disease the initial or basic lesions, wherever they appear, are inflammatory lesions strongly resembling, as noted, the lesions of eosinophilic granuloma (p. 876), in which condition the disease runs a mild course and the involvement may even be limited to a single bone area.

As already indicated, *essential familial hypercholesterolemia* (p. 528) is a hereditary disorder due to increased absorption and/or increased formation or decreased utilization of cholesterol. Total serum cholesterol values of 500 mg. per cent or more are not uncommon. Cholesterol deposits tend to appear, often bilaterally, in the various connective tissues, including fasciae and tendons about the joints,

producing the picture of so-called *xanthoma tuberosum multiplex*. Whether cholesterol tends to accumulate in the bone marrow in cases of familial hypercholesterolemia (and if so, to what extent) is not clear. At any rate, roentgenographic examination practically never reveals skeletal changes ascribable to cholesterol deposition
in the marrow. Such changes may be absent because the cholesterol (if any is
deposited) is mainly neutral cholesterol rather than cholesterol esters, which are
irritating. Altogether, then, the 2 cases described by Chester are *not* to be interpreted as instances of: (1) Schüller-Christian disease even in a relatively mild and
chronic form, or (2) clinically occult hereditary and familial hypercholesterolemia.

In regard to terminology, and in particular to the name "lipid (cholesterol)
granulomatosis," another condition which requires mention is the one which
Farber *et al.* have described under the title of "Lipogranulomatosis: A New Lipo-
Glyco-Protein 'Storage' Disease." The manifestations of that disease (sometimes
denoted as "Farber's disease") set in soon after birth, and the affected child succumbs during infancy or shortly thereafter. In these cases of lipogranulomatosis,
the significant lipid which accumulates in the tissues is, as noted, of the nature of
lipo-glycoprotein rather than cholesterol. The clinical course of so-called Farber's
disease is dominated by progressive involvement of joints and the development of
nodular swellings in the subcutaneous and periarticular tissues. Roentgenographically one may observe distention of articular capsules (especially of large joints),
some juxta-articular bone erosions, and generalized porosity of the bones (see
Schultze and Lang, and Schanche *et al.*). There is slight lymphadenopathy, but
the spleen and liver do not tend to be enlarged. Infiltration of the lungs by the
lipid supervenes, and terminally there may be severe dyspnea.

CLINICAL CONSIDERATIONS

In neither of the 2 cases described by Chester (the case of the woman of 44 and
that of the man of 69) is there any reference to clinical complaints relating to the
bones and joints. The woman died of cardiac insufficiency associated with asthma,
and the clinical history indicated that she did not have diabetes insipidus or
diabetes mellitus and had not been affected with jaundice. In the case of the man,
too, death was due to cardiac failure. The latter had been caused by very extensive
lipid granulomatous involvement of the lungs and heart, again representing the
result of the liberation of cholesterol from the foam cells. In both cases it was the
presence of small xanthomatous patches in the eyelids (xanthelasma palpebrarum)
that prompted removal of bones at the autopsy and their detailed examination.
Furthermore, it is of significance that in neither subject did the spleen show any
abnormality, although, in the man, various other viscera in addition to the lungs
and heart did present evidence of lipid granulomatosis.

In neither case was an *antemortem* serum cholesterol determination carried out.
However, in the case of the woman, a serum cholesterol determination was done on
blood removed from the cadaver. The value was found to be definitely below
normal, but the low value obtained may well be accounted for by a long lapse of
time between death and the obtainment of the blood for the examination. In any
event, it is not at all probable that there was any pronounced *hyper*cholesterolemia
before death in this case.

In the instance of lipid (cholesterol) granulomatosis (Erdheim-Chester disease)
with which the writer had had personal experience, the patient was a female. She
was 54 years of age at the time of her first admission to our hospital. She had been
under medical care at another hospital 12 years earlier—that is, when she was
42 years of age. Her clinical complaints at that time related to polydipsia and

polyuria, which had followed in the wake of a severe psychic trauma. However, roentgenographic examination of the skull failed to reveal any abnormalities in the region of the sella turcica or the cranial vault. Furthermore, clinical observation of the patient led, by the process of elimination, to the conclusion that her principal complaints (polydipsia and polyuria) had their basis in hysteria. Biochemical examination of the blood in this case revealed no evidence of hypercholesterolemia, the serum cholesterol value being 252 mg. per cent on one occasion and 230 mg. per cent on another. These values represent findings within the normal range for a female adult 54 years of age. All the other biochemical values obtained were likewise within normal limits.

ROENTGENOGRAPHIC FINDINGS

We shall consider the roentgenographic findings in lipid (cholesterol) granulomatosis only as they relate to the bones. In the case studied by the writer, the modifications found on roentgenographic examination of the skeleton were not associated with any clinical complaints referable to the bones or joints. As already noted, repeated examinations of the skull revealed no abnormalities at the base, nor any significant changes in the calvarium. It was the long tubular bones that showed the most striking alterations. These were most prominent in the radius, ulna, tibia, and fibula on both sides, and were much more prominent in these bones than in the femur and humerus on both sides. The bones of the hands presented suggestive indications of involvement, especially of the metacarpal bones. Insofar as the bones of the feet were concerned, though the calcaneus, astragalus, and bones of the midtarsus all showed changes, it was in the calcaneus that the alterations were most conspicuous.

Of interest in relation to the modifications in the long tubular bones is the fact that they were most striking in the metaphysial regions of their shafts, some of the bones failing to reveal any significant changes roentgenographically in the midportion of their shafts. Most of those long tubular bones which were severely affected showed involvement of their actual epiphysial ends, but any alterations present there were less pronounced than those in the adjacent metaphysial areas. The affected bones revealed no alterations in contour. The significant finding was a more or less diffuse and/or spotty increased radiopacity involving the spongiosa of the shafts of the long bones, especially toward their ends. In some of the affected bones, portions of the shaft cortex revealed thickening, and in these areas the cortex was usually rarefied. The increased radiodensity of the spongiosa represented intramedullary scarring and reactive new bone formation, and the changes in the cortical bone (especially the rarefaction) indicated that the compacta was being subjected to resorptive changes. (See Fig. 136.)

PATHOLOGIC FINDINGS

The presentation of the pathologic findings, like that of the roentgenographic findings, will be limited to the bones. However, it is worth noting that one of the 2 subjects described by Chester (the woman 44 years of age) presented not only skeletal changes but also extensive lipogranulomatous changes in internal organs, especially the lungs. Interestingly enough, however, the spleen was found free of involvement. The other subject (the man 69 years of age), though showing skeletal changes, did not reveal lipogranulomatous lesions either grossly or microscopically in any of the internal organs, including the spleen. Although the bones showed lipid (cholesterol) granulomatosis in both cases, the changes were much more pronounced in the woman, in whom, as noted, lipogranulomatous lesions were widely distributed in the viscera also.

In the case of the woman, many bones were removed for gross and microscopic examination. These included a humerus, both femora, a tibia and fibula, various bones of an ankle and foot, and much of the vertebral column. On sectioning these bones for gross inspection, it was noted that the humerus was the long bone least involved, while the femora and the tibia and fibula showed extensive changes. The first lumbar vertebra was the only part of the vertebral column found significantly modified.

The gross appearance presented by the sectioned tibia can serve to illustrate the advanced pathologic changes observed in the affected long bones. The interior of the shaft of the bone, except for part of its midportion, was largely occupied by closely compacted osseous tissue. Thus the original spongiosa had been substantially replaced by condensed sclerotic bone. The osteosclerosis was most conspicuous in the metaphysial areas of the bone shaft. Here and there within the sclerotic osseous tissue in the interior of the bone, one could still recognize yellowish areas presumably containing cells laden with cholesterol. However, the sclerotic osseous tissue was bordered by discrete yellowish foci representing lipid granulomata which had not yet been replaced by fibrous and/or osseous tissue. In the marrow present in the midportion of the bone shaft, some small discrete yellow foci could also be seen.

In the case of the man, a humerus, a femur, and both tibiae were removed for gross and microscopic study. When these bones were sectioned in the long axis and inspected, their shafts failed to present the large patches of osteosclerosis which had been shown by corresponding bones in the case of the woman. However, they did reveal, in the marrow occupying the midportion of the bone shafts, the presence of smaller and larger soft sulphur-yellow foci representing relatively fresh lipid granulomata, and some yellow-white firmer foci representing fibrously scarred lipid granulomata. It may well be that the differences observed between these 2 cases in respect to the gross pathologic findings in the bones reflect differences in the duration of the disease process. In particular, to judge from the absence of visceral involvement in the man, the disease was apparently of shorter duration in that case.

Figure 136

A, Roentgenograph of the distal half of the right radius and ulna in the case of lipid (cholesterol) granulomatosis studied by the writer. The left radius and ulna showed similar changes. The increased radiopacity of the bones is clearly apparent and is most striking toward the end of each bone shaft. In the region abutting on the interosseous space, the cortex of each bone shaft is thickened. The patient was a woman 54 years of age whose clinical complaints did not relate to the bones, and it was only through roentgenographic examination of the skeleton that the alterations in the bones were discovered. The other illustrations appearing on this plate show the changes manifest roentgenographically in various other bones of the same patient.

B, Roentgenograph of the proximal half of the left tibia and fibula revealing the striking radiopacity of the tibial shaft, which is largely the result of reactive intramedullary new bone formation. The right tibia and fibula were similarly affected.

C, Roentgenograph of part of the right foot and lower end of the tibia and fibula, also demonstrating increased radiopacity, most striking in the lower end of the tibia and fibula and prominent also in the os calcis. The corresponding areas of the left leg and foot showed analogous changes.

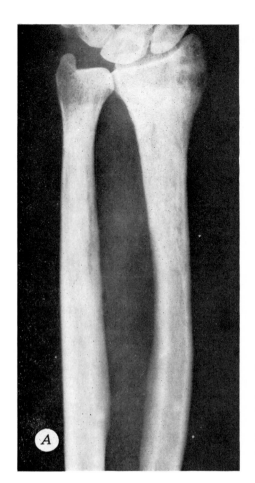

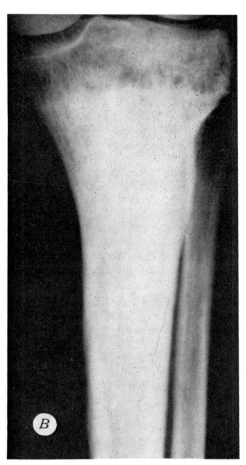

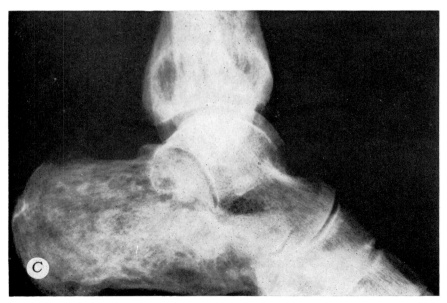

Figure 136

For *microscopic study*, tissue sections prepared from blocks of cortical and spongy bone in the case of the 44 year old woman were available to the writer, the sections having been preserved in the Erdheim collection of pathologic material. The cortical bone, though not altered in thickness, showed widening of many of its haversian canals. This was most pronounced in the deeper parts of the cortex, where many of the widened canals had also become confluent. The haversian canals, whether widened or not, and the spaces formed through confluence of several enlarged canals contained numerous and often closely packed swollen cells rich in cholesterol. These cells were nearly always uninuclear, and the nuclei were small, while the cytoplasm which composed the major part of each cell appeared delicately foamy or finely granular. Intermixed with the lipid-bearing cells were small numbers of other cells—mainly mononuclear cells, some of which were clearly lymphocytes and plasma cells. An occasional eosinophilic leukocyte was also present. In the modified cortical bone, especially where it bordered on the medullary cavity, the resorption spaces resulting from widening and confluence of neighboring haversian canals usually contained some fibrous tissue. Furthermore, in some of the spaces, collagenization of the fibrous tissue (an expression of reactive scarring) had resulted in crowding and even disappearance of the lipid-bearing foam cells.

In the spongiosa, large areas of the spongy marrow spaces were occupied by connective tissue cells which were intermingled with still-recognizable foam cells, some of which were compressed. In addition, these scarred lipogranulomatous areas contained a considerable amount of osseous tissue. Some of the latter represented spongy trabeculae thickened through the deposition of new bone on them, while elsewhere the osseous tissue had apparently formed within lipogranulomatous areas which had undergone pronounced fibrous scarring. It was in consequence of the fibrous scarring and new bone formation that had occurred in the spongiosa of the long bones (especially toward the ends of their shafts) that these bone areas appeared osteosclerotic on gross examination and rather radiopaque on roentgenographic examination. (See Fig. 137.)

As the writer has already stated, the disease picture described in this section under the title of "Lipid (Cholesterol) Granulomatosis" should be kept apart from Schüller-Christian disease. Indeed, the validity of such a distinction is clearly supported by the microscopic study of the tissue sections in one of Chester's cases, and of the biopsy material in the case which came under the writer's personal observation. However, it should be pointed out that Chiari, in his article entitled "Die generalisierte Xanthomatose vom Typus Schüller-Christian," expresses the opinion that the 2 cases described by Chester represent instances of Schüller-Christian disease—an opinion which, as noted, the writer does not share.

Figure 137

A, Photomicrograph ($\times$ 55) illustrating the appearance of the spongiosa in the lower end of a tibia in a case of lipid (cholesterol) granulomatosis. The trabeculae are thickened as the result of new bone apposition, and the intertrabecular marrow spaces show foam cells interspersed with loose filamentous connective tissue elements.

B, Photomicrograph ($\times$ 125) revealing in fuller detail the histologic pattern at a site in the tissue section where the cholesterol-bearing foam cells are fairly numerous.

C, Photomicrograph ($\times$ 125) revealing in fuller detail the histologic pattern at a site in the tissue section where the trabeculae of the spongiosa are clearly thickened in consequence of accretion of new bone, and where fibrillar connective tissue has substantially replaced the foam cells in the intertrabecular marrow spaces.

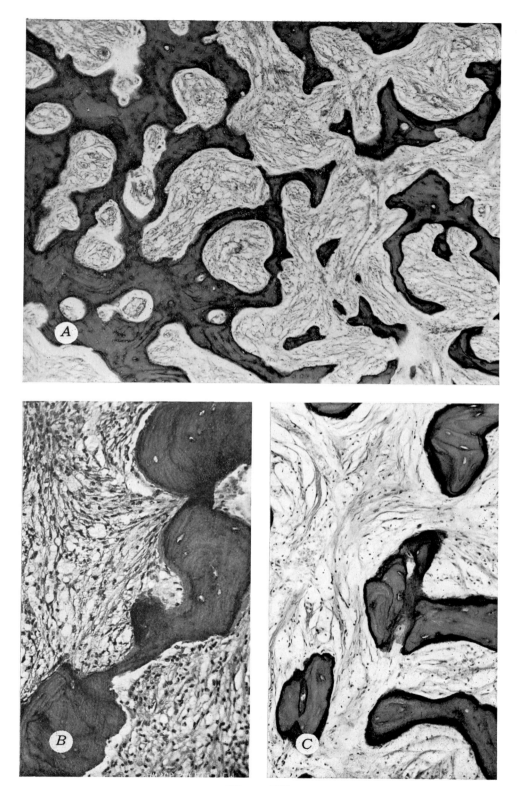

Figure 137

HURLER'S SYNDROME (GARGOYLISM)

Hurler's syndrome (Hunter-Hurler-Pfaundler syndrome) is a hereditary metabolic disorder. When the disease, which is not of rare occurrence, is present in its *florid* (or *complete*) *form*, its conspicuous clinical manifestations are: skeletal abnormalities (including stunted growth), corneal opacities, hepatosplenomegaly, and mental deficiency. When the disease is present in an *aborted* (or *incomplete*) *form* ("forme fruste"), some of the clinical abnormalities characteristic of the disease in its florid form are not striking or are absent altogether.

In regard to *nomenclature*, it is to be noted that Hurler's syndrome is also known by various other names. The principal one, *gargoylism*, emphasizes the grotesque gargoyle-like appearance presented by the subject, notably in respect to the head. The designation *"dysostosis multiplex"* draws attention to the skeletal aspects of the condition, which result from disordered osteogenesis and are expressed in dwarfing and a variety of alterations in the contour of individual bones. The term *"lipochondrodystrophy,"* now out of use, dates from the time when it was believed that the condition belonged in the category of the lipidoses—that is, before it was established that the principal metabolic disturbance relates to acid mucopolysaccharides rather than to lipids.

Hereditary Aspects.—Hurler's disease is inherited as a recessive trait—either as an autosomal recessive or as an X-chromosomal recessive (see van Pelt and Huizinga). The autosomal type of inheritance is the more common. In families in which the condition is transmitted in this way, there is often consanguinity between the parents. The offspring who are affected are as likely to be females as males, and the disease becomes manifest early in life and takes a florid form. In families in which the recessive "gargoyle gene" is carried on the X-chromosome, the affected offspring are all males, the disease tends to take an aborted or less severe form ("forme fruste"), and the clinical manifestations may even be delayed for some years.

Biochemical Findings.—The metabolic abnormality underlying the disease relates to disordered mucopolysaccharide metabolism. Normally, mucopolysaccharides are found especially in the ground substance of the various connective tissues (p. 121). The underlying aberration in mucopolysaccharide metabolism in Hurler's disease is not yet fully understood. However, there seems to be little doubt that it is rooted in congenitally disordered functioning of relevant enzymes. Mechanisms which have been inculpated include: an increased synthesis of mucopolysaccharides, a decreased catabolism of mucopolysaccharides, and/or some error in the synthesis of a mucopolysaccharide acceptor protein. In any event, the disordered mucopolysaccharide metabolism results in the accumulation of acid mucopolysaccharides (most often chondroitin sulfate B) in various organs and tissues of the affected subject, and also in an abnormally high urinary excretion of chondroitin sulfate B and/or heparitin sulfate (see Brante, Meyer *et al.*, Dorfman and Lorincz, Meyer and Hoffman, and also Berggård and Bearn).

The urine of *normal subjects* contains small quantities of chondroitin sulfate A and possibly some chondroitin sulfate C. It does *not* contain chondroitin sulfate B. Furthermore, it should be noted that, in families in which cases of Hurler's syndrome are present, the excretion of total acid mucopolysaccharides is not significantly above normal in either the carriers (the parents) or the unaffected siblings (see Campbell and Fried).

In respect to the increased urinary excretion of mucopolysaccharides, gargoylism seems to stand apart from various other diseases based on abnormal endochondral bone formation, such as achondroplasia, Morquio's disease, and dysplasia epiphysialis multiplex, in which conditions there is apparently no increase in the urinary excretion of mucopolysaccharides (see Nagel). In some cases of Hurler's disease, an abnormal glycolipid also accumulates in some of the organs and tissues, including notably the neurons of the central nervous system. It has been held that the basis for the mental deficiency so often encountered in cases of gargoylism is the accumulation of the abnormal glycolipid in the neurons of the brain. Furthermore, it has been maintained that the intracellular glycolipidosis in these cases represents a metabolic abnormality present in addition to (but distinct from) the metabolic abnormality underlying the mucopolysaccharidosis (see Wolfe *et al.*).

CLINICAL CONSIDERATIONS

The cases in which the clinical manifestations are most severe are those in which the defect relating to the metabolism of mucopolysaccharides is most pronounced. In particular, Berggård and Bearn noted that the skeletal changes were relatively slight in those patients whose urinary excretion of mucopolysaccharides related only to heparitin sulfate. On the other hand, in the patients who excreted excessive amounts of chondroitin sulfate B in addition to heparitin sulfate, the skeletal changes observed were severe and typical of the Hurler syndrome. As already noted, the affected subject may manifest the disease in either the typical complete form (florid form) or in a milder, aborted form ("forme fruste").

A stigmatized infant destined to show the disease in its *florid form* is not likely to present, at birth, any of the common clinical manifestations of the disorder. During the first few months of life, however, the face develops a coarse and ugly appearance. This is created by wide-set protruding eyes, a depressed nose, wide bulging cheeks, a large mouth and thick lips, and large ears. During the second year and thereafter, the grotesque appearance of the face, suggesting that of a gargoyle, becomes increasingly conspicuous. In addition, there may be conical distortion of the cranium (acrocephaly), or the head may show excessive length and narrowness in consequence of bulging of the forehead and occiput (scaphocephaly), or the head may present merely a generally increased size (macrocephaly). Other skeletal abnormalities which may be clinically evident in a severely affected young child include: shortness of stature, due to diminished bone growth; various bowing deformities, especially of the lower extremities; shortness of the neck; kyphosis in the lower dorsolumbar region, due to an angular deformity of one or more vertebral bodies in the area; stiffness and limitation of motion of various joints; and stubbiness of the fingers and a clawlike position of the hands.

In the florid cases of the Hurler syndrome, mental deficiency is usually already apparent during infancy, but in an occasional instance it may not set in before the second or third year of life. In any event, the mental deficiency is definitely progressive, and the mental status of the subject may come to be that of a moron, imbecile, or idiot. The mental deficiency is often accompanied by evidence of damage to the central nervous system, first manifested in muscular hypertonicity and abnormal reflexes and later in motor paralysis (see Jervis).

When the disease is present in florid form, corneal opacity is a constant finding. It is due to diffuse clouding of the deep layers of the cornea. As the opacity increases, the corneas become milky white, and total blindness may ensue. Furthermore, in these cases the liver and spleen are nearly always found enlarged on palpation. The subject usually dies in early or middle childhood.

Among the cases representing milder or aborted expressions of the disease ("*forme fruste*"), there are some in which the disorder may even escape clinical recognition. The corneal opacity which is a consistent feature of the severer expressions of the disease (complete form) is not observed in the milder cases.

Moreover, hepatosplenomegaly is encountered in only about a quarter of these cases. Though the mental and skeletal abnormalities of Hurler's disease are observed in cases representing the "forme fruste" of the disorder, they are sometimes quite inconspicuous. In those cases in which mental abnormality is clearly present, the mental status is more likely to be on the moron level than on that of imbecility or idiocy.

The subjects also show retardation of skeletal growth, but this rarely amounts to actual dwarfism, and occasionally the retardation may be so mild that the subject appears to be of normal stature. The gargoyle-like deformities of the skull which are characteristic of Hurler's disease in its florid form are not nearly so conspicuous in the cases representing the "forme fruste" of the disease. The alterations elsewhere in the skeleton are likewise less striking, though of the same general character as in the florid form. For instance, though one or more vertebral bodies may show, on roentgenographic examination, the distinctive hooklike process associated with alterations in contour, a striking kyphotic curvature is not observed. As already noted, when the mucopolysaccharide excreted in excess is only heparitin sulfate, the skeletal abnormalities are minimal (see Meyer and Hoffman). In addition, the fact that chemical analysis of the skeletal tissues in cases of the Hurler syndrome reveals only minimal amounts of heparitin sulfate seems to indicate that that mucopolysaccharide does not have a strong tendency to lodge in the skeletal tissues and thus interfere with osteogenesis.

ROENTGENOGRAPHIC FINDINGS

In a case representing Hurler's disease in its complete form, roentgenographic survey of the skeleton is likely to show striking alterations involving many bones. However, the involvement is by no means uniform, the bones of some skeletal areas (the upper extremities, for instance) being more commonly and more severely affected than those of other skeletal areas (notably the bones of the lower extremities). When the disorder is present in its milder form, the roentgenographic skeletal manifestations are of the same general character, but are, of course, less prominent. (See Reilly and Lindsay, Jervis, and also Caffey.)

A neonate in whom the disease is destined to be manifest in florid form during infancy may already reveal various skeletal changes shortly after birth, and it may be deduced that in these cases the skeletal changes must have set in before birth. Studying such florid cases, Caffey found that the tubular bones, at birth and during the first months of life, showed generalized rarefaction and widening of the metaphysial ends of their shafts. The extreme ends of the widened bone shafts also presented a slight degree of cupping and/or spurring. In addition, there was already evidence of some apposition of subperiosteal new bone on the cortex of some of the bone shafts, resulting in thickening of the cortex.

In the course of a number of months, the shafts of affected tubular bones will show an increase in diameter, ordinarily associated with thinning of the cortex and expansion of the medullary cavity. One or both ends of the expanded bone shafts will come to appear rather smoothly rounded or, in the case of the metacarpal bones and manual phalanges, even tapered. The metacarpal bones show tapering at their proximal ends, while the manual phalanges show the tapering at their distal ends. Caffey stresses the idea that an uneven increase in the girth of the shafts of the tubular bones is the finding most significant for the diagnosis of Hurler's syndrome. Indeed, he holds that without this finding the roentgenographic diagnosis remains equivocal.

Furthermore, the postnatal (secondary) epiphysial centers of ossification are somewhat delayed in their appearance and are generally smaller than they would normally be. Nevertheless, no striking or diagnostically significant changes in the junctional regions between the cartilaginous epiphyses and the bone shafts are apparent roentgenographically. That is, there are no roentgenographic changes at these sites, even though longitudinal growth is retarded and the subjects are dwarfed because of the disorganization of endochondral bone formation at the epiphysial cartilage plates in the junctional areas.

The maldevelopment of the long tubular bones results in shortness and stubbiness. In addition, a valgus angulation may be observable in relation to the head of each humerus. The femora may show coxa valga angulation of the somewhat thickened necks, and the femoral heads may be somewhat flattened or otherwise malformed. In regard to the knees, genu valgum, usually due to tilting of the distal epiphyses of the femora in consequence of their maldevelopment, is likely to be present.

In relation to the *skull*, the distortion of the shape of the calvarium, the elongation of the base of the cranium in the region of the sella turcica, and the underdevelopment of the maxilla and often of the mandibular rami contribute to the gargoyle-like appearance of the head. As to the *trunk*, the most striking changes occur in the ribs, in one or more of the thoracic and/or lumbar vertebrae, and in the acetabular areas of the innominate bones. The *scapulae* are often found broadened and thickened. The *ribs* present broad bodies, but show narrowing near their sternal ends and often narrowed and misshapen necks. The *kyphosis*, which is a feature of considerable diagnostic significance, is the result of malformation of at least one vertebral body—usually the twelfth thoracic or first lumbar. For some unknown reason, a portion of the anterior half of the affected vertebral body (or bodies) fails to ossify. The unossified portion of the body remains cartilaginous, while its ossified portion comes to present the beaklike appearance which is so conspicuous in the x-ray picture. The acetabula will be found shallow, and the ischia are disproportionately small in relation to the ilia. (See Fig. 138.)

PATHOLOGIC FINDINGS

As can be deduced from the clinical features of gargoylism and the biochemical aberration underlying the condition, one may expect to find pathologic changes not only in the skeletal tissues and other connective tissues but also in the cornea, the viscera, and various parts of the nervous system. That gargoylism represents a "storage disease" was already recognized in the early descriptions of its pathologic anatomy. In some of the early contributions relating to this aspect of the condition, it was mistakenly maintained, as already noted, that the substances accumulating in the various tissues were lipids, and that the disease thus belonged in the category of the lipid storage disorders. However, as is now well established, gargoylism actually represents a mucopolysaccharidosis rather than a lipidosis.

Some presentations relating to the pathologic anatomy of the disorder have covered the gross and microscopic findings in a variety of organs and tissues (see Kressler and Aegerter, Lindsay *et al.*, Henderson *et al.*, Strauss, and also Dawson). Others have emphasized the changes in particular tissues or organs, such as the brain (see Ashby *et al.*, and Tuthill), the liver (see Kny), and the bones (see Schmidt). In all the affected tissues, the foundation of the pathologic changes is the same—namely, the intracellular accumulation of mucopolysaccharides. This results in increased size of the affected cells, due to swelling of the cytoplasm which, on histologic examination, may be found vacuolated or granular.

In one case or another, almost all of the tissues of the body may be found involved to some extent. Of the various internal organs, the brain, liver, and spleen are almost invariably affected. The connective tissues (that is, the so-called interstitial connective tissues and the skeletal tissues) are also regularly implicated. This is natural in view of the importance of the fibrocyte in mucopolysaccharide synthesis. Here we shall stress the pathologic alterations in the bones, though some attention will also be given to the findings in nonskeletal tissues (particularly the liver and the nervous system).

Nonskeletal Tissues.—In most cases the *liver* is found at least somewhat enlarged. Its consistency is sometimes firmer than it would normally be, and when this is the case it is the result of an increase in the periportal connective tissue and of other alterations associated with a mild degree of cirrhosis. On microscopic examination the parenchymal cells of the liver appear swollen, and a large proportion of them show clear-cut vacuolation of their cytoplasm. Indeed, in many of the cells the cytoplasm is almost completely replaced by one or more large vacuoles, and the nucleus of the distended cell is shifted toward the periphery. (See Fig. 139-*A*.) In parenchymal cells without large vacuoles, tiny vacuoles are nevertheless present and tend to give the cytoplasm a foamy appearance. The Kupffer cells are usually also swollen, but the numerous vacuoles in their cytoplasm tend to be smaller than they are in the parenchymal cells. Naturally, the vacuoles represent mucopolysaccharides which have accumulated in the cells of the liver. Furthermore, it has been postulated that this accumulation is the result of exhaustion or depletion of the intracellular lysosomal enzymatic mechanism which normally brings about the degradation and/or excretion of the mucopolysaccharides (see Callahan and Lorincz, and also Callahan *et al.*).

In respect to the *nervous system*, it is clear that in florid cases the *brain*, even if it does not show pathologic changes on gross examination, almost invariably shows them on microscopic examination. Grossly, the brain is often somewhat enlarged, and it is not unusual for it to present some degree of symmetrical internal hydrocephalus. The most consistent histologic change relates to the nerve cells of the cerebral cortex, though some nerve cells in other parts of the nervous system (such

Figure 138

A, Photograph of a boy 17 years of age affected with gargoylism, and his sister who is 7 years of age and is not affected with the disease. This comparison emphasizes the boy's stunted growth and also the other external features of the disease. These are: the generally increased size of the head; the depressed nose; the wide, bulging cheeks; the large ears and thick lips; and the stubby hands. (This illustration was reproduced from the article by Nagel with his kind permission and that of the editor of the Journal of Bone and Joint Surgery.)

B, Roentgenograph showing, in lateral projection, part of the vertebral column (from the tenth thoracic to the fifth lumbar vertebra) in the case of a boy 4 years of age affected with gargoylism. The characteristic malformation of vertebral bodies is apparent, and two of the affected vertebral bodies in particular (first and second lumbar) present anteriorly a conspicuous beaklike contour whose anatomic basis is shown in Figure 139-*B*. (I am indebted to Dr. Edward Singleton of the Texas Children's Hospital, Houston, Texas, for this illustration and also for *C* and *D* on this plate.)

C, Roentgenograph showing the thickening of the body of the scapula observed in some cases of Hurler's syndrome. Note also that, for some distance proximal to the middle of the humeral shaft, the bone cortex is thin and the medullary cavity is slightly expanded. The patient in this case was a girl $2\frac{1}{2}$ years of age, stunted in height and somewhat retarded mentally.

D, Roentgenograph of the right hand and wrist of the patient mentioned in *C*. Note the tapering of the metacarpal bones at their proximal ends, and the tapering of the phalangeal bones at their distal ends.

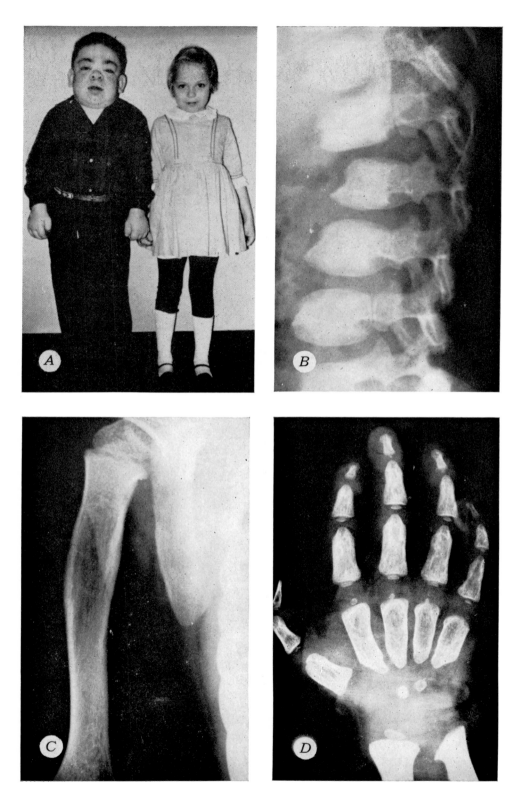

Figure 138

as the basal ganglia, brain stem, and spinal cord) are usually also found affected. Those nerve cells which are altered are swollen and tend to be rounded or oval or even ballooned out. Their nuclei are usually displaced toward the periphery, and in some cells the nuclei are found to have undergone disintegration. The cytoplasm of such nerve cells shows a diminished amount or complete absence of Nissl substance and may appear granular or vesicular. The dendrites and axons of the cortical nerve cells apparently show no consistent changes. The sympathetic ganglia tend to reveal alterations similar to those observed in the neurons of the central nervous system. In many respects, the histologic changes observed in the nerve cells of the brain and spinal cord in gargoylism are similar to the changes encountered in those cells in the infantile form of amaurotic family idiocy (Tay-Sachs disease). It was on this account that gargoylism was misinterpreted at first as being essentially a lipid storage disease.

Bones.—The more obvious changes involving the skeleton have already been covered in the sections dealing with the clinical and roentgenographic findings. These changes include notably: the various alterations in the skull bones; the stunted longitudinal growth of the tubular bones and the malformations presented by them; and the changes in bones of the trunk, including particularly the gibbus-like angulation observed in the lower part of the vertebral column, due to malformation of one or more of the lower thoracic and/or upper lumbar vertebral bodies. (See Fig. 139-*B* and *C*.)

Microscopic examination of bones of a young child affected with gargoylism in florid form reveals striking changes at all sites of endochondral bone formation. For instance, in regard to one or another long tubular bone, if one examines an epiphysis containing a secondary center of ossification, little evidence of cartilage

Figure 139

A, Photomicrograph (× 250) of a tissue section prepared from the liver removed at autopsy in the case of a child affected with gargoylism. Almost throughout, the parenchymal cells appear vacuolated, the cytoplasm of the cells having been replaced by mucopolysaccharides. The subject was a girl who was 15 months of age at the time of her death. At the age of 5 months she already exhibited some of the features of gargoylism, and these became accentuated in the course of the following months, so that she soon came to present the clinical picture of gargoylism in its florid form. In particular, she showed a large head, sunken nasal bridge, gibbus-like deformity in the lower part of the back, and also indications of mental retardation. The child died at the U. S. Naval Hospital in St. Albans, New York, and the autopsy was done there. (The present writer, as a Consultant Pathologist to that hospital, participated in the performance of the autopsy.)

B, Photograph of a part of a vertebral column, sectioned in the sagittal plane and demonstrating in one of the vertebral bodies (twelfth thoracic) the maldevelopment which is characteristic of gargoylism. In particular, because of local arrest of osteogenesis, part of the anterior half of that vertebral body is still composed of cartilage. Since the distal part of the anterior half of that vertebral body is ossified, a beaklike deformity has evolved, and in consequence the malformed vertebral body casts a beaklike shadow in the x-ray picture. The subject in this case was a boy who died when he was 13 years of age. By the time he had reached the age of 9, he manifested the typical appearance of a subject affected with Hurler's syndrome. A marked degree of mental retardation was already manifest when he was 4 years old. (This picture was reproduced, with permission, from the article by Wolfe *et al.*, and I am indebted to the authors of that article and to the editor of the American Journal of Pathology for its use.)

C, Roentgenograph showing part of the vertebral column removed at autopsy in the case of the child mentioned in *A*. The body of the second lumbar vertebra presents the characteristic beaklike deformity in its anterior portion.

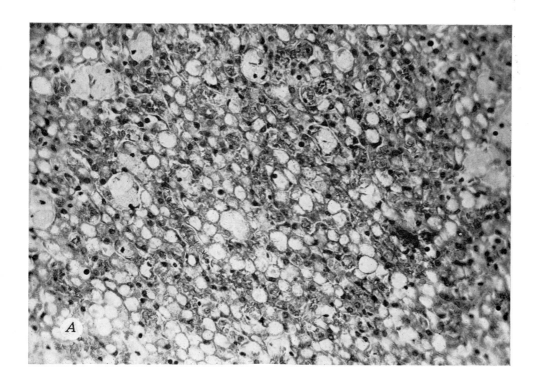

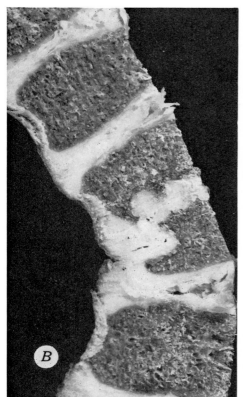
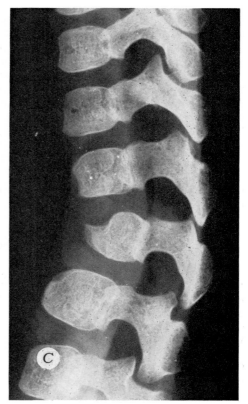

Figure 139

cell proliferation can be noted in the cartilage immediately bordering upon the center in question. Normally, such a center of ossification would be surrounded by a narrow zone of cartilage cells lined up in columns. Furthermore, there would be evidence of: disruption of these cells by capillary blood vessels breaking into them from the marrow; tonguelike spicules of calcified cartilage matrix extending toward the center of ossification; and indications of new bone deposition on the spicules of calcified cartilage matrix. On the other hand, in a florid case of gargoylism in a young child, the cartilage of the epiphysis surrounding the secondary center of ossification has a thin layer of osseous tissue apposed against it, indicating that endochondral bone formation is practically at a standstill.

The epiphysial cartilage plates show changes analogous to those observed around the ossification centers of the epiphyses. An epiphysial cartilage plate will present, on its surface abutting on the bone shaft, some cartilage cells lined up in columns, but these columns are not so wide or so regu'ar as they would normally be. Where the cartilage cells have been broken into by marrow capillaries, and calcified cartilage matrix does extend toward the shaft, the amount of such matrix is very meager and the shaft surface of the plate also has osseous tissue apposed against it. This finding again indicates the lack of active endochondral bone formation at the epiphysial cartilage plate in question. These various microscopic abnormalities at sites of endochondral ossification in a case of gargoylism simulate to some extent the findings at analogous sites in a young child affected with cretinism. However, there should be no confusion between these conditions even on a histologic basis. In gargoylism, both the region of the epiphysial cartilage plates and the cartilage which surrounds the secondary centers of ossification show foci of swollen cartilage cells in which the cytoplasm is vacuolated because of the presence of mucopolysaccharides in it. (See Figs. 140 and 141.)

In relation to the bones in cases of gargoylism, swollen cells containing mucopolysaccharides are, of course, to be found also at sites other than those of endochondral bone formation. In the bone marrow, one may note large numbers of macrophages whose cytoplasm is distinctly granular or somewhat vacuolated. In addition, many of the supporting connective tissue cells of the bone marrow likewise show granular and vacuolated cytoplasm indicating the presence of mucopolysaccharides. The periosteum of many of the bones will also reveal swollen cells containing mucopolysaccharides. This finding relates especially to the deeper layers of the periosteum and to some extent to the immediately adjacent parosteal connective tissue. In places, collections of these swollen cells in the deeper portions of the periosteum can be seen to have produced pressure defects or erosions of the underlying cortical bone.

Figure 140

A, Photomicrograph ($\times$ 6) illustrating the general histologic pattern presented by the lower end of the shaft and distal epiphysis of the right femur removed at autopsy in the case of the 15 month old child about whom clinical information is given in the legend of Figure 139-A. There is a sparsity of osseous trabeculae in the center of ossification for the epiphysis and also in the metaphysial portion of the shaft. This reflects the diminished osteogenesis which has resulted from the retarded endochondral bone formation both in the cartilage surrounding the center of ossification of the epiphysis and at the shaft surface of the epiphysial cartilage plate. In places (see arrow) one can observe focal collections of swollen cartilage cells. The swelling is due to the presence of large amounts of mucopolysaccharides in these cells (see B).

B, Photomicrograph ($\times$ 125) showing in greater detail the collection of swollen cartilage cells indicated by the arrow in A.

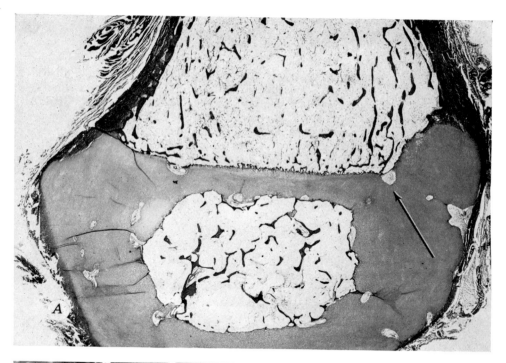

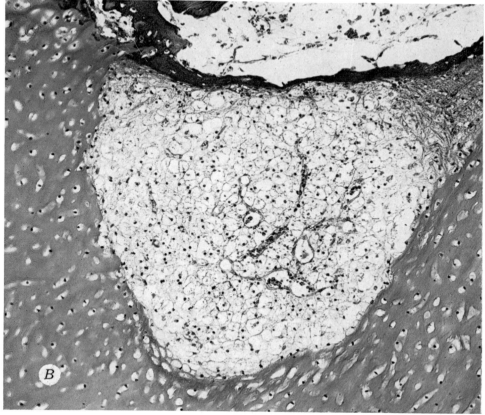

Figure 140

TREATMENT

No treatment is known which is effective against the basic metabolic disorder. In a family in which gargoylism is present in one child, the parents should be alerted to the fact that additional children may come to manifest the disorder. In a child in whom the latter has appeared, therapy has to be confined to the practical management of the various clinical problems presented. For a child showing severe mental retardation, admission to an appropriate institution is probably advisable, even if only to reduce the psychological trauma to the rest of the family. The physical difficulties created by the kyphosis, genu valgum, everted feet, etc. can be mitigated by the relevant orthopaedic appliances and/or surgical procedures.

OCHRONOSIS

Ochronosis, first described by Virchow, is a rare condition characterized *pathologico-anatomically* by abnormal pigmentation of various tissues and, in particular, of the hyaline and fibrous cartilages. The cartilages come to show yellowish, brownish, or even black discoloration. Tendons, ligaments, and joint capsules may also show the abnormal pigmentation to some extent, especially at their sites of attachment. In the course of time, the sclera of the eye, the pinna of the ear, the valves of the heart, and the walls of various blood vessels often become more or less discolored, as do fibrous scars on the surface of the body. The skin itself may show abnormal pigmentation, which is due at least in part to the presence of yellow-brown pigment granules within the walls of the blood vessels of the skin and in the sweat glands and sebaceous glands. In part also, however, it may be due to the transmission, through the epidermis, of discoloration involving the deeper tissues, such as ligaments, tendons and fascia, etc. In the present discussion, stress will, of course, be laid upon the articular sequelae of ochronosis. Numerous details relating to all aspects of ochronosis are to be found in the comprehensive review articles by O'Brien *et al.*, which summarize the pertinent world literature that has accumulated in the course of nearly four hundred years. (See also Laskar and Sargison.)

The *biochemical basis* of ochronosis is an inborn error of intermediary metabolism involving the amino acids tyrosine and phenylalanine. In the ordinary course of the metabolism of these amino acids, homogentisic acid is formed. In contrast to normal persons, those affected with the inborn metabolic error in question lack the enzyme homogentisic acid oxidase in their livers and kidneys, or at least have a

Figure 141

A, Photomicrograph ($\times$ 55) showing the epiphysial cartilage plate at the upper end of the right tibia, also from the case of the 15 month old child with gargoylism about whom clinical information was given in the legend of Figure 139-*A*. In the midportion of the plate there is a well-delimited area of swollen cartilage cells containing mucopolysaccharides. The proliferating cartilage cells of the plate are lined up in columns advancing in the direction of the shaft of the bone. It is significant, however, that there is a pronounced sparsity of tongues of calcified cartilage matrix (the primary spongiosa) extending into the shaft, such as one would see on the shaft surface of the epiphysial cartilage plate of a long tubular bone in a normal young child. Thus it is clear that endochondral ossification is greatly retarded at the plate in question.

B, Photomicrograph ($\times$ 125) illustrating the cortex of a rib in the same case, and showing the presence of swollen cells containing mucopolysaccharides (see arrows) in the deeper portion of the periosteum.

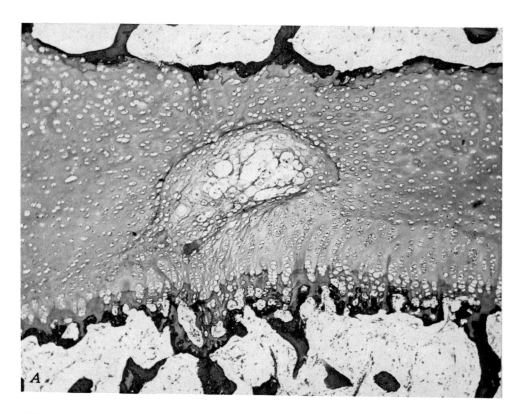

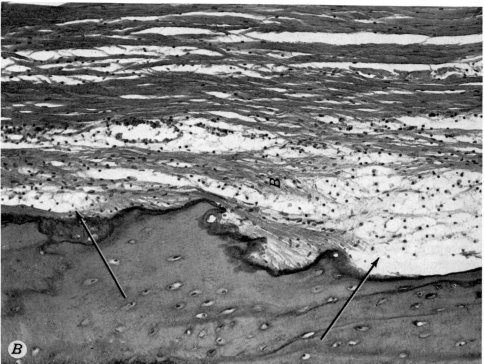

Figure 141

pronounced deficiency of it. In consequence of this gene-related enzyme deficiency, the initial step in the catabolism of homogentisic acid is substantially or completely blocked. Hence, abnormal amounts of homogentisic acid (alkapton) accumulate in the blood, and alkaptonuria (the excretion of large amounts of alkapton in the urine) results. In addition, the deposition of homogentisic acid in the various tissues is undoubtedly the basis for their subsequent pigmentation and associated pathologic changes resulting in the clinico-anatomic complex denoted as ochronosis.

In regard to the pigmentation and the evolution of the other changes leading to ochronosis, it is believed that: (1) There is a reversible physical binding of homogentisic acid to connective tissue molecules; and (2) this is followed by oxidation of the homogentisic molecules, resulting in the formation of homogentisic polymers (including benzoquinonacetic acid) which undergo irreversible chemical combination with the connective tissues, imparting the pigmentation to them and making them liable to degenerative changes. (See Garrod, Dakin, Zannoni *et al.*, La Du *et al.*, and Milch.)

Experimentally, it has been found that rats fed a diet, of which 12 per cent was tyrosine, for periods up to 40 days developed progressive dark discoloration of the articular cartilages of the hip and knee joints, and showed the presence of alkaptons in the urine (see Bondurant and Henry). It is also pertinent in this connection that injections of homogentisic acid into the knee joints of rabbits produced changes in the cartilages and synovial membrane which resembled those appearing in these structures in cases of ochronosis in man.

Of historical interest is the fact that instances of ochronosis have been observed in the past which had their basis in chronic phenol poisoning resulting, for instance, from protracted treatment of indolent ulcers with solutions or ointments containing small (noncaustic) amounts of carbolic acid (see Pope, Pick, Reid *et al.*, and also Beddard). In these cases the subjects exhibited carboluria instead of the alkaptonuria shown in the cases of ochronosis due to an inborn error of amino acid metabolism. In particular, the brown or black discoloration of the cartilages resulted from oxidation of the hydroxylated phenols deposited in these tissues (see Fishberg and Dolin).

CLINICAL CONSIDERATIONS

In regard to *inheritance*, it has long been recognized that alkaptonuria (homogentisic aciduria) is a congenital and familial disorder, and there is increasing evidence that it is transmitted as an autosomal recessive trait in most of the alkaptonuric families. On the basis of the relatively high incidence of alkaptonuria in families in which there has been intermarriage, a dominant mode of inheritance has been suggested, but actually this finding merely reinforces the concept that the condition is transmitted by an autosomal recessive gene (see Hsia). Except for its relatively high incidence in family groups in which there has been intermarriage, alkaptonuria is only rarely encountered. Furthermore, the condition is not indigenous to any one race or country and apparently does not predilect one sex over the other.

It is only exceptionally that any of the *clinical manifestations* of ochronosis become apparent during childhood or even during early adult life. Indeed, for several decades before they set in, clinical evidence of the basic metabolic disorder is nearly always limited to the finding of alkaptonuria. Because of the presence of the alkaptons in the urine, the latter tends to become brownish or even black if it is exposed to the air for many hours. The discoloration can be brought out quickly if the urine is made alkaline, and the urine may already be discolored when it is voided if its pH is on the alkaline side. The fact that an infant is affected with the disorder not infrequently comes to light shortly after birth because the urine-soaked diapers or bed linens are found discolored. In any event, there are a number of recorded instances in the literature in which alkaptonuria was noted in an infant or young child and the same person manifested ochronosis and ochronotic arthropathy many years later (see Harrold, Nägele, and Klinkert and Nauta). In fact, survival into middle life is not at all unusual in cases of ochronosis, and in some instances the subject even attains old age.

Articular Manifestations.—Complaints referable to the joints ordinarily do not set in before early middle life. In general, the clinical difficulties pertaining to joints are observed more often and are more severe in the male subjects than in the females. The initial articular complaints most commonly relate to the vertebral column. Occasionally the onset of the back pain takes the form of an acute episode ascribable to herniation of a degenerated intervertebral disk (see McCollum and Odom). As a rule, there is pain of a dull and aching character, starting in the lower part of the back and then extending upward. Gradually, the spine loses mobility, the increasing stiffness resulting from narrowing and ossification of the intervertebral disks, often associated with fusion of some contiguous vertebral bodies. The narrowing of the disks, together with a stooped posture, may lead to a significant loss in height.

In the course of time (perhaps years after the onset of back pain), one or another of the large peripheral joints becomes the site of clinical difficulties, usually after minor trauma. Of the large joints, it is the knee joint that is likely to be involved first, the shoulder and hip joints following. The affected joint is painful and swollen, the swelling being due to effusion into the articular cavity. The effusion is provoked by irritation of the synovial membrane caused by sloughing off of bits of the ochronotic articular cartilages and the incorporation of some of the cartilage fragments into the membrane. In time, the synovial membrane of the affected joint becomes greatly thickened. The severest changes are usually to be observed in the knee joints, which become sites of particularly pronounced osteoarthritis, though advanced osteoarthritis may ultimately appear in other large joints also (see Červenanský et al., and Abe et al.). It is of special interest that the small diarthrodial joints of the hands and feet seem to be spared the degenerative changes exhibited by the large diarthrodial joints. (See Fig. 142.)

PATHOLOGIC FINDINGS

In cases of long-standing ochronosis, the characteristic pigmentation (yellowish, brownish, and/or black) is widely distributed through the tissues of the body (see Kleinschmidt, Oppenheimer and Kline, Cooper and Moran, Lichtenstein and Kaplan, Puhr, and O'Brien et al.). The pigment is a melanin-like substance derived from the homogentisic acid which lodges in the tissues and which is subsequently oxidized and polymerized to form the pigment. As already mentioned in the paragraph introducing the subject of ochronosis, the sclera of the eye, the pinna of the ear, the valves of the heart, and the walls of various blood vessels may be found more or less pigmented, along with such connective tissue structures as tendons, ligaments, and joint capsules. The hyaline cartilages (the articular, costal, tracheal, and bronchial cartilages) are deeply pigmented, often being bluish black. The fibrocartilages (notably the intervertebral disks) are also deeply pigmented. In the prostate and prostatic urethra, considerable amounts of bluish black pigment may be present, and in some places the pigment may be found agglomerated into small, firm masses. The kidneys, too, may show pigmentation. If they do, microscopic examination will reveal pigment granules in the epithelium of the renal tubules and in casts within the lumens of the tubules. Our special concern in respect to the pathologic findings in ochronosis is with the changes occurring in the vertebral column and in the large diarthrodial joints.

Changes in the Vertebral Column.—The pathologic changes occurring in the various joints of the vertebral column together account for the loss of flexibility (occasionally amounting to actual rigidity) already noted as a conspicuous clinical feature of ochronosis. The evolution of the *ochronotic spondylosis* is associated with the deposition of ochronotic pigment in the components of the intervertebral disks and in the thin plates of hyaline cartilage covering the upper and lower surfaces of the vertebral bodies. This is followed by pronounced degenerative changes both in the intervertebral disks and in the cartilage plates. Disk tissue which is heavily impregnated with ochronotic pigment tends to cast a radiopaque shadow in the

Figure 142

A and B, Roentenographs in the anteroposterior and lateral projections of the lumbar vertebrae illustrating the ochronotic spondylosis which had developed in a case of alkaptonuria. The intervertebral disk spaces are very much narrowed in consequence of degenerative changes which have taken place in the disks. The lateral projection, in particular, reveals that the residual intervertebral disk tissue casts a more or less radiopaque shadow. The latter is usually interpreted as evidence of calcification of the disk tissue, but in reality is largely the result of ossification occurring in the degenerated disks. In addition, it can be seen that the alterations in the intervertebral disks are associated with the presence of spondylosis deformans characterized by the osteophytes which are extending from the vertebral bodies adjacent to the degenerated disks. The subject in this case was a man 51 years of age who died and was autopsied at the Massachusetts General Hospital. He had developed a septic arthritis of the right shoulder joint, and the immediate cause of his death was a massive hemorrhage from a duodenal ulcer. Clinical and anatomic details relating to the case in question constitute the subject of one of the Case Records of the Massachusetts General Hospital (Case 9–1966) and are reported in the New England Journal of Medicine, *274*, 454, 1966. (I am indebted to Dr. Benjamin Castleman, Pathologist at the Massachusetts General Hospital and Editor of these Case Records, for these two roentgenographs and also for the photographs illustrating various gross pathologic skeletal changes of ochronosis in this case, which appear as Figure 143.)

C, Roentgenograph of the lumbar portion of the vertebral column from a case of alkaptonuria and ochronosis showing much more advanced changes of ochronotic spondylosis than are apparent in A and B. Some of the intervertebral disk spaces appear to have been completely obliterated, and the adjacent vertebral bodies have undergone fusion in consequence of bony ankylosis between the bodies where the disks had disappeared, and also through intergrowth and union of marginal exostoses. The subject in this case was a man who was 72 years of age when this roentgenograph was taken in 1962. Twenty-four years earlier—that is, when he was 48 years of age—he attended the Out-Patient Department of our hospital, where it was recognized that he was affected with alkaptonuria. At that time, roentgenographic examination of the lumbar portion of the vertebral column already showed radiopacity of the intervertebral disks, representing an early stage in the evolution of the ochronotic spondylosis. Our hospital record also indicated that he was the father of four daughters, two of whom had alkaptonuria.

D, Roentgenograph of the right hip joint in the same case of ochronosis. This picture was taken at the same time as the picture of the vertebral column shown in C. The hip joint is the site not only of advanced changes of osteoarthritis but also of bony ankylosis. The latter undoubtedly followed in the wake of degeneration and extensive erosion of the articular cartilages of the femoral head and acetabulum, permitting osseous bridging between the bone parts in question. (I am indebted to Dr. Harold Jacobson, Chief of the Division of Diagnostic Radiology at Montefiore Hospital and Medical Center, New York City, for placing at my disposal the x-ray films from which C and D were reproduced.)

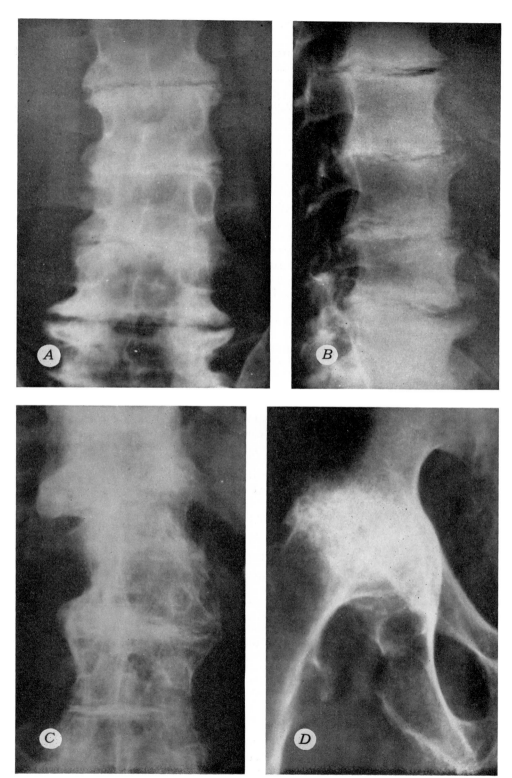

Figure 142

x-ray picture. This is the result of ossification within the disks, and to what extent calcium deposition in the altered disk tissue contributes to the intensity of the radiopacity is still open to question.

Eventually, many of the intervertebral disk spaces become narrowed because of disintegration of the degenerated disk tissue, followed by resorption of that tissue and of the ochronotic plates of cartilage covering the upper and lower surfaces of the vertebral bodies. Segments of the vertebral column where disintegration of the disks and narrowing of the spaces between adjacent vertebral bodies have proceeded slowly are likely to show osteophytes extending from the adjacent vertebral bodies and more or less surrounding the altered intervertebral disks. These exostoses, whose color is dark brown, arise as a result of traction by the longitudinal ligament at its sites of attachment to the annulus fibrosus of the disk and to the cortex of the vertebral body immediately above and below the disk. On the other hand, in segments of the vertebral column where the disk tissue and cartilage plates between adjacent vertebral bodies have undergone rapid and substantial disintegration and resorption, one may note that bony fusion has taken place (focally or more or less throughout) between apposed vertebral bodies. (See Fig. 143.)

The articular cartilages of the articular processes are also discolored by the ochronotic pigment. Thus the facet joints participate in the pathologic changes involving the vertebral column. The margins of these facet joints show exostosis formation, and the joints themselves may be bridged by exostoses.

Changes in Large Diarthrodial Joints.—It is, of course, the articular cartilages that are the sites of departure for the alterations leading to ochronotic arthropathy involving the large diarthrodial joints. The cartilages become progressively discolored because of deposition of ochronotic pigment in them. It has been found that the pigment begins to accumulate in the matrix of the deeper parts of the articular cartilage (radial and transitional zones), while the matrix of the tangential zone (that is, the surface layer of the cartilage) does not become discolored (see O'Brien *et al.*). As the amount of pigment in the cartilage matrix increases, granules of pigment are likely to be found in some of the cartilage cells. The ochronotic cartilage is brittle, and sooner or later it comes to present a somewhat shaggy, fibrillized surface in some places. In the course of continued function, fragments of the cartilage so altered become detached, and its surface now shows smaller or larger areas of superficial erosion, exposing the darkly pigmented deeper portions of

Figure 143

A, Photograph illustrating the gross appearance of the cut surface of part of the vertebral column, sectioned in the frontal plane, in the case of ochronosis to which reference was made in Figure 142-*A* and *B*. All of the intervertebral disks are narrowed and degenerated and show black pigmentation. Various degrees of marginal spurring are apparent between adjacent vertebral bodies. The two lowest intervertebral disks have undergone substantial disintegration, and the apposed portions of the vertebral bodies are sclerotic. The lighter areas in these disks and in the various other pigmented disks reflect ossification going on in them.

B, Photograph illustrating, in the same case, the gross appearance of the sternum and several costal cartilages sectioned in the frontal plane (on the left of the picture) and part of the sternum sectioned in the sagittal plane (on the right of the picture). The costal cartilages are jet-black in color. The fibrocartilage of the manubriosternal junction is also discolored black.

C, Photograph of the upper end of one of the femora in the same case. The articular cartilage is discolored black, the discoloration extending down to the bony end plate, as can be seen on the left in the sectioned specimen. Note that the ligaments and tendons in the intertrochanteric area are also discolored black.

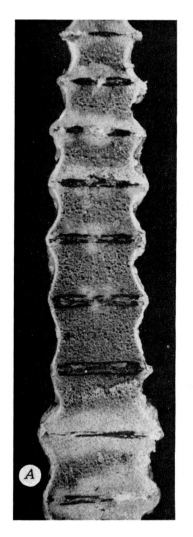

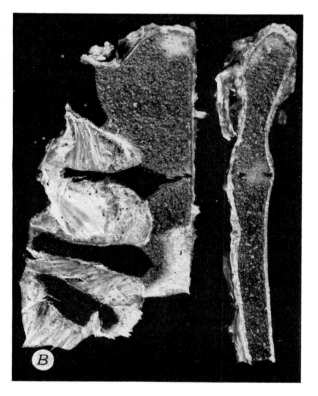

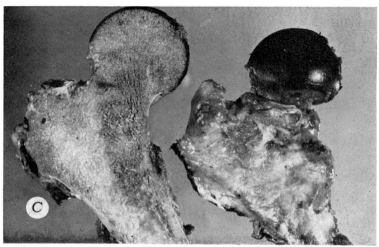

Figure 143

559

the cartilage. The erosions appear first at sites which are subjected to the greatest functional pressures, and as functional friction continues, the erosions become deeper. Furthermore, the malalignments of the articular surfaces induce the formation of additional areas of superficial erosion of the cartilages in the course of continued function.

As the alterations in the articular bone ends advance, the subchondral bone areas which are no longer covered by cartilage may present a polished, eburnated surface indicating the presence of densification and sclerosis of the bone areas in question. Various other pathologic changes of degenerative osteoarthritis, such as marginal exostoses and small subchondral bone cysts, eventually make their appearance. Many of the fragments of articular cartilage which have been sloughed off and which have entered the articular cavity become incorporated into the synovial membrane. In reaction, the latter undergoes villous proliferation. The proliferated synovial membrane shows mild, nonspecific inflammatory changes in its sublining connective tissue, and also the presence of phagocytes in the immediate vicinity of some of the bits of articular cartilage which have been taken up into the membrane.

TREATMENT

The natural basic objective in the treatment of patients affected with alkaptonuria would be to reduce the endogenous production of homogentisic acid. This could be accomplished by: (1) supplying the missing enzyme (homogentisic acid oxidase) to the subject; and (2) drastically reducing the intake of tyrosine and phenylalanine through restriction of the intake of protein. Obviously, the intake of protein cannot be severely restricted over a long period of time, and homogentisic acid oxidase in pharmaceutical form is not available. It has been suggested, but not established in relation to man, that the consumption of large amounts of vitamin C might prevent the deposition of ochronotic pigment in the connective tissues, even though, of course, it would not correct the basic enzymatic defect (see Sealock *et al.*). The orthopaedic measures appropriate against degenerative arthritis irrespective of its basis should naturally be employed against the skeletal manifestations of ochronosis.

REFERENCES

ABE, Y., OSHIMA, N., HANAKOTA, Y., AMAKO, T., and HIROHATA, R.: Thirteen Cases of Alkaptonuria from One Family Tree with Special Reference to Osteo-Arthrosis Alkaptonurica, J. Bone & Joint Surg., *42-A*, 817, 1960.

ADLERSBERG, D.: Inborn Errors of Lipid Metabolism. Clinical, Genetic, and Chemical Aspects, Arch. Path., *60*, 481, 1955.

AMSTUTZ, H. C., and CAREY, E. J.: Skeletal Manifestations and Treatment of Gaucher's Disease, J. Bone & Joint Surg., *48-A*, 670, 1966.

ARKIN, A. M., and SCHEIN, A. J.: Aseptic Necrosis in Gaucher's Disease, J. Bone & Joint Surg., *30-A*, 631, 1948.

ASHBY, W. R., STEWART, R. M., and WATKIN, J. H.: Chondro-Osteo-Dystrophy of the Hurler Type (Gargoylism), Brain, *60*, 149, 1937.

ATKINSON, F. R. B.: Gaucher's Disease in Children, Brit. J. Child. Dis., *35*, 1, 1938.

BANKER, B. Q., MILLER, J. Q., and CROCKER, A. C.: The Cerebral Pathology of Infantile Gaucher's Disease, in *Cerebral Sphingolipidoses*, edited by S. M. Aronson and B. W. Volk, New York, Academic Press, 1962 (see p. 73).

BAUMANN, T., KLENK, E., and SCHEIDEGGER, S.: Die Niemann-Picksche Krankheit, Ergebn. allg. Path., *30*, 183, 1936.

BEDDARD, A. P.: Ochronosis Associated with Carboluria, Quart. J. Med., *3*, 329, 1909–10.

BERGGÅRD, I., and BEARN, A. G.: The Hurler Syndrome. A Biochemical and Clinical Study, Am. J. Med., *39*, 221, 1965.

BIELSCHOWSKY, M.: Amaurotische Idiotie und lipoidzellige Splenohepatomegalie, J. Psychol. u. Neurol., *36*, 103, 1928.
BONDURANT, R. E., and HENRY, J. B.: Pathogenesis of Ochronosis in Experimental Alkaptonuria of the White Rat, Lab. Invest., *14*, 62, 1965.
BRANTE, G.: Gargoylism—A Mucopolysaccharidosis, Scandinav. J. Clin. & Lab. Invest., *4*, 43, 1952.
BRILL, N. E., MANDLEBAUM, F. S., and LIBMAN, E.: Primary Splenomegaly—Gaucher Type. Report on One of Four Cases Occurring in a Single Generation of One Family, Am. J. M. Sc., *129*, 491, 1905.
BRUSCO, O. J., HOWARD, R. P., JARMAN, J. B., and FURMAN, R. H.: Osseous Xanthomatosis and Pathologic Fractures in Familial Hyperlipemia (Hyperglyceridemia), Am. J. Med., *40*, 477, 1966.
CAFFEY, J.: Gargoylism (Hunter-Hurler Disease, Dysostosis Multiplex, Lipochondrodystrophy); Prenatal and Neonatal Bone Lesions and Their Early Postnatal Evolution, Bull. Hosp. Joint Dis., *12*, 38, 1951.
CALLAHAN, W. P., and LORINCZ, A. E.: Hepatic Ultrastructure in the Hurler Syndrome, Am. J. Path., *48*, 277, 1966.
CALLAHAN, W. P., HACKETT, R. L., and LORINCZ, A. E.: New Observations by Light Microscopy on Liver Histology in the Hurler's Syndrome, Arch. Path., *83*, 507, 1967.
CAMPBELL, T. N., and FRIED, M.: Urinary Mucopolysaccharide Excretion in the Sex-Linked Form of the Hurler Syndrome, Proc. Soc. Exper. Biol. & Med., *108*, 529, 1961.
ČERVEŇANSKÝ, J., SIŤAJ, Š., and URBÁNEK, T.: Alkaptonuria and Ochronosis, J. Bone & Joint Surg., *41-A*, 1169, 1959.
CHESTER, W.: Über Lipoidgranulomatose, Virchows Arch. path. Anat., *279*, 561, 1930–31.
CHIARI, H.: Die generalisierte Xanthomatose vom Typus Schüller-Christian, Ergebn. allg. Path., *24*, 396, 1931.
COOPER, J. A., and MORAN, T. J.: Studies on Ochronosis, Arch. Path., *64*, 46, 1957.
CROCKER, A. C., and FARBER, S.: Niemann-Pick Disease: A Review of Eighteen Patients, Medicine, *37*, 1, 1958.
CROCKER, A. C., and LANDING, B. H.: Phosphatase Studies in Gaucher's Disease, Metabolism, *9*, 341, 1960.
DAKIN, H. D.: The Chemical Nature of Alcaptonuria, J. Biol. Chem., *9*, 151, 1911.
DAVISON, C., and JACOBSON, S. A.: Generalized Lipoidosis in a Case of Amaurotic Familial Idiocy, Am. J. Dis. Child., *52*, 345, 1936.
DAWSON, I. M. P.: The Histology and Histochemistry of Gargoylism, J. Path. & Bact., *67*, 587, 1954.
DEMARSH, Q. B., and KAUTZ, J.: The Submicroscopic Morphology of Gaucher Cells, Blood, *12*, 324, 1957.
DORFMAN, A., and LORINCZ, A. E.: Occurrence of Urinary Acid Mucopolysaccharides in the Hurler Syndrome, Proc. Nat. Acad. Sc., *43*, 443, 1957.
EPSTEIN, E.: Beitrag zur Pathologie der Gaucherschen Krankheit, Virchows Arch. path. Anat., *253*, 157, 1924.
FARBER, S., COHEN, J., and UZMAN, L. L.: Lipogranulomatosis: A New Lipo-Glyco-Protein "Storage" Disease, J. Mt. Sinai Hosp., *24*, 816, 1957.
FISHBERG, E. H., and DOLIN, B. T.: The Biological Action of Strongly Positive Oxidation-Reduction Systems, J. Biol. Chem., *101*, 159, 1933.
FISHER, E. R., and REIDBORD, H.: Gaucher's Disease: Pathogenetic Considerations Based on Electron Microscopic and Histochemical Observations, Am. J. Path., *41*, 679, 1962.
FLEISCHMAJER, R.: Cutaneous and Tendon Xanthomas, Dermatologica, *128*, 113, 1964.
FORSYTHE, W. I., McKEOWN, E. F., and NEILL, D. W.: Three Cases of Niemann Pick's Disease in Children, Arch. Dis. Childhood, *34*, 406, 1959.
FRIED, K.: Gaucher's Disease Among the Jews in Israel, Bull. Res. Counc. Israel, *B7*, 213, 1958.
FRISELL, E.: Gauchersche Krankheit im frühen Kindesalter, Acta paediat., *30*, 470, 1942–43.
GAÁL, A.: Das Röntgenbild der Knochenveränderungen bei essentieller Xanthomatose (Diathesis xanthomatosa), Fortschr. Geb. Röntgenstrahlen, *48*, 292, 1933.
GARROD, A. E.: Inborn Errors of Metabolism. Alkaptonuria, Lancet, *2*, 73, 1908.
————: *Inborn Errors of Metabolism*, 2nd ed., London, Henry Frowde and Hodder & Stoughton, 1923.
GAUCHER, P. C. E.: De l'epithelioma primitif de la rate, hypertrophie idiopathique de la rate sans leucemie, Paris Thesis, 1882.
GEDDES, A. K., and MOORE, S.: Acute (Infantile) Gaucher's Disease, J. Pediat., *43*, 61, 1953.
GILDENHORN, H. L., and AMROMIN, G. D.: Report of a Case with Niemann-Pick Disease: Correlation of Roentgenographic and Autopsy Findings, Am. J. Roentgenol., *85*, 680, 1961.
GREENFIELD, G. B.: Bone Changes in Chronic Adult Gaucher's Disease, Am. J. Roentgenol., *110*, 800, 1970.

GROEN, J.:   The Hereditary Mechanism of Gaucher's Disease, Blood, *3*, 1238, 1948.
——————: Gaucher's Disease: Hereditary Transmission and Racial Distribution, Arch. Int. Med., *113*, 543, 1964.
——————: Present Status of Knowledge of Gaucher's Disease, Israel J. M. Sc., *1*, 507, 1965.
HAMPERL, H.:   Über die pathologisch-anatomischen Veränderungen bei Morbus Gaucher im Säuglingsalter, Virchows Arch. path. Anat., *271*, 147, 1929.
HARRIS-JONES, J. N., JONES, E. G., and WELLS, P. G.:   Xanthomatosis and Essential Hypercholesterolaemia, Lancet, *1*, 855, 1957.
HARROLD, A. J.:   Alkaptonuric Arthritis, J. Bone & Joint Surg., *38-B*, 532, 1956.
HENDERSON, J. L., MacGREGOR, A. R., THANNHAUSER, S. J., and HOLDEN, R.:   The Pathology and Biochemistry of Gargoylism, Arch. Dis. Childhood, *27*, 230, 1952.
HOFFMAN, S. J., and MAKLER, M. I.:   Gaucher's Disease, Am. J. Dis. Child., *38*, 775, 1929.
HSIA, D. Y.-Y.:   *Inborn Errors of Metabolism*, 2nd ed., Chicago, Year Book Med. Pub., Inc., 1966.
HSIA, D. Y.-Y., NAYLOR, J., and BIGLER, J. A.:   Gaucher's Disease: Report of Two Cases in Father and Son and Review of the Literature, New England J. Med., *261*, 164, 1959.
HUNTER, C.:   A Rare Disease in Two Brothers, Proc. Roy. Soc. Med., *10*, 104, 1916–17.
HURLER, G.:   Über einen Typ multipler Abartungen, vorwiegend am Skelettsystem, Ztschr. Kinderh., *24*, 220, 1919–20.
JACKSON, D. C., and SIMON, G.:   Unusual Bone and Lung Changes in a Case of Gaucher's Disease, Brit. J. Radiol., *38*, 698, 1965.
JERVIS, G. A.:   Gargoylism (Lipochondrodystrophy). A Study of Ten Cases, with Emphasis on the Formes Frustes of the Disease, Arch. Neurol. & Psychiat., *63*, 681, 1950.
KENNAWAY, N. G., and WOOLF, L. I.:   Splenic Lipids in Gaucher's Disease, J. Lipid Res., *9*, 755, 1968.
KLEINSCHMIDT, W.:   Über einen Fall von "endogener Ochronose bei Alkaptonurie," Frankfurt. Ztschr. Path., *28*, 73, 1922.
KLENK, E.:   Über die Natur der Phosphatide der Milz bei der Niemann-Pickschen Krankheit, Ztschr. physiol. Chem., *229*, 151, 1934.
——————: Über die Natur der Phosphatide und anderer Lipoide des Gehirns und der Leber bei der Niemann-Pickschen Krankheit, Ztschr. physiol. Chem., *235*, 24, 1935.
KLINKERT, D., and NAUTA, J. H.:   Demonstratie van twee patiënten met arthritis deformans als gevolg van alcaptonurie, Nederl. tijdschr. geneesk., *85*, 3063, 1941.
KNY, W.:   Zur Kenntnis der Dysostosis multiplex Typ Pfaundler-Hurler, Ztschr. Kinderh., *63*, 366, 1942–43.
KOCH, H. J., JR., and LEWIS, J. S.:   Hyperlipemic Xanthomatosis with Associated Osseous Granuloma, New England J. Med., *255*, 387, 1956.
KÖHNE, G.:   Über Morbus Gaucher mit Hirnveränderungen im Säuglingsalter, Beitr. path. Anat., *102*, 512, 1939.
KRESSLER, R. J., and AEGERTER, E. E.:   Hurler's Syndrome (Gargoylism), J. Pediat., *12*, 579, 1938.
LA DU, B. N., ZANNONI, V. G., LASTER, L., and SEEGMILLER, J. E.:   The Nature of the Defect in Tyrosine Metabolism in Alcaptonuria, J. Biol. Chem., *230*, 251, 1958.
DE LANGE, C.:   Über die maligne Form der Gaucherschen Krankheit, Acta paediat., *27*, 34, 1939.
LASKAR, F. H., and SARGISON, K. D.:   Ochronotic Arthropathy, J. Bone & Joint Surg., *52-B*, 653, 1970.
LEVIN, B.:   Gaucher's Disease. Clinical and Roentgenologic Manifestations, Am. J. Roentgenol., *85*, 685, 1961.
LICHTENSTEIN, L., and KAPLAN, L.:   Hereditary Ochronosis, Am. J. Path., *30*, 99, 1954.
LIEB, H.:   Cerebrosidspeicherung bei Splenomegalie, Typus Gaucher, Ztschr. physiol. Chem., *140*, 305, 1924.
LINDAU, A.:   Neuere Auffassungen über die Pathogenese der familiären amaurotischen Idiotie, Acta psychiat. et neurol., *5*, 167, 1930.
LINDSAY, S., REILLY, W. A., GOTHAM, T. J., and SKAHEN, R.:   Gargoylism. II. Study of Pathologic Lesions and Clinical Review of Twelve Cases, Am. J. Dis. Child., *76*, 239, 1948.
MANDLEBAUM, F. S., and DOWNEY, H.:   The Histo-Pathology and Biology of Gaucher's Disease (Large-Cell Splenomegaly), Folia haemat., *20*, 139, 1916.
MARCH, H. C., GILBERT, P. D., and KAIN, T. M.:   Hypercholesteremic Xanthomata of the Tendons, Am. J. Roentgenol., *77*, 109, 1957.
MATOTH, Y., and FRIED, K.:   Chronic Gaucher's Disease. Clinical Observations on 34 Patients, Israel J. M. Sc., *1*, 521, 1965.
McCOLLUM, D. E., and ODOM, G. L.:   Alkaptonuria, Ochronosis, and Low-Back Pain, J. Bone & Joint Surg., *47-A*, 1389, 1965.
MEDOFF, A. S., and BAYRD, E. D.:   Gaucher's Disease in 29 Cases: Hematologic Complications and Effect of Splenectomy, Ann. Int. Med., *40*, 481, 1954.

MENTEN, M. L., and WELTON, J. P.: Lipid Analysis in a Case of Niemann-Pick Disease, Am. J. Dis. Child., *72*, 720, 1946.
MERRILL, A. S.: Case of Xanthoma Showing Multiple Bone Lesions, Am. J. Roentgenol., *7*, 480, 1920.
MEYER, K., GRUMBACH, M. M., LINKER, A., and HOFFMAN, P.: Excretion of Sulfated Mucopolysaccharides in Gargoylism. (Hurler's Syndrome), Proc. Soc. Exper. Biol. & Med., *97*, 275, 1958.
MEYER, K., and HOFFMAN, P.: Hurler's Syndrome, Arthritis Rheum., *4*, 552, 1961.
MILCH, R. A.: Biochemical Studies on the Pathogenesis of Collagen Tissue Changes in Alcaptonuria, Clin. Orthop., No. *24*, 213, 1962.
MORGANS, M. E.: Gaucher's Disease without Splenomegaly, Lancet, *2*, 576, 1947.
NAGEL, D. A.: Urinary Excretion of Acid Mucopolysaccharides. A Study of Sixty-four Patients with Abnormal Enchondral-Bone Formation and Other Skeletal Abnormalities, J. Bone & Joint Surg., *47-A*, 1176, 1965.
NÄGELE, E.: Röntgenbefunde bei Alkaptonurie, Fortschr. Geb. Röntgenstrahlen, *87*, 523, 1957.
NIEMANN, A.: Ein unbekanntes Krankheitsbild, Jahrb. Kinderh., *79*, 1, 1914.
NORMAN, R. M., URICH, H., TINGEY, A. H., and GOODBODY, R. A.: Tay-Sachs' Disease with Visceral Involvement and Its Relationship to Niemann-Pick's Disease, J. Path. & Bact., *78*, 409, 1959.
OBERLING, C., and WORINGER, P.: La maladie de Gaucher chez le nourrisson, Rev. franç. pédiat., *3*, 475, 1927.
O'BRIEN, W. M., BANFIELD, W. G., and SOKOLOFF, L.: Studies on the Pathogenesis of Ochronotic Arthropathy, Arthritis Rheum., *4*, 137, 1961.
O'BRIEN, W. M., LA DU, B. N., and BUNIM, J. J.: Biochemical, Pathologic and Clinical Aspects of Alcaptonuria, Ochronosis and Ochronotic Arthropathy, Am. J. Med., *34*, 813, 1963.
OPPENHEIMER, B. S., and KLINE, B. S.: Ochronosis, Arch. Int. Med., *29*, 732, 1922.
PATRICK, A. D.: A Deficiency of Glucocerebrosidase in Gaucher's Disease, Biochem. J., *97*, 17c, 1965.
VAN PELT, J. F., and HUIZINGA, J.: Some Observations on the Genetics of Gargoylism, Acta genet., *12*, 1, 1962.
PFAUNDLER, M.: Demonstrationen über einen Typus kindlicher Dysostose, Jahrb. Kinderh., *92*, 420, 1920.
PICK, L.: Ueber die Ochronose, Verhandl. Berl. med. Gesellsch., *37*(II), 123, 1906.
————: Der Morbus Gaucher und die ihm ähnlichen Erkrankungen. (Die lipoidzellige Splenohepatomegalie Typus Niemann und die diabetische Lipoidzellenhyperplasie der Milz.), Ergebn. inn. Med. u. Kinderh., *29*, 519, 1926.
————: *Die Skelettform (ossuäre Form) des Morbus Gaucher*, Jena, Gustav Fischer, 1927.
————: A Classification of the Diseases of Lipoid Metabolism and Gaucher's Disease, Am. J. M. Sc., *185*, 453, 1933.
————: Niemann-Pick's Disease and Other Forms of So-called Xanthomatosis, Am. J. M. Sc., *185*, 601, 1933.
PICK, L., and BIELSCHOWSKY, M.: Über lipoidzellige Splenomegalie (Typus Niemann-Pick) und amaurotische Idiotie, Klin. Wchnschr., *6*, 1631, 1927.
PIPER, J., and ORRILD, L.: Essential Familial Hypercholesterolemia and Xanthomatosis, Am. J. Med., *21*, 34, 1956.
POPE, F. M.: A Case of Ochronosis, Lancet, *1*, 24, 1906.
PUHR, L.: Über Ochronose, Virchows Arch. path. Anat., *260*, 130, 1926.
REICH, C., SEIFE, M., and KESSLER, B. J.: Gaucher's Disease: A Review, and Discussion of Twenty Cases, Medicine, *30*, 1, 1951.
REID, E., OSLER, W., and GARROD, A. E.: On Ochronosis: Report of a Case, the Clinical Features, the Urine, Quart. J. Med., *1*, 199, 1907–8.
REILLY, W. A., and LINDSAY, S.: Gargoylism (Lipochondrodystrophy). A Review of Clinical Observations in Eighteen Cases, Am. J. Dis. Child., *75*, 595, 1948.
ROSENBERG, A., and CHARGAFF, E.: A Reinvestigation of the Cerebroside Deposited in Gaucher's Disease, J. Biol. Chem., *233*, 1323, 1958.
ROURKE, J. A., and HESLIN, D. J.: Gaucher's Disease. Roentgenologic Bone Changes Over 20 Year Interval, Am. J. Roentgenol., *94*, 621, 1965.
SCHANCHE, A. F., BIERMAN, S. M., SOPHER, R. L., and O'LOUGHLIN, B. J.: Disseminated Lipogranulomatosis: Early Roentgenographic Changes, Radiology, *82*, 675, 1964.
SCHMIDT, M. B.: Die anatomischen Veränderungen des Skeletts bei der Hurlerschen Krankheit, Zentralbl. allg. Path., *79*, 113, 1942.
SCHULTZE, G., and LANG, E. K.: Disseminated Lipogranulomatosis, Radiology, *74*, 428, 1960.
SEALOCK, R. R., PERKINSON, J. D., JR., and BASINSKI, D. H.: Further Analysis of the Role of Ascorbic Acid in Phenylalanine and Tyrosine Metabolism, J. Biol. Chem., *140*, 153, 1941.

SØRENSEN, E. W.: Hyperlipemia. A Report of an Unusual Case Complicated by Bone-lesions, Macrocytic Anaemia and Leukemoid Bone Marrow, Acta med. scandinav., *175*, 207, 1964.

STATTER, M., and SHAPIRO, B.: Studies on the Etiology of Gaucher's Disease, Israel J. M. Sc., *1*, 514, 1965.

STRAUSS, L.: The Pathology of Gargoylism, Am. J. Path., *24*, 855, 1948.

STRICKLAND, B.: Skeletal Manifestations of Gaucher's Disease with Some Unusual Findings, Brit. J. Radiol., *31*, 246, 1958.

SVENNERHOLM, E., and SVENNERHOLM, L.: The Separation of Neutral Blood-Serum Glycolipids by Thin-Layer Chromatography, Biochim. et biophys. acta, *70*, 432, 1963.

TENNENT, W.: Gaucher's Disease—The Early Radiological Diagnosis, Brit. J. Radiol., *18*, 356, 1945.

THANNHAUSER, S. J.: *Lipidoses. Diseases of the Intracellular Lipid Metabolism*, 3rd ed., New York, Grune & Stratton, 1958.

TODD, R. McL., and KEIDAN, S. E.: Changes in the Head of the Femur in Children Suffering from Gaucher's Disease, J. Bone & Joint Surg., *34-B*, 447, 1952.

TUCHMAN, L. R., SUNA, H., and CARR, J. J.: Elevation of Serum Acid Phosphatase in Gaucher's Disease, J. Mt. Sinai Hosp., *23*, 227, 1956.

TUCHMAN, L. R., and SWICK, M.: High Acid Phosphatase Level Indicating Gaucher's Disease in Patient with Prostatism, J.A.M.A., *164*, 2034, 1957.

TUTHILL, C. R.: Juvenile Amaurotic Idiocy, Arch. Neurol. & Psychiat., *32*, 198, 1934.

VIDEBAEK, A.: Niemann-Pick's Disease. Acute and Chronic Type? Acta paediat., *37*, 95, 1949.

VIRCHOW, R.: Ein Fall von allgemeiner Ochronose der Knorpel und knorpelähnlichen Theile, Arch. path. Anat., *37*, 212, 1866.

WHEELER, E. O., and SPRAGUE, H. B.: The Prevalence and Significance of Hypercholesterolemia Among Children and Siblings of Patients with Hypercholesterolemic Xanthomatosis, J. Clin. Invest., *32*, 611, 1953.

WILKINSON, C. F., JR., HAND, E. A., and FLIEGELMAN, M. T.: Essential Familial Hypercholesterolemia, Ann. Int. Med., *29*, 671, 1948.

WOLFE, H. J., BLENNERHASSET, J. B., YOUNG, G. F., and COHEN, R. B.: Hurler's Syndrome. A Histochemical Study. New Techniques for Localization of Very Water-Soluble Acid Mucopolysaccharides, Am. J. Path., *45*, 1007, 1964.

WOOD, H. L.-C.: Gaucher's Disease with Pseudocoxalgia, J. Bone & Joint Surg., *34-B*, 462, 1952.

YOSSIPOVITCH, Z. H., HERMAN, G., and MAKIN, M.: Aseptic Osteomyelitis in Gaucher's Disease, Israel J. M. Sc., *1*, 531, 1965.

ZANNONI, V. G., SEEGMILLER, J. E., and LA DU, B. N.: Nature of the Defect in Alcaptonuria, Nature, London, *193*, 952, 1962.

Chapter

19

Certain Disorders of Individual Epiphyses, Apophyses, and Epiphysioid Bones

This chapter treats of some of the conditions which in the past were usually grouped and discussed under the heading of *"localized osteochondritis."* The term "epiphysioid bones" denotes bones preformed in cartilage and ossified like epiphyses from a central nucleus of ossification. The term is especially convenient for referring collectively to the bones of the carpus and tarsus.

As a group, the so-called "localized osteochondritides" were at first generally interpreted as evolving on the basis of a primary or idiopathic interruption of the blood supply to the affected epiphyses, apophyses, or epiphysioid bones. The resultant partial or total ischemic necrosis of the local osseous tissue and bone marrow was held to be the factor instigating all the subsequent pathologic changes. However, most of the numerous sites in which the condition has been reported as occurring have not been studied anatomically for evidence of aseptic necrosis. Indeed, it is only as manifested in a few particular regions that the disorder is really familiar to us in its pathologic as well as in its clinical and roentgenographic aspects. These sites include notably the femoral capital epiphysis, the femoral condyle, the carpal lunate (semilunar), the second metatarsal head, the tibial tubercle, and the bodies of vertebrae. Furthermore, it is now clear that, in relation to some of these lesional sites, the aseptic bone necrosis noted is not primary but has followed upon a fracture or infraction of the bone area in question. An example of this is so-called Kienböck's disease of the lunate bone. Also, anatomic study of the lesional area in some of the other localized bone disorders discussed in this chapter (Scheuermann's disease, for example) has failed to yield evidence of aseptic necrosis even as a secondary development.

Because of these facts, the problem of *nomenclature* has been puzzling, particularly when attention has been directed toward finding a comprehensive name which would serve as a single designation for all of these conditions. Most of the general terms which have been used in the past have incorporated either the idea of "osteochondropathy" or that of "osteochondritis" or "osteochondrosis." On the other hand, reference to the condition in a particular structure is often made in such terms as "epiphysitis," "apophysitis," or "sesamoiditis." As a matter of fact, any designation which includes the root "chondro" or the suffix "itis" is inaccurate, since damage to the cartilage is not an instigating factor in the development of the disorder, and inflammation is not such a factor either. Altogether, it still seems advisable to use eponyms in designating most of the conditions discussed in this chapter. Indeed, Burrows, in a closing remark concerning this group of skeletal disorders, refers to them as "the most eponymous of affections."

LEGG-CALVÉ-PERTHES DISEASE

Legg-Calvé-Perthes disease (frequently denoted as Legg-Perthes disease or by the nonspecific descriptive term "coxa plana") is an affection of the hip joint occurring during childhood, developing on the basis of interruption of the blood supply to the ossification center of the femoral head, and resulting in partial or even complete aseptic necrosis of the center.*   In the course of time and under appropriate treatment, the necrotic ossification center of the femoral head usually becomes extensively revivified and reconstructed.   Occasionally, however, a fragment of the necrotic ossification center fails to become revascularized and hence persists as a delimited radiopaque area bordering upon the articular surface of the femoral head. This occurrence is held to represent Legg-Perthes disease complicated by osteochondritis dissecans.   Furthermore, almost from the first, the alterations in the femoral head are associated with certain changes in the juxta-epiphysial portion of the femoral neck and in the acetabulum. These changes, too, tend gradually to regress.

Nevertheless, even by the end of the growth period, the contours of the head, neck, and acetabulum in a case of Legg-Perthes disease may not be normal. In particular, they are likely to be abnormal: (1) if the patient is over 7 or 8 years of age when first coming under medical care for the condition, and has already had pertinent difficulties for some time (about a year or two); and (2) if, irrespective of the patient's age when first coming under treatment, the latter was not directed primarily toward relief from weight-bearing. Under such circumstances the femoral head, instead of having regained its spherical shape, is very likely to be irregular in contour or even flattened and/or mushroomed down upon the neck, which is shortened and broadened. Moreover, the vertical wall of the acetabulum tends to be flattened. These residual deformities expose the articular cartilages of the hip joint to functional damage, so that eventually a hypertrophic arthritis (osteoarthritis) often develops in a hip joint which has been the site of coxa plana.

CLINICAL CONSIDERATIONS

Incidence.—In regard to *general incidence* it is to be noted that Legg-Calvé-Perthes disease is not uncommon among the skeletal disorders of childhood. The *sex* of the subject is much more likely to be male than female, the proportion of affected males to females being about 4 to 1. The *age* of the child when the disorder sets in is ordinarily somewhere between 5 and 9 years. The condition is rarely encountered in children under 2 years of age, and its incidence drops abruptly from the age of 11 to the end of the growth period. There is no predilection of one hip joint over the other. In most instances (about 90 per cent) the disorder is unilateral. In those cases in which both hip joints become involved, the two joints are sometimes affected simultaneously but much more often successively (see Burrows). Occasionally, coxa plana is found in conjunction with an analogous disorder of some other epiphysis or of an epiphysioid bone.

---

* It was in 1910 that the condition in question was first recognized as a distinctive one. Legg, Calvé, and Perthes all described it in that year.   Priority probably belongs to Legg, since he seems to have distinguished the condition at least as clearly as the others and his article antedated their articles by some months. In any event, the names of these workers, separately and in various combinations, are frequently used to denote the condition. The eponymic designation most commonly used is Legg-Perthes disease. In addition to coxa plana, various other descriptive names have been applied, including osteochondritis deformans juvenilis coxae, pseudocoxalgia, and flat head.

There also seems to be a *racial difference* in the incidence of the disease, the latter being definitely uncommon among Negroes. Among the 57 cases of the disorder which were treated at the Hospital for Joint Diseases between 1929 and 1936, there was no case in which the patient was a Negro (see Sutro and Pomeranz). This finding is significant in view of the fact that Negroes constituted 15 to 20 per cent of the hospital's ward population during that period. However, it should not be inferred from this experience that Negroes are exempt from the disorder. In particular, Golding *et al.* found that the incidence of the condition among Negroes is about one tenth of the incidence in Europeans, East Indians, and Chinese. The reason for this racial difference in the incidence of Legg-Perthes disease has not been clearly established.

Clinical Manifestations and Differential Diagnosis.—The clinical complaints and findings are not dramatic, and at best only suggest the diagnosis. The latter depends upon the roentgenographic findings, which sooner or later become distinctive. The earliest and most regular clinical manifestation is an intermittent limp, which is usually noticed particularly after exertion. Not infrequently the limp is associated with some pain in the hip, in the knee on the same side, or in both regions. There may be atrophy of the soft tissues of the thigh, and muscle spasm which causes a flexion adduction contracture of the hip. Under appropriate treatment, most of these manifestations tend to wane or gradually disappear in the course of about a year or two from the time of onset of the clinical difficulties. However, it is not uncommon to find some residual limitation of the range of motion (particularly flexion, abduction, and internal rotation) due to actual incongruities between the femoral head and the acetabulum.

There are various affections which may raise problems of *differential diagnosis* from Legg-Perthes disease. It is *tuberculosis* of the head of the femur in an early stage that is most likely to create this difficulty. Indeed, in any case suspected of being tuberculosis of the head of the femur, the possibility of Legg-Perthes disease should also be considered, and vice versa. Specifically, flattening of the center of ossification of the head (coxa plana) and the appearance of areas showing increased opacity are common to the two conditions, although they deviate in their subsequent clinical and roentgenographic course. In a child affected with *Gaucher's disease,* collapse of the capital femoral epiphysis of one or both femora is a common finding. Roentgenographically the appearance of the femoral head or heads in such a case is likely to bear a close resemblance to that in some cases of Legg-Perthes disease. In Gaucher's disease the aseptic necrosis of the capital femoral epiphysis is the result of crowding of the intertrabecular marrow spaces of the epiphysis with Gaucher cells. This in turn leads to interruption of the local blood supply, and to necrosis of the Gaucher cells and also of the osseous trabeculae of the spongiosa (p. 516). In *sickle cell anemia* and its genetic variants, the occurrence of aseptic necrosis of the femoral head is not unusual. If the age of the subject falls within the age range characteristic for Legg-Perthes disease, a problem of differential diagnosis presents itself if one is not aware that the subject is affected with sickle cell anemia. This problem arises because the roentgenograph of the aseptically necrotic hip in sickle cell anemia resembles that characteristic for Legg-Perthes disease. It is well known that *slipped capital femoral epiphysis* in adolescents (p. 576) is an entity distinctly different from Legg-Perthes disease. The slipping of the femoral head is initiated not by necrosis of the head but by changes at the epiphysial cartilage plate at the site of junction between the capital epiphysis and the femoral neck. It is well recognized, however, that aseptic necrosis of the capital epiphysis may follow forcible manipulation of the hip in a case of slipped epiphysis. It may be of interest also that the writer has encountered a case in which slipping of the capital epiphysis occurred on one side and Legg-Perthes disease subsequently developed on the other.

ROENTGENOGRAPHIC FINDINGS

When the subject first comes under medical care, the history and clinical findings may already suggest the diagnosis. To clinch it, however, roentgenographic examination of the hip region is necessary. The roentgenographic findings have received attention in almost all of the very numerous articles on Legg-Perthes disease, and have been well summarized in some of the more extensive presentations (see Platt, Ferguson and Howorth, Waldenström, Ferguson, Jr., Goff, and also Meyer). Furthermore, there are a number of studies in which an attempt has been made to interpret these findings in the light of the underlying local pathologic changes (see Freund, and also Sutro and Pomeranz).

If the roentgenographic findings are not distinctive at the time of the first examination, they become so in the course of the next few months. The earliest changes which have been noted simulate those of an acute synovitis, in that the capsular shadows about the hip are distended and there is widening of the joint space. In addition, however, the proximal metaphysis of the femur will show demineralization of the femoral neck for some distance below the epiphysial cartilage plate. In time, the ossification center of the femoral head comes to present, in part (usually the anterior part) or throughout, some increase in its radiopacity (reflecting the presence of aseptic necrosis), though the center may not yet show any change in contour. At this stage there may or may not be some widening of the femoral neck.

Figure 144

A, Roentgenograph showing the left hip joint early in the course of Perthes' disease in the case of a girl who was 6 years of age when this picture was taken. For several weeks before the hip joint was roentgenographed, it was evident that the child limped, and she had also complained of some pain in the knee. Physical examination disclosed slight limitation of motion at the hip joint, due to local muscle spasm. In this picture the roentgenographic changes of Perthes' disease are still minimal, but there is widening of the joint space. The other illustrations on this plate are from the same case, and depict the progression of the pathologic alterations and the concomitant reparative changes occurring in the affected capital femoral epiphysis. The time interval between the minimal changes shown in *A* and the subsequent substantial restitution of the epiphysis manifested in *F* was 4 years.

B, Roentgenograph illustrating the status of the affected hip joint approximately 10 months after the picture shown in *A*. The femoral head is slightly flattened and reveals several clear-cut foci of radiopacity representing areas of aseptic necrosis. These are intermingled with some areas of radiolucency reflecting the revascularization of the necrotic head in the course of its repair. The femoral neck is slightly broadened.

C, Roentgenograph illustrating the status of the affected hip joint approximately 9 months after the picture shown in *B*. There has been further progress in the resorption of the necrotic tissue. Indeed, the three clear-cut foci of radiopacity seen in *B* in the general region of the fovea have now been largely replaced by areas of relative radiolucency indicative of the revascularization and repair that is taking place.

D, Roentgenograph illustrating the status of the hip joint in question approximately 3 months after the picture shown in *C*. Further progress of the repair is demonstrated by the smaller and less obvious areas of relative radiolucency which were clearly apparent in the capital epiphysis in *C*.

E, Roentgenograph demonstrating the status of the hip joint in question approximately 12 months after the picture shown in *D*. The entire capital epiphysis has clearly undergone considerable additional repair.

F, Roentgenograph of the hip demonstrating the status of the capital epiphysis 14 months after the picture shown in *E* and 4 years after the picture shown in *A*. The reconstruction of the capital epiphysis is now practically complete, as manifested by markings indicative of the presence of newly formed spongy bone.

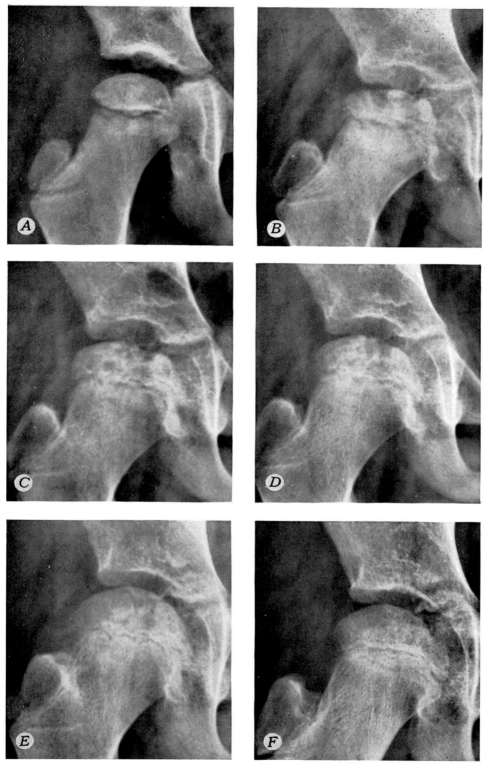

Figure 144

In some cases, when the affected hip joint is roentgenographed for the first time, the changes are even more advanced. In particular, there is already some flattening of the ossification center, an indubitable increase in its radiopacity, a clear-cut increase in the distance between it and the bottom of the acetabulum, and definite broadening of the femoral neck. In still other cases the center may present signs not only of necrosis and collapse but also of reparative changes. The reparative changes are due to revascularization, and take the roentgenographic form of areas of increased radiolucency at the poles of the center and sometimes even in the vicinity of the fovea. In the course of time, further reconstruction finds expression roentgenographically in a "fragmented" appearance of the center of ossification. The center now seems to be composed of several radiopaque foci separated by radiolucent tracts. Further progress of the revascularization and repair is associated with progressive rarefaction of the radiopaque areas and densification of the radiolucent areas, so that the shadow cast by the nucleus becomes increasingly like the normal shadow in density. The period between the onset of the disorder and the reconstruction of the necrotic ossification center of the femoral head is variable. Under appropriate treatment, a uniform radiodensity is achieved in 2 years in some cases, and not until 3 or 4 years in others. (See Fig. 144.)

Occasionally, as already noted, a fragment of the necrotic ossification center fails to become revascularized and hence persists as a delimited radiopaque area bordering upon the articular surface of the femoral head. This occurrence is held to represent Legg-Perthes disease complicated by osteochondritis dissecans (see Freehafer, Ratliff, and also Morris and McGibbon). Sooner or later the delimited necrotic fragment of the femoral head usually becomes revascularized, blends with the rest of the head, and assumes a normal radiodensity. Once in a while, however, it fails to undergo revascularization, becomes detached, enters the joint cavity as an intra-articular loose body, and may therefore have to be removed surgically.

Meanwhile, roentgenographic changes have been occurring in other parts also. In the femoral neck, one or more cystlike rarefactions, sometimes surrounded by narrow borders of increased density, may have appeared, especially just before the "fragmentation stage" in the head. These cystlike areas usually disappear while the head is undergoing reconstruction. The progress of the changes in the head and neck may be associated with narrowing, flattening, and even irregularity of the line representing the epiphysial cartilage plate. The acetabulum may also come to show roundish areas of increased radiolucency.

At the completion of the reparative process, the contours of the hip joint are usually still abnormal. The minimal degree of ultimate deformity in the femoral head is represented by some flattening without any mushrooming onto the neck. Very often, however, the head is found ovoid or altogether irregular in shape and lying partly outside of the acetabular cavity. The neck is found shortened and also broadened, especially near the head end. The acetabulum may show increased obliquity of its inner wall.

PATHOLOGIC FINDINGS AND PATHOGENESIS

Pathologic Findings.—Early contributors to our knowledge of the *pathologic anatomy* of Legg-Perthes disease include Axhausen and also Zemansky, and a particularly illuminating discussion of the pathologic changes will be found in the article by Gall and Bennett. As already noted, the basic pathologic change underlying Legg-Perthes disease is anemic infarction resulting in aseptic necrosis of part or all of the center of ossification for the femoral head. It has been maintained by some that the necrosis of the ossification center is preceded by pathologic changes involving the epiphysial cartilage plate at the junction of the femoral head and neck (see Ponseti). However, the present writer is of the opinion that the changes observed in the epiphysial cartilage plate (irregularity and disruption of the plate and also the protrusion of tongues of plate cartilage into the femoral neck) are entirely secondary to the interruption of the blood supply to the femoral head and the resultant collapse of the necrotic center. (See Fig. 145.)

The general trend of the *pathologic findings* in different stages and cases indicates that the necrosis of the ossification center takes place very rapidly and involves both the osseous tissue and the intertrabecular marrow. For some time after aseptic necrosis has occurred in the center, the contour of the femoral head remains unaltered. Sooner or later, however, the head undergoes flattening due to partial subchondral collapse of the ossification center in consequence of compression fracture. In the collapsed area the bony trabeculae are comminuted, and the spaces between them are filled by amorphous detritus. Even now it will be found that the cartilaginous portion of the head is almost completely viable and perhaps even abnormally thick. Its surface may still be smooth or may present a wrinkled, furrowed appearance, and there is usually a circular ridge in the cartilage where the head joins the neck.

If lively reconstruction has been in progress, it will be found that blood vessels are penetrating into the necrotic portion of the nucleus. The revascularization takes place especially by way of the periosteal vessels of the neck but also by way of the ligamentum teres and marrow vessels, the latter entering the head from the femoral neck through defects in the epiphysial cartilage plate. The wide differences in histologic appearance to be observed subsequently in different specimens depend upon the amount of debris to be cleared away and the briskness and duration of the reconstruction. In any event, in a case in which the reconstruction is still far from being complete, there will be evidences of new bone deposition on the necrotic and partly resorbed bony trabeculae. The extent of this bone deposition will vary from place to place. The intertrabecular marrow may still be necrotic in some areas and rather fibrovascular in others, and in yet others show evidence of substantial restitution. In the marrow abutting upon some of the necrotic trabeculae, there may be some giant cells and intraphagocytic and free blood pigment. Subchondrally one may still find a zone of detritus walled off by fibrous tissue. Furthermore, one or more fibrous-walled cystic spaces containing detritus and even necrotic trabeculae may be present elsewhere in the nucleus.

Sometimes there are fibrous-walled cysts in the juxta-epiphysial region of the neck or even extending through the plate into the head. In the juxta-epiphysial portion of the neck, the marrow also may be fibrosed, some of the trabeculae resorbed, and others even necrotic. The periosteum covering the neck may have been stimulated to new bone formation. At the plate, endochondral bone growth may be in progress in some places, while in others the plate has been disrupted and bone growth disturbed. The synovial membrane of the hip joint capsule may be somewhat injected and thickened, but shows no specific changes. The vessels of the ligamentum teres have always been found patent in the pertinent specimens examined by the present writer. Furthermore, vascular occlusion is not to be noted elsewhere in tissue specimens from cases of Legg-Perthes disease.

As the reconstruction of the head and neck progresses, their internal architecture gradually tends to approximate the normal. However, on completion of the reconstruction, the head may still be found somewhat flattened and the neck somewhat shortened and broadened if the extent of the aseptic necrosis has been considerable. The most satisfactory restoration is obtained in cases in which the condition has set in early in childhood, so that there is a long interval between the onset of the reconstruction and the physiologic fusion of the head and neck. Because of the final deformity of the femoral head and also of the acetabulum, the articular cartilages of the hip joint are subject to functional damage. It is the resultant degeneration of the articular cartilages of the joint that lays the groundwork for the development of hypertrophic arthritis, which is a common sequela of the disease. In fact, young adults affected with hip disease suggesting malum coxae senilis can frequently be shown to have developed their arthritis on the basis of Legg-Perthes disease. (See Fig. 146.)

Pathogenesis.—In regard to pathogenesis, it has been postulated that the interruption of the blood supply to the capital femoral epiphysis which leads to the aseptic necrosis is preceded by a "simple synovitis" due to inflammatory changes in the synovial membrane lining the joint capsule and the reflection of that membrane onto the periosteum of the femoral neck. This interpretation is based upon histologic examination of excised portions of the articular capsule in cases of Perthes' disease in which the tissue revealed thickening of the capsule and the presence within it of arterial blood vessels with thickened walls and small lumina (see Ferguson and Howorth). In this connection it should be borne in mind, however, that vessels with thick walls represent a normal finding in the articular capsules and para-articular soft tissues even of very young children. Thus, in the writer's opinion, the idea that the ischemic necrosis of the capital femoral epiphysis might ensue from local obliterating endarteritis is not acceptable. Nevertheless, in view of the fact that the capsule of the hip joint has been found thickened in children affected with Legg-Perthes disease, it is possible that the blood vessels within the capsular retinacula become compressed because of thickening and sclerosis of the capsular tissues. It is maintained that in children of about 3 to 8 years of age the center of ossification for the femoral head receives its blood supply from the posterior retinacular blood vessels, and in particular from the posterior-superior group of these vessels—vessels which enter the femoral head through foramina near the articular margin (see Tucker, Howe *et al.*, Trueta and Harrison, and also Trueta). Hence, constriction of the retinacular blood vessels, irrespective of its basis, could account for the interruption of the blood supply to the ossification center of the femoral head and the consequent aseptic necrosis of the center.

Figure 145

A, Photograph (somewhat enlarged) showing the upper part of a femur sectioned in the frontal plane and illustrating the gross anatomic changes of Legg-Perthes disease. The subject was a boy who died of renal insufficiency at the age of 13 and who had begun to manifest clinical evidence of Legg-Perthes disease several years before. At autopsy, as reported by Gall and Bennett (see bibliography), the head of the femur in question was found to be definitely flattened on its superior surface but covered by smooth cartilage of normal appearance. When the femur was sectioned and the cut surfaces were examined, the femoral neck was found shortened and widened, particularly near the femoral head. Flattening of the femoral head was most pronounced in an area lateral to the insertion of the ligamentum teres. The osseous tissue in the femoral head was compressed, and near the center of the head it was yellowish and appeared fragmented. (I am indebted to Dr. Edward A. Gall for permission to reproduce and use this illustration, which is Fig. 2-*A* in the article by Gall and Bennett.)

B, Photomicrograph (× 2) showing the extensiveness of the alterations in the capital epiphysis. In particular, none of the spongiosa of the femoral head has remained intact except a small area medial to the fovea. Lateral to the fovea the osseous tissue of the femoral head had largely disintegrated, and the area contained considerable granular detritus and scar tissue. (I am indebted to Dr. Gall for lending me a celloidin section of the head and neck of the femur from the case referred to in *A*. This illustration was prepared from that celloidin section.)

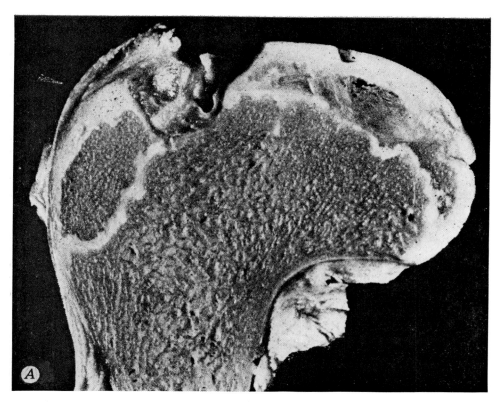

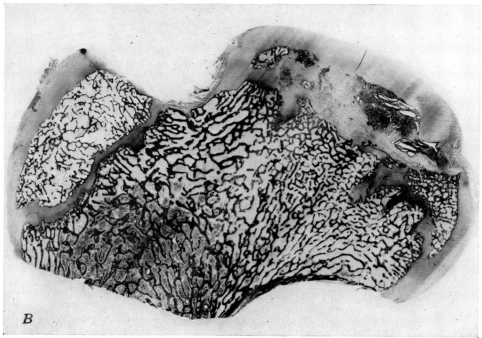

Figure 145

Axhausen's idea that the necrosis follows upon bacterial embolization which has ended in a "bland" infarction of the area can safely be rejected. Specifically, his idea was that clumps of bacteria (of one type or another) reach the ossification center and block some of its crucial vessels, but that, since no local infection develops, the thrombosis results in a noninfected "bland" infarct. Against this view is the fact that in Legg-Perthes disease neither Axhausen nor anyone else has ever observed thrombi in any of the vessels supplying the capital femoral ossification center. Various other theories have also been proposed to account for the interruption of the blood supply to the capital femoral epiphysis. These theories, too, are still unconfirmed and not generally accepted. Thus, some hold that vessels to the head may be torn by a direct blow to, or wrench of, the hip, and that the necrosis of the ossification center results from this. Others explain the interruption of the blood supply on a neurogenic basis, maintaining that a trauma causes temporary spastic contraction of the local blood vessels and throttles the local circulation in that way. A history of possibly significant trauma is noted in decidedly less than half of the cases. In any event, it is difficult to know how much importance to attach to the role of trauma. In the last analysis, we know only that in some way or other the local circulation to the capital femoral epiphysis is interrupted and

Figure 146

A, Roentgenograph showing pronounced alterations in the capital epiphysis of the left femur in a case of Perthes' disease. The patient, a boy, was 10 years of age when this roentgenograph was taken. However, he had already had clinical difficulties (pain in the hip and knee, and a limp) for about 2 years before admission to the hospital in 1937. Since conservative nonsurgical treatment for Perthes' disease was not yet generally practiced, surgery was undertaken in this case. When the hip joint was opened, the femoral head was found deformed and, in particular, flattened, widened, and depressed, especially on its anterior surface. A wedge of the anterior surface of the femoral head, extending from the fovea to the neck, was removed for anatomic study. Gross examination of the specimen revealed that the articular cartilage was irregular in thickness and detached from the subchondral bone. The latter was represented by a narrow zone of yellowish cancellous material. A cyst measuring 7.5 mm. in diameter and having a fibrous wall was present at the junction of the epiphysial cartilage plate and the articular cartilage. About half of the cyst extended into the femoral neck. Photomicrographs made from the tissue sections prepared from the excised specimen are shown in *B* and *C*.

B, Photomicrograph ($\times$ 6) giving a survey view of the histopathologic changes present in the wedge of bone removed from the capital femoral epiphysis shown in *A*. In the left portion of the picture, from above down, one can see that the articular cartilage is separated from the subchondral bone and that no endochondral ossification has been taking place on its deep surface. The marrow spaces of the subchondral spongiosa are largely filled by dark-staining material representing so-called granular detritus. (The area indicated by the arrows is shown under higher magnification in *C*.) Deep to the subchondral spongiosa, a part of the epiphysial cartilage plate is to be noted. On the metaphysial surface of the plate, endochondral ossification has been going on. In the right portion of the picture, it can be noted that the articular cartilage is disrupted at its periphery and that (as would be clearly apparent under higher magnification) the area of the defect is the site of focal hemorrhage and fibrous scarring. The epiphysial cartilage plate is likewise disrupted at its periphery, and here, too, the defect is filled by reparative scar tissue. Furthermore, a small fibrous-walled cyst can be observed in the femoral neck below the epiphysial cartilage plate.

C, Photomicrograph ($\times$ 35) showing under higher magnification the area indicated by the arrows in *B*. The intertrabecular marrow spaces on the left and right of the picture are largely filled with granular detritus. The intertrabecular marrow spaces in the central portion of the picture have been revascularized, and much of the granular detritus has been resorbed.

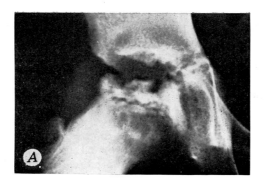

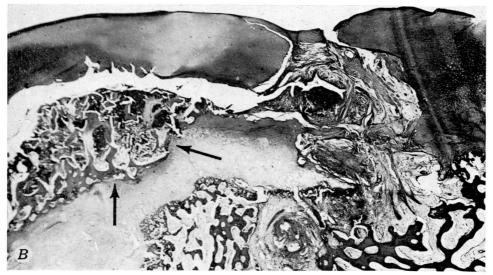

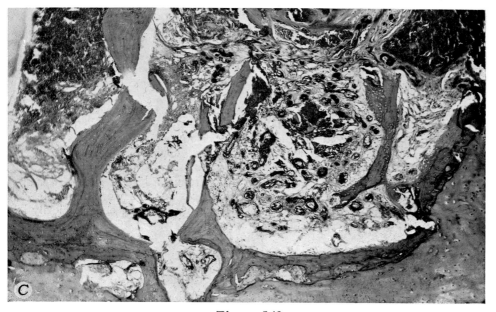

Figure 146

aseptic necrosis results. Altogether, the pathogenesis of Legg-Perthes disease is still a debated question.

A picture resembling that of Legg-Perthes disease can be produced experimentally in animals through interruption of the circulation to the femoral head by section of the ligamentum teres and concomitant severance of the blood supply to the head from the periosteal vessels of the femoral neck (see Graham, Miltner and Hu, and also Salter). In human cases of congenital dislocation of the hip, a picture like that of Legg-Perthes disease sometimes develops spontaneously or after an attempt at manual reduction of the dislocation. Furthermore, aseptic necrosis of the femoral head often follows upon traumatic dislocation at the hip joint, particularly if the head is dislocated posteriorly and the reduction is unduly delayed. Even without the occurrence of dislocation, unilateral or bilateral aseptic necrosis of the femoral head has been observed in adults who have suffered severe trauma to one or both hip regions (see Freund). In this connection, Pich reported the histopathology of a case of aseptic necrosis of the femoral head following upon a severe trauma to the hip in a boy 13 years of age, and causing changes resembling those of Legg-Perthes disease. An analogous case was also reported by Goldenberg. (Idiopathic and post-traumatic aseptic necrosis of the femoral head in adults is discussed in detail in the chapter which follows, p. 632.)

SLIPPED CAPITAL FEMORAL EPIPHYSIS

Slipping of the capital femoral epiphysis is the condition in which the femoral head begins to slip gradually off the femoral neck. This is in contrast to the abrupt dislodgment of the head from the neck, which occurs in connection with traumatic avulsion. As a disease entity, slipping of the capital femoral epiphysis has been known for about a hundred years. In the early literature relating to affections of the hip, the condition was often interpreted as an aspect of "coxa vara" or as "coxa vara traumatica." In time, it came to be recognized that the coxa vara aspect of the abnormal relationship of the head and neck of the femur to the femoral shaft in these cases was secondary to the slipping of the epiphysis. It also became established that the onset of the slipping of the femoral head was often spontaneous (that is, that the disorder frequently sets in without the agency of a traumatic incident). Nevertheless, it is clear that if the femoral head has already been somewhat dislodged from the neck, a traumatic incident can easily aggravate the slipping.

That slipping of the capital femoral epiphysis gives rise to clinical complaints and roentgenographic changes while it is in its earliest stage (the so-called preslipping stage) has been maintained by some (see Ferguson and Howorth) but denied by others (see Waldenström). In regard to the roentgenographic findings, it is rather generally accepted that if the extent of the displacement is but slight it will be seen best if the roentgenographs are taken so as to present a lateral view of the area, since the slipping of the epiphysis usually occurs first in a backward direction. For this reason the displacement is not readily demonstrable roentgenographically in a frontal view until the slipping is fairly advanced.

CLINICAL CONSIDERATIONS

Incidence.—The *general incidence* of slipping of the capital femoral epiphysis is definitely not high. Indeed, even in a hospital devoted mainly to orthopaedic disorders, the admission records are not likely to show more than a few new cases of the condition each year. Thus, Ferguson and Howorth reported in 1931 that 70 cases of slipped capital femoral epiphysis had been treated at the New York Orthopaedic Hospital during the previous 20 years. The 166 cases of slipped capital femoral epiphysis which constituted the foundation for the report by Jerre in 1950 had accumulated during the period 1917 to 1945 in three orthopaedic clinics of three different Swedish cities. Thus the average number of cases per year seen in these three clinics together was only about 6. In 1959, Billing and Severin, reporting on the cases seen at the Orthopaedic Clinic of the University of Gothenburg, Sweden, stated that, in the 4-year period extending from May 1953 to May 1957, only 50 patients (that is, about 12 per year) affected with slipping of the capital femoral epiphysis had their first admission to that clinic. Kelsey et al., reviewing the incidence of the condition in two widely separated areas of the United States (Connecticut and certain southwestern states), reported that slipped capital femoral epiphysis was almost five times more frequently encountered in the Connecticut area than in the southwestern part of the country.

In regard to *sex incidence* it has consistently been found that the condition is more common in males than in females. A statistical survey of cases of slipped capital femoral epiphysis treated in various cities of Great Britain was made by Burrows under the auspices of the British Orthopaedic Association. On the point in question the survey showed that in 60 of the 100 cases on which adequate data were available the patients were boys. The sex incidence ratio in the group of cases reported by Billing and Severin was likewise 60 per cent boys to 40 per cent girls. While the general opinion is that the condition is only somewhat more common in boys than in girls, it is of interest that, in the group of cases reported by Jerre, 83 per cent of the patients were boys and only 17 per cent girls.

The matter of the *age incidence* of slipped capital femoral epiphysis naturally brings up the question of the time from which the date of onset of the condition should be estimated. If one accepts the concept that there is a preslipping stage during which some clinical complaints may already be present, and sets the time of onset accordingly, the date is about a year earlier (on the average) than the time when clear-cut clinical and roentgenographic manifestations of slipped epiphysis become evident. The age range during which the condition develops extends from about 10.5 to 16 years for boys and about 9.5 to 13.5 years for girls. At any rate, slipping of the capital femoral epiphysis is encountered about $1\frac{1}{2}$ to 2 years earlier, on the average, in females than in males.

Clinical Complaints and Findings.—In respect to *height*, many of the subjects are at the upper limit of the normal range. That is, they tend to be tall, though not abnormally so. In regard to *weight* it has been found that many of the subjects are overweight for their age, and some of these even present the girdle-like adiposity and underdeveloped genitalia associated with the so-called Fröhlich syndrome.

When a given case first comes under medical care, the slipping of the capital femoral epiphysis may be *unilateral* or *bilateral*. If the involvement is found to be unilateral at that time, there is still considerable likelihood that the opposite femoral head will also come to be affected in the course of some months or a year or two. Synchronous slipping of the two femoral heads is certainly rare (see Burrows). Most of the statistical evaluations also indicate that, when the condition still involves only one hip, the femoral head affected is more likely to be the left than the right.

In a patient in whom slipping of a capital femoral epiphysis is still in an early stage of its evolution ("preslipping stage"), definite clinical complaints often set in after a strain, wrench, or some other minor injury. The difficulties usually consist of a feeling of tiredness or mild pain in the region of the hip or knee and some degree of limping and limitation of mobility. If a patient who has had such complaints for weeks or months suffers a severe blow or other injury to the hip, this may be followed by acute pain and pronounced limitation of mobility, and the patient may even be unable to stand on the affected lower extremity. As already implied, the onset of mild or severe clinical complaints after an injury is due merely to the fact that the traumatic incident has increased or aggravated the slipping which was already in progress and which in any event would soon have given rise to clinical complaints.

ROENTGENOGRAPHIC FINDINGS

When taken in the frontal plane, a roentgenograph of a *normal* hip region will show that, if a line is drawn along the superolateral surface of the femoral neck and is continued into the capital epiphysis, a small segment of the femoral head protrudes laterally beyond that line as a small hump.

As already indicated, when the capital epiphysis of a femur slips, the displacement takes place in the dorsal direction—that is, backward. The earliest roentgenographic evidence of displacement of the capital epiphysis consists of a reduction or even disappearance of the normal shadow representing the protruding segment of the femoral head. This is most likely to be apparent if the roentgenograph shows the hip area in the lateral projection. In any event, corresponding roentgenographs of the opposite hip should be made for purposes of comparison. (See Fig. 147.)

As the femoral head continues to slip backward, the roentgenograph will also come to show an increase in the width (and also some irregularity) of the normally present radiolucent zone between the head and neck of the bone. This widened zone of increased radiolucency is often misinterpreted as an indication that the epiphysial cartilage plate has become thickened. Actually, it merely reflects porosity of the spongy bone at the proximal end of the neck, along with any disruption of continuity at the head-neck junction which has occurred in consequence of the slipping. That is, the supposed widening of the epiphysial cartilage plate in cases of slipping of the capital femoral epiphysis is an illusion.

Figure 147

A, Roentgenograph of the left hip area from a case of slipping of the capital femoral epiphysis. The patient was a boy 13 years of age who came under medical care because of intermittent pain which had been present for 5 weeks in the region of the left knee and lower part of the thigh. The boy walked with a slight limp on the left side, and the pain in the knee was aggravated by walking. The picture shows the appearance of the affected hip joint in the frontal plane, and demonstrates the absence of the hump which would normally be present to represent the protrusion of a small segment of the head of the femur beyond the superolateral surface of the neck.

B, Roentgenograph of the same hip shown in *A.* The picture, taken on the same day as *A,* demonstrates the appearance of the affected area in lateral projection. It reveals strikingly the advantages offered by a picture showing the hip joint in the lateral projection in demonstrating the presence of slipping of the capital femoral epiphysis. The widened radiolucent zone at the juxta-epiphysial end of the neck contains small punctate radiopacities reflecting the disruption which has taken place in the epiphysial cartilage plate. The picture also suggests that a fracture has occurred at the inferior buttress of the neck of the femur.

C and *D,* Roentgenographs from another case of slipping of the capital femoral epiphysis, again demonstrating the difference apparent when one compares the pictures, taken on the same day, showing the hip joint area in the frontal plane (*C*) and in the lateral projection (*D*). The patient in this case was a girl 11 years of age whose complaints (pain in the right knee and an intermittent limp) had been present for only a few weeks.

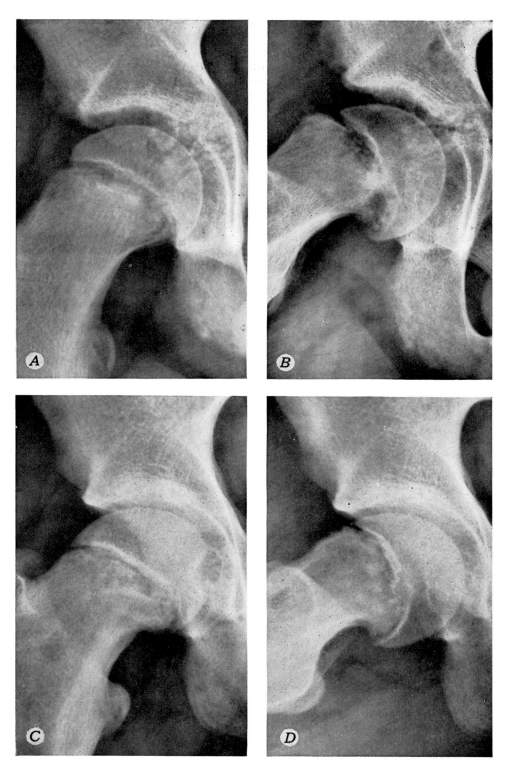

Figure 147

After the femoral head has slipped, the femoral neck undergoes a certain amount of remodeling. Resorption resulting in thinning occurs on the anterior surface of the neck, while some thickening due to new bone deposition occurs on its posterior surface. In the course of the remodeling of the neck, the projecting edge of its anterior surface becomes smoothed off, and the gap between its posterior surface and the dorsal edge of the displaced epiphysis fills in. Moreover, the femoral neck may eventually show a good deal of deformity. In particular, its longitudinal growth may have been very much impeded, especially if the extent of the slipping is considerable and if the slipping has occurred mainly in the junctional area between the epiphysial cartilage plate and the neck.

A hip joint in which slipping of the capital femoral epiphysis had taken place during the subject's late childhood or adolescence often presents roentgenographic indications of osteoarthritis even early in the subject's adult life. The factors which determine whether osteoarthritis will occur, and, if so, how severe it is likely to be, are: (1) the degree of displacement of the femoral head at the time the subject originally came under treatment; (2) the method used for treating the condition during the subject's childhood and/or adolescence; and (3) the number of years which have elapsed between the union of the head and neck of the femur and the roentgenographic examination undertaken to evaluate the local condition in respect to osteoarthritis.

In general, it may be stated that the greater the extent of the displacement of the femoral head at the time the subject first came under treatment, the greater is the likelihood that the hip joint will already show some osteoarthritis even during early adult life. Naturally, if the malalignment has laid the groundwork for an osteoarthritis, the latter can be expected to progress as the subject grows older. Furthermore, the manipulation of the hip joint during an attempt at closed reduction may aggravate the slipping. It may even result in impairment of the circulation to the femoral head and hence lead to the development of an aseptic necrosis. Certainly these complications of attempted closed reduction are potent factors favoring the occurrence of osteoarthritis, which may already be severely disabling in early middle life. Indeed, when malum coxae is present in a relatively young or middle-aged adult, it can be suspected, in the absence of some obvious other cause, that the basis for the osteoarthritis was slipping of the capital femoral epiphysis.

PATHOLOGIC FINDINGS AND PATHOGENESIS

Pathologic Findings.—The writer has examined anatomically a number of adequate specimens removed surgically in cases of slipping or slipped capital femoral epiphysis. This material includes the 3 specimens on which Sutro, working under the writer's guidance, based his description of the pathologic anatomy of the condition. In substance, his conclusion was that the slipping followed upon disruption of the epiphysial cartilage plate between the head and neck of the femur. Furthermore, he found *no histologic evidence* permitting the deduction that regressive or degenerative changes had occurred in the plate before the capital femoral epiphysis had begun to slip. The writer's subsequent experience with slipped capital femoral epiphysis is still in accord with the findings reported in 1935 by Sutro to the effect that the slipping of the capital epiphysis follows upon disruption of the plate.

However, Lacroix and Verbrugge have maintained instead that before the slipping occurs the cartilage plate undergoes fibrous transformation. This interpretation was based on the findings in a single case. Controverting the opinion of these authors is the fact that the surgical specimen (femoral head and part of the neck) on which their conclusions were based had not been removed until 3 years after the onset of clinical complaints. Indeed, one may conclude from the findings in their case that the fibrous transformation of the epiphysial cartilage plate was secondary to disruption of the plate, and that the alterations which they observed in the plate represented late changes. On the other hand, in the cases reported by Ponseti and McClintock, the anatomic findings were in line with those described by Sutro. They obtained biopsy specimens in their cases with a Phemister punch, and the core of bone removed in each case was about 1 cm. in diameter. In respect to the pathologico-anatomic changes, their most significant finding was that the epiphysial cartilage plate was disrupted and that fracture-like clefts were present in the area of the plate.

If an adequate specimen consisting of a femoral head and adjacent part of the neck is available, and if that specimen is examined after it has been cut serially on a band saw into thin slices, these will yield very illuminating findings, even to the naked eye. The present writer's total experience with the pathologic anatomy of slipped capital femoral epiphysis may be summarized as follows: In a *still-uncomplicated case* of slipped capital femoral epiphysis, the epiphysis itself is not primarily altered. On the other hand, the epiphysial cartilage plate regularly shows aberrations from the normal. Specifically, if the plate is followed through the serial sections, it will be found buckled in some places, reduplicated in others, and quite fragmented and discontinuous in still other sections (or specimens). Furthermore, in some specimens, bits of epiphysial cartilage plate, often surrounded by sclerotic bone, may be found in the capital epiphysis and even in the femoral neck at some distance from the normal plate line. Indeed, an occasional specimen will reveal, in one or more of the thin slices, that the plate looks as though it had been spattered about by some disruptive force. The articular cartilage of the femoral head is not necessarily much altered at first. Frank necrosis of the osseous trabeculae and the intertrabecular marrow is nowhere apparent. Near the disrupted plate and between the fragments of it, both toward the head and toward the neck of the affected femur, one finds areas of increased vascularization, fibrous tissue, and newly formed bone. In time, reunion (synostosis) takes place between the capital epiphysis and the femoral neck, but in a position of malalignment. (See Figs. 148 and 149.)

There are a number of *complications* which may appear in the femoral head in one case or another of slipped capital femoral epiphysis. One of these complications is the occurrence of an *ischemic necrosis* in the slipped femoral head. This may follow upon attempted closed reduction of the head. The incidence of ischemic necrosis of the head after closed reduction is rather high, particularly if one strives to obtain a good alignment of the head and neck, since such an attempt is likely to be associated with the use of excessive force in the manipulation. Ischemic necrosis of the head may also develop after such surgical procedures as fixing the head to the neck by the introduction of a nail, or after a corrective osteotomy.

Another complication—a rather rare one which is still not fully understood— is *necrosis of the articular cartilage* of the slipped femoral head. This was first brought to light by Waldenström in 1930, and its occurrence has also been recognized by others (see Jerre, Wiberg, Durbin, and also Lowe). The roentgenographic picture reflecting this complication reveals pronounced atrophy of the femoral head and of the acetabulum and surrounding skeletal parts, considerable decrease in the width of the articular space, and irregularity in the outline of the articular surface of the femoral head. The histopathologic findings relating to the necrosis of the articular cartilage are given in detail in the article by Cruess. As is well known, the articular cartilages of a joint are nourished by the synovial fluid. Since the articular cartilage of the acetabulum also undergoes acute necrosis in these cases, Cruess came to share Waldenström's opinion in regard to the basis for the necrosis. The

38

opinion is that, for some reason which is still not clear, the formation of synovial fluid by the synovial membrane of the articular capsule of the hip joint has been inadequate, and that in consequence the cartilage fails to receive sufficient nourishment and therefore undergoes necrosis.

Finally, it should be noted that in the course of time the local evidence of slipped epiphysis becomes increasingly vague, and the pathologic picture ultimately presented by the affected joint is likely to be that of a *hypertrophic arthritis* (osteoarthritis) particularly pronounced in the articular end of the femur. Indeed, it is frequently only by looking carefully into the history of the case that the arthritis which has ensued can still be connected etiologically with the slipping of the epiphysis and hence recognized as a secondary hypertrophic arthritis.

Pathogenesis.—As already noted, when a patient first comes under medical care for slipping of the capital femoral epiphysis, the involvement may be unilateral or bilateral. If the involvement is found to be unilateral at that time, there is still considerable likelihood (20 to 25 per cent) that the opposite femoral head will also come to be affected in the course of some months or a year or two. Synchronous slipping of the two femoral heads is certainly rare. If one considers these facts and also the fact that an analogous condition does not develop in relation to any of the other epiphyses (for instance, the capital epiphysis of the humerus, the distal epiphysis of the femur, or the proximal epiphysis of the tibia), one can only conclude that it must be some special local mechanical factor that underlies the slipping of the capital femoral epiphysis. One can safely exclude the possibility that some metabolic disturbance inducing an alteration in the chemical composition of the

Figure 148

A, Photograph of three thin slices cut from a specimen which included the femoral head and a small part of the femoral neck from a case of slipped capital femoral epiphysis. The patient was a boy 15 years of age who had complaints referable to the right hip for about 1 year. Roentgenographic examination of the hip showed it to be the site of a slipped epiphysis. In relation to the age of the patient, the epiphysial cartilage plate shown by these pictures is much wavier and more irregular than it would normally be. In particular, it appears buckled, fragmented, and, in some places, duplicated.

B, Photomicrograph ($\times$ 5) showing a portion of the head and neck from a case of slipping of the capital femoral epiphysis. Toward the right of the picture there is a narrow, slitlike space between the femoral head and the underlying portion of the neck. Note also that the epiphysial cartilage plate is disrupted, parts of it presenting as discrete fragments. The patient was a boy who was 16 years of age at the time of his admission to the hospital. Shortly thereafter, a wedge osteotomy was done, and this photomicrograph was made from a tissue section prepared from the specimen removed at the surgical intervention.

C, Photomicrograph ($\times$ 5) prepared from a tissue section made from a piece of bone removed in the course of a wedge osteotomy at the junction of the femoral head and neck in a case of slipped capital femoral epiphysis. The patient was a boy 10 years of age who had pain in the region of the right hip and who had been limping intermittently for about a year. The boy was considerably overweight for his age and height and showed the girdle adiposity and underdeveloped genitalia manifested by some subjects presenting slipping of the capital femoral epiphysis. Roentgenographic examination of the right hip on admission to the hospital confirmed the clinical impression that the difficulties relating to the right hip had their basis in this condition. Note that the epiphysial cartilage plate is disrupted. In particular, there is a gap between remnants of the part of the plate oriented to the neck of the femur and the part of the plate oriented to the capital femoral epiphysis. Note also that a large fragment of the plate has been dislodged into the femoral neck (see arrow).

D, Photomicrograph ($\times$ 35) illustrating in greater detail the histologic pattern in the region of the fracture through the plate shown in the lower left-hand portion of the picture in *C*.

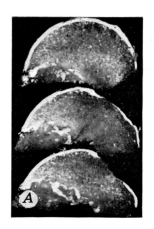

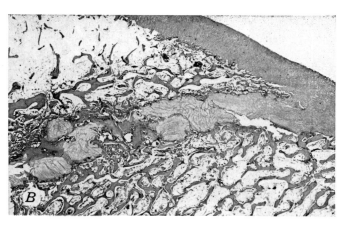

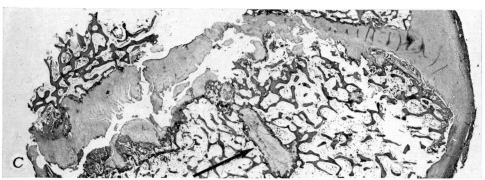

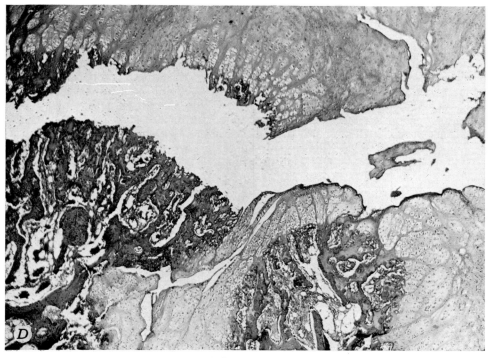

Figure 148

ground substance of the epiphysial cartilage plate might underlie the disruption of the plate and the consequent slipping of the femoral head.

With reference to mechanical influences, it is illuminating that there seem to be several anatomical factors which normally combine to prevent slipping of the capital femoral epiphysis (see Sutro). One of these is the favorable tilt of the femoral head in relation to the neck. Another is the support which the head receives from the inferior buttress of the neck of the femur. A third, and probably the most important, is the anchorage of the head to the neck by the collagenous fibers linking the periosteum of the neck to the periphery of the epiphysial cartilage plate. Abnormal pressure exerted against the head and neck of the femur (for instance, as a result of obesity) may weaken or destroy any or all of these defenses and thus initiate slipping of the epiphysis.

The mechanism of the actual slipping and of the aforementioned disruption of the epiphysial cartilage plate may be conceived somewhat as follows: In consequence of abnormal functional stress, bundles of the fibers linking the periosteum of the neck to the plate may tear at various points. Though there is as yet no actual separation of the epiphysis, the latter is now in a preslipping stage. Further functional trauma then seems to sever the periosteal fibers completely. Subsequently, various additional changes may occur, such as fracture of the atrophic buttress of the inferior cortex of the neck or compression of that projection. Finally, the activity of the muscles about the hip joint tends to sever the connections between the epiphysis and the neck. Recurrent traumatic wear and tear directed against the epiphysial cartilage plate (which remains attached to the head) accounts for the disruption and disintegration which the plate undergoes.

OSTEOCHONDRITIS DISSECANS

Osteochondritis dissecans is the condition in which a small osteochondral body (composed of articular cartilage along with a fragment of aseptically necrotic subchondral bone) is delimited and loosened from an articular end of a bone (usually a femoral condyle) and often finally extruded into the joint space. Occasionally the body is composed almost solely of articular cartilage, in which case one might even speak of "chondritis dissecans." König gave the disorder its current name in 1887, but for some time before then it was already recognized as a clinical and pathologic entity. Indeed, the case presented by Paget in 1870 (and the reports of certain others even before then) indicate this.

Figure 149

A, Photomicrograph ($\times$ 6) illustrating the changes at the epiphysial cartilage plate in another case of slipping of the capital femoral epiphysis. The patient was an obese boy 14 years of age who was admitted to the hospital with a history of pain in the left hip and thigh of 6 months' duration. In addition, it was noted that he walked awkwardly and limped slightly. Roentgenographic examination of the left hip region revealed that the femoral head had slipped downward and backward, thus confirming the clinical impression of slipped capital femoral epiphysis. A wedge osteotomy was carried out, and this was followed by the introduction of a nail to bring the head and neck into alignment. This photomicrograph was made from the wedge of bone removed in the course of the osteotomy. The epiphysial cartilage plate between the head and neck of the bone is strikingly irregular, tonguelike processes of the plate extending into the femoral neck.

B, Photomicrograph ($\times$ 25) showing in greater detail part of the epiphysial cartilage plate and the tonguelike projection from it as seen on the left in A.

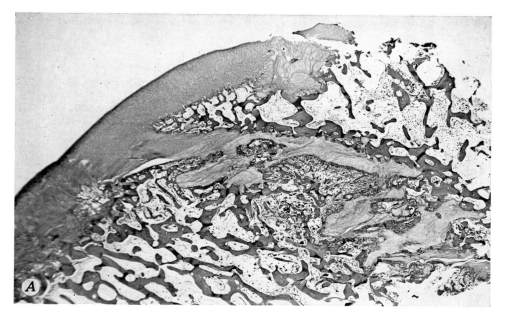

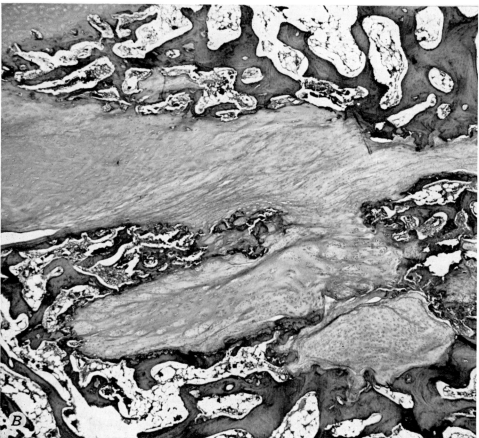

Figure 149

As used here, the term "osteochondritis dissecans" refers to the conventional instances of the condition in which the affected articular end of the bone is normal except at the site where the osteochondral body (the osteochondritis dissecans body) has become delimited. That is, we shall not be considering in this chapter those cases in which a segment of articular cartilage and necrotic subchondral bone stands out both anatomically and roentgenographically as a delimited area in an articular bone end which has undergone aseptic necrosis in large part or in its entirety. In particular, we shall *not* be dealing here with the "osteochondritis dissecans-like" lesions which an articular bone end may show in the wake of: (1) a fracture of the neck of a femur; (2) a posterior dislocation of a femoral head; (3) so-called idiopathic aseptic necrosis of the femoral head of an adult; and (4) infarction of an articular bone end appearing in association with caisson disease, sickle cell anemia, or cortisone therapy.

CLINICAL CONSIDERATIONS

Incidence.—Osteochondritis dissecans is by no means uncommon. In respect to *sex* and *age* incidence, it is of interest that the great majority of the subjects are males and that they are ordinarily between 15 and 25 years of age when they first come under medical care for the condition. The fact that the articular cartilages do not become delimited as definitive anatomic structures before the end of the growth period probably accounts for the infrequent occurrence of *clinically manifest* osteochondritis dissecans before the age of 15 and its definite rarity in young children. At the other end of the age scale, the clinical incidence of osteochondritis dissecans drops sharply after the age of 40.

There are also reports of *familial occurrence* of the disorder, and indications that in these cases one may be dealing with a predisposing hereditary or constitutional factor. Thus in 1925 Bernstein described the occurrence of osteochondritis dissecans in both knees of 2 sisters and a brother. Subsequently, Wagoner and Cohn reported on one family in which a son, father, and paternal uncle had osteochondritis dissecans of a knee, and on another family in which 2 brothers showed the condition in both knees. Osteochondritis dissecans occurring bilaterally in either the knees or the elbows in 4 members of one family (a mother and 3 of her 4 daughters) was recorded by Pick. Osteochondritis dissecans involving the medial condyle of the left knee in 3 brothers (and of the right knee also in one of them) was described by Smith. The occurrence of 9 cases of osteochondritis dissecans of one or both elbows and/or one or both knees in 3 generations of the same family is reported by Stougaard. He concluded that in these cases there was clear evidence of a dominant inheritance factor.

Clinical Manifestations.—In regard to *localization* it has long been recognized that the joint area affected is usually the knee, which is involved in about 90 per cent of the cases. Nearly always, the point of departure for the condition in the knee joint is the lateral surface of the medial femoral condyle. Sites in which osteochondritis dissecans is occasionally observed include the elbow and the hip, and rare localizations are represented by the ankle and shoulder. In respect to the knee joint, bilateral and symmetrical involvement of the femora is not unusual. In addition, an instance (apparently unique) of osteochondritis dissecans implicating the lateral and medial condyles of both femora (bilateral bicondylar osteochondritis dissecans of the knee) has been recorded (see Goldenberg and Cohen). Occasional instances of osteochondritis dissecans involving various combinations of joints have likewise been noted. In the small number of cases in which osteochondritis dissecans in multiple sites has been observed, the combined sites were most often one or both knees along with one or both elbows.

The description of the clinical manifestations of osteochondritis dissecans as they relate to the knee joint (its typical site) can serve in a general way for the other localizations also. In regard to the knee, the manifestations may be intermittent, mild, and equivocal for months. At first there is usually mere vague disability, perhaps a history of momentary "catchings" and slight swellings, and some pain. Palpation of the lateral aspect of the medial condyle of the femur is likely to elicit localized tenderness. Subsequently, there may be attacks of definite pain and locking of the joint, associated with the appearance of considerable intra-articular effusion. Under these circumstances, atrophy of the muscles of the thigh is likely to be noted. Sometimes these severer manifestations may be the presenting complaints. The definitive diagnosis can nearly always be established quite early on a roentgenographic basis.

The relation of *trauma* to the occurrence of the disorder is difficult to evaluate. Though a history of possibly causative trauma is elicited in many cases, there are also many in which it is vague or lacking. However, it is rather generally agreed that, by causing the final loosening of the osteochondral body, trauma (acute or functional) helps at least to instigate the severer clinical manifestations.

ROENTGENOGRAPHIC FINDINGS

The roentgenographic findings are determined by the phenomena of delimitation, loosening, and detachment of the osteochondral body from some place on the articular surface of the affected joint. In the knee, as already noted, the body is nearly always derived from the medial femoral condyle, and in particular from the lower part of its lateral aspect. Thus an anteroposterior view of the affected knee usually reveals some abnormality near the lower margin of the anterior aspect of the medial condyle. However, part or all of the lesion is sometimes not demonstrable in the roentgenograph taken in this way. Under these circumstances a "tunnel-view" picture taken from the back of the knee, with the latter slightly flexed, will almost certainly demonstrate the lesion. When already well delimited, the osteochondral body may still be rather firmly set in the condyle through continuity of its cartilage with the rest of the condylar cartilage. In such cases the roentgenograph shows merely a faint, narrow zone of increased radiolucency delimiting a more or less elliptical area of about the same density as the neighboring bone. When the body has come nearer to complete loosening, the delimiting zone is more conspicuous, and the density of the girdled area itself has usually increased. If the body has become completely detached, it is ordinarily found lying in the superior lateral part of the anterior compartment of the joint, and the space which it formerly occupied appears as an area of diminished density at the edge of the condyle. (See Fig. 150.)

In relation to the knee joint, the body occasionally comes from regions other than the medial condyle, and notably from the posterior surface of the patella. The writer has seen a case in which it had its origin from the medial surface of the lateral condyle. It is said that it may also come from the articular surface of the upper end of the tibia. In the elbow, the body usually separates from the capitulum of the humerus, but several instances have been reported in which it apparently arose from the medial side of the head of the radius (see Nielsen). In cases of osteochondritis dissecans involving the hip joint, the osteochondral body becomes delimited from the femoral head in the region of the fovea, and tends not to be extruded into the joint.

In connection with the roentgenographic findings in cases of *clinically manifest osteochondritis dissecans* taking its departure from a femoral condyle in an adolescent or young adult, there is an observation which is significant for purposes of comparison. This is the fact that (almost always in the *absence of pertinent clinical complaints*) infants and young children frequently show roentgenographic changes more or less suggestive of osteochondritis dissecans in the distal epiphysis of one or both femora (see Sontag and Pyle, Green and Banks, and Caffey *et al.*). In particular, these young subjects often reveal one or two small areas of irregularity in outline and/or texture somewhere along the articular margin of the ossification center for the developing condyles of one or both femora. When the ossification center shows only one area of irregularity, this is nearly always located somewhere along its medial aspect. In those instances in which the irregularity of the affected part of an ossification center amounts to a crater-like defect, there is often a clearly delimited, small, roundish or oval focus of radiopacity oriented to the crater or lying in it, and set off from it by a narrow margin of radiolucency. However, as already indicated, the infants and young children presenting the various irregularities at the margin of the ossification center of one or both distal femoral epiphyses rarely have clinical complaints referable to the affected knee area, and if there are any, these are very mild. Furthermore, the abnormalities observable on roentgenographic examination of the distal femoral epiphyses in these infants and young

Figure 150

A, Roentgenograph of a left knee area showing an osteochondritis dissecans lesion on the lateral surface of the medial condyle. The osteochondral body, although still set within its bed, appears to be composed of several fragments (or units) still held together by the covering articular cartilage. There was no history of a relevant injury to the affected knee. The patient was a girl 13 years of age who, at the time this roentgenograph was taken, complained chiefly of pain localized to the left knee area. She had been aware of the pain for about 2 weeks, and stated that it was brought on by extending the leg or arising from a sitting or squatting position. Palpation of the knee revealed tenderness localized to the anterior aspect of the medial condyle.

B, Roentgenograph of the right knee area showing a well-delineated osteochondritis dissecans lesion on the lateral surface of the medial condyle. The patient, a girl, was 14 years of age at the time this roentgenograph was taken. There was no history of relevant trauma, and no swelling or instability of the knee had been noted. The chief complaint was pain in the knee, of which the patient had been aware for about 2 years. She was also occasionally aware of a "clicking" in the knee and a feeling that movement of the knee was somewhat "blocked" from time to time. Examination revealed tenderness over the medial femoral condyle, but there was no effusion in the joint.

C, Roentgenograph of the right knee from another case of osteochondritis dissecans. Note the thin strand of radiopacity extending across the medial condyle and representing a very small amount of bone in the osteochondritis dissecans body, which undoubtedly consists largely of cartilage (see Fig. 151). The patient was a boy who was 16 years of age when this roentgenograph was taken. His chief complaint was pain localized to the anterior aspect of the knee and associated with some swelling of the joint. The first episode of swelling set in after ice skating, and subsequently swelling occurred after weight-lifting. The pain in the knee was brought on especially in the course of ascending or descending stairs and on squatting. The patient also mentioned that from time to time there was a sensation of "clicking" in the knee, but there were no episodes of locking of the knee. Examination revealed tenderness over the medial condyle and evidence of fluid in the knee joint.

D, Roentgenograph of the left knee of a boy 7 years of age showing small areas of irregularity along the articular margins of the lateral and medial condyles. It is to be noted that the lateral surface of the medial condyle, the conventional site of osteochondritis dissecans, is free of any defects suggestive of that condition. In the writer's opinion, the irregularities in the contour of the femoral condyles shown in this picture follow in the wake of local trauma (functional or acute) resulting in focal hemorrhage, scarring, and temporary disruption of endochondral ossification in the areas in question.

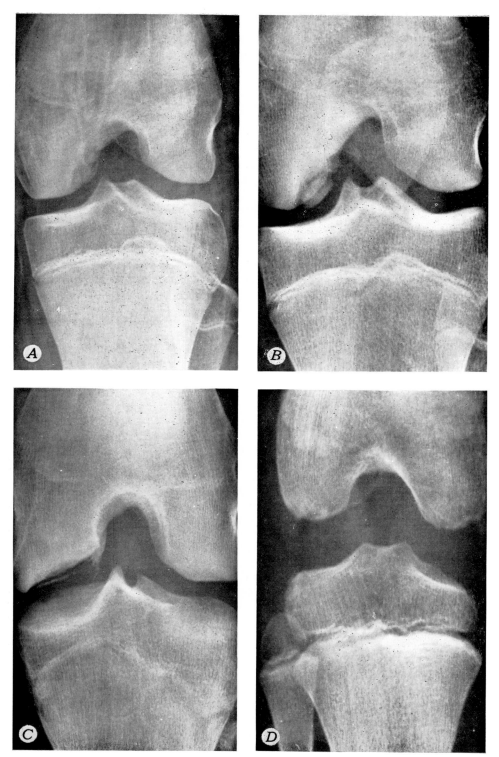

Figure 150

children tend to disappear without surgical treatment, the lesional area healing in, usually in the course of a year or two. The pathogenetic basis for these findings is considered below.

PATHOGENESIS AND PATHOLOGIC FINDINGS

Pathogenesis.—We come now to the discussion of the pathogenesis of clinically manifest osteochondritis dissecans involving the femoral condyles of adolescents and young adults. It seems advisable to consider first, however, the possible basis for the previously noted roentgenographic findings suggestive of osteochondritis dissecans which can often be observed in the distal femoral epiphyses of infants and young children, in the absence of clinical manifestations. In these young subjects, as already mentioned, the finding in question consists of one or two small areas of irregularity in outline and/or texture somewhere along the articular margin of the ossification center of one or both distal femoral epiphyses. The cartilage mass at the lower end of the femur is the body's largest epiphysial cartilage mass which is converted into an epiphysis through the appearance and growth within it of a secondary center of ossification. The rudiment of this center is nearly always already detectable at birth if the fetus is full term.

After birth, the total mass of the evolving distal femoral epiphysis, of course, increases. The increase occurs through proliferation of the cartilage cells surrounding its ossification center, and concomitant enlargement of the center itself. The growth of the center occurs through endochondral ossification taking place centrifugally around its periphery—that is, where the ossification center abuts upon a narrow zone of actively proliferating cartilage cells. Though the center increases in size throughout the growth period, it is during infancy and early childhood that the major part of its growth occurs. As is well known, wherever endochondral bone growth is taking place actively, numerous capillaries are present and penetrate the lacunae of the local swollen and degenerating cartilage cells. Also, osteoblasts which are carried in on the walls of the capillaries deposit osseous tissue on the tongues of calcified cartilage matrix which have thus become exposed.

Bordering on the ossification center there is a zone of cartilage which becomes narrower as the center increases in size in consequence of endochondral ossification. The cartilage surrounding the ossification center and bordering on the articular cavity may be regarded as articular cartilage, but it is not yet *definitive* articular cartilage. Final maturation of the epiphysis and its fusion with the femoral shaft is associated with termination of endochondral ossification on the deep surface of the cartilage bordering on the articular cavity, and closing off of this surface by arched trabeculae of spongy bone which constitute the subchondral bony end plate.

In a roentgenograph of a distal femoral epiphysis of a child, the outline of the epiphysis marks the site of the zone of provisional calcification. This is the site where endochondral ossification is taking place and, specifically, where osseous tissue is being deposited upon the tongues of calcified cartilage matrix (the primary spongiosa) to form the secondary spongiosa. The site where provisional calcification is going on is a highly vascular area. The present writer believes that, in the young children who present, roentgenographically, small areas of irregularity in outline and/or texture somewhere along the articular margin of the ossification center of a distal femoral epiphysis, there has been a focal hemorrhage, scarring, and temporary disruption of endochondral ossification in the area in question. That is, he attaches primary importance to trauma (functional or acute) as the provocative agent in the development of the roentgenographic changes under consideration. In line with this thought is the fact that, as demonstrated by the statistical studies of Köhler,

Sontag and Pyle, and Caffey *et al.*, the incidence of these defects in the distal femoral ossification centers is high in children 1 to 5 years of age and especially high in the age group 1 to 3 years. As already noted, the defects or irregularities are nearly always asymptomatic, and they tend to disappear spontaneously in the course of about 2 years from the time of their appearance. Hence, it seems clear that, if trauma is indeed the agent, the original local damage at the site of endochondral ossification must have been slight.

At any rate, it is difficult to accept the idea that these roentgenographic findings in the distal femoral epiphyses represent merely "a normal variant of ossification in children," or the related idea that they represent "a maturational disturbance of endochondral ossification of the epiphysis" instigated by accelerated growth due to heightened functioning of the thyroid gland. One reason for questioning the validity of these interpretations resides in the highly preferential localization of the abnormality in the lower epiphysis of the femur and, usually in milder form, the upper epiphysis of the tibia. It is true that roughening somewhere along the periphery of other centers of ossification is also sometimes encountered. However, its incidence in these other sites is low despite the fact that, in relation to some of these centers, endochondral ossification is likewise active. It is also on this account that one may question the idea of such factors as "a normal variant of ossification" or "a heightened functioning of the thyroid gland" in the causation of the condition. Specifically, it seems reasonable to suppose that, if these conceptions were valid, similar alterations would be found in a large variety of centers of ossification and even in many centers in the same child.

The factor of age incidence (predilection of the age group 1 to 3 years) and notably the high incidence of the condition in the lower femoral epiphysis and to a lesser degree in the upper tibial epiphysis seem to lend support to the idea of a traumatic basis. The trauma might easily consist of repeated bumping of the knees or falling on them in the process of crawling or learning to walk. It seems relevant here that the roughening and irregularity of the ossification center is observed most often on the medial aspect of the epiphysis, and that, if the lateral aspect of the epiphysis is involved, this involvement is always in addition to that of the medial aspect. If one visualizes the process of crawling or falling on the knees, it is plain that the brunt of the trauma would be taken on the medial aspect of the lower end of the femur and communicated to the medial aspect of the ossification center.

Sufficient stress has already been laid upon the great frequency with which, in infants and young children, the medial aspect (and sometimes also the lateral aspect) of the ossification center for the lower end of the femur shows irregularity of its contour. However, the likelihood is that these changes are not related to the pathogenesis of *symptomatic osteochondritis dissecans* of the knee in adolescents and young adults. The most important difference relates to the site on the condylar end of the femur where the lesion of symptomatic osteochondritis dissecans has its point of departure. Nearly always, this site is the lateral surface of the medial femoral condyle.

The pathogenesis of symptomatic osteochondritis dissecans (which is usually observed after the age of 15 and only infrequently in subjects 10 to 15 years of age) has received abundant and lively discussion. However, there is still no generally accepted hypothesis relating to the process by which the osteochondral body becomes delimited from the articular end of the affected bone, whether the site in question is the usual one (a femoral condyle) or some other articular bone end. Out of the many possibilities opened up by the statistical evaluations of cases and by the findings in experimental studies, only a few will be considered here. Special interest attaches to the following two contrasting conceptions: (1) that the basis of the condition is a circumscribed subchondral osteonecrosis, the necrotic bone area with its overlying cartilage gradually becoming loosened and often at last detached from its bed; and (2) that the basis of the condition is an acute fracture and that the suddenly detached area of subchondral bone with its overlying cartilage is extruded either immediately or after remaining *in situ* for a time.

The *primary fracture theory* has been advocated over the years by many well-known observers (see Barth, Brackett and Hall, Fisher, and also Fairbank). It seems to be clear that occasionally a joint body which comes to bear an anatomic resemblance to a conventional osteochondritis dissecans body does originate on the basis of a fracture at the lower end of a femur, and especially of the lateral condyle (see Rosenberg, and Kennedy *et al.*). An osteochondral fracture of the lateral femoral condyle occurs when the knee is in flexion, and may be accompanied by a twisting force (usually exerted by the patella), pain, and a loud snap. Altogether, the clinical features of *conventional* osteochondritis dissecans seem to stand against the assumption that acute fracture regularly plays the primary causative role.

The *primary osteonecrosis theory* has likewise had the support of many well-known observers (see Paget, König, Freiberg, and also Axhausen). Concerning the manner in which the subchondral osteonecrosis is brought about, Axhausen maintained that in many instances it is due to "bland infarction" of the area. He believed that the concept of "bland infarction" could be applied just as well to osteochondritis dissecans as, for instance, to Legg-Perthes disease, in connection with which it has already been considered (p. 574). However, the "bland infarction" concept is difficult to defend on an anatomic basis in relation to either of these conditions.

It has also been conceived that the focus of osteonecrosis may appear in consequence of traumatic squashing (without fracture) of the articular bone end, and

Figure 151

A, Roentgenograph of the right knee area of a boy 18 years of age showing an osteochondritis dissecans body *in situ* on the lateral surface of the medial femoral condyle. The medial condyle of the left femur presented a similar abnormality. The boy was admitted to the hospital for the treatment of an osteogenic sarcoma involving the upper end of the shaft of the right tibia. The presence of bilateral osteochondritis dissecans was an incidental finding, since the clinical complaints were believed to be ascribable to the sarcoma. A mid-thigh amputation was carried out for the treatment of the osteogenic sarcoma of the tibia, and thus the lower end of the right femur became available for anatomic study.

B, Photograph showing the articular surface of the condyles of the amputated femur. Note that a small area of the articular cartilage of the medial condyle projects above the rest of the cartilage and is outlined by a shallow groove. The articular cartilage of this osteochondritis dissecans body *in situ* is of the same color as the cartilage of the rest of the condyle.

C, Photograph of the lower end of the amputated femur sectioned in the frontal plane. Note that the delineated body is composed almost entirely of articular cartilage which is thicker than the neighboring cartilage—a common finding in these cases.

D, Roentgenograph of the cut specimen shown in *C*. It is clear from this picture also that the delimited body is composed largely of articular cartilage which is thicker than the rest of the cartilage of the medial condyle and also thicker than that of the lateral condyle. The streaky radiopacities present on the inner surface of the body represent fragments of subchondral bone which came away with the cartilage. The spongiosa of the condylar bed of the osteochondritis dissecans body is somewhat sclerotic.

E, Photomicrograph ($\times$ 7) illustrating the general histologic pattern presented by the lesional area in question. It is only at the right of the picture that the detached articular cartilage shows bits of subchondral bone on its deep surface. The spongy marrow spaces immediately above the detached cartilage contain granular detritus.

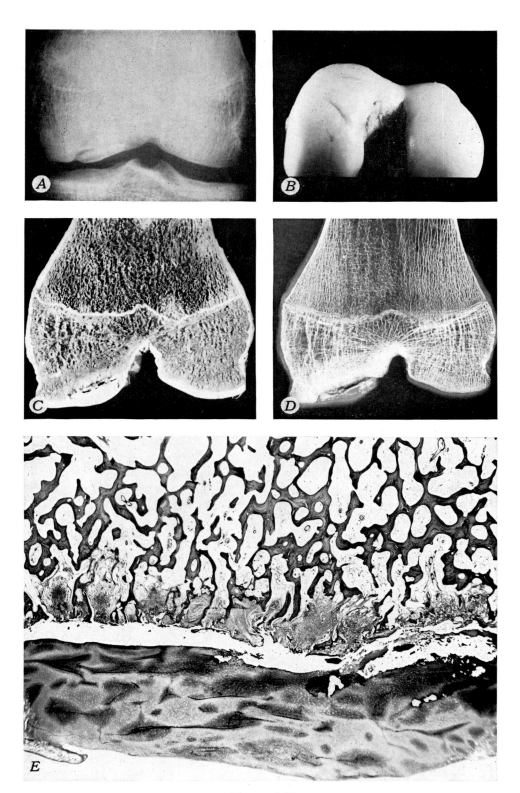

Figure 151

this idea impresses the present writer as being much more plausible. It is held that, in the knee, an excessively large medial tibial spine may act as the traumatizing agent. Furthermore, some hold that a trauma may instigate an osteonecrosis by interrupting the blood supply coming to the medial condyle by way of the posterior cruciate ligament. In general, those who favor the primary necrosis theory recognize that in any event it is usually a trauma (acute or functional) that forces the final extrusion of the loosened osteochondral body from its bed.

Pathologic Findings.—In respect to *gross pathology*, when the knee joint is opened, mere inspection of the medial femoral condyle occasionally fails to reveal the actual location of the lesional area. In particular, the site is likely to be obscure in those rare instances in which the osseous part of the delimited osteochondral body is still snugly set within its bed and the cartilaginous portion of the body still merges smoothly into the rest of the condylar cartilage. Even then, pressure exerted upon the cartilage at the site of the lesion intact in its setting is met by a certain amount of "give." Usually, however, the site of an osteochondritis dissecans body which is still *in situ* will already be revealed by inspection. In these cases the body is outlined by an encircling furrow in the articular cartilage, which may show some cracks and tears. Except along the furrow, the cartilage may be level and uniform in color with the rest of the condylar cartilage, or it may project beyond the rest and be irregularly bumpy, abnormally soft, and discolored. In other instances the entire body may be found hanging by an edge, or a part of it may still be hanging while the rest has become detached and has entered the joint cavity, or all of the body may have become detached and been extruded into the joint as a unit. (See Fig. 151.)

Whether the osteochondritis dissecans body is a unit or a mosaic of 2 or 3 fragments, it is more or less elliptical in outline and usually shaped like a segment of a shallow arc. It may measure up to 1 inch or so through its shorter axis, and somewhat more through its longer axis. Through its thickest part it measures as little as 4 or 5 mm. in some cases and as much as 15 mm. in others. The thickness in excess of 4 or 5 mm. depends mainly upon the amount of subchondral bone which has come away with the cartilage, but as a rule that amount is not great. The cartilage may be of normal thickness but is more often excessively thick. The

Figure 152

A, B, C, Photographs (somewhat enlarged) showing different views of an osteochondritis dissecans body which was well delimited and still *in situ* when it was excised from the lateral surface of the medial condyle of the right femur. The patient was a man 21 years of age. A shows the outer (or articular) surface of the osteochondral body. The covering cartilage itself is not significantly modified. B reveals the appearance of the underside (or deep surface) of the body. C illustrates the gross appearance of the cut surface of the body after the latter had been sectioned in the vertical plane. On the right the subchondral osseous tissue was yellowish in color and appeared sclerotic, while on the left it was less dense.

D, Photomicrograph (× 6) revealing the general histologic pattern of the osteochondritis dissecans body shown above. The intertrabecular marrow spaces contain granular detritus, and the subchondral osseous tissue is more compact on the right than on the left.

E, Photomicrograph (× 35) showing in greater detail the histologic pattern presented by a tissue field on the left in D. Viewing the picture from above downward, one can note that cells are present in the lacunae of the articular cartilage, indicating that the cartilage is viable. Within the marrow spaces of the subchondral spongiosa, there is necrotic fatty marrow and considerable granular detritus. In the osseous tissue of the spongiosa, practically no osteocytes can be seen in the bone cell lacunae, and there is evidence in places that the necrotic osseous tissue is undergoing disintegration. The deep surface of the body is sealed off by a layer of connective tissue.

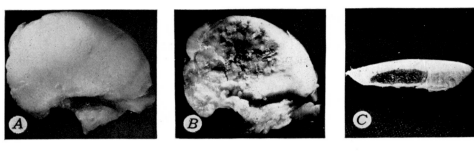

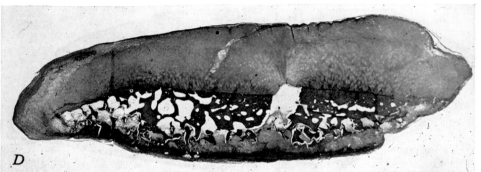

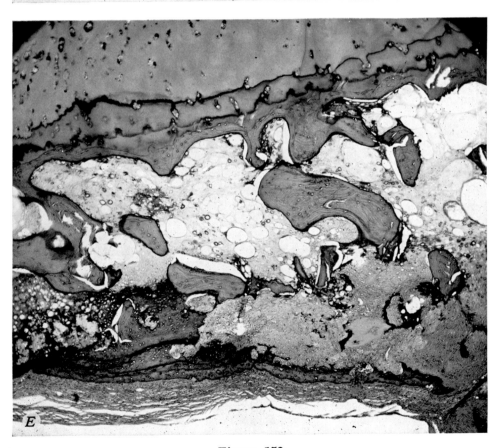

Figure 152

outer surface of the body may also show a transverse furrow, giving it a lobulated appearance. Whatever bone is present subchondrally is usually yellowish white. The deep, or condylar, surface of the body is nearly always found roughened and covered by fibrous or fibrocartilaginous connective tissue.

If the body is one that has been lying in the joint for a long time, its total size will usually indicate that it has grown since it was extruded. The writer has examined osteochondral bodies from a large number of cases of osteochondritis dissecans. In the great majority of these specimens there was no difficulty whatsoever in making the decision, on the basis of the gross appearance, that the body came from a case of this disorder. Occasionally there was difficulty, because the body, lying free in the joint, had become encased in a thick layer of calcified cartilage and fibrocartilage, taking on the contour and general outer appearance of a conventional "joint mouse." However, when such a modified osteochondritis dissecans body is sectioned, its core will still reveal its original nature on gross examination (see Freiberg and Wolley).

On *microscopic examination* of an unmodified osteochondritis dissecans body, it will be found that the cartilage covering of the body is viable on the whole. However, it is likely to show some fibrillation and degeneration toward its articular surface, and also some patches of calcification. The deepest zone of the articular cartilage (that is, its calcified zone) may be found disrupted in some places. The subchondral osseous tissue shows substantial or complete aseptic necrosis. The marrow, too, is more or less necrotic, and the intertrabecular marrow spaces ordinarily contain at least some granular detritus, which stains blue with hematoxylin. The subchondral spongy trabeculae are usually abnormally thick, whether the constituent osseous tissue is partially viable or completely necrotic. In fact, because of the excessive number of cement lines present in these trabeculae, one gains the impression that the trabeculae have been thickened through periodic deposition of new bone. The probabilities are that while the osteochondritis

Figure 153

A, Roentgenograph showing a so-called "joint mouse" in the suprapatellar bursa of a knee joint. The patient, a woman, was 24 years of age when this picture was taken. Her chief complaint was frequent locking of the right knee joint, associated with pain and swelling. There had been difficulties relating to the knee for about 9 years, but lately the episodes of pain, swelling, and locking of the knee had become more frequent. At surgery an oval, irregularly nodular, cartilage-covered body measuring $2.5 \times 1.5 \times 1.25$ cm. was removed. It presented the external appearance (see *B*) of the cartilage-covered nodular joint bodies which are often encountered in the knee in cases of osteoarthritis of long standing. However, when it was cut across and the cut surfaces were examined, it was obvious that one was dealing with an osteochondritis dissecans body whose nature was disguised by the accretion of cartilage on its surfaces (see *C*).

B, Photograph illustrating the external appearance of the joint body shown in *A*, after it had been removed from the suprapatellar bursa. This joint body had been cut through and the two parts reapposed along the line of transection.

C, Photograph of the cut surface of each half of the sectioned joint body. It is clear even to the naked eye that the core of the body consists of articular cartilage and subchondral bone (see area demarcated by arrows) and thus has the configuration of an osteochondritis dissecans body.

D, Photomicrograph ($\times$ 6) of a modified osteochondritis dissecans body removed from a knee joint in another case. The site and extent of the original osteochondritis dissecans body are demarcated by the arrows. The original articular cartilage and the narrow zone of modified subchondral osseous tissue can be discerned, even under this low magnification, beneath the newly deposited cartilage surrounding the osteochondritis dissecans body.

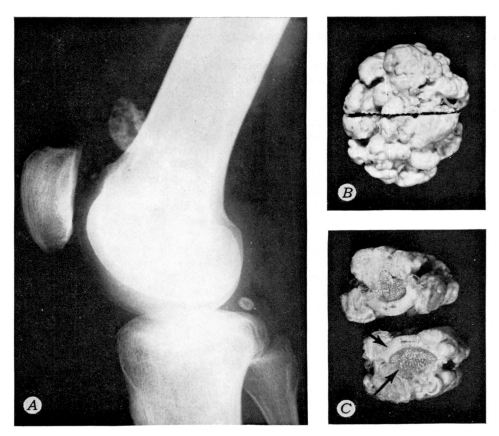

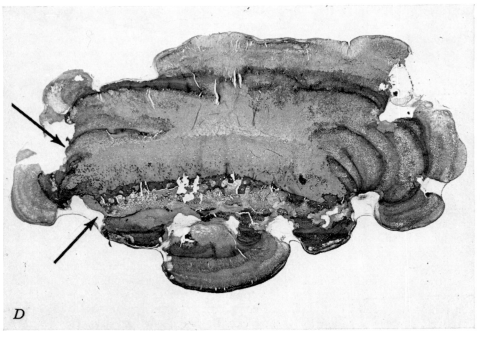

Figure 153

dissecans body is still *in situ* there are periods of partial restoration of the local blood supply, with consequent deposition of new bone on the existing trabeculae, which had been partially or completely devitalized. Indeed, it is altogether possible for a relatively small osteochondritis dissecans body which is still *in situ* to become permanently reattached and revivified (see Green and Banks).

As noted, the condylar surface of the osteochondritis dissecans body is usually covered by connective tissue. The latter may be densely fibrous or fibrocartilaginous in whole or in part. The intertrabecular spaces in the vicinity of this delimiting connective tissue may contain some granular detritus. Furthermore, if the body has been lying in the articular cavity for some time, the delimiting connective tissue on its deep surface may even show some evidence of osseous metaplasia. The condylar defect is also covered by a modified connective tissue. If a long time has elapsed since the body was extruded, it may be found that the defect has been largely filled in by connective tissue. Some have claimed that on microscopic examination the osseous tissue for a varying distance about the condylar defect may likewise be found necrotic. The articular cartilage immediately surrounding the condylar defect is undermined and frayed to some degree, but otherwise the articular surfaces of the affected joint usually present a normal appearance. (See Figs. 152 and 153.)

TREATMENT

In view of the fact that the preponderant site of osteochondritis dissecans is the articular end of a femoral condyle, our remarks on treatment will relate to osteochondritis dissecans involving the knee joint. There are several considerations which necessarily influence the course of treatment of the condition in this site. These are: (1) the age of the subject when the presence of the osteochondritis dissecans is first revealed by roentgenographic examination of the knee joint; (2) the question of whether the osteochondral body is still set in its condylar bed, irrespective of the extent to which it is delimited from the bed; and (3) whether, instead, the osteochondral body has been extruded from the bed and has entered the joint cavity.

It has long been recognized that an osteochondritis dissecans body which is intact in its setting in the condylar bed may heal in spontaneously. In particular, this often happens if the subject is an older child or an adolescent and if the knee joint is protected from functional injury. These aims may be accomplished either by merely limiting participation of the young subject in active sports or by also immobilizing the affected knee area in a plaster cylinder which holds the knee in a slightly flexed position so that weight-bearing is reduced (see Löhr, Wiberg, Müller, and also Green and Banks). Under these circumstances the conservative (nonsurgical) treatment often leads, in the course of about 3 or 4 years, to spontaneous reunion of the osteochondritis dissecans body with the rest of the condyle. On the other hand, in subjects who are about 20 years of age or older when the diagnosis of osteochondritis dissecans of the knee is first made, there seems to be little likelihood of achieving spontaneous healing by conservative nonsurgical treatment.

For these older subjects, surgery is indicated, and it is also appropriate for those younger subjects in whom reasonably prolonged conservative treatment has not been followed by relief of the clinical complaints and healing of the lesional area. Moreover, surgery is called for in any case in which part or all of the delimited osteochondral fragment has been extruded into the joint cavity. Thus, in principle, surgical treatment consists of removal of the loosened or extruded body, or an attempt to reattach the loosened or extruded body to the condylar bed.

OSGOOD-SCHLATTER DISEASE

Osgood-Schlatter disease is an affection of the developing tibial tuberosity which both Osgood and Schlatter described in 1903, and which they interpreted as the result of a partial avulsion of the tuberosity somewhere along the site of attachment of the patellar ligament to it. Confusion concerning the pathogenesis of the condition was created by the subsequent introduction of the concept that the initial pathologic change was aseptic necrosis occurring in the developing tuberosity. However, this idea has now been completely discounted, and there is general agreement that Osgood-Schlatter disease is the sequel of avulsion of part of the patellar ligament with attached cartilaginous or bony fragments from the tuberosity. The subjects are youthful and are more often boys than girls. The characteristic early clinical features include pain in the region of the knee and tenderness localized to the tibial tuberosity, and there is often also some soft-tissue swelling in the region of the tuberosity. Names in addition to Osgood-Schlatter disease which have been applied to the condition include: Osgood-Schlatter lesion, apophysitis tibialis adolescentium, football knee or Rugby knee, and osteochondritis or osteochondrosis of the tibial tubercle.

CLINICAL CONSIDERATIONS

Incidence.—In respect to *general incidence* it is to be noted that the Osgood-Schlatter lesion is by no means uncommon in orthopaedic practice, and that in particular the records of hospitals having pediatric orthopaedic services include many instances of the condition which have accumulated over the years (see Sutro and Pomeranz, Uhry, and also Ehrenborg). The *age incidence* in relation to the time of onset is determined by the postnatal development and ossification of the tibial tuberosity and the time of its fusion (synostosis) with the shaft of the tibia to form the definitive tuberosity (see p. 602). Since this whole anatomic process tends to run its course about 2 years earlier in girls than in boys, the disease sets in earlier, on the average, in girls than in boys. In the series of 170 cases of Osgood-Schlatter disease which was evaluated by Ehrenborg, he found that: (1) The age range of the patients when medical care for the condition was first sought at his hospital was 9 years and 3 months to 15 years for the girls (68 patients) and 10 years and 3 months to 15 years and 2 months for the boys (102 patients); (2) the mean age of all the patients was 12 years and 5 months; and (3) the mean age for the girls alone was 11 years and 6 months and for the boys alone it was 13 years and 3 months.

All these data make it clear that Osgood-Schlatter disease in the strict sense of the term has a very limited age range in respect to its time of onset. Apparently it does not set in before the age of 8 years in girls or before the age of 10 years in boys. Furthermore, the upper age limit for its onset in either sex is about 14 years.

As already noted, there is a difference in the *sex incidence* of the condition, boys being definitely predilected. However, the degree of difference between the sexes in regard to incidence shows considerable variation when one compares statistical compilations from various countries. This is to be expected in view of the etiologic importance of trauma in the causation of the disorder. The special predominance of boys over girls noted in some of the statistical compilations (5 to 1 in Uhry's report as contrasted with 1.5 to 1 in Ehrenborg's report) can probably be accounted for by differences in the extent to which the boys of a particular country predominate over the girls in respect to activity in strenuous sports.

The *tibia affected* in a case of Osgood-Schlatter disease may be the right or the left, or both tibiae may be involved. In some of the reports it is stated that the right tibia is more often involved, in others that the left is more often involved, and in still others that the right tibia is as likely to be affected as the left. In addition, bilateral involvement is frequently encountered, being noted in about 20 to 30 per cent of the cases in any large series.

Clinical Complaints and Findings.—The onset of the clinical complaints is often, but by no means consistently, related to a specific traumatic episode involving the affected knee. The complaints which direct the patient toward medical care are local pain and tenderness, usually of several months' duration, and are related to the general region of the knee, or more particularly to the affected tibial tuberosity. In some cases the symptoms are relatively mild, being brought on only by active exertion of the knee joint. In other cases the pain and tenderness are sufficiently severe to make the patient limp and to necessitate keeping the knee at rest to secure some relief.

Objective clinical findings include some degree of swelling in the region of the tibial tuberosity, and palpation of the tuberosity elicits rather sharply localized tenderness. Although the knee is usually completely mobile, it is very likely that the patient will complain of pain occurring toward the end of active extension or flexion of the knee. Furthermore, in cases of long duration, the region of the tuberosity is enlarged, and palpation may now reveal one or more bony-hard prominences on its anterior aspect or slightly above it. In such cases one may find, in addition, some atrophy of the calf and thigh muscles, if the pain has led to much restriction of movement.

Figure 154

A, *B*, *C*, and *D*, Roentgenographs illustrating the changes of Osgood-Schlatter disease as revealed in four different cases of the disorder.

A, The patient in this case was a boy who was 13 years of age at the time this picture was taken. For about 2 months he had been aware of pain in both knee areas after running or exercising. The illustration relates to the left knee, but the right knee, too, was the site of Osgood-Schlatter disease. Note the fragmented appearance of the tuberosity. The small, discrete radiopaque body is an ossicle of bone and cartilage avulsed from the tuberosity and apparently growing in the patellar ligament. The region of the left tibial tubercle was somewhat enlarged and was sensitive to pressure.

B, The patient in this case was a boy 13 years of age who recalled having fallen on the affected knee about 4 months before this picture was taken. However, it was only for about 2 weeks that he had been clearly aware of pain in the knee, which was aggravated by squatting. Physical examination revealed that the affected tubercle was somewhat tender to palpation and that the area was slightly enlarged. Note the defect on the anterior surface of the tubercle and the small fragment which has been avulsed from it.

C, The patient, a boy, was 13½ years of age when this roentgenograph was taken. About 15 months earlier, he had injured his left knee by falling on it in the course of jumping. Subsequently he became aware of a lump in the region of the tibial tubercle. Inquiry also revealed that the area was painful when pressure was exerted upon it. Note the irregularity in contour of the anterior surface of the tibial tubercle and the somewhat lobulated focus representing growing fragments of the tissue which had been avulsed from the anterior surface of the tuberosity. One may surmise from the roentgenographic appearances that the avulsed tissue growing in the patellar ligament is composed mainly of cartilage which has not yet been replaced by osseous tissue and whose matrix is not yet heavily calcified.

D, The patient in this case, a boy, was 13 years of age when this roentgenograph was taken. He had noted a slight swelling in the area of the right tibial tubercle, but could not recall how long it had been present and did not remember having injured the area. Squatting and ascending and descending stairs was somewhat painful, and direct pressure against the tuberosity also caused pain. The upper anterior surface of the tubercle reveals an irregularity, and a streaky, narrow strand of radiopacity extends from it into the patellar ligament.

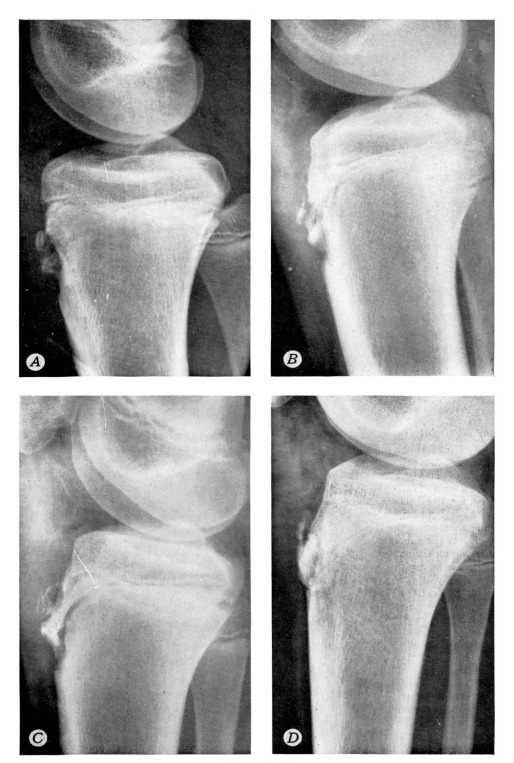

Figure 154

ROENTGENOGRAPHIC FINDINGS

Though the diagnosis of Osgood-Schlatter disease is already suggested by the clinical aspects of the case, the definitive diagnosis is dependent upon the roentgenographic findings. (See Fig. 154.) As a background for consideration of the roentgenographic features of the condition, it seems appropriate to give a brief description of the *normal course of evolution of the tibial tuberosity.* The first stage of its development (the cartilage stage) is represented by a tongue of cartilage which extends downward from the upper tibial epiphysis onto the anterior face of the tibial metaphysis. In this tongue of cartilage, a single center of ossification or two separate ossification centers which soon fuse appear, the evolution of the tuberosity thus advancing from the cartilaginous to the apophysial stage. The ossification center for the tuberosity continues to grow and, extending proximally, fuses with the ossification center for the proximal epiphysis of the tibia, the tuberosity thus entering into the so-called epiphysial stage of its development. The final stage in the evolution of the tibial tuberosity is marked by the disappearance of the epiphysial cartilage plate (apophysial cartilage plate) which had separated the evolving tibial tuberosity from the metaphysis of the tibia. Bony fusion of the tuberosity with the tibial metaphysis does not occur before the age of 15 in girls and 17 in boys. (See Hulting, Ehrenborg and Lagergren, and also Hasselwander.)

The roentgenographic findings reflect the pathologic changes resulting from the local avulsion. This nearly always implicates the evolving tibial tuberosity somewhere along the site of attachment of the patellar ligament to it. Hence it seems to be in order to consider briefly the normal anatomic relationship between these

Figure 155

A, Roentgenograph of a tissue specimen removed in a case of Osgood-Schlatter disease. From left to right, the picture shows a portion of the metaphysis of the tibia, the apophysial cartilage plate (the narrow radiolucent zone), the tibial apophysis, and the patellar ligamen with a focus of radiopacity in it representing fragments of growing bone and cartilage avulsed from the tibial tubercle. The patient was a boy 14 years of age who had pain and swelling in the region of the left knee for about 1½ years before admission to the hospital. The local difficulties were said to have set in after he had received a blow to the front of the leg, in the region of the tubercle. On physical examination he presented a walnut-sized, firm, tender swelling on the anterior surface of the tibia in the region of the tubercle.

B, Photograph illustrating the cut surface of the gross specimen represented roentgenographically in *A.* There is a close correspondence between the information conveyed by the photograph of the gross specimen and that revealed by the roentgenograph prepared from it.

C, Photomicrograph ($\times 4$) illustrating the tissue pattern presented by the Osgood-Schlatter specimen shown in *B.* From left to right, the picture reveals tibial metaphysis, apophysial cartilage plate, tibial apophysis, and patellar ligament which has some cartilage and osseous tissue embedded in it. The contour of the anterior surface of the tibial apophysis is irregular, because the fragments of cartilage and bone embedded in the patellar ligament had been avulsed from this surface of the apophysis.

D, Roentgenograph depicting the alterations in the region of the tibial tubercle in a case of Osgood-Schlatter disease. The tubercle is separated into two parts, the upper fragment being the larger one. The defect seems to extend also through the apophysial cartilage plate. The patient was a boy 14 years of age who had difficulties in the region of the left tibial tuberosity for 9 months following a fall on the knee.

E, Photomicrograph ($\times 6$) showing that the gap between the upper and lower fragments of the tibial tuberosity is filled by fibrous tissue that is highly vascularized. The laceration extends through the apophysial cartilage plate, and the defect in that region is also filled by vascular granulation tissue. The small amount of osseous tissue to the right of the upper part of the apophysial cartilage plate represents a fragment of tibia.

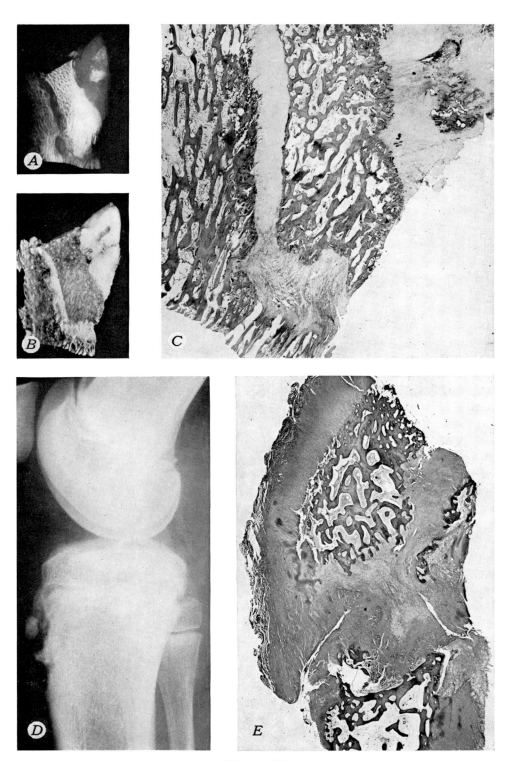

Figure 155

two structures in youthful subjects—that is, in subjects representing the age group (approximately 8 to 14 years) in which the Osgood-Schlatter lesion develops. In such subjects the major part of the patellar ligament (which also contains fibers of the quadriceps tendon) is inserted into the cartilage constituting the outer surface of the evolving tibial tuberosity. The mechanical weakness (poor tensile strength) of this ligament-cartilage attachment favors the occurrence of avulsion of fragments of cartilage and perhaps even some underlying bone, since much of the power of the quadriceps femoris muscle exerted during movement of the knee joint is supplied through those quadriceps tendon fibers which have fused with the patellar ligament (see Uhry, and also Ehrenborg and Engfeldt). Thus, in a youthful subject, an undue exertion or a traumatic incident which results in the application of an excessive force at the site of attachment of the patellar ligament to the evolving tuberosity is likely to cause avulsion of one or more fragments of the cartilaginous outer surface of the tuberosity along with attached portions of the patellar ligament. In addition, some bone representing fragments of the ossification center of the tuberosity may come away with the avulsed cartilage.

The specific roentgenographic findings in Osgood-Schlatter disease vary with the size of the avulsed fragment or fragments of cartilage and underlying bone and the duration of the condition when the affected knee was examined. To demonstrate the roentgenographic changes to best advantage, the knee should be rotated slightly inward, so that one obtains a tangential view of the affected tibial tuberosity, and attention should also be given to revealing the regional soft tissues clearly. Furthermore, in every suspected case of Osgood-Schlatter disease, a control roentgenograph of the opposite knee area, taken in the same position and exposures, is indicated for purposes of comparison. Early in the course of the disorder, swelling of the soft tissues overlying the tubercle, and thickening of the patellar ligament at the site of its insertion are almost regularly detected. In addition, the patellar ligament usually presents one or more foci of radiopacity, generally located in the immediate vicinity of the tubercle and representing fragments of cartilage and even some bits of underlying bone which have been avulsed with parts of the patellar ligament. The outer surface of the tuberosity is likely to show one or more indentations marking the site from which the fragments of cartilage, with some of the underlying bone, had been avulsed. Indeed, the tuberosity as a whole may come to present a "fragmented" appearance.

In time, the avulsed fragment or fragments increase somewhat in size through continuance of endochondral bone formation and callus formation, and may also appear more radiopaque in the roentgenograph. If more than one radiopaque fragment is present in the patellar ligament, the fragments may remain discrete or eventually enlarge and fuse. In the course of a few years the fused fragments may even become reunited with the tuberosity and present as a bony mass which extends proximally into the patellar ligament and which, if not removed, will persist into adult life.

PATHOLOGIC FINDINGS

The article by Uhry published in 1944 includes a comprehensive study of the pathology of Osgood-Schlatter disease. That part of his report was based upon examination of 23 specimens removed from 20 subjects. The material had been placed at his disposal by the present writer when Dr. Uhry was working under his direction as a Frauenthal Orthopaedic Research Fellow in the Laboratories of the Hospital for Joint Diseases. From Uhry's study of the material in question, it was evident that the fundamental pathologic change in Osgood-Schlatter disease is a traumatically induced laceration or disruption occurring most often somewhere along the site of attachment of the patellar ligament to the tibial tuberosity. His observations on this aspect of the pathology of the condition were subsequently confirmed, in their essence, by LaZerte and Rapp and by Ehrenborg and Engfeldt. Uhry also found that in some instances the site of the disruption was not at the interface of the patellar ligament and the tibial tuberosity, but in the region of the anterior or posterior surface of the cartilage plate (apophysial cartilage plate) which lies between the developing tuberosity and the tibia. In occasional instances there were histologic indications that traumatic disruption had occurred not only at the interface of the patellar ligament and the tibial tuberosity but also in the cartilage plate between the tuberosity and the metaphysis of the tibia. LaZerte and Rapp, however, observed no cases in which the site of departure for the pathologic changes was in the cartilage plate between the tuberosity and the tibia. (See Fig. 155.)

The details of the histologic findings vary with the particular interface where the laceration has occurred. As already noted, the site where it is most common is somewhere along the attachment of the patellar ligament to the anterior surface of the evolving tibial tuberosity. Under these circumstances the portion of ligament which has been avulsed from the anterior face of the tuberosity will usually have attached to it a small fragment of cartilage-covered bone derived from the ossification center of the tuberosity. In time, a zone of vascularized connective tissue, which may have embedded in it some trabeculae of osteoid and/or osseous tissue and even bits of cartilage, comes to occupy the area between the avulsed fragment of bone and the corresponding defect in the anterior cortex of the tuberosity. The fragment of bone avulsed from the tuberosity at first shows some histologic evidence of aseptic necrosis (in line with the fact that it represents a fracture fragment), and subsequently it becomes revascularized and presents histologic indications of creeping replacement. Evidence of a scarring reaction and even some aseptic bone necrosis followed by creeping replacement is also apparent along the margin of the defect (the fracture site) at the anterior surface of the tuberosity. Continued growth of the detached fragment of the tuberosity within the patellar ligament results in the development of a clearly delimited ossicle, which ultimately stands out in the roentgenograph as a clear-cut focus of radiopacity. If more than one fragment of bone has been avulsed from the anterior surface of the tuberosity, each of the growing fragments remains for some time as an individual ossicle. In the connective tissue between such ossicles, one may find one or more cleftlike spaces outlined by condensed connective tissue and suggesting pseudarthral spaces.

As already noted, there are instances of Osgood-Schlatter disease in which the point of departure for the changes is in the cartilage zone between the evolving tuberosity and the tibial metaphysis. In those instances, evidences of tissue disruption and connective tissue scar formation are to be found in the interface between the evolving tuberosity and the apophysial cartilage plate, or on the deep surface of that plate between it and the tibial metaphysis.

KÖHLER'S DISEASE OF THE TARSAL NAVICULAR

In 1908, Köhler described, on a roentgenographic basis, an affection of the tarsal navicular bone which has come to be known by his name. The pathologic changes have their foundation in an interruption of the blood supply to the developing navicular bone, resulting in partial or substantial aseptic necrosis of its ossification center. The condition is self-limited, the ossification center becoming revascularized and more or less completely reconstructed in the course of time. It is this fact, along with the crucial position of the navicular in the arch of the foot, that accounts for the sparsity of pathologico-anatomic material relating to the disorder. However, the roentgenographic findings are sufficiently distinctive to permit the diagnosis of the condition if pictures are taken at intervals in the course of the disease and are considered in the light of the clinical complaints. Like many of the other disorders discussed in this chapter, the affection in question has received a burdensome number of alternative names. Among these are: Köhler-Mouchet disease, os naviculare pedis tardum, isolated dystrophy of the tarsal scaphoid, and osteochondritis of the tarsal scaphoid.

CLINICAL CONSIDERATIONS

Incidence.—In respect to *general incidence* it is clear that the condition is not often encountered. Indeed, over a period of 10 years, only 45 cases of Köhler's disease of the tarsal navicular were treated at the Children's Hospital of Boston, Massachusetts (see Karp), and over a period of 27 years, only 62 patients affected with the disorder were treated at the Wingfield-Morris Orthopaedic Hospital and Nuffield Orthopaedic Centre in Oxford, England (see Waugh).

The *sex incidence* and the *age distribution* of Köhler's disease also present some points of special interest. The predilection for males stands out sharply, the disorder being 4 to 5 times as common in males as in females. At the time of onset of clinical complaints, the age of the subject is likely to be somewhere between 3 and 7 years. However, the age at the time of onset in any large series of cases (including both males and females) is nearer 3 than 7 years. Moreover, when the sexes are considered separately in a pertinent statistical study, it becomes evident that the disorder tends to set in somewhat earlier in girls than in boys. This finding is apparently related to the fact that the center of ossification for the tarsal navicular makes its appearance months earlier in girls than in boys. A large proportion of girls already show this center at 2 years of age, while it is only at $2\frac{1}{2}$ to 3 years of age that it has appeared in an equivalent proportion of boys.

Clinical Complaints and Findings.—The clinical manifestations are at worst not striking, and are frequently very mild. Indeed, not uncommonly, in connection with a study of the disease in one foot, roentgenographic examination of the other foot reveals its presence there also, in the absence of clinical complaints. The disease is as likely to appear in one foot as in the other, and bilateral involvement is not unusual. A history of antecedent trauma is not infrequently obtained, but more often than not the history is vague or negative in this respect.

The presenting complaint is usually pain localized to the inner aspect of the midtarsal part of the foot. The latter is likely to be held in slight varus, so that the subject walks on the outer side of the foot. When it is not so rotated, the subject may walk flat-footedly. If there is pain, there is frequently also some limp. The skin in the region of the affected navicular bone may be warm and reddened, and the soft tissues overlying this bone may be swollen. Palpation of the bone usually elicits tenderness, which is emphasized by any attempt to manipulate the midtarsal arch. If the disease is of fairly long duration, one may even note some wasting of the calf muscles. In any event, the definitive clinical diagnosis is dependent on the roentgenographic findings.

ROENTGENOGRAPHIC FINDINGS

In this connection it is important to bear in mind that it is not unusual for children who do *not* present clinical manifestations of Köhler's disease to show certain deviations in size, contour, and density of the evolving center of ossification of one or both tarsal naviculars. Furthermore, in an appreciable percentage of children, the evolving navicular bone shows more than one ossification center, these centers eventually coalescing into one. In particular, it has been stressed that such deviations are most likely to be observed if the center or centers of ossification have appeared relatively late. Under these circumstances the ossification center for one or both of the tarsal naviculars may be found irregular in outline, of increased density, and flattened or even "fragmented" (because of the presence of multiple centers), thus presenting a roentgenographic appearance suggestive of Köhler's disease. On the other hand, if the ossification center of a tarsal navicular has appeared at the normal time or somewhat early, it can be expected to show a smooth outline, a rounded shape, and a uniform density (see Karp, Ferguson and Gingrich, and also Waugh).

In clinical instances of Köhler's disease the initial roentgenograph frequently shows that the ossification center is very much narrowed (wafer-like) in the lateral projection and perhaps somewhat irregular in contour. Concomitantly the altered center usually presents a more or less uniform increase in radiopacity and lacks the normal trabecular pattern. Subsequently this stage is superseded by one in which the radiodensity of the narrowed center is somewhat patchy—that is, by a stage in which focal radiopacities are intermingled with radiolucencies. Gradually the center tends to regain its normal size, density, and trabeculated structure. This process of normalization may require 2 or 3 years or even more, and slight flattening of the center may persist for some time after this. (See Fig. 156.)

In other cases of Köhler's disease the center of ossification of the navicular, instead of appearing narrowed or even wafer-like in the original roentgenographic picture, shows no alteration in contour but merely some increased radiodensity. Thereafter, the radiodensity tends to diminish, though not uniformly, the center coming to cast a spotty shadow, and within a year or so even this spottiness has disappeared and the roentgenograph may show only a small, faint, disk-shaped focus of radiopacity representing the altered ossification center. Reconstruction of the center then begins to be apparent, the center reforming by fusion of several foci of revitalized bone and/or newly formed osseous tissue. The entire process of reconstruction may take as long as 3 years, but is often accomplished in half that time and sometimes even less.

PATHOGENESIS AND PATHOLOGIC FINDINGS

Pathogenesis.—In regard to pathogenesis it is now generally agreed that the pathologic changes follow in the wake of interruption of the blood supply to the ossification center and lead to partial or more or less complete aseptic necrosis of the center.

Normally, in an infant or a very young child, the nonarticular surfaces of the cartilaginous precursor of the navicular bone have been found to be surrounded by a dense perichondrial network of blood vessels, and from this network numerous arteries (in cartilage vessel canals) penetrate toward the center of the cartilage mass (see Waugh). This perichondrial network of vessels seems to be supplied on the dorsal surface of the developing navicular by branches from the dorsalis pedis artery, and on the plantar surface by branches from the medial plantar artery (see Velluda). When the ossification center of the navicular makes its appearance, it may be nourished, at least at first and sometimes for a year or more, by a single blood vessel. However, as the center grows, the other vessels which have penetrated into the depth of the cartilage mass also come to nourish the enlarging center of ossification.

The anatomic location of the navicular—that is, its position in front of the talus (astragalus) and behind the three cuneiforms—is such that it is practically the "keystone" in the arch of the foot, transmitting the body weight from the talus to the cuneiforms. Furthermore, it has been pointed out on the basis of actual measurements that the space between the talus and the first cuneiform is often abnormally small, so that the evolving navicular is crowded (see Scaglietti et al.). It is therefore logical to deduce that mechanical factors centering around the navicular's "keystone" position in the arch of the foot, and the narrowness of the space for that bone, may lead, under certain conditions, to interference with the blood supply to the developing navicular. If the center of ossification for the navicular is relatively late in its appearance, and if, in addition, the young subject is particularly active physically and perhaps overweight, the influence of the mechanical factors tending to interfere with the blood supply to the enlarging ossification center of the navicular is increased. Under such circumstances the enlarging ossification center is apparently subjected to pressure which is greater than that which its anatomic structure is able to withstand at a certain period during growth. In consequence, blood vessels within the center or at its periphery (where endochondral bone growth is occurring) would be compressed, and ischemic necrosis of the center may thus ensue.

Pathologic Findings.—Because of the undesirability of surgical intervention in Köhler's disease, only a few specimens of affected navicular bones have been available for study of the *pathologic anatomy* of the condition. In the few instances in which the bone was extirpated, it was found to be of normal size and shape, and its cartilage surface smooth, although perhaps somewhat lacking in luster (see Lecène and Mouchet, and Speed). However, transection of the affected navicular reveals that its ossification center is: flattened and also irregular in outline; brownish or grayish in color; and soft and pulpy instead of having the consistency of spongy bone. Furthermore, in line with the fact that growth of the center through endochondral ossification has been disturbed, the zone of cartilage surrounding the modified center is thicker than it would normally be in relation to the age of the subject. It is this excess of cartilage that accounts for the approximately normal size of the extirpated navicular as a whole.

On *microscopic examination* the few available specimens have shown that the cartilage surrounding the modified ossification center presents no abnormalities peripheral to the region where endochondral ossification has been disturbed. On the other hand, in the ossification center itself there is evidence of aseptic necrosis involving not only the osseous tissue of the spongiosa but also the intertrabecular marrow. The extent of the pathologic changes to be observed in the center is

Figure 156

A, B, and *C,* Roentgenographs illustrating the course of the changes taking place in a tarsal navicular bone which was the site of Köhler's disease. When the patient, a boy, was about $5\frac{1}{2}$ years of age, he injured his right foot. It was caught in a wheel of a tricycle.

A, A picture taken about 1 month after the injury. Note that the ossification center of the bone is somewhat narrowed and irregular in contour and presents increased radiopacity. Examination revealed definite fullness along the medial border of the foot. There was localized tenderness in the region of the scaphoid, and forceful movement of the foot caused pain.

B, Roentgenograph depicting the status of the scaphoid in this case about $5\frac{1}{2}$ months later. The bone is now narrowed to a wafer-like thinness.

C, Roentgenograph illustrating the status of the scaphoid 13 months after the picture shown in *B.* Substantial reconstruction has taken place. The time interval between the picture shown in *A* and that shown in *C* is approximately $1\frac{1}{2}$ years.

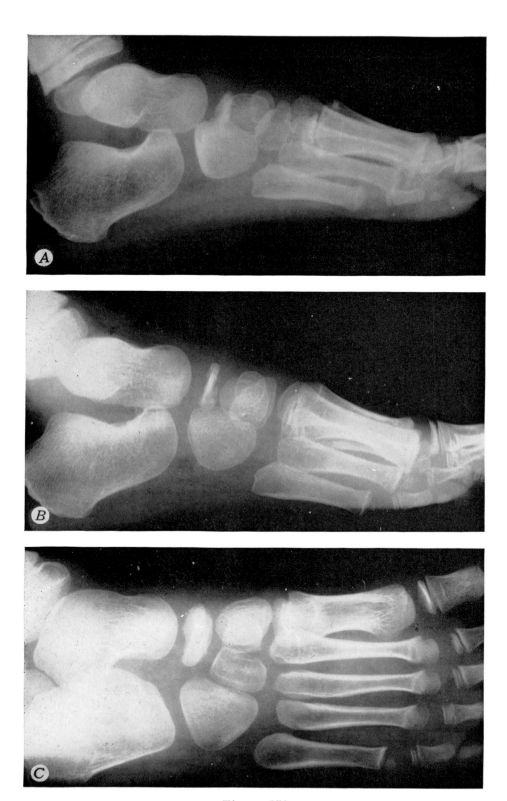

Figure 156

likely to be greatest shortly after the interference with its blood supply has set in, and also depends upon the degree of the resultant ischemia. Depending upon the extent of interruption of its blood supply, the center of ossification may manifest aseptic necrosis in part or throughout. In the necrotic areas, many of the spongy trabeculae become fragmented and undergo disintegration, which contributes to the calcific granular detritus present in the intertrabecular marrow spaces. After revascularization of the necrotic center, repair sets in, the necrotic osseous tissue being replaced through the process of "creeping substitution," and the detritus in the marrow spaces is resorbed. Eventually, as is well known, the ossification center is repaired and increases in size through the resumption of endochondral ossification at its periphery.

FREIBERG-KÖHLER DISEASE

This condition, frequently also denoted as Freiberg's infraction or as Köhler's second disease, is an affection of the head of a metatarsal bone. The bone involved is usually the second metatarsal. It was in relation to that bone that both Freiberg and Köhler discussed the condition. However, the bone affected is sometimes the third and in rare instances the fourth metatarsal. It is commonly held that the condition has its basis in aseptic necrosis involving the head of the affected metatarsal and that the necrosis weakens the resistance of the bone to functional trauma. In consequence, a part of the metatarsal head may undergo compressional collapse and become delimited as an osteochondral fracture fragment. Under these circumstances an osteoarthritis of the affected metatarsophalangeal joint may eventually ensue. However, if a compressional collapse does not occur, there is a strong likelihood that revascularization of the necrotic metatarsal head will lead to its substantial repair.

CLINICAL CONSIDERATIONS

Incidence.—Freiberg-Köhler disease is not a common disorder. In regard to its *sex incidence*, statistical evaluations indicate that females predominate among the subjects in the proportion of at least 3 or 4 to 1. In respect to *age* of the subjects, it is to be noted that a large proportion of them are between the ages of 12 and 18, though instances of the disorder are occasionally encountered in adults even up to about 40 or 50 years of age (see Cappellini and Teodorani). There can be no doubt that, in many of the cases which do not come under observation until after the end of the growth period, inquiry will reveal clinical indications that it has already been present for some years and that consequently its time of origin still fell within the growth period. Nevertheless, one should not exclude the possibility that the disorder sometimes has its inception during adult life.

Clinical Complaints and Findings.—It appears that, on the whole, the *foot involved* is as likely to be the right as the left (see Smillie). However, some reports in the literature state that the foot affected is more often the right, and others that it is more often the left. In any event, bilateral involvement is by no means uncommon.

The clinical manifestations may set in shortly after, or perhaps months after, the head of the metatarsal bone has undergone aseptic necrosis. Their onset may be abrupt or insidious, and they are not very disabling, at least at first. There is usually pain on walking, referred to the region of the head of the affected metatarsal, and with this there is often some limp. Pressure upon the head of the bone, especially from the plantar surface, elicits pain or tenderness, as does also abrupt release of this pressure. In time, a swelling tends to develop, particularly on the dorsum of the foot in the general region of the implicated metatarsophalangeal joint. This swelling is caused by broadening of the head of the metatarsal bone and often also by the formation of an adventitious bursa. The skin over the area of swelling is sometimes reddened. There is also likely to be limitation of movement (especially plantar flexion), apparently due in the main to muscle spasm or contracture. Occasionally the transverse arch of the affected foot is found flattened. There is frequently a callus on the plantar surface of the foot in the region of the affected metatarsal head. In cases showing deferred onset of clinical manifestations, the latter are frequently precipitated by some slight injury to the region in question, but are of the same general character as when they appear early.

ROENTGENOGRAPHIC AND PATHOLOGIC FINDINGS

Roentgenographic Findings.—The changes to be observed roentgenographically in Freiberg-Köhler disease reflect the progress of the destructive and reparative alterations in the affected metatarsal which occur in the wake of the aseptic necrosis of its head. In an early stage of the disease, although there may already be some local pain, the roentgenographic picture is not likely to reveal any abnormality referable to the necrosis present in the metatarsal head. In the course of time, however, the head of the metatarsal bone can be expected to present changes in radiopacity and also in contour. In particular, the head comes to show flattening and broadening. The increase in its radiopacity tends to parallel the degree of the deformation of the head. Although the head as a whole shows increased radiopacity, the latter is intermingled with some foci of radiolucency. At this stage, one can usually also note a linear transverse zone of radiolucency which is located not far from the articular surface of the head, and is generally interpreted as representing the line of the compression fracture by which an osteochondral fragment has become delimited from the rest of the head. These various changes may already be associated with slight thickening of the distal third or half of the shaft of the affected metatarsal, the thickening being due to periosteal new bone apposition.

In the further course of the disease, the flattening and broadening of the metatarsal head, the intermingling of radiopaque and radiolucent areas in it, and the thickening of the shaft all become accentuated. Subsequently the contrasts between the areas of relative radiopacity and radiolucency in the affected head tend to become more or less obliterated, so that the head of the affected metatarsal again casts a more uniform shadow. The head may be found to have fused prematurely with the shaft. It may also be noted that there has been some regression in the degree of thickening of the metatarsal shaft cortex. In those instances in which deformation of the metatarsal head persists, definite alterations may also become manifest in the contour of the base of the proximal phalanx. A pronounced osteoarthritis may ultimately supervene in the affected joint. Specifically, the joint capsule may come to show considerable thickening, and one or more calcific shadows may appear where it is attached to the bones. Exostoses may be present at the articular margins of the phalanx and metatarsal, and the articular ends of these bones may show sclerotic changes. The deformed and broadened metatarsal head sometimes projects backward and dorsally, and the bone may no longer seem to have a neck. The bursa which frequently develops over the dorsum of the head is likely to contain calcific bodies. (See Figs. 157 and 158.)

Pathologic Findings.—In connection with the pathologic findings, many satisfactory specimens in cases of Freiberg-Köhler disease have been available for detailed gross and microscopic examination (see Axhausen and also Konjetzny).

The importance of aseptic necrosis of the metatarsal head as the point of departure for the principal pathologic changes seems to be clearly established. The general course of the pathologic process, as deciphered from specimens representing various stages of the disease, may be briefly summarized as follows: In the earliest stage (while the roentgenographic findings are still negative) the head, as noted, is still normal in form but already shows, on microscopic examination, more or less complete necrosis of its osseous tissue and marrow. The articular cartilage usually reveals nothing remarkable, except that, where the head joins the shaft, the cartilage may already be found penetrated by vascular connective tissue growing into it from the neighboring periosteum. In a specimen in which the head is already flattened, the subchondral spongiosa in the region of flattening will be found collapsed and will show comminuted trabeculae and amorphous detritus.

The revascularization of the necrotic head does not take place solely through the invasion of vessels from the periosteum. It is also accomplished in part through the entrance of vessels from the metaphysis, which brings about a premature destruction of the epiphysial cartilage plate. When revascularization and regeneration are in an advanced stage, the picture presented is a highly varied one. Thus the necrotic trabeculae will display evidences of resorption and of partial replacement by new bone that is being apposed upon them. The intertrabecular marrow appears rather vascular and contains some osteoclasts, especially where trabeculae are undergoing active resorption. If a zone of subchondral detritus is still present, it is usually walled off by connective tissue. The substance of the head may contain one or

Figure 157

A, Roentgenograph illustrating the alterations in the head of the second metatarsal bone in a case of Freiberg-Köhler disease (or Freiberg's infraction). The head of the bone is flattened and broadened and is the site of a compression fracture. The patient was a girl 15 years of age. For about 2 months she had been aware of a swelling on the dorsum of the foot in the region of the affected metatarsal bone. In addition, she complained of local pain and tenderness and walked with a slight limp.

B, Roentgenograph depicting an infraction of the head of the second metatarsal bone in the case of a girl 11 years of age. She had pain in the second metatarsophalangeal joint for about 2 months before this roentgenograph was taken. Her difficulties set in when her foot was stepped on. Examination revealed enlargement of the second metatarsal head, associated with local tenderness. It is clear from this picture that a compression fracture had occurred, as indicated by the presence of the linear zone of radiolucency and the increased radiopacity of the delimited osteochondral fragment.

C, Roentgenograph of a foot from a case of Freiberg-Köhler disease involving the head of the third metatarsal bone. The medial side of the metatarsal head is somewhat flattened, and one can detect a very faint, short line of radiolucency extending obliquely in the lateral direction and marking the site of an infraction. In the central part of the proximal portion of the metatarsal head, there is a small, faint, roundish area of radiolucency representing the cyst shown in the photomicrograph made from a tissue section prepared from the resected head (see D). The patient was a young woman 21 years of age whose difficulties (pain and tenderness in the region of the third metatarsophalangeal joint) had been present for 7 years. She ascribed the onset of the difficulties to traumatization of the foot by pounding on it heavily in the course of running.

D, Photomicrograph ($\times$ 10) depicting the pathologico-anatomic changes presented by the resected metatarsal head in the case of Freiberg's disease illustrated in C. Note the delimited osteochondral fracture fragment still set in its bed. Its covering articular cartilage is thicker than the cartilage of the rest of the affected metatarsal head. When examined under higher magnification, the subchondral bone of the osteochondral fracture fragment was found to be nonviable. Just below the fragment, the metatarsal head shows a small cyst walled by fibrous tissue. At the extreme right of the picture, the head presents a small marginal exostosis.

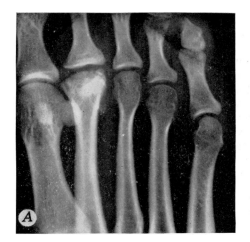

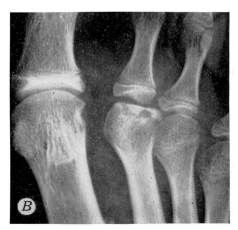

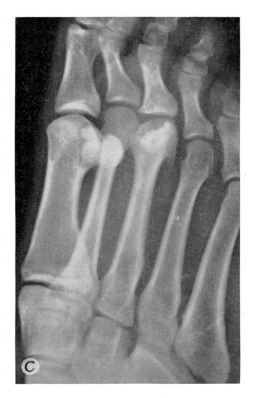

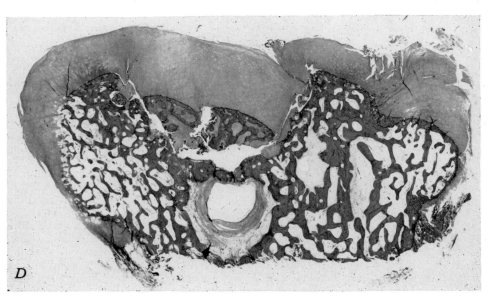

Figure 157

more foci of fibrous tissue which may have undergone central softening. Furthermore, the head is often found broadened by new bone formation in the region of the head-shaft junction. The shaft cortex, too, will be found thickened by periosteal new bone apposition.

Even after the head has undergone substantial reconstruction, its trabeculae and marrow are still likely to bear traces, here and there, of a preceding necrosis. Furthermore, the head usually remains flatter and broader than it would normally be. This happens especially in those instances in which a compression fracture has led to delimitation of a fairly large fragment of the articular bone end (articular cartilage and subchondral bone). Even if this osteochondritis dissecans-like body remains *in situ*, it is not readily revascularized. In any event, the deformity of the contour of the metatarsal head leads to damage of the articular cartilages of the joint in the course of function. The damage in turn favors the development of an osteoarthritis of the affected metatarsophalangeal joint.

In regard to the *pathogenesis* of Freiberg-Köhler disease, there can be no doubt of the importance of functional trauma. This idea is supported by the relatively high incidence of the disorder in females, in whom the wearing of high heels causes excessive functional trauma to the metatarsal heads. In this connection it has been pointed out that the second metatarsal is usually the longest and always the most fixed metatarsal, while the third metatarsal is less fixed and the fourth quite mobile (see Braddock). In tiptoeing, the metatarsals take the body weight vertically, the weight being transmitted through the talus, the three cuneiforms, and the first three metatarsals. As the most fixed and the longest metatarsal, the second one bears the heaviest share of the impact of body weight under these conditions.

Braddock conducted biomechanical experiments on fresh necropsy specimens of the second metatarsal bone and the adjacent proximal phalanx, including the capsule of the metatarsophalangeal joint. From these experiments he concluded that, in view of the fact that the second metatarsal is the longest and most fixed of the metatarsals, repeated functional trauma to the head of the bone may induce

Figure 158

A, Roentgenograph displaying the alterations in the head and neck of the second metatarsal bone in a case of so-called Freiberg-Köhler disease. Note the well-delimited radiopaque osteochondral fragment which, though separated from the rest of the metatarsal head, is still oriented to it. The focal area of radiolucency and the spur formation evident in the lateral half of the head and neck of the metatarsal in question reflect the presence of a subchondral cyst and marginal exostosis formation, both of which are shown in *C*. The patient, a man 31 years of age, was a truck driver's helper, and there was a history of painful swelling of 1 year's duration in the region of the head of the affected metatarsal bone.

B, Photograph (somewhat enlarged) showing the longitudinally sectioned head and part of the neck of the affected metatarsal bone, which had been removed surgically. The delimited osteochondral fragment measured 1.2 × 1 × 0.5 cm. The exostosis formation and the cyst with its fibrous wall are evident on the right side of the picture.

C, Photomicrograph (× 6) prepared from the sectioned specimen shown in *B*. The osteochondral fragment is covered on its outer surface by well-preserved articular cartilage. Some of the intertrabecular marrow spaces on its deep surface contain dark-staining material which, under higher magnification, can be seen to represent granular detritus. The cyst and marginal exostosis seen in *A* and *B* are apparent on the right of the picture.

D, Photomicrograph (× 25) showing in higher detail the histologic pattern of the lower central part of the osteochondral body shown in *C*. While, as noted, some of the intertrabecular marrow spaces contain dark-staining material (granular detritus), the detritus in most of the other spaces has been largely resorbed.

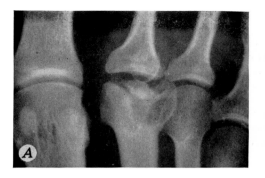

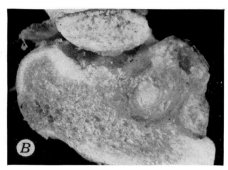

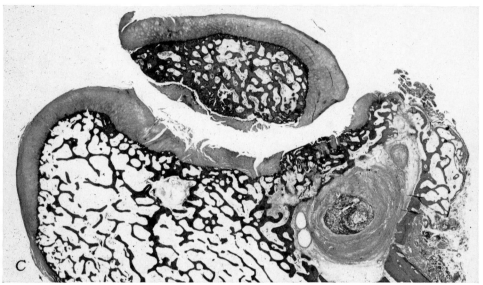

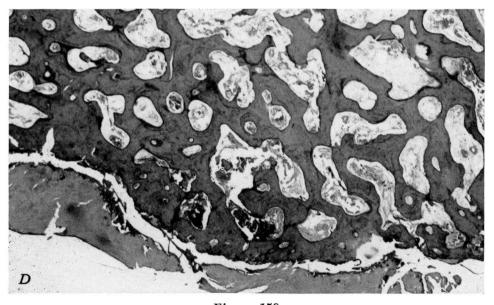

Figure 158

615

gross comminution and disruption of its articular cartilage. The disruption of the cartilage does not immediately result in alteration of the contour of the metatarsal head. However, it is held to be associated with ischemic necrosis of portions of the subchondral bone, after which the articular end of the metatarsal head is likely to become the site of a compression fracture and undergo collapse. This concept of the pathogenesis is somewhat at variance with the one proposed by Axhausen and also by Konjetzny—namely, that the osseous tissue and marrow of the head of the metatarsal first undergoes aseptic necrosis, and that all the other pathologic changes ensue from this.

KIENBÖCK'S DISEASE OF THE LUNATE (SEMILUNAR) BONE

The existence of pathologic changes involving the lunate bone had been recognized long before the introduction of roentgenography in clinical medicine. However, it was Kienböck who gave the first detailed description of the clinical and roentgenographic features of the disorder affecting the lunate bone which is now commonly denoted as Kienböck's disease and sometimes as lunatomalacia. It is held by some that the initial pathologic alteration is ischemic aseptic necrosis of the lunate (see Axhausen), and by others that it is a compression fracture of the bone, the aseptic necrosis ensuing upon the fracture (see Cordes, Ståhl, and also Rüttner). In any event, when an affected lunate bone is extirpated before substantial repair has taken place, anatomic study is likely to reveal not only evidence of aseptic necrosis of its osseous tissue and marrow but also the presence of one or more fracture lines. Thus the anatomic examination of such a specimen cannot be expected to settle the dilemma posed by the question of which came first. The problem arises because a lunate bone which has become necrotic is mechanically weakened, so that it may easily undergo compression fracture; on the other hand, a compression fracture of the lunate bone is likely to interrupt the local blood supply, so that necrosis of part or most of the bone will ensue.

An analogous affection sometimes involves one of the other carpal bones—most often the navicular. In the latter case it is denoted as Preiser's disease. The clinical complaints and findings in instances of Preiser's disease are more or less of the same kind as those given below in relation to Kienböck's disease.

CLINICAL CONSIDERATIONS

Incidence.—In regard to the incidence of Kienböck's disease it is to be noted first that the condition is not rare. The *age distribution* of the cases has a wide range, but the great majority of the patients are between 20 and 40 years of age. Furthermore, manual workers (especially laborers) predominate among the subjects, and this fact explains the difference in *sex incidence* (specifically the definite prevalence of Kienböck's disease among males). Also, the *right hand* (the usual working hand) is found implicated very much more often than the left. In an occasional instance, Kienböck's disease has been found to involve both the right and the left lunate.

Clinical Complaints and Findings.—The clinical history given by the patient often includes mention of local trauma. However, a clear-cut history of trauma is by no means the rule, and in the numerous cases in which it has been reported it has usually been mild. Indeed, the anatomic position of the lunate in itself renders it particularly susceptible to stresses applied to it, even when these do not include any violent force. Moreover, when a severe trauma to the wrist has induced a compression fracture of the lunate, the immediate appearance of a well-defined radiolucent fracture line detectable roentgenographically does not necessarily follow.

The clinical complaint which first directs attention to the condition is pain in the region of the affected bone. In the beginning, this is noted only when the wrist is used. Later, it becomes more and more persistent and annoying and is felt even when the wrist is at rest. The pain leads to increasing functional disability. There is usually also some swelling of the back of the wrist, most pronounced just over the affected bone, and indeed the wrist as a whole may be somewhat swollen. There will also be pronounced sensitiveness to direct pressure upon the lunate. The severity of these various clinical manifestations slowly regresses. However, they are still likely to reappear upon strenuous use of the wrist, even years after the onset of the condition. A common late finding is prominence of the lunate during palmar flexion of the wrist. As a sequela of the disorder, if the latter is not treated, it is not unusual to find also clinical disability resulting from a hypertrophic arthritis in the joints bordering upon the affected lunate.

ROENTGENOGRAPHIC FINDINGS

In those cases of Kienböck's disease in which the destructive changes in the lunate have already reached their full efflorescence, the *roentgenographic findings* are rather characteristic. In particular, the lunate shows flattening in the proximo-distal direction and irregularity of its proximal contour, and also presents a "fragmented" appearance. The latter is the expression of variations in radiodensity, small areas of increased radiopacity being intermingled with areas of increased radiolucency. In addition, there may even be some narrow tracts of increased radiolucency extending partly across the horizontal axis of the bone and/or in the proximodistal direction.

There is still a good deal of uncertainty about the temporal sequence of the changes culminating in this roentgenographic picture of a lunate presenting Kienböck's disease in florid form. It is often stated that, for a short time after the onset of the clinical complaints, the shadow cast by the affected lunate may still be normal in respect to its contour. Ståhl, however, reports that, even early in the course of the evolution of the changes, the lunate is somewhat flattened, and a compression fracture may be detected. The site of the fracture will be apparent roentgenographically as a "density line" (that is, a narrow zone of increased radiopacity). His experience suggested further that, since the fractured lunate is not immobilized, shearing action between the fracture fragments leads (in about a month) to replacement of the "density line" by a "rarefaction line." Beyond the "rarefaction line," each of the fracture fragments comes to present (during the next few months) foci of increased radiopacity and subsequently also some secondary fracture lines, which extend mainly in the proximodistal axis of the bone. Within a year or so after the lunate has undergone a compression fracture, some evidences of osteoarthritis may become manifest roentgenographically, especially on the volar aspect of the radiocarpal joint. This may occur even in some cases which have been treated adequately.

PATHOLOGIC FINDINGS

As a preface to discussion of the pathology of Kienböck's disease, some *anatomic and biomechanical facts* relating to the lunate and its setting in the wrist seem desirable. The major part of the bone is covered by articular cartilage, and small areas of its dorsal and volar surfaces (its nonarticular surfaces) are covered by periosteum. It receives its blood supply by way of small vessels which enter the bone on its dorsal and/or palmar aspect. Though the bone is sometimes supplied by a single dorsal or a single palmar vessel, much more often than not it is supplied by vessels which enter it both on its dorsal and its palmar aspects. Under these circumstances, branches of the dorsal and palmar vessels usually anastomose within the bone, and an anastomotic network may be present subchondrally on both the proximal and distal aspects of the bone (see Lee). There are also indications that the blood supply to the lunate is less ample than that received by the other wrist bones, and the lunate is consequently particularly vulnerable to interruption of its blood supply.

The bone articulates with the radius above, the triquetrum medially, the scaphoid laterally, the capitate below, and frequently the hamate by a narrow facet between the triquetrum and capitate. Furthermore, the lunate is hemmed in, and also set like a keystone in the arch formed by the proximal carpals. As a result, it has to withstand forces of various orders of magnitude. Indeed, it is subjected to greater pressure than any of the other carpal bones, irrespective of the position in which the hand may be held. The lines of force emanating from the hand converge to meet in the lunate, and its shape is such that all forces acting upon the bone impinge upon it at right angles to its articular surfaces (see Cordes). When the hand is clenched tightly, there is a slight ulnar deviation which will press the lunate from both sides, as well as between the capitate and the radius. This is the usual working position of the hand during heavy labor, and this position accentuates the special susceptibility of the lunate to the damaging effects of abnormal mechanical forces which may be directed against it. Another anatomic feature often mentioned as possibly contributing to the special susceptibility of the lunate to Kienböck's disease is the so-called "minus variant" in the length of the ulna compared with that of the radius, the ulna being shorter than the radius. It appears that under

Figure 159

A, Roentgenograph illustrating the changes characteristic of Kienböck's disease of the carpal lunate bone. Note that the lunate is flattened in the proximodistal direction, and that it presents a narrow tract of increased radiolucency extending horizontally across the bone, and also a short one extending in the longitudinal direction. The patient was a man who was 21 years of age when he was admitted to the hospital and this roentgenograph was taken. The history was that 4 years earlier he fell on his outstretched right hand, and the wrist then became painful. The pain subsided when the wrist was kept in a splint for a few weeks, and after that there was little difficulty with the wrist for about 3 years. Then a second traumatic incident took place, and there was a recurrence of pain in the wrist, with limitation of function.

B, Photomicrograph ($\times$ 7) prepared from a tissue section made from the excised lunate in this case. The pathologic changes are most prominent in the central and proximal portion of the affected lunate. There is a fracture line extending horizontally across the bone, and a short one extending longitudinally which involves the articular cartilage on the proximal surface of the lunate. These fracture lines correspond to those apparent in the roentgenograph.

C, Photomicrograph ($\times$ 35) showing in greater detail the histologic pattern presented by a field in the vicinity of the horizontal fracture line shown in B. In the lower right part of the picture, the intertrabecular marrow space is filled with granular detritus.

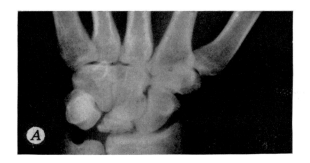

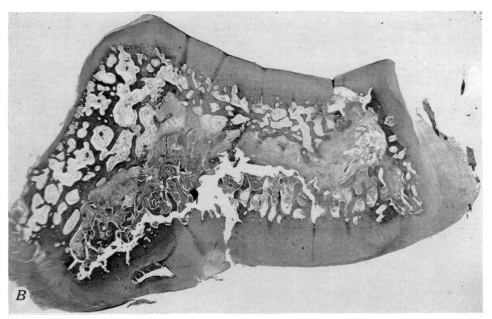

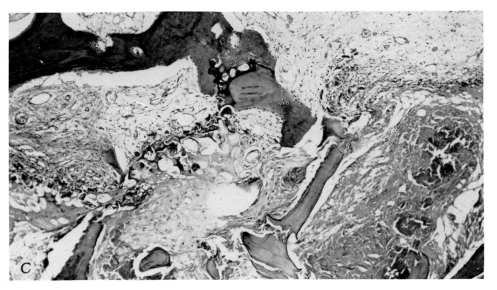

Figure 159

such circumstances a traumatic episode is more likely to cause excessive pressure contact between the lunate and the radius (see Persson).

The *pathologic changes* to be observed in an affected lunate which has been extirpated and subjected to anatomic examination are largely determined by: the extent of the original injury to the bone; additional damaging effects on the bone from continued functional use of the hand; and the length of time during which the condition was present without being appropriately treated. It is now widely accepted that the point of departure for the pathologic changes is *not* aseptic necrosis of the lunate, but a compression fracture of the bone. It also seems clear that the various other pathologic changes appearing in the wake of the original fracture represent manifestations of delayed or disturbed healing of the fracture, due to the impact of continued functional trauma directed against the already damaged, weakened, and more or less necrotic bone.

In the light of the facts just mentioned, a composite description of the pathologic changes cannot be expected to apply strictly to an individual affected lunate. In any event, the primary fracture line is usually in the subchondral spongiosa of the proximal portion of the lunate and is an incomplete fracture, not implicating at first the neighboring articular cartilage. In consequence of the fracture, a variety of additional changes emerge. These involve the spongiosa abutting upon the fracture line, parts of the spongiosa remote from the fracture line, and also the articular cartilages on the proximal and distal aspects of the bone. (See Fig. 159.)

In the immediate vicinity of the fracture line, when the condition is present in florid form, the spongy trabeculae will be found sparse, and many of those still present will show evidences of osteoclastic resorption, disintegration, and splintering. The widened intertrabecular marrow spaces in the general region of the fracture line are likely to reveal a good deal of scar tissue and granular detritus, and also some small fibrous-walled cysts containing detritus and fragments of disintegrating spongy bone. Some of the trabeculae of spongy bone remote from the fracture line may be definitely thickened, the thickening being due to the deposition of new bone, and the spongiosa so modified may appear somewhat sclerotic. Further progress of the pathologic changes is also associated with the development of "secondary" fracture lines, some of which may involve the articular cartilages and parts of the spongiosa which had not been implicated in the primary fracture. The presence of amorphous granular detritus, disintegration and fragmentation of the spongy trabeculae, and the secondary microfractures crossing through the affected lunate are all evidences of the aseptic necrosis which had ensued when the traumatic incident and the resultant primary compression fracture brought about an interruption of the blood supply to the lunate.

The scarring reaction around the amorphous detritus and the reconstruction of the necrotic osseous tissue by osteoclastic resorption and concomitant new bone deposition are manifestations of repair and regeneration, and indicate that the affected bone is being revascularized. When the regeneration has progressed further, one may no longer see detritic foci, and their former sites may be marked merely by large fibrous scars whose centers have undergone cystic softening. The volar-dorsal diameter of the bone will be found increased through periosteal new bone apposition. Even after substantial reconstruction has taken place, the trabeculae may still contain central cores of necrotic osseous tissue. At a late stage in some cases, it will also be found that the articular cartilages are fibrillized and being encroached upon by marrow vessels which are penetrating the bony end plate. Such changes in the articular cartilages lay the groundwork for the development of an osteoarthritis at the articular surfaces of the affected lunate. However, the initiation of early and appropriate treatment of Kienböck's disease can go far to circumvent this baleful sequela.

JUVENILE KYPHOSIS OF SCHEUERMANN

In 1921, under the title of *"kyphosis dorsalis juvenilis,"* Scheuermann focused attention upon a type of kyphosis involving the lower thoracic region and developing in young persons. He held that it had its basis (or point of departure) in an abnormality implicating the ringlike epiphyses (the secondary ossification centers) of the affected vertebral bodies.* Accordingly, he maintained that the resultant "round back" shown by the subjects did not have the same basis as other kyphoses, and in particular should be distinguished from the dorsal kyphosis due to muscular weakness. Names other than Scheuermann's disease which have been used to designate the condition are "vertebral epiphysitis," "osteochondrosis juvenilis dorsi," "osteochondritis deformans juvenilis dorsi," and "preadolescent and adolescent kyphosis." Analogous lesions involving vertebral bodies have now also been noted occasionally in the lumbar region of the vertebral column and sometimes even in the cervical region. Since the roentgenographic and pathologic findings relating to the condition when it affects the lumbar or the cervical region of the column are essentially similar to those in the thoracic region, the term "Scheuermann's disease" may reasonably be applied also to the affection as manifested in the former two sites.

On the assumption that the primary site of the disorder was the ringlike epiphyses of the affected vertebral bodies, it was maintained at first that the condition represented the vertebral counterpart of the disorder (aseptic necrosis) which involves the capital femoral epiphysis—that is, Legg-Calvé-Perthes disease. However, it is now clear that aseptic necrosis of the ringlike epiphyses does not play the primary role in the causation of the condition. On the other hand, it has been shown that any implication of these epiphyses follows upon prolapse of intervertebral disk tissue into the adjacent vertebral body or bodies. Furthermore, there is increasing evidence that the prolapse of the disk tissue results from the presence of structurally weak areas or actual defects in the cartilage plate covering the upper and/or lower surface of the affected vertebral body or bodies (see Schmorl and also Beadle).

CLINICAL CONSIDERATIONS

Incidence.—In regard to its *general incidence* it is to be noted that so-called juvenile kyphosis of Scheuermann is not an uncommon condition. Indeed, it was found to be present roentgenographically in about 4 to 5 per cent of 581,000 Danish recruits of conscription age (about 20 years) examined during the period of 1922 to 1939 (see Wassmann). Correspondingly it was found in 6.1 per cent of 1,000 United States naval recruits between the ages of 17 and 23 (see Dameron and Gulledge).

In respect to *age incidence* it is to be noted that juvenile kyphosis is rarely observed in persons under 10 years of age. A large proportion of the subjects are between 13 and 17 years of age when the condition is first recognized. It comes to medical attention either because of clinical manifestations or (when such manifes-

* Wedging *collapse* of the *ossification center* of a *vertebral body* of a young child was long held to be due to aseptic necrosis of the center, and was denoted as *Calvé's disease.* In recent years it has become increasingly clear that wedging collapse of a vertebral body (vertebra plana) in a child usually results from an eosinophilic granuloma (p. 877). Indeed, one may doubt whether Calvé's disease in the original sense actually exists. *Kümmel's disease* was long regarded as the adult counterpart of Calvé's disease. It is now established that in supposed cases of Kümmel's disease the basis for the collapse of the vertebral body is not a primary aseptic necrosis but rather a linear fracture of the body. This is not demonstrable in roentgenographs taken soon after the original traumatic incident. However, after a second trauma, often minor, the vertebral body collapses.

tations are absent) as an incidental finding in the course of roentgenographic examination of the vertebral column. Some of the postadolescent or young adult subjects in whom Scheuermann's disease is discovered fortuitously give a history of having previously suffered from persistent backache.

In regard to *sex incidence* it appears that, other factors such as age and occupation being equal, the disorder is as likely to develop in females as in males. That is, there seems to be *no striking inherent* sex difference in its incidence (see Sørensen). Nevertheless, most of the recorded data mention predominance of males among the subjects (see Hølund, and also Williams and Pugh). This predominance may well be related to the fact that a large proportion of the males in question had been engaged in particularly strenuous sports or heavy physical labor during their preadolescence or adolescence. Indeed, it is stressed in some articles that the incidence of Scheuermann's disease is particularly high in rural areas in which the preadolescent or adolescent children of farmers help with the heavy farm chores (see Wassmann). This finding also makes understandable the belief which has been expressed that juvenile kyphosis may have a *genetic basis*, since several members of one family may show the disorder. However, it is much more probable that in such families one is dealing not with a hereditary factor but merely with similar external conditions, notably in respect to the effects exerted on the vertebral column by heavy physical labor undertaken years before the subjects have attained physical maturity. A contrary opinion is expressed by Sørensen, who minimizes the importance of heavy physical farm labor done by youthful subjects in the causation of juvenile kyphosis.

Clinical Complaints and Findings.—Ordinarily the *site of involvement* of the vertebral column in juvenile kyphosis is the thoracic part of the column and particularly the lower thoracic part. In a small percentage of any large series of cases, the site of the involvement may be the thoracolumbar or the lumbar region alone, and occasionally the site may even be the cervical region of the column (see Butler, Fried, and also Edgren and Vainio). Juvenile kyphosis affecting the thoracic part of the column (its typical site) usually involves several vertebral bodies—most often two to four—but may involve only one or, on the other hand, as many as six or seven. When the condition is present in the lumbar part of the column, it may again involve only one or several of the regional vertebral bodies. Furthermore, when one or more lumbar vertebrae are affected, it is not unusual to find one or more thoracic vertebrae also implicated. In those rare instances in which it is the cervical part of the column that is affected, the regional involvement may again be multiple.

In a youthful subject (characteristically 14 to 19 years of age) in whom the condition has developed recently or within a year or so, it may still be asymptomatic. Somewhat more often, however, it is *pain* that calls attention to its presence. When there is pain, the latter is usually limited to the affected part of the vertebral column, which, as noted, is ordinarily the thoracic area. However, when the lesion is in the lumbar part of the column, the pain is usually referred to the lumbosacral area. Even in cases in which the lesion is in the lumbar part of the column, the pain rarely if ever radiates down the thighs, as it would do if there were compression of the sciatic nerve.

The pain is generally of an aching character. It is usually aggravated by physical exertion, by working in a stooping position, and sometimes even by standing or sitting for long periods of time. It is also likely that the affected area of the vertebral column will be somewhat tender to palpation.

In relation to the subjects who are somewhat older, it is only in occasional instances that there are complaints of pain in the back at the time roentgenographic examination of the vertebral column discloses the presence of the condition. Among the rest of these older subjects there are some who will recall having had persistent backache at some time during their adolescence. Actually, then, in most of the cases of Scheuermann's disease first detected during the third decade of life, one does not elicit a history of previous backache.

When the site of involvement is the lower thoracic part of the vertebral column, a mild degree of *kyphotic deformity* (not infrequently associated with some scoliosis) is a common finding. Even if some degree of scoliosis is present, this is not accompanied by torsion of the column. Furthermore, the thoracic kyphotic curvature is a gentle one, ordinarily representing only an exaggeration of the curve which is normal for the thoracic area. When the thoracic kyphosis becomes fixed, as it usually does, the subject is merely round-shouldered, and the presence of an angulation (gibbus formation) is evidence against a diagnosis of Scheuermann's disease. On the other hand, *some flattening of the normal lumbar lordosis* is the characteristic change in contour of the column when the site of involvement is the lumbar region.

ROENTGENOGRAPHIC AND PATHOLOGIC FINDINGS

The development and anatomic structure of the vertebrae (and particularly of the vertebral bodies) has been described and illustrated in Chapter 1 (p. 20 and Figures 8 and 9). The information conveyed there in regard to the normal conditions supplies a background for interpretation of the roentgenographic and pathologico-anatomic findings in cases of adolescent kyphosis. It is logical, in discussing these aspects of so-called Scheuermann's disease, that we should give primary consideration to the abnormalities observed in the vertebral column of youthful subjects (preadolescents, adolescents, or those just past adolescence). When such subjects reach middle age or old age, they may present roentgenographic and anatomic residua and sequelae of the condition as it appeared during their youth.

Roentgenographic Findings.—Roentgenographic examination of a preadolescent subject in whom it is the *lower thoracic* part of the column that is affected may reveal only a mild accentuation of the curve which is normal for the thoracic area. In particular, at this time the roentgenograph taken in the lateral projection is likely to show merely that some of the thoracic vertebral bodies are slightly narrowed anteriorly. Defects in the cartilage plates which cover the proximal and distal surfaces of the vertebral bodies may have permitted small herniations of intervertebral disk tissue into a given body. However, at this stage in the evolution of the changes, the herniated disk tissue has usually not as yet modified or altered the roentgenographic appearance of the apophysial ossification centers. These, of course, are growth zones developing in the cartilaginous marginal ridge which extends around the upper and lower border of each growing vertebral body.

In a preadolescent in whom the condition has been present for several years and has progressed, or in an adolescent in whom it is already present in florid form, it is likely that the dorsal kyphosis will be quite pronounced. Furthermore, a number of the vertebral bodies will now show definite narrowing anteriorly. Also, the outlines of the upper and/or lower surfaces of some of these thoracic vertebral bodies will have lost their normal smoothness. Those so affected present smaller or larger, single or multiple indentations or defects on their upper and/or lower surfaces, representing sites where intervertebral disk tissue has prolapsed into the bodies after penetrating their covering cartilage plates. The prolapse of large foci of intervertebral disk tissue may also be observed anteriorly, and in some places the extruded disk tissue may even extend beneath the apophysial centers of ossification and come to appear submarginally beneath the anterior longitudinal ligament. Under such circumstances a portion of the proximal and/or distal ringlike apophysial centers of ossification of the vertebral body may have become separated from the body proper by disk tissue, so that the subsequent development of the apophysis is disordered. Also, disk tissue which has protruded between the anterior surface of the vertebral body and the longitudinal ligament may produce a pressure defect on the anterior surface of that vertebral body. In consequence of the pathologic changes which have involved the intervertebral disks and the adjacent vertebral bodies, including the apophysial ossification centers, the intervertebral disk spaces are often found substantially narrowed. (See Fig. 160.)

Much of what has been said in regard to the roentgenographic findings relating to involvement of the lower thoracic region of the vertebral column applies also to the less common but by no means infrequent involvement of the lumbar portion of the column. If it is the thoracolumbar region that is affected, there may be a slight degree of kyphotic curvature at the proximal end of the implicated area. However, when the condition is localized to the lumbar region, that part of the back appears flat instead of showing the normal lordotic curve. This flattening is the result of narrowing of the intervertebral disk spaces. In the lumbar region the defects produced in the vertebral body or bodies by the protrusion of the intervertebral disk tissue into them tend to be large. They are usually located anteriorly, extend submarginally, and often separate part of the ringlike apophysial ossification center from the main part of the vertebral body (see Butler). Bradford and Garcia described the case of a 16 year old boy affected with Scheuermann's disease and kyphosis in the thoracic region of the column. The subject developed spastic paraplegia secondary to a herniated disk which caused pressure on the spinal cord in the region of the apex of the kyphosis.

Pathogenesis and Pathologic Findings.—The pathologic changes in the part of

Figure 160

A, Roentgenograph illustrating, in lateral projection, five thoracic vertebral bodies from a case of juvenile kyphosis. The patient, a boy, was 13 years of age when this picture was taken. The intervertebral disk space between the two uppermost vertebral bodies is narrowed. The lower surface of the upper body shows alterations in its contour, reflecting depressions caused by disk tissue which has deformed the cartilage plate and apparently penetrated into the vertebral body to a slight degree. The third vertebral body from the top is somewhat narrowed anteriorly, and its appearance is also greatly modified otherwise. Specifically, disk tissue from the intervertebral disks above and below that body has apparently penetrated into the latter and extended below the anterior longitudinal ligament to deform the anterior surface of the body. The disk tissue has also distorted the position of the small island of ossification representing part of the ringlike secondary ossification center of the body. The other vertebral bodies are also more or less modified.

B, Roentgenograph showing, in lateral projection, four thoracic vertebral bodies from the same case as A, the present picture having been taken 1 year later. The uppermost of these four vertebral bodies corresponds to the third, or middle, one shown in A. The intervertebral disk between the second and third bodies shown in this roentgenograph reveals herniation of the disk into the adjacent vertebral bodies.

C, Roentgenograph showing a number of the lower thoracic vertebrae in a case of Scheuermann's disease. The patient was a boy 19 years of age who participated in various forms of athletics, including weight-lifting. The disk space between the eighth and ninth vertebral bodies is greatly narrowed, and there is clear-cut evidence of herniation of the disk into the eighth vertebral body on the left of the picture.

D, Roentgenograph showing, in lateral projection, part of the lower thoracic portion of the vertebral column in this case. This picture was taken 2 years after the picture shown in C. The eighth vertebral body is narrowed anteriorly, and there are indications that the intervertebral disk tissue has also protruded under the anterior ligament and has deformed the anterior contour of that vertebral body.

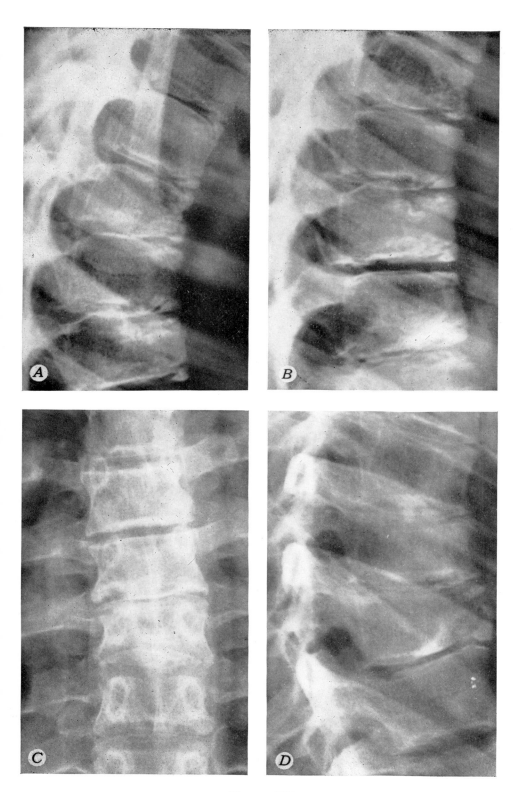

Figure 160

the vertebral column affected in a case of so-called Scheuermann's disease consist of alterations involving: (1) intervertebral disks, (2) the cartilaginous growth plates covering the proximal and distal surfaces of the vertebral bodies abutting on the altered intervertebral disks, and (3) the regional vertebral bodies themselves (not infrequently including their apophysial ossification centers).

As we know from the basic pathologico-anatomic studies carried out by Schmorl, the point of departure for the pathologic changes is in the intervertebral disks of the affected part of the column. Commonly, the first change consists of some degree of biconcave bulging of one or more of the disks. This bulging, which is mainly in the direction of the contiguous bodies, deforms their contour somewhat, exerts pressure against the cartilage plates covering the bodies which abut on the altered disk, and causes thinning of the plates. The pressure, in turn, interferes more or less with the endochondral bone formation which normally takes place on the deep surface (the growth surface) of the plate. This aberration may result in the appearance of focal areas of degeneration in the affected plates, and consequent lowering of resistance of the areas in question to the turgor of the expanded intervertebral disk. It is the presence of these areas of mechanical weakness, permitting the formation of small gaps in the cartilage plates, that is the basis for herniation of

Figure 161

A, Photomicrograph (× 4) showing parts of two thoracic vertebrae and the corresponding portion of the intervertebral disk from the case of a boy who died when he was 17 years of age and came to autopsy. The picture illustrates the earliest pathologic change of juvenile kyphosis of Scheuermann. The anterior longitudinal ligament is at the extreme left. The expansion of the anterior portion of the disk has deformed the contour of the corresponding parts of the cartilage plates covering the vertebral bodies and has resulted in thinning of the plates, which is more clearly apparent in relation to the upper one. Examination of the latter area under higher magnification would also show that there has been some interference with endochondral bone formation on the growth surfaces of the thinned and depressed portion of the cartilage plate.

B, Photomicrograph (× 4) showing parts of two thoracic vertebrae and the corresponding portion of the intervertebral disk in the case of a girl who died when she was 18 years of age and came to autopsy. The anterior portion of the disk is expanded, and in the region of the altered disk the cartilage plates of the contiguous vertebral bodies have been penetrated by the nucleus pulposus, and small amounts of disk tissue have prolapsed into the vertebral body above and below the disk. This anatomic finding was an incidental one, but it is clearly indicative of the presence of juvenile kyphosis.

C, D, E, and F, Photomicrographs prepared from tissue sections illustrating different areas of the lower thoracic column in the case of a girl 16 years of age presenting juvenile kyphosis. C shows expansion of the anterior part of an intervertebral disk and penetration of the upper contiguous cartilage plate by disk tissue which has herniated into the vertebral body. D illustrates the general histologic pattern presented by an intervertebral disk and the two abutting vertebral bodies in another part of the column. On the right side of the picture, it is clearly evident that disk tissue has deformed, penetrated, and partially destroyed the cartilage plate of the upper vertebral body. E depicts even more advanced changes characterizing the pathologic anatomy of juvenile kyphosis. In this picture it can be seen that the disk has herniated, mainly into the lower vertebral body. There has been extensive destruction of the cartilage plate of that body, and a large amount of disk tissue has penetrated into it and advanced to the anterior ligament. F reveals the changes of juvenile kyphosis in still another site and in even more advanced form than that shown in E. There has been massive penetration of the disk tissue into the upper vertebral body, and much of the latter's cartilage plate has been destroyed. Anteriorly, the disk has penetrated into the lower vertebral body and has extended across the body beneath the deep surface of its cartilage plate.

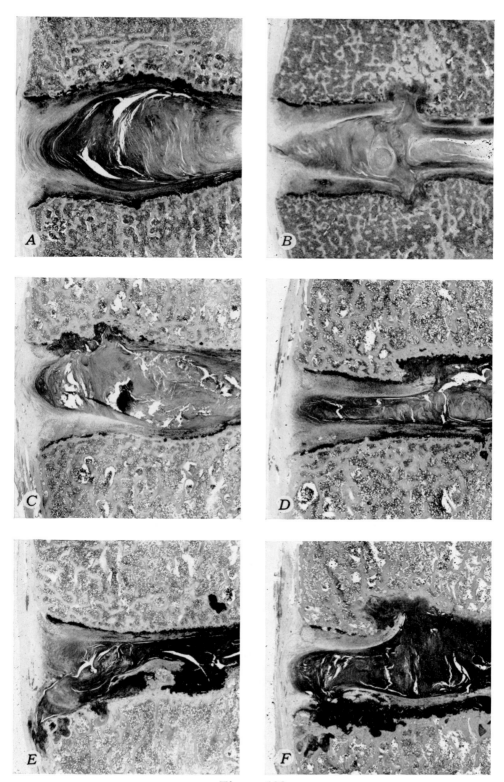

Figure 161

intervertebral disk tissue into the vertebral bodies.   This is particularly likely to occur under the influence of special strain from arduous labor or from vigorous activity in sports during the second decade of life.

The prolapsed disk tissue usually consists of parts of both the nucleus pulposus and the annulus fibrosus.   When a large amount of the disk tissue has prolapsed, it is not unusual to find that a part of the cartilage plate in the vicinity of the prolapse has also been dislodged into the body.   In general, microscopic examination may reveal: (1) that a bulbous mass of disk tissue has protruded into one or both contiguous vertebral bodies; (2) that the herniated disk tissue extends in a narrow zone for a considerable distance beneath one or another cartilage plate; and/or (3) that the herniation of the disk tissue into the body often occurs near the apophysial ossification center, the disk tissue inserting itself beneath the apophysis, isolating the latter from the vertebral body proper, and perhaps even continuing under the anterior longitudinal ligament.   In the course of time, the prolapsed disk tissue is walled off by a thin layer of osseous tissue, and a bulbous mass of extruded tissue (Schmorl's node) hence comes to stand out as an area of radiolucency in the roentgenographic picture of the affected body.   (See Fig. 161.)

In consequence of these various changes, the intervertebral disk loses some of its mass, along with some of its resiliency.   In time, ingrowth of connective tissue may render the disk extensively fibrotic.   These various alterations of the disk tissue tend to induce narrowing of the disk space.   The narrowing is usually more prominent anteriorly than posteriorly, and results in increasing pressure upon the anterior portions of the contiguous vertebral bodies.   This pressure impedes the longitudinal growth of the anterior portions of these bodies, thus contributing to their narrowing in this region.

REFERENCES

Axhausen, G.:   Der Krankheitsvorgang bei der Köhler'schen Krankheit der Metatarsalköpfchen und bei der Perthes'schen Krankheit des Hüftkopfes, Zentralbl. Chir., *50*, 553, 1923.
————:   Nicht Malacie, sondern Nekrose des Os lunatum carpi! Arch. klin. Chir., *129*, 26, 1924.
————:   Über den Abgrenzungsvorgang am epiphysären Knochen (Osteochondritis dissecans König), Virchows Arch. path. Anat., *252*, 458, 1924.
————:   Die aseptische Knochennecrose und ihre Bedeutung für die Knochen- und Gelenkchirurgie, Acta chir. scandinav., *60*, 369, 1926.
Barth, A.:   Zur pathologischen Anatomie der Gelenkmäuse, Zentralbl. Chir., *22*, 977, 1895.
Beadle, O. A.:   *The Intervertebral Discs.   Observations on their Normal and Morbid Anatomy in Relation to Certain Spinal Deformities,* Medical Research Council, Special Report Series, No. 161, London, His Majesty's Stationery Office, 1931.
Bernstein, M. A.:   Osteochondritis Dissecans, J. Bone & Joint Surg., *7*, 319, 1925.
Billing, L., and Severin, E.:   Slipping Epiphysis of the Hip, Acta radiol., Suppl. 174, 1959.
Brackett, E. G., and Hall, C. L.:   Osteochondritis Dissecans, Am. J. Orthop. Surg., *15*, 79, 1917.
Braddock, G. T. F.:   Experimental Epiphysial Injury and Freiberg's Disease, J. Bone & Joint Surg., *41-B*, 154, 1959.
Bradford, D. S., and Garcia, A.:   Neurological Complications in Scheuermann's Disease, J. Bone & Joint Surg., *51-A*, 567, 1969.
Burrows, H. J.:   Coxa Plana, with Special Reference to its Pathology and Kinship, Brit. J. Surg., *29*, 23, 1941.
————:   Slipped Upper Femoral Epiphysis, J. Bone & Joint Surg., *39-B*, 641, 1957.
————:   Osteochondritis Juvenilis, J. Bone & Joint Surg., *41-B*, 455, 1959.
Butler, R. W.:   The Nature and Significance of Vertebral Osteochondritis, Proc. Roy. Soc. Med., *48*, 895, 1955.
Caffey, J., Madell, S. H., Royer, C., and Morales, P.:   Ossification of the Distal Femoral Epiphysis, J. Bone & Joint Surg., *40-A*, 647, 1958.
Calvé, J.:   Sur une forme particulière de pseudo-coxalgie greffée sur des déformations caractéristiques de l'extrémité supérieure du fémur, Rev. chir., *42*, 54, 1910.

CAPPELLINI, O., and TEODORANI, G.: Considerazioni sulla malattia metatarsale di Köhler, Ann. radiol. diag., *29*, 81, 1956.

CORDES, E.: Über die Entstehung der subchondralen Osteonekrosen. A. Die Lunatumnekrose, Bruns' Beitr. klin. Chir., *149*, 28, 1930.

CRUESS, R. L.: The Pathology of Acute Necrosis of Cartilage in Slipping of the Capital Femoral Epiphysis, J. Bone & Joint Surg., *45-A*, 1013, 1963.

DAMERON, T. B., JR., and GULLEDGE, W. H.: Adolescent Kyphosis, U. S. Armed Forces M. J., *4*, 871, 1953.

DURBIN, F. C.: Treatment of Slipped Upper Femoral Epiphysis, J. Bone & Joint Surg., *42-B*, 289, 1960.

EDGREN, W., and VAINIO, S.: Osteochondrosis Juvenilis Lumbalis, Acta chir. scandinav., Suppl. 227, 1957.

EHRENBORG, G.: The Osgood-Schlatter Lesion, Acta chir. scandinav., *124*, 89, 1962.

EHRENBORG, G., and ENGFELDT, B.: Histologic Changes in the Osgood-Schlatter Lesion, Acta chir. scandinav., *121*, 328, 1961.

————: The Insertion of the Ligamentum Patellae on the Tibial Tuberosity, Acta chir. scandinav., *121*, 491, 1961.

EHRENBORG, G., and LAGERGREN, C.: Roentgenologic Changes in the Osgood-Schlatter Lesion, Acta chir. scandinav., *121*, 315, 1961.

FAIRBANK, H. A. T.: Osteo-chondritis Dissecans, Brit. J. Surg., *21*, 67, 1933–34.

FERGUSON, A. B., and HOWORTH, M. B.: Slipping of the Upper Femoral Epiphysis, J.A.M.A., *97*, 1867, 1931.

————: Coxa Plana and Related Conditions at the Hip, J. Bone & Joint Surg., *16*, 781, 1934.

FERGUSON, A. B., JR.: Synovitis of the Hip and Legg-Perthes Disease, Clinical Orthopaedics, *4*, 180, 1954.

FERGUSON, A. B., JR., and GINGRICH, R. M.: The Normal and the Abnormal Calcaneal Apophysis and Tarsal Navicular, Clinical Orthopaedics, *10*, 87, 1957.

FISHER, A. G. T.: A Study of Loose Bodies Composed of Cartilage or of Cartilage and Bone Occurring in Joints, Brit. J. Surg., *8*, 493, 1920–21.

FREEHAFER, A. A.: Osteochondritis Dissecans Following Legg-Calvé-Perthes Disease, J. Bone & Joint Surg., *42-A*, 777, 1960.

FREIBERG, A. H.: Infraction of the Second Metatarsal Bone. A Typical Injury, Surg. Gynec. & Obst., *19*, 191, 1914.

————: Osteochondritis Dissecans, J. Bone & Joint Surg., *5*, 3, 1923.

————: The So-called Infraction of the Second Metatarsal Bone, J. Bone & Joint Surg., *8*, 257, 1926.

FREIBERG, A. H., and WOOLLEY, P. G.: Osteochondritis Dissecans: Concerning Its Nature and Relation to Formation of Joint Mice, Am. J. Orthop. Surg., *8*, 477, 1910.

FREUND, E.: Zur Deutung des Röntgenbildes der Perthesschen Krankheit, Fortschr. Geb. Röntgenstrahlen, *42*, 435, 1930.

FRIED, K.: Cervical Juvenile Osteochondrosis (Scheuermann's Disease), Fortschr. Geb. Röntgenstrahlen, *105*, 69, 1966.

GALL, E. A., and BENNETT, G. A.: Osteochondritis Deformans of the Hip (Legg-Perthes Disease) and Renal Osteitis Fibrosa Cystica, Arch. Path., *33*, 866, 1942.

GOFF, C. W.: *Legg-Calvé-Perthes Syndrome*, Springfield, Charles C Thomas, 1954.

GOLDENBERG, R. R.: Traumatic Dislocation of the Hip Followed by Perthes' Disease, J. Bone & Joint Surg., *20*, 770, 1938.

GOLDENBERG, R. R., and COHEN, P.: Bilateral Bicondylar Osteochondritis Dissecans of the Knee, Bull. Hosp. Joint Dis., *26*, 84, 1965.

GOLDING, J. S. R., MACIVER, J. E., and WENT, L. N.: The Bone Changes in Sickle Cell Anaemia and Its Genetic Variants, J. Bone & Joint Surg., *41-B*, 711, 1959.

GRAHAM, R. V.: Experimental Considerations in Perthes's Disease, M. J. Australia, *17*, 207, 1930.

GREEN, W. T., and BANKS, H. H.: Osteochondritis Dissecans in Children, J. Bone & Joint Surg., *35-A*, 26, 1953.

HASSELWANDER, A.: Bewegungssystem, in *Handbuch der Anatomie des Kindes*, Munich, J. F. Bergmann, *2*, 1938 (see p. 557).

HØLUND, T.: Kyphosis Juvenilis Scheuermann, Ugesk. laeger, *105*, 389, 1943.

HOWE, W. W., JR., LACEY, T., II, and SCHWARTZ, R. P.: A Study of the Gross Anatomy of the Arteries Supplying the Proximal Portion of the Femur and the Acetabulum, J. Bone & Joint Surg., *32-A*, 856, 1950.

HULTING, B.: Roentgenologic Features of Fracture of the Tibial Tuberosity (Osgood-Schlatter's Disease), Acta radiol., *48*, 161, 1957.

JERRE, T.: A Study in Slipped Upper Femoral Epiphysis, Acta orthop. scandinav., Suppl. 6, 1950.

KARP, M. G.: Köhler's Disease of the Tarsal Scaphoid, J. Bone & Joint Surg., *19*, 84, 1937.

41

Kelsey, J. L., Keggi, K. J., and Southwick, W. O.: The Incidence and Distribution of Slipped Capital Femoral Epiphysis in Connecticut and Southwestern United States, J. Bone & Joint Surg., *52-A*, 1203, 1970.

Kennedy, J. C., Grainger, R. W., and McGraw, R. W.: Osteochondral Fractures of the Femoral Condyles, J. Bone & Joint Surg., *48-B*, 436, 1966.

Kienböck, R.: Über traumatische Malazie des Mondbeins und ihre Folgezustände: Entartungsformen und Kompressionsfrakturen, Fortschr. Geb. Röntgenstrahlen, *16*, 77, 1910.

Köhler, A.: Ueber eine häufige, bisher anscheinend unbekannte Erkrankung einzelner kindlicher Knochen, München. med. Wchnschr., *55*, 1923, 1908.

————: Eine typische Erkrankung des 2. Metatarsophalangealgelenkes, München. med. Wchnschr., *67*, 1289, 1920.

————: Typical Disease of the Second Metatarsophalangeal Joint, Am. J. Roentgenol., *10*, 705, 1923.

————: *Röntgenology*, New York, William Wood and Company, 1928.

König, F.: Ueber freie Körper in den Gelenken, Deutsche Ztschr. Chir., *27*, 90, 1887–88.

Konjetzny, G. E.: Zur Pathologie und pathologischen Anatomie der Perthes-Calvé'schen Krankheit, Acta chir. scandinav., *74*, 361, 1934.

Lacroix, P., and Verbrugge, J.: Slipping of the Upper Femoral Epiphysis, J. Bone & Joint Surg., *33-A*, 371, 1951.

LaZerte, G. D., and Rapp, I. H.: Pathogenesis of Osgood-Schlatter's Disease, Am. J. Path., *34*, 803, 1958.

Lecène, P., and Mouchet, A.: La scaphoidite tarsienne (anatomie pathologique et pathogénie), Rev. d'orthop., *11*, 105, 1924.

Lee, M. L. H.: The Intraosseus Arterial Pattern of the Carpal Lunate Bone and its Relation to Avascular Necrosis, Acta orthop. scandinav., *33*, 43, 1963.

Legg, A. T.: An Obscure Affection of the Hip-Joint, Boston M. & S. J., *162*, 202, 1910.

Löhr, W.: Dauererfolge bei der Behandlung der Osteochondritis Dissecans, Arch. klin. Chir., *157*, 752, 1929.

Lowe, H. G.: Avascular Necrosis Complicating Slipped Upper Femoral Epiphysis, J. Bone & Joint Surg., *41-B*, 618, 1959.

————: Necrosis of Articular Cartilage After Slipping of the Capital Femoral Epiphysis, J. Bone & Joint Surg., *52-B*, 108, 1970.

Meyer, J.: Treatment of Legg-Calvé-Perthes Disease, Acta orthop. scandinav., Suppl. 86, 1966.

Miltner, L. J., and Hu, C. H.: Osteochondritis of the Head of the Femur, Arch. Surg., *27*, 645, 1933.

Morris, M. L., and McGibbon, K. C.: Osteochondritis Dissecans Following Legg-Calvé-Perthes' Disease, J. Bone & Joint Surg., *44-B*, 562, 1962.

Müller, U.: Spontanheilung der Osteochondrosis dissecans, Ztschr. Orthop., *81*, 377, 1951.

Nielsen, N. A.: Osteochondritis Dissecans Capituli Humeri, Acta orthop. scandinav., *4*, 307, 1933.

Osgood, R. B.: Lesions of the Tibial Tubercle Occurring During Adolescence, Boston M. & S. J., *148*, 114, 1903.

Paget, J.: On the Production of some of the Loose Bodies in Joints, St. Bartholomew's Hosp. Rep., *6*, 1, 1870.

Persson, M.: Pathogenese und Behandlung der Kienböckschen Lunatummalazie, Acta chir. scandinav., *92*, Suppl. 98, 1945.

Perthes, G.: Über Arthritis deformans juvenilis, Deutsche Ztschr. Chir., *107*, 111, 1910.

Pich, G.: Histopathologic Study in a Case of Perthes' Disease of Traumatic Origin, Arch. Surg., *33*, 609, 1936.

Pick, M. P.: Familial Osteochondritis Dissecans, J. Bone & Joint Surg., *37-B*, 142, 1955.

Platt, H.: Pseudo-Coxalgia (Osteochondritis Deformans Juvenilis Coxae: Quiet Hip Disease.), Brit. J. Surg., *9*, 366, 1921–22.

Ponseti, I. V.: Legg-Perthes Disease, J. Bone & Joint Surg., *38-A*, 739, 1956.

Ponseti, I. V., and McClintock, R.: The Pathology of Slipping of the Upper Femoral Epiphysis, J. Bone & Joint Surg., *38-A*, 71, 1956.

Preiser, G.: Eine typische posttraumatische und zur Spontanfraktur führende Ostitis des Naviculare carpi, Fortschr. Geb. Röntgenstrahlen, *15*, 189, 1910.

Ratliff, A. H. C.: Osteochondritis Dissecans Following Legg-Calvé-Perthes' Disease, J. Bone & Joint Surg., *49-B*, 108, 1967.

Rosenberg, N. J.: Osteochondral Fractures of the Lateral Femoral Condyle, J. Bone & Joint Surg., *46-A*, 1013, 1964.

Rüttner, J. R.: Beiträge zur Klinik und pathologischen Anatomie der Kienböckschen Krankheit (Lunatummalacie), Helvet. chir. acta, *13*, Suppl .1, 1946.

Salter, R. B.: Experimental and Clinical Aspects of Perthes' Disease, J. Bone & Joint Surg., *48-B*, 393, 1966.

SCAGLIETTI, O., STRINGA, G., and MIZZAU, M.: Plus-Variant of the Astragalus and Subnormal Scaphoid Space, Two Important Findings in Koehler's Scaphoid Necrosis, Acta orthop. scandinav., *32*, 499, 1962.

SCHEUERMANN, H.: Kyphosis dorsalis juvenilis, Ztschr. orthop. Chir., *41*, 305, 1921.

SCHLATTER, C.: Verletzungen des schnabelförmigen Fortsatzes der oberen Tibiaepiphyse, Beitr. klin. Chir., *38*, 874, 1903.

SCHMORL, G.: Die Pathogenese der juvenilen Kyphose, Fortschr. Geb. Röntgenstrahlen, *41*, 359, 1930.

——————: Über Verlagerung von Bandscheibengewebe und ihre Folgen, Arch. klin. Chir., *172*, 240, 1932.

SMILLIE, I. S.: Freiberg's Infraction (Köhler's Second Disease), J. Bone & Joint Surg., *39-B*, 580, 1957.

SMITH, A. DEF.: Osteochondritis of the Knee Joint, J. Bone & Joint Surg., *42-A*, 289, 1960.

SONTAG, L. W., and PYLE, S. I.: Variations in the Calcification Pattern in Epiphyses, Am. J. Roentgenol., *45*, 50, 1941.

SØRENSEN, K. H.: *Scheuermann's Juvenile Kyphosis*, Copenhagen, E. Munksgaard, 1964.

SPEED, K.: Köhler's Disease of the Tarsal Scaphoid Bone, Tr. Am. S. A., *45*, 179, 1927.

STOHL, F.: On Lunatomalacia (Kienböck's Disease), Acta chir. scandinav., *95*, Suppl. 126, 1947.

STOUGAARD, J.: The Hereditary Factor in Osteochondritis Dissecans, J. Bone & Joint Surg., *43-B*, 256, 1961.

——————: Familial Occurrence of Osteochondritis Dissecans, J. Bone & Joint Surg., *46-B*, 542, 1964.

SUTRO, C. J.: Slipping of the Capital Epiphysis of the Femur in Adolescence, Arch. Surg., *31*, 345, 1935.

SUTRO, C. J., and POMERANZ, M. M.: Osgood-Schlatter's Disease, Arch. Surg., *31*, 807, 1935.

——————: Perthes' Disease, Arch. Surg., *34*, 360, 1937.

TRUETA, J.: The Normal Vascular Anatomy of the Human Femoral Head During Growth, J. Bone & Joint Surg., *39-B*, 358, 1957.

TRUETA, J., and HARRISON, M. H. M.: The Normal Vascular Anatomy of the Femoral Head in Adult Man, J. Bone & Joint Surg., *35-B*, 442, 1953.

TUCKER, F. R.: Arterial Supply to the Femoral Head and its Clinical Importance, J. Bone & Joint Surg., *31-B*, 82, 1949.

UHRY, E., JR.: Osgood-Schlatter Disease, Arch. Surg., *48*, 406, 1944.

VELLUDA, C.: Sur la vascularisation du scaphoide du tarse, Ann. anat. path., *5*, 1016, 1928.

WAGONER, G., and COHN, B. N. E.: Osteochondritis Dissecans, Arch. Surg., *23*, 1, 1931.

WALDENSTRÖM, H.: On Necrosis of the Joint Cartilage by Epiphyseolysis Capitis Femoris, Acta chir. scandinav., *67*, 936, 1930.

——————: Necrosis of the Femoral Epiphysis Owing to Insufficient Nutrition from the Ligamentum Teres. A Clinical Study Mainly Based on Experiences of the Treatment of Epiphyseolysis Capitis Femoris, Acta chir. scandinav., *75*, 185, 1934.

——————: The First Stages of Coxa Plana, J. Bone & Joint Surg., *20*, 559, 1938.

——————: Slipping of the Upper Femoral Epiphysis, Surg. Gynec. & Obst., *71*, 198, 1940.

WASSMANN, K.: Kyphosis Juvenilis Scheuermann—An Occupational Disorder, Acta orthop. scandinav., *21*, 65, 1951.

WAUGH, W.: The Ossification and Vascularisation of the Tarsal Navicular and their Relation to Köhler's Disease, J. Bone & Joint Surg., *40-B*, 765, 1958.

WIBERG, G.: Spontanheilung von Osteochondritis dissecans im Kniegelenk, Acta chir. scandinav., *85*, 421, 1941.

——————: Considerations on the Surgical Treatment of Slipped Epiphysis with Special Reference to Nail Fixation, J. Bone & Joint Surg., *41-A*, 253, 1959.

WILLIAMS, H. J., and PUGH, D. G.: Vertebral Epiphysitis: A Comparison of the Clinical and Roentgenologic Findings, Am. J. Roentgenol., *90*, 1236, 1963.

ZEMANSKY, A. P., JR.: The Pathology and Pathogenesis of Legg-Calvé-Perthes' Disease (Osteochondritis Juvenilis Deformans Coxae), Am. J. Surg., *4*, 169, 1928.

Chapter

20

Idiopathic and Post-Traumatic Ischemic Necrosis of the Femoral Head

IN THIS chapter we are concerned mainly with the consequences of ischemic necrosis of the marrow and osseous tissue of the femoral head ensuing upon interruption of its blood supply under certain circumstances. Specifically, we are concerned with the short-term and ultimate changes in the femoral head (and the rest of the hip joint) which appear in connection with: (1) so-called idiopathic ischemic necrosis of the femoral head; (2) dislocation at the hip joint; and (3) fracture of the proximal end of the femur but especially of the neck of the femur. Since in all these conditions the necrosis occurs without the agency of an infection, the general term "aseptic necrosis" of the femoral head may appropriately be interchanged or combined with "ischemic necrosis." As a background for consideration of aseptic ischemic necrosis of the femoral head, a brief survey of pertinent aspects of the normal anatomic structure and blood supply of the proximal end of the femur seems appropriate.

For detailed visualization of the *gross anatomic structure* of the upper end of the femur, it is necessary to examine a specimen which has been macerated by one method or another, so that it has been cleared of all the adherent soft tissues and also of the bone marrow in the major marrow cavity and the intertrabecular marrow spaces. In regard to the external configuration of the proximal end of the femur, it will be recalled that: (1) The head of the bone is almost spherical in shape (actually about two thirds of a sphere); (2) the neck of the femur, connecting the head of the bone with the shaft, is somewhat flattened and thus more rectangular than cylindrical in shape; and (3) the neck ends at the lesser trochanter medially, while laterally the greater trochanter projects above the junction of the shaft with the neck.

If one examines the proximal end of a femur which has been sectioned in the frontal plane and also macerated, it will be evident that the cortex of the femoral neck is strikingly thin in comparison with the cortex of the shaft distal to the neck. The proximal part of the neck and also the head of the femur contain large quantities of spongy (cancellous) bone, in comparison with the sparsity of spongy bone in the interior of the upper end of the femoral shaft. The spongy trabeculae distributed over the surface of the sectioned head (the compression trabeculae) merge with the compacted osseous tissue on the medial side of the shaft. Trabeculae curving upward from the lateral aspect of the shaft (tension trabeculae) spread through the head, cross the compression struts at right angles, and fix them into position. Thus the arrangement of the trabeculae of the spongy bone is such that they resist stresses and strains and indeed may be regarded as constituting the internal weight-bearing system in the head and neck of the femur (see Garden).

In harmony with its obvious importance, the *blood supply* of the head and neck of the femur has been the subject of many studies (see Trueta and Harrison,

Tucker, Judet *et al.*, Claffey, Sevitt and Thompson, and also Crock). The arteries which enter the head by way of the ligamentum teres (round ligament) are derived from branches of the obturator artery or of the medial femoral circumflex artery. However, the main blood supply for the femoral head and neck is derived from branches of the arteries encircling the base of the femoral neck, at the level of attachment of the capsule of the hip joint to the base of the neck. The anterior component of this arterial ring consists of a number of branches derived from the *lateral* femoral circumflex artery. The posterior component is usually a rather large and well-defined branch of the *medial* femoral circumflex artery. In the process of supplying blood to the head and neck of the femur, branches from this encircling ring of arteries in the region of the capsular attachment penetrate the capsule. Some of the arterial branches extend upward under the superior and inferior retinacula—that is, the synovial reflection of the capsule covering the neck of the femur. Some of these subsynovial blood vessels penetrate the cortex of the neck and thus come to represent metaphysial vessels supplying blood to the local spongiosa. Other subsynovial arterial branches (the lateral epiphysial vessels) continue further along the neck to the head-neck junction, where they enter the head of the femur and thus contribute to its blood supply.

Crock suggests the following simplified terminology for the blood vessels supplying the head and neck of the femur: (1) the arterial ring of the femoral neck; (2) the ascending cervical branches of this ring; and (3) the arteries of the round ligament. At any rate, after entering the head and neck of the femur, these various blood vessels anastomose freely with each other. However, in a case of fracture of the femoral neck, disruption of the ascending cervical branches of the ring which enter the femoral head (branches also denoted as the lateral epiphysial vessels) play a considerable part in the occurrence of ischemic necrosis of the head.

IDIOPATHIC (PRIMARY) NECROSIS OF THE FEMORAL HEAD IN ADULTS

The term *"idiopathic (primary) necrosis of the femoral head in adults"* relates to those instances of ischemic aseptic necrosis of the femoral head in which the necrosis not only occurs in an adult but in which: (1) The interruption of the blood supply to the femoral head is not conditioned by a pre-existing disease process (such as sickle cell anemia, caisson disease, or Gaucher's disease) which may in itself be the basis for the development of an aseptic necrosis, and (2) the interruption of the blood supply and the consequent necrosis of the femoral head was not preceded by a fracture of the femoral neck or by a dislocation at the hip joint. These conditions explain why the disorder is also denoted simply as *"primary aseptic necrosis"* of the femoral head.

In 1926, Freund gave what appears to be the first detailed description of the pathologico-anatomic findings in a case representing the condition under consideration. The subject was a woman 77 years of age in whom, at autopsy, the necrosis was found to be present in both femoral heads. Although the clinical, roentgenographic, and pathologic aspects of idiopathic aseptic necrosis of the femoral head in adults have been well elucidated, the reason for the interruption of the blood supply remains obscure. It is true that there is a tendency to implicate *corticosteroid therapy* as a common cause of idiopathic aseptic necrosis of the femoral head, and as the basis for its recent increased incidence. That corticosteroid therapy (particularly cortisone therapy) may give rise to aseptic necrosis of the femoral head or some other articular bone end is now well recognized (p. 635). However, it is also clear that the condition in question is encountered at least as often in subjects who have not received cortisone therapy as in those who have. Also relevant is the fact that the development of Legg-Calvé-Perthes disease, the childhood counterpart of idiopathic aseptic necrosis of the femoral head in adults, has never been linked with steroid therapy. Other possible etiologic influences leading to the interruption of the blood supply to the affected femoral head are mentioned below.

The pertinent literature has increased considerably since Freund made his contribution to the subject. Those who have been intrigued by the problem and have contributed clinical and anatomic information on the condition as a whole include Chandler, Phemister, Serre and Simon, Mankin and Brower, Patterson *et al.*, Merle d'Aubigné *et al.*, Hastings and Macnab, and also Duse *et al.* Chandler's reference to the disorder as *"coronary disease of the hip"* probably accounts for the occasional designation of it as *"Chandler's disease."* It has also sometimes been denoted as *"osteochondritis dissecans"* of the femoral head.

CLINICAL CONSIDERATIONS

Incidence.—The *general incidence* of idiopathic aseptic necrosis of the femoral head is certainly low in comparison with the incidence of necrosis of the femoral head following upon fracture of the femoral neck. In line with the general rarity of the condition is the report by Mankin and Brower to the effect that only 5 cases were observed by them at the University of Pittsburgh Medical Center over a period of 4 years. Again, Patterson *et al.* report that 52 cases were seen at the Mayo Clinic during the period extending from 1935 to 1960 inclusive—that is, an average of only about 2 cases per year. Merle d'Aubigné *et al.* report observing 139 cases during the 5-year period 1959 to 1963. They thus saw about 28 cases per year, on the average, during that period. Included among these cases were many in which the patient had been given cortisone therapy before the onset of clinical complaints relating to the affected femora. In the writer's opinion, it is questionable whether cases of necrosis of the femoral head developing after cortisone therapy should actually be included in the category of idiopathic (or primary) aseptic necrosis.

In regard to the *age and sex incidence*, it is clear that in any large series of cases about 80 per cent of the patients are likely to be between 30 and 60 years of age, and also that about 80 per cent of all of them will be males.

Localization.—As already indicated, *one or both* femoral heads may be the site of the disorder in a given case. Not uncommonly, both femoral heads are already found involved when the patient first comes under medical care. If only one femoral head is found necrotic at this time, there is considerable likelihood that the other femoral head will come to show aseptic necrosis within a year or so. The over-all incidence of bilateral involvement as recorded in the literature naturally varies with the number of cases in the reported series, the promptness with which the patients first came under treatment for the relevant clinical complaints, and the length of the total period during which the patients were observed. About 50 per cent seems to represent a reasonable approximation of the averaged proportion of cases in which both hips are ultimately involved.

Clinical Complaints and Findings.—The initial clinical complaint is nearly always pain. This is usually localized to the region of the hip joint, but occasionally the pain is first referred to the region of the knee joint. In some cases the initial pain is mild, but in other instances there is sudden severe pain in the hip joint which incapacitates the subject for several days, necessitating bed rest. In any event, whether the pain took this acute form at first or was not very severe at the start, the pain tends to become intermittent, but its general course is progressive. While the pain is still intermittent, it is felt mainly when the patient is ambulatory. As the pathologico-anatomic changes in the hip become more pronounced, the pain increases in severity, tends to become more or less constant, and is usually no longer relieved by bed rest. The clinical progress of the condition is often characterized by bouts of acute exacerbation of the pain, associated with striking impairment of function of the affected hip joint, due to muscle spasm. Apart from the latter, the actual range of motion of the hip joint is only slowly impaired. Lateral and medial rotation tend to become restricted earlier than flexion and extension. Eventually, however, a flexion contracture does develop, and this is manifested in a short-stepped, shuffling gait.

Possible Etiologic Factors.—As already indicated, cases in which the interruption of the blood supply to the femoral head can be assigned to an established and well-recognized cause should be excluded from the category of idiopathic (primary) aseptic necrosis of the femoral head in adults. In this connection, consideration should be given first to the ischemic necrosis of the femoral head which may follow upon a course of *systemic administration of steroids* (most often cortisone) either in large doses or over a long period of time (see Pietrogrande and Mastromarino, Heimann and Freiberger, Serre and Simon, and also Sutton *et al.*). When necrosis of the femoral head occurs in these cases, it becomes clinically evident within several months or even a year or two after the beginning of the therapy, or even after the steroid administration has been discontinued. In all these cases the steroid had been administered in the course of treatment of various diseases (rheumatoid arthritis, pemphigus, etc.) which are known not to lead in themselves to the occurrence of aseptic necrosis of the femoral head or other articular bone ends.

The mechanism by which steroid (or corticosteroid) therapy brings about the interruption of the blood supply to the femoral head has not been clearly established. It has been postulated that, since the administration of corticosteroids induces an osteoporosis, a trauma or traumata acting upon the region of the hip but not sufficiently severe to produce a femoral neck fracture might nevertheless result in necrosis of the femoral head. Another mechanism which has been proposed is represented by the idea that the corticosteroids cause intra-osseous hyperpressure resulting in obstruction of the venous return from the femoral head. It is supposed that this in turn interferes with the flow of arterial blood to the femoral head, and that it is this interference with the arterial circulation that results in the ischemic necrosis. Altogether, the precise mechanism by which steroid therapy interrupts the blood supply to the femoral head is still obscure. However, since we know that such therapy sometimes leads to the appearance of aseptic necrosis of the femoral head, it is problematical, as already indicated, whether such cases strictly belong in the category of idiopathic ischemic necrosis.

Another etiologic factor frequently mentioned in the literature is *alcoholism*. The incidence of alcoholism is apparently higher among persons affected with the aseptic necrosis in question than in the population at large. It is suggested by Mankin and Brower that the reason for the high incidence of alcoholism among these subjects may be "that alcohol provides some relief from the severe, unremitting pain of 'Chandler's Disease'." In any event, it is well known that an inebriated person often undergoes traumata. A particular trauma may even be severe, but the subject may nevertheless fail to recall it when he is questioned about a history of trauma. At any rate, it is to be doubted that there is an adequate basis for holding that a reduced blood flow to the femoral head, such as might be associated with the increased peripheral circulation characteristic of the state of inebriation, is the basis for the ischemic necrosis in these cases.

Among the other suggested etiologic factors are lesions involving the blood vessels supplying the femoral head. This question is considered in the section dealing with the microscopic pathologic findings (p. 639).

Figure 162

A, Roentgenograph of the right hip region in the case of a man 27 years of age who, on admission to the hospital, gave a history of pain in the hip and knee of $3\frac{1}{2}$ months' duration. The pain, which was felt particularly during ambulation, had been increasing in severity. He related his difficulties to the repeated bumping of his buttocks while he was being subjected to the recoil from a howitzer. However, since these episodes occurred 5 years before the onset of his clinical complaints, it does not seem likely that they played a causative role in the necrosis of the femoral head, which was interpreted clinically as an idiopathic necrosis. The picture shows a very narrow curved line of diminished radiodensity immediately beneath the bony end plate and to the left of the fovea. This line of diminished radiodensity represents the site of an infraction extending through the necrotic femoral head and resulting in separation of the articular cartilage, along with bits of the necrotic subchondral bone, from the rest of the femoral head (see *C*). Lateral to the fovea, one can observe a somewhat wedge-shaped delineated area of more or less uniform radiopacity. On histologic examination of the resected head, it was apparent that in this region the osseous tissue of the head was completely necrotic, that the intertrabecular marrow was also necrotic and showed some granular detritus, and that the necrotic marrow was being replaced by fibrous tissue. In the direction of the neck, and abutting upon the wedge-shaped zone, small, irregular patches of increased radiopacity can be observed in the roentgenograph. Microscopic examination revealed that these foci of increased radiopacity were sites where the pre-existing necrotic spongy trabeculae were thickened through the deposition of new bone upon them, or were sites where heavily calcified connective tissue was present in the intertrabecular marrow spaces.

B, Roentgenograph showing the head of the right femur from a case in which both femoral heads were sites of idiopathic aseptic necrosis. The patient was a man 27 years of age who stated that 2 years before admission to the hospital he experienced the sudden onset of pain in both hips. The pain also radiated down both thighs, and shortly before admission to the hospital the man had become aware of what he described as a feeling of "crackling" in the hips. The roentgenograph of the hip illustrated was taken on the day of the subject's admission to the hospital. For the interpretation of the roentgenographic changes present, see *D*.

C, Roentgenograph of a slice cut from the femoral head shown in *A* after the head had been resected and replaced by a prosthesis. The separation of the articular cartilage, along with a sliver of necrotic subchondral bone, is clearly shown.

D, Roentgenograph of a slice cut from the femoral head shown in *B*, the head having been resected and replaced by a prosthesis. This picture reveals in greater detail many of the roentgenographic features shown by the clinical roentgenograph. In the upper midportion of the picture, it can be seen that the articular cartilage and some bits of subchondral bone are separated from the underlying part of the head. Beneath the separated articular cartilage there is a roughly oval focus of bone which, on histologic examination, was found to consist of completely necrotic osseous tissue. Beyond the focus of necrotic bone there is a zone which is more or less radiolucent and which, on histologic examination, was found to consist of a band of more or less vascularized connective tissue. The close-meshed spongiosa beyond this relatively radiolucent zone consists of necrotic spongy trabeculae which have been thickened through the deposition of new bone upon them. The histologic basis for the roentgenographic features shown in this picture is represented in *E*.

E, Photomicrograph ($\times$ 5) of part of a tissue section prepared from the slice of femoral head illustrated in *D*. Most of the articular cartilage with some tiny fragments of subchondral bone can be seen to be separated from the underlying area of necrotic bone which appeared in the roentgenograph as a well-delineated ovoid focus. On microscopic examination under higher magnification, it was apparent that the osseous tissue of the trabeculae was nonviable, that the marrow in the intertrabecular spaces had undergone necrosis, and that a considerable amount of blue-staining granular detritus was also present between the trabeculae. The band of vascularized fibrous tissue which was the basis for the zone of relative radiolucency stands out even under this low magnification. At the extreme right of the picture, thick, close-meshed spongy trabeculae account for the zone of increased radiopacity beyond the band of fibrous tissue.

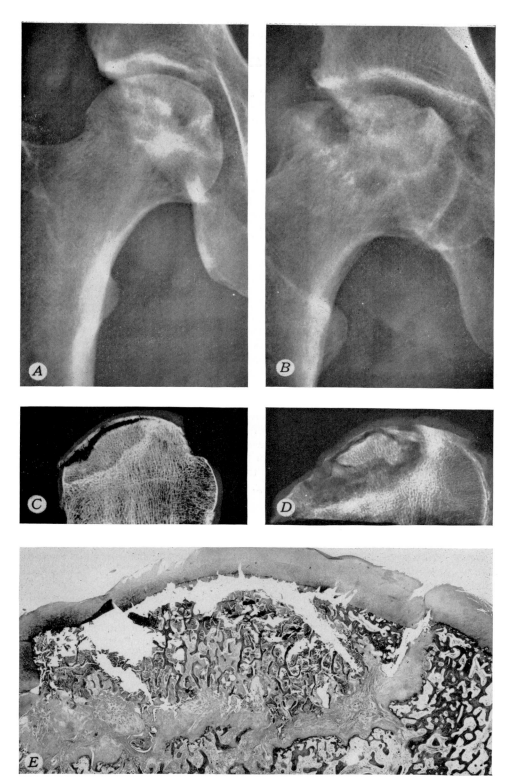

Figure 162

ROENTGENOGRAPHIC FINDINGS

The femoral head may already be the site of the necrosis and be the source of some clinical complaints for several months before the first roentgenographic indication of the presence of the condition becomes evident. At this early stage, the general contour of the femoral head is still normal. However, if the roentgenograph is taken to show the femoral head in a lateral projection, it is often already possible to detect a very narrow, faint, curved line of *diminished radiodensity* immediately beneath the bony end plate abutting upon the deep surface of the articular cartilage. It is ordinarily on the anterior aspect of the proximal part of the femoral head that this narrow zone of diminished density is located.

In the course of further progress of the changes, a smaller or larger focus of *increased radiodensity* becomes delimited in the anterosuperior segment of the head. This radiopaque focus, which may vary somewhat in shape from lesion to lesion, represents an area of the femoral head which is completely necrotic. The area in question may appear crescent-shaped or ovoid, or present as a broad-based wedge, the base of which is directed toward the articular surface of the femoral head. In any case, the margin delimiting this radiopaque focus from the rest of the femoral head is likely to be quite irregular, and it may be set off from the rest of the head by an irregular zone of radiolucency. Eventually the femoral head becomes flattened in the region of this focus of necrotic bone, and the latter may come to appear fragmented in the roentgenograph. The appearance of fragmentation is the result of foci of radiopacity intermingled with areas of radiolucency. The rest of the femoral head may likewise come to show increased radiopacity—a fact which is accounted for by revascularization of the femoral head and the deposition of new bone on the pre-existing, more or less devitalized spongy trabeculae. In the course of 2 or 3 years from the time of onset of the necrosis, the great majority of the femoral heads in any large pertinent series of cases will be found to have collapsed. Consequently it is not surprising that, in these cases, roentgenographic evidences of osteoarthritis become engrafted upon the roentgenographic changes characterizing the aseptic necrosis *per se*. (See Fig. 162.)

PATHOLOGIC FINDINGS

Gross Pathology.—The details of the gross pathologic findings in a given necrotic femoral head naturally vary with the extent of the necrosis and the length of time which has elapsed between its onset and the anatomic examination of the head. If the condition has been present for a relatively short time, the external configuration of the head will still be normal, and the articular cartilage will probably still be found smooth and appear unaltered. Nevertheless, palpation of the anterosuperior surface of such an affected head is likely to reveal an area of the articular cartilage which yields if pressure is applied to it. Where the articular cartilage can be depressed, it will be found that the immediate subchondral bone is necrotic and has become delimited as a sequestrum *in situ* from the rest of the necrotic part of the head. When the changes have advanced further and the anterosuperior part of the head has collapsed and flattened, the articular cartilage may be found discolored and irregularly buckled, and even show some slitlike cracks and areas of degeneration.

If a necrotic head in which advanced changes are present is sectioned in the frontal plane, the alterations to be noted on gross examination are striking. The completely necrotic portion of the head stands out as a yellowish white area in the upper part of the head. It is of special interest that the inferior part of the head and the part of the head in the immediate vicinity of the fovea are not at all likely to be implicated in the necrosis. The articular cartilage overlying the necrotic area is usually found separated from the latter and may have some small fragments of necrotic bone adherent to its deep surface. The portion of the head which is obviously necrotic eventually comes to be bordered by a zone of fibrous tissue which, on microscopic examination, may still be found rather rich in blood vessels. Beyond this fibrous zone the remaining spongiosa of the head and part of the neck may be found sclerotic. The obviously necrotic portion of the head may eventually consist of several adjacent fragments resulting from fractures through the necrotic area.

Finally, it should be noted that the gross pathologic findings outlined above in relation to idiopathic aseptic necrosis of the femoral head in adults are not distinctive of this condition. Entirely analogous appearances are to be observed in a femoral head which has undergone infarction in an instance of caisson disease, or in a femoral head in which ischemic necrosis has followed upon a dislocation at the hip joint. Furthermore, the ischemic aseptic necrosis of the femoral head which may ensue upon the therapeutic administration of steroids likewise presents essentially the same gross pathologic appearance as does the ischemic necrosis of the femoral head in cases still classifiable as "idiopathic."

Microscopic Pathology.—Like the gross findings, the microscopic pathologic findings in the affected femoral head vary with the extent of the necrosis, the time which has elapsed since the onset of the condition, and the amount of repair which has occurred as a result of revascularization. Since the articular cartilage receives its nourishment from the synovial fluid, those portions of the cartilage which are still smooth and not discolored are viable and do not reveal any significant histologic changes, though the cartilage may be thicker in some places than it would normally be. On the other hand, where the articular cartilage is buckled and discolored and has been subjected to abnormal functional pressure, it shows evidences of degeneration. The degeneration is expressed in the appearance of splits in the cartilage matrix at right angles to the surface of the cartilage (fibrillation), focal necrosis of the fibrillized cartilage, and even erosion of areas of cartilage which have been altered in these ways. In the areas of necrotic subchondral bone, osteocytes are naturally absent from the bone cell lacunae, and the intertrabecular marrow is likewise found to be necrotic. In addition, the spongy marrow spaces contain a variable amount of blue-staining granular material (granular detritus) representing disintegrated marrow and disintegrated bits of the spongy bone.

Microscopic examination also reveals that, beyond the frankly necrotic portions of the femoral head, reparative changes are taking place. At the border between the necrotic and the viable bone there may be a narrow zone of more or less vascularized connective tissue. The spongy trabeculae of the necrotic bone immediately adjacent to the zone of vascularized connective tissue may show evidences of active osteoclastic resorption. The marrow spaces of the spongiosa of the viable bone contain numerous blood vessels, and newly formed osseous tissue is being deposited on the pre-existing spongy trabeculae. In consequence, these trabeculae are thickened, and it is on this account that the non-necrotic osseous tissue of the femoral head and even of the adjacent part of the neck becomes sclerotic. (See Fig. 163.)

The *synovial membrane* of the articular capsule of the joint ordinarily does not show anything remarkable. In advanced cases it presents at most a mild degree of nonspecific synovitis, such as one would expect to find in the synovial membrane of any joint which is the site of degenerative changes of long standing.

In an effort to discover whether the ischemic necrosis of the femoral head in these cases is to be related to lesions in the *capsular blood vessels*, Merle d'Aubigné *et al.* removed the ligaments of the joints, together with the femoral head, in the course of surgical intervention in 6 of their cases. They report that, in 4 of the 6 cases, vascular lesions were found. In 2 of these cases they noted perivascular inflammatory changes. In the other 2 cases they report finding alterations in the walls of the arteries supplying the anterosuperior pedicle of the femoral head. In particular, they noted changes in the media, and even more in the intima, of the arteries present in the pathologic area. The intima was thickened and also showed rupture of its elastic layer. Since these changes were found in the anterosuperior artery, which is the main nutrient artery to the head, and since the arterial lesions observed resembled those of temporal arteritis, they were held to play a significant causal role in the development of the ischemic necrosis. It is to be emphasized, however, that these changes were observed in only 2 of the 6 cases in which the capsular blood vessels were examined. Indeed, it may well be that the findings described by Merle d'Aubigné *et al.* in relation to the main nutrient artery to the femoral head might have been secondary to the necrotic changes in the head rather than a cause of those changes. Mankin and Brower, commenting on the possible role of endarteritis (also suggested by others) as an etiologic agent in the development of the necrosis of the femoral head in these cases, summarized their reaction to the possible role of endarteritis as follows: "The remarkable predilection of an arteritis to both femoral heads, sparing the rest of the body in an otherwise healthy individual, taxes the imagination." Finally, it should be pointed out that the capillaries, venules, and even the arterioles of the capsular and pericapsular tissues of a joint normally have thick hyaline walls and narrow lumina, even in young subjects. Therefore, one must be particularly wary about attributing disease processes in joints to such thick blood vessels.

Figure 163

A, Roentgenograph illustrating the advanced changes of idiopathic necrosis in both femoral heads. There is also evidence of bilateral osteoarthritis, which developed as a complication of the pathologic alterations in the femoral heads. The *left femur* is shown on the *right* side of the picture, and the other illustrations in this figure pertain to the left femoral head, which was resected and replaced by a prosthesis. The patient, a man, was 50 years of age at the time he was admitted to the hospital and this roentgenograph was taken. The history was that he had had pain in both hip regions for about 3 years. The pain was more pronounced on the left side, and was felt particularly during walking. There was no history of injury or of working under compressed air, and no evidence of any hematological disease.

B, Photograph of the cut surface of the resected head of the left femur, the head having been sectioned in the frontal plane. The gross pathologic changes revealed in this picture can be correlated with the modifications shown on the right in *A*, the clinical roentgenograph. Note the well-delineated and somewhat wedge-shaped necrotic portion of the head. This is bordered below by fibrous tissue, and its articular surface is covered by cartilage which is adherent only in part. This portion of the head is clearly identifiable in the clinical roentgenograph. Beyond the zone of fibrous tissue bordering upon this focus of residual necrotic bone, there is a wide zone of rather closely compacted osseous tissue. This is apparent in the clinical roentgenograph as a band of radiopacity. The marginal exostoses visible on the left and on the right of the specimen photograph are also recognizable in the clinical roentgenograph.

C, Roentgenograph of the part of the gross specimen illustrated in *B*. It reveals in even clearer detail the correlation between the gross pathologic picture and the alterations observable in the clinical roentgenograph.

D, Photomicrograph ($\times 4$) of a tissue section prepared from part of the gross specimen shown in *B*. In the upper and central part of the picture, the delineated necrotic portion of the femoral head is clearly apparent. Its articular surface is covered in part by cartilage. Its deep surface is marked off from the rest of the head by a thick band of tissue which, under higher magnification, is found to be fibrous connective tissue.

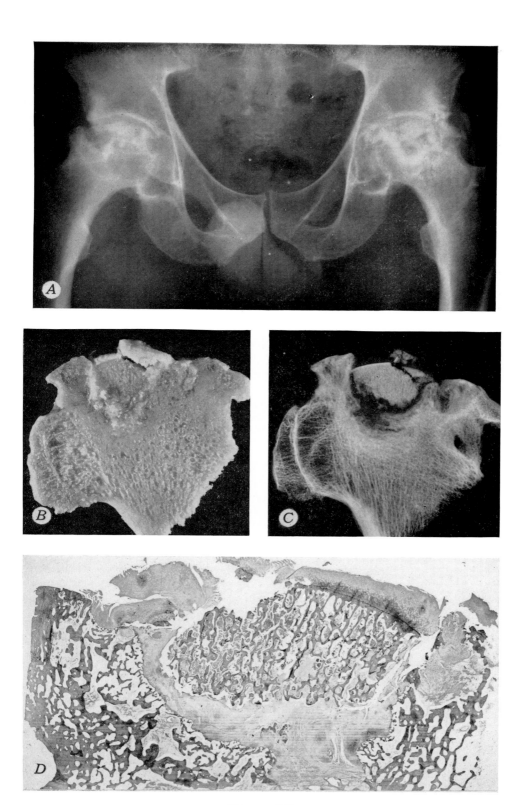

Figure 163

TREATMENT

The results of *conservative nonsurgical treatment* of adults affected with idiopathic aseptic necrosis of the femoral head compare *unfavorably* with the results to be expected from this type of treatment in children manifesting Legg-Perthes disease, in which the femoral head is likewise the site of aseptic necrosis. Indeed, in the adult it is not to be expected that conservative nonsurgical treatment will ultimately result in spontaneous regeneration and restoration of the head to a condition even approximating the normal, while in children such a result is frequently achieved by means of conservative treatment. The best results that can be hoped for under conservative nonsurgical treatment in the adult subjects are that, in a small percentage of the cases, the alterations in the femoral head will not progress and the clinical difficulties will remain tolerable.

It is for these reasons that one or another *surgical procedure* is ordinarily employed in the treatment of these cases. The procedures used vary in accordance with the severity of the changes in the diseased head, the presence of pathologic changes in the acetabulum, and the presence or absence of involvement of the opposite hip.

TRAUMATIC DISLOCATION OF THE FEMORAL HEAD

Dislocation of the femoral head often represents merely one aspect of the pathologic changes created by traumatic disruption of the hip joint. In the present section of this chapter, we shall be concerned mainly with the alterations taking place in the dislocated femoral head, and specifically with the occurrence of ischemic aseptic necrosis of the femoral head, and the sequelae of the condition as a whole.

CLINICAL CONSIDERATIONS

Incidence.—The most common causes of traumatic disruption of the hip joint are traumata sustained in the course of skiing or other athletic activities, but particularly as a result of motor vehicle accidents. In respect to the latter, one is usually dealing with the effect of a so-called "dashboard injury." In a dashboard injury, the knee of the affected limb is propelled with great force against the dashboard, and if the thigh is in a position of adduction, the likelihood of a dislocation is considerable. Traumatic dislocations at the hip joint, with or without fractures involving that joint, constituted 7.3 per cent of all the dislocations treated in the Surgical Clinic of the University of Zurich during the years 1919 to 1958 (see Germann and also Eberle). In the estimate made by Brav, traumatic dislocation at the hip joint comprised about 5 per cent of all traumatic dislocations. His study represented a statistical evaluation of pertinent cases treated in United States Army hospitals during the 12 years from 1947 through 1958. In that statistical evaluation, covering 523 dislocations of the femoral head, 84.7 per cent were reported as having been caused by accidents involving civilian or military motor vehicles. In the remaining 15.3 per cent of the cases, the cause of the dislocation included such incidents as a fall from a height, an athletic injury, a blow from a falling object, the impact of an automobile, or a motorcycle crash.

As to *age incidence*, the proportion of children among subjects affected with traumatic dislocation of the femoral head is rather small. Indeed, for a long time, this condition was held to be a rarity among children, but its occurrence is apparently not so unusual as it was once thought to be. It was also formerly held that the common or typical cause of dislocation of the femoral head in a child was the impact of a heavy object falling upon the back while the child was in a crouching or squatting position. However, more recent experience has tended to minimize the importance of this mode of injury as the typical one in the causation of the condition in children. Other accidents which have been shown to be responsible for the injury in individual children include: falls from some height; falls incurred while running or while riding a bicycle or tricycle; or a trauma sustained when the subject was struck by an automobile or some other type of vehicle (see Choyce, Goldenberg, Morton, and also Freeman). It has also been maintained that a slighter trauma is sufficient to cause the dislocation of the femoral head in children than is required in adults (see Glass and Powell, and also Donaldson *et al.*).

Clinical Findings and Complications.—In the course of traumatic disruption of the hip joint in any particular case, the head of the femur may merely be dislodged from the acetabulum and dislocated, sometimes anteriorly but much more often posteriorly. The proportion of anterior to posterior dislocations is about 1 to 10. With a posterior dislocation of the femoral head, detachment of one or more fracture fragments from the posterior rim of the acetabulum may also occur. Furthermore, the head of the femur, instead of being dislocated from the acetabulum, may be driven in toward the pelvic cavity as a result of a fracture (sometimes comminuted) of the acetabular floor (central dislocation). Again, the disruption of the hip joint may have led to a combination of the pathologic changes cited, including, for instance, fracture of the rim of the acetabulum along with the floor of the acetabulum, and even a fracture of the dislocated femoral head (see Armstrong and also Thompson and Epstein). Mention should also be made of the fact that if, in the course of a traumatic incident, a fracture of the femoral shaft has occurred and a dislocation at the hip joint has taken place at the same time, the presence of the dislocation may be temporarily overlooked because attention has been concentrated upon the fracture (see Helal and Skevis).

The immediate and late complications of the disruption of the hip joint depend upon the severity of the disruption, the promptness with which the dislocation of the femoral head is corrected (by closed and/or open reduction), and the removal or refixation of any fracture fragments, especially of the acetabulum. The most serious early complication is injury to the sciatic nerve, resulting in some degree of *sciatic palsy*. This occurs in about 10 to 15 per cent of the cases, and is nearly always caused by damage to the nerve from the displaced femoral head or possibly from a displaced fracture fragment. If the pressure on the nerve is not promptly released, recovery from the paralysis may fail to take place.

Next in importance as a complication is *ischemic necrosis of the femoral head*. The incidence of the necrosis depends upon whether the femoral head is merely dislocated (anteriorly or posteriorly), or whether the dislocation is associated with fracture of the rim and/or floor of the acetabulum, and also upon whether the femoral head itself has been fractured. A very important additional factor is certainly the time interval between the occurrence of the dislocation and its reduction. Of course, necrosis of the femoral head is least likely to occur (and probably rarely occurs) when one is dealing with cases of mere anterior dislocation of the femoral head (uncomplicated by fracture or fractures of the acetabulum) and when the reduction of the dislocation is carried out within about 6 to 8 hours of its occurrence. The incidence of ischemic necrosis of the femoral head rises sharply when the dislocation is posterior and is associated with fracture or fractures of the acetabular rim and/or floor. Necrosis of the femoral head is almost certain to occur if the dislocated head has also undergone a fracture. The crucial baleful effect of the aseptic necrosis of the femoral head following upon a traumatic dislocation is collapse of the head if the subject is permitted to bear weight upon the affected limb before substantial repair of the necrosis has had a chance to take place.

One of the postdislocation complications frequently mentioned in the earlier literature is the appearance of a focus of *myositis ossificans*, but the incidence of this occurrence is minimized in the more recent literature.

Some degree of *osteoarthritis* is a common sequela in cases of traumatic dislocation of the femoral head, even if the dislocation is not associated with a fracture either of the acetabulum or of the head. However, the incidence of postdislocation arthritis is definitely higher in cases in which there has been a complicating fracture, and is highest if the fracture involves the floor of the acetabulum.

ROENTGENOGRAPHIC AND PATHOLOGIC FINDINGS

In our consideration of traumatic disruption of the hip joint, we are concerned principally, as already indicated, with the changes occurring in the femoral head,

Figure 164

A, Roentgenograph revealing, in the head of the left femur, the alterations following upon a dislocation at the hip joint. The dislocation, which occurred about 1 year before this roentgenograph was taken, was the result of an injury sustained while the subject (a man of 27) was playing football. In the course of that traumatic incident, he also sustained injury to his left knee and the lower part of his back. The immediate disability was so severe that he had to be carried from the playing field. He gave no clear indication of the time interval between the accident and the reduction of the dislocation, but stated that he remained in bed for about 8 weeks. Although no roentgenograph taken shortly after the accident was available for examination at the time of his admission to our hospital, it seems highly probable that it was a posterior dislocation that he had suffered, since he indicated that he had also sustained a fracture, presumably of the acetabulum. Note the rather well-delineated and somewhat depressed segment of the femoral head, representing that part of the head which is still completely necrotic. The roentgenograph also shows that the hip joint is already the site of an osteoarthritis, which is indicated by the presence of marginal exostoses, especially in relation to the femoral head.

B, Photograph illustrating the appearance of the cut surface of the femoral head in this case, the head having been resected and replaced by a prosthesis about 3 months after the roentgenograph shown in *A* was taken (about 1 year and 3 months after the dislocation). That portion of the head which is still completely necrotic is clearly apparent in the upper central part of the picture. Note also that the articular cartilage, over part of its extent, is separated from the completely necrotic subchondral bone. Distal to this still-necrotic area, revascularization and some repair of the necrosis has been taking place.

C, Roentgenograph of the portion of the femoral head which is shown in *B*. Note that the deep surface of the articular cartilage, where the latter is separated from the necrotic subchondral bone, has a thin layer of necrotic bone adherent to it.

D, Roentgenograph of a thin slice cut from the part of the femoral head represented roentgenographically in *C*. The details visible in *C* stand out even more clearly here. The area demarcated by the arrows corresponds to that represented by the photomicrograph shown in *E*.

E, Photomicrograph ($\times$ 4) of a tissue section prepared from part of the thin slice of femoral head illustrated in *D* and, specifically, from the area indicated by the arrows. One can see, on the left, that the articular cartilage is not separated from the necrotic subchondral bone, while on the right it is so separated and has adherent to it some fragments of necrotic bone. It is also evident that fibrous connective tissue is interposed between the necrotic subchondral bone and the deeper-lying portion of the head which has already undergone repair. This zone of fibrous tissue is represented by the narrow, irregular radiolucent area present in *D* between the still-necrotic portion and the reconstructed portion of the femoral head. Where substantial repair has occurred (see the lower left part of this photomicrograph), the spongy trabeculae are thick and even closely compacted, and this, too, stands out well in the roentgenograph (see *D*).

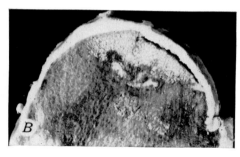

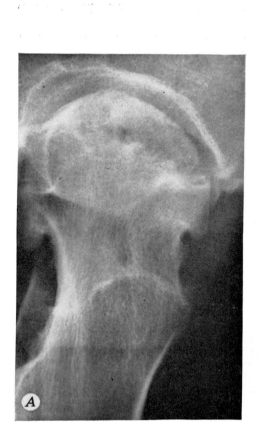

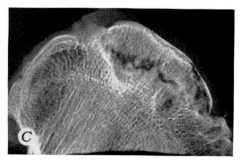

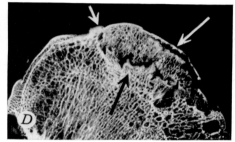

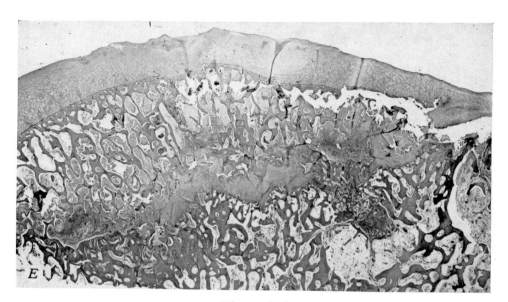

Figure 164

and specifically with the manifestations of ischemic necrosis. It is well recognized that if one is dealing merely with an anterior dislocation which has been reduced rather promptly, there is little likelihood that necrosis of the femoral head will develop. With a posterior dislocation, on the other hand, necrosis of the femoral head is to be expected, especially when the dislocation is associated with a fracture of the rim or floor of the acetabulum, and particularly when there has been a delay in the reduction of the dislocation and also of the fracture of the acetabular rim, if one has occurred. (See Fig. 164.)

If the dislocated femoral head does undergo ischemic necrosis, it is because the local blood supply is compromised at the time of the dislocation, and in consequence the necrosis of the osseous tissue and bone marrow of the head ensues. The blood supply to the femoral head is derived from arteries which enter the head by way of the round ligament and, more importantly, from branches of the lateral and medial circumflex arteries which are present in the joint capsule. As is well known, reflec-

Figure 165

A, Roentgenograph showing aseptic necrosis and collapse of the capital epiphysis of the right femur in the case of a boy 13 years of age who, a year before, had suffered an injury to the hip joint on that side. The trauma was a fall of 8 to 10 feet. Immediately after the accident he was hospitalized (at another institution) because he was unable to walk or put weight on the right limb. He remained in that hospital for 2½ months. On discharge, he was free from complaints for about 3 weeks, but then began to experience pain in the hip joint and walked with a limp. Insofar as we could ascertain, he had not suffered a dislocation. The roentgenographic changes, which suggest those of Legg-Perthes disease, are apparently attributable to aseptic necrosis resulting from the direct trauma to the hip.

B and *D*, Roentgenograph (*B*) of one of the thin slices into which the resected head and part of the neck of the femur had been cut, and photograph (*D*) of the cut surface of this slice, enlarged about 2½ ×. The roentgenograph and the photograph of this tissue slice complement each other in regard to the pathologic changes which they illustrate. Note that the articular cartilage covering the right half of the tissue slice has become separated from the underlying bone. On the right in the photograph, part of the femoral head appears white. The area in question represents a portion of the femoral head which has not yet undergone revascularization and which is hence still completely necrotic. Microscopic examination of a tissue section which included this area showed that bone cells were absent from the bone cell lacunae of the spongy trabeculae, and that the marrow in the intertrabecular spaces was completely necrotic. The osseous tissue of the femoral head, immediately to the left of the completely necrotic focus, is composed of close-meshed spongiosa. Microscopic examination of a tissue section which also included this area revealed that the osseous tissue consisted of thick spongy trabeculae and that most of this osseous tissue was viable. The spongy trabeculae had become thickened through new bone deposition on the pre-existing necrotic trabeculae, and the necrotic osseous tissue had been largely resorbed by so-called "creeping replacement." In the viable osseous tissue of the trabeculae, practically all the bone cell lacunae showed the presence of osteocytes. Microscopic examination of the epiphysial cartilage plate area revealed that endochondral ossification was in progress on the surface of the plate where the latter abutted on the femoral neck.

C and *E*, Roentgenograph (*C*) of another of the thin slices into which the resected head and part of the neck of the femur had been cut, and photograph (*E*) of the cut surface of this slice, enlarged about 2½ ×. Again, the roentgenograph and photograph of this tissue slice complement each other in regard to the pathologic changes which they illustrate. Note that the articular cartilage covering the left half of the tissue slice has become separated from the underlying bone. In the photograph it can be seen that a portion of the femoral head (a roundish focus) is still necrotic, and this necrotic area also stands out in the companion roentgenograph (*C*). Immediately to the right of this portion of the necrotic head, the spongy bone is rather thickened and compacted, in consequence of revascularization and repair. This reconstructed area of the femoral head appears in the companion roentgenograph as an area of increased radiodensity. (See also Fig. 166.)

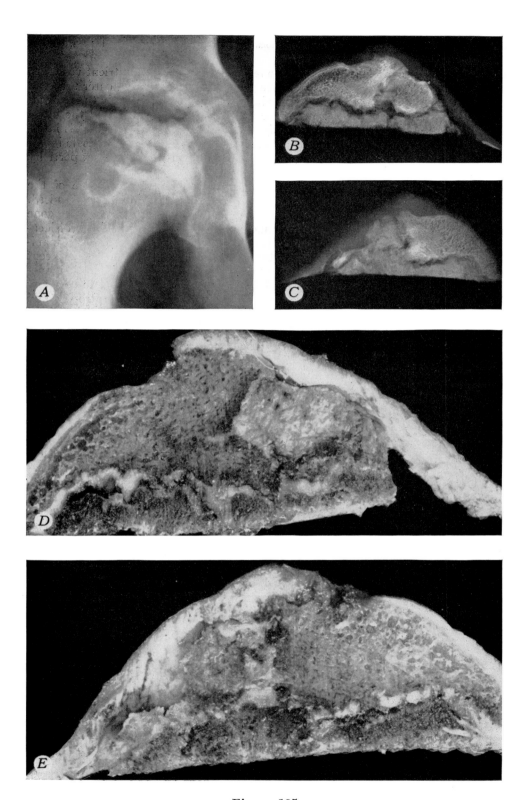

Figure 165

tions of the joint capsule extend onto the femoral neck, and the nutrient vessels in the capsular reflections on the femoral neck extend along the neck, enter the head at the head-neck junction, and are the main source of the blood supply to the head. When the femoral head is dislocated, the round ligament is torn, and the blood supply to the head which would normally come from the round ligament is interrupted. Furthermore, when the femoral head is dislocated, the joint capsule is also commonly torn, and the blood supply to the head is likely to be at least partially interrupted on this account also.

Anatomic examination of the dislocated head would reveal evidence of the ischemic necrosis shortly after the blood supply to the head had been compromised. However, roentgenographic indications that the femoral head has undergone necrosis are usually not apparent until some months have elapsed after the dislocation took place. Roentgenographic evidence of the presence of necrosis is manifested by differences in radiodensity between the necrotic head and the adjacent viable bone of the femoral shaft and the pelvis. Since the affected limb is immobilized, and the patient, even if not confined to bed, is not permitted to bear any weight on that limb, the viable osseous tissue undergoes disuse atrophy and becomes relatively more radiolucent. On the other hand, the necrotic part of the head, which has not yet undergone revascularization, retains its normal radiodensity or is even abnormally radiopaque. That is, the necrotic part of the head presents normal or increased radiodensity, thus standing out from the adjacent viable osseous tissue, which shows reduced radiodensity (see Phemister and also Banks).

If strict deloading of the affected hip is maintained over a period of about 6 months, through the use of crutches or a brace, substantial regeneration and revivification of the necrotic femoral head may be expected to become evident roentgenographically. It is also recognized that the likelihood of attaining a substantial or even complete reconstruction of the femoral head is much greater in a child than in an adult, especially if the latter is of middle age or older. On the other hand, if, after a period of only a month or two of immobilization of the limb, the bearing of weight upon it is allowed because there is already a good range of motion and the subject is free from pain, there is a possibility that, sooner or later, the still-devitalized head will collapse. Under such circumstances the affected femoral head is often irreparably damaged, and the hip joint may become the site of a seriously incapacitating osteoarthritis.

Occasionally, in a child, a severe trauma to the region of the hip may be followed by ischemic necrosis of the femoral head, even in the absence of a dislocation. A case in point observed by the writer is illustrated in Figures 165 and 166. A similar case has been reported and illustrated by Pich.

Figure 166

A and B, Roentgenograph (A) of another of the thin slices into which the head and neck of the femur from the case illustrated in Figure 165 had been cut. The articular cartilage on the left side of the picture is separated from the underlying bone. As is shown in the photograph (B) of this slice, immediately beneath the loosened articular cartilage a rather clearly delimited necrotic portion of the femoral head can be seen. Just to the right of the area of necrosis, the spongy trabeculae of the femoral head are close-meshed, indicating that revascularization and repair of the necrosis has been going on.

C, Photomicrograph ($\times$ 5) which supplements the gross pathologic findings demonstrated by B. The completely necrotic portion of the head is present on the left. The intertrabecular marrow spaces in this area are filled with granular detritus. The thickened and more compacted spongy trabeculae apparent in B to the right of the area of necrosis likewise stand out well in the photomicrograph.

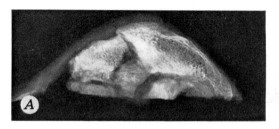

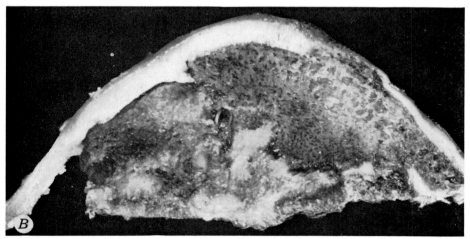

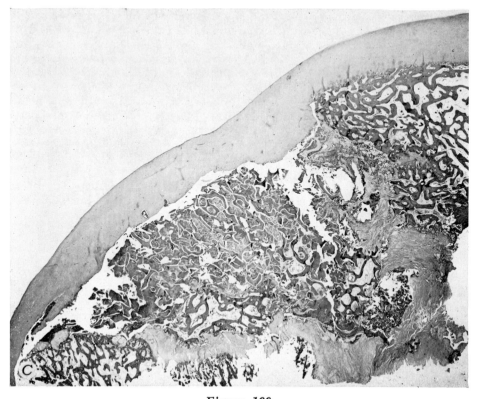

Figure 166

TREATMENT

As already indicated, the best results are to be expected in cases in which the dislocation of the femoral head is not associated with a fracture, and the outlook for complete recovery is most favorable when one is dealing merely with an anterior dislocation of the femoral head. In cases in which the dislocation of the femoral head is not associated with a fracture (uncomplicated dislocation), closed reduction of the dislocation as soon as possible (preferably within a few hours) after the accident is the treatment of choice.

The prospects for complete recovery are unfavorable when the dislocation is associated with a fracture, and the prognosis is particularly poor if the fracture involves the floor of the acetabulum. In these cases the aims of treatment are: to reduce the dislocation; to refix any large fracture fragments; and to remove any small loose fracture fragments which cannot be reattached. To accomplish these aims, surgical exploration of the joint is, of course, necessary. The specific object is to correct incongruity of the articular surfaces, in the hope of avoiding the ultimate development of a disabling osteoarthritis. Despite all precautions, the dislocation of the femoral head (with or without associated fractures) may result in collapse of the head and the ultimate development of an incapacitating post-traumatic arthritis of the hip joint.

FRACTURE OF THE FEMORAL NECK

Fractures involving the proximal end of the femur may be subclassified into two groups: (1) fractures of the actual anatomic neck of the femur, and (2) fractures involving the trochanters. Those implicating the actual anatomic neck (intracapsular fractures) may be located just below the head (subcapital fractures) or may extend across the neck at a site more or less distal to the head (transcervical fractures). Fractures involving the trochanters (extracapsular or pertrochanteric fractures) may be further classified on the basis of the fracture line as follows: (1) those in which the fracture line extends obliquely through the trochanters; (2) those which, in addition to the oblique fracture line, show some comminuted fracture fragments; and (3) those which extend more or less transversely across the respective distal ends of the trochanters. It is in connection with subcapital and transcervical fractures that ischemic necrosis and late segmental collapse of the femoral head represents a fairly common complication. Therefore our primary concern in this section of the chapter will be with fractures of the actual anatomic neck of the femur.

CLINICAL CONSIDERATIONS

The special aspects of fractures involving the femoral neck include: (1) the high incidence of the condition among elderly persons (mainly women); (2) the frequency with which a relatively slight injury (or mere functional trauma) suffices to cause the fracture in women manifesting postmenopausal osteoporosis; (3) the likelihood of inadequate union or even nonunion of the fracture, particularly if the fracture fragments are not impacted and have not been properly aligned and kept in alignment by internal fixation; and (4) the rather grave danger of ultimate collapse of the weight-bearing segment of the femoral head in consequence of inadequate repair of the ischemic necrosis ensuing upon the fracture.

Incidence.—Fractures of the femoral neck are occasionally encountered in children and, somewhat more often, in young adults. However, they occur predominantly in elderly persons—more commonly in women than in men. In respect to *age*, about half of the patients are 70 years of age or older. In regard to *sex* the proportion of women to men among patients with fractures of the neck of the femur is about 3 to 1. This ratio increases with advancing age of the patients. On the basis of large statistical compilations, it also is evident that the incidence of fractures of the femoral neck is, on the whole, somewhat higher than that for pertrochanteric fractures. However, the ratio of femoral neck (intracapsular) fractures to pertrochanteric (extracapsular) fractures tends to vary with the age of the subjects. In particular, with advancing age—that is, in subjects over 70 years and especially over 80 years of age—the proportion of extracapsular to intracapsular fractures tends to rise, the former even coming to exceed the latter. (See Nyström, Spotoft, Odén, and also Leikkonen.)

Precipitating Factors.—In this discussion of fractures involving the proximal end of the femur, we are not, of course, concerned with so-called pathologic fractures— that is, with fractures occurring at the site of a tumor (primary or metastatic) or occurring in a bone area whose viability has been lowered by external or internal radiation. In elderly persons, especially women, a subcapital fracture of the femoral neck or a fracture of the neck more distal to the head frequently follows upon a trivial injury. The slight trauma in question often occurs during walking and may consist merely of a slip or misstep, or a sudden twist of the pelvis while the lower extremity is stationary and the foot is more or less fixed to the floor or ground. Under these circumstances the subject falls, but actually the fall occurs because a fracture has already taken place, instead of being the cause of the fracture. On the other hand, in some cases a fracture follows upon a definite trauma to the part, incurred in the course of a fall. In the latter cases the structural weakness of the neck of the femur may have been due only to the presence of some degree of osteoporosis before the fracture occurred. However, in those older subjects in whom a subcapital fracture follows upon a trivial injury (a misstep, for instance), a stress fracture may already have been present. The stress fracture is represented by a line of cleavage extending from the proximal cortical surface of the neck across the local spongy trabeculae to the inferior cortex of the neck. As long as the fracture line does not extend through the inferior cortex of the neck, and the dissolution of continuity of the spongy trabeculae has not occurred in depth, there may be no displacement along the line of cleavage, and the stress fracture may even undergo spontaneous healing. It is when the inferior cortex of the neck is actually fractured that the cleavage line is complete and separation of the fracture fragments takes place (see Garden).

In relation to stress (or fatigue) fractures of the femoral neck, it should be noted that these are also known to take place even in youthful subjects. There have been several reports on their occurrence in young men undergoing basic military training. Furthermore, it is not at all unlikely that occasionally a stress fracture of the neck of the femur occurs in other youthful subjects who are subjecting themselves to what, for them, is exceptional physical exertion. (See Watson and Berkman, Ernst, Devas, and also Blickenstaff and Morris.)

Clinical Complaints and Findings.—The clinical manifestations to be noted in subjects with fractures of the femoral neck naturally vary in accordance with the recency of the fracture and the amount of displacement of the fracture ends. Immediately after the occurrence of the fracture, there is considerable pain in the region of the groin (or pain referred to the thigh and knee). Movement of the extremity is restricted by the pain and muscle spasm, and, if the fracture fragments are displaced, the pain and muscle spasm are likely to be so severe that movement of the extremity cannot be endured and walking even with a support is impossible. Under these conditions it may be noted that the affected extremity is short in relation to the opposite one, and that it is in a position of external rotation. On the other hand, if the fracture fragments are not displaced, some movement at the hip joint is tolerable, since pain and spasm are likely to become evident only at the extremes of motion. Also, if the fracture fragments are impacted, use of the limb is possible. The subject walks with a limp and also needs some support. However, days or weeks may elapse before medical care is sought and the presence of the fracture is discovered.

As is generally recognized, a fracture of the femoral neck is almost regularly followed by more or less complete ischemic necrosis of the femoral head, due to interruption of its blood supply. Even though the femoral head becomes necrotic, a definite majority of the fractures treated by internal fixation unite, undergoing sound bony union, sometimes within a few months. During the same period, the necrotic head is usually undergoing revascularization and repair. However, the repair of the necrotic femoral head usually lags far behind the healing of the fracture of the neck. Therefore it is not surprising that collapse of the upper, weight-bearing segment of the femoral head constitutes a fairly common ultimate complication of fractures of the femoral neck. This complication often does not develop until about $1\frac{1}{2}$ years after the occurrence of the fracture, and sometimes appears 2 years or more after the fracture (see Catto). The patient may have been ambulatory and free of pain for months before the segmental collapse of the femoral head

Figure 167

A, Roentgenograph showing the hip joint and proximal end of the left femur in the case of a woman 43 years of age who had sustained a fracture of the neck of the femur 2 years previously. She came under care for the fracture at another hospital, where the treatment consisted of internal fixation, a Smith-Petersen nail having been inserted. About 2 years after the internal fixation of the fracture, she was admitted to our hospital with the complaint of pain and stiffness in the hip of 6 months' duration. The Smith-Petersen nail was removed, and an obturator neurectomy was performed for the relief of the pain. This relief was achieved, but was temporary. The patient was readmitted about 1 year later because of return of the pain. This roentgenograph, taken at the time of her readmission, reveals that a rather large, wedge-shaped section of the femoral head is still necrotic. The femoral head was resected and replaced by a prosthesis.

B, Roentgenograph of a thick slice cut in the longitudinal plane from the resected head. The orientation is the same as in the clinical roentgenograph. Part of the articular cartilage and a narrow rim of necrotic subchondral bone can be seen to have separated from the rest of the head. The delimited area of necrosis shown in the clinical roentgenograph is again apparent, though less striking. On the right, the articular surface of the head shows a small marginal exostosis.

C, Photograph of the cut surface of the femoral head illustrated in *B*. For orientation, it should be noted, however, that this picture represents a mirror image in relation to the changes shown in *A* and *B*. (That is, the right and left are the opposite of what they are in *A* and *B*.) The large, necrotic area of the femoral head stands out clearly, as does the detached articular cartilage and the adherent narrow rim of necrotic subchondral bone. The small marginal exostosis apparent on the right in *B* is clearly visible on the left in this picture.

D, Photomicrograph ($\times 4\frac{1}{2}$) presenting a survey view of a tissue section prepared from a part of the specimen shown in *C*. The necrotic portion of the head shows the presence of granular detritus in the intertrabecular marrow spaces and also separation of the articular cartilage from the still-necrotic portion of the head. On the extreme left of the picture, the spongy trabeculae are thick and rather compacted. This is evidence that that portion of the femoral head has undergone revascularization and repair.

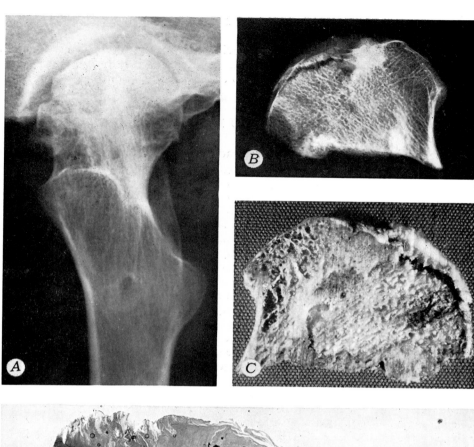
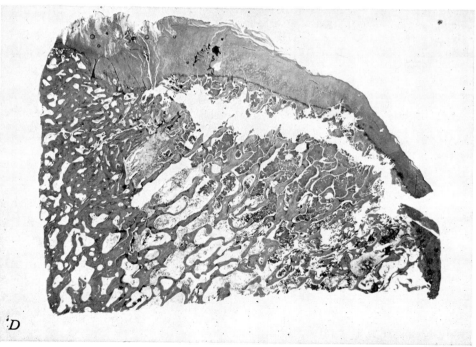

Figure 167

set in. The occurrence of the collapse is evident on roentgenographic examination of the hip. It is accompanied by pain, which increases in severity, and by progressive functional disability in relation to the affected hip joint.

ROENTGENOGRAPHIC AND PATHOLOGIC FINDINGS

Immediately after the occurrence of a fracture of the femoral neck, its presence is usually easy to demonstrate on roentgenographic examination, provided that the fracture fragments have become separated. If the fracture fragments are not displaced, a roentgenograph showing the hip in the anteroposterior projection may fail to demonstrate the fracture line. However, the latter is very likely to be apparent in pictures revealing the hip in a lateral view or in a position of rotation.

The roentgenographic and pathologic changes taking place in the femoral head after the occurrence of the fracture naturally shed light upon each other and will be considered together. (See Figs. 167 and 168.) It should be noted that the roentgenographic and pathologic changes recorded in the literature on fractures of the neck of the femur have to be considered in relation to the treatment employed for the subjects in question. A highly salutary change in the management of these cases was the introduction (about 1930) of osteosynthesis by means of a metal nail or pins. This greatly reduced the incidence of nonunion, permitted earlier ambulation of the patients, and thus obviated the occurrence of inactivity atrophy at the hip joint, previously engendered by prolonged immobilization of the patient in bed. There is no doubt that the roentgenographic and pathologic findings recorded in the earlier literature, when juxtaposed against those in the more recent literature, reflect mainly differences relating to the methods of treatment employed (see Phemister and also Sherman and Phemister).

One of the most comprehensive recent studies of the pathologic changes in the femoral head after fracture of the femoral neck was made by Catto. Her report

Figure 168

A, Photograph of the cut surface of the femoral head which was resected and replaced by a prosthesis in the case of a woman 64 years of age who had sustained a fracture of the neck of the femur 4 years previously. The fracture was treated at another hospital by internal fixation. The patient was allowed full weight-bearing about 8 months after the fracture. She stated that, since she had begun to bear weight on the injured hip again, she had never been completely free from pain in the hip, and that, in the course of the year prior to admission to our hospital, the pain had become progressively worse. Note the large, well-delineated necrotic portion of the head and the slight depression of the articular surface in that area.

B, Roentgenograph of a thick slice cut from the femoral head illustrated in *A.* The portion of the necrotic head which is somewhat depressed stands out clearly. The large radiolucent area to the right of the necrotic area represents the focus of connective tissue visible in the corresponding area in *A.*

C, Photomicrograph ($\times$ 5) presenting a survey view of part of the articular end of the femoral head in this case. On the left in this picture is an area which is still covered for the most part by intact articular cartilage, though the subchondral bone can be seen to be completely necrotic (see *D*). On the right, there are indications that reparative changes have been taking place in the necrotic subchondral bone.

D, Photomicrograph ($\times$ 25) showing in greater detail the histologic features presented by the area blocked out in *C.* The intertrabecular marrow spaces contain granular detritus. On the extreme right in the picture there is also some evidence of fragmentation and disintegration of the necrotic spongy trabeculae.

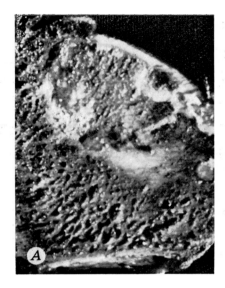

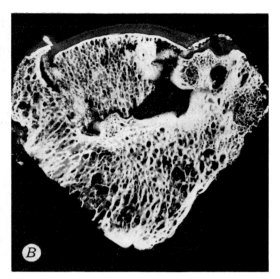

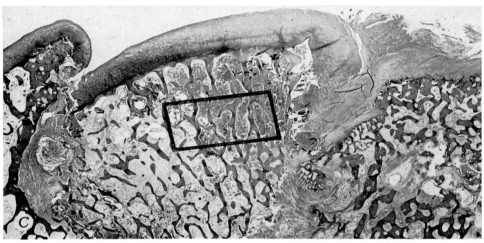

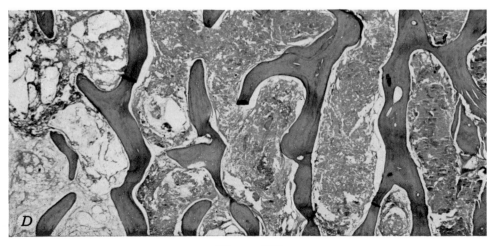

Figure 168

655

was based on findings relating to 168 femoral heads. Of these, 59 were obtained (through surgery or at necropsy) from cases in which the fracture had taken place within 16 days before the removal of the head. The remaining 109 femoral heads had been obtained (through surgery or at necropsy) from cases in which the fracture had taken place more than 16 days before the head was removed. Though fracture of the femoral neck usually leads to partial or even complete ischemic necrosis of the femoral head, there are some cases in which the finding of necrosis is limited to the fracture line. In those rarer cases in which the femoral head had remained viable, the head continued to be nourished by blood vessels of the ligamentum teres and sometimes by retinacular arteries, usually of the inferior group.

As pointed out by Catto and also by Barnes, the earliest histologic indication of the ischemia, as shown in the femoral heads removed within 16 days after the fracture, was necrosis of the hematopoietic and fatty components of the inter-trabecular marrow. However, in respect to loss of viability of the osseous tissue itself, it was observed that osteocytes were rarely completely absent from the bone cell lacunae of the trabeculae until 3 or 4 weeks after the fracture had occurred.

Despite these early histologic changes, the roentgenographic shadow cast by the head is not likely to show any deviation from the normal for several months after the occurrence of the fracture. The minimal time elapsing between the fracture and the appearance of the first related roentgenographic alterations is about 2 months, but in some cases the interval may be a few months longer. The initial modification visible roentgenographically is focal or more or less widespread increased radiopacity of the femoral head. This is evident only if the necrotic head is being revascularized and is undergoing repair, and the increased radiopacity shows up specifically where this has been taking place. Where the femoral head reveals increased radiopacity, the latter is mainly the result of thickening of the necrotic (nonviable) pre-existing spongy trabeculae, due to the deposition of new bone upon them in the course of the repair (see Hulth, Bohr and Larsen, Coleman and Compere, and also Catto).

The revascularization of the necrotic head occurs by way of: the vessels entering it from the ligamentum teres; any retinacular vessels that have not been disrupted— especially those of the inferior retinaculum; and blood vessels entering the head from the femoral neck, especially after union of the fracture fragments. In the course of revascularization, vascular granulation tissue comes to permeate the intertrabecular marrow spaces of the femoral head. In consequence, micro-scopic examination reveals a varied histologic picture characterized by: resorption of some of the osseous tissue composing the spongy trabeculae; concomitant deposi-tion of newly formed osseous tissue on the surface of some of the necrotic trabeculae; and the formation of loose-meshed fiber bone in the osteogenetic connective tissue which has developed in the spongy marrow spaces (see Sevitt).

It is because new bone deposition is in ascendancy over resorption during the early phases of repair of the necrotic femoral head that focal or more or less wide-spread increased radiopacity is usually the initial change observable roentgeno-graphically. Later, areas of radiolucency make their appearance in the head. They are found intermingled with the more radiopaque areas, so that the necrotic head in the process of revascularization presents a mottled appearance roentgenograph-ically. The areas of distinct radiolucency are the sites where considerable amounts of the osseous tissue of the head have been resorbed and replaced by fibrous tissue.

Collapse of the upper, weight-bearing segment of the femoral head (late seg-mental collapse) seems to occur because repair of the necrosis through the agency of blood vessels entering the head by way of the ligamentum teres has failed to take place. Altogether, the revascularization and repair of the upper segment of the necrotic femoral head tends to lag behind repair of the rest of the head. When collapse of the upper, weight-bearing segment of the femoral head occurs, the roentgenograph usually reveals a somewhat triangular area whose articular surface is depressed in relation to the contour of the rest of the femoral head. As Catto and others have pointed out, segmental collapse of the incompletely revitalized femoral head may occur despite the fact that the fracture of the femoral neck has healed. Also, the segmental collapse often does not take place until about $1\frac{1}{2}$ years after the occurrence of the fracture, and sometimes even later.

REFERENCES

ARMSTRONG, J. R.: Traumatic Dislocation of the Hip Joint, J. Bone & Joint Surg., *30-B*, 430, 1948.

BANKS, S. W.: Aseptic Necrosis of the Femoral Head Following Traumatic Dislocation of the Hip, J. Bone & Joint Surg., *23*, 753, 1941.

BARNES, R.: The Diagnosis of Ischaemia of the Capital Fragment in Femoral Neck Fractures, J. Bone & Joint Surg., *44-B*, 760, 1962.

——————: Fracture of the Neck of the Femur, J. Bone & Joint Surg., *49-B*, 607, 1967.

BLICKENSTAFF, L. D., and MORRIS, J. M.: Fatigue Fracture of the Femoral Neck, J. Bone & Joint Surg., *48-A*, 1031, 1966.

BOHR, H., and LARSEN, E. H.: On Necrosis of the Femoral Head after Fracture of the Neck of the Femur, J. Bone & Joint Surg., *47-B*, 330, 1965.

BRAV, E. A.: Traumatic Dislocation of the Hip, J. Bone & Joint Surg., *44-A*, 1115, 1962.

CATTO, M.: A Histological Study of Avascular Necrosis of the Femoral Head after Transcervical Fracture, J. Bone & Joint Surg., *47-B*, 749, 1965.

——————: The Histological Appearances of Late Segmental Collapse of the Femoral Head after Transcervical Fracture, J. Bone & Joint Surg., *47-B*, 777, 1965.

CHANDLER, F. A.: Observations on Circulatory Changes in Bone, Am. J. Roentgenol., *44*, 90, 1940.

——————: Coronary Disease of the Hip, J. Internat. Coll. Surgeons, *11*, 34, 1948.

CHOYCE, C. C.: Traumatic Dislocation of the Hip in Childhood, and Relation of Trauma to Pseudocoxalgia: Analysis of 59 Cases Published up to January, 1924, Brit. J. Surg., *12*, 52, 1924.

CLAFFEY, T. J.: Avascular Necrosis of the Femoral Head, J. Bone & Joint Surg., *42-B*, 802, 1960.

COLEMAN, S. S., and COMPERE, C. L.: Femoral Neck Fractures: Pathogenesis of Avascular Necrosis, Nonunion and Late Degenerative Changes, Clinical Orthopaedics, *20*, 247, 1961.

CROCK, H. V.: A Revision of the Anatomy of the Arteries Supplying the Upper End of the Human Femur, J. Anat., *99*, 77, 1965.

DEVAS, M. B.: Stress Fractures of the Femoral Neck, J. Bone & Joint Surg., *47-B*, 728, 1965.

DONALDSON, W. F., JR., RODRIQUEZ, E. E., SKOVRON, M., and GARTLAND, J. J.: Traumatic Dislocation of the Hip Joint in Children, J. Bone & Joint Surg., *50-A*, 79, 1968.

DUSE, G., LANZETTA, A., and PARRINI, L.: Necrosi idiopatica della testa femorale, Arch. ortop., *78*, 301, 1963.

EBERLE, H.: Traumatische Hüftgelenksluxation und Femurkopfnekrose, Schweiz. med. Wchnschr., *95*, 326, 1965.

ERNST, J.: Stress Fracture of the Neck of the Femur, J. Trauma, *4*, 71, 1964.

FREEMAN, G. E., JR.: Traumatic Dislocation of the Hip in Children, J. Bone & Joint Surg., *43-A*, 401, 1961.

FREUND, E.: Zur Frage der aseptischen Knochennekrose, Virchows Arch. path. Anat., *261*, 287, 1926.

GARDEN, R. S.: The Structure and Function of the Proximal End of the Femur, J. Bone & Joint Surg., *43-B*, 576, 1961.

——————: Low-angle Fixation in Fractures of the Femoral Neck, J. Bone & Joint Surg., *43-B*, 647, 1961.

GERMANN, W.: Über die traumatischen Luxationen und Luxationsfrakturen des Hüftgelenkes, Helvet. chir. acta, *28*, 672, 1961.

GLASS, A., and POWELL, H. D. W.: Traumatic Dislocation of the Hip in Children, J. Bone & Joint Surg., *43-B*, 29, 1961.

GOLDENBERG, R. R.: Traumatic Dislocation of the Hip Followed by Perthes' Disease, J. Bone & Joint Surg., *20*, 770, 1938.

HASTINGS, D. E., and MACNAB, I.: Spontaneous Avascular Necrosis of the Femoral Head, Canad. J. Surg., *8*, 68, 1965.

HEIMANN, W. G., and FREIBERGER, R. H.: Avascular Necrosis of the Femoral and Humeral Heads after High-Dosage Corticosteroid Therapy, New England J. Med., *263*, 672, 1960.

HELAL, B., and SKEVIS, X.:   Unrecognised Dislocation of the Hip in Fractures of the Femoral
    Shaft, J. Bone & Joint Surg., 49-B, 293, 1967.
HULTH, A.:   Necrosis of the Head of the Femur, Acta chir. scandinav., 122, 75, 1961.
JUDET, J., JUDET, R., LAGRANGE, J., and DUNOYER, J.:   A Study of the Arterial Vascularization
    of the Femoral Neck in the Adult, J. Bone & Joint Surg., 37-A, 663, 1955.
LEIKKONEN, O.:   Fractures in the Femoral Neck, Ann. chir. et gynaec. Fenniae, 51, Suppl. 110,
    1962.
MANKIN, H. J., and BROWER, T. D.:   Bilateral Idiopathic Aseptic Necrosis of the Femur in
    Adults: "Chandler's Disease," Bull. Hosp. Joint Dis., 23, 42, 1962.
MERLE D'AUBIGNÉ, R., POSTEL, M., MAZABRAUD, A., MASSIAS, P., and GUEGUEN, J.:   Idiopathic
    Necrosis of the Femoral Head in Adults, J. Bone & Joint Surg., 47-B, 612, 1965.
MORTON, K. S.:   Traumatic Dislocation of the Hip in Children, Brit. J. Surg., 47, 233, 1959.
NYSTRÖM, G.:   Further Experiences with Osteosynthesis of Medial Fractures of the Femoral
    Neck with the Aid of Three Nails ("Multiple Nailing"), Acta chir. scandinav., 107, 89, 1954.
ODÉN, G.:   Final Results of Osteosynthesis of Fractures of the Femoral Neck ad Modum Sven
    Johansson, Acta chir. scandinav., Suppl. 131, 1947.
PATTERSON, R. J., BICKEL, W. H., and DAHLIN, D. C.:   Idiopathic Avascular Necrosis of the
    Head of the Femur, J. Bone & Joint Surg., 46-A, 267, 1964.
PHEMISTER, D. B.:   Fractures of Neck of Femur, Dislocations of Hip, and Obscure Vascular
    Disturbances Producing Aseptic Necrosis of Head of Femur, Surg. Gynec. & Obst., 59, 415,
    1934.
————————: The Pathology of Ununited Fractures of the Neck of the Femur with Special
    Reference to the Head, J. Bone & Joint Surg., 21, 681, 1939.
————————: Changes in Bones and Joints Resulting from Interruption of Circulation: I. General
    Considerations and Changes Resulting from Injuries, Arch. Surg., 41, 436, 1940.
PICH, G.:   Histopathologic Study in a Case of Perthes' Disease of Traumatic Origin, Arch. Surg.,
    33, 609, 1936.
PIETROGRANDE, V., and MASTROMARINO, R.:   Osteopatia da prolungato trattamento cortisonico,
    Ortop. e traumatol., 25, 791, 1957.
SERRE, H., and SIMON, L.:   Aspects cliniques des nécroses parcellaires aseptiques primitives de la
    tête fémorale chez l'adulte, Montpellier méd., 56, 193, 1959.
————————: Le rôle de la corticothérapie dans l'ostéo-nécrose primitive de la tête fémorale
    chez l'adulte, Presse méd., 69, 1995, 1961.
SEVITT, S.:   Avascular Necrosis and Revascularisation of the Femoral Head after Intracapsular
    Fractures, J. Bone & Joint Surg., 46-B, 270, 1964.
SEVITT, S., and THOMPSON, R. G.:   The Distribution and Anastomoses of Arteries Supplying the
    Head and Neck of the Femur, J. Bone & Joint Surg., 47-B, 560, 1965.
SHERMAN, M. S., and PHEMISTER, D. B.:   The Pathology of Ununited Fractures of the Neck of
    the Femur, J. Bone & Joint Surg., 29, 19, 1947.
SPOTOFT, J.:   Osteosynthesis Colli Femoris, Copenhagen, E. Munksgaard, 1944.
SUTTON, R. D., BENEDEK, T. G., and EDWARDS, G. A.:   Aseptic Bone Necrosis and Corticosteroid
    Therapy, Arch. Int. Med., 112, 594, 1963.
THOMPSON, V. P., and EPSTEIN, H. C.:   Traumatic Dislocation of the Hip, J. Bone & Joint Surg.,
    33-A, 746, 1951.
TRUETA, J., and HARRISON, M. H. M.:   The Normal Vascular Anatomy of the Femoral Head in
    Adult Man, J. Bone & Joint Surg., 35-B, 442, 1953.
TUCKER, F. R.:   Arterial Supply to the Femoral Head and its Clinical Importance, J. Bone &
    Joint Surg., 31-B, 82, 1949.
WATSON, F. C., and BERKMAN, E. F.:   Fatigue (March) Fracture of the Femoral Neck, J. Bone
    & Joint Surg., 26, 404, 1944.

Chapter

21

Skeletal Manifestations of Decompression Sickness

Decompression sickness represents the baleful consequences of the liberation of gas bubbles (notably nitrogen) in the tissues and blood of subjects who have undergone decompression too rapidly after a period of exposure to a hyperbaric environment—that is, to an environment in which the ambient pressure was considerably above the usual atmospheric pressure. At pressures within the normal range, various gases constituting the atmosphere (mainly nitrogen, oxygen, and carbon dioxide) are in solution in the blood and body tissues in amounts corresponding to the saturation point for those pressures. In a subject who is exposed to a hyperbaric environment, greater amounts of these various gases go into solution until a state of saturation of the blood and tissues has been reached in respect to these gases at the higher pressures. The time required for saturation is not the same for all the tissues. Those which are rich in fat and have a relatively poor blood supply may require hours before the saturation point for nitrogen in particular is reached. Indeed, nitrogen is about 5 times more soluble in fat than in water, and this fact explains why a number of hours may elapse before the fatty tissues have become saturated with nitrogen. When the blood and all the tissues have become saturated with the various atmospheric gases at the new pressure, a new state of gaseous equilibrium is reached (see Walder).

If a person whose blood and tissues are saturated with the gases of the atmosphere in a high pressure environment passes too quickly from the hyperbaric environment to one of normal atmospheric pressure, the various gases come out of solution, and a state of supersaturation of the blood and tissues for the gases ensues. By ventilation, the body readily disposes of the excess of oxygen and carbon dioxide which has thus accumulated. On the other hand, the nitrogen which has come out of solution and which is not ventilated by the lungs forms bubbles. Nitrogen bubbles present in the circulating blood may act as air emboli, partially or completely blocking terminal vascular channels at a distant site or sites, and give rise to manifestations consistent with impairment of circulation at those sites. The accumulation of bubbles of nitrogen in various tissues (extravascular bubbles) is greatest in tissues rich in fat. In consequence of the extravascular pressure upon the regional blood vessels, the local blood supply may be obstructed and the baleful effects of decompression sickness be brought about in this way also.

The *acute manifestations* of decompression sickness are: (1) the *bends*, consisting of pain which may be limited to large joint areas (most often the knees) and which is not associated with systemic complaints and findings; and (2) *injury to vital organs* (central nervous system, heart, lungs, etc.) due to bubbles of nitrogen arising or lodging in these organs, the damage sometimes leading to permanent disability or even death. The *late* (or *chronic*) *skeletal aspects* of decompression sickness are observed particularly in bone sites which are rich in fatty marrow, and are the result of ischemic aseptic necrosis. These skeletal changes are commonly denoted as *caisson disease of bone*. Months or even years may elapse between the occurrence of the underlying bone infarction and the appearance of clinical and/or roentgenographic evidence of the bone necrosis.

Decompression sickness has been most frequently observed among men working in hyperbaric environments during the construction of tunnels under rivers or other bodies of water. Since the early part of this century, a large and world-wide literature has accumulated on the subject of bone infarction occurring in compressed air workers. This literature has been carefully evaluated and interpreted by McCallum and Walder (and their associates) in the light of their experience with bone lesions occurring in men engaged in the construction of the Clyde Tunnels during 1958 to 1963. Occasionally, bone lesions analogous to those occurring in caisson workers have also been noted among deep sea divers (see Dale, and also Sartor). Furthermore, such bone lesions have been found in men of a submarine crew years after they had been rescued from their submarine which had sunk in deep water. Each rescued sailor had suffered a severe attack of the bends in the course of the rescue (see James). That medical personnel directly involved in hyperbaric oxygen therapy may be subjecting themselves to the hazards of decompression sickness has been pointed out by Walder.

Evidence has also accumulated that exposure to *reduced pressures* (a hypobaric environment) sometimes results in decompression sickness, usually denoted as *"dysbarism"* when it occurs under these circumstances (see Behnke, Berry and King, Berry and Hekhuis, and also Markham). It has been observed in the course of high altitude flights and during work in low pressure chambers simulating such aeronautical conditions. Thus a pilot in flight at an altitude of 30,000 to 40,000 feet for an hour or more is exposed to dysbarism if pressurization of the cabin is not adequate. While the condition may be manifested in bends, its more serious immediate effects may consist of such neurological disturbances as unconsciousness, paresthesias, and even hemiparesis. The occurrence and actual incidence of ischemic bone necrosis similar to that encountered in caisson workers has still to be clarified in subjects who have suffered from attacks of dysbarism.

As already noted, at atmospheric pressures within the normal range, various gases constituting the atmosphere (notably nitrogen, oxygen, and carbon dioxide) are in solution in the blood and body tissues in amounts corresponding to the saturation point for these gases. The basis for the dysbarism associated with exposure to subatmospheric pressures is the liberation of these gases from the blood and the tissues, resulting in their supersaturation with these gases. Hence, bubbles of nitrogen accumulate in the tissues and in the blood and spinal fluid, and this leads to the manifestations of dysbarism. In addition, it has been maintained that in airmen who have suffered from decompression shock and have recovered, or who have died in consequence of it, there has also been embolization of liver fat to the lungs and brain (see Rait).

In this chapter the discussion of the skeletal aspects of decompression sickness will relate solely to the changes observed in the bones of men who worked in the construction of tunnels. However, it is of special interest that, in cases in which one or several bones show areas of infarction of *undetermined* origin, the changes are indistinguishable roentgenographically and anatomically from the infarcts observed in the bones (at the articular ends or in the shafts) of men who have worked under hyperbaric conditions (see Kahlstrom *et al.*). For instance, the roentgenographic and pathologic changes observed in cases of so-called *idiopathic* aseptic necrosis of the femoral head illustrate this point (p. 638). Examples of bone infarction likewise of undetermined origin but involving areas other than the femoral head are described in the following chapter (p. 674).

CLINICAL CONSIDERATIONS

Incidence.—Reported estimates of the incidence of bone infarction in compressed air workers have ranged from about 5 to 75 per cent. This wide range is understandable on the basis of: (1) differences between one project and another in respect to the procedure of decompression employed and the care with which it is carried out; and (2) statistical differences relating to the compressed air "population." In regard to the statistical differences, one must consider such factors as: the total number of men working on a particular project and the period over which they had been engaged upon it; the number of men eventually followed up by means of roentgenographic survey of their bones, in search of lesions; and the period elapsing between the time the subjects began work under compressed air and the time their bones were roentgenographed in a search for relevant bone damage. It is true that bone infarction may eventually be found in a man who has had only one exposure or only a few exposures to compressed air. It is also true that there is a relationship between the occurrence of attacks of bends and the eventual discovery of bone infarction, but experience has shown that some compressed air workers tend *not* to report mild attacks of the bends.

Individual factors which seem to favor the occurrence of bone infarcts in a compressed air worker include: relatively advanced age (over 40); obesity; and lack of regularity in the pursuit of compressed air work. In general, the incidence of bone infarction in compressed air workers is highest: (1) in groups in which the men have been engaged for a long time in work under hyperbaric conditions; (2) where the procedures for decompression have not been meticulous; and (3) where a large percentage of such workers have been examined after an interval of at least several years from the time they began work on the project. However, even under carefully controlled management of the decompressions as currently practiced, it is to be expected that evidences of caisson disease of bone will eventually be detectable on long-term follow-up in about 10 to 20 per cent of the men working for a long period on any particular tunnel project (see Walder, and also McCallum *et al.*).

Localization and Clinical Complaints.—Our knowledge relating to caisson disease of bone pertains mainly to its occurrence in long tubular bones and specifically in the femur, humerus, and tibia. In these bones the infarct may be located in the proximal or the distal part of the bone and/or in the shaft. An infarct limited to the shaft of one of these long bones is unlikely to give rise to clinical complaints. In the humerus, the infarct usually involves the proximal portion of the bone, and in the tibia also it is usually this part of the bone that is affected. In the femur, the area involved is usually the proximal portion but may be the distal portion of the bone, and sometimes both of these areas are affected.

It is when the involvement of the proximal or distal portion of the bone is associated with extension of the area of infarction to the bony end plate abutting on the deep surface of the articular cartilage that collapse of the articular surface may occur. When this happens, the affected joint becomes the site of pain and disability, and eventually a secondary osteoarthritis develops. Because of functional trauma associated with weight-bearing, the collapse of the articular surface occurs most often after infarction of the head of one or both femora. (See Fig. 169.)

ROENTGENOGRAPHIC FINDINGS

In a caisson worker, an area of bone which has become the site of ischemic aseptic necrosis may not present roentgenographic alterations indicative of caisson disease for several months or even a year or more after the necrosis has set in. This fact

43

apparently accounts in part for the differences in the details of the roentgenographic findings relating to a lesion in a given bone site in one case as compared with a lesion in the same site in another case. For instance, an area of ischemic necrosis involving an articular end of a bone (or the shaft of a bone) which was already apparent roentgenographically 6 months after the area became infarcted will probably present more striking changes 1½ years later than will lesions in similar

Figure 169

A, Roentgenograph showing the upper third of the right humerus and also the corresponding shoulder joint of a caisson worker 58 years of age. The man had been a caisson worker for 30 years and had suffered many attacks of bends. Practically the entire humeral head is the site of ischemic necrosis, as shown by the striking and more or less uniformly increased radiopacity, which clearly extends to the subchondral cortex. A small spherical focus of radiopacity can be seen in the region of the greater tuberosity, and a few such foci can also be discerned in the region of the anatomical neck of the humerus. In the upper portion of the shaft of the humerus, there are indications of ischemic necrosis, as evidenced by a small area of increased radiolucency partially demarcated by a narrow border of increased radiopacity. On its medial aspect the articular surface of the humerus is slightly flattened. This flattening is the result of local subchondral collapse of the necrotic bone. The shoulder joint in question also presents some evidence of osteoarthritis, represented by the presence of a marginal exostosis protruding from the rim of the glenoid fossa. In addition to the changes relating to the right shoulder area, as demonstrated in this picture, a roentgenographic survey of the skeleton revealed evidence of caisson disease in the upper end of the left humerus, in both hip joints, and in the lower portion of each femoral shaft.

B, Roentgenograph of the upper third of the right humerus and also the corresponding shoulder joint of a caisson worker who was 46 years of age when he was admitted to the hospital and this picture was taken. His history indicated that he had had pain in this shoulder for about 3 years. Prior to the onset of his clinical complaints, he had an attack of bends necessitating decompression. Despite his difficulties, he continued to work under compressed air, but discontinued his tunnel work about 2 years after the onset of his pain. Note that much of the humeral head shows increased radiopacity, representing the presence of ischemic necrosis. However, in addition, there are clear-cut indications that subchondral fractures have led to the delimitation of several osteochondral fragments which are still *in situ* in the necrotic humeral head.

C and *D*, Roentgenographs showing the upper third of the left and right humerus, respectively, and the corresponding shoulder joints of a caisson worker who was 55 years of age at the time these pictures were taken. He had worked for many years on various tunnel projects, and had had a number of attacks of the bends. On admission to the hospital he stated that during the previous 6 years he had been suffering from progressive pain and stiffness of both shoulders, more pronounced on the right than on the left. During this interval he also had pain and stiffness in the right hip joint, and not long before admission the left hip joint had also become painful. In *C* the roentgenographic appearances presented suggest those shown in *A*, but are much more striking. A large part of the humeral head shows radiopacity, in accordance with the presence of necrosis involving the local osseous tissue and intertrabecular marrow. On the other hand, part of the head and the region of the greater tuberosity are radiolucent, and this appearance suggests that the necrotic osseous tissue and marrow in these sites have been resorbed and the area has become cystified. An area of cystlike rarefaction is also present in the shaft cortex on the left side of the picture. The neck and the proximal part of the shaft of the bone show the presence of streaky, curlicue radiopacities constituting evidence that ischemic necrosis had occurred in the spongiosa of that region also. In *D* the roentgenographic changes are much more advanced than in *C*. This is in line with the fact that, in the shoulder in question (the right), the clinical difficulties were more severe than in the opposite shoulder. In particular, the right shoulder joint shows an advanced degree of osteoarthritis and much more pronounced evidence of ischemic necrosis in the proximal portion of the humerus.

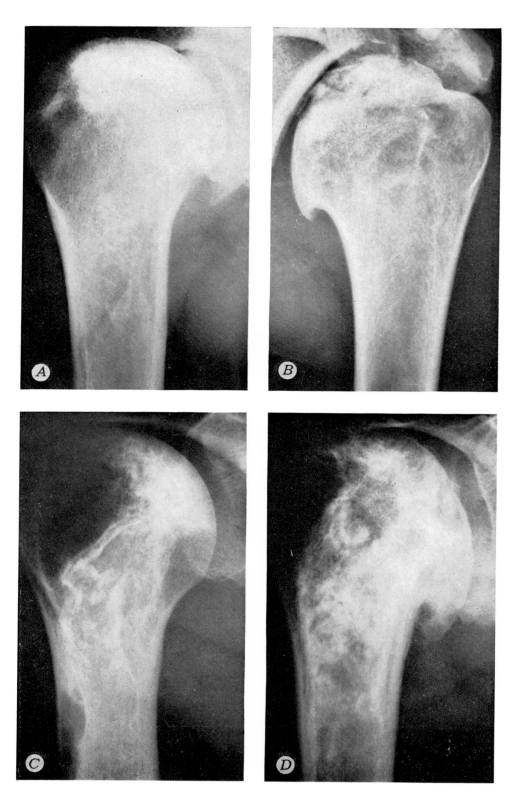

Figure 169

sites which became manifest roentgenographically only a year or so after the areas in question had become infarcted.

Insofar as the articular ends of long bones are concerned, the most striking changes are to be observed in the head of the humerus and of the femur. In one case or another, the heads of both humeri and/or both femora may be affected. In these bone sites, an early indication of infarction is the presence of a rather

Figure 170

A, Roentgenograph of the right hip joint region of a caisson worker in whom the joint had come to present an osteoarthritis in the wake of ischemic necrosis of the femoral head. The subject was 69 years of age at the time this picture was taken. He had been a caisson worker for 15 years (from the age of 36 to 51) and had suffered numerous attacks of the bends. During the years after he had stopped working on tunnel projects, he began to experience pain in various joints. In particular, the pain and associated disability related to both shoulder joints, both knee joints, and the right hip joint. A roentgenographic skeletal survey revealed that, in addition to the pathologic changes demonstrated by the illustrated right hip joint, there were evidences of ischemic necrosis involving both shoulder joints, and signs of extensive infarction of the lower portion of the shaft of each femur. (See *D* and *E*.)

B, Roentgenograph illustrating the region of the right hip joint in another caisson worker. Ischemic necrosis and structural collapse of the femoral head have taken place, and osteoarthritis has developed in consequence. The subject was 36 years of age at the time of his admission to the hospital, when this picture was taken. It was not possible to obtain satisfactory information about the period or periods during which he had been a caisson worker. The site of the fovea is indicated by the arrow, which serves as a marker permitting correlation of the roentgenographic changes present in the femoral head with the gross pathologic changes revealed by the cut surface of the head as shown in *C*. In addition to the roentgenographic alterations in the illustrated right hip joint, a skeletal survey revealed clear indications of intramedullary ischemic necrosis in the lower portions of both femoral shafts.

C, Photograph of the cut surface of the femoral head shown in *B*. The head had been resected and replaced by a prosthesis. The site of the fovea is again indicated by an arrow. The spongy osseous tissue abutting upon the fovea is close-meshed, and it is on this account that the osseous tissue in question appears rather opaque in the roentgenograph. Lateral to the fovea, the roentgenograph presents a narrow serpiginous tract of relative radiolucency. The photograph of the sectioned femoral head reveals that this tract of radiolucency is occupied by fibrous tissue. The latter marks the farthest advance of the reparative process that had been taking place in the necrotic femoral head. Distal to the tract of fibrous tissue, the spongy osseous tissue of the head is, for the most part, close-meshed, and this fact is represented in the roentgenograph by an area of relative radiopacity. Proximal to the tract of fibrous tissue, a clearly delineated ovoid focus of whitish osseous tissue can be observed. The overlying articular cartilage is separated from this ovoid focus. Microscopic examination would reveal that the area of spongy osseous tissue under consideration is composed of completely necrotic spongy trabeculae, and that the intertrabecular spaces contain necrotic marrow and considerable amounts of granular detritus.

D and *E*, Roentgenographs presenting in anterior and lateral projection, respectively, the alterations in the shaft of a femur which are characteristic of ischemic aseptic necrosis of long duration when it involves the shaft of a long bone. The roentgenographic changes in the head of this femur are illustrated in *A*, whose pertinent legend includes the essential clinical data in the case. Note that the area of infarction presents a vaguely multiloculated appearance. Some of the loculi are roundish, others are oval, and some are irregularly elongated. Many of the loculi are clearly outlined by narrow radiopaque borders. Experience with comparable infarcts of long standing in femoral shafts of persons who were not caisson workers has revealed that the radiopaque shadows outlining the loculi represent walls of calcified fibrous tissue. These develop about the necrotic spongiosa, which may have undergone resorption in some places by the time the lesional area became available for anatomic study (see Fig. 174).

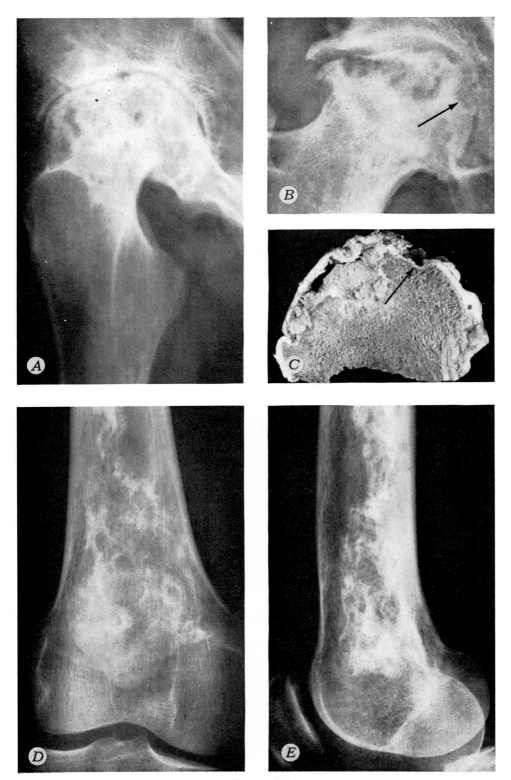

Figure 170

large subchondral area of pronounced and more or less uniform radiopacity. With further progress of the changes, the originally rather uniform radiopaque area may come to show alterations in the contour of the articular surface, due to focal collapse of the surface which is caused by the occurrence of subchondral fractures. As a result, the shadow of the necrotic humeral or femoral head will appear "fragmented." In addition, especially in relation to the humerus, there may be few or many delicate or rather thick streaks of radiopacity extending from the head into the adjacent part of the shaft. Further advance of the changes in the articular end of the humerus or femur is associated with increasingly sharp delineation of the osteochondral fragments, which appear as sequestra *in situ*. When the changes are as advanced as this, the articular cartilages of the affected shoulder or hip joint are naturally subjected to attrition. The resultant degenerative changes in the articular cartilages, and the malalignment of the articular surfaces, form the basis for the development of an osteoarthritis.

Infarcts in the shafts of the long bones affect the spongiosa and are likely to be most conspicuous in the lower part of the shaft of the femur. The ischemic necrosis of the marrow and osseous trabeculae of the spongiosa of the shaft is followed in the course of time by resorption of the necrotic marrow and osseous tissue and the formation of irregular cavities in the interior of the affected shaft. These spaces come to be lined by calcified fibrous tissue. In the roentgenographic picture the calcified fibrous tissue appears radiopaque, so that the site of the modified infarct in the shaft now casts a somewhat multiloculated shadow. (See Kahlstrom *et al.*, Deák and Rózsahegyi, Fournier and Jullien, Taylor, and also Golding.) (See Fig. 170.)

PATHOLOGIC FINDINGS

There seem to be no reports in the literature which describe the pathologic changes in the head and/or shaft of a humerus or femur in men who have died shortly after first starting work under compressed air and who, in the course of this short period of tunnel work, had suffered one or more attacks of the bends. That is, in respect to the pathologic anatomy of caisson disease of bone, we lack information relating to the gross and microscopic appearances presented by an area of recent or fresh infarction in a previously normal bone site. On the other hand, abundant anatomic material has now accumulated which reveals the late and advanced changes of caisson disease of bone. Pertinent specimens have become available, for instance, as a result of reconstructive surgery at the hip joint, necessitated by destructive changes in the femoral head. Relevant material has also been obtained in the course of autopsies. In particular, studies have been made of affected bones removed at autopsy from subjects who had worked for a long time under compressed air, but in whom the cause of death was not directly related to work under hyperbaric conditions.

It is recognized that several years may elapse after the occurrence of bone infarction in the head of the humerus and/or femur before the development of severe destructive changes (notably osteochondral fractures and collapse of the articular surface) at these bone sites. This is illustrated in the case described by Bennison *et al.* The subject in question was a man who had been employed intermittently in compressed air work for 14 years and who was 33 years of age at the time of his death, which occurred while he was under treatment for an attack of decompression sickness. Inquiry revealed that he had also suffered several attacks of bends within the period of $1\frac{1}{2}$ to 2 years before his death. At the autopsy in this case, the left humerus and right femur were removed and studied anatomically by Catto (see McCallum and Walder and their associates). Neither bone presented anything unusual in respect to contour or general external appearance. However, when these bones were sectioned longitudinally in the frontal plane, it was evident on gross examination that there were areas of necrosis in the humeral head and shaft and in the femoral head. From histologic study of tissue sections prepared from the head of the humerus and femur, it could be deduced that the extent of the necrosis must have been greater in the past. This was evident from the fact that, though considerable revascularization and repair of the necrosis had taken place, there were still cores of nonviable osseous tissue within many of the reconstructed spongy trabeculae. Though much of the head of the humerus and femur had been revascularized, a shallow zone of completely necrotic spongiosa was still present subchondrally. Between this necrotic zone and the revascularized portion of the head of the bone, there was a tract of collagenous fibrous tissue. The spongy trabeculae adjacent to this fibrous tissue in the revascularized portion of the head tended to be thick. These trabeculae showed necrotic cores, and their thickening had resulted from the deposition, in the course of revascularization and repair, of a good deal of viable osseous tissue upon the pre-existing trabeculae, which were now represented by the necrotic cores.

The time which elapsed in this case between the occurrence of the ischemic necrosis of the head of the humerus and of the femur and the death of the subject is problematical. In view of the fact that extensive repair and reconstruction had already taken place by the time the man died, it seems reasonable to surmise that the bone infarction antedated his death by about $1\frac{1}{2}$ to 2 years—that is, to the time he suffered several attacks of bends.

In a humeral or femoral head showing such pathologic changes, the tract of collagenous fibrous tissue interposed between the still-necrotic subchondral bone and the reconstructed and thickened spongy trabeculae in the deeper portion of the head of the bone represents a barrier to further repair. The necrotic subchondral portion of the head is under a mechanical disadvantage in relation to the reconstructed and sclerotic spongiosa deep to the tract of fibrous tissue. In the course of continued functional use of the joint, one or more fractures may occur. Where this happens, the fracture line extends between the still-necrotic subchondral bone and the underlying zone of collagenous fibrous tissue. In consequence of the appearance of one or more osteochondral fractures, the head of the bone in question will eventually come to show an irregularly bumpy and, in places, even grooved articular surface. The articular cartilage will be found more or less brownishly discolored, fibrillized in places, and, in some sites, even eroded. These changes in the articular surface lay the foundation for the subsequent development of a degenerative (secondary) osteoarthritis. (See Figs. 171 and 172.)

In recent years there have appeared in the literature several reports to the effect that, on rare occasions, a fibrosarcoma may develop in a bone area which is the site of an infarct (see Furey et al., Johnson et al., and Dorfman et al.). The case reported by Dorfman seems to be the only recorded instance of a fibrosarcoma developing in a bone infarct of a caisson worker. In that case the infarct was located in the shaft of the right femur. The present writer had the opportunity of examining the roentgenographic pictures and the pathologic material in that case, and likewise interpreted the tumor as a fibrosarcoma. However, for reasons which will be stated presently, he doubted that there was a cause-and-effect relationship between the bone infarct in that case and the sarcoma.

It is now over 50 years since the roentgenographic aspects of bone infarction in caisson workers came to be recognized. During that half century, there must have been thousands of caisson workers throughout the world who had developed bone infarcts. Certainly, many of these workers must have continued to live for many years (with or without skeletal disabilities), whether or not they had given up their trade. In view of this fact, it is the writer's opinion that in the case cited above it can safely be held that the development of the sarcoma in the infarcted femur represented merely a coincidence—that is, that there was no causal relation between the infarct and the sarcoma. To justify the conception that there is a cause-and-effect relationship, the incidence of this complication would obviously have to be much higher than one case in several thousand. For instance, in Paget's disease of bone, the development of a sarcoma in an affected bone is definitely related to the basic bone disease. The pathogenetic interconnection between the presence of a focus of radiation osteitis and the occurrence of a sarcoma in the affected bone area is likewise unequivocal. The statistical frequency of sarcoma appearing as a complication in cases of Paget's disease and at sites of radiation osteitis is in itself evidence of a cause-and-effect relationship. On the other hand, the rarity of a sarcoma appearing in the general region of a bone infarct makes such a relationship in that connection highly questionable.

Figure 171

A, Roentgenograph of the right hip region of a caisson worker who was 51 years of age at the time this picture was taken. Ten years before, he had suffered several attacks of the bends. About 6 weeks after the last of these attacks, roentgenographs were taken of both hip joints, because he had some pain referable to these joints, particularly the right. At that time the roentgenographs showed nothing remarkable. During the following years, however, progressive changes became visible in both hip joints, and this picture represents the appearance of the right femoral head prior to its resection and replacement by a prosthesis. It is evident that an advanced degree of osteoarthritis was already present at this time. In relation to the deep part of the acetabulum, one can also note a clearly delineated osteochondral fracture fragment which has become detached from the femoral head, in the general region of the fovea, but has remained *in situ.* Lateral to that fragment, another osteochondral fracture fragment was found to be present when the cut surface of the resected femoral head (*B*) was examined anatomically. This one, however, is hardly discernible in the clinical roentgenograph.

B, Photograph illustrating the gross anatomic appearance of the cut surface of the resected femoral head in this case. The gross anatomic changes presented by the femoral head are clearly reflected in the clinical roentgenograph. For orientation, one must realize that the gross picture represents a mirror image of the roentgenographic picture. The osteochondral fracture fragment in the general region of the fovea stands out clearly and matches the corresponding area in the roentgenograph. The osteochondral fracture fragment on the superior surface of the femoral head, though hardly discernible in the clinical roentgenograph, can be identified there if one compares the roentgenograph with the picture of the cut specimen. Below this osteochondral fragment the specimen photograph shows that a portion of the head is somewhat darkly discolored. This is a part of the femoral head which is being revascularized and repaired, and the corresponding portion of the femoral head appears in the clinical roentgenograph as a more or less loculated area of relative radiolucency. Lateral to the osteochondral body in the region of the fovea, the shadow cast by part of the femoral head is rather radiopaque. In the photograph of the specimen, this portion of the femoral head appears whitish, since in that area the osseous tissue is necrotic and the intertrabecular marrow spaces contain granular detritus. In the direction of the femoral neck, the rest of the head seems to be composed of close-meshed spongy bone which apparently represents an area that has undergone revascularization and reconstruction.

C, Roentgenograph of the anatomic specimen shown in *B.* Correlations similar to those made between the findings presented by the gross specimen and the clinical roentgenograph can be made between the photograph of the specimen and this roentgenograph.

D, Photomicrograph ($\times$ 25) illustrating a field from the femoral head in which the spongy trabeculae are necrotic and disintegrating and the intertrabecular marrow is also necrotic and contains granular detritus in some places.

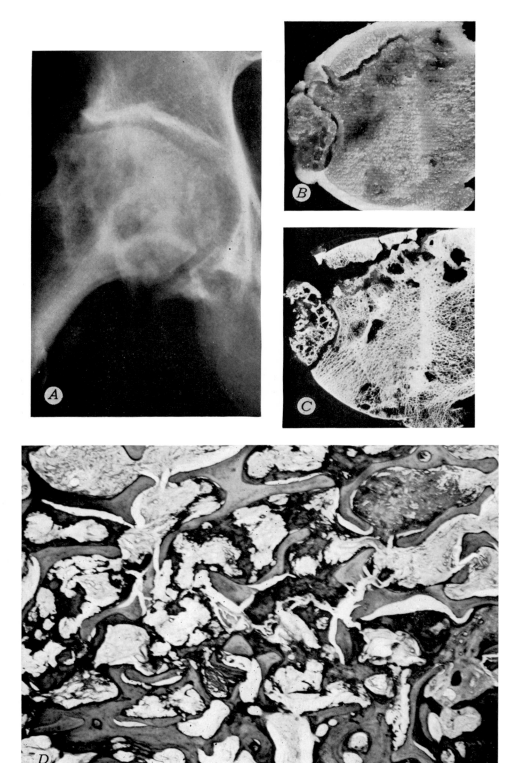

Figure 171

TREATMENT

As yet there seems to be no way of completely preventing the occurrence of bone lesions in caisson workers. In respect to *prophylactic measures*, it is known that the incidence of these lesions can be reduced by careful adherence to decompression procedures appropriate for the particular working conditions. When decompression is carefully controlled, the number of workers suffering from attacks of bends severe enough to require treatment by recompression is much lower than it is when decompression control is less meticulous. Furthermore, as already noted, there is a direct relationship between attacks of bends and the appearance of foci of ischemic aseptic necrosis of bone in caisson workers. The likelihood that bone lesions will develop is greatest when the attacks of bends have been severe. However, it is also known that bone lesions may be found in caisson workers who had the bends in so mild a

Figure 172

A, Roentgenograph of the right hip region of a caisson worker 39 years of age who had suffered several attacks of bends about $3\frac{1}{2}$ years before this picture was taken. Note the loss of the normal trabecular architecture of the femoral head, its increased radiopacity, and the presence of an osteochondral fracture fragment, which is clearly delineated but still *in situ* on the superolateral surface of the head (see arrow). As recorded in the hospital chart, the patient's clinical complaints began about 6 months after he had experienced the attacks of the bends. More specifically, these complaints, which were now of 3 years' duration and progressive, consisted of pain, stiffness, and limitation of motion of both shoulders and hips and also of the lower part of the back. The man walked awkwardly and with the suggestion of a double waddle. He sat down with difficulty and had to support himself with his upper extremities. He was unable to sit properly because of lack of flexion at both hip joints, and was also unable to raise his arms over his head. Rotation to the right and left was relatively painless. Forward bending was greatly restricted, and he was able to reach only slightly below the knee joints with the tips of his fingers. On arising from a sitting position, he had to raise himself with his hands.

B, Photograph of the cut surface of the right femoral head, which was resected and replaced by a prosthesis. The osteochondral fracture fragment *in situ*, indicated by the arrow in *A*, stands out clearly. Its articular cartilage is smooth, but the yellow-white color of the subchondral bone of the fracture fragment is an indication that the spongy osseous tissue is necrotic and that the intertrabecular marrow spaces contain considerable granular detritus. The rest of the cut surface of the femoral head showed large areas in which the spongy osseous tissue was strikingly yellow or yellow-white, in accordance with the presence of ischemic necrosis (see arrow on the right). In other places the spongiosa of the head appeared grayish, and in these areas in particular the osseous tissue was found close-meshed. Such areas represent tissue fields which had been the site of a good deal of repair, the necrotic osseous tissue having become thickened through the apposition of new bone (see arrow on the left).

C, Roentgenograph of the sectioned gross specimen shown in *B*, but representing the latter in a mirror image. The close-meshed spongiosa indicated by the arrow on the left in *B* is evident on the right in this picture. The yellow necrotic spongiosa indicated by the arrow on the right in *B* is evident on the left in this picture.

D, Photomicrograph ($\times$ 6) illustrating the histologic architecture of part of the articular end of the femoral head in the region of the osteochondral fracture fragment *in situ*. Note that the articular cartilage is smooth, for the most part, and that the fragment of subchondral bone which has separated from the head shows granular detritus in some of the intertrabecular marrow spaces. Between the osteochondral fracture fragment and the rest of the femoral head, there is a zone of collagenous fibrous tissue which marks the farthest advance of the reparative process that has been going on in the head. (This was one of several instances of aseptic necrosis of the femoral head reported by Laufer, who held a Fellowship grant from the Dazian Foundation for Medical Research and worked under the direction of the writer in the Laboratories of the Hospital for Joint Diseases.)

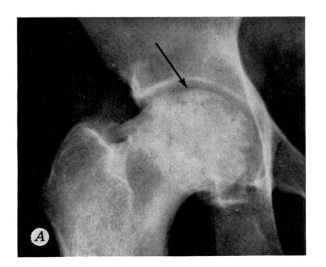

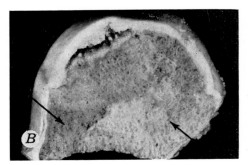

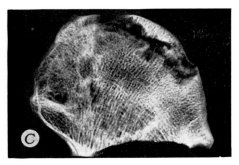

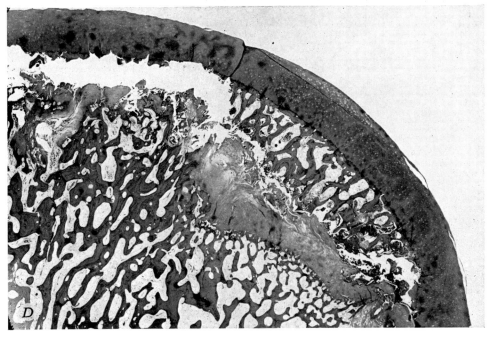

Figure 172

form that they were not reported, or even in some workers who had not experienced the bends at all.

As is well known, a caisson worker may show one or more bone lesions on roentgenographic examination, in the absence of any clinical complaints referable to these lesions. When such asymptomatic lesions are present in the juxta-articular portion of the head of a humerus or femur, there is a strong possibility that serious clinical difficulties will eventually appear as an aftermath of collapse of the affected articular bone end. A caisson worker who shows evidence of ischemic necrosis of one femoral head may develop ischemic necrosis of the opposite femoral head if he continues working under compressed air. If this happens, and the articular ends of both femoral heads collapse, the man may become seriously disabled. Thus, if one femoral head has developed juxta-articular changes which create the possibility of its future collapse, the man should be strongly advised to discontinue work under compressed air.

If a femoral head shows evidence of juxta-articular ischemic necrosis, it is to be doubted that protection of the femoral head from functional trauma by conservative (nonsurgical) measures, such as traction and rest in bed, is likely to result in complete repair of the necrotic area. Furthermore, even if conservative measures are undertaken, there is no assurance that ultimate collapse of the head will be prevented. It is for these reasons that management of ischemic necrosis of a femoral head, for instance, in a caisson worker usually consists of surgical procedures. The choice among such procedures will depend upon the presence or absence of collapse of the femoral head, and the presence or absence of involvement of the opposite femoral head.

REFERENCES

BEHNKE, A. R.: Decompression Sickness Incident to Deep Sea Diving and High Altitude Ascent, Medicine, *24*, 381, 1945.

BENNISON, W. H., CATTON, M. J., and FRYER, D. I.: Fatal Decompression Sickness in a Compressed-Air Worker, J. Path. & Bact., *89*, 319, 1965.

BERRY, C. A., and KING, A. H.: Severe Dysbarism in Actual and Simulated Flight, United States Air Force M. J., *10*, 1, 1959.

BERRY, C. A., and HEKHUIS, G. L.: X-Ray Survey for Bone Changes in Low-Pressure Chamber Operators, Aerospace Med., *31*, 760, 1960.

DALE, T.: Bone Necrosis in Divers, Acta chir. scandinav., *104*, 153, 1952–53.

DEÁK, P., and RÓZSAHEGYI, I.: Osteoarthropathie der Caissonarbeiter, Fortschr. Geb. Röntgenstrahlen, *84*, 312, 1956.

DORFMAN, H. D., NORMAN, A., and WOLFF, H.: Fibrosarcoma Complicating Bone Infarction in a Caisson Worker, J. Bone & Joint Surg., *48-A*, 528, 1966.

FOURNIER, M., and JULLIEN, G.: Aspects radiologiques de la maladie des caissons, J. radiol. et électrol., *40*, 529, 1959.

FUREY, J. G., FERRER-TORELLS, M., and REAGAN, J. W.: Fibrosarcoma Arising at the Site of Bone Infarcts, J. Bone & Joint Surg., *42-A*, 802, 1960.

GOLDING, C.: Radiology and Orthopaedic Surgery, J. Bone & Joint Surg., *48-B*, 320, 1966.

JAMES, C. C. M.: Late Bone Lesions in Caisson Disease, Lancet, *2*, 6, 1945.

JOHNSON, L. C., VETTER, H., and PUTSCHAR, W. G. J.: Sarcomas Arising in Bone Cysts, Virchows Arch. path. Anat., *335*, 428, 1962.

KAHLSTROM, S. C., BURTON, C. C., and PHEMISTER, D. B.: Aseptic Necrosis of Bone. I. Infarction of Bones in Caisson Disease Resulting in Encapsulated and Calcified Areas in Diaphyses and in Arthritis Deformans, Surg. Gynec. & Obst., *68*, 129, 1939.

LAUFER, A.: Aseptic Necrosis of the Femoral Head, J. Mt. Sinai Hosp., *24*, 957, 1957.

MARKHAM, T. N.: Aseptic Necrosis in a High-Altitude Flier, J. Occup. Med., *9*, 123, 1967.

McCALLUM, R. I., WALDER, D. N., BARNES, R., CATTO, M. E., DAVIDSON, J. K., FRYER, D. I., GOLDING, F. C., and PATON, W. D. M.: Bone Lesions in Compressed Air Workers, J. Bone & Joint Surg., *48-B*, 207, 1966.

RAIT, W. L.: The Etiology of Postdecompression Shock in Aircrewmen, United States Air Force M. J., *10*, 790, 1959.

SARTOR, E.: Skelettförändringar vid tryckluftsjuka, Nord. med., *35*, 1551, 1947.

TAYLOR, H. K.: Aseptic Necrosis in Adults: Caisson Workers and Others, Radiology, *42*, 550, 1944.

WALDER, D. N.: Some Problems of Working in an Hyperbaric Environment, Ann. Roy. Coll. Surgeons England, *38*, 288, 1966.

Chapter

22

Ischemic Necrosis of Bone Observed in Various Other Disorders

In Chapter 20, the first of the chapters dealing with ischemic necrosis of bone, the presentation was limited to: (1) so-called idiopathic ischemic necrosis of the femoral head; (2) ischemic necrosis of the femoral head which may follow upon trauma to the hip joint (with or without a dislocation of the head); and (3) ischemic necrosis of the femoral head appearing in the wake of a fracture of the femoral neck. Chapter 21 was devoted to the skeletal manifestations of decompression sickness which are the result of ischemic necrosis of bone, and whose most baleful consequences relate to one or both humeral heads or one or both femoral heads.

In the present chapter, attention will be directed toward ischemic necrosis of bone developing under circumstances different from those already discussed. In particular, consideration will be given to ischemic necrosis of bone observed in: (1) cases in which an individual bone or a number of bones other than the femoral head show evidence of ischemic necrosis in the absence of any known etiologic factor (this group of cases will be discussed in the subsection entitled "Idiopathic Ischemic Necrosis in Bone Sites Other than the Femoral Head"); (2) cases of acute and chronic recurrent pancreatitis; (3) cases of systemic lupus erythematosus; and (4) instances of occlusive peripheral vascular disease—particularly of the lower extremities.

The ischemic necrosis of bone observed in subjects who suffer from various hemoglobinopathies will be considered in the following chapter (Chapter 23). In that chapter the numerous skeletal alterations which occur in association with certain of the anemias will be presented together, since ischemic necrosis of bone is only one of these.

IDIOPATHIC ISCHEMIC NECROSIS IN BONE SITES OTHER THAN THE FEMORAL HEAD

Occasionally one encounters instances of solitary (monostotic) and also of multiple (polyostotic) foci of idiopathic ischemic necrosis of bone in sites other than the femoral head. The condition in the latter location has already been discussed (p. 632). In the writer's experience, idiopathic ischemic necrosis in bone sites other than the femoral head is encountered somewhat more often in women than in men. The age range of the subjects was rather wide, but the average age for the entire group was about 45 years. In respect to localization, most of the lesions (whether monostotic or polyostotic) were in the shaft of a long tubular bone. In such a bone the major portion of the lesion was more often in the upper or lower part of the shaft than in the midportion of the shaft. Among the cases studied by the writer, there were also several in which the lesion was located in an ilium, usually in the vicinity of the sacroiliac joint.

In some cases the lesion or lesions were asymptomatic, and their presence was discovered fortuitously in the course of a roentgenographic examination. In the other cases the *principal complaint* was intermittent pain of variable severity and duration. In those subjects in whom the lesions were located in the upper part of the shaft of a femur or in an ilium, there was usually pain in the region of the hip and the lower part of the back, and these patients also limped. In those in whom the lesion was located in the upper part of the shaft of one or both tibiae, pain was usually referred to the region of the knee and was associated with a limp.

The details of the *roentgenographic appearance* presented by the area of ischemic necrosis in these cases are by no means always the same. In some instances the lesional area appears as a small or large patch of radiopacity (mottled or more or less uniform) from which one or more irregular streaks of radiopacity may project. If present for a long time, the area of ischemic necrosis tends to become walled off from the uninvolved portion of the bone, usually by a border zone of calcified fibrous tissue. As the delimitation progresses, the necrotic osseous tissue in the interior of the infarcted area disintegrates and is slowly resorbed. Thus, in the course of time, the site of infarction may come to present, on gross examination, the appearance of a multiloculated cyst, the walls of the loculi consisting of calcified fibrous tissue. It is on this account that infarcts (in the shafts of long bones in particular) eventually cast a loculated shadow in the roentgenograph. (See Figs. 173, 174, and 175.)

CERTAIN DISORDERS OF THE PANCREAS

It is well established, though not generally known, that intramedullary fat necrosis and ischemic necrosis of the local spongy trabeculae may appear: (1) in cases of pancreatitis, and (2) in cases of carcinoma of the pancreas in which metastases are present in one or more visceral organs and/or in bones, and in which the metastatic cancer cells are producing pancreatic enzymes (especially lipase).

Pancreatitis.—Intramedullary fat necrosis of bone has been observed both in cases of acute pancreatitis and in cases of chronic relapsing (recurrent) pancreatitis (see Scarpelli, Gerle *et al.*, and Immelman *et al.*). The most familiar and obvious pathologic changes associated with an attack of pancreatitis are those involving the pancreas itself and the immediate peripancreatic tissues. It is also recognized that foci of fat necrosis are usually to be found in such other intra-abdominal sites as abdominal fat deposits, the mesentery, and the peritoneum. In a small proportion of cases, fat necrosis has also been noted in such extra-abdominal sites as the pericardium and mediastinum, beneath the parietal pleura, and even in the subcutaneous and para-articular tissues.

An attack of pancreatitis is associated with irritation of the peritoneum and the consequent exudation of an increased amount of peritoneal fluid, which, of course, contains large quantities of pancreatic enzymes that have seeped out of the damaged pancreas. The presence of foci of fat necrosis at sites remote from the pancreas (including the fatty marrow of the bones) is usually attributed to the pancreatic enzymes (especially lipase) which have gained entry to the vascular system. The abdominal fluid containing the pancreatic enzymes is absorbed by the peritoneal and transdiaphragmatic lymphatic channels, drains into the thoracic duct, and then enters the vascular system (see Allen, and also Perry). On lodging in various fat deposits, the still-active pancreatic lipase induces lipolysis, in the course of which fatty acids are liberated. Sooner or later, calcium becomes fixed to the fatty acids, and the disintegrated and necrotic fat comes to contain fatty acid soaps.

As is to be expected, intramedullary fat necrosis is most likely to occur and is most obvious in bone sites in which the marrow is essentially fatty marrow. Thus the most striking changes are to be found in the marrow within the shafts of long tubular bones. In middle-aged and elderly subjects the intertrabecular marrow of the upper ends of the humerus and femur, for instance, is essentially fatty marrow. Consequently, in such subjects, obvious foci of necrosis of the fatty marrow may also be observed in these bone sites. In the marrow within vertebrae and ribs, on the other hand, foci of necrosis are few and usually so small as to be visible only microscopically. This is in accordance with the fact that the marrow in those bone sites has only a small fat content, being essentially myeloid (hematopoietic) marrow.

Metastatic Pancreatic Carcinoma.—Intramedullary fat necrosis was observed in a humerus, femur, and tibia removed at autopsy in a case of carcinoma of the pancreas in which the metastases were limited to the liver (see Jackson *et al.*). In that case there was also widespread necrosis of the subcutaneous fat. The metastatic tumor was producing pancreatic enzymes, as was indicated by the high serum lipase level. The excess of circulating serum lipase was apparently the main factor in the occurrence of the fat necrosis. Hegler and Wohlwill described a case of carcinoma of the pancreas in which intramedullary fat necrosis was noted in various long tubular bones and also in the subcutaneous fatty tissues. In that case, metastases were present in the femur but not in any of the other long tubular bones which were examined and which also showed necrosis of their fatty marrow.

ROENTGENOGRAPHIC AND PATHOLOGIC FINDINGS

Our interest here relates only to those changes in the bones which represent the local effects of the intramedullary fat necrosis. The roentgenographic and pathologic changes observed in the affected bones vary in accordance with the time

Figure 173

A, Photograph of the cut surface of the lower end of the right tibia showing a large area of infarction. Actually, the infarct shown (appearing more or less white in the picture) was only part of the total infarcted area, which, indeed, occupied almost the entire shaft of the bone. The patient was a woman 66 years of age who was admitted to the hospital for treatment of a focus of osteomyelitis. This developed after surgical plating of a fracture which had occurred in the midshaft of this tibia about one year before admission. The fracture had failed to unite, and it was apparent on gross examination that the osteomyelitis was more or less localized to the region of the fracture site. The osteomyelitis extended for only a few centimeters upward and downward from the fracture line. That the extensive infarction of this tibia had antedated the fracture and the superimposed osteomyelitis was established by the fact that a roentgenograph of this tibia, taken on the day of the fracture, already showed an infarct involving almost the entire shaft of the bone. It was also supported by the finding that the shaft of the opposite tibia (the left tibia) was likewise the site of an infarct. Since the right lower extremity was functionally useless and the osteomyelitis and nonunion of the fracture were persisting, a supracondylar amputation was carried out. Detailed examination of the limb failed to reveal an anatomic basis for the infarction. Hence, the case was recorded in the writer's files as an instance of idiopathic ischemic necrosis of bone in a site other than the femoral head.

B, Roentgenograph of the part of the tibia shown in *A*. The infarct presents as a vaguely loculated and variegated area of radiopacity. The more intensely radiopaque regions correspond to those which appear strikingly white in *A*. In these areas the intertrabecular marrow spaces contain considerable amounts of calcific granular detritus. The histologic appearance of part of the small area blocked out in this picture is shown in *C*.

C, Photomicrograph ($\times$ 25) of part of the area blocked out in *B*. Many of the necrotic spongy trabeculae have undergone more or less disintegration, and the intertrabecular marrow spaces are largely filled with calcific granular detritus which stains dark in the picture.

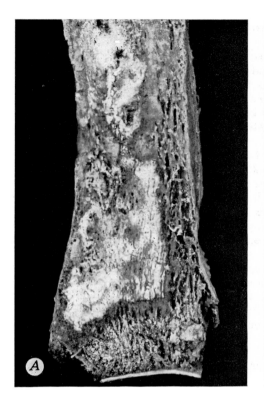

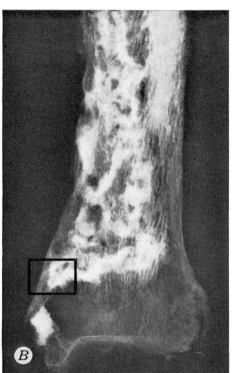

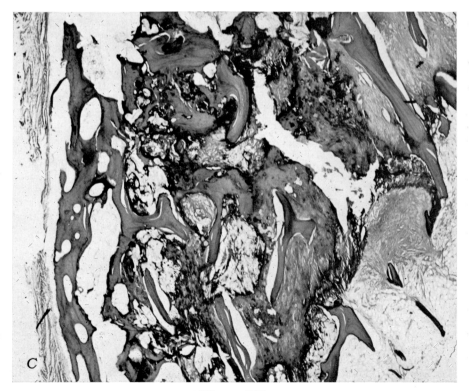

Figure 173

which has elapsed between: (1) the occurrence of the intramedullary fat necrosis and the concomitant necrosis of the local osseous tissue and (2) roentgenographic and/or pathologic study of the bones in question.   Naturally, it is in the cases of pancreatitis, and notably in cases of chronic relapsing pancreatitis, that the relevant pathologic changes can be expected to be visible roentgenographically.   Indeed, in a case of acute hemorrhagic pancreatitis in which the subject develops intra-medullary fat necrosis but dies within a week or two after the onset of the pan-creatitis, evidence of the necrosis will be absent roentgenographically, although already apparent anatomically.   For instance, in a long tubular bone removed at autopsy and sectioned longitudinally in such a case, the major medullary cavity in particular is likely to show a large area in which the fatty marrow appears yellow-white (rather than definitely yellow) because it has undergone necrosis.

In cases of pancreatitis (acute or chronic recurrent) in which large foci of intra-medullary fat necrosis have appeared in one or more bones and in which the subject continues to live for at least a few years, roentgenographic evidence of the necrosis will become apparent.   Under these circumstances the shafts and/or the articular ends of some of the long bones may present roentgenographic and pathologic find-ings similar to those encountered in caisson workers who have developed ischemic bone necrosis as a consequence of decompression sickness.   Thus the shaft of one or both femora, for instance, may present small or large, vaguely multiloculated

Figure 174

A, Photograph of the cut surface of the upper end of a right femur which was sectioned in its long axis.   Note the multilocular cystic area in the femoral neck and intertrochanteric region.   Detailed study of the specimen indicated that, in the distant past, the area in question must have been the site of an infarct which, in the course of time, underwent cystic softening.   The subject was a man 72 years of age who was admitted to the hospital because of general weakness and various neurological complaints.   However, there was nothing in his clinical record to indicate that he had ever been a caisson worker or had otherwise been subjected to hyperbaric conditions.   The lesion in the upper end of the right femur was a fortuitous finding in the course of a roentgenographic skeletal survey, and it was the only skeletal lesion present.   The patient died 2 weeks after admission.   An autopsy disclosed the classic lesions of periarteritis nodosa widely distributed through the various organs of the body.   The neurological complaints which the subject presented were the result of lesions of periarteritis nodosa involving the blood vessels within the supporting connective tissue of the peripheral nerves.   The upper end of the right femur was removed at autopsy for the purpose of determining the anatomic nature of the lesion present there.   In view of the gross and microscopic appearance of the affected area, the lesion could not have been of recent origin, and it certainly antedated the periarteritis nodosa by some years.   Since the cause of the underlying bone infarction was obscure, the lesion was recorded in the writer's files as an instance of so-called idiopathic ischemic necrosis.

B, Roentgenograph of the sectioned upper end of the femur shown in *A.*   As is to be expected, there is a clear-cut correlation between the roentgenographic appearance of the lesional area and the appearance of the sectioned gross specimen.   The individual cystic spaces are delimited by a border of radiopacity which, even in relation to the same cyst, may be thin in some places and thick in others.   The border of radiopacity may contain some osseous tissue but consists mainly of calcified collagenous connective tissue.

C, Photomicrograph ($\times$ 17) showing the histologic structure of the cyst wall in the general area blocked out in *B.*   For orientation, it should be noted that the inner surface of the cyst is at the right side of the picture.   From right to left, one can observe a thin lining layer which consists of acellular collagenous tissue, the deeper part of which is calcified. Immediately to the left, there is a zone of nonviable and disintegrating osseous tissue. Further to the left, there is an area of collagenous tissue which is poor in cells and heavily calcified in some places.

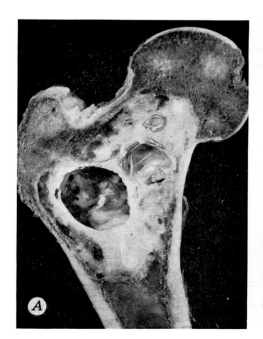

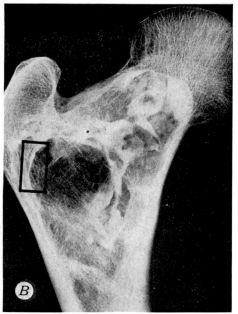

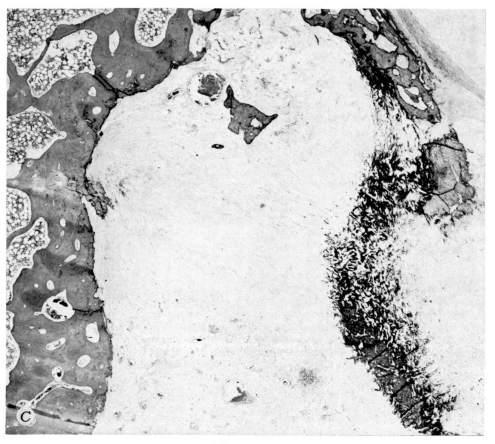

Figure 174

intramedullary cystlike shadows. These roentgenographic findings represent the anatomic presence of calcified collagenous fibrous tissue which surrounds and delimits the areas of necrotic fatty marrow and spongy bone.

In addition, since the humeral and femoral heads of an adult also contain fatty marrow between the spongy trabeculae, one or both femoral or humeral heads may also become sites of fat necrosis. In consequence, the nutrition of the local spongy trabeculae is disturbed, and the affected femoral or humeral head will present evidence of ischemic aseptic necrosis, likewise similar to that observed in caisson workers or in instances of so-called idiopathic ischemic necrosis. In an affected femoral head, for instance, the cumulative mechanical effects of weight-bearing will lead to the occurrence of one or more subchondral fractures extending for variable distances through the necrotic osseous tissue. The resultant alterations in the contour of the articulating surface of such a hip joint may be the basis for the subsequent development of a disabling osteoarthritis.

The writer has had an opportunity of examining the upper end of a femur in a

Figure 175

A, Roentgenograph showing an area of ischemic necrosis in the left iliac bone, in the vicinity of the sacroiliac joint. The patient was a woman 33 years of age whose complaints relating to this lesion had been present for about 2½ years before this roentgenograph was taken. At the time of onset of her difficulties, she was 3 months pregnant. Her presenting complaint was pain involving mainly the lower part of the back but also radiating down the left lower extremity to the foot. The attacks of pain were intermittent, and when present, the pain was aggravated by physical exertion. The woman went through her pregnancy and had a normal delivery. After this, however, she was experiencing more or less constant dull pain in the back, interspersed with attacks of acute pain. She then entered the hospital for surgery. At the surgical intervention, an irregular cystlike space in the iliac bone was unroofed. The wall of this cavity was defined by the outer and inner cortical tables of the iliac bone. Adherent here and there to the cortical walls and also present in the space between them was some whitish yellow osseous tissue. Bits of the posterior wall of the ilium, and curettings from the cavity within it, were submitted for histologic examination.

B, Photomicrograph (× 25) showing a fragment of osseous tissue from the posterior (outer) cortical wall of the iliac bone in the vicinity of the cystlike space found in the interior of the bone shown in *A*. The darkly discolored area represents osseous tissue which is undergoing granular disintegration and which appeared whitish or yellow-white on gross inspection. Further to the left, the disintegrating osseous tissue is lined in part by a thin layer of collagenous connective tissue.

C, Roentgenograph of the upper part of the *right* tibia showing two well-delineated cystlike areas, between which there are some irregular foci of radiopacity and also some very small, vaguely delineated cystlike areas. The part of the tibia illustrated is the site of ischemic necrosis of long duration. The upper part of the *left* tibia in this case was also the site of ischemic necrosis. The patient was a woman 62 years of age who, for a number of years, had been receiving physiotherapy for relatively mild pain in the lower part of the back and also in both knees. About 6 months before her admission to the hospital, the pain in the knees had become worse, and roentgenographs were taken which revealed pathologic changes in both tibiae. After her admission, a biopsy specimen was taken from the lesional area in the right tibia. On entering the medullary cavity in the general region of the tibial tubercle, a large cystic cavity was encountered which extended upward almost to the subchondral cortex. The wall of the cavity was smooth in some places, while in other areas gritty material could be curetted from it. Exploration of the medullary cavity distal to the aforementioned cyst revealed a considerable amount of soft, yellow-white, gritty granular material and disintegrated spongy trabeculae.

D, Photomicrograph (× 25) showing the general architecture presented by part of the wall of one of the cystic spaces shown in *C*. Note the disintegrated spongy trabeculae which, at the left of the picture, are bordered by a layer of collagenous connective tissue poor in cells.

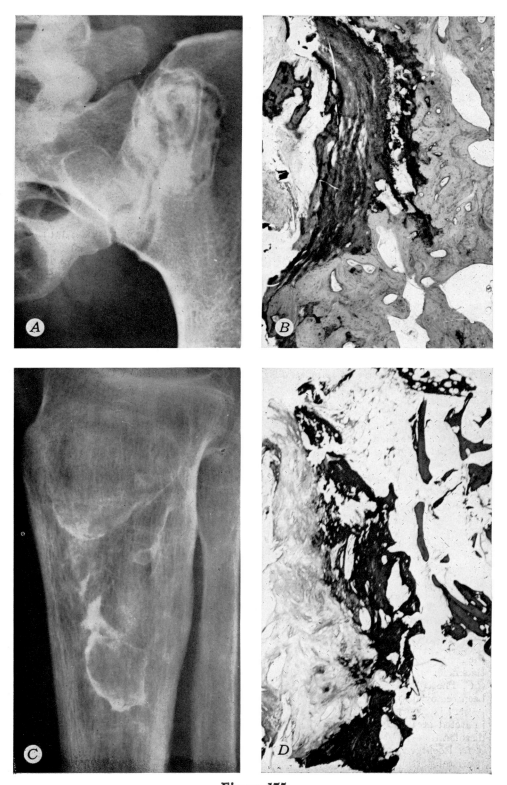

Figure 175

case in which the subject, a 34 year old man, developed intramedullary fat necrosis and ischemic necrosis of the local spongy trabeculae as a result of pancreatitis. The pathologic and roentgenographic changes in that case resembled those illustrated in Figure 170.

SYSTEMIC LUPUS ERYTHEMATOSUS

Systemic lupus erythematosus is a connective tissue disorder presenting a variety of clinical manifestations. Approximately 80 to 90 per cent of the subjects are females. The disease may appear in young children or in adults well beyond middle life. However, fully half of all the subjects (male and female) in any large series of cases are between 20 and 40 years of age at the time the disease sets in.

The *clinical complaints and findings* in cases of systemic lupus erythematosus in the early stages of its evolution are highly diverse. Indeed, in a given case, it is often difficult to recognize the condition at this stage. An important though by no means infallible criterion of the presence of the disease is a positive L. E. cell test result. A diagnostic cue is also afforded by the complaint of pain (often rather

Figure 176

A, Photograph showing the cut surface of the lower part of the left femur removed at autopsy in a case of disseminated lupus erythematosus. Note the presence of a rather large and apparently recent intramedullary infarct in the shaft. An ante-mortem clinical roentgenograph of the lower end of the femur, taken 8 weeks before death, failed to reveal the presence of the infarct. Thus, the discovery of the latter on sectioning the femur was an unexpected finding. The subject was a woman who was 42 years of age at the time of her death. She had had clinical manifestations of the disease for about 4 years. Her complaints at the time of her first admission to the hospital were migratory pain involving many joints, especially those of both hands, and she was also aware that she had fever from time to time. Despite the fact that, on her first admission, no L. E. cells were found in the sternal marrow puncture smears, lupus erythematosus was considered the most plausible diagnosis, and steroid therapy was started. Subsequent admissions to the hospital revealed the presence of pleural effusion, anemia and leukopenia, and also L. E. cells both in the bone marrow puncture smears and in blood smears. On her final (seventh) admission she still complained of migratory polyarthritis and also presented an erythematous eruption on various parts of the body. About 2 months thereafter she died of bronchopneumonia, and an autopsy was performed. Because of the pain which had been present in the left knee joint, it was decided to remove that joint at autopsy, along with a large part of the femur and tibia. The capsule of the knee joint was found slightly thickened but otherwise not remarkable. The synovial membrane showed no striking changes, and the articular cartilages of the femur and tibia did not reveal any erosion by synovial pannus, such as one would encounter in an affected knee joint in a case of rheumatoid arthritis of long duration.

B, Roentgenograph of a slice cut from the surface of the femur shown in *A*. This picture reveals that in the general region of the infarct there are focal areas lacking spongy trabeculae, the latter apparently having undergone disintegration. The cortex of the bone is of normal thickness, and the subchondral spongiosa shows nothing remarkable.

C, Photograph of the cut surface of the upper part of the tibia, which, as noted, had also been removed at autopsy in this case. A large, irregularly contoured area of infarction is present in the shaft of the bone. Except in the uppermost portion of the infarct, where the infarcted area appears whitish, the infarct shows a dark peripheral zone of hemorrhagic discoloration.

D, Roentgenograph of a slice cut from the surface of the tibia shown in *C*. In the most proximal portion of the infarcted area, spongy trabeculae are lacking, apparently having undergone disintegration. The roentgenographic changes shown in this illustration were not evident in the ante-mortem roentgenograph of the tibia.

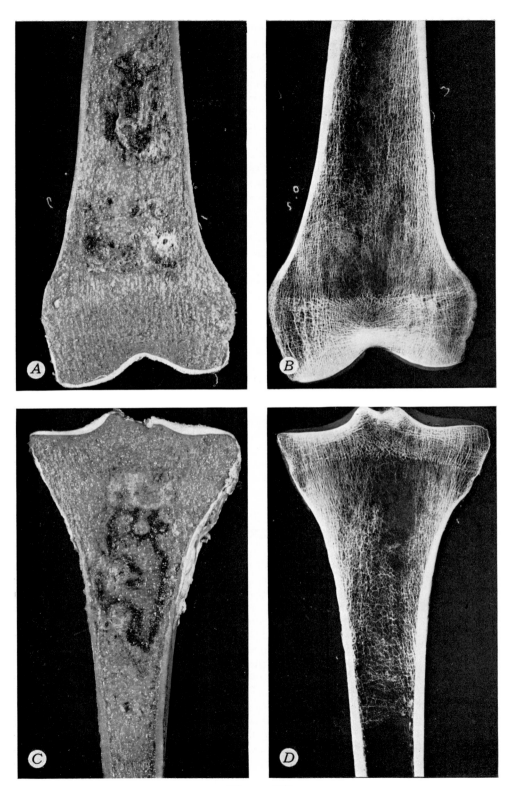

Figure 176

severe) relating to various joints. In the course of time, a symmetrical polyarthritis, clinically resembling that of rheumatic fever or early rheumatoid arthritis, frequently becomes evident. The polyarthritis involves the small joints of the hands and wrists and such large joints as those of the shoulder, knee, and ankle. The polyarthritis frequently precedes the other clinical findings, sometimes by months.

The presence of cutaneous lesions enhances the diagnostic value of the articular findings. An erythematous eruption (ephemeral or persistent) frequently appears on the face, neck, front or back of the chest, sometimes on the tips of the fingers, and even on the palms. With further progress of the disease, various hematologic abnormalities may develop. These include indications of depression of bone marrow function (such as leukopenia, anemia, and thrombopenia) and also certain hemorrhagic phenomena (such as purpura, petechial hemorrhages, and also bleeding from various viscera). In addition to the articular complaints due to changes in the synovial membrane of the affected joints, there may be complaints and findings indicative of polyserositis resulting from involvement of the pleura, peritoneum, and pericardium.

Other systemic manifestations are derived from pathologic changes in the heart, the kidneys, the gastrointestinal tract, and even the central and peripheral nervous systems. Indeed, before the introduction of adrenal steroid therapy in the treatment of the disease, its clinical aspects were so manifold and varied as to be bewildering, and the mortality rate was extremely high. The most ominous factor in the prognosis was, and remains, involvement of the kidneys (see Ginzler and Fox, and also Klemperer *et al.*).

The *skeletal manifestations* of systemic lupus erythematosus with which we are essentially concerned here are those relating to the ischemic necrosis now sometimes encountered in the shafts and/or articular ends of long bones. A case in point is illustrated in Figure 176. However, before considering the occurrence and pathologic aspects of this recently reported finding, it seems appropriate to give some attention to the more familiar pathologic alterations observed in those joints which have been the site of arthritic manifestations suggestive of rheumatic fever or rheumatoid arthritis (see Bennett and Dällenbach, Cruickshank, and also Nesgovorova).

PATHOLOGIC SKELETAL FINDINGS

"Rheumatic" Joints.—In a case of lupus erythematosus, when one examines a joint which has been the site of clinical manifestations suggestive of rheumatic fever or early rheumatoid arthritis, the *gross findings* are usually not striking. In particular, one is likely to note only that the synovial membrane is somewhat swollen and congested, and that the amount of fluid in the articular cavity is increased. The articular cartilages of the joint usually also fail to reveal striking changes, although some synovial pannus may be observed extending from the periphery for a variable distance over the articular surfaces.

On *microscopic examination* of the synovial membrane of the affected joint, the most conspicuous findings are a diminution in the number of synovial lining cells and the presence of patches of fibrin-like (fibrinoid) material on the lining surface. At sites where synovial lining cells are absent, fibrinoid material may also be found in the sublining tissue. Such synovial cells as are still present often have pyknotic nuclei. Intermingled with the pyknotic nuclei of the synovial cells, but distinguishable from them, so-called "hematoxylin bodies" are to be observed. These bodies can also be noted in the sublining layer of the synovial membrane. There is ordinarily no evidence of acute inflammation of the synovial membrane, such as would be expressed by the presence of polymorphonuclear leukocytes. However, the membrane does tend to show a slight to moderate infiltration with lymphocytes and plasma cells.

On the basis of histologic and histochemical examinations, Gueft and Laufer report that the fibrinoid material in systemic lupus erythematosus includes a protein residue of nuclear origin. Furthermore, they maintain that the fibrinoid material represents the result of a degradation of nucleoprotein, initiated by an aberration of desoxyribose nucleic acid metabolism, and that this metabolic aberration plays a basic role in the pathogenesis of the disease. The presence of the so-called "hematoxylin bodies" encountered in the synovial membrane (and various other tissues of the body) is likewise held to be the result of a disturbance of nucleic acid metabolism. By cytochemical methods it has been determined that the hema-toxylin-staining bodies contain partially depolymerized desoxyribose nucleic acid (see Klemperer et al.).

In a joint in which the articular cartilages are affected, synovial pannus will be found to have extended from the articular margin onto the surface of the cartilage. The latter is eroded by the pannus, but usually the erosion is limited to the periph-ery. Extensive erosion of the articular cartilage sometimes occurs, but is excep-tional. Intra-articular fibrous adhesions and/or bony ankylosis do not tend to develop, as they are likely to do in cases of rheumatoid arthritis.

Ischemic Necrosis of Bone.—As already indicated, the finding of ischemic necrosis of bone in cases of systemic lupus erythematosus represents a rather recent observation. Attention was called to this finding in 1960 by Dubois and Cozen, who noted its presence roentgenographically in 11 of 400 cases of systemic lupus erythematosus which they reviewed. In all of the 11 patients in question, the ischemic necrosis involved one femur or both femora. More particularly, in 8 of the patients, both femoral heads showed evidence of ischemic necrosis; in another case, only one femoral head was involved; and in the 2 remaining cases there was bilateral involvement of the femoral condyles. Since 1960, additional reports of the occurrence of ischemic necrosis of bone in cases of systemic lupus erythematosus have appeared (see Siemsen et al., Ruderman and McCarty, and also Velayos et al.). The roentgenographic and pathologic changes noted in the femoral head in these cases are indistinguishable from those to be found in instances of idiopathic ischemic necrosis of the femoral head or in subjects in whom the femoral head has undergone necrosis in consequence of decompression sickness resulting in caisson disease of bone.

Opinion is still divided as to the basic cause and pathogenesis of ischemic necrosis of bone in cases of systemic lupus erythematosus. Since subjects affected with the disease are now surviving for many years and are being maintained on steroid therapy, the question naturally arises whether the bone necrosis is to be attributed to the corticosteroid therapy. It is true that a few cases have been reported in which the ischemic necrosis of bone developed in patients with disseminated lupus erythematosus who had not received corticosteroid therapy. It is known, however, that in this disease there is a predisposition toward vascular lesions (arteritis). Hence, it might well be that, in those instances in which the necrosis of bone occurred in the absence of corticosteroid therapy, the intrinsic vasculitis was the sole factor in the pathogenesis of the necrosis. However, since it has come to be recognized that an existing vasculitis may be indirectly aggravated by corticosteroid therapy, one may be dealing in some cases with a combination of the two factors in the causation of the ischemic necrosis of bone (see Johnson et al., and also Schmid et al.). Indeed, it is well recognized that corticosteroid therapy may lead to ischemic bone necrosis in subjects not affected with systemic lupus erythematosus. It is quite possible that corticosteroid therapy results in periarterial and perivenal edema, and that this induces compression of the blood vessels of the marrow (see Uehlinger). Altogether, the possibility that corticosteroid therapy plays at least a contributory role in the development of ischemic necrosis in cases of systemic lupus erythematosus cannot be excluded (see Heimann and Freiberger, and also Burrows).

OCCLUSIVE VASCULAR DISEASE

In this section of the chapter we shall be concerned mainly with the changes to be observed in bones of lower extremities in subjects: (1) in whom an extremity has been amputated because of gangrene of part of the foot, ensuing upon thrombotic occlusion of peripheral blood vessels which were the site of arteriosclerosis of long duration; and (2) in whom the arterial occlusion was acute and located higher up, involving the distal end of the aorta and the common iliac arteries or the iliac arteries alone at the site of bifurcation of the aorta (saddle thrombus). More specifically, we are interested in presenting the status of the bones high above the

Figure 177

A and B, Photograph and roentgenograph showing an area of infarction in the posterior third of the right astragalus in a case of occlusive peripheral vascular disease of long duration. On gross examination this area of infarction appeared as a yellow-white focus which was definitely demarcated from the neighboring part of the bone. On microscopic examination the area of infarction was found to be composed of nonviable spongy trabeculae. The local intertrabecular marrow was also necrotic, and there was no evidence of reparative vascularization. The osseous tissue of the rest of the astragalus was extremely atrophic, as was that of the calcaneus. The area of infarction stands out clearly in the roentgenograph because, unlike the spongy trabeculae of the rest of the astragalus, the necrotic spongy trabeculae had not undergone atrophy to any significant extent. The patient, a man 68 years of age, had had clinical difficulties relating to the right lower extremity for about 2 years. These difficulties consisted of slowly progressive gangrene of the toes, and culminated in an infection of the foot, necessitating a midthigh amputation. For almost a year before the amputation, the man had been confined to bed.

C, Roentgenograph of the lower half of the left femur in the case of a man 69 years of age who, on his first admission to the hospital, gave a history of intermittent claudication of 4 years' duration. In neither extremity was pulsation detectable in the popliteal, posterior tibial, and dorsalis pedis arteries. At the time of admission the roentgenographs of both lower extremities revealed evidence of bone infarction in the lower part of the shaft of each femur and in the upper portion of the shaft of the left tibia. Since there was no evidence of gangrene of the toes of either foot at this time, a two-stage bilateral sympathectomy was performed, and this brought about some temporary amelioration of the intermittent claudication. However, about 5 months later, the patient was readmitted to the hospital with evidence of impending gangrene of the left foot, and a *midleg amputation* was carried out. About 2 months after this, since the amputation stump had failed to heal and was also the site of necrosis and gangrene of the soft tissues, a *midthigh amputation* was performed. This roentgenograph shows the status of the infarct in the shaft of the left femur shortly before the midthigh amputation was carried out. The infarcted area appears as a multiloculated tract, the locules (small and large) being outlined by relatively narrow radiopaque borders.

D, Photograph of the cut surface of the lower half of the left femur in this case. The bone has been sectioned in the frontal plane. The anatomic basis for the loculated appearance presented by the infarct in the roentgenograph (C) is apparent in this photograph. The necrotic spongy bone and marrow are walled off by calcified collagenous fibrous tissue. The latter varies in thickness from place to place and is serpentine in configuration. In some of the resultant locules, residual areas of necrotic spongiosa and fatty marrow can be seen.

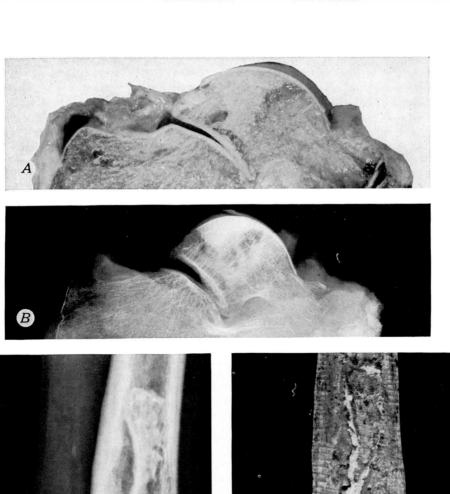

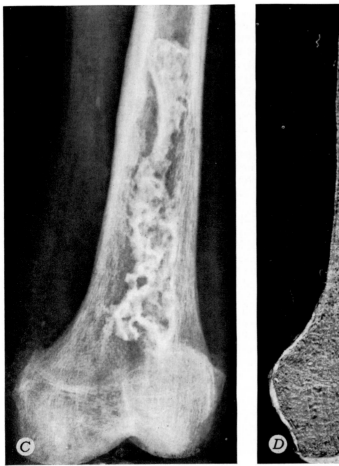

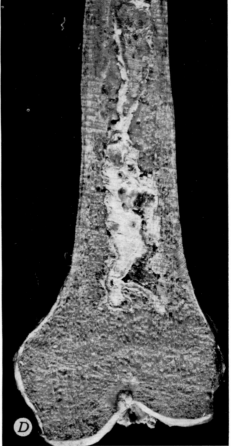

Figure 177

level of the gangrene and any complicating local infection involving the soft tissues and/or bones in the general area of the gangrene.

Protracted Peripheral Vascular Insufficiency.—In some instances of occlusive vascular disease based on arteriosclerosis of long duration, the changes which have occurred in the bones above the level of the gangrene are detectable only on microscopic examination Indeed, they may be limited to *widespread disappearance of osteocytes* (due to their death) from the interstitial lamellar osseous tissue of the cortical bone. Under these circumstances the osteocytes of the haversian lamellae of the cortical bone as well as those of the ground lamellae (especially the inner ground lamellae) may still be viable. Furthermore, the osteocytes of the spongy trabeculae are likely to be viable, and no abnormalities are ordinarily revealed by the marrow in the intertrabecular spaces and the major marrow cavity.

Figure 178

A, Photograph showing the distal portion of the aorta, the right and left common iliac arteries, and the corresponding external and internal iliac arteries in the second of the two cases of high vascular occlusion discussed in the text. A thrombus is to be seen in the aorta extending for several inches above its bifurcation. Furthermore, it is evident that the thrombus also extends into the common iliacs and their branches. The subject was a man 66 years of age who was admitted with the clinical complaint of pain and swelling, of 6 months' duration, in the region of the left ankle. On admission the pain was acute and the left ankle and foot were found discolored. Pulsation of the dorsalis pedis and tibial arteries could not be felt in either the left or the right extremity. Though the bones of the lower extremities showed pronounced rarefaction roentgenographically, the blood vessels of these extremities revealed no evidence of calcification. Because of gangrene of the toes of the left foot, the extremity was amputated above the knee. One week after the left lower limb was amputated, the patient went into coma, had convulsions, and died. The autopsy revealed that this saddle thrombus in the lower end of the aorta was the basis for the circulatory difficulties relating to the lower limbs.

B, Photograph showing the cut surface of part of the shaft of the tibia which was removed in the course of dissection of the amputated limb in this case. Over a large area, the midshaft of the bone shows necrosis of the fatty marrow. Note in addition that the bone cortex in the general vicinity of the necrotic marrow is thinned in some places, and that it is also rather porous.

C, Photomicrograph ($\times$ 75) showing the altered architecture of the femoral cortex in the first of the two cases of high vascular occlusion mentioned in the text. The subject was a man 45 years of age who experienced the sudden onset of pain in the right lower extremity. This was promptly followed by a feeling of numbness from the knee down. As the patient expressed it, the extremity "felt dead," and he was unable to bear weight on it. Five months after the onset of these complaints, he was admitted to the hospital, and all the indications pointed to the existence of a thrombus in the left common iliac artery, possibly at the bifurcation of the aorta. Approximately one month after that, several of the toes came to show dry gangrene, and a midthigh amputation was then performed. The muscles and periosteum were stripped from the amputated portion of the femur, and the bone was sectioned longitudinally. It was then clearly apparent that the marrow cavity was enlarged on the endosteal side, and that the cortex of the bone was thinned and less compact than it would normally have been. The spongy trabeculae were sparse, and those present were thin. The histologic basis for the porosity of the cortex is evident in this photograph. In particular, it can be seen that many of the haversian canals are enlarged and that fusion of the enlarged canals has led to the formation of wide haversian spaces. These changes had followed upon revascularization of the previously necrotic cortical bone. In the wake of this process, much of the nonviable cortical osseous tissue was resorbed. However, when the tissue field shown was examined under higher magnification, it was apparent that the revascularization which was going on in the cortex was associated with the deposition of rings of new bone on the nonviable osseous tissue surrounding the enlarged haversian spaces.

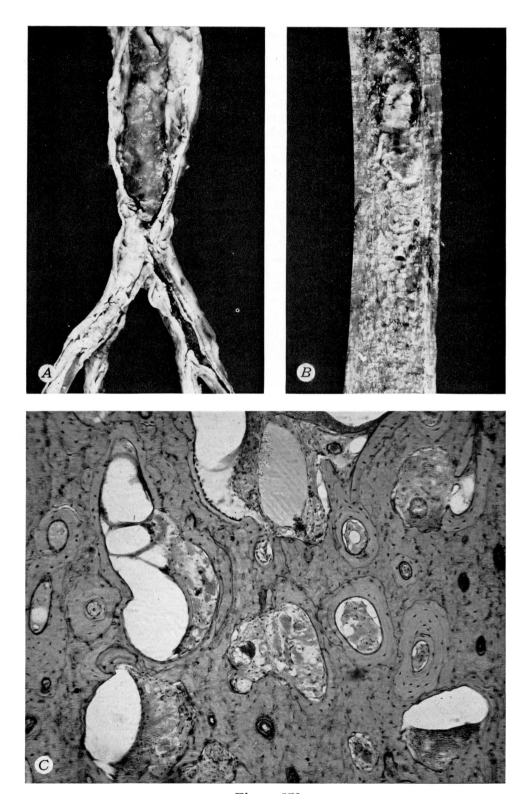

Figure 178

689

In regard to these findings it should be emphasized that the absence of viable osteocytes in the interstitial lamellar osseous tissue is also to be noted (though to a much lesser degree) in cortical bone of persons not affected with occlusive vascular disease and gangrene of the extremities. In particular, the nature, the mode of formation, and the location of the interstitial lamellar osseous tissue of normal cortical bone are the basis for the inherent disposition favoring the death and disappearance of osteocytes and the consequent finding of empty bone cell lacunae. Interstitial lamellae are fragments of old and splintered haversian systems; in the disintegration of these systems, interstitial lamellae form an important supporting mass for newer haversian systems and, as a result, become disadvantageously placed for the receipt of nutrition. This is not the fate of the osteocytes of the interstitial lamellae of compact bone alone; wherever osteocytes are disadvantageously situated for the receipt of nutrition, they tend to die. Thus, to a slight extent, degeneration and death of the bone cells of deeply placed lamellar osseous tissue of compact bone are normal manifestations even in young adults. With increasing age of the subject, the presence of empty bone cell lacunae in the interstitial lamellar osseous tissue becomes a more common finding. However, in cases of arteriosclerosis with gangrene, the absence of osteocytes in the interstitial osseous tissue is much more pronounced, and is to be observed in the bones high above the level of the gangrene. If, under these circumstances, the cortical bone remains compact, the roentgenographic shadow cast by the bone will present a normal appearance even if there is extensive absence of osteocytes from the interstitial osseous tissue (see Jaffe and Pomeranz, Müller, and Sherman and Selakovich).

When chronic vascular disease has persisted for any length of time before gangrene evolves, the pronounced innate disposition toward the development of collateral circulation frequently reduces to secondary importance the factor of vascular obstruction *per se* in regard to the pathologic and roentgenographic changes in the bones. Although therapy may have staved off for months the necessity for amputation, the long interval of time permits such additional factors as infection, inactivity, and so-called trophoneurotic influences to exert themselves on the bones. Thus the roentgenographic changes apparent in the bones depend upon the extent to which these various influences have been brought into play, even though the bones show definite histologic changes (especially extensive aseptic necrosis) of the interstitially located osseous tissue. If a devitalized bone undergoes revascularization through circulatory readjustments, the resorption and reconstruction will be demonstrated roentgenographically by punctate shadows of increased radiolucency. These are the result of enlargement of pre-existing vessel canals in the cortex, and also of cortical erosion, particularly from the periosteal side.

Furthermore, in a case of protracted peripheral vascular insufficiency, detailed gross examination of the bones occasionally reveals the presence of clearly delimited areas of intramedullary infarction. In one instance, the writer encountered a delimited area of ischemic necrosis in a talus of an amputated lower extremity in which the femur, tibia, fibula, and calcaneus, though profoundly altered in other ways, failed to show areas of bone infarction. In another case of arteriosclerotic gangrene, the lower half of the interior of the shaft of a femur was the site of an extensive infarct involving the spongy bone and marrow. The infarcted area was found to be walled off by a thick zone of poorly vascularized and also calcified connective tissue. In the roentgenograph the shadow cast by the affected part of the femur simulated the appearance presented by a large intramedullary infarct of the shaft of a bone, such as may be encountered in instances of caisson disease. The upper part of the tibial shaft of that limb also showed a focus of intramedullary infarction. (See Fig. 177.)

Acute High Vascular Occlusion.—The writer has studied the bones from two lower extremities amputated from two patients who had developed gangrene in those extremities after the occurrence of an acute high vascular occlusion. In one of the cases, the gangrene was the result of a thrombus which had formed in the right common iliac artery, and the amputation was done about 6 months after the onset of the clinical complaints, which for 5 months were not associated with clinical indications of gangrene of the foot. Collateral circulation was adequate to prevent immediate gangrene, though not sufficient for normal nutrition of the limb.

Roentgenographs of the bones of the extremity 5 months after the onset of the vascular occlusion revealed extensive changes. In particular, there were areas of rarefaction disseminated throughout and exhibited in round or somewhat elongated radiolucencies. Histologic examination of bone areas high above the level of gangrene disclosed the presence of widespread necrosis. For instance, the original compacta of the femur was almost entirely necrotic. Revascularization of the necrotic bone was in evidence. Accordingly, numbers of haversian canals were greatly widened, especially where some of them had fused. The enlarged spaces were lined by newly deposited bone and contained loosely cellular tissue with numerous blood vessels. Extensive necrosis of the compacta of the other bones was likewise manifest. The roentgenographic findings essentially reflected the revascularization of the necrotic cortical bone.

In the other case, the gangrene of the toes of the left foot was related, as autopsy disclosed, to the presence of a thrombus in the lower part of the aorta and extension of the thrombus into the common iliacs and, to a lesser degree, into their branches. In this case there was an interval of 6 months between the onset of clinical complaints referable to the affected extremity and the appearance of clinical indications of gangrene in the foot (see Fig. 178).

REFERENCES

ALLEN, L.: The Peritoneal Stomata, Anat. Rec., *67*, 89, 1936.

BENNETT, G. A., and DÄLLENBACH, F. D.: Synovial Membrane Changes in Disseminated Lupus Erythematosus, Mil. Surgeon, *109*, 531, 1951.

BURROWS, F. G. O.: Avascular Necrosis of Bone Complicating Steroid Therapy, Brit. J. Radiol., *38*, 309, 1965.

CRUICKSHANK, B.: Lesions of Joints and Tendon Sheaths in Systemic Lupus Erythematosus, Ann. Rheumat. Dis., *18*, 111, 1959.

DUBOIS, E. L., and COZEN, L.: Avascular (Aseptic) Bone Necrosis Associated with Systemic Lupus Erythematosus, J.A.M.A., *174*, 966, 1960.

GERLE, R. D., WALKER, L. A., ACHORD, J. L., and WEENS, H. S.: Osseous Changes in Chronic Pancreatitis, Radiology, *85*, 330, 1965.

GINZLER, A. M., and FOX, T. T.: Disseminated Lupus Erythematosus: A Cutaneous Manifestation of a Systemic Disease (Libman-Sacks), Arch. Int. Med., *65*, 26, 1940.

GUEFT, B., and LAUFER, A.: Further Cytochemical Studies in Systemic Lupus Erythematosus, Arch. Path., *57*, 201, 1954.

HEGLER, C., and WOHLWILL, F.: Fettgewebsnekrosen in Subcutis und Knochenmark durch Metastasen eines Carcinoms des Pankreasschwanzes, Virchows Arch. path. Anat., *274*, 784, 1929–30.

HEIMANN, W. G., and FREIBERGER, R. H.: Avascular Necrosis of the Femoral and Humeral Heads after High-Dosage Corticosteroid Therapy, New England J. Med., *263*, 672, 1960.

IMMELMAN, E. J., BANK, S., KRIGE, H., and MARKS, I. N.: Roentgenologic and Clinical Features of Intramedullary Fat Necrosis in Bones in Acute and Chronic Pancreatitis, Am. J. Med., *36*, 96, 1964.

JACKSON, S. H., SAVIDGE, R. S., STEIN, L., and VARLEY, H.: Carcinoma of the Pancreas Associated with Fat-Necrosis, Lancet, *263*, 962, 1952.

JAFFE, H. L., and POMERANZ, M. M.: Changes in the Bones of Extremities Amputated Because of Arteriovascular Disease, Arch. Surg., *29*, 566, 1934.

JOHNSON, R. L., SMYTH, C. J., HOLT, G. W., LUBCHENCO, A., and VALENTINE, E.: Steroid Therapy and Vascular Lesions in Rheumatoid Arthritis, Arthritis Rheum., *2*, 224, 1959.

KLEMPERER, P., GUEFT, B., LEE, S. L., LEUCHTENBERGER, C., and POLLISTER, A. W.: Cytochemical Changes of Acute Lupus Erythematosus, Arch. Path., *49*, 503, 1950.

MÜLLER, W.: Über das Verhalten des Knochengewebes bei herabgesetzter Zirkulation und das Bild von Nekrose der Zwischenlamellen, Bruns' Beitr. klin. Chir., *138*, 614, 1926.

NESGOVOROVA, L. I.: Lupus Polyarthritis (Clinical and Morphological Investigation), Rheumatism, *22*, 99, 1966.

PERRY, T. T., III: Role of Lymphatic Vessels in the Transmission of Lipase in Disseminated Pancreatic Fat Necrosis, Arch. Path., *43*, 456, 1947.

RUDERMAN, M., and McCARTY, D. J., JR.: Aseptic Necrosis in Systemic Lupus Erythematosus, Arthritis Rheum., *7*, 709, 1964.

SCARPELLI, D. G.: Fat Necrosis of Bone Marrow in Acute Pancreatitis, Am. J. Path., *32*, 1077, 1956.

SCHMID, F. R., COOPER, N. S., ZIFF, M., and McEWEN, C.: Arteritis in Rheumatoid Arthritis, Am. J. Med., *30*, 56, 1961.

SHERMAN, M. S., and SELAKOVICH, W. G.: Bone Changes in Chronic Circulatory Insufficiency, J. Bone & Joint Surg., *39-A*, 892, 1957.

SIEMSEN, J. K., BROOK, J., and MEISTER, L.: Lupus Erythematosus and Avascular Bone Necrosis, Arthritis Rheum., *5*, 492, 1962.

UEHLINGER, E.: Aseptische Knochennekrosen (Infarkte) nach Prednisonbehandlung, Schweiz. med. Wchnschr., *94*, 1527, 1964.

VELAYOS, E. E., LEIDHOLT, J. D., SMYTH, C. J., and PRIEST, R.: Arthropathy Associated with Steroid Therapy, Ann. Int. Med., *64*, 759, 1966.

Chapter

23

Skeletal Manifestations of Certain Anemias

THIS chapter will be devoted mainly to *sickle cell anemia, thalassemia, erythro-blastosis fetalis,* and *myelosclerotic (osteomyelosclerotic) anemia.* The first two of these disorders have their basis in qualitative and quantitative aberrations, respectively, relating to the hemoglobin of the red blood cells. On the other hand, erythroblastosis fetalis (hemolytic disease of the newborn) results from the action of iso-antibodies acquired by the fetus from the maternal circulation and causing hemolysis of the red blood cells of the fetus. Myelosclerotic anemia differs from the aforementioned diseases in that it is not a hemolytic anemia. Instead, it is the consequence of replacement of much of the bone marrow by connective tissue in which a good deal of osseous tissue may also be laid down.

NORMAL AND ABNORMAL HEMOGLOBINS

To supply a background for the consideration of the *abnormal* hemoglobins present in the red blood cells of persons affected with sicklemia, sickle cell anemia, or thalassemia, it seems appropriate to make brief mention of the hemoglobins present in the red blood cells of normal persons. Those found in normal persons (the normal hemoglobins) have been denoted as F, A_1, and A_2. Hemoglobin F is the so-called fetal hemoglobin, and hemoglobins A_1 and A_2 are the so-called adult hemoglobins. Fetal hemoglobin usually begins to be replaced by adult hemoglobin during the final month of fetal life and has usually been completely or almost completely replaced by the end of the seventh month of extra-uterine life.

In considering the manner in which the abnormal hemoglobins are formed, it should be pointed out first that the protein portion of hemoglobin consists of 4 coiled polypeptide amino acid chains. In *hemoglobin A_1* (by far the major fraction of normal adult hemoglobin), 2 of the 4 polypeptide chains are alpha chains and 2 are beta chains. In *hemoglobin A_2* (the definitely minor fraction of adult hemoglobin), 2 of the polypeptide chains are alpha chains and 2 are delta chains. In normal *fetal hemoglobin* (hemoglobin F), beta chains are absent, and the 4 polypeptide chains consist of 2 alpha and 2 gamma chains.

Each polypeptide chain is a coiled string of amino acids whose specific identity, precise number, and order of arrangement are governed by the genetic constitution of the individual. It has been ascertained that the alpha chain has 141 amino acids, while the beta, gamma, and delta chains each have 146 amino acids (see Hutchison). Under normal conditions, the individual amino acids line up in an established pattern (as though on a template) to form normal hemoglobin. However, if there is a mutation in the genetic template of the individual, one or more of the amino acids may be deleted, or the order of arrangement of the amino acids may be disturbed. Even if the disturbance consists of entrance of a single amino acid at the wrong place in one or more of the chains, an abnormal hemoglobin results. For instance, the only difference between hemoglobin A (normal adult hemoglobin) and hemo-globin S (the hemoglobin of sicklemia and sickle cell anemia) is that the amino acid group sixth from the end of the beta chain is glutamic acid in hemoglobin A and valine in hemoglobin S.

A large number of abnormal hemoglobins (approximately 50) have been identi-fied since Pauling *et al.* discovered that sickle cell anemia was a molecular disease and designated the pertinent abnormal hemoglobin as *hemoglobin S*. In particular, it is now held that in sickle cell anemia about 80 to 85 per cent (or even more) of the hemoglobin is hemoglobin S, and that the rest of it consists almost solely of hemo-globin F. In subjects affected with sickle cell anemia in whom the hemoglobin S content of the erythrocytes is not much less than 100 per cent, there seems to be an increased tendency toward sickling of the red blood cells, and consequently an increased likelihood that the clinical manifestations will be severe (see Jackson *et al.*). In cases representing merely the sickle cell trait (sicklemia), definitely less than half of the hemoglobin content of the red blood cells is hemoglobin S, the remainder being normal hemoglobin.

Furthermore, abnormal hemoglobin may result from variations in the combina-tions of the polypeptide chains in the hemoglobin molecule, as, for instance, in the presence of beta chains *only*, in hemoglobin H. As already noted, fetal hemoglobin (hemoglobin F) contains *no* beta chains. In the thalassemias, the hemoglobinopathy results *not* from abnormalities in the amino acid sequences of the polypeptide chains, but from a lack of synthesis of certain of the polypeptide chains constituting the globin moiety of normal hemoglobin (p. 704).

Genetic Considerations.—The *genetic mechanisms* involved in the formation of normal and abnormal hemoglobins have been intensively studied. Genes for hemoglobin production are inherited from both parents. Individual genes control the formation of the various polypeptide chains, including the precise sequences of the amino acids in the chains, and these genes have been denoted as "structural genes." Furthermore, it has been postulated that there are also "regulator genes" which control the rate of synthesis of the individual polypeptide chains and, in addition, the type of polypeptide chain (alpha, beta, gamma, or delta) to be produced.

After infancy, the hemoglobin of the red blood cells in a person who has inherited normal genes is normal adult hemoglobin (hemoglobin A_1 and A_2), and the genetic constitution of that person in respect to hemoglobin may be denoted as AA. Muta-tions relating to either the structural or the regulatory genes may give rise to a variety of hereditary abnormalities. These mutations may implicate the amino acid sequences of the polypeptide chains, the types of chains that are synthesized, or the relative rates at which the synthesis of the chains takes place.

If one inherited structural gene is abnormal (representing the *heterozygous state*), the hemoglobins present in the subject's red blood cells are of two types—normal adult hemoglobin, and one or more of the various abnormal hemoglobins (S, C, E, etc.). The proportion of the abnormal hemoglobins may range from about a quarter to almost a half of the total hemoglobin. In accordance with the type of abnormal hemoglobin present, the genetic constitution of the heterozygous subject in respect to hemoglobin may be denoted as AS, AC, AE, etc. Such subjects are usually designated as *trait carriers*. In general, the trait carriers do not present clinical manifestations of hemolytic disease. However, there are some trait carriers in whom the abnormal hemoglobin is unstable, and this instability may result in the appearance of relevant clinical manifestations.

In the *homozygous state* the structural mutation often involves only one of the polypeptide chains of hemoglobin A (usually the beta chain), so that only a single abnormal adult variety of hemoglobin is produced. Concomitantly, in cases of homozygous hemoglobin disease, elevated levels of fetal hemoglobin are often also present. In accordance with the type of abnormal hemoglobin produced, the genetic constitution of the homozygous subject may be denoted as SS, CC, or EE, for instance. Furthermore, since the alpha and beta chains of hemoglobin are under independent genetic control, it is possible for mixtures of abnormal hemoglobins to be formed. In any event, the homozygous subject usually presents anemia and also serious clinical manifestations, as strikingly exemplified in sickle cell anemia (SS disease). In that disease, infarction of bone is a common finding.

There are also genetic variants of sickle cell anemia. One of these is hemoglobin SC disease, which results from the presence of hemoglobin S and hemoglobin C in the red blood cells. Sickle cell-hemoglobin C disease is clinically milder than ordinary sickle cell anemia (SS disease), but tends like the latter to present, as one of its manifestations, ischemic necrosis of bone due to infarction ensuing upon thrombosis of local blood vessels. Another variant is hemoglobin S-thalassemia, and in that condition, too, bone infarction occasionally occurs. Furthermore, the sickling phenomenon has also been observed in a variety of conditions involving combinations of hemoglobin S with still other abnormal hemoglobins.

SICKLEMIA AND SICKLE CELL ANEMIA

Sickle cell anemia, which is practically limited to Negroes, is one of the most common and clinically serious hemoglobinopathies. It is characterized by variable numbers of sickle-shaped red blood cells and by an anemia which varies considerably from case to case and from time to time in the same case. When the presence of sickle-shaped cells in the blood is not associated with anemia, the condition is known as "sicklemia" or "the sickle cell trait."

CLINICAL CONSIDERATIONS

Incidence.—It is estimated that about 8 per cent of North American Negroes have the sickle cell trait (the heterozygous form of sickle cell hemoglobinopathy). However, at most about 1 in 40 North American Negroes whose red blood cells sickle actually has sickle cell anemia (the homozygous form of the disorder). Naturally, the incidence of sickle cell trait and sickle cell anemia varies among the Negro population in different parts of the United States. In regard to the incidence of the condition in Central and South America, it has been reported that as large a proportion as 9 per cent of the Negroes in that area who have the sickle cell trait actually suffer from sickle cell anemia (see Tomlinson). This finding is in striking contrast to the observation that, though there is an exceedingly high incidence of the sickle cell trait among the Negro population extending more or less across the middle third of Africa, the incidence of sickle cell anemia is exceedingly low among those African Negroes exhibiting the sickle cell trait (see Raper, and also Neel).

Inheritance.—As already noted, a person affected merely with sicklemia represents genetically the *heterozygous* manifestation of an abnormal gene (for hemoglobin production) derived from one of the parents, who is likewise heterozygous in respect to the sickle cell trait. The parent in question has one normal and one abnormal gene, while in the other parent both of the pertinent genes are normal. Of the offspring resulting from the mating of such parents, one half will be heterozygotes, since they will have one normal and one abnormal gene for hemoglobin formation. The other half of the offspring will have two normal genes and thus be normal in respect to their hemoglobin formation, and specifically will be free of sicklemia. On the other hand, if both parents are heterozygous in regard to the trait, the offspring may inherit two abnormal genes for hemoglobin formation. Under those circumstances they will be *homozygous* for the abnormal trait and will be victims of the actual disease, sickle cell anemia. In any event, the vast majority of cases of sickle cell anemia result from the mating of two persons having the sickle cell trait rather than from the mating of persons affected with sickle cell anemia. Indeed, the latter subjects either die before reaching maturity or, if they do reach maturity, are not likely to have offspring, since their fertility is very low.

Clinical Complaints and Findings.—In persons affected with *sicklemia* (that is, with the sickle cell trait alone), the sickling of the red blood cells can be demonstrated in the course of a hematological examination by subjecting a drop or more of the blood to reduced oxygen tension. Ordinarily, as noted, sicklemia is not associated with any special or characteristic clinical complaints; that is, it is essentially a benign condition. However, if a person affected with the sickle cell trait is exposed for an appreciable period of time to an atmosphere abnormally low in oxygen, serious clinical manifestations may ensue. These include hematuria, hemorrhage into, and/or infarction of, various tissues. In addition, the sinusoids, notably those of the spleen, become filled with masses of sickled red blood cells. Hypoxia due to pneumonia or to some cardiopulmonary disease has been known to induce *acute sicklemia*, occasionally resulting in the death of the subject (see Tseng).

Clinical manifestations of *sickle cell anemia* only infrequently set in before the end of the first year of life. Even in those instances in which they do appear so early, the infant is usually more than 6 months of age. This finding is in conformity with the fact that the presence of fetal hemoglobin (hemoglobin F) in the erythrocyte reduces the tendency of the red blood cells toward sickling. In a normal infant, fetal hemoglobin has usually been completely replaced by adult hemoglobin by the end of the seventh month of extra-uterine life. During the first few months of life, therefore, the erythrocytes of an infant destined to develop sickle cell anemia probably still contain considerable amounts of hemoglobin F, and this may explain the usual delay in the appearance of clinical indications of the disease until the infant in question is over 6 months old. Nevertheless, a large proportion of the stigmatized infants die during the first year of life, and many of those who live on into childhood die before the age of 10.

In those who continue to survive into later childhood and adulthood, sickle cell anemia is characterized by alternating exacerbations and remissions of the clinical manifestations. Thus a surviving affected subject may be remarkably free of complaints for long periods of time, despite the persistent presence of a definite anemia, a slight icteric tint of the sclerae, and, of course, evidence of sickling of the red blood cells. Then, spontaneously and at unpredictable intervals, there occurs an exacerbation of the disease (a "crisis"), during which the anemia may become gradually or rapidly worse. Sudden exacerbation of the anemia, characterized by rapid destruction of erythrocytes, is likely to be associated with fever, increased icterus, nausea, vomiting, abdominal pain, and severe prostration. The crisis is often precipitated by an infection, and it is well known that patients affected with sickle cell anemia have an increased susceptibility to infections, especially in relation to the respiratory tract. Occasionally an osteomyelitis appears as a complication, and in these cases the responsible organism is usually one of the Salmonella group. (See Engh *et al.*, and also Barrett-Connor.)

During an exacerbation, the anemia may be very severe. The red cell count may even drop to a million and the hemoglobin be proportionately reduced. In addition to the sickle cells, the blood smears may show some red blood cells of the "target" type. Nucleated red blood cells (chiefly normoblasts) are a common finding and increase with the severity of the anemia, as do reticulocytes. In addition, one may note polychromatophilia and basophilic stippling. Neutrophilic leukocytosis is regularly present in sickle cell anemia, and during a crisis the total leukocyte count may reach 30,000 or more.

Other clinical features of the disorder which may evolve in the course of time include: enlargement of the liver, enlargement of the spleen (usually only in the younger patients), cardiac hypertrophy and cardiovascular manifestations, recurrent chronic ulcers of the legs (especially in the region of the ankles), and episodes of pain referred to the chest, abdomen, and/or bones and joints. Even though the patient may survive for several decades, the chronic anemia, the leg ulcers, the cardiac complaints, and the recurrent crises make sickle cell anemia a consistently serious disease. Death may result from an intercurrent infection, a rapidly developing severe anemia leading to cardiac decompensation and the occurrence of thromboses and infarction in various organs—especially the lungs and brain.

The *treatment* of patients affected with sickle cell anemia is largely directed toward preventing or ameliorating the clinical manifestations which appear in the course of exacerbations (crises) of the disease. Since, as already noted, such crises are often precipitated by an infection, the latter should be carefully guarded against, and vigorously combated if it does appear. For a subject who is already in a clinical crisis when observed, the appropriate treatment is largely supportive (including bed rest and relief of pain) but is also directed against specific clinical difficulties. In particular, the intravenous administration of fluid is indicated to combat dehydration. Transfusion of normal blood is advisable even if the clinical exacerbation of the disease is not severe, and is certainly indicated when there has been a sudden increase in the anemia, due to a rapid destruction of erythrocytes.

ROENTGENOGRAPHIC AND PATHOLOGIC FINDINGS

We shall limit our consideration of these findings to the various abnormalities relating to the bones. The subjects may present evidence of retarded growth, attributable in large part to the anemia itself (see Whitten). The more specific changes in the bones result from: (1) hyperplasia of the erythroblastic elements of the bone marrow; (2) plugging (thrombosis) of local blood vessels by masses of sickle cells; and (3) a complicating infection (most often by bacteria of the Salmonella group) involving one or another bone which is usually already the site of an infarct.

The *hyperplasia of the erythroblastic elements* of the bone marrow represents their response to the long-standing hemolytic anemia. As a consequence of the hyperplasia, rarefaction of the local osseous tissue occurs. This is most conspicuous in relation to the bony trabeculae of the spongiosa, and results in widening of the intertrabecular marrow spaces and even in complete resorption of many of the trabeculae. In addition, the marrow hyperplasia may even lead to thinning of the cortical bone and widening of the major marrow cavity. Even in youthful subjects, the short and long *tubular bones* in cases of sickle cell anemia often already show the widened trabecular pattern attributable to erythroid hyperplasia, and the *innominate bones* and *ribs* may show more. (See Fig. 179.)

Roentgenographic changes representing the effects of erythroid hyperplasia are also to be found in the *bones of the skull* and particularly in the mandible and calvarium. The diagnostic importance of the roentgenographic findings in these sites has been stressed by Reynolds. In the *mandible* the numerous delicate trabecular markings which would normally be present are lacking, and the medullary portion of the mandible shows increased radiolucency, and the trabeculae traversing it are sparse and coarse. With further advance of the changes in the mandible, the lamina dura appears more prominent, and the inferior cortex becomes thinned. The significant changes observed in the *calvarium* include thinning of the cortical tables, widening of the diploic zone, and a coarsely granular roentgenographic appearance, especially of the superolateral aspect of the parietal zone. The so-called "hair-on-end" pattern commonly noted in the calvarium in cases of thalassemia major is rarely observed, even in a very attenuated form, in classic cases of sickle cell anemia.

As is well known, the *vertebral bodies* are composed largely of spongy bone, have thin cortices, and are also one of the main sites of erythropoiesis. The upper and lower surfaces of each vertebral body consist not of cortical bone but of a thin plate of cartilage resting upon the spongiosa. The intervertebral disk between two adjacent vertebral bodies is contiguous with these cartilage plates. During the growth period of the subject, the cartilage plates contribute to longitudinal growth of the vertebral bodies through endochondral bone formation occurring at the surface of each plate where the latter abuts upon the spongiosa.

On the basis of this anatomic background, one can proceed to consider the alterations in the vertebral bodies which are frequently observed in cases of sickle cell anemia. Since, as noted, the vertebral bodies are one of the main sites of erythropoiesis, it is not surprising that extensive rarefaction of the spongiosa of the vertebral bodies can follow in the wake of the erythroid hyperplasia which occurs in sickle cell disease. The resultant porosity of the bodies is due to the thinning

Figure 179

A, Roentgenograph illustrating the characteristic changes of sickle cell anemia in the bodies of several thoracic vertebrae. The upper three vertebral bodies pictured show the cuplike depression (or somewhat squared-off indentation) implicating the midportion of the upper and/or lower surfaces of the involved bodies. The patient, a woman, was 23 years of age when she was admitted to our hospital and this roentgenograph was taken. Her clinical history revealed that the presence of sickle cell anemia had been discovered when she was 17 years old, and that her mother and a younger brother were also affected with the disease. Physical examination disclosed that her spleen and liver were both enlarged.

B, Roentgenograph depicting the alterations not infrequently encountered in the ribs in cases of sickle cell anemia. Note the widened trabecular pattern (attributable to the erythroid hyperplasia) and the thinning of the cortices of the ribs. The patient was a man who was 32 years of age at the time this roentgenograph was taken. From his clinical history one could date the onset of the manifestations of sickle cell anemia in his case to the time when he was about 20 years of age. These manifestations consisted of sporadic attacks of abdominal pain representing "crises" of the disease, and the hematological findings were consistent with sickle cell anemia. Roentgenographic examination of various other skeletal areas also yielded evidence of the disease.

C, Roentgenograph showing the condylar area of the left femur and the upper parts of the corresponding tibia and fibula in a case of sickle cell anemia. The bone areas illustrated show large and small patches of increased radiopacity. These represent the results of ischemic necrosis of the spongiosa and the reparative reaction occurring within the affected bone areas. This roentgenograph was taken during the patient's twenty-first admission to the hospital, when she was 45 years of age. Her first admission took place 11½ years earlier. Nearly all her admissions, both before and after the one in question, were occasioned by the occurrence of acute clinical episodes, almost always represented by a so-called sickle cell crisis.

D and *E*, Anteroposterior and lateral roentgenographic views of the bones of the left leg in another case of sickle cell anemia. The patient was a girl 5 years of age who had been underweight and in poor health since birth. The fibula is the site of an osteomyelitis. The clinical manifestations of the osteomyelitis were relatively mild, and the clinical course was torpid. No surgery was performed, and in about 2 years the osteomyelitic process had undergone substantial regression.

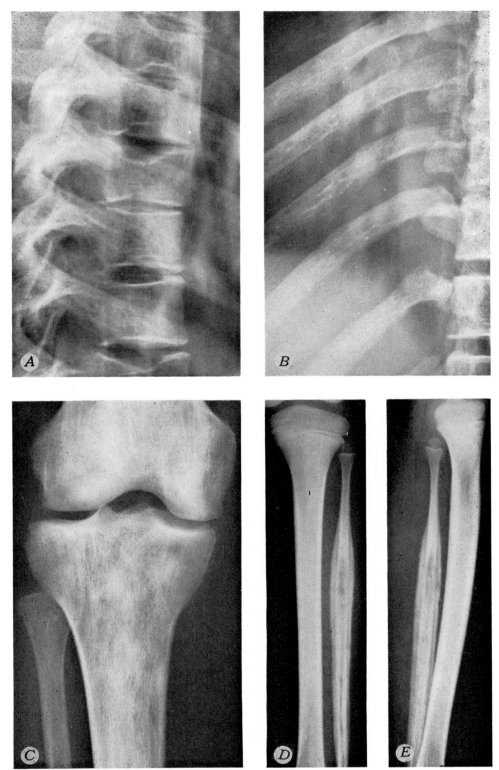

Figure 179

and/or resorption of the trabeculae of the spongiosa and the enlargement of the intertrabecular marrow spaces. There can be no doubt that such vertebral bodies present a reduced resistance to the impact of mechanical forces. However, it has been questioned that the compression and deformity of vertebral bodies so commonly observed in sickle cell disease (in about 30 per cent of affected adults) is due merely to expansion of the intervertebral disks against vertebral bodies made porous by the effect of erythroid hyperplasia. In particular, it has been emphasized that the deformity of the vertebral bodies in sickle cell disease is different both in contour and in mode of development from the familiar type of biconcave deformity

Figure 180

A, Roentgenograph of the right hip joint from a case of sickle cell anemia. The femoral head is the site of ischemic necrosis and also presents postnecrotic alterations. The subchondral portion of the head, which is still completely necrotic, casts a radiopaque shadow. The radiolucent crescent extending over a large part of the head represents an area in which the articular cartilage and fragments of the bony end plate have become separated from the rest of the head in consequence of fracture (see *B*). The part of the head distal to the still completely necrotic subchondral zone also casts a shadow of increased radiopacity (see *C*). In this portion of the head the increased radiopacity is largely the result of the reparative process which followed the revascularization of the necrotic osseous tissue. In particular, it is the deposition of new osseous tissue upon the pre-existing necrotic trabeculae that accounts for the increased radiopacity of this part of the head. Naturally, such trabeculae are thick, and the repaired spongiosa is more compact (see *E*). The patient was a Negress 29 years of age. Sickle cell anemia was also known to be present in other members of her family. Her clinical history in regard to the right hip joint indicated that for about 10 months before admission to the hospital she had been suffering from progressive pain in the hip and limitation of motion. The pain was most pronounced on walking, but there was some local pain even when she was in bed. The treatment for the hip disability consisted of resection of the femoral head and its replacement by a prosthesis.

B, Photograph showing the cut surface of part of the resected femoral head in this case. It reveals the gross pathologic changes which are so well reflected in the roentgenograph. The detachment of the articular cartilage and bits of the bony end plate is the basis for the radiolucent crescent apparent in the clinical roentgenograph. The irregular white zone located beneath the detached articular cartilage represents that portion of the femoral head in which repair has not taken place. The spongy trabeculae are still necrotic and the intertrabecular marrow spaces are filled with granular detritus (see *D*). Below this completely necrotic portion of the head, there is a bandlike gray zone of spongiosa which has undergone repair. Here the trabeculae are thick and closely set and the intertrabecular marrow spaces contain vascularized connective tissue (see *E*).

C, Roentgenograph illustrating the part of the femoral head portrayed in *B*. From above down, the picture shows the articular cartilage and fragments of subchondral bone which have become detached from the head. The immediately subchondral radiopaque area represents the still completely necrotic spongiosa. The more intensely radiopaque area distal to the completely necrotic spongiosa is the part of the head in which repair has occurred. Here the trabeculae are thick, and the spongiosa is close-meshed.

D, Photomicrograph ($\times$ 4) illustrating the general histologic architecture of part of the femoral head in this case. The necrotic spongiosa, containing granular detritus in the intertrabecular marrow spaces, stands out in sharp contrast to the spongiosa below it. The latter has been the site of revascularization and repair, and its trabeculae are relatively thick.

E, Photomicrograph ($\times$ 16) presenting in higher detail the histologic appearance of the area blocked out in *D*. In the upper part of this picture, the intertrabecular marrow spaces reveal granular detritus, and the trabeculae themselves are still necrotic. In the lower part of the picture, the intertrabecular marrow spaces are occupied, for the most part, by vascularized connective tissue, and many of the spongy trabeculae are thick. The thickening is due to the deposition of new osseous tissue on the cores of the still-necrotic original osseous tissue.

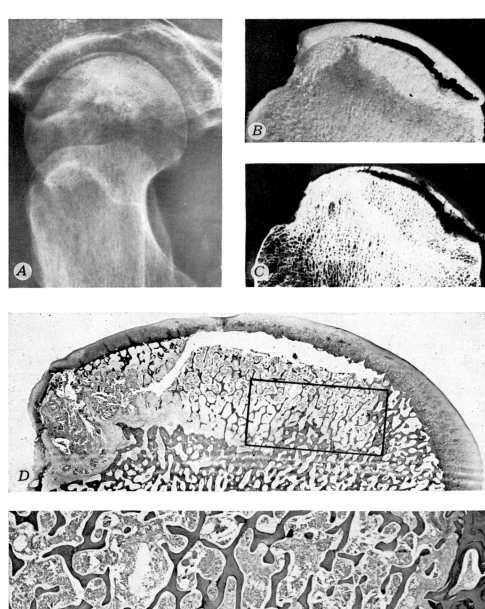

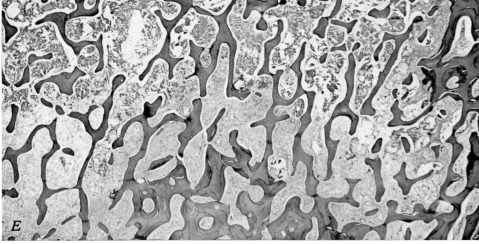

Figure 180

of vertebral bodies (so-called "fish vertebrae") so frequently encountered in cases of osteoporosis of the senescent and/or postmenopausal state (p. 371).

As is well known, the deformity of the vertebral bodies in instances of osteoporosis of the senescent and/or postmenopausal state is ordinarily characterized by a smooth, concave depression of the entire upper and lower surfaces of the affected vertebral bodies, the concavity usually being deepest in the midportion of the affected body. In contrast, as Reynolds points out, the deformity of the vertebral bodies which is encountered in cases of sickle cell disease begins as a cuplike depression or somewhat squared-off indentation implicating the midportion of the upper and lower surfaces of the vertebral bodies involved. Thus, at least at first, these surfaces, peripheral to the indented areas, tend to retain their normal flat contour. It is held that the significant pathogenetic factor underlying the cuplike deformation of the vertebral bodies in sickle cell anemia is not porosity of the spongiosa due to erythroid hyperplasia. Instead, it is maintained that this factor is blocking of the blood vessels, resulting in ischemia and hence in diminished endochondral ossification at the cartilage plates covering the upper and lower surfaces of the vertebral bodies. Apparently the effect of the ischemia is most pronounced in the central portion of the vertebra and interferes with endochondral ossification at the cartilage plates in this area, and this is therefore the area where the plate yields to the turgor of the intervertebral disks.

Infarction of bone, as observed in sickle cell anemia and its genetic variants, is the result of occlusion of small local blood vessels by thrombi consisting of masses of sickle cells. It is in those cases in which the subject has suffered from repeated clinical crises, representing periods of exacerbation of the disease, that one encounters the roentgenographic and pathologic alterations indicative of foci of bone infarction. The infarcts (sites of ischemic bone necrosis) are not necessarily limited to any particular bone site or type of bone. While they are most commonly observed in the short and long tubular bones, they have also been noted in vertebral bodies and (though rarely) in a scapula, one or another bone of the carpus or tarsus, or even one of the skull bones.

In cases of sickle cell anemia and its genetic variants, it is particularly in infants and very young children that phalanges, metacarpal bones, and/or metatarsal bones are the sites of infarction. It is not unusual for several of the short tubular bones of a hand or foot to be found involved at the same time. In these bones it is the shaft that is the site of infarction. The reparative response is represented by: (1) a slight amount of focal periosteal new bone formation; (2) patches of increased radiolucency expressing the resorption of the necrotic osseous tissue consequent upon the occurrence of revascularization in the vicinity of the infarct; and (3) the subsequent appearance of radiopaque patches resulting mainly from the deposition of new osseous tissue upon the pre-existing necrotic osseous tissue because of the progress of the reparative vascularization in the affected part of the involved bone (see Middlemiss and Raper, and also Burko *et al.*).

The long tubular bones are common sites of ischemic necrosis. In one or another long tubular bone, the site of the infarction may be the shaft of the bone, one or the other of its articular ends, or the shaft along with one articular bone end. The articular bone end most likely to be the site of an infarct is the upper end of a femur, and in some cases the upper ends of both femora show evidence of infarction (see Chung and Ralston). A somewhat less common site is the upper end of a humerus.

If the capital femoral epiphysis of the subject has not yet united with the shaft, the roentgenographic appearance of the involved area simulates that of Legg-Perthes disease. However, children manifesting ischemic necrosis of the capital femoral epiphysis in cases of sickle cell anemia or one of its variants are nearly always several years older than those affected with typical Legg-Perthes disease. In addition to this age difference there is the fact that Legg-Perthes disease as such is of rare occurrence in Negroes. In adults affected with sickle cell anemia and its variants, ischemic necrosis of the head of the femur is also encountered. (See Fig. 180.) In these cases the roentgenographic and pathologic findings are essentially similar to those observed in so-called idiopathic ischemic necrosis of the femoral head and in instances of necrosis of the femoral head in caisson disease (see Cockshott, and also Reich and Rosenberg). Despite this similarity, the etiologic differential diagnosis among cases of ischemic necrosis involving the femoral head in adults can usually be made merely on the basis of the clinical history and clinical findings. Hemorrhage into the joint related to the infarcted articular bone end provokes a chronic synovitis, and the cartilage of the infarcted articular bone end may come to be eroded by synovial pannus (see Sherman).

In the shaft of a long bone, the roentgenographic and pathologic changes resulting from the infarction are variable. In one bone shaft or another, the roentgenographic changes may be reflected in the form of multiple small patches of radiopacity, or mainly as a large irregular focus of radiopacity substantially filling the medullary cavity of the shaft. These changes in the direction of bone sclerosis represent a reparative response to infarction of the marrow and contiguous osseous tissue, following in the wake of local vascular obstruction. In the sclerotic bones from the patient studied by Graham, there was evidence of focal necrosis of the marrow and of the osseous tissue. The necrotic marrow was being replaced by a loose granulation tissue, and in this tissue a good deal of reparative new bone was being laid down. Furthermore, along the inner surface of the cortex of affected long bones, there was a layer of lamellated new bone. The sclerotic long bones studied by Diggs et al. likewise showed new bone formation within the shafts. This usually took the form of delicate linear trabeculae traversing the marrow, but in some instances the new bone was also found deposited against the inner surface of the cortex. In some places the new bone formation was so abundant as to have obliterated the regional marrow cavity. The tibia and fibula are among the long bones which may present this endosteal sclerosis. In addition to medullary sclerosis, or sometimes without it, these bones may show thickening of the external surface of the cortex. This is due to subperiosteal new bone apposition and usually represents a response to local infection related to the presence of leg ulcers.

Independently of infections spreading to the regional bones and joints from chronic ulcers of the soft tissues in the vicinity of the ankle, a *blood-borne infection* of one or more bones or joints may occur. Not infrequently the bacterial agent belongs to the Salmonella group. The Salmonella bacteremia often follows in the wake of a clinical crisis, and the osteomyelitis develops as the result of settlement of the bacteria at the site of a bone infarct. Clinically, the Salmonella osteomyelitis tends to run a benign and torpid course, and in particular it is not associated with any severe constitutional disturbance. Roentgenographically, an affected bone shows evidence of subperiosteal new bone formation, but the severe destructive alterations which characterize a full-fledged staphylococcal pyogenic osteomyelitis are absent (see Golding *et al.*, Barton and Cockshott, and Middlemiss and Raper).

THALASSEMIA

This form of hemolytic anemia is found mainly, though not exclusively, in persons of Italian and Greek descent. On this account it has frequently been denoted in the past as "Mediterranean anemia," in accordance with the geographic area to which it was first thought to be indigenous. However, it should be noted that the disease is rare or nonexistent among natives of pure stock on the French and Spanish Mediterranean shores. Actually, thalassemia is much more widely distributed geographically and racially than the term "Mediterranean anemia" would suggest (see Rucknagel). It was particularly through the efforts of Cooley that the severe form of the disease (now known as thalassemia major) was delineated from the omnibus category of "infantile pseudoleukemia," and for this reason the disease is still often designated as "Cooley's anemia" (see Cooley and Lee, and Cooley *et al.*). Other designations include "erythroblastic anemia" and "target cell anemia."

BIOCHEMICAL AND GENETIC CONSIDERATIONS

When present in pure form (that is, when not associated with other hemoglobinopathies), thalassemia has its basis in the absence of certain polypeptide chains normally present in the protein fraction of the hemoglobins, and their replacement by certain other chains. Thus, in thalassemia, in contrast to what one finds in sickle cell disease, there are no abnormalities relating to the amino acid sequences in those polypeptide chains which are formed. In accordance with the fact that there are alpha, beta, gamma, and delta polypeptide chains in the various hemoglobins, one might expect a number of biochemical types of thalassemia due merely to aberrations relating to these chains. Actually, however, only two pertinent types of thalassemia (alpha and beta thalassemia) have been identified. In the alpha type the synthesis of alpha polypeptide chains is partially or completely suppressed, and in the beta type the aberration relates to the beta polypeptide chains.

As has already been pointed out, the 4 coiled polypeptide amino acid chains are represented: in hemoglobin A_1, by 2 alpha chains and 2 beta chains; in hemoglobin A_2, by 2 alpha chains and 2 delta chains; and in hemoglobin F, by 2 alpha and 2 gamma chains. Thus, in beta thalassemia, in which there is an inherited defect of beta chain synthesis, there is an increased production of hemoglobin A_2 and/or hemoglobin F—hemoglobins which do not possess the beta chains. In alpha thalassemia, in which the pertinent inherited defect relates to the alpha chain, there is a consequent interference with the formation of hemoglobin F, which is vital for the survival of the fetus (see Hsia, and also Hutchison).

It has become clear that both of these biochemical types of thalassemia may be present in different degrees of severity. This range in the clinical gravity of the condition is apparently related in part to the heterozygous or homozygous inheritance of it. In addition, there seem to be intrinsically mild and intrinsically severe forms of the disorder, each transmittable on a heterozygous or on a homozygous basis. When inherited on a homozygous basis, both alpha thalassemia and beta thalassemia appear in the severe clinical form known as *thalassemia major*. When inherited on a heterozygous basis, the condition takes the clinical form of *thalassemia minor*, or the subject is merely a thalassemia trait carrier. Between these two expressions of the disease, there are instances of so-called *thalassemia intermedia*, and in these cases the genetic background of the condition may be somewhat obscure.

There are also cases of thalassemia in which the hemoglobin defect of thalassemia is combined with the defect characterizing some other hemoglobinopathy. The most common and clinically serious mixed, or hybrid, form of thalassemia is sickle cell thalassemia disease (hemoglobin S-thalassemia).

CLINICAL CONSIDERATIONS

Thalassemia minor tends to be mild in its clinical expression, the subject presenting at most a moderate anemia and splenomegaly. In many cases there are no clinical manifestations at all, the disorder coming to light only because the subject has been examined as a member of a family group in which thalassemia is known to exist. Also, in a particular family, one may encounter children or adults affected with thalassemia minor who have or had siblings showing the disease in its grave form—thalassemia major. Despite the fact that in cases of thalassemia minor the degree of the anemia may be very slight, striking morphologic abnormalities in the red cells are encountered. In particular, some of these cells may appear as so-called "target cells," or they may show stippling or be ovoid in shape. In addition, there is an increased resistance of the red blood cells to hemolysis in hypotonic salt solution.

Thalassemia major is a serious illness seen chiefly in infants and young children, few of whom survive beyond adolescence. The first clinical indication of its presence is pallor, which may already be noticeable during early infancy. In general, the clinical picture of thalassemia major is characterized by progressive anemia, yellowish discoloration of the skin (in consequence of hemolysis), and enlargement of the spleen and often of the liver. Frequently the child is stunted in growth and presents a mongoloid facies (due to expansion of the facial bones), along with other skeletal aberrations which are demonstrable roentgenographically and which are of considerable diagnostic value. In thalassemia major the anemia is likely to be pronounced. In blood smears the red cells show considerable variety in size, many being larger and many smaller than the mean. The large cells tend to be extremely pale. Most of their hemoglobin is concentrated around the periphery, and sometimes the center shows an additional mass of hemoglobin, so that the cell has the appearance of a target (hence the name "target cell anemia"). The resistance of the red blood cells to hypotonic saline is increased. Normoblasts (varying in respect to maturity) are likely to be found in the circulating blood, sometimes appearing in showers. The immaturity of the red blood cells is manifested also by polychromasia, basophilic stippling, and an increase in the number of reticulocytes. Frequently the number of leukocytes is found increased, especially by the addition of immature forms.

In a case of Cooley's anemia (thalassemia major) in which the manifestations set in during early infancy, the affected child often dies within the first year of life, usually from an intercurrent infection. In cases in which the presence of the disease has not become apparent until the second or third year of life, the child may survive for several years longer. Occasionally a case is also encountered in which the subject has survived into adolescence or even into adult life. In those instances of thalassemia major in which the patient lives on for some years, it may be cardiac failure that is responsible for death.

In regard to the *treatment* of thalassemia, it is to be noted that the disease does not seem to yield to any of the various antianemic therapeutic agents. Furthermore, transfusion has only temporary value. If the spleen is inordinately large, splenectomy is sometimes indicated.

ROENTGENOGRAPHIC AND PATHOLOGIC FINDINGS

Consideration will be given to the roentgenographic and pathologic findings only as they relate to the bones in cases of thalassemia major. (See Fig. 181.) That the roentgenographic findings are of considerable diagnostic value was already recognized by the early contributors to our knowledge of the disease (see Cooley *et al.*, Vogt and Diamond, Baty *et al.*, and also Caffey). Even if the disease is present in the severe form, the skeletal changes are at most only slight during the first year of life. During the next few years, they are often found well developed and may even be so pronounced and characteristic as to suggest the diagnosis by themselves. Although, in a severe case, practically all the bones may come to show alterations, the latter are by no means of uniform severity throughout the skeleton. Of the long tubular bones, the femora are likely to be most affected; of the short tubular bones, the metacarpals and metatarsals; and of the skull bones, those of the calvarium (see Baker).

In the calvarium, as Caffey points out, the changes tend to begin in the upper portion of the frontal bone and to spread backward, eventually involving the occipital bone. In the early stages of the disease or in milder cases, the cranial vault shows only a slight thickening and an increased porosity of the bones, with thinning of the tables—especially the outer table. Further progress of the changes is represented by increased (though not uniform) thickening of the calvarium and by the appearance of a "hair-on-end" feature. Specifically, one now notes dense, fuzzy, radial striations traversing the thickened calvarium, which seems actually devoid, at least anteriorly, of a clear-cut outer table. This radial alignment of the diploic spongiosa is held to represent an arrangement tending to compensate for the weakened or deficient outer table. In connection with the calvarial changes described above, interest attaches to the "symmetrical osteoporosis" which has frequently been noted by physical anthropologists in the skulls of ancient American Indians

Figure 181

A, Roentgenograph showing, in lateral projection, part of the skull in a case of thalassemia major. There is thickening of the calvarium, particularly in the frontal and parietal areas. Note also that the inner table is still clearly defined, while the outer table is not clearly delimited, especially in the anterior part of the calvarium. In that area, faint, fuzzy radial striations are apparent which represent the "hair-on-end" feature of the calvarial changes commonly observed in thalassemia major (see *C*). The patient, a woman of Italian ancestry, was 25 years of age when this roentgenograph was taken. Though she was aware of the fact that she had anemia, she sought admission to the hospital primarily because of large, persistent ulcers on the inner aspect of each ankle. Her father was known to have had a large spleen, and he died at the age of 35. Her mother was alive and well at the time of the patient's admission to the hospital, and did not have an enlarged spleen. The patient had 5 sibs. One of them died at the age of 12, and of the remaining sibs she and 2 brothers had enlarged spleens. Her spleen was very much enlarged, reaching down to the level of the umbilicus, and her liver was somewhat enlarged. Examination of her blood revealed anemia and the presence of numerous so-called "target" red blood cells. (See also *D* and *E*.)

B and *C*, Photograph of a slice of bone from a macerated calvarium, and roentgenograph of the same slice. These illustrations were prepared from a fragment of a skull excavated in New Mexico and believed to date back to about 1000 to 1100 A.D. The paleopathologic details relating to this skull are presented in the article by Jarcho *et al.* In that article it was the present writer who contributed the description of the pathologic features of the specimen. He concluded that the pathologic changes presented by the specimen could justifiably be interpreted as the effects of some type of hemolytic anemia—most probably Mediterranean anemia (thalassemia major). The "hair-on-end" feature is strikingly demonstrated in *C*. It is clear that this appearance is created by osseous trabeculae which were deposited by the pericranium on the outer table. These trabeculae are directed more or less at right angles to the surface of the calvarium.

D, Roentgenograph of part of a hand and forearm in the case of thalassemia major whose clinical aspects were noted in the legend concerning *A*. It is evident that the cortices of the illustrated bones are abnormally thin and are permeated by small, roundish radiolucencies. In addition, the spongiosa of these bones is wide-meshed—an appearance reflecting atrophy and distortion of the spongy trabeculae.

E, Roentgenograph illustrating the changes found in the ilium in the same case. Note the wide-meshed spongiosa and the distorted architecture of the trabeculae.

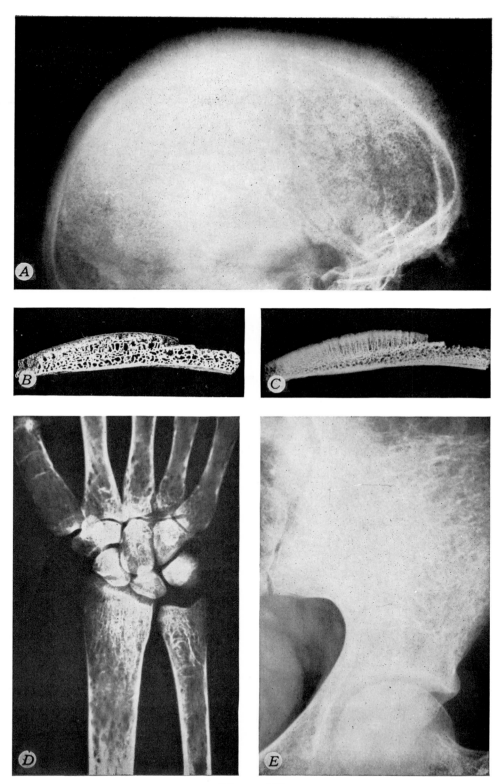

Figure 181

(see Hrdlička, and also Williams). The changes found on roentgenographic examination in these osteoporotic skulls resemble very strikingly those seen in severely
altered skulls in cases of thalassemia major (see Jarcho *et al.*). However, that these
calvarial changes actually had their basis in a hemolytic anemia such as thalassemia
major has been questioned (see Moseley).

At autopsy in a case of thalassemia major in which the calvarium presented a
roentgenographic picture of this kind, Whipple and Bradford found that when the
scalp was reflected the thickened calvarium presented a mulberry-red color. This
is due, of course, to the fact that deficiency of the outer table permits the color of
the marrow to show through the periosteum. The anatomic basis for the radial
markings seen in the roentgenograph was found to consist of spicular osseous
trabeculae interspersed with dark brownish red marrow. It seems worth noting
here that Dykstra and Halbertsma have described the case of a child suffering from
polycythemia vera in whom the calvarium showed changes similar to the pronounced
alterations of the skull in thalassemia major.

In the presence of advanced changes in the calvarium, the bones of the rest of the
skull tend to show increased porosity and irregular trabeculation. As a result of
expansion of the temporal and nasal bones, the air spaces in the temporal bones
and paranasal sinuses may be found encroached upon and even obliterated. In
some instances there is also expansion of the zygomas, which makes the cheek bones
stand out and contributes to the mongoloid facies presented by some of the patients.
Furthermore, one sometimes finds expansion of the upper and lower jaws, with
consequent malposition of the teeth and malocclusion of the jaws.

The vertebral bodies, too, may be found porotic, and may be cupped, relatively
shortened in vertical height, and also widened. When this is the case, anatomic
examination of the vertebral column shows thinning of the cortical shells of the
affected vertebrae, pronounced reduction in the number of trabeculae, and an
abundance of marrow, which is dark brown in color. The ribs, also, may be found
altered through thinning of the cortices and reduction in spongy trabeculae. Some
of the ribs may be found expanded, but the widening tends to be limited to the
posterior part, usually not extending beyond the axillary line. Abundant red bone
marrow fills the medullary cavity of such affected ribs, and in some places the
thinned cortex may even have yielded and marrow be found underneath the periosteum. The same anatomic background of marrow hyperplasia and bone atrophy
underlies the exaggerated trabecular markings which may be observed also in the
iliac bones, the scapulae, and the clavicles.

The roentgenographic picture presented by a strikingly altered tubular bone is
likewise that of a widened marrow cavity, a thinned cortex, and an abnormally
wide-meshed spongiosa with atrophic, distorted trabeculae. This picture is a
reflection of the anatomic findings noted by Whipple and Bradford in a femur of a
young child coming to autopsy. They observed that the shaft cortex was very
much thinned, the spongy trabeculae were sparse, and the marrow cavity was
enlarged. Dark, cellular, chocolate-red bone marrow filled the entire space inside
the cortical shell, but no marrow was found between the periosteum and cortex.

In association with striking cortical thinning observed roentgenographically, one
occasionally also notes small, punched-out radiolucent areas in the cortex. On the
other hand, instead of a coarse, trabeculated spongiosal pattern, the affected
tubular bones may present a swollen, homogeneously porotic appearance. Also,
some of the tubular bones may show alterations in contour, the normally concave
outline of the shaft region being replaced by one which is much more shallow,
straight, or even convex. Thus the femoral shafts may even come to take on, at
their lower ends, a shape suggesting an Erlenmeyer flask, and metacarpal bones, in
particular, may show convex contours. Near the ends of the long bone shafts, one

may find irregular transverse lines suggestive of the so-called "growth lines." Occasionally, supervening pathologic fractures are encountered, particularly in the femur.

In severe cases of long duration, it is found that maturation and growth of the skeleton have been retarded. In addition, premature fusion of epiphyses of long tubular bones has been observed in cases of thalassemia major. Such fusion has been found to occur most often at the proximal end of one or both humeri and in the distal end of one or both femora. The premature fusion is associated in some instances with a tilting of the epiphysis in question. When this occurs, the head of the humerus is usually found tilted medially, and the distal epiphysis of the femur tilted either anteriorly or posteriorly (see Currarino and Erlandson).

Histologic examination of bones from a child who has died of the disease shows that the thinning and atrophy of the osseous tissue is not associated with active osteoclastic resorption or significant marrow fibrosis. The red marrow is very cellular and few fat cells remain anywhere. Nests of parent marrow cells are conspicuous, as are nucleated red cells and myelocytes. Megakaryocytes are likely to be present in considerable numbers. Phagocytes may be found in moderate amounts, and some of these contain iron-staining pigment. Iron-containing pigment is also found widely distributed in the various other tissues of the body. Also, one may see islands of foam cells in the marrow (as also in the spleen), and some of these may be fairly large. Nests of metaplastic marrow are usually to be observed in the spleen and sometimes in the liver and in some lymph glands.

As to *pathogenesis*, it is to be noted that the porosity of the bones, as it evolves in the actively growing skeleton of the young child in cases of Cooley's disease (thalassemia major), is usually attributed to the pressure exerted by the hyperplastic myeloid marrow against the osseous tissue. Specifically, it is generally held that: (1) Excessive destruction of red blood cells leads to compensatory overgrowth of the bone marrow; (2) pressure atrophy of the spongiosa and cortical bone ensues, resulting in enlargement of the major and minor marrow spaces; and (3) some yielding of the contours of the severely affected bones may take place in consequence of the increased pressure from the hyperplastic marrow. The concept that porosity of the bones results from the pressure effect of hyperplastic myeloid marrow is supported by the following: In those bones in which the myeloid marrow is normally replaced by fatty marrow during childhood (for instance, the metacarpal and metatarsal bones and the phalanges), roentgenographic changes which may have been present in early childhood may substantially disappear from these bones in later childhood or during adolescence.

ERYTHROBLASTOSIS FETALIS

Erythroblastosis fetalis (also denoted as erythroblastosis neonatorum and hemolytic disease of the newborn) is a hemolytic disorder characterized by excessive destruction of erythrocytes beginning during fetal life. A fetus in whom the hemolysis of the red blood cells has set in during early fetal life usually dies *in utero* near the end of the gestation period. If born alive, a severely affected neonate ordinarily does not survive for more than a few days. However, those neonates who are less gravely affected have increasingly good chances for longer survival and even recovery under modern therapy—especially exchange transfusion.

The *pathogenetic basis* for erythroblastosis fetalis is usually Rh incompatibility between the blood of the fetus and that of the mother. About 85 per cent of the white population of the United States have the Rh factor in their red blood cells and are therefore to be denoted as Rh-positive, while those lacking this factor are denoted as Rh-negative (see Levine *et al.*). The Rh factor is inherited as a men-

46

delian dominant. If, therefore, even one of the parents transmits this factor, the fetus will be Rh-positive. When the blood of the mother is Rh-negative and that of the fetus is Rh-positive, the intermingling of the fetal and maternal blood leads to immunization of the mother against the Rh-positive red blood cells of the fetus and to the appearance of an abnormal hemagglutinin in the serum of the mother. This anti-Rh agglutinin is an antibody which passes by way of the placenta into the circulation of the fetus, and causes the hemolysis of the fetal red blood cells which underlies the various clinical manifestations and anatomic alterations characterizing the disease. If the mother is Rh-negative and the fetus or neonate shows evidence of erythroblastosis fetalis, both the child and the father are invariably Rh-positive. It should also be noted that mothers who are Rh-positive only infrequently bear children affected with the disease.

The Rh incompatibility between the blood of the mother and that of the fetus, resulting in anti-Rh agglutinin formation in the mother, represents the usual pathogenetic mechanism underlying the disease. However, anti-Rh agglutinin may also be present in the mother's blood if she is Rh-negative and has received, even years before the pregnancy, one or more transfusions of Rh-positive blood. Under such circumstances the first fetus conceived may not be severely affected, but in subsequent pregnancies the fetuses may show the disease in grave form.

CLINICAL CONSIDERATIONS

Incidence.—The over-all incidence of erythroblastosis fetalis is difficult to state categorically. It is certainly not a very common disease. Its incidence correlates with the proportion of Rh-negative individuals in a given population. The frequency with which it is encountered in maternity hospitals also varies with the geographical location of the institution and the racial distribution of its population. In particular, it has been found that the condition is relatively uncommon among Negroes. In accordance with variations in all these factors, there may be only one affected fetus or neonate among 400 or 500 deliveries in a given maternity hospital, while in another maternity hospital the over-all incidence may be higher or lower.

In contrast, if one considers only those pregnancies in which there is Rh incompatibility between the blood of the mother and that of the fetus, the incidence of erythroblastosis fetalis in maternity hospitals is very much higher. The occurrence of the disease in an individual family is also influenced by the position of a given child in the sequence of births in the family. When an Rh-negative mother is pregnant with an Rh-positive fetus as her first child, the latter is very rarely affected with the disease, and sometimes the first two or three fetuses are spared. However, when the disease has once made its appearance among the offspring, the likelihood of its occurrence increases from pregnancy to pregnancy, as does also the gravity of its manifestations (see Javert, and also Wintrobe). In the past few years, anti-Rh gamma globulin has been found to immunize the Rh-negative mother, so that the incidence of erythroblastosis fetalis is expected to diminish markedly in time (see Freda *et al.*, Pollack *et al.*, and also Levine).

Clinical Findings.—The hemolysis of the red blood cells of the fetus leads to the development of a severe anemia. This comes to be associated with the occurrence of large numbers of nucleated red blood cells in the circulating blood (erythroblastosis), extensive extramedullary hematopoiesis, hepatomegaly, splenomegaly, and often icterus. The principal and most conspicuous clinical findings are: edema, jaundice, pallor, and enlargement of the spleen and liver. In any individual case the clinical picture of erythroblastosis fetalis is likely to be dominated: by hydrops of the serous cavities and edema of the organs (*hydrops fetalis*); by intense icterus appearing within the first day or two after birth (*icterus gravis neonatorum*); or by profound anemia and/or a hemorrhagic diathesis (*congenital anemia of the newborn*). The most gravely affected fetuses are usually born before term and dead, and are often macerated. If not dead at birth, a severely affected neonate usually dies within the first 2 weeks after birth. In neonates who are less seriously affected, the chances for continued survival, and even cure, under appropriate treatment, become increasingly good. These neonates are notably the ones who do not present edema at birth, and in whom the jaundice and anemia are at least not severe at birth and show no rapid increase afterward.

Treatment.—The treatment of the affected *neonate* centers around blood transfusions, and exchange transfusion is preferable to repeated simple transfusion (see Pickles, and also Wiener *et al.*). For an Rh-positive infant, Rh-negative blood is used.

Wintrobe states that: *"Exchange transfusion is recommended* (1) whenever there is clinical evidence of disease at the time of birth as manifested by enlargement of the spleen and liver or by anemia (hemoglobin of cord blood less than 15 gm per 100 ml); (2) when there is a history of severe disease or of kernicterus in a previous baby; (3) in all premature erythroblastotic infants (because of their marked tendency to become severely jaundiced); (4) when the maternal titer of anti-Rh is 1:64 or higher (since there is a marked tendency for severe jaundice to occur in such cases); (5) if exchange transfusion is not done at birth, (*a*) it should be carried out if jaundice becomes apparent before the infant is 6 hours of age, (*b*) if the serum bilirubin level reaches 10 mg per 100 ml or more in the first 12 hours even though the hemoglobin is above 15 gm but is less than 17.5 gm. Exchange transfusion should be repeated within the first 12 to 24 hours if the serum bilirubin still rises; it should not be permitted to exceed 20 mg per 100 ml. A third exchange transfusion is rarely necessary if the first two are done early."

ROENTGENOGRAPHIC AND PATHOLOGIC FINDINGS

The pathologic findings in the viscera, the brain, and the various soft tissues in erythroblastosis fetalis are conditioned by the protracted anemia and jaundice and include edema and also effusions into the serous cavities. In consequence of the protracted hemolysis characterizing the condition, the bone marrow will be found hyperplastic, and extramedullary hematopoiesis will be demonstrable in the various organs removed at autopsy (for instance, in the spleen, liver, and kidneys). Splenomegaly and hepatomegaly are consistent findings. The jaundice is associated with icteric discoloration of various tissues and with kernicterus (intensive icteric staining of the spinal cord and of the basal nuclei of the brain by bile pigment). However, we are naturally most concerned here with the changes relating to the bones.

Alterations in the *bones* have been noted in some cases of erythroblastosis fetalis, though in other cases, including even severe ones, they have not been found. Follis *et al.*, reporting on 5 cases representing various clinical forms of the disease, found, on the basis of both roentgenographic and anatomic study, that the bones were abnormally dense. Anatomically, in regard to long bones, for instance, they noted that the cartilaginous epiphyses were not abnormal and there was no irregularity at the epiphysial-shaft junctions. Also, there was no abnormal thickening of the shaft cortex through abnormal periosteal new bone deposition. The increased roentgenographic and anatomic density of the bones seemed to be related only to an increase in the number and thickness of the spongy trabeculae in the interior of the bone shafts. In the abnormally thickened trabeculae, cores of calcified cartilage matrix were found persisting even toward the middle of the bone shaft. The marrow between the abnormally thickened trabeculae was found hyperplastic, and there was no evidence of excessive osteoclastic activity. Because of the thickening of the spongy trabeculae and the resultant densification of the spongiosa, the affected bones presented increased radiopacity. This was more or less uniform throughout the bone shaft in some instances. In others, the ends of the shaft (metaphyses) were less radiopaque than the rest of the shaft. In one case there were transverse bands of alternating diminished and increased radiopacity in the metaphysial portions of the shafts of the affected long bones. The bones in the case of erythroblastosis fetalis studied by the writer (see Fig. 182) showed changes in line with those described by Follis *et al.*

Caffey, too, stressed the finding of alternating radiopaque and radiolucent bands at the ends of long bone shafts in some cases of fetal erythroblastosis. However, he does not appear to have found anything strikingly abnormal about the bone shafts as a whole in respect to radiopacity. Others, too, have reported observing band formation in the metaphyses of the shafts of long bones, but no evidence of significant radiopacity elsewhere in the shaft (see Brenner and Allen).

The *pathogenesis* of the disordered endochondral ossification in fetal erythroblastosis is by no means clear. Densification of the spongiosa and abnormal persistence of calcified cartilage cores in the spongy trabeculae are also a striking feature in osteopetrosis (marble bone disease). Furthermore, it is to be noted that alternating bands of increased and diminished radiopacity at the ends of the long bone shafts, such as are seen in some cases of fetal erythroblastosis, are observed also in occasional cases of congenital syphilis. Of course, in fetal erythroblastosis there is no sign of syphilitic inflammation in the juxta-epiphysial portions of the bone shaft. Altogether, it must be left for further investigation to discover what, if any, are the skeletal changes specific for fetal erythroblastosis.

MYELOSCLEROTIC ANEMIA

Occasionally a case is encountered in which, for reasons not yet clear, the bone marrow of much of the skeleton has come to be more or less replaced by connective tissue in which a good deal of osseous tissue may also have been laid down. Roentgenographically, in accordance with the deposition of osseous tissue in the fibrotic marrow, the affected bones show increased radiopacity, along with disorganization of the original trabecular architecture but without cortical thickening. The choking out of the functioning bone marrow leads to an anemia (often with immature cells in the peripheral blood) and to extensive compensatory myeloid metaplasia. The

Figure 182

A, Roentgenograph of the distal two thirds of the femur and the proximal two thirds of the tibia and fibula of a somewhat premature fetus, born dead, and affected with erythroblastosis fetalis. Note the presence of alternating radiopaque and radiolucent bands in the distal metaphysis of the femur and the proximal metaphysis of the tibia.

B, Photomicrograph ($\times$ 3) of a tissue section prepared from the tibia shown in *A*. The spongiosa in the interior of the bone is close-meshed, and the dark-staining tract extending part way across the spongiosa represents an area in which the trabeculae are particularly thick. The roentgenographic reflection of this tract of spongiosa corresponds to one of the relatively radiopaque bands in the tibial metaphysis shown in *A*.

C, Photomicrograph ($\times$ 12) revealing in somewhat fuller detail the more or less transverse tract of thick spongy trabeculae shown in *B*. Even this low magnification permits one to deduce that calcified cartilage matrix is present in the cores of the thickened trabeculae.

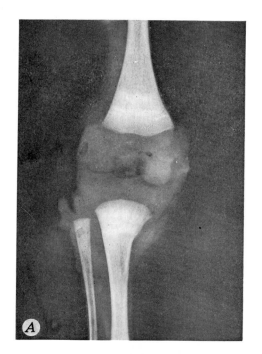

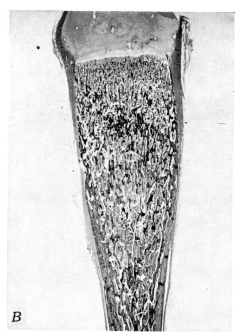

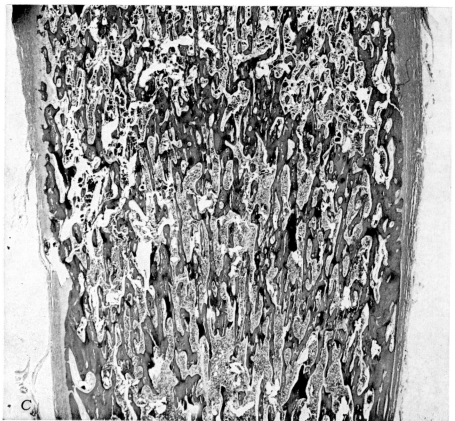

Figure 182

spleen in particular may become massively enlarged as it assumes an increasingly important role in hematopoiesis.

It is to cases presenting this general clinical and anatomic picture that the name "osteosclerotic anemia" was originally applied (see Assmann). In the past the condition has also been denoted as "pseudoleukemic osteosclerosis," "chronic nonleukemic myelosis," and "aleukemic megakaryocytic myelosis." The common current designations include: "osteomyelosclerosis," "myelofibrosis," and "primary (idiopathic) myelofibrosis" (see Oechslin, Goldberg and Seaton, Pitcock *et al.*, and also Fresen). Because none of these designations takes into account the anemia which is such an important facet of the disease, the writer prefers the designation "myelosclerotic anemia." One might use, as an alternate term, "osteomyelosclerotic anemia," but since the compensatory foci of *extra*medullary hematopoiesis may also come to undergo sclerosis, the more neutral term "myelosclerotic anemia" seems preferable.

CLINICAL CONSIDERATIONS

Myelosclerotic anemia occurs mainly in people of middle age or older. It is observed more often in males than in females, in a proportion of about 2 to 1 (see Fresen). The disease runs a chronic course marked by weakness, dyspnea, bouts of fever, refractory anemia, splenomegaly, hepatomegaly, hemorrhagic phenomena (petechiae and ecchymoses), and sometimes also bone pains. It is ultimately fatal because of the progressive intramedullary marrow fibrosis and the fibrosis occurring at sites of compensatory extramedullary bone marrow formation. The survival time from the onset of the condition is shorter for subjects beyond middle age than for younger subjects.

Hematological examination in any large series of cases reveals that the degree of anemia is quite variable. Furthermore, some cases even present a moderate polycythemia in the early phases of the disease. The anemia may be normochromic or hypochromic, and a pronounced poikilocytosis can usually be noted. Many of the misshapen red blood cells have the form of teardrops. The white blood cell count may be normal, below normal, or increased. If increased, the white cell count rarely exceeds 50,000 per cu. mm., and the differential count does not usually deviate much from the normal. The platelet count may be normal or moderately increased, and thrombocytopenia may be present even when the leukocyte count is normal.

Various numbers of immature leukocytes of the myeloid series, as well as nucleated red blood cells, are also usually present in the circulating blood. If the number of myelocytes and myeloblasts is high, subleukemic leukemia may be suspected. Apparently, also, as already noted, some cases of myelosclerotic anemia actually terminate with frank leukemic blood pictures. In such cases one may have difficulty in deciding, at least without autopsy, whether one is dealing with a case of myelosclerotic anemia dominated by myeloid metaplasia or with a case of leukemia associated with extensive fibrosis and sclerosis of the marrow. However, it is important to make every effort to distinguish between these two conditions clinically, since chemotherapy and radiation therapy are definitely contraindicated for myelosclerotic anemia.

The *treatment* is necessarily directed toward maintaining the patient's general well-being as much as possible, since the disorder cannot be cured. If the disease has progressed to a stage in which the subject presents a severe anemia, blood transfusions are indicated. Splenectomy is not advisable as a therapeutic procedure except under special circumstances, and in any event involves certain hazards. The special circumstances include abdominal discomfort from a very large spleen, and the presence of hemorrhagic phenomena due to thrombocytopenia. Irradiation of the spleen as an alternative to splenectomy may be advisable in cases in which the circulating blood shows a very high white cell count and many immature cells.

ROENTGENOGRAPHIC AND PATHOLOGIC FINDINGS

We are concerned here with the roentgenographic and pathologic aspects of myelosclerotic anemia mainly as they relate to the bones. (See Fig. 183.) Though the pathogenesis of the condition has by no means been clarified, mention will also be made of some of the relevant hypotheses which have been proposed.

Roentgenographic Findings.—Roentgenographically, severely affected bones appear abnormally radiopaque. The shadow cast by the bones may be uniformly radiopaque or of a patchy nature, even including small areas of relative radiolucency. The anatomic basis for the altered radiopacity is thickening and distortion of the original spongy trabeculae and the deposition of new osseous tissue on and between them. Thus, the roentgenographic abnormalities relate mainly to alterations in the cancellous bone. In affected long bones the cortex may not be thickened, but if it is, the thickening is due to the deposition of new bone on its medullary rather than on its periosteal surface. Especially if thickened, the cortex may be somewhat more porous (that is, less radiopaque) than it would normally be, or even somewhat lamellated.

Pathologic Findings.—In relation to the bones, the point of departure for the *pathologic changes* in myelosclerotic anemia is in the bone marrow. In an adult it is those bones or bone areas which are still the sites of active hematopoiesis that are the first to reveal the changes characterizing the disease, and these are also the sites in which the pathologic changes are most pronounced when the disease process is well advanced. It is for these reasons that the bones of the trunk tend to be more severely altered than the long tubular bones, and the latter in turn more severely altered than the calvarium or the short tubular bones.

In the vertebrae, ribs, and innominate bones, which are still the sites of active hematopoiesis in the adult, the first pathologic alteration to be noted is the appearance of focal areas of fibrosis in the myeloid marrow. As the fibrous replacement of the hematopoietic marrow of these trunk bones advances, foci of hematopoietic marrow make their appearance in certain other bone sites in which the marrow is largely fatty marrow. Ordinarily, in persons of middle age or older, the marrow in the spongiosa of the proximal and distal ends of the humeri, femora, and tibiae is already fatty marrow. In cases of myelosclerotic anemia, foci of hematopoietic marrow appear in the fatty marrow in the ends of these long bones, in compensation for the replacement of the hematopoietic marrow of the trunk bones by fibrous tissue. The hematopoietic marrow in these long bone sites is likewise subjected to fibrous replacement, and the stage is thus set in these sites also for the development of the other pathologic changes characteristic of myelosclerotic anemia.

Even in a case in which the pathologic alterations are well advanced, *gross examination* of the affected bones reveals little or no alteration of their cortices. As already noted, the abnormalities center mainly in the spongy bone and its intertrabecular marrow spaces (see Wolf, Sussman, and also Oechslin). In severely altered bones which have been cut open, the spongiosa is likely to be found gray-white in color, reflecting the sparsity of functioning myeloid tissue and the presence of fibrous tissue and new bone in the marrow spaces. The spongy trabeculae are thickened and irregular, and, in accordance with the deposition of new osseous tissue, the spongiosa is much more close-meshed than it would normally be. In the ribs, sternum, and vertebrae, the distortion and compaction of the spongiosa tend to be more pronounced toward the periphery than centrally. In long bones, in addition to alterations in the spongiosa along the lines already indicated, one may also find that grayish fibrous or fibro-osseous tissue fills the major marrow cavity.

The course of evolution of the *histopathologic changes* underlying such gross findings will now be briefly outlined. The initial alterations in the myeloid marrow consist of the appearance of foci of loose-meshed reticulum composed mainly of fibers, reticulum cells, and fibroblasts, and also including some osteoclasts. In time, the spongy trabeculae present evidence of osteoclastic resorption, and collagen fibers become manifest in increasing numbers between the fibroblasts. The resorption defects (the Howship's lacunae) on the surfaces of the spongy trabeculae are gradually filled in by new bone. In the fibrous tissue which has crowded out and replaced the myeloid marrow, trabeculae of nonmineralized matrix (osteoid) come to be laid down, but these osteoid trabeculae soon undergo mineralization, thus becoming converted into coarse-fibered osseous tissue. Some of these newly formed trabeculae of osseous tissue will be found to have become attached to the preexisting spongy trabeculae.

In regard to the osteoclastic resorption which occurs in the initial phase of the evolution of the pathologic changes, it is also of interest that, after the fibrous tissue has replaced the myeloid tissue and has undergone metaplastic bone formation, there is no further evidence of osteoclastic resorption. That is, even if the pathologic process continues to advance, what remains of the original osseous trabeculae or of the newly formed trabeculae of osseous tissue is not subjected to osteoclastic resorption.

Here and there in the spongiosa, one can find persisting islands of myeloid marrow. In this marrow, however, erythrocytes and myeloid cells tend to be sparse, but megakaryocytes are abundant and may be found disposed in small clumps. Why the megakaryocytes persist is not known, but it has been suggested that they may be more resistant to destruction than the other myeloid elements. It is interesting that, in myelosclerotic anemia, megakaryocytes (or, at any rate, cells resembling them) are prominent also in the extramedullary foci of hematopoiesis, and notably in the spleen. Some may even be present in lymph nodes not exhibiting other evidences of myeloid metaplasia.

Pathogenesis.—Various interpretations of the pathogenesis of myelosclerotic anemia (osteomyelosclerosis) have been proposed. Although none of them can yet be held to be necessarily valid, the principal ones will be briefly summarized below.

It has been maintained by some that the obliteration of the bone marrow which underlies the clinical and pathologic picture of myelosclerotic anemia follows in the wake of persistent toxic damage to the bone marrow (see Gall, Mallory *et al.*, and also Wyatt and Sommers). In the early stages of myelosclerotic anemia, they found scattered minute foci of marrow necrosis, associated with hyperplasia of the undamaged marrow. Later, presumably after the noxious agent has acted over a long

Figure 183

A, Roentgenograph showing more or less diffuse increased radiopacity in the proximal halves of the tibiae in a case of myelosclerotic anemia. In the corresponding portions of the fibulae, there is only a slight degree of increased radiopacity, and this is largely limited to the metaphysial portions of their shafts.

B, Photomicrograph ($\times$ 65) illustrating the histopathologic pattern of the spongiosa in a case of myelosclerotic anemia. There are focal areas of fibrosis in the myeloid marrow, and much of the marrow has been crowded out in consequence. Note also that trabeculae of nonmineralized matrix are present in the focal areas of fibrosis. In some places this osteoid matrix has already undergone mineralization and even become attached to the pre-existing spongy trabeculae.

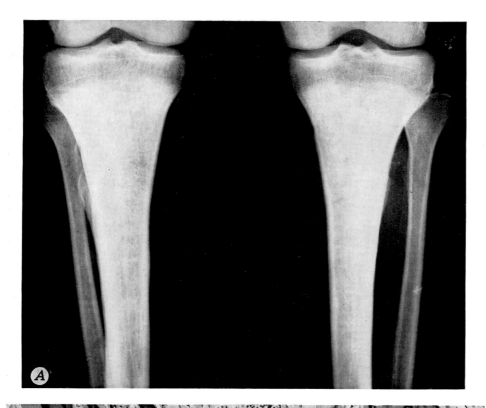

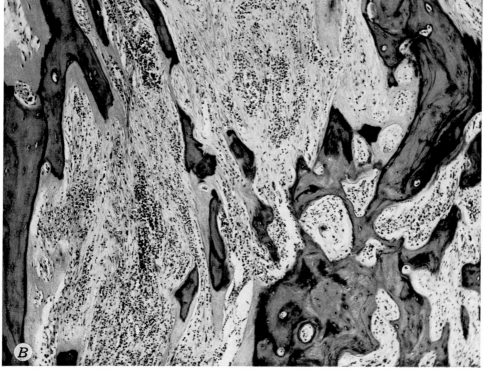

Figure 183

period of time, the marrow comes to show proliferation of its connective tissue, replacement of the myeloid elements by connective tissue, and, eventually, even calcification and ossification of this replacement tissue. The idea is that the myelo-fibrosis and sclerosis and the concomitant chronic marrow failure may be provoked by one or another of a variety of toxic agents, and that the reason these are toxic to the bone marrow is that they have not been conjugated by the liver and excreted as they would normally have been.

Another pathogenetic concept which has been proposed relates the disease to injury of the bone marrow capillaries by toxins. In particular, it is postulated that damage to the bone marrow capillaries by the toxins instigates focal serous inflammatory changes in the marrow, and that these are followed by connective tissue scarring and the subsequent formation of osseous tissue in the scarred marrow (see Apitz, and also Stodtmeister and Sandkühler).

Still another point of view about the pathogenesis is represented by the idea that myelosclerotic anemia (osteomyelosclerosis) follows in the wake of a chronic neoplastic reticulosis involving the reticulum cells of the bone marrow (see Rohr). On the basis of this concept, an analogy is drawn between the skeletal changes of myelosclerotic anemia (or, as Rohr calls it, osteomyeloreticulosis) and those characterizing the osseous form of Hodgkin's disease, as described by Krumbhaar.

REFERENCES

APITZ, K.: Zur Histogenese der Knochenveränderungen bei osteosklerotischer Anämie, Verhandl. deutsch. path. Gesellsch., *31*, 486, 1938 (published 1939).

ASSMANN, H.: Beiträge zur osteosklerotischen Anämie, Beitr. path. Anat., *41*, 565, 1907.

BAKER, D. H.: Roentgen Manifestations of Cooley's Anemia, Ann. New York Acad. Sc., *119*, 641, 1964–65.

BARRETT-CONNOR, E.: Bacterial Infection and Sickle Cell Anemia, Medicine, *50*, 97, 1971.

BARTON, C. J., and COCKSHOTT, W. P.: Bone Changes in Hemoglobin SC Disease, Am. J. Roentgenol., *88*, 523, 1962.

BATY, J. M., BLACKFAN, K. D., and DIAMOND, L. K.: Blood Studies in Infants and in Children: I. Erythroblastic Anemia; A Clinical and Pathologic Study, Am. J. Dis. Child., *43*, 667, 1932.

BRENNER, G., and ALLEN, R. P.: Skeletal Changes in Erythroblastosis Foetalis, Radiology, *80*, 427, 1963.

BURKO, H., WATSON, J., and ROBINSON, M.: Unusual Bone Changes in Sickle-Cell Disease in Childhood, Radiology, *80*, 957, 1963.

CAFFEY, J.: The Skeletal Changes in the Chronic Hemolytic Anemias (Erythroblastic Anemia, Sickle Cell Anemia and Chronic Hemolytic Icterus), Am. J. Roentgenol., *37*, 293, 1937.

————: Syphilis of the Skeleton in Early Infancy: The Nonspecificity of Many of the Roentgenographic Changes, Am. J. Roentgenol., *42*, 637, 1939.

————: Cooley's Anemia: A Review of the Roentgenographic Findings in the Skeleton, Am. J. Roentgenol., *78*, 381, 1957.

CHUNG, S. M. K., and RALSTON, E. L.: Necrosis of the Femoral Head Associated with Sickle-Cell Anemia and Its Genetic Variants, J. Bone & Joint Surg., *51-A*, 33, 1969.

COCKSHOTT, W. P.: Haemoglobin SC Disease, J. Fac. Radiologists, *9*, 211, 1958.

COOLEY, T. B., and LEE, P.: A Series of Cases of Splenomegaly in Children, with Anemia and Peculiar Bone Changes, Tr. Am. Pediat. Soc., *37*, 29, 1925.

COOLEY, T. B., WITWER, E. R., and LEE, P.: Anemia in Children, with Splenomegaly and Peculiar Changes in the Bones, Am. J. Dis. Child., *34*, 347, 1927.

CURRARINO, G., and ERLANDSON, M. E.: Premature Fusion of Epiphyses in Cooley's Anemia, Radiology, *83*, 656, 1964.

DIGGS, L. W., PULLIAM, H. N., and KING, J. C.: The Bone Changes in Sickle Cell Anemia, South. M. J., *30*, 249, 1937.

DYKSTRA, O. H., and HALBERTSMA, T.: Polycythaemia Vera in Childhood: Report of a Case with Changes in the Skull, Am. J. Dis. Child., *60*, 907, 1940.

ENGH, C. A., HUGHES, J. L., ABRAMS, R. C., and BOWERMAN, J. W.: Osteomyelitis in the Patient with Sickle-Cell Disease, J. Bone & Joint Surg., *53-A*, 1, 1971.

FOLLIS, R. H., JR., JACKSON, D., and CARNES, W. H.: Skeletal Changes Associated with Erythroblastosis Fetalis, J. Pediat., *21*, 80, 1942.

FREDA, V. J., GORMAN, J. G., and POLLACK, W.: Successful Prevention of Experimental Rh Sensitization in Man with an Anti-Rh Gamma₂-Globulin Antibody Preparation: A Preliminary Report, Transfusion, *4*, 26, 1964.

FRESEN, O.: On Osteomyelosclerosis, Acta path. jap., *11*, 87, 1961.

GALL, E. A.: Benzene Poisoning with Bizarre Extramedullary Hematopoiesis, Arch. Path., *25*, 315, 1938.

GOLDBERG, A., and SEATON, D. A.: The Diagnosis and Management of Myelofibrosis, Myelosclerosis and Chronic Myeloid Leukaemia, Clin. Radiol., *11*, 266, 1960.

GOLDING, J. S. R., MACIVER, J. E., and WENT, L. N.: The Bone Changes in Sickle Cell Anaemia and Its Genetic Variants, J. Bone & Joint Surg., *41-B*, 711, 1959.

GRAHAM, G. S.: A Case of Sickle Cell Anemia with Necropsy, Arch. Int. Med., *34*, 778, 1924.

HRDLIČKA, A.: Anthropological Field Work in Peru in 1913, with Notes on the Pathology of the Ancient Peruvians, Smithsonian Misc. Collect., *61*, 57, 1914.

HSIA, D. Y.-Y.: *Inborn Errors of Metabolism*, 2nd ed., Chicago, Year Book Med. Pub., Inc., 1966.

HUTCHISON, H. E.: *An Introduction to the Haemoglobinopathies*, London, Edward Arnold Ltd., 1967.

JACKSON, J. F., ODOM, J. L., and BELL, W. N.: Amelioration of Sickle Cell Disease by Persistent Fetal Hemoglobin, J.A.M.A., *177*, 867, 1961.

JARCHO, S., SIMON, N., and JAFFE, H. L.: Symmetrical Osteoporosis (Spongy Hyperostosis) in a Prehistoric Skull from New Mexico, El Palacio, *72*, 26, 1965.

JAVERT, C. T.: Erythroblastosis Neonatorum, Surg. Gynec. & Obst., *74*, 1, 1942.

KRUMBHAAR, E. B.: Hodgkin's Disease of Bone Marrow and Spleen without Apparent Involvement of Lymph Nodes, Am. J. M. Sc., *182*, 764, 1931.

LEVINE, P.: Prevention and Treatment of Erythroblastosis Fetalis, Ann. New York Acad. Sc., *169*, 234, 1970.

LEVINE, P., KATZIN, E. M., and BURNHAM, L.: Isoimmunization in Pregnancy: Its Possible Bearing on the Etiology of Erythroblastosis Foetalis, J.A.M.A., *116*, 825, 1941.

LEVINE, P., VOGEL, P., and ROSENFIELD, R. E.: Hemolytic Disease of the Newborn, in *Advances in Pediatrics*, Vol. VI, p. 97, Chicago, The Year Book Publishers, Inc., 1953.

MALLORY, T. B., GALL, E. A., and BRICKLEY, W. J.: Chronic Exposure to Benzene (Benzol). III. The Pathologic Results, J. Indust. Hyg. & Toxicol., *21*, 355, 1939.

MIDDLEMISS, J. H., and RAPER, A. B.: Skeletal Changes in the Haemoglobinopathies, J. Bone & Joint Surg., *48-B*, 693, 1966.

MOSELEY, J. E.: The Paleopathologic Riddle of "Symmetrical Osteoporosis," Am. J. Roentgenol., *95*, 135, 1965.

NEEL, J. V.: Data Pertaining to the Population Dynamics of Sickle Cell Disease, Am. J. Human Genet., *5*, 154, 1953.

OECHSLIN, R. J.: Osteomyelosklerose und Skelett, Acta haemat., *16*, 214, 1956.

PAULING, L., ITANO, H. A., SINGER, S. J., and WELLS, I. C.: Sickle Cell Anemia, a Molecular Disease, Science, *110*, 543, 1949.

PICKLES, M. M.: *Haemolytic Disease of the Newborn*, Springfield, Ill., Charles C Thomas, 1949.

PITCOCK, J. A., REINHARD, E. H., JUSTUS, B. W., and MENDELSOHN, R. S.: A Clinical and Pathological Study of Seventy Cases of Myelofibrosis, Ann. Int. Med., *57*, 73, 1962.

POLLACK, W., GORMAN, J. G., and FREDA, V. J.: Prevention of Rh Hemolytic Disease, Progr. Hemat., *6*, 121, 1969.

RAPER, A. B.: Sickle-Cell Disease in Africa and America—A Comparison, J. Trop. Med., *53*, 49, 1950.

REICH, R. S., and ROSENBERG, N. J.: Aseptic Necrosis of Bone in Caucasians with Chronic Hemolytic Anaemia due to Combined Sickling and Thalassemia Traits, J. Bone & Joint Surg., *35-A*, 894, 1953.

REYNOLDS, J.: An Evaluation of Some Roentgenographic Signs in Sickle Cell Anemia and Its Variants, South. M. J., *55*, 1123, 1962.

————: A Re-evaluation of the "Fish Vertebra" Sign in Sickle Cell Hemoglobinopathy, Am. J. Roentgenol., *97*, 693, 1966.

ROHR, K.: Myelofibrose und Osteomyelosklerose (Osteomyeloretikulose-Syndrom), Acta haemat., *15*, 209, 1956.

RUCKNAGEL, D. L.: On the Geographical Distribution and Ethnic Origin of Thalassaemia, New Zealand M. J., *65*, 826, 1966.

SHERMAN, M.: Pathogenesis of Disintegration of the Hip in Sickle Cell Anemia, South. M. J., *52*, 632, 1959.

STODTMEISTER, R., and SANDKÜHLER, S.: Knochenmarkatrophie und Knochenmarkfibrose, Deutsche med. Wchnschr., *76*, 1431, 1951.

————: *Osteosklerose und Knochenmarkfibrose*, Stuttgart, Georg Thieme, 1953.

SUSSMAN, M. L.: Myelosclerosis with Leukoerythroblastic Anemia, Am. J. Roentgenol., *57*, 313, 1947.

Tomlinson, W. J.: The Incidence of Sicklemia and Sickle Cell Anemia in 3000 Canal Zone Examinations Upon Natives of Central America, Am. J. M. Sc., *209*, 181, 1945.

Tseng, H. L.: Fatal Cases of Acute Sicklemia, Arch. Path., *67*, 339, 1959.

Vogt, E. C., and Diamond, L. K.: Congenital Anemias, Roentgenologically Considered, Am. J. Roentgenol., *23*, 625, 1930.

Whipple, G. H., and Bradford, W. L.: Mediterranean Disease—Thalassemia (Erythroblastic Anemia of Cooley). Associated Pigment Abnormalities Simulating Hemochromatosis, J. Pediat., *9*, 279, 1936.

Whitten, C. F.: Growth Status of Children with Sickle-Cell Anemia, Am. J. Dis. Child., *102*, 355, 1961.

Wiener, A. S., Wexler, I. B., and Brancato, G. J.: Treatment of Erythroblastosis Fetalis by Exchange Transfusion, J. Pediat., *45*, 546, 1954.

Williams, H. U.: Human Paleopathology, with Some Original Observations on Symmetrical Osteoporosis of the Skull, Arch. Path., *7*, 839, 1929.

Wintrobe, M. M.: *Clinical Hematology*, 6th ed., Philadelphia, Lea & Febiger, 1967 (p. 826).

Wolf, C.: Über einen Fall von osteosklerotischer Pseudoleukämie. Beitrag zur Frage der Osteosklerosen, Beitr. path. Anat., *89*, 151, 1932.

Wyatt, J. P., and Sommers, S. C.: Chronic Marrow Failure, Myelosclerosis and Extramedullary Hematopoiesis, Blood, *5*, 329, 1950.

Chapter

24

Hemophilia

HEMOPHILIA is a constitutional anomaly of blood coagulation characterized by a tendency toward protracted hemorrhage associated with deficiency of a specific clotting factor in the plasma. Among hemophiliacs (especially those in whom the deficiency of the clotting factor is pronounced), repeated intra-articular hemorrhage eventually leads to destructive changes in various large joints. The resultant *arthropathy* is one of the most common causes of protracted disability connected with hemophilia. Occasionally the nonarticular part of one or another bone becomes grossly expanded, most plausibly in consequence of the pressure effects of intramedullary hemorrhage. The supervening bone lesion is usually denoted as a *hemophilic pseudotumor*. Two rather uncommon aspects of hemophilia which are pertinent to skeletomuscular disease are *femoral neuropathy* and *Volkmann's contracture*.

Hemophilia is a *sex-linked inherited disorder*, transmitted as a recessive mendelian trait. The disease is manifested exclusively (or almost exclusively) by males, but it is transmitted within a family from one generation to the next by the females, who themselves are outwardly normal. That is, the disease is transmitted from an affected male through an unaffected but trait-carrying daughter to his grandsons. More particularly, half of the sons of the daughter or daughters of a hemophilic male can be expected to present evidence of the disease. Moreover, half of the daughters of the trait-carrying females, while not presenting any clinical evidence of hemophilia, are also capable of transmitting hemophilia or the hemophilic trait to their offspring. On the other hand, the sons of a hemophilic father are normal themselves and also do not pass the disorder on to their children. Furthermore, note should also be taken of the fact that the disease may appear *de novo* in a family as a result of a spontaneous mutation. Indeed, it has been estimated that about a third of all cases of hemophilia are of this type (see Soulier). Hemophilia resulting in hemophilic arthropathy has also been found to occur in dogs, but in canine hemophilia the disease does not seem to be limited to males (see Swanton).

Hemophilia has been a subject of medical interest for many centuries. However, the *biochemical basis* for the abnormally slow coagulability of the blood, which clearly underlies the protracted bleeding, has only recently been elucidated (see Patek and Taylor, and also Bendien and van Creveld). Relevant biochemical studies have also made it clear that hemophilia as a disease complex comprises hemophilia A and hemophilia B. In hemophilia A (classical hemophilia) the bleeding and delayed coagulation of the blood are due to a deficiency of a plasma factor denoted as "antihemophilic globulin" (AHG or factor VIII). In hemophilia B (also denoted as Christmas disease, after the surname of one of the families in which it was first recognized), the bleeding and delayed coagulation of the blood are the result of a deficiency of the plasma factor denoted as "plasma thromboplastin component" (PTC or factor IX). Hemophilia A appears to be the more common form of the disease, but the clinical and pathologic features are essentially the same in hemophilia B as in hemophilia A (see Moseley). Occasionally a case is encountered in which the plasma deficiency relates to both factor VIII and factor IX, the subject thus being affected with both hemophilia A and hemophilia B.

CLINICAL CONSIDERATIONS

In addition to occurring within joints, the frequent and stubborn *hemorrhages* which characterize hemophilia may take place at any other site of trauma—under the skin, in the subcutaneous tissues, and in and about the muscles. Particularly in young subjects, trauma to the head may be followed by subdural, epidural, or intracerebral hemorrhage. The hemorrhages may also appear without obvious cause, issuing apparently spontaneously from various parts of the body, especially the mucous membranes of the nose, the gums, and the lips. Hematuria due to hemorrhage from the kidneys and the urinary bladder is also frequently encountered. Intraperitoneal and gastrointestinal hemorrhage may likewise occur.

Femoral neuropathy is a rather infrequent but striking nonskeletal manifestation of hemophilia (see Brower and Wilde). As summarized by them, "the condition consists in severe pain of rapid onset in the groin, on the superior aspect of the thigh, and deep in the hip region. The pain is extremely intense and usually lasts about one week. A pronounced contracture of the hip in acute flexion and slight external rotation results. The slightest movement of the hip causes severe pain. A tender swelling appears in the iliac fossa and groin and over the superior medial aspect of the thigh. There is a depression in the center of this swelling corresponding to the inguinal ligament. After a few days the skin overlying these areas becomes ecchymotic. Later a flaccid paralysis of the quadriceps femoris, diminution or absence of sensation in the anteromedial aspect of the thigh and proximal portion of the leg, and a depressed or absent patellar reflex are discovered." It is proposed as a conjecture by Brower and Wilde that the syndrome of femoral neuropathy is the result of hemorrhage in the iliopsoas muscle at the musculotendinous junction beneath the iliacus fascia, and that the femoral nerve becomes compressed beneath the unyielding inguinal ligament superiorly and the iliopectineal ligament medially. (See Goodfellow *et al.*)

Volkmann's contracture has occasionally been observed in hemophiliacs (see Thomas, and also Newcomer). It is generally maintained that the most likely cause of this contracture is massive hemorrhage into the volar muscles of the forearm.

It is, of course, with the *skeletal manifestations* of hemophilia and in particular with the changes relating to the joints that we are mainly concerned here. Nevertheless, though *hemophilic pseudotumor* is a relatively uncommon lesion, it acquires clinical significance because of the potential danger of misinterpreting that lesion, on a roentgenographic basis, as a malignant tumor of bone (see Firor and Woodhall, Ghormley and Clegg, Nelson and Mitchell, Abell and Bailey, Stiris, and also Ahlberg).

The two bones in which a hemophilic pseudotumor has been observed most often are the femur and the ilium. When present in an ilium, the lesional area usually appears roentgenographically as a large, ballooned-out, multilocular shadow representing the effects of intra-osseous hemorrhage. Under these circumstances the lesion might be misinterpreted as a benign or malignant neoplasm if one was unaware that the patient had hemophilia. When the hemophilic pseudotumor involves the end of the shaft of a long bone, the site of the lesion may be represented roentgenographically by a large area of radiolucency, associated with expansion of the contour of the affected part of the bone and even with a pathologic fracture. On the other hand, a hemophilic pseudotumor may be located in relation to the midportion of the shaft of a long bone. In such a case it may appear in the roentgenograph as a tumor mass resulting from elevation of the periosteum by hemorrhage which has provoked some subperiosteal new bone formation. Again, the hemophilic pseudotumor may evolve following a massive hemorrhage into the soft tissues surrounding the shaft of a long bone. Under such circumstances the regional bone cortex undergoes more or less extensive pressure erosion by the fibrous soft-tissue mass resulting from organization of the extravasated blood. Several instances of hemophilic pseudotumor have also been observed in which the lesion was located in one or another short tubular bone of a hand or foot—usually a terminal phalanx.

Arthropathy.—Statistical surveys have shown that in a particular subject the number of joints involved and the extent of articular damage occurring in the course of time correlate to a considerable degree with the severity of the biochemical defect relating to the clotting mechanism in the case in question (see Ahlberg). In hemophilia based on deficiency of factor VIII, it is recognized that there are 4 grades of severity of the condition. These are: (1) severe (classical) hemophilia; (2) moderate hemophilia; (3) mild hemophilia; and (4) subhemophilia. The grade of severity of the disorder correlates with the findings relating to the per cent of factor VIII in the plasma. Assays for plasma factor VIII in cases ranging from severe hemophilia (grade 1) down to subhemophilia (grade 4) have demonstrated respectively 0 per cent, below 3 per cent, below 16 per cent, and 20 to 30 per cent. For comparison, it is useful to know that the normal value for factor VIII in the plasma is 70 per cent or above (see Brinkhous, and also Wintrobe).

The over-all *incidence* of articular lesions among "bleeders" is high. As already noted, the incidence and severity of the articular lesions rise with the degree to which the specific clotting factor in the plasma is deficient. As to *age distribution*, the first evidence of articular involvement seldom appears before the second year of life, but not infrequently does appear during that year and the next. Initial articular involvement is perhaps less common during the next few years, but its occurrence rises again in subjects between 8 and 13 years of age. In regard to *localization*, it is clear that the knee joint is by far more often affected than any other. The elbow and ankle joints are also rather often involved, while the hip, shoulder, and wrist joints are relatively infrequently implicated. Small joints, such as those of the fingers and toes, are only rarely the site of hemophilic arthropathy. In some hemophiliacs a single joint tends to be affected repeatedly, while other joints are spared. In other subjects, various joints are involved from time to time. Implication of both knee joints is fairly common in cases in which the hemophilia is of the severe (classical) type. On the other hand, bilateral involvement of the hip is by no means common.

Frequently the arthropathy is initiated by trauma, which is often so slight that in a normal person it might have passed unnoticed. The incidence of recurrent hemarthrosis is higher in children than in adults, because the latter are more fully aware of the threat of trauma to their joints and hence more likely to avoid it. In addition, if the subject is a young child and the deficiency of the plasma factor is considerable, even the physiological "trauma" of weight-bearing may sometimes be sufficient to induce an episode of hemarthrosis.

One of the first to describe the articular aspects of hemophilia was König, who listed 3 progressive clinical stages of hemophilic joint involvement. Among the older discussions of the pathologic and/or roentgenographic features of hemophilic arthritis are those by Freund, Doub and Davidson, Reinecke and Wohlwill, and also Petersen. Among the early review articles on the subject are those by Schloessmann and by Key. The 3 progressive stages of hemophilic joint involvement listed by König are: (1) the stage of the initial intra-articular hemorrhage, characterized by uncomplicated hemarthrosis; (2) the stage of reactive inflammation (pan-arthritis), distinguished particularly by proliferation of the synovial membrane, sometimes developing as a response to the initial hemorrhage but usually repre-senting a cumulative reaction to successive hemorrhages; and (3) the stage of greatly advanced articular changes, in which contraction and permanent deformity of the joint have appeared.

As long as the hemorrhage or hemorrhages in a hemophilic joint are resorbed completely, and as long as no permanent damage has developed in the joint, the latter is still in the first stage of involvement (that is, the one of acute simple hemarthrosis). The second and third stages merge into each other and together present the picture of chronic hemophilic arthritis. In the earlier phases of the chronic stage, the clinical course may still be marked by repeated acute hemorrhages into the joint. It should be recognized that König's observations relating to the progressive stages in the evolution of the articular changes in cases of hemophilia were presented in 1892—that is, 3 years before Roentgen's discovery of the X ray (roentgen ray). This explains why König's description of the articular changes in hemophilia could not include a correlation of the clinical and pathologic findings with radiographic findings relating to the affected joints.

Clinically, especially in a child or adolescent, the occurrence of a sudden derange-ment of a large joint, appearing without apparent adequate cause, should suggest the possibility of an *acute simple hemarthrosis* due to an underlying hemophilia. The patient may be seen during the first attack of acute hemarthrosis, or there may be a history of previous acute swelling of the involved joint or of other joints. The amount of intra-articular bleeding may be moderate or considerable. The resultant enlargement of the joint often develops with great rapidity (within half an hour) but may require 10 to 12 hours for its evolution. If there has been a large amount of bleeding, the affected joint is greatly swollen, and the capsule is tense and dis-tended. The joint is held in a deloaded position, motion being abolished because of pain and spasm. The joint may be acutely tender and the tenderness may radiate. If, on the other hand, there has been little hemorrhage, the degree of swelling is slight and there may be little or no pain or limitation of motion. Thus, the clinical findings in the involved joint vary with the amount of intra-articular hemorrhage and the consequent tension on the capsule.

Local redness and heat are not present except when the joint is greatly distended with blood. In the latter case, there is also a complaint of increasing pain until the swelling has reached its limit. Afterwards (within a day or two), the pain gradually subsides even if the swelling persists. If, in addition to bleeding into the joint, there has been hemorrhage into the periarticular and subcutaneous tissues, large ecchymoses may be apparent early or may become evident 3 or 4 days later through greenish discoloration of the skin. The hemarthrosis is likely to be followed in a few days by slight rises in body temperature, usually not greater than 1° to 3° F. There is also a slight increase in the polymorphonuclear leukocyte count.

Generally after the first attack of acute hemarthrosis, and often after subsequent attacks, the blood is resorbed and the joint regains a normal appearance. The blood exudate disappears rather slowly—ordinarily within 3 to 6 weeks. Sooner or later, perhaps only after some years, the affected joint may become the site of a *chronic hemophilic arthritis*. After one of the hemorrhages, the swelling may not regress completely. The joint remains enlarged, tender, and painful. The condi-tion is often aggravated by further attacks of acute swelling and pain, usually associated with minor injuries. The swellings are mainly the result of acute hemor-rhage. After each attack, although there is some degree of restoration of function, the arthropathy nevertheless worsens. In this later stage of its evolution, the affected articulation is found enlarged, and the details of its outline are obscured.

The frequency of the acute swellings with their associated pain and tenderness on motion decreases. On examination the affected joint shows capsular thickening, diminished mobility, crackling or grating on movement, deformation of the bony contours, and atrophy of the muscles. Finally a state of permanent articular disability develops. This is characterized by forced contraction positions, muscular atrophy, subluxations, and ankylosis caused, in large measure, by shriveling of the capsule and periarticular tissues. It is obvious that if several crucial joints are affected in this way the patient will be severely crippled.

ROENTGENOGRAPHIC AND PATHOLOGIC FINDINGS

Roentgenographic Findings.—A frequently cited classification of hemophilic arthropathy which takes the roentgenographic as well as the clinical findings into consideration is the one proposed by DePalma and Cotler. They distinguished 4 grades of hemophilic arthropathy. In *grade 1*, representing the earliest form of involvement, the intra-articular hemorrhage or hemorrhages have not yet resulted in any functional impairment of the joint. Such joints show minimal roentgenographic changes expressed by slightly diminished radiopacity of the articular bone ends and some increased radiopacity of the capsular tissue of the joint. In *grade 2* the affected joint presents a slightly reduced range of mobility. The joint space is still well preserved, and there is no irregularity of the articular surfaces nor any subchondral cysts. However, the spongy trabeculae of the epiphysial ends of the bones entering into the formation of the joint may be somewhat more prominent than they would normally be. In *grade 3* the articular involvement is such that there is a fixed deformity of the joint, manifest in at least one plane. The combined changes in the soft tissues and articular bone ends are of sufficient severity to have produced an appreciable degree of articular dysfunction. For instance, the muscles connected with the motor activity of the joint show pronounced atrophy, and this is associated with pericapsular and capsular thickening and with knobbiness of the bone ends. The latter show irregularities of the articular surfaces, small or large cystlike rarefactions in the bone ends, and some marginal spur formations. In *grade 4*, in which the affected joint presents the most advanced changes, the deformity is likely to be pronounced and fixed (partly in consequence of fibrous ankylosis), and palpation of the joint reveals striking knobbiness. The articular bone ends are irregular and deformed and show increased radiopacity in some places, while in other places focal areas (sometimes large) of radiolucency may be apparent. Roentgenographic examination will reveal narrowing of the joint space and even obliteration of part of the articular cavity. Articular changes of grade 4 severity are nearly always noted in hemophilic adults in whom many episodes of acute intra-articular hemorrhage had occurred in the past, but in whom the episodes of acute bleeding have been infrequent during the past few years.

In general, the roentgenographic features of hemophilic arthritis can be summarized as follows: For years a hemophilic joint may remain essentially intact, so that it presents no noteworthy changes visible roentgenographically. Paralleling disturbed mobility and functional disability, radiographic indications of bone atrophy gradually become evident. With further progression of the chronic arthritis, the joint space narrows and the articular contours become irregular. The space may even be substantially obliterated in the course of destruction of the articular cartilages. The bone ends tend to flatten and spread, and subluxations are common. In some cases of unusually long duration, bony ankylosis may be apparent in the affected joint or joints. There is also a rather strong tendency

47

toward the formation of marginal exostoses similar to those of hypertrophic arthritis (osteoarthritis).

Two roentgenographic manifestations which are regarded as characteristic of chronic hemophilic arthritis, though they are not always present, are: (1) roundish cystlike areas of radiolucency in the bone ends of the joint, and (2) shadows of increased radiopacity in the soft tissues about the joint. The anatomic basis for these particular shadows is explained below in the discussion of the pathology of hemophilic arthritis. (See Figs. 184 and 185.)

Pathologic Findings.—The resorption of the hemorrhagic exudate is more and more delayed with each recurrence of acute hemarthrosis. Finally, persisting blood and organizing blood clots create conditions favoring the development of severe changes. The anatomic alterations, depending on the severity and chronicity of the condition, range from slight reactive proliferation and brownish discoloration of the synovial membrane to severe destructive osteoarticular changes.

There are few anatomic studies of the earliest changes in hemophilic joints. If an articulation which has suffered a single acute hemorrhage is opened before the exudate has been completely resorbed, it will be found to contain blackish fluid blood with some clots. These may be free, adherent to the capsule, or located in recesses of the joint space. The synovial membrane is discolored by the blood, and the capsule and periarticular tissues may also present evidences of the recent hemorrhage.

In a joint in which the hemorrhages have been repeated, the synovial membrane will be found moderately or even strikingly thickened, and will show more or less intense brownish discoloration by absorbed blood pigment. The fibrous portion of the capsule may also be so discolored. If bloody fluid from the last acute episode is still present in the joint space, small clots may be in evidence and fibrin deposits may be found on the articular cartilages and the synovial membrane.

Figure 184

A, Roentgenograph of a knee joint which is the site of hemarthrosis in the case of a hemophilic boy 8 years of age. The intra-articular hemorrhage has greatly distended the joint capsule, as evidenced by the pronounced fullness of the suprapatellar bursa, the outward displacement of the patella, and the prominence of the posterior compartment of the joint. Note the slightly frayed appearance of the articular surface of the patella.

B, Roentgenograph illustrating the left knee joint of a hemophilic boy who was 14 years of age at the time of his admission to our hospital. The first episode of intra-articular bleeding occurred when he was 7 years of age. In the course of the succeeding years, there were several additional intra-articular hemorrhages into that knee joint. The difficulties which led to the boy's admission to the hospital were pain and swelling of the left elbow joint (due to intra-articular hemorrhage), hematuria of sudden onset, and frequent bouts of epistaxis. Note that the spongy trabeculae of the epiphysial ends of the bones are prominent. In the epiphysis of the tibia, a small cystlike rarefaction is present in the vicinity of the lateral tubercle. The articular surface of the medial half of that epiphysis is no longer smooth.

C, Roentgenograph of part of the shafts of a tibia and fibula of an adolescent boy from a family in which there were several hemophiliacs. There had been an injury to the leg in question, but the trauma to the tibia had been rather slight. However, it had resulted in subperiosteal hemorrhage and elevation of the periosteum of the tibia, and this had been followed by subperiosteal new bone formation.

D, Roentgenograph of the right elbow region in the case of a boy 8 years of age who was known to have hemophilia. The elbow joint had been the site of a chronic effusion. The olecranon of the ulna presents a deeply grooved defect, and the regional margin of the trochlea is also slightly indented. Note also that the epiphyses of the bones entering into the formation of the elbow joint show a state of maturation appropriate to an age several years beyond 8.

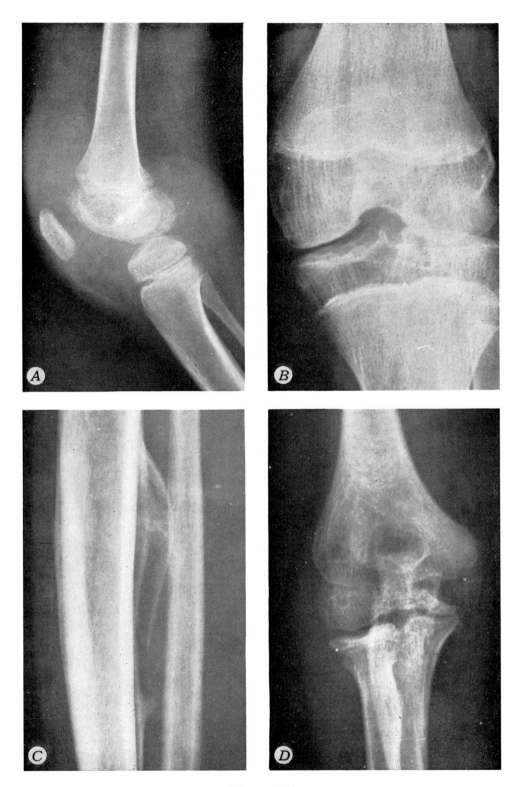

Figure 184

Progress of the arthritis is characterized by more marked reactive inflammation of the synovial membrane, resulting in considerable proliferation of the membrane. The latter may then present numerous vascular, brownishly discolored villi, some of which may be very long and thin. By this time, the articular cartilage is also modified, having lost its gloss and become gray-brown in color. As the arthropathy advances, areas of degeneration, necrosis, fibrillation, and obvious erosion appear in the articular cartilage. The defects present in the cartilage may reach down to the bony end plate. Thus, in a joint which is the site of chronic hemophilic arthritis, the articular cartilages come to show, sooner or later, numerous small and larger serrated erosions. Some of these cartilage defects may be partly filled in by discolored connective tissue, and in other sites they become filled in by regenerated cartilage. Elsewhere the bone exposed by the cartilage erosion may be found ground down and eburnated. The changes in the synovial membrane are associated with induration and shriveling of the subsynovial and capsular connective tissues, which also contain accumulations of free and phagocytosed blood pigment. It is the superficial layers of the synovial membrane, however, that show the greatest concentration of hemosiderin pigment. The relatively radiopaque roentgenographic shadows sometimes appearing in the capsular and periarticular tissues of a joint affected with chronic hemophilic arthritis do not represent calcium deposits in these tissues, but represent, at least in part, the accumulation of large amounts of iron-containing pigment (hemosiderin), especially in the synovial membrane.

In hemophilic joints in which the changes have advanced further, the articular ends of the bones are likely to become strikingly misshapen, and may also present alterations involving the spongiosa (see Freund, and Rodnan et al.). The photomicrographs (Figs. 186 and 187) illustrating the histologic changes presented by the right knee joint in a pertinent case of hemophilic arthropathy were made from tissue slides prepared from that joint, which had been removed at autopsy. The subject was a man 53 years of age who had had clinical manifestations of hemophilia since childhood. The autopsy in this case was performed by the eminent pathologist, the late Professor Erdheim of Vienna, and it is his description of the gross findings relating to this knee joint that are summarized below from the autopsy protocol available to the present writer.

The condylar surface of the right *femur* presented deep grooves, marginal exos-

Figure 185

A, Roentgenograph of the right knee joint of a hemophilic boy 10 years of age illustrating destructive changes which are rather advanced in view of the relative youth of the subject. There are subchondral erosions of the articular surfaces of the femur and tibia. The interosseous space is narrowed, the epiphyses are increased in width and present diffuse demineralization, and the intercondylar notch of the femur is strikingly widened.

B, Roentgenograph of a knee joint of a young hemophilic adult. The changes are much more advanced than those to be seen in *A*. Numerous subchondral cystlike rarefactions are present. Those in the upper end of the tibia are the most conspicuous. Such foci of rarefaction can also be seen in the lateral condyle of the femur, as well as in the patella. The intercondylar notch is widened, and small areas of radiopacity representing sclerotic spongiosa are present in the articular end of the femur and of the tibia.

C and *D*, Roentgenographs illustrating the changes of advanced hemophilic arthropathy in a shoulder joint and an ankle joint of a middle-aged man. The shoulder joint (*C*) shows numerous subchondral cysts in the head of the humerus and also in the spongiosa of the scapula in the vicinity of the glenoid fossa, along with increased radiopacity of both these areas. The ankle joint (*D*) presents evidence of destruction of the articular surfaces of the tibia and astragalus. The joint space is narrowed, there are numerous subcortical cystlike rarefactions, and there is pronounced sclerosis of the articular surfaces of the bones.

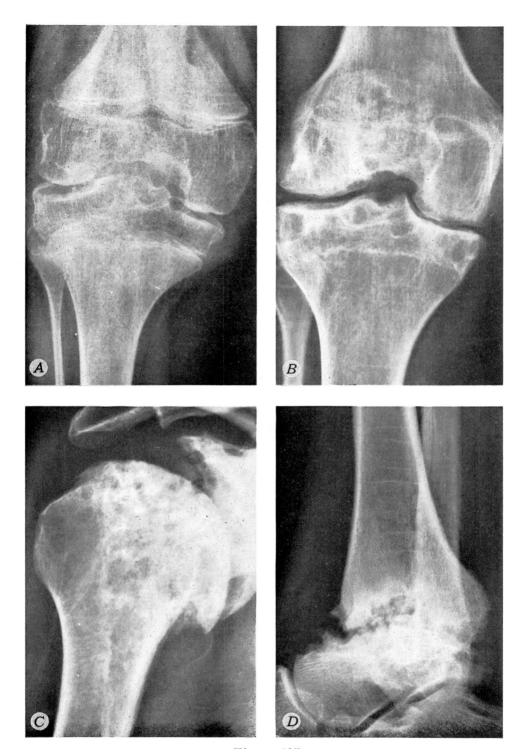

Figure 185

toses, and extensive destruction of the articular cartilage. The capsule of the joint was thickened and showed focal areas of hemorrhage in various stages of organization. The synovial lining of the capsule had undergone widespread proliferation and showed long discrete villi and also matted masses of villi, all of which were rust brown in color. Interspersed between the discrete or matted villi, some blood was still present as evidence of unresolved hemorrhage. On gross sectioning of the articular end of the femur, it was evident that in some areas the subchondral spongiosa was close-meshed or sclerotic, while in other areas it was loose-meshed or porotic. Near the articular surface, the subchondral spongiosa also showed a number of cystlike cavities, some of which clearly communicated with the joint space. Some of the cavities contained loose gelatinous tissue, others rather collagenous fibrous tissue, and still others brownishly discolored connective tissue and/or clotted blood.

The articular surface of the right *tibia* likewise showed extensive degenerative changes of the cartilage, particularly centrally, and also a girdle of marginal exostoses. Changes entirely analogous to those observed in the condylar region of the femur were also noted in the tibia. An additional feature here was the presence of a large organizing hematoma located in the recess of the attachment of the capsule to the tibia. This had caused bulging of the capsule and a gouged-out defect in the condylar area of the tibia, due to the effect of mechanical pressure from the encapsulating and partly organized blood clot.

Figure 186

A, Photomicrograph ($\times$ 12) illustrating the histologic pattern of a representative area from the synovial membrane of the right knee joint which had been removed at autopsy. The subject was a hemophilic man 53 years of age who had had clinical manifestations of hemophilia since childhood. Note that the proliferated synovial villi are plump, and that in many places they are matted together. The sections were stained with hematoxylin and eosin, and the intense black coloration of the tissue reflects the presence of large amounts of hemosiderin pigment. Examination under higher magnification revealed that the synovial lining cells contained granules of hemosiderin pigment. However, the most deeply pigmented cells are macrophages which were present in large numbers in the supporting connective tissue of the membrane. Considerable amounts of hemosiderin pigment could also be found lying free in the connective tissue. Furthermore, detailed microscopic study of the altered synovial membrane showed that it was heavily permeated by capillaries, and that the pericapillary mesenchymal cells were also heavily impregnated with hemosiderin pigment.

B, Photomicrograph ($\times$ 4) demonstrating the histologic changes at the periphery of the articular surface of the upper end of the tibia in the case mentioned in *A*. The dark, wedge-shaped tissue mass at the top of the picture represents one of the menisci. To the right of the meniscus there is a small fragment of modified articular cartilage. Between the meniscus and that fragment of cartilage, the articular cartilage has been destroyed, and the surface of the bone is covered by a layer of fibrous pannus heavily infiltrated with hemosiderin. Since the arthropathy was of long duration, it is not surprising that a marginal exostosis is present (see arrows). The villously proliferated synovial membrane has eroded the cartilaginous surface of the exostosis and burrowed into the spongiosa at the site between the arrows. The cartilage of the upper part of the exostosis is covered by a fibrous pannus which is heavily infiltrated with hemosiderin (see *C*). At the lower edge of the marginal exostosis there is a deep indentation which is filled with heavily pigmented connective tissue. The latter has apparently been formed as the result of organization of hemorrhage. The dark-staining area at the lower edge of the picture represents a mass of deeply pigmented connective tissue which is adherent to the periosteum and which has resulted from the organization of hemorrhage.

C, Photomicrograph ($\times$ 8) showing a part of the tissue field illustrated in *B*, with particular emphasis on the alterations relating to the marginal exostosis.

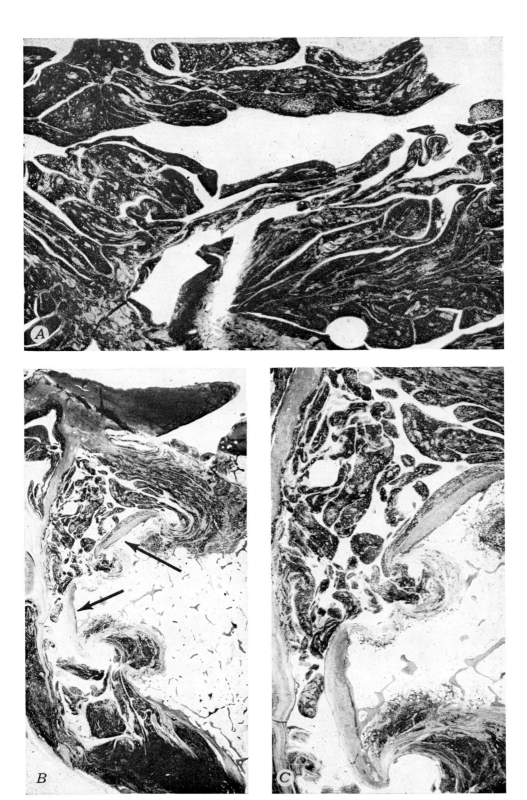

Figure 186

There are differences of opinion in regard to the manner in which the subchondrally located cystlike cavities develop in cases of chronic hemophilic arthropathy. Some maintain that the cystic cavities form in the subchondral bone as a result of focal mucoid degeneration of the bone marrow, and that subsequently the cyst comes to communicate with the articular cavity. However, it seems more plausible to the present writer that they are the result of the intrusion of hemorrhagic synovial fluid into the subchondral bone through areas where the articular cartilage has become ulcerated. At any rate, the response at these sites consists of the proliferation of connective tissue which becomes collagenized, and eventually the reparative connective tissue may undergo mucoid degeneration. Subsequently there may also be bleeding from the fibrous lining of the cyst into the cyst cavity.

TREATMENT

The genetic aberration underlying hemophilia cannot, of course, be corrected. The incidence of the disease is subject to control, and could be greatly reduced by *prophylactic measures* such as pertinent marriage counseling in families in which the disease is known to be present. Such counseling would take into consideration the fact that, as already noted, the disease is transmitted from an affected male through an unaffected but trait-carrying daughter or daughters (p. 721). The sons of a hemophilic father are normal themselves and do not pass either the disease or the hemophilic trait on to their children. On the other hand, half of the sons of a trait-carrying daughter of a hemophiliac will be affected with the disease, and half of the daughters of that trait-carrying daughter will also inherit the capacity to transmit the disease to half of their sons, and the hemophilic trait to half of their daughters. Since there is no way of knowing which of the daughters or granddaughters of a hemophilic male carry the hemophilic trait, elimination of the disease within a given family tree can be assured only if the lineage is continued by way of propagation of its unaffected males with females who do not have the hemophilic trait.

The control and actual management of the clinical problems raised by hemophilia are essentially the same in hemophilia A (classical hemophilia) and hemophilia B (Christmas disease). As is well known, the underlying plasma factor deficiency in classical hemophilia relates to "antihemophilic globulin" (AHG or factor VIII), while in Christmas disease the underlying plasma deficiency relates to the "plasma thromboplastin component" (PTC or factor IX). In both classical hemophilia and

Figure 187

A, Phomicrograph ($\times$ 4) showing a large, deeply pigmented mass representing an organizing hematoma which is situated between the articular capsule on the left (see arrow) and the upper end of the tibia on the right. It is clear that the contour of the upper end of the tibia has been deformed by pressure erosion from the hematoma, which, in the course of its organization, has undergone some degree of collagenization. The articular surface of the part of the tibia illustrated is devoid of normal articular cartilage, and in one small area the cartilage is entirely absent.

B, Photomicrograph ($\times$ 4) of part of the articular surface of the femur. The articular cartilage has been completely destroyed, and in its stead the surface of the bone has a covering of pigmented collagenous connective tissue. On the right there is a large, organizing hematoma which is eroding into the spongiosa.

C, Photomicrograph ($\times$ 12) showing, in some detail, a part of the articular end of the femur pictured in *B*. The pigmented collagenous fibrous tissue covering the articular surface of the bone is well demonstrated, as are the periosteum and parosteal connective tissues on the left, which are likewise heavily discolored by hemosiderin, in consequence of hemorrhage.

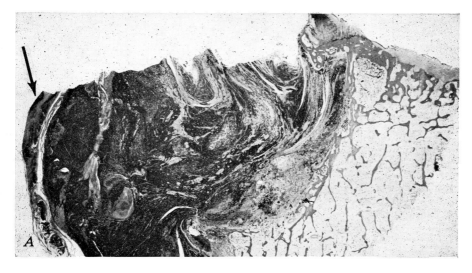

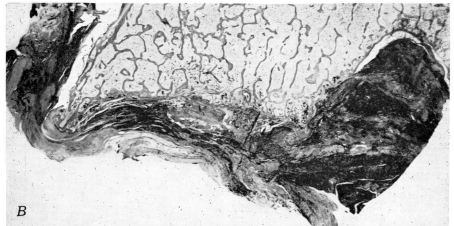

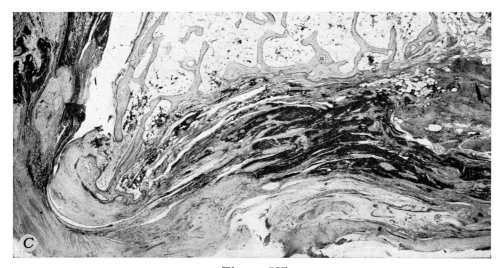

Figure 187

Christmas disease the subject must be cautioned to avoid undue physical exertion and traumatic incidents which might result in a wound. Special importance attaches to the avoidance of surgical procedures (including extraction of teeth) unless it is imperative that they be carried out. In any case, they should not be undertaken without preliminary treatment directed toward increasing the coagulability of the subject's blood by ameliorating the specific plasma factor deficiency before and for some time after the surgical intervention. (See George and Breckenridge, Rayne, and also Mazza *et al.*)

REFERENCES

ABELL, J. M., JR., and BAILEY, R. W.: Hemophilic Pseudotumor, Arch. Surg., *81*, 569, 1960.

AHLBERG, Å.: Haemophilia in Sweden. VII. Incidence, Treatment and Prophylaxis of Arthropathy and other Musculo-skeletal Manifestations of Haemophilia A and B, Acta orthop. scandinav., Suppl. 77, 1965.

BENDIEN, W. M., and VAN CREVELD, S.: On Some Factors of Blood Coagulation, Especially with Regard to the Problem of Hemophilia, Acta med. scandinav., *99*, 12, 1939.

BRINKHOUS, K. M.: Hemophilia, Bull. New York Acad. Med., *30*, 325, 1954.

BROWER, T. D., and WILDE, A. H.: Femoral Neuropathy in Hemophilia, J. Bone & Joint Surg., *48-A*, 487, 1966.

DEPALMA, A. F., and COTLER, J.: Hemophilic Arthropathy, Clinical Orthopaedics, *8*, 163, 1956.

DOUB, H. P., and DAVIDSON, E. C.: Roentgen-ray Examination of the Joints of Hemophilics, Radiology, *6*, 217, 1926.

FIROR, W. M., and WOODHALL, B.: Hemophilic Pseudotumor: Diagnosis, Pathology and Surgical Treatment of Hemophilic Lesions in the Smaller Bones and Joints, Bull. Johns Hopkins Hosp., *59*, 237, 1936.

FREUND, E.: Die Gelenkerkrankung der Bluter, Virchows Arch. path. Anat., *256*, 158, 1925.

GEORGE, J. N., and BRECKENRIDGE, R. T.: The Use of Factor VIII and Factor IX Concentrates During Surgery, J.A.M.A., *214*, 1673, 1970.

GHORMLEY, R. K., and CLEGG, R. S.: Bone and Joint Changes in Hemophilia. With Report of Cases of So-called Hemophilic Pseudotumor, J. Bone & Joint Surg., *30-A*, 589, 1948.

GOODFELLOW, J., FEARN, C. B. d'A., and MATTHEWS, J. M.: Iliacus Haematoma, J. Bone & Joint Surg., *49-B*, 748, 1967.

KEY, J. A.: Hemophilic Arthritis, Ann. Surg., *95*, 198, 1932.

KÖNIG, F.: Die Gelenkerkrankungen bei Blutern mit besonderer Berücksichtigung der Diagnose, Klin. Vorträge, N.F., No. 36, 233, 1892.

MAZZA, J. J., BOWIE, E. J. W., HAGEDORN, A. B., DIDISHEIM, P., TASWELL, H. F., PETERSON, L. F. A., and OWEN, C. A., JR: Antihemophilic Factor VIII in Hemophilia. Use of Concentrates to Permit Major Surgery, J.A.M.A., *211*, 1818, 1970.

MOSELEY, J. E.: Patterns of Bone Change in Classic Hemophilia and Christmas Disease, J. Mt. Sinai Hosp., *29*, 5, 1962.

NELSON, M. G., and MITCHELL, E. S.: Pseudo-Tumour of Bone in Haemophilia, Acta haemat., *28*, 137, 1962.

NEWCOMER, N. B.: The Joint Changes in Hemophilia, Radiology, *32*, 573, 1939.

PATEK, A. J., JR., and TAYLOR, F. H. L.: Hemophilia. II. Some Properties of a Substance Obtained from Normal Human Plasma Effective in Accelerating the Coagulation of Hemophilic Blood, J. Clin. Invest., *16*, 113, 1937.

PETERSEN, O. H.: Das Blutergelenk und seine Beziehungen zu den deformierenden Gelenkerkrankungen, Arch. klin. Chir., *126*, 456, 1923.

RAYNE, J.: Multiple Dental Extractions in Patients with Severe Hemophilia, J. Oral Surg., *26*, 381, 1968.

REINECKE, and WOHLWILL: Über hämophile Gelenkerkrankung, Arch. klin. Chir., *154*, 425, 1929.

RODNAN, G. P., BROWER, T. D., HELLSTROM, H. R., DIDISHEIM, P., and LEWIS, J. H.: Postmortem Examination of an Elderly Severe Hemophiliac, with Observations on the Pathologic Findings in Hemophilic Joint Disease, Arthritis Rheum., *2*, 152, 1959.

SCHLOESSMANN, H.: Die Hämophilie, Neue Deutsche Chir., No. 47, 1930.

SOULIER, J.-P.: Étude génétique des syndromes hémorragiques, Sang, *25*, 355, 1954.

STIRIS, G.: Bone and Joint Changes in Haemophiliacs, Acta radiol., *49*, 269, 1958.

SWANTON, M. C.: The Pathology of Hemarthrosis in Hemophilia, in *Hemophilia and Hemophilioid Diseases*, edited by K. M. Brinkhous, The University of North Carolina Press, 1957.

THOMAS, H. B.: Some Orthopaedic Findings in Ninety-eight Cases of Hemophilia, J. Bone & Joint Surg., *18*, 140, 1936.

WINTROBE, M. M.: *Clinical Hematology*, 6th ed., Philadelphia, Lea & Febiger, 1967 (p. 944).

Chapter

25

Degenerative Joint Disease

DEGENERATIVE joint disease (osteoarthritis) is by far the most common form of arthritis. In relation to large or small diarthrodial (synovial) joints, its point of departure is generally held to be the articular cartilage of the affected joint or joints. In relation to the vertebral column, degenerative arthritis involves not only the synovial joints between articular facets but also the fibrocartilaginous joints formed by the intervertebral disks between the vertebral bodies.

This chapter will be devoted mainly to the clinical and anatomic features of degenerative joint disease as expressed in implication of: (1) the large diarthrodial joints, with particular emphasis on involvement of the *hip joint* (malum coxae); (2) the diarthrodial joints of the fingers and especially of the terminal interphalangeal joints, in regard to which the fully evolved arthritic changes are usually denoted as *Heberden's nodes;* and (3) the bony protuberances developing at the upper and/or lower margins of vertebral bodies as a consequence of alterations taking their departure in the intervertebral disks, the resultant condition being known as *spondylosis deformans.*

Degenerative joint disease, especially as it relates to the large diarthrodial joints, is usually subclassified as *primary* and *secondary* osteoarthritis. *Primary osteoarthritis* is the type in which the degeneration of the articular cartilage is the initial change and is intrinsic. This change is commonly held to be related to deterioration of the articular cartilages of the affected joint, occurring as a result of "biological" aging—that is, the changes associated with senescence (see Sokoloff, and also Bunim). The deterioration of the cartilage may have its basis in alterations relating to the rate of production and chemical composition of the matrix of the cartilage. As is well known, the cartilage matrix is produced by the chondrocytes and is composed of chondromucin enmeshed in a network of collagen fibers (see Mankin and Baron, Barland *et al.*, Mankin and Laing, and also Mankin). On the other hand, there are those who maintain that, in the evolution of primary osteoarthritis, remodeling of the contours of the subchondral articular cortex of the bones entering into the formation of the affected joint is the initial alteration, and that it is the resultant change in the articular contours that subjects the articular cartilages to degenerative changes (see Johnson, and also Moffett *et al.*). At any rate, it is clear that, in addition to degenerative changes in the articular cartilages, superimposed local mechanical or functional stress (induced, for instance, by weight-bearing or excessive motion) is needed to create the full gamut of the pathologic changes characterizing osteoarthritis (see Larson). By contrast, it is of interest that adults manifesting residual paralysis of lower limbs years after having suffered from anterior poliomyelitis show, in comparison with age controls, a low incidence of osteoarthritis involving the hip and knee joints of the affected limbs. This is to be attributed to the reduced activity of those limbs (see Glyn *et al.*).

Secondary osteoarthritis is the type in which the alterations of the articular tissues are secondary to minor anatomical variations in the joint, a traumatic incident, or some pre-existing inflammatory or even noninflammatory disease process involving one or both articular bone ends (see Murray). In previous chapters, reference has already been made to secondary osteoarthritis, notably of the hip joint, developing as a result of Legg-Perthes disease, Gaucher's disease, ochronosis, caisson disease, slipped capital femoral epiphysis, dislocation of the femoral head, fracture of the femoral neck, and sickle cell anemia. Indeed, the hip joint, which is such a common site of *primary* osteoarthritis, is by far the most common site of *secondary* osteo-arthritis.

Another sequence of events favoring the development of secondary osteoarthritis is inflammation of the synovial membrane of a joint (resulting in some injury to its articular cartilages), subsequent subsidence of the inflammatory process, and continued functional use of the joint. Still another cause of secondary osteoarthritis is the continued use of a joint after its surfaces have become malaligned following a

Figure 188

A, Roentgenograph of the right ankle region in a case in which the joint had become the site of advanced osteoarthritic changes secondary to a severe local trauma which had resulted in a fracture of the astragalus. The subject was a man who was 54 years of age at the time he was admitted to our hospital and this picture was taken. His clinical record indicated that during his childhood he had sustained an injury to the right ankle. The record also revealed that 14 years prior to admission to the hospital he had fallen off a scaffold and injured his back and right lower extremity, particularly the right knee area. It was because of pain in the lower part of his back, and incapacitating pain in the right knee and ankle, that he entered the hospital. A fusion of that knee joint was carried out. Unfortunately, however, this surgical intervention was followed by the development of gangrene of the toes, and one month after the knee fusion a midthigh amputation was done. The amputated extremity was dissected, and the ankle joint was exposed (see *B*).

B, Photograph of the opened ankle joint from the case in question. The articular surface of the astragalus is deformed and pitted. Much of the articular cartilage has been destroyed. Toward the left side of the picture, the astragalus shows marginal exostosis formation. Sectioning of the astragalus revealed the presence of an old but healed fracture site. The articular surface of the tibia is even more modified. Almost all of the articular cartilage has been eroded, and the articular surface is extensively pitted. Marginal exostoses are present, large ones being observable on the medial border of the lower end of the tibia.

C, Roentgenograph showing advanced changes of osteoarthritis involving a left hip joint. The articular space is narrowed, and the femoral head is somewhat displaced laterally. The displacement is due to a very large marginal exostosis which is present on the medial surface of the head, and which occupies a considerable part of the acetabulum. There is also an exostotic projection extending outward from the lateral margin of the acetabulum. In addition, the picture presents evidence of considerable subchondral sclerosis involving part of the acetabulum and the corresponding part of the femoral head. The patient, a woman, was 54 years of age when this roentgenograph was taken. She was admitted to the hospital with a 20-year history of pain and disability relating to the hip. She had been receiving conservative treatment for many years, but her condition became progressively worse and ultimately she found it difficult to walk. The degenerative arthritis in this case was a secondary osteoarthritis which had its basis in a congenital dislocation at the hip joint.

D, Photograph of the head and part of the neck of the femur from the case illustrated in *C*, the specimen having been obtained in the course of a replacement arthroplasty. At no site did the articular cartilage of the femoral head present a normal appearance. In particular, it was fibrillated and eroded in some places. In addition, the contour of the femoral head was modified by the presence of bumpy elevations and also marginal exostoses, one of which (on the right side of the picture) was very large.

E, Photograph showing, in the frontal plane, the cut surface of the femoral head illustrated in *D*. Note that the dome of the femoral head is virtually devoid of articular cartilage. The architecture of the large marginal exostosis on the right is clearly apparent.

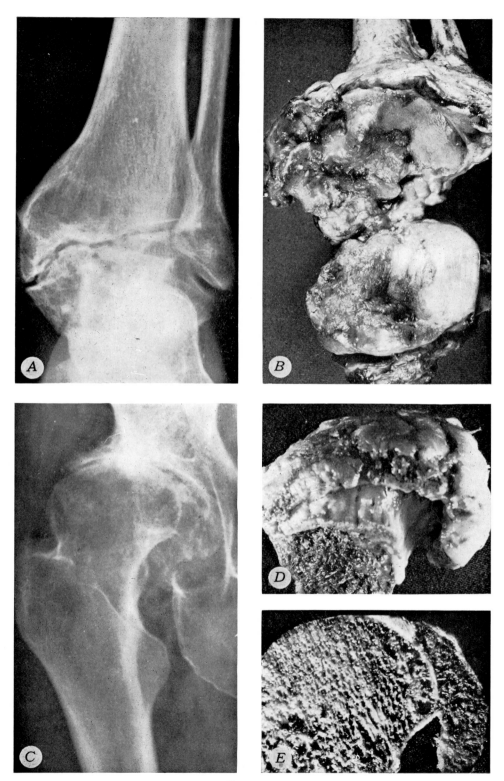

Figure 188

fracture through the shaft or through an articular bone end of one of the bones entering into the formation of the joint. (See Fig. 188.) The destructive neuropathic arthropathies occurring in cases of tabes dorsalis and syringomyelia, and in some instances of diabetes mellitus, are discussed together in a later chapter (p. 847).

In respect to *terminology*, the arthropathy being considered in this section of the chapter has also been denoted by such names as "arthritis deformans," "osteoarthritis" (without a modifying adjective), "hypertrophic arthritis," and "degenerative arthritis." "Arthritis deformans" as used especially in the Germanic literature is a collective concept. It embraces arthritides which may have had different origins although they present the same ultimate pathologic picture of a "hypertrophic joint." The British have long preferred "osteoarthritis," and the term "hypertrophic arthritis" was long preferred in the United States. Finally, the term "degenerative arthritis," which was also rather often employed, is too comprehensive. This designation could include instances of mere senile articular degeneration, since it omits the factor of reactive (hypertrophic) changes in the articular bone ends—equally essential in the concept of the arthropathy under discussion.

One may ask why the arthropathy we have been defining is being denoted as an *arthritis* instead of an *arthrosis*. The use of the suffix "osis," it must be conceded, would emphasize the factor of degeneration, to which so much attention has been directed. The use here of "itis," with its implication of inflammation, is open to some objection. Inflammation is not the primary change and does not become prominent clinically or pathologically. Nevertheless, the suffix "itis" is justifiable on the basis of custom and facility of recognition.

ARTICULAR CHANGES OF SENESCENCE

Ordinarily the *articular changes of senescence*, even if they are rather far advanced, do not in themselves give rise to clinical complaints. There is no doubt, however, that the "creakiness" so often noted in one or more large joints by elderly or old people is often ascribable to these changes. The proportion of those persons in whom large joints manifest the articular changes of senescence and who subsequently develop primary osteoarthritis is, after all, relatively small. In those who do, the advanced articular changes of senescence merge imperceptibly into those of primary osteoarthritis. The additional influences which contribute toward the development of primary osteoarthritis on the foundation of the changes of senescence include constitutional factors, occupational factors, conditions of stance and balance, and the continued functional activity of the altered joint. Complaints of pain, stiffness, and limited motion in a joint of an elderly or old person mark the presence there of changes exceeding those of senescence. At any rate, the following description of the articular changes of senescence may well serve as a background for the description of the pathologic changes characterizing primary osteoarthritis.

The pathologico-anatomic studies by Weichselbaum dealt with the articular changes of senescence as observed in a variety of joints. More often, pertinent studies have been limited to the changes as they appear in some particular joint— usually a large one. As a rule, this has been the knee, since it is in this region that the articular changes of senescence occur most regularly (see Nichols and Richardson, Keefer *et al.*, and Bennett *et al.*). Altogether, the various pathologico-anatomic studies have indicated clearly that both the frequency and the severity of the articular changes tend to increase with advancing age. This generalization applies above all to some of the large joints, and especially to the knee (see Heine, and also Chung).

The *articular cartilage* is the joint tissue which usually shows the most striking gross and microscopic changes with advancing age. In the course of senescence, this cartilage almost regularly becomes somewhat thinned and discolored. It tends to acquire a brownish gray or gray-yellow cast. The thinned and discolored cartilages may remain smooth and glossy. Frequently, however, they come to manifest more definite evidence of degeneration. This is revealed particularly in certain parts of the cartilage of an affected joint. On *gross examination* of these areas, the cartilage may appear roughened, in some places only superficially and in others more deeply and coarsely. Where the roughening is pronounced, the cartilage has a definitely naplike or finely villous feel. This is due to the fact that the degenerated cartilage has broken up into closely meshed perpendicular strands of varying depth and thickness. That is, it has undergone gross fibrillation. Near the edges of grossly fibrillated areas, the cartilage may present irregular cracks penetrating to various depths.

In the wake of gross fibrillation, erosion of the articular cartilage may appear. This, of course, is a more advanced change. It is the result of gradual rubbing away of the fibrillized cartilage, especially where it comes into functional contact with the apposed articular surface. After the superficial surface has become eroded, the fibrillation extends deeper into hitherto intact cartilage, and further erosion follows it. In this way, all the cartilage may eventually be worn away in some places, and the subchondral bone may be exposed. However, the erosion or ulceration of the articular cartilage does not necessarily go deep enough to expose the bone. The margins of an ulcerated area are likely to be irregular in outline. At the sites of erosion, a certain degree of repair of cartilage sometimes takes place. The base of the ulcer often comes to be lined by a pearly white thin membrane, generally composed of connective tissue, although various cartilaginous elements may enter into it. If subchondral bone has been exposed and remains so, the friction of function may stimulate the development of some degree of sclerosis in this bone area. (See Fig. 189.)

Microscopic examination reveals that the changes of senescence in the articular cartilage start in the interstitial substance (matrix). If an area is studied which is not as yet grossly fibrillated but which is already somewhat modified, focal swelling of the interstitial substance may be noted. At this stage, the included cartilage cells also appear swollen. The dissolution and disappearance of the chondromucoid of the cartilage matrix from a region in which the latter is swollen unmasks the collagen fibers present in the matrix. This dissolution is followed by further degeneration, and by the perpendicular splitting and cracking of the cartilage, which induces the naplike, grossly fibrillated appearance noted above. The fibrillated cartilage undergoes erosion and ulceration, even down to the subchondral bone. Along with the erosion, some evidences of repair may appear.

The *synovial membrane* usually remains smooth during the evolution of the degenerative changes in the articular cartilages. Sometimes, especially if the changes in question are pronounced, there may be concomitant changes in the synovial membrane. The simplest aberration there is the appearance of fine villous hypertrophy at the synovial reflections. Occasionally this hypertrophy may become rather extensive and may spread over a considerable part of the membrane. Rarely, a strand of connective tissue may be found to have spread from the synovial membrane into nearby hollows and grooves created by the erosion of the cartilage. Accessory articular structures, such as *menisci, ligaments*, and *tendons*, may likewise show alterations. In joints in which menisci are present, these usually become thinned and discolored and even split up as the changes of senescence advance. Ligaments, both intra-articular and extra-articular, and tendons, especially in joint regions, also show degenerative changes, becoming more or less brownish. For instance, the cruciate ligaments of the knee, the long head of the biceps, and the supraspinatus tendon are often found to be thinned and frayed and, in older persons, sometimes even torn.

Against this background of the anatomic aspects of the articular changes relating to senescence, we are now prepared to consider the clinical features and the anatomic alterations relating to large joints which are the site of primary osteoarthritis.

PRIMARY OSTEOARTHRITIS OF LARGE JOINTS

Primary osteoarthritis of large joints usually evolves, or at least attains real intensity, in only a single joint, a few joints, or a locally limited group of joints. Its general incidence is about the same for males as for females, but osteoarthritis of the hip joint is encountered much more often in females than in males. Furthermore, osteoarthritis seems to be more often the source of clinical complaints in females than in males. It is not likely to be seriously incapacitating or debilitating, except in relation to the hip or the knee joint. An affected articulation in its early stage may show definite enlargement, but is ordinarily not obviously inflamed, and mobility is not usually much impaired. As noted, the condition is characterized anatomically by degenerative changes in the articular cartilages, combined with hypertrophic changes in the bone ends, leading to deformation of the articular surfaces. Inflammatory phenomena in the synovial membrane, so conspicuous in rheumatoid arthritis, are insignificant in this condition.

On the whole, the disease in a particular joint evolves gradually. Nevertheless, it shows wide variations in severity and in the speed with which it develops. After evolving to a certain stage, both the pathologic condition and the clinical manifestations may become stabilized. It is well known that the severity of the clinical symptoms is not necessarily coordinate with that of the pathologic changes. For example, a person complaining about one knee may have equally severe pathologic changes but relatively few complaints in the opposite knee.

Figure 189

Photographs of the articular surfaces of the bones of a knee joint illustrating the changes of senescence. The patient was a woman 69 years of age who was admitted to the hospital with clinical indications of bronchopneumonia. She died a few weeks after admission, and this knee joint was removed at autopsy. As is usual in regard to the knee joint, the changes of senescence are most striking in the articular cartilage of the patella and in the cartilage on the patellar surface of the condyles. The articular cartilage covering the condyles of the tibia likewise shows changes of senescence, but these are ordinarily much less striking than in the patella and the femoral condyles.

In *A*, note that the articular cartilage of the patella is not smooth anywhere. Indeed, its entire surface is roughened, and it presents small areas of superficial ulceration in the midzone, especially on the left. The articular cartilage of the femoral condyles is roughened and ulcerated, almost exclusively on the left side of the so-called patellar surface. The roughening and ulceration in this area correspond to the most altered area of the articular cartilage of the patella.

In *B*, the articular cartilage covering the tibial condyles shows changes of senescence, especially on the left, but these are by no means so conspicuous as they are on the patella and femoral condyles. Close inspection will reveal that, in the direction of the intercondylar area, the articular cartilage presents a number of delicate linear cracks and also an area in which the cartilage has lost its smoothness, apparently because it has undergone fibrillation.

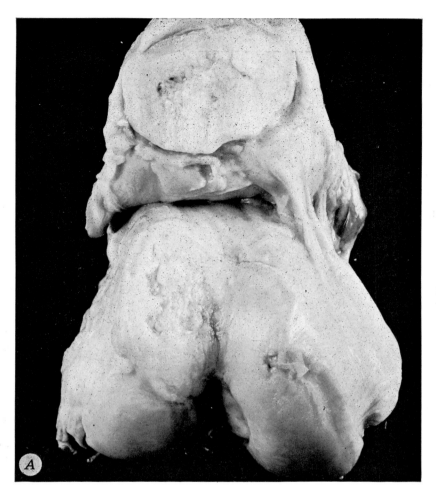

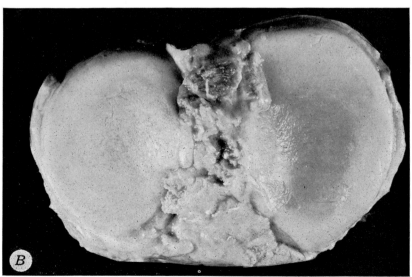

Figure 189

CLINICAL COMPLAINTS AND FINDINGS

Unless precipitated by some definite traumatic incident, the clinical onset of primary osteoarthritis in a large joint is usually insidious. With a mild degree of involvement of a large joint, the patient may complain merely of some early morning *stiffness*. This often diminishes in the course of daily motion, only to increase again toward the end of the day. When it is the hip joint that is affected, rapid fatigability may be complained of, even before stiffness. There may be some *pain*, especially if weight-bearing joints are involved. If present, this is definitely aggravated by prolonged use of the joint. Even if severe, however, the pain may subside or disappear during rest.

In the early stages of the disease, disturbances of *mobility* are not prominent

Figure 190

A, Roentgenograph of the right hip joint area showing an advanced degree of osteoarthritis. The patient was a man 65 years of age who was admitted to the hospital mainly because of the presence of a large retroperitoneal tumor. However, the clinical record revealed that he had had difficulties relating to both hip joints for a number of years. A roentgenographic skeletal survey disclosed the presence of osteoarthritis involving both hip joints. In particular, the picture shows: narrowing of the articular space; marginal exostosis formation at the border of the acetabulum; marginal exostosis formation involving the femoral head; a small cystlike rarefaction in the femoral head; and subchondral sclerosis of both the acetabulum and the femoral head. The patient died 4 weeks after admission, and an autopsy was performed. The tumor proved to be a liposarcoma which had metastasized widely. Since it was known that both hip joints were the site of osteoarthritis, the pelvis and femora were removed at autopsy for anatomic study.

B, Photograph of part of the right innominate bone and the upper end of the femur demonstrating some of the osteoarthritic changes represented in *A*. Note that much of the femoral head projects beyond the acetabular socket. The projecting part consists mainly of a large marginal exostosis at the head-neck junction.

C, Roentgenograph of the right hip joint area, which is the site of advanced osteoarthritis. The patient was a man 58 years of age who, for a number of years, had had pain and disability in this hip. In respect to the femoral head, the picture reveals: a very large, cystlike area of rarefaction occupying a considerable part of the head; two prominent exostoses, the larger of which is oriented toward the inferior surface of the femoral neck; and a large, crescent-shaped area of subchondral sclerosis. In relation to the acetabulum, the picture shows: a small, roundish, cystlike area of rarefaction near the outer border of the acetabulum; a large area of subchondral sclerosis; and a marginal exostosis at its lower lip.

D, Photograph of the cut surface of the femoral head and part of the femoral neck illustrated in *C*. The specimen became available for anatomic examination because a replacement arthroplasty had been done for the treatment of the osteoarthritis. Examination of the uncut specimen revealed that the head was definitely increased in its transverse diameter in consequence of the presence of exostoses both laterally and medially. Over most of its articular surface the femoral head was denuded of its articular cartilage, and where this was so, the subchondral bone appeared sclerotic. In those areas in which the cartilage was still present, it was fibrillated and more or less pitted. When the specimen was cut in its long axis, it was found that the cyst measured approximately $4 \times 4 \times 3$ cm. in its greatest dimensions. The cyst contained a small amount of yellowish fluid, and the wall was lined in some places by a distinct layer of fibrous tissue which was in the process of mucoid degeneration. The cut surface also revealed the anatomic basis for the other features presented by the roentgenograph. From above down, this surface shows in particular: the osteocartilaginous exostosis at the upper surface of the head; the densely sclerotic osseous tissue neighboring on the proximal end of the cyst; and, below, the larger of the two osteocartilaginous exostoses.

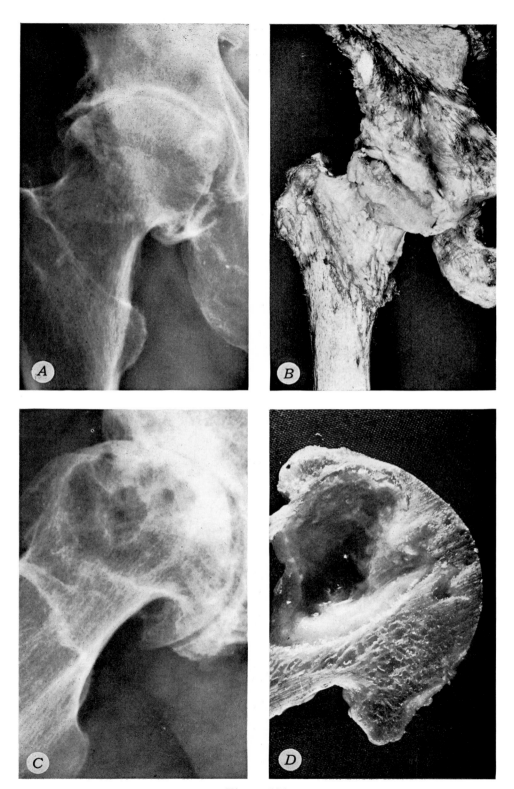

Figure 190

among the clinical manifestations, since the joint space is seldom obliterated in this form of arthritis. Nevertheless, in severe cases, and especially in the hip and knee joints, the range of motion may become very much limited. This limitation is due mainly to incongruity of the joint ends or blocking by exostoses. Some restriction of joint movement may, at first, be induced directly by *muscle spasm*. Degeneration of ligaments (such as the cruciate ligaments of the knee or the ligamentum teres of the hip) and the tearing and fraying of degenerated menisci or of tendons near the affected joints can further handicap movement. Motions in the hip joint quite often become limited, even in an early stage of the arthritis.

The muscles at their points of attachment to the periosteum are often the seat of pain. Such *muscle pain* is especially likely to appear if the pathologic condition in the affected joint is aggravated by a deformity of the bone ends. When the knee is involved, spasm of the hamstrings often constitutes a rather serious clinical problem. The muscle pain is sometimes referred, as, for instance, along the obturator nerve when the arthritis is in the hip. *Muscle atrophy* may be present in the early stages, but becomes more pronounced as the articular changes progress. However, it does not achieve the high degree of muscle wasting encountered in the inflammatory arthritides.

As the arthritic changes advance, *crepitations* are apparent on palpation and may even be audible. *Tenderness* may be noted early and becomes pronounced, especially over marginal exostoses and thickened synovium. When the arthritic changes have become advanced, the joint region may show obvious enlargement. Even at this stage, however, inflammatory phenomena, such as redness and heat, are lacking. The marginal exostoses may be felt on examination, and even the presence of joint bodies may be suggested when the capsule is carefully palpated. Occasionally, pain in a knee joint may be brought about by the jamming of tabs of hypertrophied synovial tissue or the breaking off and jamming of bits of cartilage or bone between the articulating ends of the joint.

In the *hip joint*, some degree of primary osteoarthritis has been encountered in 34 per cent of persons over 55 years of age. More often than not, the involvement is limited to one hip (see Gofton and Trueman). In the affected hip, the degenerative changes involve mainly the cartilage at the margins of the femoral head, those parts of the cartilage that border on the boss, and the cartilage covering the inner segment of the head. In the acetabulum, it is the cartilage in the vicinity of the rim that is most likely to show degenerative changes. (See Fig. 190.)

The development of primary osteoarthritis in the hip joint is associated with such severe and exuberant manifestations that the condition in that site has acquired a special name—*malum coxae senilis*. The arthritis in question is likely to be highly incapacitating. Very early, there may be restriction of adduction and rotation, and eventually movement in the joint may become limited to flexion. However, even when the arthritic changes are advanced, there may be little pain in the hip, the pain being referred largely to the corresponding knee. It has been postulated that the pain may be the result of impaired outflow of venous blood from the altered femoral head (see Hulth). As the fixation of the hip usually occurs in a position of medium flexion and adduction, lordosis of the lumbar region and tilting of the pelvis may appear.

The head of the femur may be found ovoid or mushroom-shaped, and striking changes may also be apparent in the acetabulum. Its hollow may become so shallow that subluxation of the femoral head may occur. On the other hand, the acetabulum may become deeper, acquiring a more or less oval shape. When the deformation is extreme, the rim of the acetabulum may clamp the upper end of the femur and completely inhibit motion, which may also be limited by the presence of marginal exostoses on the head and acetabulum and even by bony outgrowths at the upper end of the greater trochanter. In a late stage of malum coxae senilis, a high degree of muscle atrophy may also develop.

The articular cartilages of the *knee joint* are by far the most frequently and gravely involved by degenerative changes. After young adulthood, the frequency of regressive changes in the cartilages increases rapidly with advancing age. In persons over 60, the knee joints have almost always undergone well-defined changes of senescence. As to the particular areas of the cartilage most likely to degenerate, there is fairly close agreement among those who have investigated knee joints of older people. Parker *et al.* found that the patella showed alterations in 81 per cent of their cases, the intercondylar groove in 65, the lateral condyle of the tibia in 64, the medial condyle of the tibia in 55, the medial condyle of the femur in 43, and the lateral condyle of the femur in 36 per cent. This distribution agrees essentially with that reported by Weichselbaum.

The term *chondromalacia of the patella* has been applied to an internal derangement of the knee joint occurring in younger people and characterized mainly by fissural degeneration of the patellar cartilage. There is pain, usually in the patella itself, and there may be intermittent hydrops, patellar pressure tenderness, and subpatellar crepitus.

With advanced osteoarthritic involvement of the knee, not only the cartilages and subchondral bone but also the menisci and cruciate ligaments are usually severely altered. In contrast to the hip joint, the knee joint only very rarely shows much limitation of movement by bony obstructions. Nevertheless, muscle spasm may limit movement considerably. (See Fig. 191.)

Primary degenerative arthritis is definitely less common in the joints of the *shoulder girdle* than in the hip or the knee. In the *shoulder joint* itself, it is mainly the cartilage near the tubercles of the humeral head that is likely to present the degenerative changes of senescence. However, the cartilage of the articular portion of the glenoid cavity also sometimes manifests such changes. Primary osteoarthritis of the shoulder joint rarely attains the severity of the condition in the hip joint. The *acromioclavicular* and *sternoclavicular joints* have a certain anatomic similarity to each other. In both of these joints there is a thick meniscus and relatively thick articular cartilages. Nevertheless, these joints, and particularly the acromioclavicular joints, are fairly common sites of senescent changes in osteoarthritis (see Silberberg *et al.*).

PATHOLOGIC AND ROENTGENOGRAPHIC FINDINGS

The *pathologic condition* of large joints affected with primary osteoarthritis is characterized by alterations in the cartilage and subchondral bone, leading to deformation of the contour of the articular surfaces. These changes consist essentially of: (1) erosion of portions of the articular cartilages, (2) sclerosis of, and various other changes in, the bone underlying the damaged cartilage, (3) grinding down of exposed subchondral bone, (4) formation of bony overgrowths at the margins of the articular cartilages (marginal exostoses), and, in some places (5) shifting and reduplication of the bone-cartilage border, resulting in bumpiness of the articular surface. In contrast to the changes in the cartilage and subchondral bone, those in the *synovial membrane* are usually slight and incidental. Even when the articular changes are quite extensive, intra-articular adhesions sufficient to interfere with motion are insignificant, the joint space is usually not obliterated, and in general the mobility of the joint is usually preserved.

The *roentgenographic findings* are likely to be surprisingly prominent in comparison with the clinical manifestations. If the osteoarthritis is well developed, the roentgenographs will show that some of the cartilage has been destroyed and the joint space reduced in size. The marginal exostoses stand out clearly in the roentgenograph. These findings, taken in conjunction with the absence of bone atrophy, the presence of bone sclerosis corresponding to areas of eburnation, and sometimes the existence of joint bodies, are strong evidence in favor of the diagnosis of osteoarthritis. There may be cystlike cavities beneath the articular surfaces. Rarely, there may be evidence of calcification and ossification at the points of attachment of ligaments and tendons. The presence of marginal exostoses alone by no means justifies a diagnosis of osteoarthritis. In relation to the hip joint in particular, the development of osteophytes may constitute an aspect of alterations representing merely senescence. Indeed, the roentgenographic diagnosis of osteoarthritis of the

Figure 191

A and *B*, Photographs of the lower end of a femur which is the site of advanced osteoarthritis. The specimen came from a man 58 years of age whose left lower extremity had been amputated because of arteriosclerotic gangrene involving the toes. In *A* the femoral condyles are shown in the frontal view. The articular cartilage covering the intercondylar groove is severely altered in consequence of fibrillation and ulceration. Extending upward from each condyle there is a projection representing the proximal end of a large marginal exostosis. *B* presents a lateral view of the large marginal exostosis shown on the left in *A*. The extent to which this exostosis projects outward from the femoral condyle is emphasized by the deep hollow, or trough, between the outer edge of that exostosis and the rest of the condyle.

C, Photograph of the surface of the condyles of the right femur of a patient whose knee joint was the site of degenerative arthritis. The subject was a man 58 years of age who was admitted to the hospital for treatment of an adenocarcinoma of the colon. The osteoarthritis of the right knee was noted in the course of a roentgenographic skeletal survey. The patient's clinical history does not contain any reference to the right knee joint. This lack of reference may be due to the fact that, on admission, the subject was already seriously ill because of widespread metastases of his carcinoma. Indeed, he died 16 days after admission to the hospital. At the autopsy, the right knee joint was opened and inspected, and the lower end of the femur was excised. As this photograph shows, much of the articular surface of the femur is devoid of articular cartilage, and whatever articular cartilage is present does not appear normal. Where articular cartilage is lacking, the exposed subchondral bone presents a polished, eburnated surface.

D, Photograph of the articular surface of a patella which was excised because it was considered to be the site of chondromalacia. The patient was a man 28 years of age who had been aware for a number of months of difficulties relating to the left knee. Clinical examination of the joint revealed crepitation on movement, evidence of a small amount of intraarticular effusion, and pain when pressure was made over the patella. Note that the articular cartilage of the patella is not normal anywhere. In the upper half of the patella the cartilage is degenerated and, in places, more or less eroded. Surgical exploration of the knee revealed not only alterations of the articular surface of the patella but also considerable degenerative changes in the articular cartilage covering the intercondylar groove. Inspection of the rest of the joint failed to disclose any abnormalities relating to the synovial membrane, the menisci, or the articular cartilage lining the tibial condyle.

E, Photograph of the articular surface of a patella in which the manifestations of chondromalacia are much more advanced than those revealed in *D*. The patient was a woman 60 years of age who had difficulty in fully extending the knee, and who also presented evidence of intra-articular effusion. Note that, over a large area, the articular cartilage has been completely worn away and the exposed subchondral bone appears polished and ridged. The articular cartilage neighboring upon the polished subchondral bone (especially on the right) is fibrillated and partly ulcerated. A very large marginal exostosis can be seen on the left side of the picture. At surgery, extensive degeneration of the cartilage covering the intercondylar groove of the femur was also noted.

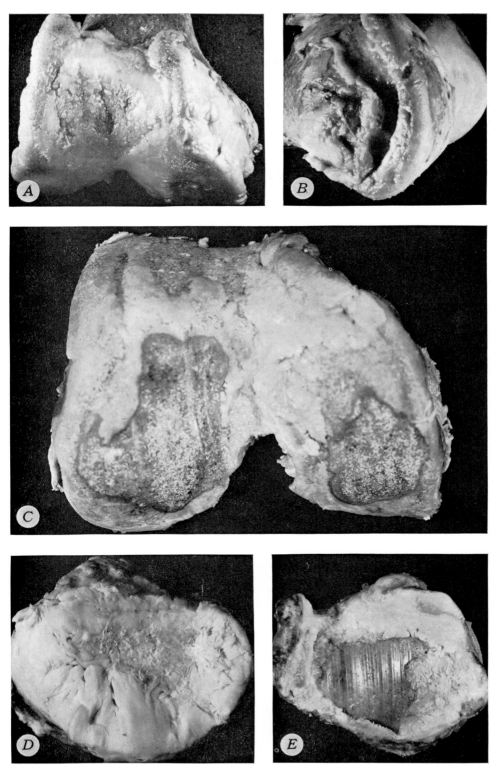

Figure 191

hip joint must be based upon changes in the joint space and structural alterations in the articular bone ends (see Danielsson).

Articular Cartilage.—In most ways, as already noted, the cartilage changes of primary osteoarthritis in its early stages are of the same general character as those observed in joints which have merely undergone the changes of senescence. Thus, grossly, the cartilage shows varying degrees and amounts of fibrillation or fissuring and areas of erosion. In some places the cartilage may have disappeared com-

Figure 192

Photomicrographs from different cases illustrating the histopathologic sequence of the alterations occurring at the femoral condyles or at the proximal surface of various tibiae at different stages in the course of the evolution of osteoarthritis.

In *A* (× 18) it is apparent that the degenerative changes are still limited to the surface of the articular cartilage of the tibia and correspond to what one would also observe in the tibia of a knee joint presenting the articular changes of senescence. In particular, the surface of the cartilage is frayed, and one can note shreds of degenerated cartilage, some lying free and some still attached. This appearance is the result of fibrillation, and in some places linear slits can be observed between the fragments of altered cartilage which are still attached. The subject in this case was a man 64 years of age—a diabetic whose knee joint became available for anatomic examination when a supracondylar amputation was done because of the development of arteriosclerotic gangrene of the toes. In addition to degenerative changes involving the articular cartilage of the proximal end of the tibia, there were similar changes in the articular cartilage of the patella and especially in the intercondylar groove of the femur.

In *B* (× 5), much of the upper two thirds of the articular cartilage can be seen to have lost its staining qualities. Note, on the left, the slit extending down through this part of the cartilage and then across toward the right. The area of cartilage delimited in this way is necrotic and would eventually have been sheared or sloughed off. This section was prepared from a femoral condyle of a woman 56 years of age. More advanced degenerative changes were present in other parts of the femoral condyles (see *C*).

In *C* (× 5) one can note much more advanced degenerative changes than those illustrated in *B* Proceeding toward the right side of the picture, it can be observed that the upper third of the articular cartilage is fibrillated and degenerated and is in the process of being sloughed off. Further to the right, the cartilage is necrotic throughout its thickness and is fragmented. In this area of the section, one can no longer discern a clearly delineated calcified cartilage zone. Also, it is apparent that the bony end plate has been disrupted, and the marrow spaces of the spongiosa in that particular area seem to contain fibrous tissue.

In *D* (× 7) the histopathologic changes are still more advanced. The section was prepared from the femoral condyle of a woman 73 years of age who had had pain and disability referable to the right knee joint for many years. At the top of the left half of the picture, one can note small fragments of obviously degenerated articular cartilage. To the right, the surface of the bone presents almost no articular cartilage at all. At the extreme right, a small area of sclerotic subchondral bone can be seen. The arrow on the left points to a subchondral focus of fibrous tissue which is apparently beginning to undergo cystic softening at its center. The arrow on the right points to a focus of cartilage in the subchondral spongiosa. This cartilage probably reached the site in question after being dislocated and depressed into the subchondral region through a minute fracture defect at the cartilage-bone border.

E and *F* (× 5) illustrate the histopathologic changes present at two different sites of the articular surface of a tibia. The specimen came from the left knee joint in the case of a man 82 years of age. In *E* the central portion of the articular surface is completely denuded of cartilage, and the subchondral bone is sclerotic. The articular cartilage at each side of the sclerotic subchondral bone appears degenerated and has been undergoing erosion. In *F* it can be seen that the articular surface is devoid of cartilage except for two minute nubbins, one of which is visible on each side of the center of the picture. There is also a moderate degree of subchondral sclerosis.

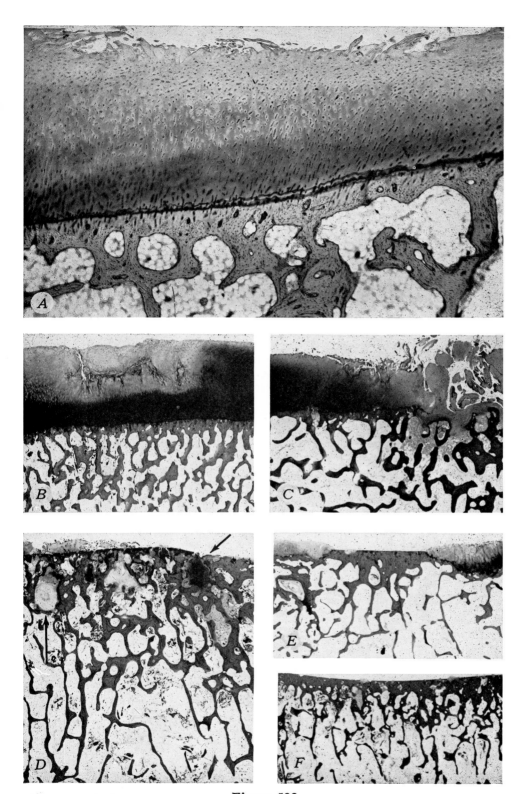

Figure 192

pletely, so that the subchondral bone has been exposed. Even before the cartilage becomes fibrillated or eroded, the appearance of acidophilic staining tendencies in swollen interstitial substance can be noted microscopically. As the chondromucoid of the interstitial substance disappears, the fibrillar basis of this substance becomes apparent. As for the cartilage cells, these tend first to swell and then to disappear.

As a rule, the grossly damaged articular cartilage presents no obvious evidence of repair. Nevertheless, there are usually some microscopic indications of attempts at regeneration in the cartilage. Thus, newly formed cartilage cells clustering in groups may appear, especially in the superficial layers of the articular cartilage that is undergoing fibrillation (see Meachim and Collins). Where the cartilage has been partly eroded, its deeper portions, in spite of necrosis, may also show such clusters of newly formed cartilage cells. Even where the cartilage has been completely eroded, the denuded bone may come to be covered, or the gap in the cartilage filled in, by connective tissue. The latter is usually derived either from the sub-chondral marrow, through the medium of penetrating blood vessels, or from remnants of the original cartilage. Such connective tissue may even become transformed into cartilage—usually fibrocartilage. Re-covering of the denuded bone can, of course, occur only where the formerly opposed joint surfaces have ceased to rub against each other. (See Mankin and Lippiello, and Mankin et al.)

In the presence of advanced changes, numerous blood vessels may be seen penetrating into the calcified zone of the articular cartilage. They come from the subchondral marrow spaces and may penetrate into the deeper portions of the original or regenerating articular cartilage. Pommer has attached crucial importance to this phenomenon in connection with the microscopic diagnosis of the early stages of primary osteoarthritis.

Subchondral Bone.—In primary osteoarthritis the subchondral region is likely to undergo pronounced modification. In the course of erosion of the articular cartilage, the underlying bone is exposed. Friction against each other of opposed bone ends that have been denuded of their cartilage is followed by *sclerosis* of such bone. This is essentially the result of the deposition of new bone on already existing bone trabeculae. Compression of the trabeculae against each other may also play some role in the sclerosis. Under continued friction, the articular surface of the sclerotic subchondral bone becomes quite compact and polished. Such eburnated bone will usually show some surface necrosis, and, in places, shallow grooves due to grinding down of the sclerotic bone may appear. Even the deeper-lying subchondral bone may be modified if the arthritic alterations are severe. This bone will show thickening of the trabeculae in consequence of the apposition of additional lamellar bone. (See Fig. 192.)

The intertrabecular marrow, too, is modified in accordance with the severity of the arthritis. Instead of being quite fatty, as it normally is in the subchondral regions of the joints of middle-aged or older adults, it acquires varying degrees of vascularity and cellularity. For some distance below the articular surfaces, quite cellular fiber marrow may develop, in which trabeculae of new bone may also form. The cellular fiber marrow may contain phagocytes filled with blood pigment, and even collections of plasma cells and lymphocytes. It is worthy of note that, in cases in which the arthritis is no longer actively evolving, the intertrabecular marrow may be quite fatty and only slightly fibrous.

Minute cystic spaces (*detritus cysts*) lined by dense fibrous tissue may likewise appear between the trabeculae, especially in the vicinity of the joint end. These spaces may communicate with the joint cavity through narrow channels resembling bottle necks. Occasionally (especially in cases of advanced primary osteoarthritis of the hip joint), a very large cyst develops in the femoral head or, perhaps independently, in the ilium adjacent to the acetabulum. Furthermore, in an adult with a painful hip, a large cyst in the iliac acetabulum is not infrequently encountered, even before the hip joint shows roentgenographic evidence of osteoarthritis (see Eggers *et al.*).

In places where the cartilage has been ground down, the articular surface may reveal, even on gross inspection, tiny, projecting grayish or whitish *cartilage nodules*. They are usually of about pinhead size or smaller, but occasionally larger. Their significance is not clear, but they seem to be one of the manifestations of repair. In any case, they have only a limited capacity for growth. In addition, microscopic examination of the subchondral region also often reveals fragments of cartilage, sometimes as much as a centimeter or more below the articular surface. Such bits of cartilage are frequently fixed like minute islands between bone trabeculae, or lie on the surface of trabeculae. The character of this cartilage varies from fibrous to hyaline.

There are conflicting opinions as to the source of the deeply placed cartilage. Some hold that most often it is derived from articular cartilage which has become dislocated and depressed into the subchondral region through fracture defects at the cartilage-bone border. There can be no doubt that portions of the calcified cartilage zone and bits of the bony end plate may become herniated into the subchondral region. Nevertheless, as a number of observers have shown, some deeply placed bits of cartilage apparently arise solely on the basis of cartilaginous metaplasia of subchondral fiber marrow. Ultimately the cartilage nests may become calcified and even undergo transformation into bone. Or, instead, they may succumb to mucinous and cystic degeneration.

Marginal Exostoses.—These appear so commonly in primary osteoarthritis that they constitute a characteristic feature of its pathologic anatomy. (They are apparently not a specific feature, however, since, as Heine points out, they are occasionally seen at the head of the humerus or at the condyles of the femur in the absence of all other manifestations of osteoarthritis.) It is at the periphery of articulating surfaces of the affected large joints that marginal exostoses are found. That is, they tend to appear in the general region where the articular cartilage becomes continuous with the local periosteum. Marginal exostoses overhang the periphery of the articulating surfaces more or less like lips, or ledges. As sectioning of the involved part of the bone will show, the marginal exostosis is usually continuous with the adjacent bone area. Ordinarily the exostosis is composed of spongy trabeculae and fatty intertrabecular marrow. Toward the joint surface, a marginal exostosis is usually delimited by a layer of bone continuous with the bony end plate. Often, this bony layer is covered partly by fibrocartilage and/or periosteum. Not infrequently, however, especially at the hip joint, the fibrocartilaginous covering of a marginal exostosis has been partially or wholly worn away. Where this happens, a bony surface is exposed which usually becomes more and more eburnated and polished. There has been considerable speculation in regard to the mode of origin of marginal exostoses. The conception most generally favored is that they represent outgrowths from the subchondral bone (see Pommer, Heine, Lang, and also Knaggs).

This interpretation implies that such exostoses start where an area at the periphery of the articular cartilage has become vascularized from the direction of the subchondral marrow. The cartilage around the vascularized region becomes calcified. In this way the formation of new endochondral bone at the margin of the cartilage is stimulated. The direction of growth of the osseous tissue is determined by molding pressure upon the articular surface. In the course of the growth of this new bone, a marginal exostosis develops, for the bone pushes outward along the line of least resistance. That is, it grows outward from the undermined cartilage toward the margin of the articulating surface. Finally, the spongy bone of the exostosis becomes entirely continuous with the adjacent subchondral spongy trabeculae. (See Fig. 193.)

While not entirely rejecting the view that the exostoses are outgrowths from the subchondral bone, Keefer *et al.* maintain that at times the exostoses seem to be the result of a mechanical mushrooming outward of tissue in this region, due to forcible flattening of the articular surface. Under these circumstances, however, one would expect to find fiber marrow, splintered trabeculae, and signs of previous hemorrhage. The concept of Nichols and Richardson is that the exostoses originate as new bone appositions formed from periosteal, perichondrial or capsular tissue at the margin of the articular surface. The point of view expressed by Axhausen is somewhat similar. He maintained that exostosis formation begins with synovial hyperplasia at the margins of the articular cartilage, and interpreted the exostoses as reactive-regenerative sequelae of cartilage damage.

Figure 193

A, Photomicrograph ($\times$ 2) of a femoral head illustrating the characteristic histopathologic changes of degenerative arthritis. The patient was a man 49 years of age who worked as a laborer, and who was admitted to the hospital because of pain in the lower part of his back and in the region of the right hip joint. His clinical record also indicates that, though these pains had been present for several years, it was during the year before admission to the hospital that the condition relating to the hip became incapacitating. The patient experienced severe pain when he walked even a short distance, and he now also limped. A roentgenographic skeletal survey revealed osteoarthritic changes in both hip joints and also pronounced spondylosis deformans, particularly in the lumbar region. The right femoral head became available for anatomic study when it was removed in the course of prosthetic replacement arthroplasty. The specimen consisted of the head and upper part of the neck of the femur. The head was deformed and appeared broadened and somewhat flattened. Nowhere on its surface did it present cartilage of normal appearance. Over part of the convexity of the head, the articular cartilage had been eroded and the subchondral bone was exposed. Where this had happened, several small islands of whitish tissue could be seen. On microscopic examination, these proved to be small foci of cartilage located in the intertrabecular spaces of the subchondral spongiosa (see arrow on the left). As the picture also demonstrates, there is a large exostosis on the right. To some extent, this is a marginal exostosis, but for the most part it is a so-called flat exostosis resulting from invasion of the articular cartilage by blood vessels carrying osteogenetic cells. In consequence, a thick layer of spongy osseous tissue has formed between the original calcified zone of the articular cartilage (see arrow on the right) and the original and/or newly formed covering cartilage.

B, Photomicrograph ($\times$ 5) illustrating the histopathologic changes presented by a tissue section prepared from the head of the right femur from another case of degenerative arthritis of the hip joint. The patient was a man 49 years of age who had been experiencing disability in that hip for several years. The hip was painful, and the patient walked with a marked limp on the right side. Roentgenographic examination confirmed the presence of pronounced osteoarthritis involving the right hip joint, and also the presence of osteoarthritis of milder degree in the left hip. On the left side of the picture, the articular surface shows a small amount of fibrillated and degenerated residual articular cartilage. On the right side of the picture, the surface of the bone is denuded of cartilage, and on the extreme right a small area of sclerotic subchondral bone is to be observed. In the midportion of the picture one can note a subchondral focus of fibrous tissue with a small cystlike cavity in it, and an adjacent focus of poorly cellular fibrous tissue presenting *no* evidence of cystic softening.

C, Photomicrograph ($\times$ 4) of a tissue section prepared from another part of the femoral head in the case mentioned in *B*. Except for the small amount of degenerated articular cartilage to be seen on the left, the surface of the bone is devoid of cartilage. The most striking feature of this picture is the presence of many large and small cysts located close together. All the cysts have fibrous linings, in part or throughout. Though none of the cysts open onto the surface of the bone to communicate with the articular cavity, the likelihood is that sections taken at another level would have revealed such communication.

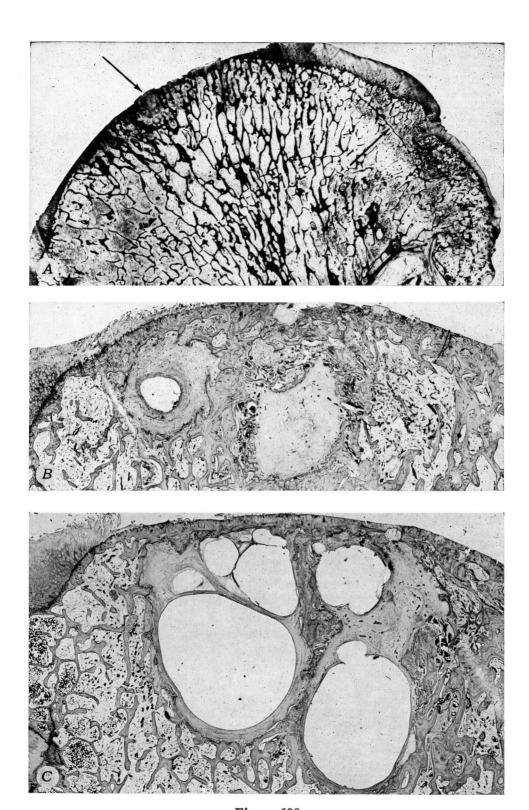

Figure 193

Shifting and Reduplication of the Bone-Cartilage Border. —These changes produce what the present writer denotes as "flat exostoses." They are created on a basis quite similar to that underlying the generally favored conception of the formation of marginal exostoses. It is in the hip joint, and specifically in the head of the femur, that the flat exostoses attain their greatest prominence. The shifting and reduplication take place only where the surface of the joint still retains some covering cartilage. They seldom if ever appear in those parts of the joint surface which are subject to friction through functional contact, since in such areas the cartilage is often rubbed down. Mere inspection of the articular surfaces will not reveal the shifting and reduplication. However, in longitudinal sections of the affected

Figure 194

A, Photomicrograph (× 6) illustrating the histopathologic pattern presented by the articular surface of an osteoarthritic femoral head in an area in which the cartilage had been completely eroded and the immediate subchondral bone is highly sclerotic. In the central part of the picture, below the sclerotic subchondral bone, there is a large focus of loose vascularized connective tissue. Ultimately, a cyst probably would have developed at this site. To the left of this focus of connective tissue, one can note two small cysts surrounded by rather sclerotic spongiosa. The patient was a woman 67 years of age whose difficulties relating to the hip in question (the right hip joint) had been of 2 years' duration at the time of her admission to the hospital. She complained of progressive stiffness of the hip joint, associated with some pain and much difficulty in walking. The femoral head was removed in the course of a prosthetic replacement arthroplasty. It showed extensive alteration of the articular cartilage, which was roughened, fibrillated, pitted, and eroded in various areas. Where the cartilage had been completely worn away, the subchondral bone appeared polished. Furthermore, in the vicinity of the head-neck junction there were large and small marginal exostoses.

B, C, and *D,* Photomicrographs illustrating the histopathologic basis for the formation of flat exostoses and/or the appearance of small bumps on the surface of an osteoarthritic femoral head where that surface is not subject to functional friction.

In *B* (× 4) the articular surface shows two small bumps representing flat exostoses. Proceeding from the left, one can see that a small area of the articular surface is covered by highly fibrillated and degenerated articular cartilage. Beyond the latter there is a small, humplike projection of osseous tissue. Its articular surface seems to be covered by fibrocartilage. It is also evident that the original bony end plate and calcified zone of the articular cartilage underlying the modified articular cartilage to the left of this projecting area does not continue across the base of the osseous hump. Further to the right, there is another bony projection. It is clear that the latter has formed as the result of the invasion of blood vessels and osteoblasts through the bony end plate into the articular cartilage. Note also that much of the deeply located portion of the articular cartilage is still present, and that the bump of osseous tissue seems to be covered by fibrocartilage.

In *C* (× 6) the histopathologic architecture of a flat exostosis is demonstrated. The articular cartilage had been invaded by blood vessels carrying osteoblasts on their walls. This invasion had resulted in the replacement of much of the articular cartilage by spongy bone and fatty and myeloid marrow. Proceeding from above down, one can note a layer of cartilage, a zone of spongy bone and marrow, and then, extending across the picture, a thin, bandlike zone composed of some of the original bony end plate and some fragments of the calcified zone of the original articular cartilage. At the extreme left of the picture, a small island of deeply placed original articular cartilage is still present, though it is being penetrated by blood vessels.

In *D* (× 8) the articular cartilage is of irregular thickness and appears undulated. The spongy osseous tissue is sparse and atrophic. The illustrated area of the arthritic femoral head had not, of course, been subjected to functional pressures. The head had come from an elderly subject whose affected hip joint had been immobile for a long time, as evidenced by the atrophy of the spongy bone.

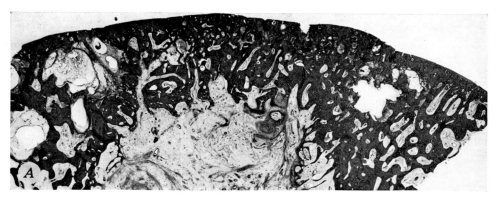

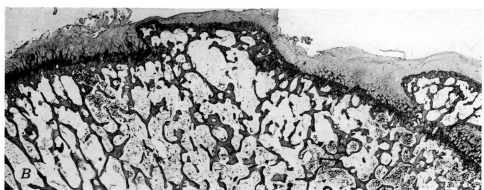

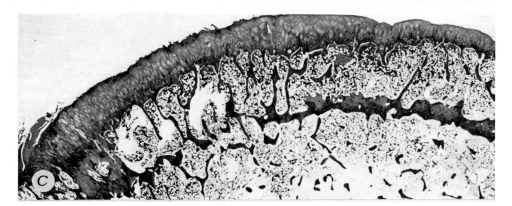

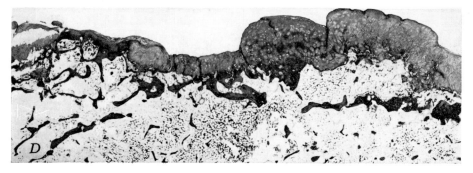

Figure 194

articular bone end, the abnormalities are quite apparent microscopically and even grossly. The picture which they present microscopically is highly complex.

In consequence of the *shifting* of the bone-cartilage border, a *bumpy irregularity* may be created in the contour of the articular surface. The inception of this irregularity depends upon the penetration of blood vessels from the subchondral marrow through the calcified zone of the articular cartilage into the deeper part of the cartilage. As a result of endochondral ossification within the articular cartilage, the frontier between the cartilage and subchondral bone tends to shift.

The *reduplications* of cartilage and bone occasionally found at the articular ends present even more bizarre pictures. These reduplications differ from the bumpy elevations described above, in that the original calcified cartilage zone does not shift forward toward the joint. The reduplications are the result of the appearance of new bone between the original calcified cartilage zone and a newly formed one above it. The latter in turn becomes covered by a layer of regenerated articular cartilage which may be deposited on eroded remnants of the original articular cartilage.

Microscopic examination, proceeding downward in the direction of the sub-chondral bone, will reveal in such an area: (1) a layer of regenerated articular cartilage, and then, successively, (2) a new zone of calcified cartilage, (3) spongy bone, (4) some original articular cartilage, often showing a considerable degree of regeneration, (5) the original calcified cartilage zone and bony end plate, and finally (6) the subchondral bone. The bone formed between the more superficially located cartilage and the original calcified cartilage zone may eventually communi-cate and coalesce with the subchondral bone. Where this happens over an extensive area, the appearance of such an area will ultimately resemble that of the bumpy irregularities. (See Fig. 194.)

Periosteal Osteophytes.—It is on the neck of the femur and on the neck of the humerus that such overgrowths are most likely to be found. They arise through irritative stimulation of periosteum to new bone formation or, on the neck of the femur, from synovial membrane, which in this site is the counterpart of periosteum. On the neck of the femur, osteophytes also occasionally arise where articular cartilage extending down the neck is stimulated by irritation to endochondral activity.

Synovial Membrane.—The alterations in this tissue are ordinarily very slight in comparison with those in the cartilage and bone of the joint ends. However, if the changes in the cartilage and bone are severe, the synovial membrane is usually at least congested and somewhat hypertrophied. It is especially likely to show hyper-trophy where it reflects off the bone. Here this condition is expressed in the forma-tion of villi, sometimes delicate and sometimes rather coarse. As the hyperplasia of the synovial membrane becomes more pronounced, the villi tend to spread and may come to line the membrane almost completely.

When it has undergone considerable hypertrophy and hyperplasia, the membrane may show: (1) islands of cartilage proliferation; (2) small pedunculated fatty and fibrous polyps containing cartilage, which may come to be partly ossified; (3) villi which have become necrotic through having been caught and compressed between the bones; and (4) large, bulbous, fatty villi. Sometimes the synovial membrane contains bits of cartilage and bone that have broken off from the joint ends and become incorporated in the membrane. These bits may irritate the synovial mem-brane to proliferation. Sometimes, too, the membrane becomes inflamed in response to traumatic injury.

In the joint space, or in recesses of the synovial membrane, there may be *free joint bodies*. Some of these may be composed of compressed masses of fibrin, others of masses of cartilage, and still others of cartilage undergoing bony meta-plasia. The *joint capsule* may show distortion and even some thickening and, rarely, some bony metaplasia at points of attachment. The *ligaments* and *tendons* may also show fraying and degeneration. Once in a great while, there may be some calcification at the site of attachment of tendons. Generally the amount of *synovial fluid* is so slightly increased that the increase is not perceptible or is only barely perceptible clinically. If it is sufficient to be so detectable, aspiration will usually show the fluid to be yellow and clear. The cell count is low—usually not over several hundred cells per cubic millimeter. Whether or not polymorphonuclear leukocytes predominate will depend on the rapidity with which the fluid has accumulated and on how long it has been in the joint cavity. The protein content of the joint fluid will not be much above that of the blood serum. (The structure of the synovial membrane, and the chemical composition and cell content of the synovial fluid, are discussed in Chapter 4.)

OSTEOARTHRITIS OF THE
TERMINAL INTERPHALANGEAL JOINTS

Osteoarthritis involving the *terminal interphalangeal joints* of the hands is a very common disorder. It is characterized by the presence of small, hard, nodular swellings in the vicinity of the affected joints, particularly on their dorsolateral surfaces. It was Heberden who first focused attention on the condition, which is now usually denoted as *Heberden's nodes*. Though he was uncertain about the nature of the nodular swellings, he stressed the point that they were not to be confused with the tophi to be found in the region of finger joints in cases of gout. (See Fig. 195.)

In the great majority of instances, the nodes represent marginal exostoses and osteophytes developing in the course of *primary osteoarthritis* which had its origin in degenerative changes in the articular cartilages of the affected interphalangeal joints. In such cases the condition is commonly denoted as *idiopathic* Heberden's nodes. *Secondary osteoarthritis* of interphalangeal joints is also encountered, and takes the form of knobby swellings resembling the Heberden nodes of primary osteoarthritis. However, the nodes appearing in cases of secondary osteoarthritis ordinarily involve only one or two interphalangeal joints, and their origin can clearly be traced to a severe traumatic incident. Thus they may develop as the result of striking the joint or joints forcefully, for instance, with a hammer, or having them struck by a slamming door or window. In such cases the condition is commonly denoted as *traumatic* Heberden's nodes.

CLINICAL CONSIDERATIONS

Incidence and Inheritance.—We are concerned here only with the *idiopathic Heberden nodes*. The vast majority (about 90 per cent) of the affected subjects are women. Furthermore, when the condition does appear in men, it seldom manifests itself in the florid form so common in women. Those men who do develop Heberden's nodes are older than the women, on the average, when the condition begins to evolve. The women are usually in middle life when the disorder sets in, and its onset commonly dates from about 3 years after the menopause. With advancing age, the incidence of Heberden's nodes increases. Penetrance becomes complete (that is, maximum incidence is reached) at the age of 80 years, when about 30 per cent of women and 3 per cent of men show the condition.

Statistical evidence has accumulated to the effect that there is a *hereditary factor*

49

in the occurrence of the condition.   In studying the pedigrees of families in which
Heberden's nodes were present, and comparing the incidence of the condition in
those families with the incidence in women in the general population, Stecher found
that the disorder was twice as common in mothers of affected women, and three
times as common in sisters of affected women.   On the other hand, he also noted
4 families in which the mother was not affected and in which therefore the trait for
Heberden's nodes seemed to be transmitted to the offspring through the unaffected
father.   On investigation of the pedigrees of these 4 families, it was found that in
2 of them the paternal grandmother had Heberden's nodes, and in the 2 others a
paternal aunt was so affected.   Thus the condition seems to be inherited as a single
autosomal chromosome factor, sex influences being dominant in women and recessive
in men.

Clinical Complaints and Findings.—At the time of examination of an individual
patient, Heberden's nodes may be present on one finger or on several or all of the
fingers of both hands.   In the majority of cases, Heberden's nodes are limited to the
terminal interphalangeal joints, but there are also cases in which some of the
proximal interphalangeal joints are involved in addition to the terminal interphalangeal joints.   Idiopathic Heberden's nodes evolve gradually, without known
predisposing local cause.   The condition usually takes its departure in the terminal
interphalangeal joint of one finger—ordinarily a forefinger or a middle finger.   Sooner
or later, other fingers become involved successively, and in time many or even all
of the terminal interphalangeal joints of both hands may become affected.

At first, an involved articular area is somewhat tender.   The overlying skin may
show some reddish discoloration, but remains movable.   In the course of some
months or even a year or so, an affected joint area ceases to be tender, and the
reddish discoloration of the local skin disappears.   Now small, hard, knobby protuberances representing fully evolved Heberden's nodes are palpable and also
visible.   At this stage the articular ends of the bones entering into the formation of
the affected terminal interphalangeal joints are grossly distorted, and the ends of
the fingers usually deviate from the normal straight line.   In a subject in whom the

Figure 195

A, Photograph of the hands of an elderly woman showing, in the fingers of both hands,
nodular deformities characteristic of Heberden's nodes.   The changes are most obvious at
the terminal interphalangeal joints of the little finger and the index finger of both hands.
Note that the end of the right index finger deviates toward the middle finger, and that there
is no obvious involvement of the interphalangeal joint of either thumb.   That joint is often
the last to become implicated.

B, Roentgenograph of the left hand of another elderly woman illustrating narrowing of
the terminal interphalangeal joints of that hand and distortion of the contour of these
joints as a result of the development of marginal projections.   The proximal interphalangeal
joints appear to be free of involvement, and the metacarpophalangeal joints are certainly not
implicated.

C and *D*, Photographs illustrating the gross appearance of Heberden's nodes as presented by the terminal interphalangeal joint areas of the index finger and middle finger
of the right hand of a woman 53 years of age.   After these bones were removed at autopsy,
the specimens were macerated to free them from the overlying soft tissues, so that the
changes at the interphalangeal joint areas would be clearly visible.   In *C*, spurlike and dentate
projections are apparent at the base of the distal phalanx.   In *D*, one can note an apron-like
exostosis extending more or less uniformly around the base of the distal phalanx and the
distal end of the proximal phalanx.

E, Roentgenographs presenting, in anteroposterior and lateral projections, the changes at
the terminal interphalangeal joint illustrated in *D*.

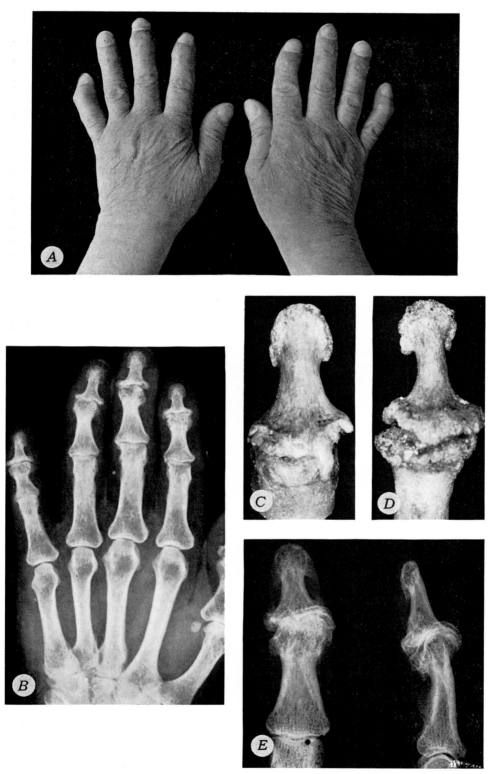

Figure 195

759

interphalangeal joints show Heberden's nodes, degenerative arthritis (primary osteoarthritis) of other diarthrodial joints may also be present. Of the large joints, those of the knee and hip are most likely to be concomitantly affected.

Gross deformities of several or all of the fingers, simulating those characteristic of Heberden's nodes but involving the proximal interphalangeal joints more strikingly than the terminal joints, are occasionally encountered. Such cases have been described under a variety of names, and the general term *"familial osteoarthropathy of the fingers"* serves to set the condition apart from Heberden's nodes (see Shaw, and also Allison and Blumberg). Familial osteoarthropathy of the fingers is a genetically determined abnormality which makes its appearance during late childhood or adolescence. It is reported to have its basis in ischemic necrosis of the epiphyses of the affected phalanges (see Dessecker). However, the pertinent article does not present any illustrations of the pathologic findings (either gross or microscopic) to support that interpretation. The mode of inheritance of the disorder is dominant, with strong penetrance, and the appearance of the abnormality is controlled by a single autosomal gene which manifests itself in nearly all persons who are heterozygous for it.

Figure 196

A, Photomicrograph ($\times$ 4) illustrating the general architecture of a normal terminal interphalangeal joint of a middle-aged woman. Note that the articular cartilage covering the base of the distal phalanx and the head of the middle phalanx is smooth and of almost uniform thickness. Juxtaposed against the bony end plate of each phalanx, the calcified zone of the articular cartilage stands out clearly as a thin, dark line.

B, Photomicrograph ($\times$ 5) illustrating the general architecture of the terminal interphalangeal joint of an index finger in the case of a woman 78 years of age who presented Heberden's nodes. The articular cartilage at the base of the distal phalanx is, for the most part, very thin, having undergone erosion. The immediate subchondral bone is somewhat sclerotic. The articular cartilage over the head of the middle phalanx is also thinned and eroded, notably in its midportion. On the right, the terminal phalanx shows an exostotic projection, and the middle phalanx reveals exostosis formation both on the left and on the right side, but particularly on the right. These exostoses have developed in the same manner in which marginal exostoses develop in primary degenerative arthritis involving large synovial joints.

C, Photomicrograph ($\times$ 5) of the terminal interphalangeal joint of a forefinger in the case of a woman 70 years of age. The articular cartilage covering the base of the terminal phalanx has undergone substantial erosion. A large, bony projection (a traction osteophyte) extends on the right from the base of the phalanx into the site of attachment of the articular capsule. The middle phalanx also shows, on the right, a large marginal exostosis of conventional architecture.

D, *E*, and *F* are photomicrographs of three terminal interphalangeal joints from the case of a woman 73 years of age who presented Heberden's nodes on both hands. Specimens were taken from the left hand of this subject. In *D* ($\times$ 12), one can see that the articular cartilage at the base of the distal phalanx and the head of the middle phalanx has been substantially eroded. On the right, there is a small focus of ossification in the joint capsule, at the site of attachment of the capsule to the terminal phalanx. Also on the right, below this traction osteophyte, the head of the middle phalanx shows a marginal exostosis of conventional architecture. In *E* ($\times$ 10), a large traction osteophyte is visible on the right at the site of attachment of the capsule to the base of the terminal phalanx. On both of the phalanges, the articular cartilage has been substantially eroded. In *F* ($\times$ 4), it is apparent that the articular cartilages of the interphalangeal joint are almost completely eroded. Small traction osteophytes are visible, both on the right and on the left, at the sites of attachment of the capsule to the base of the terminal phalanx. The illustration also reveals, on the left, a small joint "mouse" in a recess of the articular cavity—an unusual finding in cases of Heberden's nodes.

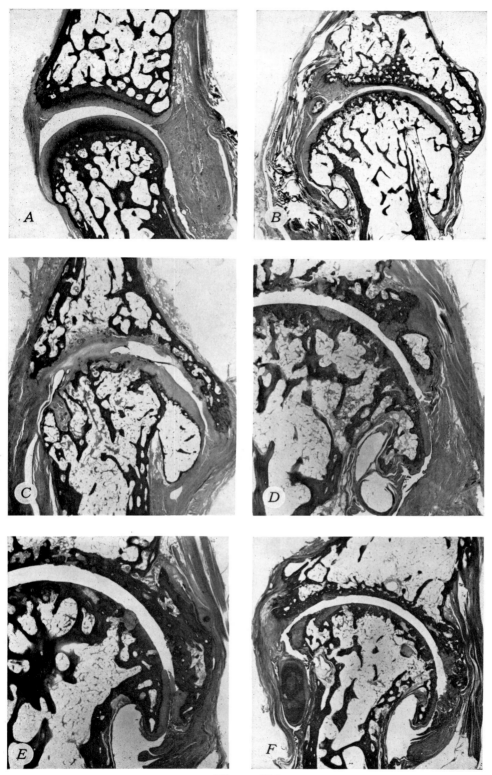

Figure 196

ROENTGENOGRAPHIC AND PATHOLOGIC FINDINGS

In the course of evolution of Heberden's nodes, the earliest *roentgenographic* change to be observed (for instance, in relation to an affected distal interphalangeal joint) is narrowing of the joint space, following upon erosion of the articular cartilages. After partial or substantial erosion of these cartilages has occurred, continued functioning of the joint leads to reactive sclerosis of the exposed subchondral bone, expressed in increased radiopacity. Concomitantly, smaller or larger marginal projections become manifest. Eventually, roentgenographs of affected terminal interphalangeal joints reveal that the contours of those joints are strikingly distorted.

As *pathologico-anatomic* examination reveals, the marginal projections may take the form of apron-like exostoses extending more or less uniformly around the proximal end of the distal phalanx and/or the distal end of the middle phalanx. One may also find spurlike and dentate projections extending proximally from the margin of the articular surface of the distal phalanx. It is stated in the literature that these projections are the result of traction exerted on the tendons (extensor and/or flexor) at the site of their attachment to the base of the distal phalanx. However, on the basis of histologic examination of terminal interphalangeal joints showing Heberden's nodes, the present writer doubts that this is actually the manner in which they usually arise. Instead, it is his opinion that some of them develop through traction at the site of attachment of the joint *capsule* to the base of the distal phalanx, and that many of them develop in the manner in which marginal exostoses usually evolve in other instances of primary (degenerative) osteoarthritis. (See Fig. 196.)

SPONDYLOSIS DEFORMANS

Spondylosis deformans is a common disorder of the vertebral column characterized by the presence of ledges (or buttresses) of new bone which start their development at the junction of the cortex of the affected vertebral bodies with the upper and/or lower marginal ridges of these bodies. The ledges of bone (which may also be designated as osteophytes) tend to grow toward each other and sometimes even fuse. In the course of their growth, they gradually compress between them, and may eventually pinch off, the intervertebral disk tissue which has protruded between the ledges of new bone. Under these circumstances the severed portion of the disk is destroyed when the adjacent ledges fuse.

The term "spondylosis deformans" was popularized by Schmorl. Like Rokitansky and also Beneke, he recognized that the condition had its point of departure in changes occurring in the intervertebral disks. However, Schmorl stressed in particular the idea that spondylosis deformans ensues upon avulsion of annulus fibrosus fibers of the intervertebral disk from the marginal ridges of the vertebral bodies bordering on the intervertebral disk in question (see Pathogenesis below).

In respect to *terminology*, "spondylosis deformans" is clearly preferable to "spondylitis deformans," a name previously used to designate the condition. That name was undesirable and confusing, because it suggested that the disorder had its basis in inflammation. Other names which have been used in the past but have been discarded include: "spondylitis osteoarthritica" and "polyspondylitis marginalis osteophytica." An alternative name introduced by Collins and also frequently used by others for spondylosis deformans is "spinal osteophytosis." In the opinion of the present writer, however, the name "spondylosis deformans" is to be preferred to the other names which have been suggested.

In discussing spondylosis deformans in this chapter, which is devoted to degenerative arthritis (osteoarthritis), the writer is aware that there are those who would restrict the designation "degenerative arthritis" or "osteoarthritis" to degenerative changes involving diarthrodial joints. The reason given for this restriction is that in these joints the articular bone ends are covered by hyaline cartilage in which degenerative changes are the point of departure for the osteoarthritis. It is on this account that one finds statements in the literature to the effect that spondylosis deformans should not be regarded as a manifestation of degenerative arthritis. Those who favor this idea would limit the occurrence of osteoarthritis involving the vertebral column to the apophysial (facet) joints and the costovertebral joints, since these are synovial joints whose articular bone ends are covered by hyaline cartilage. However, in the opinion of the present writer, the exclusion of spondylosis deformans from the general category of degenerative arthritis for the reasons cited does not appear justified on anatomic grounds. Indeed, it is reasonable to regard spondylosis deformans as belonging in the category of secondary osteoarthritis, since the condition follows in the wake of avulsion of fibers of the annulus fibrosus of the intervertebral disk from the site of anchorage of these fibers in the marginal ridge of the vertebral body.

CLINICAL CONSIDERATIONS

Incidence.—Spondylosis deformans is a common disorder whose occurrence is conditioned by such factors as age, sex, and occupation (see Schmorl and Junghanns). In regard to *age*, the disease process is sometimes already present in persons 40 years old. After that age, its incidence rises, and after the age of about 60 almost all subjects are likely to present some evidence of spondylosis deformans. In relation to *sex* incidence, there can be no doubt that the condition is found more often in males than in females. However, there is some variance among the reports in respect to the extent of the sex difference. In those reports in which it is stated that the sex difference is small, that finding is probably related to the background of the surveyed women in regard to physical work. In particular, women doing heavy work on farms could be expected to show a relatively high incidence of spondylosis deformans. The role played by *occupation* in the occurrence of the disorder in males has been recognized for a long time. Thus Gantenberg, in a survey of a large series of cases, found that in miners there was a particularly high incidence of spondylosis deformans of severe and medium degree; in factory workers the incidence was much lower; and in artisans it was found still lower.

Localization and Clinical Complaints.—Spondylosis deformans is not limited to any one portion of the vertebral column. Clinically (through roentgenography) it is certainly noted most often in the lower thoracic and lumbar regions and the lumbosacral joint. Indeed, the condition is often discovered as an incidental finding in the course of roentgenographic examination of the thorax and/or abdomen for some unrelated disorder. Furthermore, in a middle-aged or elderly subject coming to autopsy, if the entire vertebral column is removed and the condition is searched for by palpation and roentgenographic examination, the presence of some degree of spondylosis may also be revealed in the cervical and upper thoracic portions of the column. (See Fig. 197.)

Spondylosis deformans *per se* is usually asymptomatic. Obviously, not everyone having spondylosis deformans has complaints arising from it, since otherwise an overwhelming proportion of the older population would have back pain. When the latter does develop, it is usually mild at first and consists of transient but recurrent local aching and stiffness. However, in consequence of related local anatomic changes, radiating pain (radiculitis) may set in because of narrowing of one or more intervertebral foramina and compression of the spinal nerve root within them. Radiculitis most commonly involves one or both upper or lower extremities, and it is important to realize that radiculitis often occurs as the result of intervertebral disk protrusion or extrusion in the complete absence of spondylosis deformans.

The local anatomic changes which may result in radiculitis consist of: (1) advanced intervertebral disk degeneration, permitting posterior protrusion of the affected disk or extrusion of its nucleus pulposus; (2) exostosis formation about the periphery of a facet joint, resulting in narrowing of the intervertebral foramen by one or more exostotic spurs protruding into it; and (3) narrowing of the intervertebral foramen by a shift in the alignment of two adjacent vertebrae, due to slipping at the facet joints between them (see Barr and Mixter, and also Badgley).

Whether associated with spondylosis deformans or not, radiculitis may be induced by excessive strain upon, or direct trauma to, the vertebral column. This is most likely to occur if the strain or traumatic force is superimposed on a vertebral column in which the intervertebral disks are already compressed by the action of a loading force, and/or in which the disks have previously undergone degenerative changes, usually in consequence of senescence (see Hirsch).

In the *cervical region* the intervertebral foramina are small in comparison with those of the lower thoracic and lumbar regions. Therefore it is not surprising that a relatively slight degree of narrowing of one or more cervical intervertebral foramina may irritate and/or compress the pertinent cervical nerve roots and produce the so-called *cervical syndrome* (see Rydén, and also Jackson). The intervertebral foramina between the fourth, fifth, and sixth cervical vertebrae are the ones most subject to narrowing. The narrowing is usually brought about by a sprain injury of the ligamentous and capsular structures of the part of the cervical spine in question. Most commonly, sprain injury to the cervical spine is the result of vehicular crash accidents, in the course of which there is a sudden forceful movement of the neck in one direction and recoil in the opposite direction. Such sprain

Figure 197

Roentgenographs of parts of four vertebral columns, removed at autopsy, which illustrate the progressive changes of spondylosis deformans. The subjects were all beyond middle age, and none had pertinent clinical complaints.

In *A*, a small, hooklike projection (osteophyte) is apparent at the upper and/or lower anterior margin of each vertebral body. The intervertebral disk between the two fully outlined vertebral bodies in the uppermost part of the picture is definitely narrowed. Several small radiopacities are oriented to the lower margin of the upper of these two vertebral bodies. These radiopacities probably represent osteophytic projections somewhere along the lateral surface of that body. The vertebral body at the bottom of the picture reveals a small osteophyte projecting downward from its lateral surface.

In *B* the anterior margins of the illustrated vertebral bodies reveal more conspicuous osteophytic projections. In the upper part of the picture, the osteophyte projecting from the lower margin of the uppermost vertebral body appears to have fused with the osteophyte projecting from the upper margin of the adjacent body.

In *C*, proceeding from above downward, one can note that the osteophytic projections are still more prominent and are in various stages of fusion. A large, girdle-like osteophyte extends along the lateral surface of a vertebral body in the lower part of the picture. The facet joints show nothing remarkable.

In *D* there is even more striking evidence of fusion of osteophytic outgrowths. It is only in the midportion of the picture that the osteophytes of two adjacent vertebral bodies are not yet completely fused.

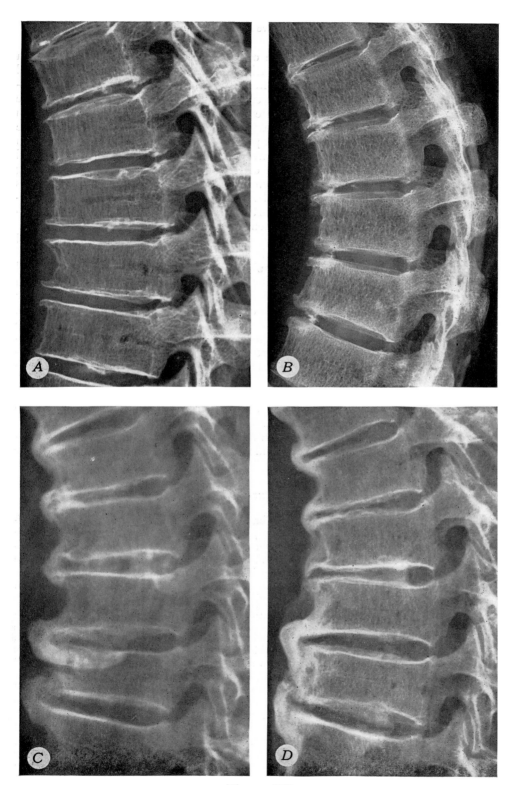

Figure 197

injuries may induce narrowing of one or more cervical intervertebral foramina because of: (1) a slight degree of subluxation of one or more of the cervical vertebral bodies, or (2) damage to one or more intervertebral disks, resulting in local degenerative changes and narrowing of intervertebral disk spaces. Degeneration of the disk tissue may be associated with a posterolateral tear of the annulus fibrosus of an affected disk and protrusion or even extrusion of a small amount of disk tissue (mainly nucleus pulposus), resulting in pressure against the local nerve root. In addition to narrowing of the cervical intervertebral foramina, sprain injuries tend to lead ultimately to the development of ledges of new bone between adjoining cervical vertebral bodies (spondylosis deformans) and also to degenerative arthritis of the facet joints of implicated cervical vertebrae. Occasionally, also, the protrusion of a marginal exostosis of an osteoarthritic facet joint may result in some narrowing of the local intervertebral foramen.

In the *thoracic part* of the column, degenerative joint disease may be associated with radiating pain (radiculitis), likewise due to narrowing of the intervertebral foramina and impingement on thoracic spinal nerves. The ventral rami of the third to the sixth thoracic spinal nerves are the typical intercostal nerves. Compression of these intercostal nerves sometimes results in chest pain suggesting that caused by coronary artery disease, and may lead to the erroneous diagnosis of angina pectoris. In the absence of abnormal electrocardiographic tracings, it merely needs to be borne in mind that in these cases the pains suggestive of angina pectoris can be provoked by pressure against the dorsal vertebrae, and can be relieved by proper management, including postural correction, use of a bed board, and traction upon the cervicodorsal spine (see Davis). Much less frequently, precordial pain simulating that of coronary heart disease may even be produced by rupture of an intervertebral disk in the lower cervical region and consequent pressure on local nerves (see Nachlas, and also Josey and Murphey).

Spondylosis deformans is encountered most frequently in the *lumbar* and *lumbosacral region* of the vertebral column, and it is also in these areas that the anatomic

Figure 198

A, Roentgenograph of the cervical vertebrae showing spondylosis deformans and specifically the presence of small, hooklike bony projections emanating from the bodies of the fifth and sixth vertebrae. The patient was a woman 67 years of age who had been experiencing intermittent stiffness and mild pain in the neck for about 8 years. Three weeks before this clinical roentgenograph was taken, the pain became severe, and it also started to radiate to the vertebral border of the right scapula. The patient did not associate the exacerbation of the clinical complaints with any specific injury. Except for pain in the neck on extension of the cervical spine, and tenderness on the right side of the C5–C6 interspace, the physical examination yielded only negative findings.

B, Roentgenograph of the lumbar vertebrae taken in the course of physical examination of a man 54 years of age who, not long after this roentgenograph was taken, died of Hodgkin's disease. He had had no clinical complaints referable to his back, despite the presence of spondylosis deformans (of moderate degree) as revealed in this picture.

C and *D*, Roentgenographs showing, in anteroposterior and lateral projections, advanced changes of spondylosis deformans involving the lumbar part of the vertebral column. The subject was a man 77 years of age who had worked as a laborer until he was 71 years old. His clinical complaints were of only 6 years' duration and consisted mainly of stiffness and intermittent pain in the lower part of his back. The striking alterations revealed in *C* might lead one to suspect that those changes had their basis in a neurological disorder, such as tabes dorsalis. However, the possibility of a tabetic arthropathy was ruled out by repeated serological tests. Analysis of the urine and biochemical study of the blood also eliminated the possibility that the condition represented a diabetic arthropathy.

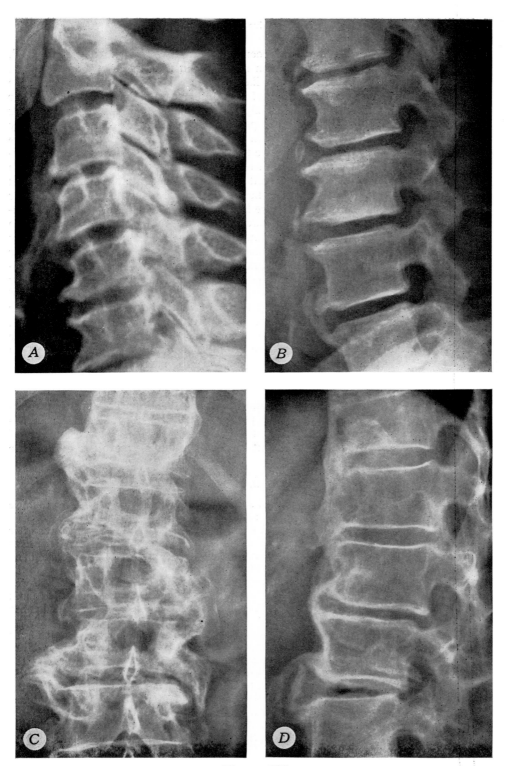

Figure 198

changes of spondylosis as revealed roentgenographically are most pronounced. However, complaints of low back pain and/or pain radiating down one or both extremities should not hastily be ascribed to nerve root compression related to changes involving intervertebral disks of the lumbar or lumbosacral portion of the spine. A variety of disease conditions implicating the pelvic organs, the soft tissues of the floor of the pelvis, the bones comprising the pelvis, and even the femur may be the basis for low back pain and/or pain radiating down one or both lower extremities. When low back pain is ascribable to intervertebral disk degeneration, it frequently has its basis in a sprain implicating the lumbosacral region. When the pain radiating down one or both lower extremities (sciatica) is ascribable to intervertebral disk changes, it is usually the result of nerve root compression due to protrusion or extrusion of disk tissue into one or more lumbar intervertebral foramina (occasionally between L_3 and L_4 and usually between L_4 and L_5 and L_5 and S_1) or even into the spinal canal. Under these circumstances, neurological examination will usually elicit evidence of various neurologic abnormalities, and the results of myelographic examination may also support the diagnosis of nerve root compression. Furthermore, it should be borne in mind that, especially in persons over the age of 45, low back pain may have its morphologic basis in osteoarthritis of the facet joints of several of the lumbar vertebrae and/or the facet joints between the fifth lumbar vertebra and the sacrum. In the presence of osteoarthritis of lumbar facet joints, osteophytes developing around the margins of the articular facets may narrow the local intervertebral foramina and hence impinge on emerging spinal nerves. In addition, lumbar intervertebral foramina may also be narrowed by encroachment upon them of the bony protuberances characterizing spondylosis deformans (see Lewin, and also Epstein).

From what has already been said and demonstrated, it is obvious that *roentgenographically* the condition does not present a diagnostic problem. In an advanced case of spondylosis deformans, the bony protuberances at the margins of the affected vertebral bodies stand out clearly. Since they are present on the

Figure 199

A, Photograph (anterior view) of part of a vertebral column showing the lower thoracic and lumbar vertebrae. The specimen was removed at autopsy in the case of a laborer 63 years of age who was known to have had hypertension, and who died a few hours after suffering a cerebral hemorrhage. The protuberances characteristic of spondylosis deformans are present in the general region of the intervertebral disks between all the vertebrae illustrated. In the thoracic region the protuberances are most prominent on the left side of the picture. In the lumbar region they are larger than in the thoracic region, and are well developed on both sides of the column. The spinal column was sectioned in the frontal plane, and *B* and *C* show the appearance of the cut surface of some of the thoracic and lumbar vertebral bodies and the intervening disks.

B, Photograph illustrating the gross appearance of the sectioned surface of part of the thoracic vertebral column pictured in *A*. On the left side, the protuberance which has developed at the lower margin of the uppermost vertebral body and the protuberance at the upper margin of the adjacent body have fused, and at the site of the fusion the local intervertebral disk tissue has disappeared. The two vertebral bodies just below reveal, on the left side, lateral protrusion of the intervertebral disk and the presence of buttresses of new bone which have formed in consequence of traction upon the anterior ligament and underlying periosteum.

C, Photograph illustrating the gross appearance of the sectioned surface of the lumbar part of the vertebral column shown in *A*. The two intervertebral disks between the upper three vertebral bodies are narrowed, discolored, and degenerated. The ledges, or buttresses, of new bone stand out prominently. In the midportion of the picture, the protrusions both on the left and on the right are fusing (see Fig. 200-*A*).

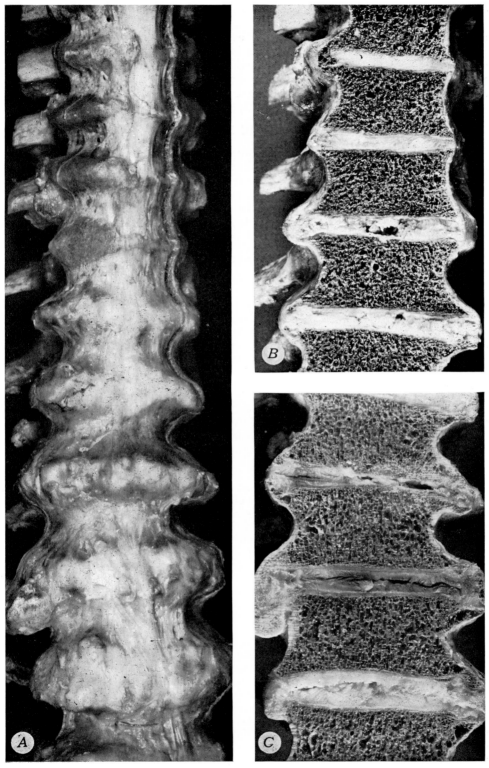

Figure 199

anterior and anterolateral borders, the exostotic protuberances can be readily visualized in clinical roentgenographs showing the column in the anteroposterior or, even better, in the lateral view. Extremely striking roentgenographic pictures are presented by specimens prepared from affected vertebral columns removed at autopsy and sawed into thin sections. (See Fig. 198.)

PATHOLOGIC FINDINGS

Gross Pathology.—Since the space between adjacent vertebral bodies is regarded anatomically as a joint, and since the point of departure of spondylosis deformans resides in certain changes in the intervertebral disks, some orienting remarks relating to the general anatomy of these joints are in order. It is well known that vertebral bodies are firmly united by the intervertebral disks and also by the anterior and posterior longitudinal ligaments. Along their course, the ligaments are attached to

Figure 200

A, Roentgenograph illustrating the appearance of the left side of the lumbar vertebral area shown in Figure 199-*C*. The roentgenograph was prepared from a thin slice of bone cut from that specimen. The large knobby protuberance apparent in the photograph stands out prominently in the roentgenograph as two almost fused bony projections originating from the lower and upper margins, respectively, of the adjacent vertebral bodies. Note also the smaller, hooklike protuberances present at the junction of the marginal ridge and cortex of the other vertebral bodies shown. Some of these protuberances can also be discerned in the photograph of the specimen in question.

B, Photograph of the cut surface of five contiguous thoracic vertebral bodies (T_6–T_{10}) which are bridged anteriorly by very large, highly sclerotic, and closely apposed but still unfused protuberances. Between these adjacent protuberances, there is degenerated intervertebral disk tissue which eventually would have been completely destroyed, so that the apposed protuberances would have undergone bony fusion. The subject was a woman 58 years of age who, for many years before emigrating to the United States, had done heavy physical labor on a farm. Her first admission to our hospital was for a carcinoma of the left breast, and a radical mastectomy was performed. Subsequently she came to manifest metastases, and died 3 years after the mastectomy. In the course of the autopsy, palpation of the vertebral column revealed the presence of spondylosis deformans, and the portion of the column extending from the fifth thoracic vertebra to the sacrum was removed for further study. Sectioning of the column in the sagittal plane revealed not only spondylosis deformans but also a small focus of metastatic carcinoma in the body of the tenth thoracic vertebra (see arrow).

C, Roentgenograph of the specimen illustrated in *B* demonstrating strikingly the protuberances and other changes apparent grossly in the specimen. Several of the intervertebral disks in the general vicinity of the protuberances show punctate radiopacities representing calcification in the degenerated disk tissue. In contrast, note the complete absence on the posterior surface of the vertebral bodies of new bone formation which characterizes spondylosis deformans.

D, Photograph presenting two views of part of a sectioned and macerated vertebral column from a subject about whom the writer has no clinical information. On the left of the picture, the outer surface of the specimen illustrates the presence of various degrees of spondylosis deformans within the same vertebral column. It also emphasizes the fact that the pathologic changes, even when not pronounced, do tend to be present laterally. If the macerated specimen is viewed from above downward, it can be seen that the small juxtaposed exostotic protuberances often have a dentate configuration (see arrows). The large adjacent protuberances present near the bottom of the picture were in the process of fusion. Immediately above these protuberances is one in which fusion has already taken place. The intervertebral foramen second from the top is distinctly narrowed, in consequence of osteoarthritis of the local facet joint.

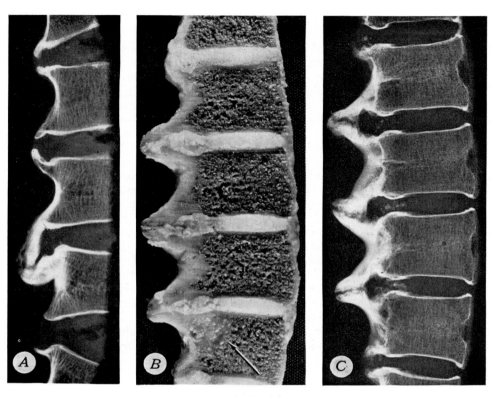

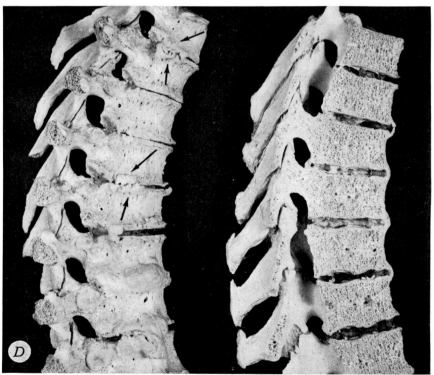

Figure 200

the periphery of the individual intervertebral disks and to the adjacent margins of the vertebral bodies. Beyond these sites of attachment of the ligaments, the anterior ligament in particular blends with the periosteal covering of the vertebral bodies. The intervertebral disks are squat fibrocartilaginous structures, each of which is adherent to the thin layer of hyaline cartilage covering the upper and lower surfaces of the adjacent vertebral bodies. In an adult these plates of hyaline cartilage may be regarded as the analogues of the articular cartilage of synovial joints. In a young subject the interior of a disk (the nucleus pulposus) is composed of glistening, semigelatinous tissue consisting mainly of bundles of collagenous fibers, fibroblasts, cartilage cells, and considerable amounts of amorphous intercellular material—mainly mucoprotein consisting of a protein polysaccharide complex. In a mature or older adult, the nucleus pulposus no longer appears glistening and semi-gelatinous, since the water and polysaccharide content is greatly reduced in amount and the constituent tissue is more collagenous (see Hirsch *et al.*, and Mitchell *et al.*). In consequence, the nucleus pulposus, though still soft and elastic, now appears yellowish. The more peripheral part of an intervertebral disk (the annulus fibrosus) consists largely of concentric lamellae of collagenous fibrous tissue. The fibers of the annulus fibrosus are anchored mainly in the bony marginal ridge at the periphery of the contiguous vertebral bodies above and below the intervertebral disk. Some fibers of the annulus are also anchored to the margin of the hyaline cartilage plates covering the upper and lower surfaces of these vertebral bodies. The outermost fibers of the annulus fibrosus intertwine with the fibers of the anterior and pos-

Figure 201

A, Photomicrograph ($\times$ 7) showing part of the lower portion of the twelfth thoracic vertebral body and the upper portion of the first lumbar body, along with part of the corresponding intervertebral disk. The subject was a young adult male. The histologic pattern presented is a normal one, and this picture is intended to serve for comparison of the normal pattern with the histopathologic changes observed in spondylosis deformans. Note on the left the smoothly arched contours presented by the upper and lower margins, respectively, of the two adjacent vertebral bodies. These arched contours represent the narrow bony marginal ridges which encircle the periphery of the upper and lower surfaces of each vertebral body. As is apparent from the picture, these ridges are important sites of anchorage for the fibers of the annulus fibrosus (see arrows). To the left, it can be seen that the fibers of the annulus fibrosus fuse with the anterior longitudinal ligament. The ligament is also adherent to the outer coat of the periosteum covering the cortices of the vertebral bodies.

B, Photomicrograph ($\times$ 5) illustrating histologic changes to be observed early in the course of the evolution of spondylosis deformans. Note that the marginal ridge of the lower vertebral body is no longer smooth in contour, appearing uneven and ragged. In addition, it is evident that the annulus fibrosus fibers are no longer anchored in this altered marginal ridge, apparently having been torn away from it. In the upper vertebral body, it is only at the extreme left that the marginal ridge is irregular in contour and that fibers of the annulus fibrosus are severed from it. In addition to the histologic findings just described, it is to be noted that the intervertebral disk has bulged forward to a slight degree and is exerting pressure against the anterior longitudinal ligament and, in turn, on the periosteum where the ligament blends with it.

C, Photomicrograph ($\times$ 4) demonstrating further advance of the histopathologic alterations characterizing spondylosis deformans. As a result of laceration of the annulus fibrosus fibers and forward protrusion of the disk against the anterior ligament, traction has evidently been exerted in turn upon the local periosteum. This traction has provoked the deposition of subperiosteal new bone and specifically the formation of apposed hooklike exostoses (or osteophytes), one directed downward and the other upward from the margins of the adjacent vertebral bodies.

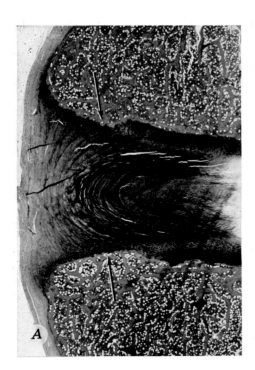

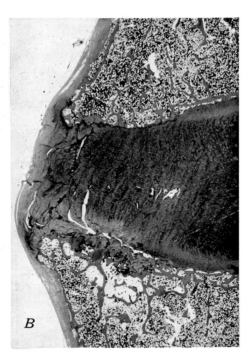

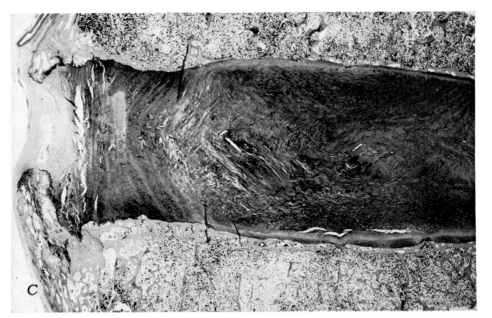

Figure 201

terior longitudinal ligaments where these ligaments become attached to the periphery of the intervertebral disks and the adjacent margins of the vertebral bodies.

Early in the course of their evolution, the bony excrescences characterizing spondylosis deformans present as small serrations somewhere along the junction of the upper and/or lower marginal ridge of the involved vertebral body with the cortex of that body. If present at the distal margin of one vertebral body and the proximal margin of the adjacent body, the bony serrations may interdigitate. As they grow larger, they present as prominent knobby bony protrusions, or ledges, which may ultimately fuse and bridge the neighboring intervertebral disk spaces. The excrescences are most prominent far over laterally and not just a little to the side of the midline, as they are often stated to be. As the result of encroachment of the osteophytic outgrowths onto the surface of individual vertebral bodies, such bodies may come to have a configuration suggestive of an hourglass, because the transverse diameter of the midportion of the body is much less than that of the upper and lower portion of the body, where the osteophytes are present. (See Fig. 199.)

Finally, it is to be noted that, even when the osteophytic outgrowths are large and prominent on the anterolateral surface of many of the vertebral bodies, osteophytic outgrowths (even very small ones) are rarely to be found on the posterior surface of any of the vertebral bodies—that is, on the surface which borders on the spinal canal. In those exceptional instances in which osteophytes have been observed in this location, they are tiny bony projections which never significantly compromised the diameter of the spinal canal and hence caused no pressure upon the spinal cord or the cauda equina. The rarity and smallness of osteophytes on the posterior surface of the vertebral bodies is apparently related to the anatomic factors underlying the attachment of the posterior longitudinal ligament to the vertebral bodies. The posterior ligament is a much thinner structure than the anterior ligament, and is also less intimately attached to the vertebral bodies than is the anterior ligament. Most of the fibers of the posterior ligament are attached to the intervertebral disks, and only a few thin fibers from it blend with the periosteum on the posterior surface of each vertebral body. Consequently, the periosteum of the posterior surface of the vertebral bodies is not subject to traction strong enough to provoke subperiosteal new bone formation (osteophyte formation). (See Fig. 200.)

Pathogenesis and Microscopic Pathology.—In considering the sequence of events in the pathogenesis of spondylosis deformans, one must remember that, as already pointed out, the most important anchorage of the annulus fibrosus is at the bony marginal ridge, and also that the outer fibers of the annulus are fused with the anterior longitudinal ligament. A tearing of some of the fibers of the annulus from

Figure 202

A, Photomicrograph ($\times$ 4) illustrating large and conspicuous apposed buttress-like osteophytic outgrowths from the margins of two adjacent vertebral bodies. That part of the intervertebral disk which has moved outward and is gripped between the osteophytes is obviously in the process of degeneration and collagenization. This can be deduced from the fact that the small amount of disk tissue present to the right of the disk area that has undergone these changes has retained its normal staining properties.

B, Photomicrograph ($\times$ 4) again showing two large apposed buttress-like osteophytic outgrowths. The protruded part of the intervertebral disk which is clamped between these bony outgrowths is substantially degenerated.

C, Photomicrograph ($\times$ 3) revealing the histopathologic pattern produced when two apposed osteophytic outgrowths fuse, in the course of which the intervening intervertebral disk tissue is destroyed.

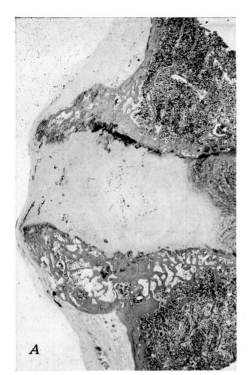
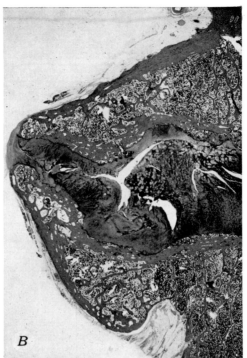
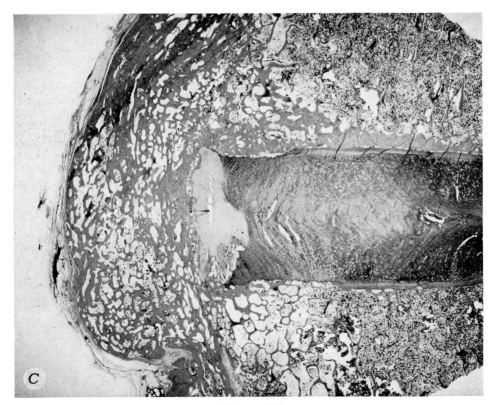

Figure 202

the marginal ridge permits a forward protrusion of the nucleus pulposus against the anterior longitudinal ligament. In the course of physical labor or other functional activity, the resultant traction on the anterior ligament provokes subperiosteal new bone formation at the ridge-cortex junction where the ligament is firmly attached to the periosteum covering the cortex of the vertebral bodies.

It is now clearly established that the alterations of spondylosis deformans are not initiated by degeneration, narrowing, and forward protrusion of the disk *per se*— that is, in the absence of avulsion of fibers of the annulus fibrosus from the bony marginal ridge. It is for this reason that one may encounter instances in which there is pronounced degeneration of the intervertebral disk and only very slight evidence of spondylosis deformans. On the other hand, one may also encounter instances in which evidence of spondylosis deformans is not only present but conspicuous, while the intervertebral disks appear to be free or almost free of degenerative changes. In support of the importance of avulsion of fibers of the annulus fibrosus from the marginal ridge in the instigation of spondylosis deformans, one can also cite the absence of spondylosis deformans in certain key instances. These are cases in which the intervertebral disks have been replaced by fibrous tissue and in which the adjacent vertebral bodies have consequently become clamped together and rendered practically immobile, so that almost no traction is exerted on the anterior ligament in the course of physical labor or other functional activity (see Güntz).

As already noted, avulsion of some of the fibers of the annulus fibrosus from the marginal ridge permits a forward protrusion of the intervertebral disk against the anterior longitudinal ligament. In the course of physical labor or other functional activity, the resultant traction on the anterior ligament provokes subperiosteal new bone formation at the ridge-cortex junction where the ligament is firmly attached to the periosteum covering the cortex of the vertebral bodies.

If enough pertinent specimens are studied microscopically to permit evaluation of the sequence of the anatomic changes, it becomes evident that, following avulsion of the annulus fibrosus fibers, the earliest demonstrable alteration is a slight irregularity and/or humping of the marginal ridge. This may already be associated with the presence of a small exostotic projection at the ridge-cortex junction. As the exostosis formation progresses, well-developed ledges (or buttresses) of new bone, of variable size, are to be observed at the ridge-cortex junction. These bony protuberances tend to grow toward each other, sometimes fusing, and compress between them, or even pinch off, the drawn-out disk tissue. Fragments of disk tissue which have been clamped between opposed exostotic ledges are eventually destroyed when the latter fuse. The progressive microscopic changes are illustrated in Figures 201 and 202.

REFERENCES

ALLISON, A. C., and BLUMBERG, B.: Familial Osteoarthropathy of the Fingers, J. Bone & Joint Surg., *40-B*, 538, 1958.

AXHAUSEN, G.: Neue Untersuchungen über die Rolle der Knorpelnekrose in der Pathogenese der Arthritis deformans, Arch. klin. Chir., *104*, 301, 1914.

BADGLEY, C. E.: The Articular Facets in Relation to Low-Back Pain and Sciatic Radiation, J. Bone & Joint Surg., *23*, 481, 1941.

BARLAND, P., JANIS, R., and SANDSON, J.: Immunofluorescent Studies of Human Articular Cartilage, Ann. Rheumat. Dis., *25*, 156, 1966.

BARR, J. S., and MIXTER, W. J.: Posterior Protrusion of the Lumbar Intervertebral Discs, J. Bone & Joint Surg., *23*, 444, 1941.

BENEKE, R.: Zur Lehre von der Spondylitis deformans, 69. Versam. deutsch. Naturf. u. Ärzte, Braunschweig, 1897.

BENNETT, G. A., WAINE, H., and BAUER, W.: *Changes in the Knee Joint at Various Ages*, New York, Commonwealth Fund, 1942.

Bunim, J. J.: Arthritis in the Elderly Patient (Osteoarthritis), Bull. New York Acad. Med., *32*, 102, 1956.

Chung, E. B.: Aging in Human Joints. I. Articular Cartilage, J. Nat. M. A., *58*, 87, 1966.

Collins, D. H.: *The Pathology of Articular and Spinal Diseases*, Baltimore, The Williams & Wilkins Company, 1950.

Danielsson, L. G.: Incidence and Prognosis of Coxarthrosis, Acta orthop. scandinav., Suppl. 66, 1964.

Davis, D.: Spinal Nerve Root Pain (Radiculitis) Simulating Coronary Occlusion: A Common Syndrome, Am. Heart J., *35*, 70, 1948.

Dessecker, C.: Zur Epiphyseonekrose der Mittelphalangen beider Hände, Deutsche Ztschr. Chir., *229*, 327, 1930.

Eggers, G. W. N., Evans, E. B., Blumel, J., Nowlin, D. H., and Butler, J. K.: Cystic Change in the Iliac Acetabulum, J. Bone & Joint Surg., *45-A*, 669, 1963.

Epstein, J. A.: Diagnosis and Treatment of Painful Neurological Disorders Caused by Spondylosis of the Lumbar Spine, J. Neurosurg., *17*, 991, 1960.

Gantenberg, R.: Zur klinischen Bedeutung deformierender Prozesse der Wirbelsäule, Fortschr. Geb. Röntgenstrahlen, *42*, 740, 1930.

Glyn, J. H., Sutherland, I., Walker, G. F., and Young, A. C.: Low Incidence of Osteoarthrosis in Hip and Knee after Anterior Poliomyelitis: A Late Review, Brit. M. J., *2*, 739, 1966.

Gofton, J. P., and Trueman, G. E.: Unilateral Idiopathic Osteoarthritis of the Hip, Canad. M. A. J., *97*, 1129, 1967.

Güntz, E.: Versteifung der Wirbelsäule durch Fibrose der Zwischenwirbelscheiben, Mitt. Grenzgeb. Med. u. Chir., *42*, 490, 1931.

Heberden, W.: De nodis digitorum. In *Commentarii de morborum historia et curatione*, London, T. Payne, 1802.

Heine, J.: Über die Arthritis deformans, Virchows Arch. path. Anat., *260*, 521, 1926.

Hirsch, C.: The Reaction of Intervertebral Discs to Compression Forces, J. Bone & Joint Surg., *37-A*, 1188, 1955.

Hirsch, C., Paulson, S., Sylvén, B., and Snellman, O.: Biophysical and Physiological Investigations on Cartilage and other Mesenchymal Tissues. VI. Characteristics of Human Nuclei Pulposi during Aging, Acta orthop. scandinav., *22*, 175, 1952.

Hulth, A.: Circulatory Disturbances in Osteoarthritis of the Hip, Acta orthop. scandinav., *28*, 81, 1958.

Jackson, R.: *The Cervical Syndrome*, 3rd ed., Springfield, Charles C Thomas, 1966.

Johnson, L. C.: Kinetics of Osteoarthritis, Lab. Invest., *8*, 1223, 1959.

Josey, A. I., and Murphey, F.: Ruptured Intervertebral Disk Simulating Angina Pectoris, J.A.M.A., *131*, 581, 1946.

Keefer, C. S., Parker, F., Jr., Myers, W. K., and Irwin, R. L.: Relationship Between Anatomic Changes in Knee Joint with Advancing Age and Degenerative Arthritis, Arch. Int. Med., *53*, 325, 1934.

Knaggs, R. L.: A Report on the Strangeways Collection of Rheumatoid Joints in the Museum of the Royal College of Surgeons, Brit. J. Surg., *20*, 113, 309, 425, 1932–33.

Lang, F. J.: Osteo-Arthritis Deformans Contrasted with Osteo-Arthritis Deformans Juvenilis, J. Bone & Joint Surg., *14*, 563, 1932.

Larson, C. B.: The Wearing-Out of Joints, J. Am. Geriatrics Soc., *10*, 558, 1962.

Lewin, T.: Osteoarthritis in Lumbar Synovial Joints, Acta orthop. scandinav., Suppl. 73, 1964.

Mankin, H. J.: The Effect of Aging on Articular Cartilage, Bull. New York Acad. Med., *44*, 545, 1968.

Mankin, H. J., and Baron, P. A.: The Effect of Aging on Protein Synthesis in Articular Cartilage of Rabbits, Lab. Invest., *14*, 658, 1965.

Mankin, H. J., and Laing, P. G.: Protein and Ribonucleic Acid Synthesis in Articular Cartilage of Osteoarthritic Dogs, Arthritis Rheum., *10*, 444, 1967.

Mankin, H. J., and Lippiello, L.: Biochemical and Metabolic Abnormalities in Articular Cartilage from Osteo-Arthritic Human Hips, J. Bone & Joint Surg., *52-A*, 424, 1970.

Mankin, H. J., Dorfman, H., Lippiello, L., and Zarins, A.: Biochemical and Metabolic Abnormalities in Articular Cartilage from Osteo-Arthritic Human Hips. II. Correlation of Morphology with Biochemical and Metabolic Data, J. Bone & Joint Surg., *53-A*, 523, 1971.

Meachim, G., and Collins, D. H.: Cell Counts of Normal and Osteo-arthritic Articular Cartilage in Relation to the Uptake of Sulphate ($^{35}SO_4$) *in Vitro*, Ann. Rheumat. Dis., *21*, 45, 1962.

Mitchell, P. E. G., Hendry, N. G. C., and Billewicz, W. Z.: The Chemical Background of Intervertebral Disc Prolapse, J. Bone & Joint Surg., *43-B*, 141, 1961.

Moffett, B. C., Jr., McCabe, J. B., and Askew, H.: Histologic Age Changes in Adult Human Temporomandibular Joints, Anat. Rec., *142*, 259, 1962.

MURRAY, R. O.: The Aetiology of Primary Osteoarthritis of the Hip, Brit. J. Radiol., *38*, 810, 1965.

NACHLAS, I. W.: Pseudo-Angina Pectoris Originating in the Cervical Spine, J.A.M.A., *103*, 323, 1934.

NICHOLS, E. H., and RICHARDSON, F. L.: Arthritis Deformans, J. Med. Research, n.s. *16*, 149, 1909.

PARKER, F., JR., KEEFER, C. S., MYERS, W. K., and IRWIN, R. L.: Histologic Changes in the Knee Joint with Advancing Age: Relation to Degenerative Arthritis, Arch. Path., *17*, 516, 1934.

POMMER, G.: Zur Kenntnis der Ausheilungsbefunde bei Arthritis deformans, besonders im Bereiche ihrer Knorpelusuren, nebst einem Beitrag zur Kenntnis der lakunären Knorpel-resorption, Virchows Arch. path. Anat., *219*, 261, 1915.

————: Über die mikroskopischen Kennzeichen und die Entstehungsbedingungen der Arthritis deformans (nebst neuen Beiträgen zur Kenntnis der Knorpelknötchen), Virchows Arch. path. Anat., *263*, 434, 1927.

ROKITANSKY, C.: *Lehrbuch der pathologischen Anatomie*, Wien, W. Braumüller, 1855.

RYDÉN, Å.: Spondylitis Deformans of the Cervical Spine as a Cause of So-called Brachial Neuralgia and other Neuralgiform Pains. A Contribution Specially to the Question of Treatment, Acta orthop. scandinav., *5*, 49, 1934.

SCHMORL, G.: Beiträge zur pathologischen Anatomie der Wirbelbandscheiben und ihre Beziehungen zur den Wirbelkörpern, Arch. orthop. u. Unfall-Chir., *29*, 389, 1931.

SCHMORL, G., and JUNGHANNS, H.: *Die gesunde und kranke Wirbelsäule im Röntgenbild*, Leipzig, Georg Thieme, 1932.

SHAW, E. W.: Avascular Necrosis of the Phalanges of the Hands (Thiemann's Disease), J.A.M.A., *156*, 711, 1954.

SILBERBERG, M., FRANK, E. L., JARRETT, S. R., and SILBERBERG, R.: Aging and Osteoarthritis of the Human Sternoclavicular Joint, Am. J. Path., *35*, 851, 1959.

SOKOLOFF, L.: The Biology of Degenerative Joint Disease, Perspect. Biol. Med., *7*, 94, 1963.

STECHER, R. M.: Heredity of the Joint Diseases, Reumatismo, *11*, 1, 1959.

————: Osteoarthritis and Old Age, Geriatrics, *16*, 167, 1961.

WEICHSELBAUM, A.: Über die senilen Veränderungen der Gelenke und deren Zusammenhang mit der Arthritis deformans, Sitzungsb. Kais. Akad. Wissensch. Math.-natur. Classe. Wien, *75-76*, 193, 1877.

Chapter

26

Inflammatory Arthritis of Undetermined Etiology

MUCH of this chapter will be devoted to the classic form of rheumatoid arthritis, which affects adults, but it will also deal with various other inflammatory arthritides of uncertain etiology, including specifically: (1) juvenile rheumatoid arthritis (Still's disease); (2) polyarthritis associated with splenomegaly and leukopenia (Felty's syndrome); (3) psoriatic arthritis; (4) the triad of arthritis, urethritis, and conjunctivitis (Reiter's syndrome); and (5) ankylosing spondylitis.

There are various other arthritides of undetermined etiology, but these will not be discussed in detail. They include the arthritides which sometimes appear with diseases of the intestinal tract. In that connection, it is now well established that a small but not inconsiderable proportion of persons affected with *regional enteritis* present articular manifestations, especially in relation to peripheral joints and sometimes in relation to the vertebral column, alone or in addition to the peripheral joints (see Ansell and Wigley). There is usually an interval of months or years between the onset of the regional ileitis and the involvement of joints in these cases. A small percentage of subjects affected with *ulcerative colitis* likewise develop arthritis of peripheral joints and also joints of the vertebral column. However, with ulcerative colitis (in contrast to regional ileitis), the articular involvement ordinarily sets in within a few weeks after the onset of the colitis, and the arthritis sometimes leads to permanent damage of the affected peripheral joints and even to ankylosing spondylitis (see Ford and Vallis, McEwen *et al.*, and also Soren). However, the reported incidence of ankylosing spondylitis in cases of ulcerative colitis is increased by the fact that subjects affected with ankylosing spondylitis may have ulcerative colitis but still be free of complaints referable to the gastrointestinal tract (see Jayson and Bouchier). Furthermore, a very large proportion of patients affected with *Whipple's disease* (intestinal lipodystrophy) complain of acute, intermittent, often migratory polyarthritis. Not infrequently, the arthritis becomes evident even before the diagnosis of Whipple's disease is indicated by the presence of diarrhea or steatorrhea. Residual articular deformities are rare in subjects affected with Whipple's disease, and, though many show involvement of the sacroiliac joints, full-fledged ankylosing spondylitis does not evolve (see Kelly and Weisiger).

RHEUMATOID ARTHRITIS

Rheumatoid arthritis in its *usual* (or *classic*) *form*—that is, the form affecting adults—is the articular expression of a chronic systemic disease (sometimes denoted as *rheumatoid disease*). The latter usually involves various nonarticular tissues and organs in addition to joints. The arthritis which constitutes the central feature of rheumatoid disease is initiated by nonsuppurative inflammation in the synovial membrane of affected joints. The cause of the disease has not yet been fully elucidated, but much evidence points to the importance of a hypersensitivity mechanism in its etiology (p. 784).

The clinical course is variable, but the condition tends to be chronic and progressive, resulting in disability and characteristic articular deformities. Almost always, many of the peripheral joints come to be involved, those of the knees and hands being predilected. The early intra-articular inflammatory changes in the synovial membrane, together with periarticular soft-tissue swelling, cause stiffness of the affected joint or joints, and this feature is prominent among the initial complaints. In the further progress of the arthritis, the articular bone ends and the adjacent musculature usually become highly atrophic. Articular deformity and ankylosis are likely to develop as the result of muscular contractures and intra-articular adhesions. In cases in which the course is protracted and many joints have become implicated, sometimes even including those of the vertebral column, the general well-being of the patient is often seriously affected. This happens not only because of the pathologic changes relating to the joints, but because of nonarticular pathologic alterations (vascular, cardiac, and pulmonary, for instance).

CLINICAL CONSIDERATIONS

Incidence.—The prevalence of rheumatoid arthritis, and the severe, crippling deformities to which it often gives rise make it the most important disorder in the group of so-called connective tissue diseases. That rheumatoid arthritis occurs much more often among females than among males is well established, the proportion of affected females to affected males being about 3 to 1. It is sometimes postulated that this sex difference in the incidence of the disease is based upon a hereditary factor. Though the disease may set in during childhood, adolescence, or very early adult life, it is most likely to make its appearance in adults between 30 and 45 years of age and occasionally sets in even in later life. Since the disease pursues a chronic course, its over-all incidence in a given population rises with increasing age of the subjects, being highest among those in the sixth and seventh decades (see Lawrence *et al.*, and Bunim *et al.*). On the basis of a combined survey of several urban and rural populations in northern Europe, Lawrence *et al.* reported that 4 per cent of male subjects and 16 per cent of female subjects over 65 years of age presented probable or definite evidence of rheumatoid arthritis. With respect to the factor of *climate*, rheumatoid arthritis in severe form is observed much less often in countries having a warm climate than in countries of the temperate zone—especially those bordering on the North Sea and the Baltic Sea (see Méndez-Bryan *et al.*, and also Laine). On the other hand, there is as yet no evidence of a statistically valid difference in the incidence of rheumatoid arthritis between rural and urban populations. Furthermore, the results of various studies indicate that the occurrence of rheumatoid arthritis in a given population bears no special relation to the occupations pursued by the subjects, or to the physical conditions under which they live and work (see Kellgren *et al.*, and also Miall).

It also seems worth noting that during the course of a pregnancy the subject tends to show clinical improvement in respect to her arthritis. It may be conjectured that this improvement is the result of an inhibitory effect (possibly mediated by hormones) on the immune mechanism responsible for the production of rheumatoid factor. However, within 4 months after childbirth, there is likely to be an exacerbation of the arthritic manifestations. This may persist for several months, but in most cases the general course of the arthritis does not seem to be significantly altered (see Oka and Vainio).

Distribution of the Articular Lesions.—Even before the onset of difficulties relating to the joints, persons affected with rheumatoid arthritis commonly complain of general weakness, fatigue, and discomfort. When the manifestations of the arthritis set in, the pain related to the inflamed joints soon dominates these general complaints. Concomitantly, the patient may have some fever, and, sooner or later, anemia (usually of a mild degree) is likely to develop. Indeed, anemia is the most common nonarticular feature in cases of rheumatoid arthritis.

There is a definite tendency toward symmetry in the distribution of the lesions. It is the joints of the hands that are most likely to be affected and most often affected first. Specifically, the second and third metacarpophalangeal and the proximal interphalangeal joints are the ones most frequently implicated, though the intercarpal joints are also very often involved early in the course of the disease. Of the large joints, it is the knee joints that are most commonly affected. Indeed, they almost rival the joints of the hands in frequency as well as in earliness of involvement. The tarsal and metatarsophalangeal joints are somewhat less often affected than are the corresponding joints of the hand. The joints of the toes are less often involved than those of the fingers (see Serre *et al.*).

The wrist, ankle, shoulder, and elbow joints are fairly common sites of the disease, though implicated considerably less often than the knee joints and those of the hands. The temporomandibular joint is fairly often involved. In particular, Archibald Garrod reported that it was affected in about 25 per cent of 500 cases of rheumatoid arthritis, and stressed the significance of involvement of that joint in the differential diagnosis of the condition. Implication of the sternoclavicular joints has also been noted (see Epstein). Strikingly often (indeed, in more than half of the cases in any large series of *non-hospitalized* patients), the hip joint is spared. In fact, of all the large joints, the hip joint is the one least often affected. When it is found involved, both hips are likely to be implicated, and the rheumatoid arthritis is usually already in an advanced stage in which many other joints are also affected. In this respect, the hip joint contrasts with the knee joint, which is often the first large joint to be involved and may remain the only one affected for some time.

The joints of the vertebral column (especially the cervical region) are often affected. When they become involved, the complaints may be limited to pain and stiffness in the cervical region, probably due to inflammation in the local small intervertebral joints (facet joints). A much more serious group of clinical manifestations may follow upon atlanto-axial subluxation, which is by no means a rare finding in cases of rheumatoid arthritis (see Sharp and Purser, and also Robinson). Atlanto-axial subluxation (a separation of about 2.5 to 3.0 mm.) frequently gives rise to pain in the upper part of the neck and in the occipital region, and the pain is aggravated by movement of the head backward. Neurological difficulties may follow. These are due to disturbance of the normal anatomic relations of the odontoid process of the axis (C_2) to the atlas (C_1). The tip of the odontoid process is anchored by the alar and apical ligaments to the anterior margin of the foramen magnum. The odontoid process is separated by a bursa from the transverse ligament of the atlas. The spinal canal and cord are located posteriorly to this ligament. Rheumatoid inflammatory changes involving the bursa and the ligaments in question result in laxity of these ligaments and are the basis for the subluxation. In particular, the atlas (together with the skull) may move forward far enough to cause pressure by the odontoid process upon the spinal cord. The neurological complaints depend, of course, upon the extent and precise location of the neural injuries. Specifically, there may be paresthesia, weakness of the upper extremities, and occasionally also clear-cut evidence of compression of the cord. In addition, there are some reports to the effect that the compression of the cord may lead to paraplegia and even tetraplegia (see Whaley and Dick). The subluxation may also cause compression of one or both vertebral arteries as they ascend through the foramina transversaria. An instance of death ensuing upon compression and resultant thrombosis of both vertebral arteries in a case of rheumatoid arthritis has also been reported (see Webb *et al.*).

The sacroiliac joints and the facet joints other than those of the cervical region may also become implicated in a case of rheumatoid arthritis. Estimates of the frequency of extensive involvement of the spinal column in rheumatoid arthritis depend on whether ankylosing spondylitis (spondylitis ankylopoietica) as expressed in Marie-Strümpell disease *per se* actually represents rheumatoid spondylitis. Spondylitis ankylopoietica is a chronic inflammatory disease of the sacroiliac, intervertebral, and costovertebral joints, leading to ankylosis of the affected joints and associated with ossification of the spinal ligaments and intervertebral disks, and rather often with inflammatory arthritis of the large proximal joints of the limbs. There are many reasons for holding that ankylosing spondylitis (spondylitis ankylopoietica) as represented by so-called Marie-Strümpell disease is a disease entity separate from rheumatoid arthritis (p. 828). However, an occasional instance of extensive involvement of the spinal column is encountered in cases of rheumatoid arthritis, and in these instances the spondylitis *per se* is not readily distinguishable from the ankylosing spondylitis of Marie-Strümpell disease (see Martel and Duff).

Clinical Course and Findings.—The inflammation in an affected joint may develop gradually, though not infrequently it appears rather abruptly. In either case, the further course of the disease in that joint and the spread of the rheumatoid inflammation to other joints is likely to be slow. Thus the evolution of the full-fledged polyarticular picture of rheumatoid arthritis usually requires many years. Sometimes, however, especially in young adults, the disease runs a full course, with fever, quite rapidly. When it does, the interval between the initial involvement of the joints of the fingers, for example, and pronounced disease of many joints elsewhere in the body may be only a few months. These cases may closely resemble those in which chronic polyarthritis develops on the basis of rheumatic fever. However, involvement of the heart is not a characteristic part of the picture in these cases as it is in rheumatic fever.

When the disease pursues the typical slow, protracted course, the joints of the fingers are frequently the first to be implicated. The arthritis may remain limited to these, but generally many other joints, including large ones, become inflamed. However, it is sometimes a large joint, such as the knee or shoulder, that is the first to be involved. Furthermore, after the onset of the arthritis in a large joint, it may be many months, and even years, before other joints are affected. Possibly there are cases in which they never come to be implicated at all, and in which the paradox of a rheumatoid arthritis which has remained monarticular may hence be observed.

The course of the disease, when the latter is of long duration, is usually marked by periods of regression of the articular inflammation and by spurts of exacerbation. During remissions, pain and swelling in some or all of the affected joints may subside for months or years. During the exacerbations, previously unaffected joints may become involved, or joints already affected may show recrudescences of inflammation. However, even if the condition has been quiescent for a long time, new spurts of inflammation may appear in one joint or another. This explains the differences in the severity of the arthritis in different joints of the same patient.

Finally, when the disease is protracted, a terminal stage may be reached in which the more acute inflammatory changes have receded and the clinical picture has come to be dominated by ankyloses and subluxations. Thus, when rheumatoid arthritis has persisted for years and many joints have become involved, the foundations for serious disability have been laid. When such crucial joints as those of the hip, knee, and/or spinal column are implicated, the patient will finally be severely, if not completely, incapacitated.

In cases of rheumatoid arthritis of long duration, some degree of *laryngeal obstruction* due to arthritis involving the cricoarytenoid joints is not unusual. The clinical manifestations of arthritis implicating both of these joints include sensations of fullness and tightness in the throat, dysphagia, pain during speech, dyspnea, and stridor. Permanent relief of these clinical difficulties may require tracheostomy (see Vassallo). A rare instance has been reported in which laryngeal obstruction related to inflammation and limitation of motion of the cricoarytenoid joints actually *preceded* by 5 months the onset of inflammatory changes in peripheral joints (see Pinals). Involvement of the *eyes* is also sometimes encountered in cases of rheumatoid arthritis, and may affect the cornea of one or both eyes, taking the form of marginal furrows. These usually present as small arcs, seldom encircling the cornea completely. The furrows tend to be superficial and not to progress, but sometimes they do progress and result in thinning and even perforation of the cornea (see Brown and Grayson). In addition, uveoscleritis (essentially a recurrent scleritis with anterior chamber signs of uveal inflammation) is occasionally observed in patients affected with rheumatoid arthritis (see Kimura *et al.*).

Rheumatoid arthritis in any particular joint first manifests itself objectively in periarticular soft-tissue swelling. However, for some weeks before swelling appears, there may be feelings of numbness, tension, or prickling, or intermittent and fleeting pains in the joint or its vicinity. The affected joint is usually painful, at least on movement or on functional loading. Motion is ordinarily limited, even early in the course of the inflammation, but the early limitation is slight, and due merely to soft-tissue swelling, muscle spasm, or pain. The skin over the joint, though pale as a rule, feels warm, particularly if the articular inflammation is active. Subfebrile rises in temperature are not infrequent, especially when several joints are inflamed.

The contour of certain joints, at the height of the inflammatory phase of their involvement, may be obscured by the periarticular soft-tissue swelling and by effusion into the joint space. It is usually in joints which are superficially located (like those of the fingers) or which have large joint spaces (like those of the knee and elbow) that this is most easily observed. The amount of fluid that accumulates in the inflamed joint varies with the activity of the synovial inflammation. Especially in the knee, and also in the finger and elbow joints, the fluid may be clinically detectable by palpation. Notably in the case of the fingers and of the elbows, the joint region often becomes spindle-shaped. In other areas, such as the shoulder and hip, swelling and exudation are less prominent features, and the arthritis makes itself noticeable mainly in pain and disturbances in mobility. The fluid may persist in the joint for a long time. Even if it does, however, it may ultimately be resorbed.

On the other hand, a persisting effusion, especially in an affected knee joint, may result in massive enlargement of a synovial cyst in the popliteal space (a so-called Baker's cyst) whose presence antedated the onset of the rheumatoid inflammation in the knee. Also, the effusion may be the basis for a rupture of the popliteal cyst and/or the joint capsule, resulting in the escape of the rheumatoid synovial fluid into the tissue planes. The site of the capsular rupture may be anterior, the synovial fluid draining into the thigh; or, as happens more often, the rupture may occur in the posterior part of the capsule, usually between the semimembranosus and the median head of the gastrocnemius, where the capsule has been thinned and weakened. The causes underlying the rupture of the articular capsule of the knee in cases of rheumatoid arthritis are: (1) the presence of considerable fluid in the joint, and (2) a resultant striking increase in intra-articular pressure in the course of use of the knee, and in particular with active extension of the knee during weight-bearing and concomitant sudden hyperextension of the joint (see Maudsley and Arden, Dixon and Grant, Hall and Scott, and Perri *et al.*). The extrusion of fluid from the joint posteriorly is the basis for pain at the back of the knee and calf, swelling, and tenderness due to widespread deep cellulitis. These clinical manifestations may suggest a deep-seated thrombophlebitis and hence lead to an erroneous diagnosis. In rare instances a rheumatoid synovial cyst develops in relation to the hip joint. In this location, the cyst extends anteriorly into the inguinal region and presents as a mass in the groin, but may be painless (see Coventry *et al.*). A synovial cyst developing in relation to an elbow joint has, on rare occasions, caused compression of the ulnar nerve (see Palmer). Rupture of a synovial cyst at the elbow has been known to result in edema, swelling, and pain of the forearm, the elbow, and even the arm (see Goode). Linquist and McDonnell have described a case of chronic rheumatoid arthritis in which a rheumatoid cyst extended from the joint between the articular processes of the third lumbar vertebra on the left into the epidural space, compressed the cauda equina, and also extended posteriorly into the subcutaneous tissues.

Even quite early in the course of involvement of a joint, some degree of atrophy is usually manifest in the adjacent *muscles* and also in the bone ends. Especially if the articular inflammation is active and the arthritis is progressive, both the osseous and the muscular atrophy tend to increase. When the arthritis is well established, functional disability may become greatly increased by severe and lasting changes in the articular and periarticular structures.

Another feature of rheumatoid arthritis is the not infrequent presence of juxta- and periarticular *subcutaneous nodules*. These have been the subject of considerable discussion. Further details regarding these nodules will be found in the section dealing with the pathologic findings (p. 799). Swelling of regional lymph nodes is another rather common extra-articular change. Sometimes this is associated with slight enlargement of the spleen.

In the *terminal stage*, when the inflammation has burned itself out but severe articular damage remains, the joints may be contracted into various more or less deforming and incapacitating positions. The hands, for instance, may be quite distorted as a result of ulnar deviation of the fingers and of dislocations and subluxations (or various combinations of the two) at the interphalangeal and metacarpophalangeal joints (see Smith and Kaplan). Rather infrequently, the terminal interphalangeal joints become flail joints instead of being contracted. Often, the wrist becomes fixed, usually in flexion—a position which is very inconvenient. Ankylosis of the elbow joint in flexion, which also occurs fairly frequently, is, of course, less of a handicap. When the shoulder is ankylosed, it is usually fixed in a position of adduction and internal rotation. In the knee joints, the disease may lead to ankylosis in the position of flexion contracture. This, especially if combined with flexion contracture of one or both hip joints, is particularly disabling. If the joints of the midtarsus have been severely affected, rigid metatarsal arches and painful flat feet may develop. Hallux valgus, too, may appear in the course of rheumatoid arthritis involving the feet. If the small joints of the vertebral column have been extensively implicated, a large area of the spine is likely to become stiffened and even distorted into a kyphotic position.

ETIOLOGY

As already noted, it is currently held that a hypersensitivity mechanism underlies the etiology of rheumatoid arthritis. The so-called "rheumatoid factor" detectable in the serum of about 70 to 80 per cent of patients with unequivocal rheumatoid arthritis is an antibody. Specifically, it is a macrogammaglobulin, and is believed to be produced as part of a generalized immune response by sensitized plasma cells in the inflamed synovial membrane, and by the cells of the germinal centers of the regional lymph nodes draining the affected joints. The mechanism of production of the rheumatoid factor, and the precise nature of the antigenic stimulus have not yet been unequivocally established.

However, evidence is accumulating which suggests that rheumatoid arthritis develops: (1) on the basis of autoimmunity which is the consequence of a reaction to the subject's own gamma globulin, the latter having been altered in some unknown manner; or (2) as an abnormal response of the subject's connective tissue cells to one or another bacterial component (see Abruzzo and Christian, Vaughan and Butler, Schwab *et al.*, and also Hamerman).

In harmony with the second possibility, Hamerman has proposed that the sequence of events which could initiate or perpetuate rheumatoid arthritis is as follows: (1) *Oligosaccharide* or *glycopeptide fragments* derived from bacterial cell walls or capsules are the inciting agents. (2) Predisposed connective tissue cells (represented in relation to joints by the lining cells of the synovial membrane) take up increased amounts of the bacterial components, fail to digest them completely, and incorporate them into the proteinpolysaccharide normally synthesized by these cells. (3) Subsequently, there is an accelerated cycle of synthesis, degradation, and reutilization of the altered proteinpolysaccharide. The cycle of increased synthesis, elaboration, and phagocytosis of the altered proteinpolysaccharide by the synovial lining cells results in a series of biochemical, biological, and pathologicoanatomic alterations characterizing rheumatoid arthritis. The successive phenomena involved have been schematized by Hamerman, and his chart summarizing the processes in question is herewith reproduced.*

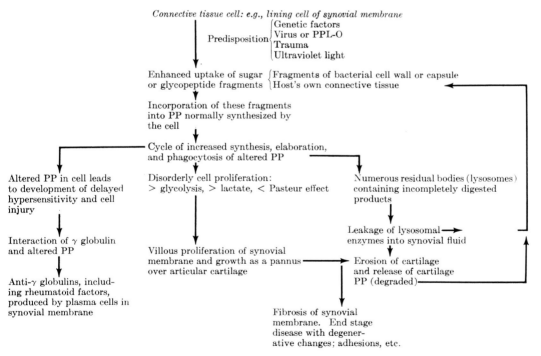

* This chart is reproduced with the kind permission of Dr. David Hamerman and also Dr. Alexander Gutman, the Editor of the American Journal of Medicine.

LABORATORY FINDINGS

The laboratory findings in cases of rheumatoid arthritis are in accordance with the chronic inflammatory nature of the disease. Nevertheless, there is no laboratory test or finding which is diagnostically specific for the disease. The demonstration of the presence of the *rheumatoid factor* in the blood plasma is a valuable indication of the presence of the disease, when taken in conjunction with the clinical findings. The belief that the rheumatoid factor is an antibody has received much support. Evidence is accumulating which suggests that the appearance of the rheumatoid factor is a secondary phenomenon, perhaps representing a reaction to the subject's own gamma globulin which has been altered in some unknown manner (see Milgrom and Witebsky, and also Milgrom *et al.*). Various studies indicate that the rheumatoid factor is produced by sensitized plasma cells in the inflamed synovial membrane and by the cells of the germinal centers of the regional lymph nodes draining the affected joints. The rheumatoid factor has also been demonstrated in the plasma cells present in subcutaneous rheumatoid nodules (see Mellors *et al.*).

Rheumatoid Factor.—The so-called rheumatoid factor is found in the serum of about 70 to 80 per cent of patients affected with unequivocal rheumatoid arthritis. However, serological tests for the rheumatoid factor have also yielded positive findings for it, by one test or another, in cases of: subacute bacterial endocarditis (at least 27 per cent), infectious hepatitis (20 per cent), and chronic pulmonary tuberculosis (7 to 13 per cent), in accordance with the particular test employed for detecting the rheumatoid factor (see Alexander and McCarthy). The factor has also been reported to be present in the serum in cases of leukemia. Tests for the rheumatoid factor were positive in 43 per cent of a series of cases of acute leukemia (lymphatic or myelogenous) and in 22 per cent of a series of cases of chronic leukemia (see Sherry). It should also be pointed out that positive test results for the rheumatoid factor have been obtained in up to about 4 per cent of controls (persons in good health) selected at random, the incidence being even somewhat higher among elderly controls.

The *two tests* commonly used to determine the presence of the rheumatoid factor in the serum are the *sheep cell agglutination test* and the *latex fixation test*. Both of these tests depend on the ability of the rheumatoid factor in the serum to combine with denatured gamma globulin. In the sheep cell agglutination test, the rheumatoid factor is demonstrated by the agglutination of sheep cell erythrocytes lightly coated with rabbit amboceptor. In the latex fixation test, the latex particles (to which heated human gamma globulin has been adsorbed) are clumped in the presence of the rheumatoid factor. In respect to a series of cases of rheumatoid arthritis in which both of these tests were carried out in each case, Greenbury reported agreement between the tests in 90 per cent of the cases, but indicated that he preferred the sheep cell agglutination test.

For several months after the onset of rheumatoid arthritis, tests for the rheumatoid factor are likely to yield negative results in most cases of a given series. In such a series, the proportion of positive test results for the rheumatoid factor usually rises sharply during the first years of the disease. Nevertheless, in some of the patients in any large group of cases, the test results for the rheumatoid factor will continue to be negative. It has been maintained that in these cases the rheumatoid factor is actually present in the plasma and that the test result is negative because of the concomitant presence of an inhibitor in the plasma (see Ziff *et al.*). With remission of the inflammatory phase of rheumatoid arthritis, the plasma of a subject in whom the test results for the rheumatoid factor had been positive may come to yield negative test results. The continuance of negative test results is usually associated with an improved prognosis (see Duthie *et al.*).

Other Laboratory Findings.—The presence of the disease in an active form is likely to be associated with various laboratory findings reflecting the fact that one is dealing with an inflammatory process. The most consistent and reliable of these findings (albeit a nonspecific response) is an *elevated erythrocyte sedimentation rate*. The latter is elevated in most instances in which the inflammatory manifestations are still mild, and in practically all those in which they are moderate or severe. In an individual case, clinical exacerbation or remission of the disease activity is usually accompanied by a corresponding elevation or reduction of the erythrocyte sedimentation rate. In instances in which the articular inflammation is still present, even in mild form, the sedimentation rate may remain elevated, but if the inflammatory process has subsided completely, the sedimentation rate tends to become normal.

Another nonspecific response to the inflammatory process in rheumatoid arthritis is the finding that the patient's serum yields a positive test result for *C-reactive protein* during the active inflammatory phases of the disease. The reactive protein is not present in the serum of normal persons and, unlike other abnormal proteins, is associated with the albumin fraction rather than with the globulin fraction of the serum. The C-reactive titer of the serum is maximal in the active inflammatory stage of the disease and decreases as the inflammatory activity recedes. An important diagnostic advantage of the C-reactive protein test over the erythrocyte sedimentation rate is that the test result for C-reactive protein is not much influenced by such factors as anemia, congestive heart failure, or hyperglobulinemia, which do influence the erythrocyte sedimentation rate.

The presence of *anemia* is a common finding in rheumatoid arthritis. The anemia is usually moderate in degree but refractory, and is ordinarily of the normocytic hypochromic type, although occasionally it is of the macrocytic (megaloblastic) type. There is no conclusive evidence that the anemia is to be related to hemolysis (see Mongan and Jacox). In any event, the absorption of iron from the intestinal tract appears to be normal, and there are indications that the anemia is to be related to an unknown factor that was interfering with the utilization of iron for the synthesis of hemoglobin (see Gardner and Roy). The leukocyte count is ordinarily within the normal range, but slightly elevated leukocyte counts are not unusual. In adult patients, leukocyte counts above 14,000 may be ascribed to a superimposed infection or to the effects of steroid therapy upon the bone marrow. However, in juvenile rheumatoid arthritis (Still's disease), leukocytosis is a common finding, and occasionally the leukocyte count is extremely high. On the other hand, in rare instances, adult patients exhibit leukopenia and splenomegaly, associated with polyarthritis (Felty's syndrome). In regard to the differential white cell count in *classic* rheumatoid arthritis of adults, it is to be noted that this is usually within normal limits, but occasionally one encounters a case in which the differential count reveals an inordinately high neutrophilic leukocyte value, or in which, on the contrary, that value is far below normal and is associated with a high lymphocyte value. In some cases the differential count also shows abnormally high values for eosinophilic leukocytes.

PATHOLOGIC FINDINGS

Rheumatoid arthritis is a systemic disease in which the significant changes center in the joints, but in which pathologic changes are likely to be present also in auxiliary skeletal tissues (tendon sheaths and bursae) and even nonskeletal tissues (striated muscles, lymph nodes, spleen, heart, blood vessels, skin, and subcutaneous tissues). The alterations to be found in a particular joint vary both with the severity and with the duration of the arthritis.

Charcot, in 1853, gave a good account of the pathology of rheumatoid arthritis in his thesis on "primary chronic articular rheumatism." Weichselbaum, in 1877, in discussing "arthritis deformans," emphasized the inflammatory changes in the synovial membrane which are found in what we now call rheumatoid arthritis. Nichols and Richardson, in 1909, presented the first comprehensive discussion in the American literature of the pathology of this disease, which they called the "proliferative type of arthritis deformans." In 1932, Knaggs published a survey of the pathology of rheumatoid arthritis based upon the Strangeways Collection in the Museum of the Royal College of Surgeons. In the monograph by Collins, published in 1950, dealing with the pathology of articular and spinal diseases, he gave a comprehensive presentation of the pathologic features of rheumatoid arthritis.

Figure 203

A, Photograph of the inflamed synovial membrane from the region of the quadriceps pouch of the right knee joint in the case of a woman 39 years of age affected with rheumatoid arthritis. The specimen was obtained in the course of a synovectomy, which had been carried out 3 weeks after the patient's admission to the hospital. Her clinical record indicates that the articular difficulties began with pain and swelling of both knee joints 5 months before admission to the hospital. The first joint to be affected was the right knee, and a few days later she became aware of pain and swelling of the left knee joint. About 1 month after this, both shoulder joints became painful. Soon thereafter, pain and swelling were noted in both wrists, in the metacarpophalangeal joints, and in some of the interphalangeal joints of both hands. Some degree of ulnar deviation became apparent. In addition, the ankle joints were swollen. However, the hip joints and the vertebral column were as yet not involved.

In the course of the surgical intervention on the right knee joint, both menisci were found to be loose and covered on their anterior ends by thickened and inflamed synovial membrane. The anterior cruciate ligament also was covered by synovial pannus. The articular cartilage of the joint was thin, and presented evidence of erosion on the patella and on the medial condyle of the tibia. The extirpated synovial membrane was 4 or 5 times as thick as it would normally be. The inner surface was moderately trabeculated, and in some places it was covered by fibrin. In sites where the fibrin was removed, the lining was, for the most part, smooth and glistening. Tissue sections prepared from the synovial membrane showed that the lining surface was represented by a granulation tissue layer containing polymorphonuclear leukocytes and also lymphocytes and plasma cells.

B, Photograph of the thickened and inflamed synovial membrane removed from the right knee joint in the course of surgical intervention in the case of a 51 year old woman who had had pain, swelling, and disability in that knee joint for 4 years, but in whom the rheumatoid arthritis was still limited to a few large diarthrodial joints. The serological examinations supported the diagnosis of rheumatoid arthritis. At the surgical intervention on the right knee joint, the articular space was found to contain a considerable amount of rather thick fluid. The articular cartilage covering the lower end of the femur and upper end of the tibia was roughened and eroded in some places. The semilunar cartilages were substantially destroyed.

As the photograph shows, the synovial membrane is thickened, and indeed it measured up to 1 cm. in thickness in some places, and was edematous. The membrane shown in this picture represents practically the entire lining of the quadriceps pouch, and much of the surface is covered by shaggy tags and masses of fibrin. Where the fibrin is not adherent to the surface, the synovial membrane presents a distinctly brownish discoloration. At the extreme right of the picture, a small portion of the membrane shows definite villus formation. On microscopic examination, representative areas of the actively inflamed part of the membrane revealed that it was extensively vascularized and densely infiltrated with polymorphonuclear leukocytes and numerous lymphocytes and plasma cells. Where the membrane showed villous proliferation, the round cells (the lymphocytes and plasma cells) tended to be aggregated in some places into follicle-like clusters.

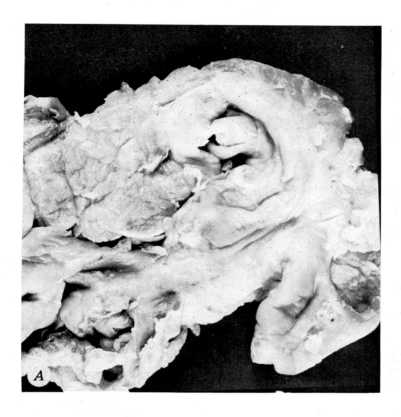

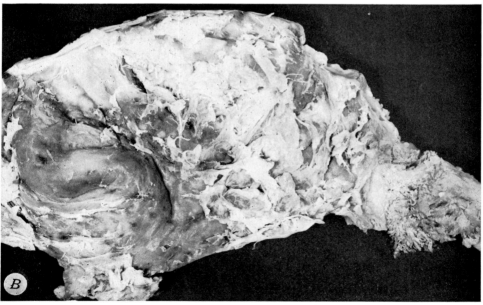

Figure 203

Synovial Membrane.—Inflammation of the synovial membrane is the initial and fundamental alteration underlying the evolution of the articular changes. The actual inflammatory changes, as distinct from periarticular soft-tissue swelling, tend to be limited to the synovial membrane or, in any event, not to trespass beyond the joint capsule. If they do go beyond, they are likely to be much milder in the periarticular tissues and to recede from them as the condition progresses. The inflammation involving the synovial membrane also constitutes the point of departure for the other articular alterations occurring in the course of the disease. (See Fig. 203.)

The synovial membrane of an inflamed joint from a case of rheumatoid arthritis shows itself, on *gross inspection*, to be thickened and injected. If the inflammation has been developing insidiously, the membrane will present a moderate degree of villous hypertrophy. On *microscopic examination* the succulent villi will be found to consist of a highly vascular connective tissue strongly infiltrated with plasma cells, lymphocytes, and macrophages (some of which are multinuclear), and to be lined by hypertrophied synovial cells. Often, the lymphocytes are also present in the form of small foci. Polymorphonuclear leukocytes are rather sparse. Occasionally a multinuclear giant cell can be observed near the surface of a villus. (See Fig. 204.)

The synovial membrane of an actively inflamed joint will usually show necrotic fibrinoid material spread over its surface in patches of varying thickness, compactness, and extent. This material often adheres so firmly that it can be removed only by scraping. Synovial recesses may contain free or loosely attached masses of the fibrinoid material. At this stage, in contrast to that of mild inflammation, the membrane shows practically no villous hypertrophy, except perhaps a very slight amount in some places where the membrane reflects from the articular cartilage. The superficial portion of an acutely inflamed membrane appears microscopically as a thick layer of cellular and moderately vascular granulation tissue. This proliferated fibroblastic tissue is infiltrated—in some places quite heavily—with various types of cells. Where the inflammatory process is very active, these infiltrating cells include numerous polymorphonuclear leukocytes, which are located especially at the surface of the membrane. Furthermore, in inflamed portions, the granulation tissue layer will usually reveal areas of fibrinoid dissolution, which may be continuous with the necrotic fibrinoid surface material mentioned above.

Where the inflammatory process is less active, organization of the granulation layer is to be observed. The latter may then be covered by several thicknesses of connective tissue spindle cells, while the number of polymorphonuclear leukocytes

Figure 204

A, Photomicrograph ($\times$ 20) showing the histologic pattern of a tissue section prepared from the synovial membrane removed from the right knee joint of a 34 year old man whose rheumatoid arthritis had been present for about 5 years at the time of his admission to the hospital. A synovectomy was done and the synovial membrane was found thickened and villously proliferated. Inspection of the articular surfaces of the bones revealed considerable erosion of the articular cartilages, and in various places the surface of the cartilage was covered by villously proliferated pannus. On a subsequent admission, the patient presented arthritis of the left knee and also of the left elbow. Even under this low magnification, it is evident that the thickened synovial villi are heavily infiltrated with cells which in places are even aggregated into follicles (see *B*).

B, Photomicrograph ($\times$ 150) showing the hypertrophied synovial cells lining the villi; the infiltration of the sublining layer of the villi by macrophages and small round cells (most of which are lymphocytes); and, deeper, an aggregation of the small round cells into a follicle-like formation.

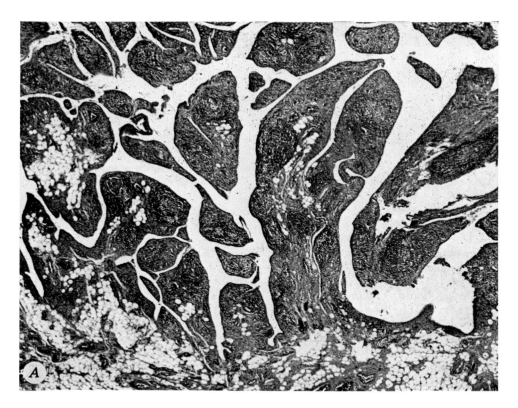

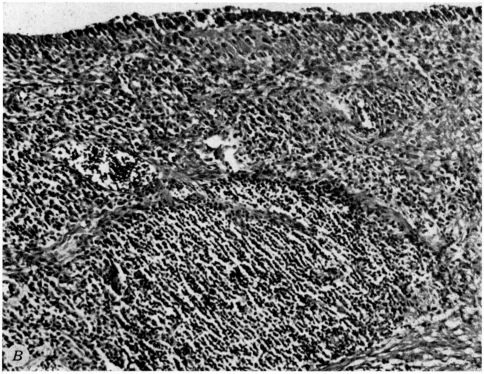

Figure 204

diminishes. In such an area, plasma cells, lymphocytes, and mononuclear phago-cytes predominate. Some of the latter may contain brownish (blood) pigment. Some phagocytes which have undergone hyaline degeneration may also be seen. Further regression of the inflammatory process in the granulation layer is followed by further increase in the number of lymphocytes and plasma cells, and these may have accumulated in nests.

Below the granulation layer, the synovial membrane becomes thickened through proliferation of the pre-existing connective tissue and through edema and vasculari-zation. Collections of lymphocytes and plasma cells may be found deep down even in the subjacent capsule. The lymphocytes and plasma cells often cluster around smaller blood vessels, but may be sparsely distributed between layers of connective tissue instead. In the knee, for instance, in the deeper portions of the synovial membrane and in the subjacent capsule, metaplasia of the fibrous connective tissue may occur in some areas. This connective tissue may show all stages of transition to fibrocartilage, hyaline cartilage, and occasionally even metaplastic bone. Stiffen-ing and toughening of the capsule is likely to result from these changes, and often in itself constitutes the basis for contracture of the knee joint. (See Fig. 205.)

Synovial Fluid.—The amount and character of the synovial fluid which accumu-lates vary with the severity of the inflammatory process. The fluid is likely to be turbid, yellow-green, and of decreased viscosity. In *normal* synovial fluid, the al-bumin-globulin ratio is about 2:1, and globulins, such as prothrombin, profibrinoly-sin, and fibrinogen, which are involved in blood coagulation and clot lysis, are present only in small amounts or are absent. In cases of rheumatoid arthritis, the synovial fluid shows an increase of both albumin and globulin, and their ratio is about 1:1. This change in ratio is due to the fact that the synovial fluid comes to contain relatively large amounts of the globulins mentioned above because of increased vascularization and permeability of the membrane. In subjects affected with rheumatoid arthritis, these globulins in the synovial fluid attain amounts approaching their values in the plasma (see Bluhm *et al.*). In addition, the synovial fluid eventually also shows a relatively high content of gamma globulin, most of which is produced by the plasma cells which are present in great numbers in the inflamed synovial membrane (see Johansen). The gamma globulin value of the synovial fluid may be even higher than that of the serum. Furthermore, it should be noted that the synovial fluid often yields a positive test result for the rheumatoid factor and C-reactive protein.

If the inflammatory process is relatively mild, there may be merely several

Figure 205

A, Photomicrograph ($\times$ 20) illustrating the appearance, in a case of rheumatoid arthritis, of an area of synovial membrane which is the site of active inflammatory changes. The patient was a woman 47 years of age whose presenting articular difficulty related to the right ankle. The next joint to become affected was the right knee, which was painful on ambula-tion, and swollen in consequence of the presence of fluid in the joint. Shortly before the syno-vectomy was done, the knee joint was aspirated twice, and 140 cc. and 85 cc., respectively, of synovial fluid were withdrawn. The largest piece of the excised synovial membrane measured 8 x 7 cm. in length and width and as much as 1.5 cm. in thickness. The synovial membrane was edematous, and much of its surface was covered by fibrin, which was soft and stringy in some places and adherent in others. In those areas where fibrin was absent, the synovial membrane showed a moderate degree of hypertrophy.

B, Photomicrograph ($\times$ 150) showing in higher detail the histologic field indicated by the arrows in *A*. Under still higher magnification, the concentration of cells near the upper part of the picture was found to be composed of lymphocytes, plasma cells, and polymorpho-nuclear leukocytes. Indeed, in some fields, polymorphonuclear leukocytes predominated.

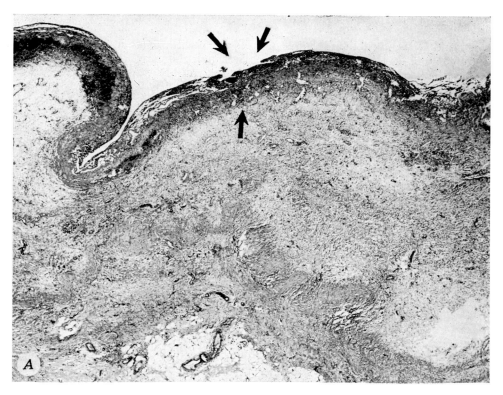

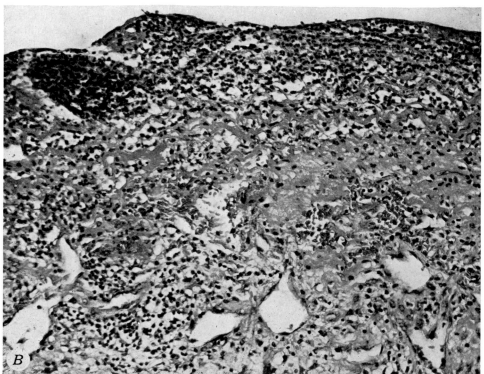

Figure 205

thousand cells per cubic millimeter of fluid, while with severe inflammations there may be 20 or 30 times that number. In particular, the percentage of polymorphonuclear leukocytes in the synovial fluid is likewise roughly proportional to the severity of the inflammation. It has been reported that, in any individual case, a small or large percentage of the leukocytes in the synovial fluid contain cytoplasmic inclusion bodies (see Hollander *et al.*, and Astorga and Bollet). These inclusion bodies are believed to result from the *in vivo* phagocytosis of precipitates containing rheumatoid factor. Evidence for this is furnished by the fact that homogenates of inclusion-containing cells from the synovial fluid almost always yielded a positive latex fixation reaction.

Articular Cartilage.—The inflammatory changes in the synovial membrane may recede, sometimes without having involved the articular cartilage. However, a partial or temporary recession of the synovial inflammation is usually followed by exacerbations or recrudescences. Chronicity of the inflammatory process in the synovial membrane is nearly always associated with damage to the articular cartilage. In contrast to the rapidly destructive effects of suppurative infections of joints upon the cartilage, those of rheumatoid arthritis are slow in evolving. At first the injury is mild, and usually limited to the periphery of the cartilage. Here (where it meets the inflamed synovial membrane), small foci of ulcerated cartilage covered by fibrinoid material may be found. Such mildly altered areas may also be observed elsewhere on the articular surface.

The damage to the cartilage may ultimately be severe. It is due largely to the action of hydrolytic enzymes released from the lysosomes (intracellular particles) contained within the synovial lining cells of the inflammatory pannus. The latter grows out from the synovial membrane and creeps over the cartilage from its periphery, or lies on the cartilage surface apparently detached from the synovial membrane. Inflammatory pannus may also be seen extending (in appropriate joints) onto such intra-articular structures as ligaments, menisci, and tendons. (See Fig. 206.)

Figure 206

A, Photograph of the articular surfaces of both femoral condyles (the right is above and the left is below) from the case of a woman 70 years of age who had been affected with rheumatoid arthritis. The articular cartilage of the medial condyle of the right femur has been extensively eroded, and the exposed subchondral bone is covered with connective tissue representing more or less organized pannus. In places, this connective tissue pannus presents evidences of having undergone transformation into fibrocartilage. The articular cartilage of the medial condyle of the left femur likewise shows evidence of erosion by pannus, as does the patellar surface of the condyle.

B, Photograph of the articular surfaces of the tibial condyles (the right is above and the left is below) from the case illustrated in *A*. The cartilage covering the medial condyle of the right tibia has been extensively eroded by pannus. The articular cartilage of the medial condyle of the left tibia shows a small area of erosion anteriorly.

C, Photomicrograph ($\times$ 12) from the same case illustrating part of the articular surface of the medial condyle of the left femur. In the left half of the picture, it can be seen that the articular cartilage has been almost completely eroded and replaced by fibrovascular pannus. In the right half of the picture, practically all of the articular cartilage is still present, but its surface is coated by an extremely thin, sheetlike layer of pannus, which as yet has caused minimal superficial erosion.

D, Photomicrograph ($\times$ 16) showing part of the articular surface of the medial condyle of the right tibia. A thin layer of fibrovascular pannus can be seen to have advanced along the articular cartilage and to have replaced much of the latter. In the left half of the picture, one can note a small amount of residual, though modified, articular cartilage, and in the right half, a small fragment of only slightly modified articular cartilage is apparent.

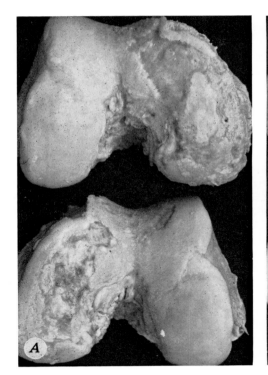

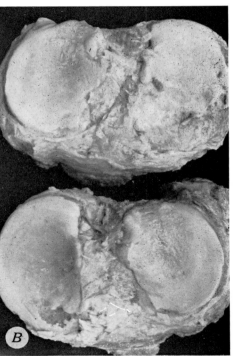

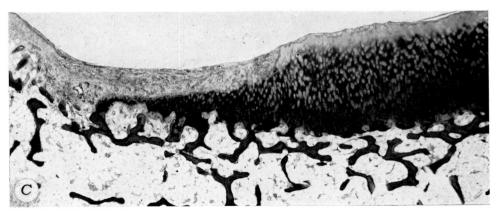

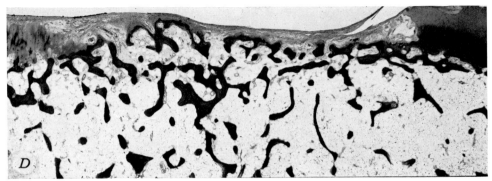

Figure 206

That the degradation of cartilage matrix in rheumatoid arthritis was to be related to the activity of lysosomal enzymes present in the synovial lining cells was proposed by Dingle. It seems well established that one of the several enzymes released by the lysosomes is acid phosphatase. The various enzymes gain access to the cartilage and apparently degrade and/or dissolve the proteinpolysaccharide of its matrix. Fragments of the altered proteinpolysaccharide are phagocytosed by the synovial lining cells of the inflammatory pannus. In consequence, the lysosomes of these cells are further altered and activated and release additional lysosomal enzymes (see Barland et al.). Evidence that the hydrolytic enzymes are *not* the result of dissolution of polymorphonuclear leukocytes contained in the synovial fluid is also furnished by the fact, established by Kream, that rheumatoid synovial fluid contains high levels of acid phosphatase but normal levels of alkaline phosphatase—an enzyme localized in the leukocyte granules (see Lehman et al.).

Beneath pannus that is highly vascular and cellular, erosion of the cartilage is conspicuous. With remission of the inflammatory activity, the pannus tends to become more organized. Beneath organized pannus, some degree of regeneration of the cartilage is regularly observed. If the inflammatory activity reappears, erosion of the cartilage tends to recur. As the pannus extends and penetrates, large areas of the articular cartilage come to be eroded. The pannus may reach the subchondral bony end plate in those places in which the cartilage has been entirely destroyed. In time, the inflammatory pannus which has replaced the articular cartilage shows evidence of organization in the direction of more or less fibrovascular granulation tissue. Ultimately, intra-articular fibrovascular adhesions develop which connect the organized granulation tissue covering the articular surfaces of the joint. Such strandlike adhesions also form between various parts of the inflamed synovial membrane not in contact with the articular surfaces.

Subchondral Bone.—The precise nature of the subchondral changes depends largely upon the severity of the inflammation in the synovial membrane and the degree of damage undergone by the articular cartilage. In the early phases of the

Figure 207

A, Photomicrograph ($\times$ 5) showing the metacarpophalangeal joint of the right index finger in a case of rheumatoid arthritis of about 2½ years' duration. The patient was a man 75 years of age who died of pulmonary tuberculosis. Roentgenographically, this joint showed relatively meager changes, and histologically, too, the changes are not very pronounced. As a reflection of the presence of osteoporosis, the proximal end of the phalanx and the distal end of the metacarpal bone reveal relatively few spongy trabeculae, and show thinning of the subchondral end plate of each of these bones. Even under this low magnification, it is evident that the articular cartilage of the metacarpal bone, both on the left and on the right side of the picture, is being eroded by synovial pannus extending over its surface. In the right side of the picture, it is apparent that synovial pannus is also eroding the articular cartilage of the proximal phalanx. The details of these changes are clearly visible in *C*.

B, Photomicrograph ($\times$ 5) demonstrating the histologic changes which have taken place at the proximal interphalangeal joint of an index finger in the case of a man 58 years of age who had been affected with rheumatoid arthritis for 14 years. He also presented evidence of rheumatoid arthritis in other diarthrodial joints, the involvement being most pronounced in the knee joints. Even under this low magnification, it is apparent that the articular cartilage at the base of the middle phalanx has been almost completely eroded, and that very little of the articular cartilage of the head of the proximal phalanx remains. In addition, it can be seen that the immediate subchondral area of the head of the proximal phalanx presents two small foci of vascularized fibrous tissue. The details stand out in *D*.

C and *D*, Photomicrographs ($\times$ 14) illustrating in greater detail the histologic changes of rheumatoid arthritis presented in the metacarpophalangeal joint shown in *A* and the proximal interphalangeal joint shown in *B* and described under those captions.

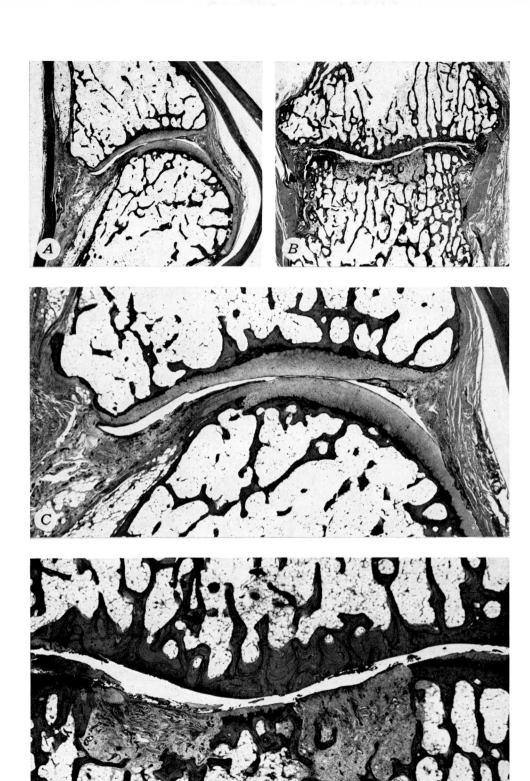

Figure 207

articular involvement, associated with active inflammatory changes in the synovial membrane, the subchondral marrow may be converted into a loose fiber marrow containing scattered or agglomerated lymphocytes. Very soon, the subchondral spongy trabeculae show simple (smooth) atrophy, which may be progressive. Where the articular cartilage has been extensively eroded, the subchondral spongy trabeculae will present surface lacunae and osteoclasts—evidences of active resorption. Vascular sprouts may also be found extending from the marrow into remnants of articular cartilage and/or into the pannus. (See Fig. 207.) If the joint has been severely affected and function has been very much limited, the bone atrophy may become extreme and extend along the shaft considerably beyond the immediate subchondral region. The bone atrophy is associated with atrophy of the muscles in the vicinity of the joint. In brief, then, the atrophy of the ends of the bones entering into the formation of the affected joint results from the combination of disuse of the joint and osteoclastic resorption of the subchondral spongy trabeculae. The bone atrophy (osteoporosis) may be the basis for the occasional occurrence of fractures of long or short tubular bones after minimal trauma (see Baer). However, the introduction of corticosteroid therapy for rheumatoid arthritis has been followed by reports of the occurrence of multiple stress fractures of long and short tubular bones, and also of fracture and collapse of vertebral bodies (see Miller *et al.*).

Course of the Articular Changes.—The pathologic changes are not necessarily progressive in all affected joints in any given case. Indeed, early in the course of rheumatoid arthritis, a joint in which the inflammatory changes are still limited to the synovial membrane may show practically complete regression of these changes, and the joint in question may even become normal in appearance and function. On the other hand, it is important to realize that a joint which has been the site of rheumatoid inflammation may eventually manifest the changes of *osteoarthritis* and thus come to represent a *secondary osteoarthritis* (p. 735).

The prerequisites for the secondary development of osteoarthritis in these cases are: subsidence of the inflammation in the synovial membrane; the occurrence of damage to the articular cartilage; and continued functional use of the joint, leading to alteration of the articular ends by friction. Under these conditions, a joint previously the site of rheumatoid inflammation will develop erosion of the articular cartilages, subchondral sclerosis, and marginal exostoses—the cardinal pathologic features of osteoarthritis. In an individual case, it may be difficult to prove that the osteoarthritis has been superimposed upon a joint which was originally the site of rheumatoid inflammation. This is notably true if but one joint—especially a large one—was affected by the rheumatoid inflammatory process. The difficulty is increased by the fact that at this late stage there may no longer be any active inflammation in the synovial membrane. In studying obscure cases showing osteoarthritic articular changes, the possibility of a rheumatoid precursor should always be considered, however.

In cases in which various joints have been the site of protracted involvement due to repeated flare-ups of the rheumatoid inflammation, such joints often ultimately show striking gross pathologic changes. The latter include *flexion and hyperextension deformities and also subluxations, dislocations, and ankyloses*. The resultant distortions caused by the subluxations and dislocations are most striking in the joints of the hands and also of the wrists. The distortions at the phalangeal and metacarpophalangeal joints are due to muscular contractures, and are aggravated by the deformity of the articular bone ends and by laxity of the capsule and ligaments of the joints. The laxity results from protracted distention of these structures by the synovial fluid which had accumulated in the joints.

A joint in a late or an advanced stage of rheumatoid arthritis is likely to have lost much or all of its mobility. *Ankylosis* is particularly apt to occur if, notably because of pain, the joint is kept at rest. One way in which ankylosis may take place is through progressive destruction of the articular cartilages and the development of abundant intra-articular fibrous adhesions. In consequence, the articular space may be narrowed and even completely obliterated. Specifically, the opposed pannus-covered joint surfaces fuse, inflamed portions of synovial membrane grow together, and intra-articular masses of fibrin become organized into connective tissue. The adhesions inducing the immobilization are at first loosely cellular and vascular, but later become tough and rigid through organization. If blood vessels from the adjacent marrow penetrate these adhesions, cartilage or bone may develop in them. If that occurs, the joint becomes rigid or even completely immobile because of bony ankylosis. (See Fig. 208.)

Not all ankyloses in rheumatoid arthritis are due to intra-articular processes. When residual inflammatory changes are present in the capsule and periarticular tissues, the ankylosis may arise essentially through capsular contraction. In such instances, although the articular cartilages may not have been severely injured originally, they are now subjected to secondary injury because of excessive loading due to static abnormalities. Not only the joints of the extremities but also those of the vertebral column may become ankylosed. Stiffening of the spine in consequence of either fibrous or bony adhesions of the small intervertebral joints may produce an ankylosing rheumatoid spondylitis.

In rheumatoid arthritis, inflammation occasionally occurs in the linings of such auxiliary skeletal structures as *tendon sheaths* and *bursae mucosae*. The tendon sheaths on the back of the hand are particularly likely to be affected (see Potter and Kuhns). Fluid may accumulate between the tendon and the inflamed sheath. Of the bursae, it is especially those in the region of the tuberosity of the ischium and the back of the calcaneus that are likely to be inflamed.

Subcutaneous Rheumatoid Nodes.—A common and diagnostically significant finding is the presence of subcutaneous nodes. The first detailed description of "rheumatic" subcutaneous nodes was given by Meynet in 1875 in relation to a case of recurrent rheumatic fever. Not long thereafter, it was established that subcutaneous nodes appear fairly often in both rheumatic fever and rheumatoid arthritis. The *incidence* of these nodes in rheumatoid arthritis and rheumatic fever as reported in different accounts shows a wide range of variation (see Fahr, Coates and Coombs, Freund, Clawson and Wetherby, Dawson, and also Swift). Dawson found subcutaneous nodes in 25 per cent of his patients with rheumatoid arthritis, but others have reported an incidence of only about 5 per cent. For rheumatic fever, the estimates of the frequency of occurrence of the nodes range from about 10 to as much as 50 per cent.

The *site of origin* of the nodes in the juxta- and periarticular tissues is in joint capsules, in the walls of bursae, in tendons or tendon sheaths, or in periosteum. Extending outward, such nodes may come to lie under the cutis, or, working inward from a joint capsule, they may penetrate the synovial membrane. In both rheumatoid arthritis and rheumatic fever, the most common site for the juxta- and periarticular nodes is the region of the elbow. Within this region, it is in the area beginning a few centimeters below the olecranon that they are most likely to develop, although they may also be found at the tip of the olecranon. The joint in the vicinity of which they appear is not necessarily diseased. Furthermore, it should be pointed out that rheumatoid nodules identical with those found in subcutaneous tissues, tendon sheaths, and bursae, for instance, have also been noted at autopsy on rare occasions in vertebral bodies, but much more often in the pleura, pericardium, and meninges, or within the parenchyma of various organs, such as the lungs, heart, and spleen. The rheumatoid nodules located on the surface of viscera or within them may be clinically silent or, on the other hand, may be the basis for serious clinical difficulties (pleural effusion, heart block, etc.). The presence of rheumatoid nodules within one or more vertebral bodies is likely to result in necrosis of the osseous tissue of the affected vertebral body and its subsequent collapse (see Glay and Rona).

There are definite *clinical similarities* between the nodes of rheumatoid arthritis and those of rheumatic fever. In both conditions, when the nodes first appear, they are rather soft, but they gradually harden somewhat. They are not usually spontaneously painful, but may be painful to pressure. They are frequently palpable under the skin and may even elevate it to a visible degree. The skin over the node is almost always movable, and the node itself is usually movable on its base. When rheumatic nodes appear in the vicinity of a joint, they are found predominantly on the extensor side of the joint. They are also occasionally seen on the flexor side, however, notably when they appear in the region of the wrist. There is a strong tendency toward symmetrical distribution. That is, when nodes develop near one joint they are likely to be found also near the corresponding opposite joint.

There are also certain consistent *clinical differences* between the nodes in the two conditions. Thus, in rheumatoid arthritis, they predilect juxta- and periarticular tissues, especially in the region of the elbow, while in rheumatic fever they occur in nonarticular regions also, especially the scalp. Furthermore, in rheumatoid arthritis the nodes generally evolve slowly and persist for months or years, while in rheumatic fever they usually evolve very rapidly, if not abruptly, and may disappear almost as quickly. The nodes are more likely to appear in large numbers in a case of rheumatic fever, however, than in one of rheumatoid arthritis, though the number varies considerably from case to case. The nodes are usually not so large in rheumatic fever as in rheumatoid arthritis. In the latter they may attain the size of pigeon eggs, while in rheumatic fever they are ordinarily only as large as lentils or peas, and may be even smaller.

As *microscopic examination* will reveal, a soft subcutaneous node only recently formed is composed mainly of what appears to be fibrinoid material. In the connective tissue that has undergone the fibrinoid dissolution, polymorphonuclear leukocytes are sometimes present. The blood vessels in the affected region or in its immediate vicinity also show fibrinoid degeneration of their walls and even occlusion of lumina. The sparsity of cellular elements is a striking feature of these nodes in an early stage of their development. In a later stage, as their cellularity increases, the nodes become firmer. As noted by Freund, by Dawson, and others, such mature

Figure 208

A, Photomicrograph ($\times$ 5) illustrating the histopathologic changes in a terminal interphalangeal joint in the case of a woman 65 years of age who suffered from rheumatoid arthritis for many years and showed the disease in advanced form anatomically. It is evident even at this magnification that the articular cartilage at the base of the distal phalanx has been completely eroded and replaced by inflammatory pannus. Furthermore, the spongy trabeculae are very sparse, indicating the presence of osteoporosis. The articular cartilage of the distal end of the middle phalanx is substantially eroded, and where such erosion has occurred, the articular surface is covered by synovial pannus. The spongy trabeculae in this bone, too, are sparse and thin (see *C*).

B, Photomicrograph ($\times$ 5) illustrating fibrous ankylosis of the terminal interphalangeal joint of the left index finger in the case of a woman 78 years of age who had suffered from rheumatoid arthritis for many years. The bones are somewhat subluxated and are fixed in a position of moderate flexion. The picture also shows the presence of advanced osteoporosis. For the details, see *D*.

C and *D*, Photomicrographs ($\times$ 14) revealing in fuller detail the changes which have occurred in the interphalangeal joints illustrated and described in *A* and *B*.

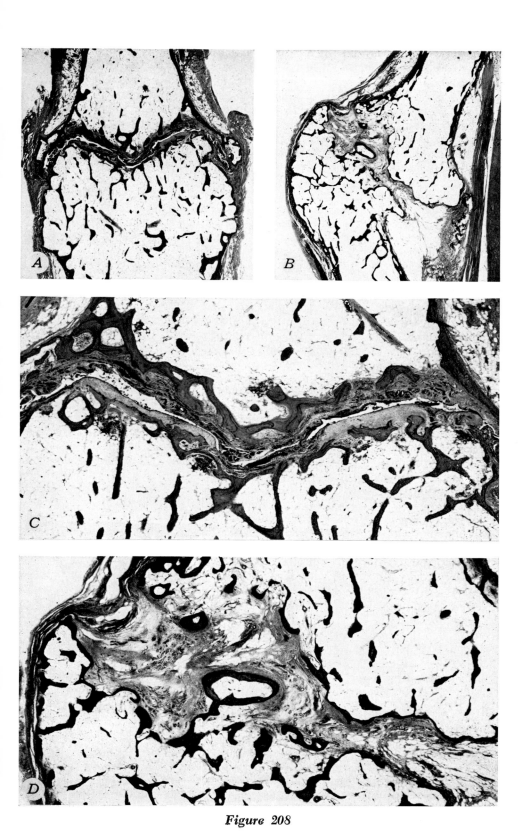

Figure 208

nodes contain zones or irregular cores of fibrinoid necrosis surrounded by richly cellular tissue arranged in a sort of palisade. This tissue is infiltrated by inflammatory cells quite similar in character to those found in Aschoff bodies. Lymphocytes may be present in various quantities, or may be absent. The outer wall of the node consists of a capsule of rather dense and avascular fibrous tissue. (See Fig. 209.)

In rheumatoid arthritis, as contrasted with rheumatic fever, the subcutaneous nodes tend to persist for years. Nevertheless, they are capable of complete regression even after existing for many years. The slowly involuting nodes eventually contain large amounts of fibrous scar tissue. Rarely, calcium is deposited in the scar tissue, or metaplasia of scar tissue into cartilage and bone may occur. Even more rarely, a rheumatic node undergoes necrosis, and its center, which is cystic, comes to contain thick creamy material representing tissue detritus intermixed with calcium phosphate and various lipids.

It is also to be noted that subcutaneous nodes similar to those of rheumatoid arthritis and rheumatic fever are occasionally encountered, especially in children, in cases in which neither rheumatoid arthritis nor rheumatic fever is present. These *pseudorheumatoid* subcutaneous nodules resemble the nodules associated with rheumatic fever in regard to localization and, to a lesser extent, in regard to histologic structure. In relation to microscopic structure, the pseudorheumatoid nodules differ from the rheumatoid nodules in that they tend to show a greater number of histiocytes, a lesser degree of peripheral collagenization, and less central fibrinoid necrosis (see Mesara *et al.*).

Nonskeletal Tissues.—The *muscles* about an inflamed joint are regularly and conspicuously affected in rheumatoid arthritis. Even when a joint has only recently become involved, and is still functioning, pronounced muscle atrophy may already be evident. The actual atrophy may be preceded by muscle spasm. A certain amount of replacement of muscle by fibrous tissue occurs if the atrophy has been present for a long time. When the joint assumes, or is kept in, an abnormal position, the muscles may become permanently contracted. This contraction, in turn, increases the fixity of the joint in the abnormal position. The pathogenesis of the muscle atrophy is a problem that has long intrigued and puzzled investigators. This problem is created by the fact that the severity of the atrophy does not depend entirely upon the degree or duration of functional inactivity of the part. Inactivity probably results in poor circulation and hence poor local nutrition. In this way, it certainly favors the development of the atrophy. We still do not know, however, why the atrophy associated with rheumatoid arthritis should be so much more

Figure 209

A and B, Photographs of the right hand and forearm illustrating the presence of several rheumatoid nodules. On the hand, the largest nodule is located on the dorsum of the fifth finger, at the metacarpophalangeal joint. On the extensor surface of the forearm, near the elbow joint, two large rheumatoid nodules can be seen. The patient was a woman 45 years of age whose rheumatoid arthritis, which involved many joints, was of about 8 years' duration. These photographs were taken at the time of her admission to the hospital. At that time, in addition to the rheumatoid nodules, she presented a polyarthritis with pronounced deformity of the feet (notably the toes), hands, elbows, and knees.

C, Photomicrograph ($\times$ 20) of a rheumatoid nodule removed from the region of the right elbow in the case of a man 58 years of age who had been suffering from rheumatoid arthritis for 2 years. The nodular pattern of the agglomerated individual nodules entering into the formation of the rheumatoid nodule as a whole is clearly evident. Many of the small nodules show a central area of fibrinoid degeneration surrounded by a zone of cells which, under higher magnification, would demonstrate the palisade formation characterizing the delimiting peripheral zone.

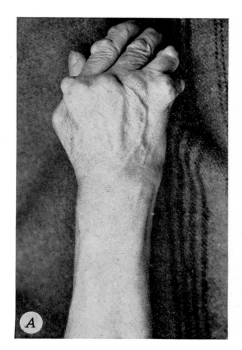

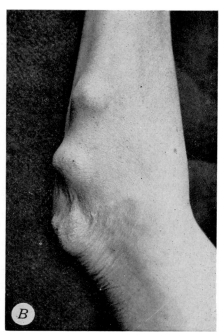

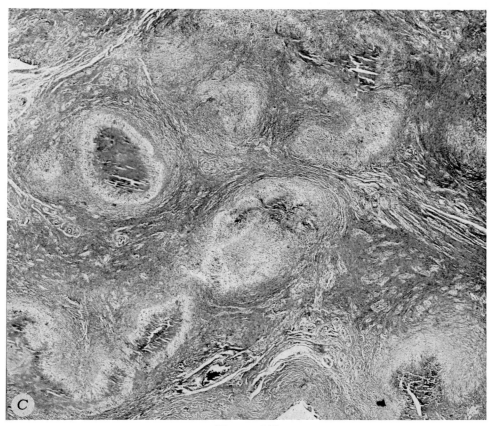

Figure 209

severe than that found in other conditions in which there is the same degree of in-activity. We do not know, either, why the same degree of inactivity should be associated with much more severe atrophy in some cases of rheumatoid arthritis than in others.

It should be pointed out, however, that the voluntary muscles in cases of rheuma-toid arthritis often show small collections of lymphocytes and plasma cells, with occasional macrophages and/or polymorphonuclear cells (neutrophilic or eosino-philic) between individual muscle fibers and/or between muscle bundles. These minute "granulomata" are commonly oriented to small blood vessels. Nevertheless, it is to be doubted that this focal interstitial myositis is the basis for the atrophy of the voluntary muscles in rheumatoid arthritis (see de Forest *et al.*, Clawson *et al.*, and Desmarais *et al.*). In any event, it has been found that electromyographic changes of polymyositis are common in rheumatoid arthritis, and that the electro-myographic changes bear no constant relation to the wasting and weakness of the muscles or to the functional activity of the regional joints (see Steinberg and Parry).

In the region of inflamed joints, the endoneurium and perineurium of *peripheral nerves* sometimes show perivascular aggregates of lymphocytes and other mono-nuclear cells—"granulomata" like those encountered in the voluntary muscles. The peripheral nerves most often involved are the ulnar, radial, median, lateral popliteal, and posterior tibial, but usually only one or two of the peripheral nerves are affected in a given case. The resultant peripheral neuropathy may be expressed in sensory and/or motor changes. Similar perivascular cellular infiltrates have also been observed occasionally in tissue sections prepared from the sympathetic ganglia and also from the peripheral postganglionic autonomic fibers (see Freund *et al.*, Ferguson and Slocumb, and also Bennett and Scott).

In cases of rheumatoid arthritis, *vascular lesions* are common and play an im-portant role in the disease complex. In particular, the vascular lesions include focal venular and capillary dilatation and also arteritis. It has been maintained that the *venular and capillary dilatation* results in exudative leakage, and is thus one of the factors underlying the inflammatory changes in the synovial membrane and the proliferation and necrosis of the connective tissue in various sites. The presence of *disseminated arteritis* (in an active stage or in a healing or healed form) has been observed in a fairly large percentage of cases of rheumatoid arthritis coming to autopsy (see Cruickshank, Kulka, and also Sokoloff and Bunim). The arteritis tends to be localized to sites where other nonarticular lesions of rheumatoid arthritis are likely to occur, such as the heart, lungs, skeletal muscles, and peripheral nerves. The arteritis typically involves isolated segments of arterioles and small arteries, but almost any portion of the arterial system may be implicated.

The affected blood vessels show a variety of histologic changes and may exhibit inflammatory thickening and/or focal necrosis of the vessel wall. In addition, some amorphous fibrin-like material (fibrinoid) may be present in the wall of the vessel, along with some leukocytes (especially lymphocytes). If the rheumatoid disease is present in the severe (so-called malignant) form, the affected arteries or arterioles may show a variety of changes, including: the presence of large numbers of neutro-phils or even eosinophils in their walls; necrosis of the arterial wall; intramural thrombi; and even focal dilatations (aneurysms) of the vessel walls. It is now es-tablished that necrotizing arteritis may develop in consequence of hypercortisonism induced by steroid therapy. Nevertheless, arteritis may occur in cases of rheuma-toid arthritis in which there had been *no* corticosteroid therapy. In cases of rheuma-toid arthritis in which corticosteroid therapy has been given, the arteritis tends to be somewhat more pronounced and widespread than in those cases in which the arteritis has occurred in the absence of corticosteroid therapy (see Johnson *et al.*).

In respect to the *viscera*, it is now well established that the *heart* is not infrequently the site of pathologic changes and, in particular, may present rheumatoid coronary arteritis, pericarditis, myocarditis, or valvulitis, either separately or occasionally (in the course of severe rheumatoid disease) as a pancarditis. The anatomic manifestation of rheumatoid disease in the various sites in question has not infrequently been found to consist of rheumatoid granulomata and sometimes also rheumatoid nodules (see Bywaters, and also Sinclair and Cruickshank). Involvement of the *respiratory tract* also occurs. In some cases this is limited to the upper respiratory tract, and is expressed in diminished secretion by the mucous membranes of the pharynx, larynx, and bronchi, leading to a dry, irritating cough, associated with dryness of the mouth and nose. In addition to, or independent of, these features of the sicca syndrome (Sjögren's syndrome), there may be rheumatoid lesions involving the pleura and/or the parenchyma of the lungs. In particular, one may encounter pleuritis with pleural effusion and also rheumatoid nodules in the pulmonary parenchyma. Nodular pulmonary fibrosis and massive pulmonary fibrosis (*pneumoconiosis*) have been observed in coal miners, and a high incidence of rheumatoid arthritis was also found among these miners. It was deduced from these findings that the development of rheumatoid arthritis was related to the presence of the pneumoconiosis (see Caplan, and also Caplan *et al.*). However, additional epidemiological studies have shown that neither exposure to coal dust nor the pulmonary changes of advanced pneumoconiosis have any etiologic significance in the development of rheumatoid arthritis (see Miall).

Regional *lymph nodes* not infrequently become enlarged in rheumatoid arthritis, and it is especially during the active stage of the articular involvement that they are likely to become prominent. The swollen lymph nodes are found most often in the axilla, the cubital region, and the groin. Microscopically, such nodes show merely prominent lymphoid follicles and simple hyperplasia. When the acute inflammation in the pertinent joints subsides, the enlargement of the lymph nodes usually also regresses.

Enlargement of the *spleen* in rheumatoid arthritis is rather rare as compared with enlargement of lymph nodes. When present, splenomegaly is usually associated with lymphadenopathy. In cases of Still's disease, though lymphadenopathy is prominent, the splenomegaly is not striking. On the other hand, in instances of Felty's syndrome, splenomegaly is a conspicuous finding, while lymphadenopathy is not.

Amyloidosis is not uncommon in cases of rheumatoid arthritis and is frequently the basis for the splenomegaly. In a case of rheumatoid arthritis complicated by amyloidosis, amyloid deposits may be present not only in the spleen but also in the kidneys, liver, adrenals, intestinal mucosa, lymph nodes, and occasionally other organs. The over-all incidence of amyloidosis in *unselected clinical cases* of rheumatoid arthritis is somewhere between 5 and 10 per cent (see Fearnley and Lackner, and also Arapakis and Tribe). However, in *selected cases*, as represented by those which had come to autopsy, the reported incidence of amyloidosis is much higher. Thus, amyloidosis was found by Fingerman and Andrus in 13 of 61 instances of rheumatoid arthritis (21 per cent) coming to autopsy at the University of Minnesota and affiliated local hospitals. On the other hand, Teilum and Lindahl found *histologic* evidence of amyloidosis in 17 of 28 cases (61 per cent) of rheumatoid arthritis which had come to autopsy, and in 10 of these 17, the amyloidosis was moderate or pronounced.

Albuminuria is a common though not invariable finding when amyloidosis is present. Clearly, the diagnosis may be missed if albuminuria is used as the sole screening test for amyloidosis. While *renal biopsy* has been done to establish the presence of amyloidosis, it should be stressed that renal biopsy is not devoid of risk and is rarely warranted solely for diagnosis (see Tribe). Instead, *rectal biopsy* is ad-

52

vocated, since this is a relatively simple procedure causing little discomfort to the patient, is almost devoid of danger, and nearly always yields a positive result in the presence of visceral amyloidosis. Indeed, if amyloid is detected in a rectal biopsy specimen, it is almost certain that a considerable amount of amyloid is also present in the kidneys (see Arapakis and Tribe).

The presence of amyloidosis in patients affected with rheumatoid arthritis is often manifested clinically by renal involvement sufficiently pronounced to have produced renal insufficiency resulting in uremia. Generalized amyloidosis leading to death of the patient in uremia is particularly common in juvenile rheumatoid arthritis (see Portis).

TREATMENT

It is rarely possible to forecast the course and ultimate prognosis in an individual case of rheumatoid arthritis, particularly while the disease is still in an early stage. However, there are certain general principles of treatment which, on a long-term basis, are useful in all instances of the disease, irrespective of the stage of its development. To exert their full value, these measures must be applied early in the course of the disease. This plan of treatment necessarily includes the following objectives: (1) the control of the pain, inflammation, and systemic manifestations; (2) the prevention of deformity, and the reduction of existing deformities; and (3) improvement and maintenance of function.

JUVENILE RHEUMATOID ARTHRITIS

The designation "juvenile rheumatoid arthritis" is ordinarily applied to rheumatoid arthritis having its onset in children who are almost always under 14 years of age. In the past, cases of juvenile rheumatoid arthritis in which the articular involvement has been preceded by systemic manifestations (notably spiking fever and toxemia) have usually been denoted as instances of *Still's disease*. Additional nonarticular features characterizing Still's disease include: pericarditis, lymphadenopathy, splenomegaly, and a transient rash (see Still). However, the eponym "Still's disease" is now no longer restricted to cases presenting conspicuous systemic features but is also often used as an alternate designation for "juvenile rheumatoid arthritis" as a whole.

CLINICAL CONSIDERATIONS

Incidence.—There are no satisfactory statistics bearing on the *over-all incidence* of the disease. The reason for this is that many children affected with juvenile rheumatoid arthritis in mild form are not hospitalized, and they are therefore not included in the statistical evaluations of the incidence of the disorder. It is known, however, that in hospitals devoted to the treatment of rheumatoid arthritis (both juvenile and adult) only about 5 per cent of the patients represent instances of juvenile rheumatoid arthritis. In regard to *sex distribution*, it seems to be clear that only about twice as many females as males are affected, while in classic rheumatoid arthritis setting in during adult life the proportion of females to males is about 3 to 1. In cases of juvenile rheumatoid arthritis, the *family history* not uncommonly reveals that a parent, a sibling, or a more distant relative is or was affected with rheumatoid arthritis and, much less often, that one or more of the persons in question had had rheumatic fever. It is often stated that such findings indicate a *hereditary factor* in the occurrence of juvenile rheumatoid arthritis. However, in the writer's opinion, the familial incidence of the disease may be ascribable to environmental or other influences rather than to a hereditary factor.

Age and Mode of Onset.—It is known that, though juvenile rheumatoid arthritis occasionally sets in during infancy, it is only exceptionally that the subject is under 6 months of age. In about half of the cases in any large series, the *age* of the subjects at the time of onset of the disease is somewhere between $1\frac{1}{2}$ and 8 years. In the other approximate half, the incidence is highest in the age group 11 to 14 years—that is, when the subjects are approaching puberty (see Ansell and Bywaters, and also Laaksonen).

The *mode of onset* varies considerably. It is especially in the youngest subjects that the disease is likely to set in with systemic manifestations. In particular, the young child may have a spiking fever, feel extremely ill, and present a skin rash and even clinical evidence of iridocyclitis, pericarditis, and pneumonitis, along with pronounced leukocytosis. Though arthralgia may be present early, weeks or months may elapse before clear-cut arthritis appears. In the interim, the diagnosis is often uncertain, especially in those occasional instances in which the constitutional expressions of the disease subside spontaneously for a time. When, after an interval, the systemic manifestations reappear, now in association with arthritic involvement, the nature of the disease becomes apparent.

In other cases, especially in older children, arthritis affecting one or many joints is the dominant clinical feature from the beginning, and the constitutional reactions are few or may even be absent. The articular involvement usually becomes evident initially through pain on movement (arthralgia), which is ordinarily not yet associated with obvious alterations in the external appearance of the affected joints. Sometimes, however, the painful joints are already somewhat swollen, but their mobility does not tend to be greatly restricted at first.

Clinical Course and Findings.—Whether rheumatoid arthritis in children and in adults has the same basic cause or not, the course of the disease and many of its clinical features are quite different in children from what they are in adults. In regard to the *nonarticular aspects* of juvenile rheumatoid arthritis, it is to be noted that in an affected child presenting systemic manifestations the fever tends to show diurnal spiking. In particular, the temperature may be as high as 105° F. in the evening, but is likely to return to normal by the following morning, only to rise again in the course of the day. The rash (an erythematous maculopapular eruption) may be present on the trunk and extremities and may even involve the face. It is usually fleeting, occurs mainly in children who have bouts of fever, and is present most often in the evening, when the fever is at its peak.

The *lymphadenopathy* is a much more prominent clinical feature in juvenile rheumatoid arthritis than in adult (classic) rheumatoid arthritis. It tends to become apparent early in the course of the disease, and in the youngest subjects the cervical and axillary lymph nodes may eventually be so large as to be visible on external examination. However, when the various other systemic manifestations recede, the lymphadenopathy is likely to become less prominent. The presence of *splenomegaly* is less common than that of lymphadenopathy. However, if a child affected with juvenile rheumatoid arthritis for a year or more does have an enlarged spleen, the possibility must be borne in mind that the enlarged spleen is the site of amyloid deposition. As to *cardiac involvement*, it is to be noted that this nearly always takes the form of pericarditis, but the latter is often not sufficiently pronounced to be detectable clinically. *Iridocyclitis* of long standing used often to lead to blindness of one or both eyes, and *uveitis* is another serious ophthalmic complication.

While the *nonarticular* features of the disease (spiking fever, rash, lymphadenopathy, etc.) may suggest that one is dealing with a case of Still's disease even in the absence of clear-cut implication of joints, it is not until *articular involvement* becomes evident that a definitive diagnosis can be made. For an unequivocal diagnosis of Still's disease, Ansell and Bywaters require that the child present a polyarthritis affecting more than four joints for a minimum period of 3 months. However, if the child shows involvement of fewer than four joints, a diagnosis of Still's disease may nevertheless be justified if a biopsy of the synovial membrane of one of these joints shows histologic changes compatible with those presented by the synovial membrane of an affected joint in a case of classic (adult) rheumatoid arthritis. The pertinent histologic criteria are hyperplasia of the synovial membrane, increased vascularization, and the presence of focal collections of lymphocytes and plasma cells.

The *articular involvement* is often first evident in one joint, and in a small percentage of cases it remains monarticular. When it does not remain monarticular, several months may elapse before additional joints become implicated. The joint most often affected at first is a knee joint or both knee joints. In time, almost any joint may become involved. In the series of cases reported by Martel *et al.*, in which the arthritis was already polyarticular, the joints most often found implicated were (in descending order of frequency) those of the knee, ankle, wrist, hand, elbow, hip, foot, shoulder, and cervical spine. The high frequency of involvement of the knee is stressed in all the reports on large series of cases (see Cassidy *et al.*). However, there is no close agreement about the order of frequency in relation to the other joints mentioned above.

Early in the course of the disease, an arthritic *large peripheral joint*, such as a knee, usually appears swollen, has reduced mobility, and feels warm, but is not necessarily red or ordinarily tender to palpation. The intra-articular exudate varies, the amount being very small in some joints (dry type of involvement) and rather large in others (wet type of involvement). If the amount of intra-articular effusion is considerable but the capsule has not been stretched enough to permit subluxation, the chances for eventual recovery of the joint in question are improved, since the exudate tends to protect the articular cartilages from erosion. If the amount of the intra-articular effusion is meager, there is a likelihood of erosion of the articular cartilages, the formation of intra-articular adhesions, and the appearance of muscle spasm, together resulting in contracture of the joint. Eventually, even though the inflammatory process subsides, the joint may become ankylosed, or, if it retains its mobility, a *secondary osteoarthritis* may supervene.

The *small diarthrodial joints* of the hands and feet are not uncommonly affected. Indeed, the distal interphalangeal joints of the hands are frequently implicated in juvenile rheumatoid arthritis, in contrast to the relatively low incidence of involvement of those joints in adult (classic) rheumatoid arthritis. Symmetrical involvement of the metacarpophalangeal joints, so common in the affected adults, is unusual in the children. In the wrists, implication of the carpal joints is frequently associated with effusion under the dorsal sheath and eventually with ankylosis of the intercarpal joints and carpometacarpal joints. In consequence of the changes in the bones of the hands and wrists in cases of Still's disease, the hands of the affected children show radial deviation, in contrast to the ulnar deviation observed in the adults. In the feet, juvenile rheumatoid arthritis may lead to progressive hallux valgus, hammer toes, and prominence of the metatarsal heads. Rheumatoid inflammation of the Achilles bursa and of the sheath of the Achilles tendon may lead to local soft-tissue swelling and eventually to small erosions of the calcaneus where it abuts on the inflamed local bursa and tendon sheath. (See Fig. 210.)

Early in the course of Still's disease, there are often indications that the *vertebral column* has been affected. It is generally in the cervical region that the manifestations of Still's disease first appear in the column. In a young child the earliest clinical evidences that changes have taken place in the cervical vertebrae are limitations in extension and rotation of the neck, due to retarded growth of these vertebrae and at least partial ankylosis of some of the local apophysial joints. In an older child—that is, one in whom the disease has already been present for some years—the alterations in the cervical vertebrae may have progressed to a stage in which the apophysial joints (especially the more proximal ones) are completely ankylosed, the intervertebral disk spaces have become narrowed, and some of the vertebral bodies have even fused. Aside from these changes, atlanto-axial subluxation sometimes occurs. It has been described, in an unusual case, as the first clinical evidence of the presence of Still's disease (see Nathan and Bickel).

Changes in the *sacroiliac joints* are fairly common. They are observed more often in the affected males than in the females, and especially in those cases in which Still's disease has set in after the age of 10. The sacroiliitis is usually asymptomatic, and consequently its presence is ordinarily first recognized on the basis of roentgenographic examination of the area in question. However, there are indications that, though the roentgenographic examination may fail to reveal sacroiliitis, the latter may nevertheless be present, as demonstrated by autopsy findings (see Carter, and also Carter and Loewi).

Clinical complaints relating to arthritis of the *temporomandibular joints* are not common. When these joints do become involved, the arthritis tends to persist, and in rare instances one or both of the joints may become ankylosed. However, even in the absence of erosion of the articular surfaces and ankylosis, there may be roentgenographic evidence of changes in the mandible and the articular fossae. In particular, the body of the mandible may be small, the rami abnormally short, the mandibular notches excessively wide, and the articular fossae broad and shallow.

In Still's disease, *rheumatoid nodules* are sometimes encountered, but not nearly so often as in classic (adult) rheumatoid arthritis or in rheumatic fever. When present, they are usually few in number, and they are observed most often in the region of the elbow. Histologically, the nodules in children generally resemble more closely those of rheumatic fever than those of adult rheumatoid arthritis (see Bywaters *et al.*).

In juvenile rheumatoid arthritis, *aberrations relating to skeletal development and growth* are not at all uncommon. These may have their basis in: (1) the disordered general metabolism associated with the disease, and (2) the effects of the local inflammatory processes upon the time of appearance and growth of some of the secondary centers of ossification and also upon the epiphysial cartilage plates, which contribute to the growth of the bones through endochondral ossification. In particular, certain secondary centers of ossification (epiphysial ossification centers) may appear prematurely, and this occurrence sometimes leads to accelerated maturation and eventual overgrowth of the epiphyses in question. Furthermore, in consequence of the disturbed endochondral ossification at the epiphysial cartilage plates, some of these epiphyses may fuse prematurely with the adjacent bone shafts. In rare instances the retardation of growth associated with rheumatoid arthritis beginning in childhood is so extreme as to induce a state of dwarfism characterized especially by shortness of the long tubular bones and even short tubular bones. Conversely, in some cases there may be overgrowth in the length of tubular bones, especially the long bones, and if this overgrowth is uneven in regard to adjacent bones, such as the tibia and fibula, a bowing deformity may result.

Laboratory Findings.—The *laboratory findings* ordinarily yield little pertinent diagnostic information. *Leukocytosis* and *anemia* are likely to be present in those children in whom the disease is in the active stage and is associated with systemic manifestations. In such subjects the leukocyte counts are generally in the range of 15,000 to 25,000, and the increased white cell count reflects a neutrophilic leukocytosis. The anemia, which is of the normocytic hypochromic type, is ordinarily of a moderate degree, the hemoglobin value rarely being below 60 per cent of the normal. In cases in which the disease is in a very active phase, the erythrocyte sedimentation rate is generally increased, as is to be expected, and the test result for C-reactive protein is positive. Tests for the *rheumatoid factor* have not proved to be helpful in the diagnosis of juvenile rheumatoid arthritis. Indeed, nearly all young children affected with Still's disease fail to show positive test results for the rheumatoid factor. On the other hand, positive test results for the presence of the rheumatoid factor have been obtained in a significant proportion of the cases in which the disease had been present for some time and had set in when the subjects were about 10 years old (see Cassidy and Valkenburg, and also Schierz *et al.*).

Prognosis and Ultimate Status.—From what has been said already concerning the clinical course and findings in Still's disease, it might be inferred that the prognosis for the affected subjects is uniformly unfavorable. However, experience has shown that, in contrast to what happens in rheumatoid arthritis setting in during adult life, many subjects affected with juvenile rheumatoid arthritis do recover completely under current methods of treatment. A prerequisite for recovery without any residual arthritis is reasonably prompt initiation of treatment in the form of general care, steroid therapy, analgesics, physiotherapy, and orthopaedic measures directed toward counteracting the development of contractures which result in deformities.

It has been reported by Ansell and Bywaters that, in the large series of cases which they followed, nearly half of the affected children who came under their care within a year of the onset of the disease showed no residual lesions of the joints 5 years later. Favreau and Laurin report that, of 102 cases which they followed and

Figure 210

A, Roentgenograph of the left hand and wrist of a 10 year old girl who had been affected with polyarthritis since the age of 7. According to our hospital records, the patient's manifestations of Still's disease consisted mainly of articular difficulties, and the constitutional aspects of the disease were inconspicuous. On her admission to the hospital, physical examination revealed flexion contractures of many joints. The bones of the hand are highly porotic. The intercarpal joints are largely obliterated, and some of the carpal bones have become ankylosed. The carpometacarpal joints are largely obscured, and some of these joints, too, appear to be ankylosed. Of the carpal bones articulating with the metacarpals, the capitate is the one in which the osteoporosis is most severe. The metacarpophalangeal joints are also involved, but the proximal interphalangeal joints show striking changes, and these joints are in a position of flexion contracture.

B, Roentgenograph of the region of the right hip joint in the same case. The bones are porotic, and the articular surfaces of the acetabulum and femoral head no longer present the normal smooth contour. Instead, both surfaces are slightly pitted, apparently in consequence of erosion of the cartilage by synovial pannus. The femoral head appears somewhat enlarged and flattened, possibly as a result of disordered endochondral bone growth, which is often an aspect of juvenile rheumatoid arthritis.

C, Roentgenograph of the region of the right knee joint in the same case. Clinically, the knee was held in a position of approximately 90° of flexion, but it could be passively flexed and extended somewhat. The bones are highly porotic and present abnormal contours, and their articular surfaces are irregular. A roentgenograph showing the joint in a lateral position revealed that the tibia was somewhat subluxated.

D, Roentgenograph of the right foot, in lateral projection, in this case. The tarsal bones are highly porotic. All of the joints between the tarsal bones are narrowed, and some of the tarsometatarsal joints are obliterated.

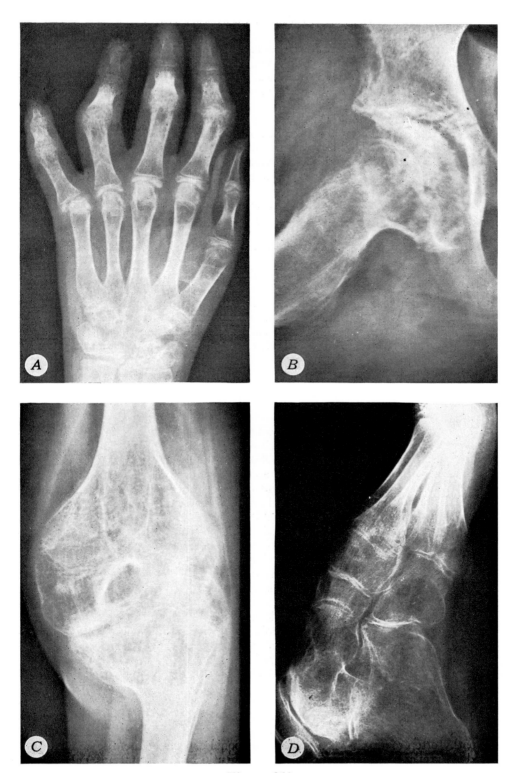

Figure 210

reviewed and in which adequate treatment was undertaken early, 50 per cent of the patients made a complete recovery, while 25 per cent had mild residual disability and 25 per cent became severely crippled. In contrast, subjects who did not come under intensive medical care until more than one year had elapsed from the time of onset of the disease showed a much lower rate of remission for the arthritis. When there has been a remission of the inflammatory changes in the joints, some children make a complete recovery and present no residual arthritis. Thus, in some cases there is only one period of active disease, and this is followed by recovery; in others there are several remissions and recurrences of the articular inflammation; and in still others the disease pursues an uninterrupted active course even into adult life. In such cases the clinical state becomes progressively worse, and the subject is seriously disabled by contractures and deformities (see Schlesinger). In cases of Still's disease pursuing a protracted course into late childhood or into adult life, the clinical, roentgenographic, and pathologic findings are similar, on the whole, to those encountered in cases of advanced classic (adult) rheumatoid arthritis (see Jeremy *et al.*).

In regard to *survival*, it is to be noted that some subjects affected with juvenile rheumatoid arthritis live to middle age or even longer, while others die in early or middle childhood or early in adult life. The survival rate is, of course, unfavorably influenced by severe systemic manifestations (including notably pericarditis), the occurrence of intercurrent infections, and renal failure due to amyloidosis. In general, however, the mortality rate has been much lowered in recent years by current therapeutic approaches.

PATHOLOGIC FINDINGS

There are relatively few detailed accounts of autopsy findings in cases of Still's disease. Pirani and Bennett have described the clinical histories and the pathologic findings (gross and microscopic) in 3 cases of juvenile rheumatoid arthritis which had set in at the ages of 5, 6, and 3 years and had continued for 40, 16, and 5 years, respectively, to the time of death of the subjects in question. Portis detailed the clinical histories and necropsy findings in 2 cases of juvenile rheumatoid arthritis in which the disease had set in when the subjects were 7 and 11 years of age and which had continued for 5 and 8 years, respectively, to the time of death. Portis and also Pirani and Bennett correlated the pathologic findings in their cases with the autopsy findings in cases already recorded in the literature.

A fairly common finding at autopsy is amyloidosis, which may have been present for some years before death. While amyloid deposition may occur in the spleen and/or liver, its most ominous site is the kidney. The presence of *splenomegaly*, especially if the enlargement of the spleen is striking, should suggest, on a clinical basis, that the spleen is the site of amyloid infiltration. Pronounced *renal amyloidosis* is very likely to induce renal insufficiency and eventually uremia, and hence to lead to, or at least be a factor in, the death of the subject.

If the *spleen* is only moderately enlarged, microscopic examination will reveal such nonspecific changes as an increase in the cellular elements of the pulp and in the fibrous stromal elements of the spleen. The *lymphadenopathy* which may be observed even in the absence of splenomegaly involves most commonly the superficial lymph nodes (cervical, axillary, and inguinal). As already noted, the lymphadenopathy often regresses when the constitutional aspects of the disease have subsided. However, with recurrence of the constitutional manifestations, enlargement of the lymph nodes will again become apparent, and if the patient dies and an autopsy is performed, one may also find enlarged internal lymph nodes (in the mediastinum, the mesentery, and the region of the hilus of the liver). Microscopically, the enlarged lymph nodes, like the spleen, show merely nonspecific hyperplasia.

In 1 of the 3 cases studied in detail by Pirani and Bennett, *cardiac and aortic lesions* were found at autopsy. In that case, the arthritis set in at the age of 3, and the child died at the age of 8. At autopsy, the heart was found enlarged, the mitral valve was slightly thickened, and the aortic valve leaflets were moderately thickened and showed rolled edges and adhesions at the commissures. The aortic sinuses were very deep, and in this region the aorta presented two irregular outpouchings above the anterior cusp. These outpouchings were associated with thinning and dilatation of the aortic wall. On microscopic examination, sections through the wall of the aorta, near the aortic valve, disclosed a pronounced infiltration with lymphocytes and plasma cells, especially around the vasa vasorum. There was definite fibrosis and hyalinization involving all layers of the aortic wall. The vasa vasorum were prominent and showed varying degrees of hyalinization, with narrowing of their lumina. Sections from other segments of the aorta and from the pulmonary artery showed no noteworthy changes. Pirani and Bennett held that the cardiac and aortic lesions described above actually represented changes due to the Still's disease, since cardiovascular lesions are known to be part of the autopsy findings in some cases of classic (adult) rheumatoid arthritis (see Gruenwald).

The *articular lesions* of juvenile rheumatoid arthritis are basically the same as those of rheumatoid arthritis setting in during adult life (p. 787). As in the adult form, the involvement of a joint begins with inflammatory proliferation of the synovial membrane, associated with the accumulation of synovial fluid in the affected joint. In a child in whom a particular affected joint contains a relatively large amount of synovial fluid but not so much as to stretch the capsule excessively, the articular cartilages are afforded some protection from erosion, and the joint is not likely to be the source of much pain or spasm. Under these conditions, there may be complete though temporary remission of the articular inflammation. In a joint in which the inflammation of the synovial membrane is not associated with an amount of accumulated synovial fluid sufficient to separate the articular surfaces, the articular cartilages are subjected to pannus erosion and ultimately to the formation of intra-articular adhesions, abetted by spasm of the local muscles. Badly damaged joints tend to lose their mobility and may finally become ankylosed. When many joints have become involved and ankylosed, the child may be completely and permanently crippled. Because of disuse, the bones will then show very pronounced atrophy. In addition to ankylosis, one may find striking deformities at the articular ends of various bones (especially long tubular bones) because of aberrations in the formation and growth of the epiphysial centers of ossification and disordered endochondral ossification at the epiphysial cartilage plates. This disorder is due in part to increased growth activity at the plates but mainly to premature disappearance of the plates and premature fusion of the epiphyses with the shafts.

FELTY'S SYNDROME

The eponym "Felty's syndrome" is applied to those cases of rheumatoid arthritis in which, sooner or later: (1) the spleen becomes enlarged (moderately as a rule but in rare instances massively); and (2) the peripheral blood reveals a more or less pronounced leukopenia, especially in regard to the neutrophilic polymorphonuclear leukocytes. It is clear that relatively few cases of rheumatoid arthritis develop splenomegaly and leukopenia sufficiently pronounced to justify classification of these cases as instances of the Felty syndrome. Short *et al.*, reviewing 293 cases of rheumatoid arthritis which they followed for 20 to 25 years, found that only 3 of the cases (that is, about 1 per cent) had developed the manifestations characteristic of the syndrome.

CLINICAL CONSIDERATIONS

As in ordinary rheumatoid arthritis, the subjects are much more likely to be females than males. Indeed, in some reported series of cases, the proportion of affected females to males is much greater than the 3 to 1 proportion commonly noted in connection with ordinary rheumatoid arthritis. The patients are usually middle-aged or older at the time the diagnosis of Felty's syndrome is made, and the rheumatoid arthritis has generally been present for some years and often for many years by that time (see de Gruchy and Langley, and also Ruderman *et al.*). The arthritis may still be an active polyarthritis or may be in a quiescent stage, with residual articular deformities.

A persistent low grade febrile state evolves and is associated with chronic infections which tend to be refractory to antibiotics. In consequence of the toxic systemic aspects of the disease, the subjects often manifest anorexia, weight loss, easy fatigability, and generalized malaise. Other less common features include hepatomegaly, pigmentation of the skin, lymphadenopathy, and the development of a chronic ulcer of the skin of one or both legs.

In regard to the *spleen* in particular, it should be pointed out that, even in the rare instances in which the spleen is not palpable clinically, it is at least somewhat enlarged when removed in the course of splenectomy. In such cases the weight of the spleen may be only about 250 to 275 gm. When the spleen is very much enlarged, it has sometimes been found to extend to or below the umbilicus. In a survey of the pertinent literature, Mason and Morris noted the weight of the spleen as recorded in 45 out of 82 cases of Felty's syndrome in which splenectomy was done or the spleen was examined at autopsy. In these cases the weight of the spleen ranged from 260 to 2,070 gm., and averaged 910 gm. In only 5 of the cases, however, did the spleen weigh more than 1,500 gm., and the case in which it weighed 2,070 gm. was the only one in which it weighed more than 2,000 gm. The article by Mason and Morris also deals in detail with a case of Felty's syndrome which they themselves studied and in which the spleen was massively enlarged and was found, after splenectomy, to weigh 2,420 gm.

The occurrence of *lymphadenopathy* in Felty's syndrome is not of diagnostic significance, since it is also not an uncommon finding in classic rheumatoid arthritis affecting adults. The pathogenesis of the *leg ulceration* occasionally noted in Felty's syndrome remains obscure. The arthritis has usually been present for a long time before ulcerations make their appearance on the skin of the legs. Along with ulceration of the skin on one or both legs, or independently of it, the patient may present one or more of the following: stomatitis, multiple painful buccal ulcerations, sinusitis, bronchitis, pharyngitis, furunculosis, conjunctivitis, iritis, and corneal ulceration. Though these various lesions are refractory to antibiotics, there are indications that healing is favored by splenectomy (see Peden, and also Hutt *et al.*). These clinical aspects of the disease, and the fact that splenectomy tends to ameliorate them, are indications that their causation is related to the neutropenia (and consequent lowered resistance to infection) induced by the hypersplenism.

LABORATORY AND PATHOLOGIC FINDINGS

Hematologic Features.—Often, though not always, a mild degree of *anemia* is present. This is usually of the normocytic and hypochromic variety, and the values for hemoglobin and red blood cells are in fairly close accord with those commonly noted in cases of uncomplicated rheumatoid arthritis affecting adults. In the rare instances in which the anemia is pronounced, its severity is attributable to some complicating or associated factor, such as an acquired hemolytic anemia or chronic blood loss. The *platelet count* is ordinarily within normal limits. In those cases in which it is somewhat depressed, the mild thrombocytopenia is *not* usually associated with evidence of a tendency toward bleeding.

The most significant hematologic finding relates to the *white blood cells*. The generally accepted value for the leukocyte count in the peripheral blood of the normal adult is somewhere between 5,000 and 10,000 cells per cu. mm., and the average count is about 7,000. Segmented neutrophilic leukocytes normally constitute 54 to 62 per cent of the total number of leukocytes, thus numbering approximately 4,000 if the total leukocyte count is around 7,000. Leukocyte counts above 10,000 per cu. mm. are usually regarded as representing leukocytosis, while counts below 5,000 are held to be indicative of a leukopenia.

In cases of the Felty syndrome, a leukopenia, as already noted, is one of the three principal diagnostic features characterizing the condition. In most cases the leukopenia tends to become more pronounced in the course of time. An eventual total leukocyte count well under 3,000 cells per cu. mm. is not unusual, and the count may even come to be less than 1,000. Furthermore, when the total white blood cell count is well below 3,000, and especially if it is less than 1,000, the proportion of neutrophilic leukocytes drops sharply below the normal figure of 54 to 62 per cent. In some cases in which the total leukocyte count is less than 1,000, a differential count may even fail to reveal the presence of any neutrophilic leukocytes. Furthermore, the presence of an infection, even a severe one, is not usually associated with a rise in the neutrophil count.

The relation of the leukopenia (and particularly the neutropenia) to the splenomegaly is evidenced by the fact that, after splenectomy, the total leukocyte count and also the percentage of neutrophilic leukocytes is likely to rise, usually within a few days, to values which are normal or slightly above normal. If the neutrophil count has risen to a value above normal, it then tends to recede to a value within the normal range and to remain at that value. Sometimes, however, the neutrophil count drops to a level near where it was before splenectomy, and if this has occurred, the count only occasionally rises again to a normal value. In this connection, it seems pertinent that an *accessory spleen* is by no means an unusual finding in adults who have come to autopsy. Though the possibility seems not to have been expressed in the literature, it occurs to the present writer that the postsplenectomy drop in the neutrophil count in some cases of Felty's syndrome might have its foundation in enlargement of an accessory spleen.

The hematologic abnormalities observed in cases of the Felty syndrome are related to the effects of the *hypersplenism on the bone marrow* and consequently on the cells of the circulating blood. The cellularity of the bone marrow has been found to vary among the cases. Usually, the marrow is hyperplastic. Sometimes, however, its cellularity is normal, and occasionally it is decreased. In any event, the marrow shows an increased proportion of erythroid and myeloid cells and a pronounced diminution in the number of segmented neutrophils—that is, neutrophilic granulocytes. In brief, then, the characteristic findings relating to the bone marrow in Felty's syndrome are generally held to be: (1) pronounced myeloid hyperplasia; (2) arrest of myeloid maturation between the metamyelocyte stage and the stage of mature segmented neutrophil formation; and (3) moderate erythroid hyperplasia (see de Gruchy and Langley, and also Hutchison and Alexander).

The concept of myeloid maturation arrest resulting in a reduction in the number of segmented polymorphonuclear leukocytes entering the circulation has been proposed by Dameshek and Welch. Specifically, their thesis is that the spleen produces a humoral substance which, acting upon the bone marrow, inhibits the maturation and release of granulocytes from the bone marrow into the blood stream. However, others have postulated that hypersplenic leukopenia is due to sequestration, destruction, and phagocytosis of the cellular elements of the blood (particularly the granular leukocytes) by the reticuloendothelial cells of the spleen (see Wiseman and Doan, and also Gibberd et al.). On the whole, most investigators favor the concept that maturation arrest in the bone marrow is the basis for the reduction in the number of neutrophilic polymorphonuclear leukocytes present in the circulating blood in cases of Felty's syndrome. However, there are also those who favor the idea that maturation arrest in the bone marrow and destruction of the leukocytes in the spleen *both* play a part in the development of the leukopenia.

Various Other Laboratory Findings.—Tests for the rheumatoid factor generally yield positive results. In a small percentage of cases, a positive L.E. test result is also obtained (see Ruderman et al.). As determined by paper electrophoresis, the total globulin value of the serum is generally elevated, while the albumin fraction is likely to be somewhat reduced. Of the individual globulins, it is the gamma globulin that tends to show the highest percentile rise.

Pathologic Findings.—The pathologic changes in the joints and the nonarticular tissues in Felty's syndrome are essentially like those encountered in cases of advanced rheumatoid arthritis of the classic type (p. 787). The articular changes are usually pronounced, and severe deformities may be present. In addition to the splenomegaly, the nonarticular findings in cases of Felty's syndrome commonly include rheumatoid nodules and often lymphadenopathy and hepatomegaly.

Our discussion of the pathologic aspects of the disorder will be limited, however, to the findings relating to the spleen, in view of the importance of splenomegaly in the triad of features (rheumatoid arthritis, leukopenia, and splenomegaly) characterizing the syndrome. As already noted, the spleen may be only slightly enlarged or very much enlarged, and the weight of the individual spleens in the series of cases collected by Mason and Morris from the literature was found to range from 260 gm. to 2,070 gm. The averaged weight of the spleens in that series was 910 gm.

Apart from its size and weight, the spleen usually presents no abnormal gross features. It is of normal consistency, and neither its external surface nor its cut surface ordinarily shows anything remarkable. In most instances, *microscopic examination* of the spleen reveals an increase in the reticular connective tissue, lymphoid hyperplasia, congestion of the red pulp, and hypertrophy of the cells lining the sinuses. In particular, the malpighian corpuscles are found prominent, because their germinal centers are hyperplastic in consequence of an increase in the lymphoid cells. In spite of its congestion, the red pulp does not reveal evidence of myeloid metaplasia, but in some instances, small groups of plasma cells and, less often, eosinophils are present. Hutchison and Alexander report finding iron pigment, chiefly in the hypertrophied cells lining the sinuses but also in some of the cells of the pulp and in some of the connective tissue cells of the trabecular framework of the spleen. Though they found few polymorphonuclear leukocytes in the spleen, they did not find evidence of phagocytosis of these leukocytes, which other workers have reported. In brief, then, the histologic structure of the spleen may be interpreted as having undergone nonspecific changes compatible with an idiopathic hypersplenism.

TREATMENT

In regard to the treatment of patients affected with Felty's syndrome, the therapeutic considerations relate to the leukopenia and associated splenomegaly, the rheumatoid arthritis, and intercurrent infection. Corticosteroids and/or ACTH have been administered mainly with the aim of correcting the leukopenia. However, the results do not indicate consistent or lasting benefit from such treatment. In some cases the polymorphonuclear leukocyte count fails to rise on a rather low corticosteroid dosage but does rise if a large dose is administered. In other cases, cortisone, prednisone, or ACTH in ample doses induces a gradual rise in the polymorphonuclear leukocyte count to an approximately normal level within a few weeks. However, the rise in the leukocyte count is only temporary, and there is usually a subsequent drop in the count to the pretreatment level. Furthermore, the rise in the leukocyte count is usually not associated with correction of any infections which may be present.

In the absence of infection, *splenectomy* is an indicated therapeutic procedure against the leukopenia and the subsequent development of infections. In the presence of significant infection, splenectomy cannot necessarily be expected to be of benefit, the patients often succumbing to the infection despite the usual improvement in the leukocyte count. The influence of splenectomy on the leukocyte count, and particularly on the neutrophil count, has already been discussed. The rheumatoid arthritis *per se* is not an indication for splenectomy, and should be given the same treatment that would be administered if one were dealing with chronic rheumatoid arthritis not complicated by leukopenia and significant splenomegaly.

PSORIATIC ARTHRITIS

As a disease complex, psoriatic arthritis is represented by a combination of psoriasis and inflammatory polyarthritis, in the absence of rheumatoid nodules and the so-called rheumatoid factor in the serum. In a case of polyarthritis in which the patient also exhibits psoriasis and is seropositive for the rheumatoid factor, one is dealing with a coincidental combination of rheumatoid arthritis and psoriasis (both fairly common diseases). (See Fig. 211.)

CLINICAL CONSIDERATIONS

In regard to the *sex incidence* of psoriatic arthritis, the statistics recorded in the literature are not in agreement. The differences probably are influenced by variations in the sex distribution of the population in the out-patient departments and/or hospitals from which the reports have emanated. In particular: Some workers found the incidence of the disease in the cases they studied to be approximately the same for the two sexes (see Krebs, and also Lassus *et al.*); others found males to be more frequently affected (see Coste and Solnica, Zellner, Reed, and also Sherman); and in still other reports it is stated that the condition was found to be much more common in females than in males. In the latter connection, it is reported by Baker *et al.* that in their series of cases the ratio of affected females to affected males was approximately 5 or 6 to 1. The preponderance of females over males as noted by them would thus be about twice what it is in connection with so-called classic rheumatoid arthritis.

In respect to the *temporal relation* between the two principal manifestations of the disease, it has been found that, more often than not, the psoriasis precedes the arthritis. Indeed, the skin lesions may already have been present for some years or even several decades before the polyarthritis sets in. However, in a small percentage of cases, the arthritis has already been present for a number of years before the psoriasis appears. Under these circumstances, it is quite likely that an erroneous diagnosis of rheumatoid arthritis will be made at first. As noted, either the psoriasis or the arthritis may set in first, and a long time may elapse between the appearances of these two aspects of psoriatic arthritis. However, there are cases in which the psoriasis and the polyarthritis appear almost synchronously—that is, within a few months of each other. In some instances, though the subject already has pronounced polyarthritis, the skin lesions are clinically mild or inconspicuous. In these cases the absence of a rheumatoid factor in the subject's serum is nevertheless sufficient to justify their classification in the category of psoriatic arthritis.

In some cases of psoriatic arthritis the *articular involvement* is limited to one joint at first, but more frequently the arthritis is polyarticular from the start. The mode of onset of the arthritic manifestations tends to be insidious but is sometimes acute. When it is insidious, the patient may complain first of transient morning stiffness in some of the large diarthrodial joints. Pain and stiffness in the cervical and/or lumbar region of the vertebral column may also be present. In brief, the initial arthritic manifestations are essentially the same in psoriatic arthritis as in classic rheumatoid arthritis.

In a series of cases of psoriatic arthritis, the joints most often found involved at the time the diagnosis is established are the small joints of the hands and of the feet—especially the distal interphalangeal joints. Next in order of frequency of involvement in such a series of cases are the shoulder joints, the knee joints, and the wrist, elbow, and ankle joints. The hip joints and temporomandibular joints are

Figure 211

A and *B*, Photographs of the severely deformed hands and of the distal ends of the forearms from the case of a man who was 55 years of age at the time of his first admission to our hospital. According to the clinical record, he had been suffering from arthritis for 4 years prior to admission. At that time, physical examination revealed clear-cut evidence of arthritis involving the proximal interphalangeal joints, the metacarpophalangeal joints, and both knee joints. The patient also presented a skin lesion which two dermatologists of the hospital staff diagnosed as psoriasis. Since there were nodule formations in the region of the metacarpophalangeal joints and in the region of the olecranon at both elbow joints, it was decided to remove the nodule from the right elbow for histopathologic examination. Microscopically, the excised tissue was found to be a rheumatoid nodule. This finding helped to establish the diagnosis of rheumatoid arthritis associated with a superimposed psoriasis, and thus to negate the diagnosis of psoriatic arthritis *per se*. The patient had two additional admissions to the hospital during the next 6 years. It was evident that the arthritic deformities were becoming worse, and these pictures of the hands were taken at the time of his third admission, when the arthritis had already been present for 10 years. At that time, reconstructive surgery was done on the left hand, the intervention consisting of resection of the proximal phalanges of the fourth and fifth fingers. At the same time, a local soft-tissue mass was removed, which proved to have the histologic architecture of a rheumatoid nodule.

C, Roentgenograph of the hands shown in *A*. Note the obliteration of almost all the intercarpal joint spaces, the advanced changes at the metacarpophalangeal joints, associated with subluxations, and the relatively slight involvement of some of the interphalangeal joints.

D, Roentgenograph of the right hand, wrist, and part of the forearm of a woman 45 years of age who had been affected with rheumatoid arthritis for 15 years. Note the pronounced osteoporosis of all the bones; the ankylosis of the carpal bones, resulting in obliteration of the intercarpal joints; the ankylosis of the radiocarpal joints; the absence of the distal end of the ulna; and the absence (due to resorption) of the distal portions of the second, third, and fourth metacarpal bones and almost the entire fifth metacarpal. Analogous roentgenographic changes were present in the left hand of this patient and, to a lesser degree, also in both feet. Such advanced destructive changes in the hands are generally denoted as representing "arthritis mutilans," which is most often seen in cases of psoriatic arthritis.

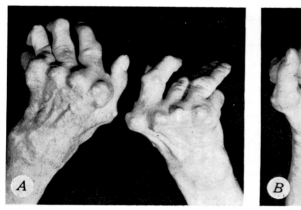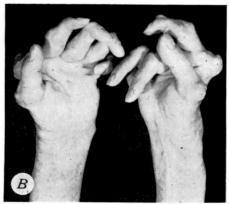

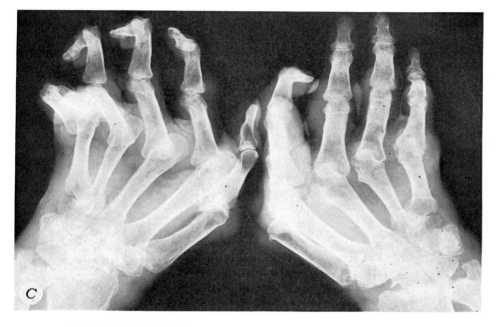

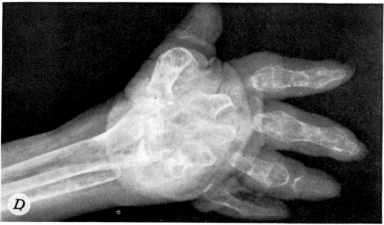

Figure 211

only infrequently found involved at the time the diagnosis is established. However, later in the course of the disease, radiographic examination frequently discloses erosive changes in the temporomandibular joints (see Lundberg and Ericson). It has been reported in the literature that it is not unusual to encounter cases of psoriatic arthritis in which the articular involvement is limited to the terminal interphalangeal joints. Actually, however, such cases seem to be exceptional.

As already noted, rheumatoid nodules do not develop in cases of psoriatic arthritis. In a supposed case of this disease, the finding of a rheumatoid nodule negates that diagnosis, since under these circumstances one is dealing merely with the coexistence of two independent diseases—psoriasis and rheumatoid arthritis—in the same subject. Furthermore, pulmonary and cardiac lesions, such as are encountered in cases of classic rheumatoid arthritis (p. 804), are not observed in persons affected with psoriatic arthritis. There are clear indications that, in those cases in which the psoriasis and the polyarthritis appeared more or less synchronously (or within a few months of each other), both of these manifestations of the disease tend to be more severe than in those cases in which there is a significant time interval between the onset of the psoriasis and the polyarthritis, irrespective of which appeared first. In addition, in those cases in which the arthritis is severe, it is likely that the psoriasis will also be severe. Another feature of the psoriasis is the frequent presence of changes involving the nails of the fingers, such as pitting, ridging, and subungual keratosis. The changes to be found in the nails of the toes usually consist of thickening of the nails and subungual keratosis, while pitting and ridging are uncommon findings in the toe nails.

ROENTGENOGRAPHIC AND PATHOLOGIC FINDINGS

The *roentgenographic features* characterizing psoriatic arthritis center around the destructive changes involving the distal interphalangeal joints of the hands and feet (see Avila *et al.*, and also Wright). The proximal interphalangeal joints of the fingers are not likely to be found affected. In contrast, the corresponding joints of the toes (especially the interphalangeal joint of the large toe) usually show destructive changes roentgenographically, along with bony proliferation at the base of the

Figure 212

A, Photograph of the hands of a woman affected with psoriatic arthritis associated with destructive changes in the short tubular bones of the hands. These changes had resulted in pawlike deformities of the hands. This type of deformity has also been denoted as "main en lorgnette"—a name suggested by the very conspicuous overlapping of the skin of the fingers because of shortening of the fingers as a result of destruction and overriding of its bones. The patient was a woman 57 years of age who had had psoriatic arthritis for 20 years. The arthritis involved many joints and had led to the appearance of mutilating deformities of both hands and both feet.*

B, Roentgenograph demonstrating the destruction of the proximal ends of the proximal phalanges and the distal ends of the metacarpal bones. The shortening and overriding of these bones demonstrates clearly the basis for the overlapping of the skin of the individual fingers ("opera-glass" appearance).

C, Photograph of the feet in this case. The toes are markedly shortened, and the phalanges and metacarpal bones presented changes comparable to those apparent roentgenographically in the hands.

* The details relating to this case have been described in the article by Shlionsky and Blake entitled "Arthritis Psoriatica; Report of a Case" (see Ann. Int. Med., *10*, 537, 1936). The authors of that article consulted the present writer about the nature of the condition before they presented the case. At that time, permission was given to reproduce these illustrations.

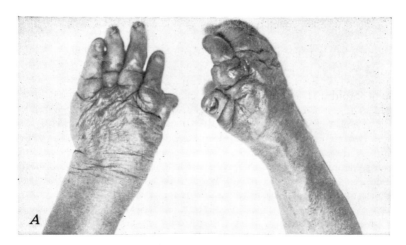

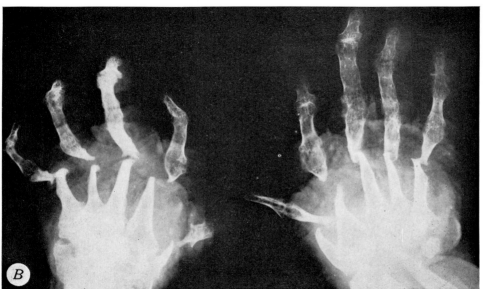

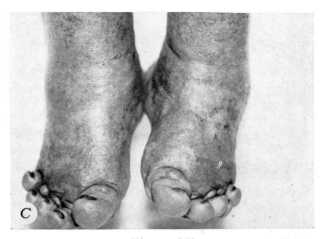

Figure 212

distal phalanx of that toe. However, involvement of the metacarpophalangeal and metatarsophalangeal joints is uncommon in cases of psoriatic arthritis, compared with the frequency of the implication of these joints in classic rheumatoid arthritis. Also, the carpal, radionavicular, and radio-ulnar joints are less often affected in psoriatic arthritis than in rheumatoid arthritis. The terminal interphalangeal joints may undergo bony ankylosis. In contrast, some of the subjects come to present massive bone destruction, resulting in loss of portions of the phalangeal shafts, and ultimately show the crippling changes of the hands and feet (especially the hands) commonly denoted as *"arthritis mutilans."* (See Fig. 212.)

In addition to small joints of the hands and feet, large diarthrodial joints may be sites of the arthritis (see Black and O'Brien). The cervical spine, too, may present roentgenographic alterations (see Kaplan *et al.*). In particular, the apophysial joints often show narrowing, and the apophyses themselves may be sclerotic. Changes involving the sacroiliac joints are not unusual, but one does not often find the full gamut of changes characterizing ankylosing spondylitis as a separate entity (see Jajić). Calcification of the anterior longitudinal ligament is sometimes observed. Paravertebral ossification in cases of psoriatic arthritis has been reported. This consisted of extensive paraspinal ossification in the lumbar and thoracic areas, differing from the changes characterizing ankylosing spondylitis and advanced spondylosis deformans (see Bywaters and Dixon).

A comprehensive and detailed presentation of the *pathologic findings* relating to 33 involved joints is given in the article by Sherman. In most of these cases the tissue was obtained in the course of a biopsy, but in several instances the tissue became available in the course of reconstructive surgery necessitated by articular deformities, notably in relation to the feet. The pathologic findings were nonspecific (that is, not pathognomonic) and varied greatly among the cases, apparently being influenced by the evolutionary age of the lesion.

On exploration of interphalangeal joints which had been affected for only 2 to 8 weeks, Sherman found that the synovial membrane had the gross appearance of pale edematous granulation tissue. At this early stage, the tissue in question was seen to extend for a few millimeters along the shaft of one or both phalanges and had eroded the cortex somewhat, so that the latter appeared roughened. The articular cartilages of these interphalangeal joints still appeared normal, and in particular no synovial pannus was as yet demonstrable on them. On microscopic examination, the synovial membrane from an interphalangeal joint still in the early stages of the arthritis showed a fairly pronounced edema and considerable fibrosis, not only in the immediate sublining area but even well below the lining layer.

In cases in which the arthritis has been of somewhat longer duration, the synovial membrane is found thickened and injected. In some areas the membrane shows proliferation of the synovial lining cells and also villus formation, while in other areas the membrane may be rather fibrotic. Not infrequently, the synovial membrane is found diffusely infiltrated with round cells, or the latter are agglomerated into small foci. There may also be evidence of erosion along the periphery of the articular cartilages, but the remainder of their surfaces is free of pannus.

In time, the erosive process extends onto the cortices of the bone shafts, in the general vicinity of the joint, and it is these erosions of the cortical bone that are reflected in the roentgenographs as "gnawed out" defects. As the inflammatory and destructive changes progress, the articular ends of the bones entering into the formation of the affected interphalangeal joint may come to be represented merely by stubs of cancellous bone or slender spicules of bone embedded in thick fibrous tissue, which also obliterates the articular cavity. In consequence of these various changes, the articular bone ends usually become subluxated and/or dislocated, but ankylosis of the bone ends is not likely to take place.

TREATMENT

In the treatment of psoriatic arthritis, the management of the arthritis *per se* is essentially the same as that appropriate for rheumatoid arthritis. However, care must be taken in the treatment of the condition to avoid drugs which might induce skin reactions. For instance, chloroquine phosphate and the antimalarial drugs should not be used, since the skin lesions have been known to flare up during their administration. It has been claimed that, if steroid therapy is to be used, triamcinolone is the steroid drug of choice, since it has been held to be of value against both the arthritis and the psoriasis. However, it appears that steroid therapy should be restricted to those patients in whom both the psoriasis and the arthritis are severe and have proved intractable, since calculated risks are involved in the prolonged use of steroid therapy. One of these risks is that, even though the withdrawal of the steroid is done gradually and carefully, there may be a severe flare-up of the psoriasis and/or arthritis at the end of the withdrawal period.

REITER'S SYNDROME

The term *"Reiter's syndrome"* represents the clinical triad of urethritis, conjunctivitis, and arthritis, in the absence of gonococci in direct smears and/or bacteriologic cultures prepared from the urethral and conjunctival discharge and also from the synovial fluid of an inflamed joint. Even if the bacteriologic studies fail to reveal the presence of gonococci, the diagnosis of Reiter's syndrome in a given case is not applicable unless the subject shows the above-mentioned three principal clinical aspects of the condition concurrently at some time in the course of the disease. In addition, the affected subjects may present one or more of the following manifestations: iritis, hyperkeratotic dermatitis (often denoted as keratosis blennorrhagica), circinate balanitis, and shallow ulcerations of the buccal mucosa.

The syndrome in question was described in 1916 (on the basis of one case) by Reiter, who held that it was caused by spirochetes and denoted it as "Spirochaetosis arthritica." It is not generally recognized that, almost a century earlier (in 1818), Brodie described 5 cases representing classic examples of the condition which has come to be denoted as Reiter's syndrome. Reiter's idea that the syndrome resulted from an infection by spirochetes has not been confirmed by subsequent investigators. Indeed, the cause of the condition is still obscure, although there are some reports to the effect that it may be due to an infection by a Mycoplasma, a pleuropneumonia-like organism (see Claus *et al.*), or a member of the Bedsonia group of organisms, such as psittacosis-lymphogranuloma venereum-trachoma (see Schachter *et al.*). Of the 344 cases of Reiter's syndrome reported from Finland by Paronen, practically all had a history of bacillary dysentery (due to the Shigella of Flexner), and in two thirds of these cases the syndrome appeared within 11 to 30 days after the onset of the dysentery. In this connection, Noer has reported the occurrence of 9 cases of Reiter's syndrome among 602 sailors who had suffered an attack of bacillary dysentery contracted while they were on board ship. The initial symptoms of the syndrome in these cases followed the onset of the dysentery within 9 to 24 days. Approximately 600 other sailors on the ship did not contract dysentery, and none of these sailors developed Reiter's syndrome.

Despite these various bacteriologic findings, it has not been established that any one of the suggested bacteriologic agents bears an unequivocal etiologic relationship to Reiter's syndrome. It is pertinent in this connection that Mycoplasmas have also been isolated from normal persons, as well as from patients affected with gonococcal urethritis who did not present the full Reiter syndrome. It is recognized that a member of the Bedsonia group of organisms (psittacosis-lymphogranuloma venereum-trachoma) can be the cause, under natural conditions, of polyarthritis in sheep, and that sheep inoculated with this organism in the course of experimental studies also develop polyarthritis. However, the animals do not show the full Reiter's triad, though some of the sheep do manifest conjunctivitis in addition to the polyarthritis (see Norton and Storz). In any event, though there is no clear evidence linking either Mycoplasmas or Bedsoniae agents to Reiter's syndrome, Ford is of the opinion that one or the other of these two classes of microorganisms is most likely to be established eventually as the etiologic factor in the disease.

CLINICAL CONSIDERATIONS

The reports in the literature on Reiter's syndrome have increased considerably since 1942, when the article by Bauer and Engleman appeared. The accounts representing extensive reviews of the literature and/or studies of large numbers of cases include those by Touraine and Ruel, Paronen, Peters, Engleman and Weber, and also Buchan. A comprehensive description of the clinical and pathologic features of Reiter's syndrome, based on long-term observation of 16 patients and also some data on 19 additional cases, is given by Weinberger *et al.* The present writer has drawn extensively upon their presentation for his account of the syndrome.

As to *general incidence*, while Reiter's syndrome is not a common condition, it is by no means rare. The occurrence of the disease is not confined to any geographical area, typical cases having been observed in widely separated parts of the world. In regard to *age* and *sex incidence*, the subjects are mainly adult males between 20 and 40 years of age. The disease is definitely uncommon in females, even in that age group. Furthermore, it is only rarely encountered in persons under 15 years of age, and those in that age category who are affected are very likely to be males.

In connection with the *order of appearance* of the three diagnostic clinical features (urethritis, conjunctivitis, and arthritis) essential for the diagnosis of Reiter's syndrome, it is to be observed that the condition may set in with any one of these three manifestations, or with two, or (though infrequently) all of them. The urethritis is by far the most common initial symptom, and it is only in a small percentage of the cases that conjunctivitis is the presenting feature. When two of the diagnostic aspects of the triad appear simultaneously, these are usually urethritis and arthritis, and less often conjunctivitis and arthritis.

In any event, in the course of a month or so after the condition has set in, most of the subjects come to present the complete triad. In those cases in which this pattern is not followed, one or another of the diagnostic features may fail to appear for many months. There are also some cases in which one or two of the significant clinical manifestations appear, disappear, and reappear in the course of many months before all three are present together. On the other hand, in many cases in which the full triad of Reiter's syndrome had been manifest during the initial attack, there may be exacerbations involving one or another component of the triad. In addition, the subject now tends to present certain constitutional reactions, and in particular a slightly elevated temperature, malaise, and anorexia, the latter two usually subsiding when the temperature returns to normal.

Among patients exhibiting the full triad of the syndrome, the time elapsing between the onset and the subsidence of the initial attack varies from about 2 to about 6 months, and in an occasional instance the articular manifestations may persist alone for many months. Despite the long continuance of the arthritis in these cases, eventual complete recovery from the initial attack can be expected.

In a large proportion of the cases, the *further clinical course* of the disease is marked by one or more recurrences after the initial attack has subsided. In some cases the first recurrence becomes evident within a few months, but in others it takes place only after an interval of several years. The clinical manifestations associated with the recurrence may consist of the complete clinical triad or be limited to one or two aspects of it. The clinical expressions of the disorder during the recurrences tend to be less severe and of shorter duration than those characterizing the original attack (see Weinberger *et al.*). Details relating to the various diagnostic findings will now be presented. The discussion of the pertinent pathologic changes will be confined to the articular aspects of the triad, and is given below.

Urethritis.—The penile discharge resulting from the urethritis is usually moderate in amount. It may be frankly purulent (that is, thick and mucoid) or slightly purulent (that is, rather thin and watery). Ordinarily, the discharge is associated with burning on urination. There is considerable variation among the patients in respect to the amount of the discharge and its duration. Sometimes the discharge is intermittent at first, and it usually subsides in about a month, though occasionally it persists for a number of months. In association with the urethritis, some of the patients present other genitourinary difficulties. Of these, the most common is prostatitis, and such other local urogenital abnormalities as seminal vesiculitis and hemorrhagic cystitis have also been reported. The latter occasionally leads to obstruction of the ureters, and hydronephrosis may result.

Conjunctivitis.—This is usually the only ocular manifestation of the disorder, and it is ordinarily of short duration, lasting only a few days or weeks at a time. As a rule, it is expressed in a mild degree of irritation of both eyes and a slight amount of conjunctival discharge. Because of the usual mildness of the conjunctivitis, the patient may not bring it to the attention of the physician, and it may even be overlooked in the course of the physical examination. *Iritis* and less often *keratitis* have been observed, and even more rarely a recurrent *retinitis* and *retrobulbar neuritis* have been noted. However, despite these various ocular changes, actual blindness rarely develops, though permanent impairment of vision may ensue.

Lesions of the Skin and Oral Mucous Membrane.—Thickened and horny growths of the *skin* (especially of the palms and soles and sometimes of the trunk and extremities) are frequently observed in cases of the Reiter syndrome. These dermal lesions are denoted as "keratosis blennorrhagica" or, more precisely, "keratoderma blennorrhagica." Some of the subjects so affected also present subungual hyperkeratosis, expressed in the accumulation of friable cornified material beneath the nails, which may become detached from the nail bed. The lesions of the skin evolve rather rapidly in consequence of the coalescence of small papules, and healing occurs after several weeks, without scar formation, despite the fact that the hyperkeratotic skin on the soles of the feet may have presented in the form of heaped-up crusts and fissured plaques. On the glans penis, circular or ringlike superficial ulcerations of the skin have been observed in some cases, and when such ulcerations are limited to the glans, and in particular not associated with hyperkeratotic changes elsewhere on the skin of the penis, this local condition is denoted as *balanitis circinata*. The ulcerations characterizing circinate balanitis may heal, and the skin of the glans may become somewhat keratotic. In relation to the *oral cavity*, small superficial ulcerations and/or small thickened areas of the mucous membrane are sometimes present. They may be observed on the mucous membrane of the lips, cheeks, and palate. They usually do not give rise to clinical complaints, and tend to clear up within a short time.

Arthritis.—The articular component of the triad often dominates the clinical picture. The arthritis is sometimes monarticular but is usually polyarticular. In the course of an initial or recurrent attack of the arthritis, the weight-bearing joints are the ones most often involved, and among these it is the knee joint and ankle joint that are predilected. Of the other articulations, it is the small joints of the feet and hands that are most often implicated. Somewhat less frequently, the joints of the wrist and midtarsus are found affected. Furthermore, roentgenographic examination not infrequently reveals changes in one or both sacroiliac joints, but the involvement of these joints is usually asymptomatic.

In an initial attack, the onset of the arthritis is ordinarily acute and accompanied by malaise, fever, and an increased erythrocyte sedimentation rate. If the knee joints are affected, effusion into these joints is common. The duration of the arthritis varies considerably, persisting in some cases for only a few days, but in the majority of the cases continuing for some months. Although generalized swelling of an affected joint is not a common finding, palpation reveals localized swelling and tenderness of the periarticular tissues in some area of the joint. These localized areas of tenderness have been ascribed to periostitis, tendinitis, myositis, and/or bursitis.

Spontaneous and complete recovery is the rule in regard to most of the affected joints, but relapses are frequent. Usually the relapses, too, are followed by recovery, but in the feet permanent abnormalities are likely to develop eventually after repeated attacks of the arthritis. These abnormalities include: calcaneal spurs, pes cavus or planus, and dorsiflexion and fibular deviation of the toes at the metatarsophalangeal joints (see Weldon and Scalettar, Buchan, and also Peterson and Silbiger). After repeated attacks, progressive articular damage may ultimately be evident in the bones of the hands and wrists. In particular, the phalanges, metacarpal bones, and carpal bones are likely to present roentgenographic evidence of subchondral atrophy and narrowing of the articular spaces. Eventually the carpal bones may even undergo bony ankylosis. However, such advanced and permanent alterations are only infrequently encountered elsewhere than in the hands and feet. Altogether, involvement of joints is the most disabling and persistent feature of Reiter's syndrome.

The *synovial fluid* obtained from an inflamed large diarthrodial joint (whether in the course of an initial or a recurrent attack) tends to appear cloudy and clots readily, and its mucin content is very likely to be somewhat lowered. The leukocyte count per cubic millimeter ranges from as little as 1,000 to many thousands, and about two thirds of the leukocytes are neutrophils. Another significant finding is the presence of macrophages containing leukocytes (see Pekin *et al.*). In about half of such cases, the glucose content of the synovial fluid is somewhat less than the glucose content of the serum. On repeated examination of synovial fluid from an inflamed joint, it will be found that these various aberrations relating to the cytological and chemical aspects of the synovial fluid become more pronounced if the inflammatory process is severe and persists for a long time. Cytological and chemical alterations in the reverse direction are indications that the inflammatory process is subsiding.

As already noted, the presentation of the *pathologic findings* in cases of Reiter's syndrome will be limited to the articular alterations. The latter are largely confined to the synovial membrane, and consist of hyperemia, edema, and thickening of the membrane. In a rather early acute phase of the arthritis, the thickened and edematous membrane may appear deep red. In cases in which the arthritis is of somewhat longer duration, the periphery of the articular cartilage may present a narrow zone of erosion by synovial pannus. In addition, the inflamed synovial membrane may have patches of fibrin adhering to its surface.

On *microscopic examination* it is apparent that the histologic changes presented by an affected synovial membrane vary with the clinical activity and duration of the articular inflammation. If the latter has been present for only a few weeks, the edematous synovial membrane will show increased vascularity, some degree of infiltration with leukocytes (both neutrophils and lymphocytes) and sometimes also some plasma cells. The synovial lining cells are increased in number and tend to show a palisade arrangement. In the sublining layer of the membrane, the connective tissue cells are likely to have undergone proliferation. In cases in which the articular inflammation is of long standing, the synovial membrane may show changes practically indistinguishable from those manifested by the synovial membrane in cases of rheumatoid inflammation of long duration—i.e., hyperemia, edema, perivascular round cell collections, and large focal collections of lymphocytes.

DIFFERENTIAL DIAGNOSIS

Differential Diagnosis.—In arriving at the diagnosis of Reiter's syndrome in a given case, a number of other conditions must be considered and eliminated. Foremost among these is *gonococcal infection*, since some subjects in whom the latter is present come to show the triad of manifestations (urethritis, conjunctivitis, and arthritis) characteristic of Reiter's syndrome. The possibility of a gonococcal infection can be almost eliminated if repeated cultures from the penile discharge due to the urethritis fail to reveal the presence of gonococci. In addition, the possibility that one is dealing with a gonococcal infection can be minimized or even eliminated on clinical grounds. In contrast to a patient affected with Reiter's syndrome, a patient in whom urethritis, conjunctivitis, and arthritis are the result of gonococcal infection presents severe constitutional symptoms (including chills).

A problem of differential diagnosis may also arise in a subject affected with *classic rheumatoid arthritis* who has also developed a gonococcal urethritis and a conjunctivitis. The diagnostic problem in such a case is resolved in favor of rheumatoid arthritis with a superimposed gonococcal infection, if the urethritis and conjunctivitis yield to antibiotic therapy but the arthritis does not. Occasionally it is quite difficult to decide whether a particular case should be classified as one of Reiter's syndrome or one of *psoriatic arthritis*. In this connection, a finding which would favor a diagnosis of Reiter's syndrome is the presence of small, superficial ulcerations of the mucous membrane of the oral cavity, since such lesions are rarely observed in a case of psoriatic arthritis. However, there are reports of cases in which psoriatic arthritis and Reiter's syndrome were present in the same patient (see Wright and Reed).

ANKYLOSING SPONDYLITIS

Ankylosing spondylitis is a progressive inflammatory polyarthritis affecting principally the vertebral column, though some of the large peripheral joints may also be involved. The clinical complaints are referable mainly to the pathologic changes in the sacroiliac joints, the synovial (apophysial) joints of the spine, and the costovertebral articulations (which are likewise synovial joints). In addition, pathologic alterations develop in various soft tissues associated with the vertebrae, including notably the intervertebral ligaments, the intervertebral disks, the anterior longitudinal ligament, and the paraspinal muscles, and these changes, too, contribute to the clinical difficulties. (See Fig. 213.)

The anatomic aspects of the disease were recognized and described more than a hundred years ago, on the basis of findings relating to macerated skeletons or skeletal parts preserved in museums. Some of the specimens in question came from persons who had died several thousand years before. Subsequent clinical descriptions of the disease complex led to designation of the condition under a wide variety of names, some of which were descriptive terms while others were eponyms. These names include: spondylitis rhizomelica, Marie-Strümpell disease, von Bechterew's disease, spondylarthritis ankylopoietica, spondylitis ossificans ligamentosa, adolescent and/or juvenile spondylitis, pelvospondylitis ossificans, and also rheumatoid spondylitis. Although, in cases of classic rheumatoid arthritis, some degree of spondylitis (especially in the cervical region) is a common finding, it is now almost universally held that ankylosing spondylitis, with which we are dealing in this section of the chapter, should be regarded as a distinct disease entity, and not as an expression of rheumatoid arthritis (see Gofton).

CLINICAL CONSIDERATIONS

Incidence.—Estimates of the *general incidence* of ankylosing spondylitis in the adult population vary with the source of the case material. The incidence of the disorder in the city of Bristol (England) has been stated to be 1 case per 2,000 of the general population (see West). A much higher incidence was reported by Sharp. Specifically, he noted an incidence of 6 cases per 1,000 adult males under treatment in the "spondylitis clinic" of his institution. It may well be that this relatively high incidence, which would suggest that the condition is not uncommon, merely reflects the special composition of the population from which his figures were de-

Figure 213

A, Photograph of a macerated specimen showing part of the thoracic region of the vertebral column from a case of ankylosing spondylitis. The ribs are fused to the vertebral bodies as a result of ankylosis of the costovertebral joints. Even in this view, there is some evidence that the costotransverse articulations are also ankylosed, and this is more clearly apparent in *B*. The patient was a man who was 43 years of age at the time he died and came to autopsy. Nineteen years earlier, when he was 24, he began to have pain in the lower part of the back. In the course of 5 years, the pain gradually increased in severity and finally was associated with rigidity and kyphotic curvature of the vertebral column. Coincidentally, flexion gradually became limited in both hips. The patient was first admitted to our hospital at the age of 29, and subsequently he had three other admissions. Between admissions, he was in a nursing home, where he received custodial care. On his final admission to our hospital, he manifested renal insufficiency, and he died of uremia. In addition to the ankylosing spondylitis, the autopsy revealed the presence of generalized amyloidosis. Amyloidosis of the kidneys was the cause of the renal insufficiency and of the patient's death. The other illustrations presented in this figure are from the same case.

B, Photograph showing bony ankylosis of the costotransverse articulations.

C, Photograph revealing the external surface of the lumbosacral area of the macerated spine, including a part of the ilium. The lumbar facet joints are completely ankylosed, and the periphery of most of the intervertebral disks is osseous tissue resulting from ossification of the annulus fibrosus of the disks.

D, Photograph showing the cut surface (sectioned in the sagittal plane) of the lumbosacral portion of the vertebral column shown in *C*. The intervertebral disks between the second, third, fourth, and fifth lumbar vertebrae clearly reveal the presence of osseous tissue, and osseous tissue is also present in the disk between the body of the fifth lumbar vertebra and the first sacral segment. As already noted, some of the intervertebral disks also show bone formation at their periphery.

E, Roentgenograph of the lumbosacral region of the spine shown in *D*. It demonstrates the presence of osseous tissue in the intervertebral disks and the ankylosis of the facet joints of the lumbar vertebrae.

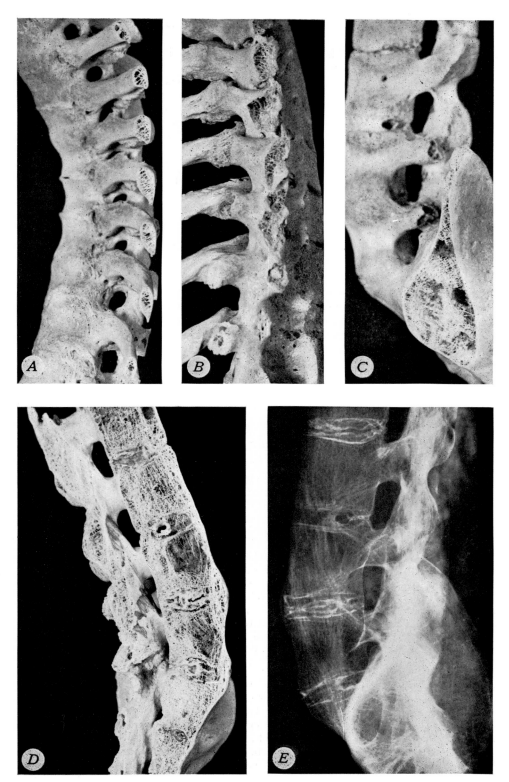

Figure 213

rived. In support of this inference, it can be pointed out that, among 10,000 cadavers coming to autopsy at the City Hospital of Dresden (a general hospital), Schmorl and Junghanns encountered only 6 to 8 clear-cut instances of spondylitis ankylopoietica, and they felt satisfied that at most only a few early cases had been overlooked. Furthermore, the incidence of ankylosing spondylitis as based on these autopsy findings is not much out of line with the incidence of 1 case per 2,000 of the general population of Bristol as reported by West.

The *sex and age incidence* are more clearly established than the general incidence, and in regard to these two aspects, ankylosing spondylitis presents striking contrasts to classic rheumatoid arthritis. In classic rheumatoid arthritis the affected subjects are predominantly females in the proportion of about 3 to 1, while in ankylosing spondylitis this sex ratio is more than reversed, and in some series of cases the proportion of males to females has been found to be as high as 4 or 5 or even 8 or 9 to 1. In regard to the *age at onset*, it is known that in a large proportion of the cases the disease has set in at some time between the ages of 16 and 30.

Clinical Complaints and Findings.—In a large majority of the cases, the presenting complaints consist of discomfort in the lower part of the back (including the buttocks, groins, and thighs) or even actual pain in that part of the back, sometimes associated with sciatic radiation but not associated with paresthesias. All these early complaints are at their worst in the morning and may have awakened the patient, but they tend to subside in the course of ordinary morning activity. These presenting complaints may become progressively worse, and in the course of months or years the patient may come to suffer from pain relating to the cervical, dorsal, and lumbar portion of the spine, associated with progressive limitation of movement of the spine. As the disease advances, involvement of peripheral joints tends to become evident. However, in an occasional instance, implication of these

Figure 214

A, Roentgenograph of the cervical region of the spine in a case of ankylosing spondylitis showing a pronounced exaggeration of the cervical curve, in accordance with the appearance of the neck in B. The facet joints are ankylosed.

B, Photograph of a 31 year old man affected with ankylosing spondylitis. The photograph shows, in lateral projection, the stance characteristic of this disorder when it is present in an advanced form. The patient was first admitted to our hospital when he was 17 years of age. The clinical history relating to that admission indicates that he had been having pain in the lower part of the back for about 1½ years. In that area the pain was first localized to the right side of the back, but within a year or so it was also felt on the left side. On his readmission to the hospital 14 years later (at age 31), it was evident that, when he stood, the trunk was bent forward at an angle of about 60°. When he was sitting, a posterior curve was apparent in the dorsal region, while the head and neck projected forward. When he was sitting or standing, the lumbar region of the spine was flat. He walked with difficulty, because his hips were ankylosed both in flexion and in adduction. Roentgenographic examination revealed ankylosis of the facet joints (in the cervical, dorsal, and lumbar regions), along with other evidences of ankylosing spondylitis, including notably ankylosis of the sacroiliac joints, narrowing and ossification of many of the intervertebral disks, and fusion of the lumbar vertebrae in particular, as a result of the formation of syndesmophytes.

C, Roentgenograph in lateral projection of the thoracic vertebrae. The facet joints in this region of the spine are also ankylosed. All the intervertebral disks are narrowed, with the exception of the one at the bottom of the picture. The narrowed disks show streaks of radiopacity, to a greater or lesser extent, and these represent ossification within them.

D, Roentgenograph of the lumbar vertebrae in the anteroposterior projection. The intervertebral disks show streaks of radiopacity. The adjacent vertebral bodies are anchored to each other because of bone formation (ossification) which has occurred in the peripheral part of the annulus fibrosus of the disks.

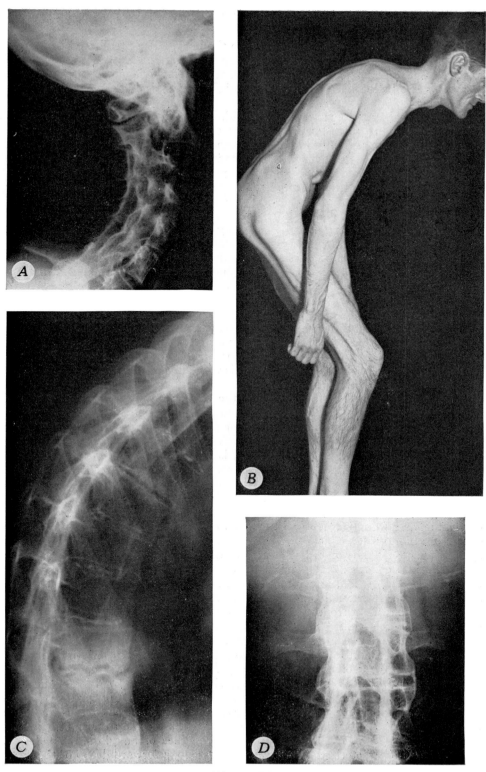

Figure 214

joints antedates the complaints referable to the back. The predilected peripheral joints are the hip joints, shoulder joints, and knee joints. Not uncommonly, the sternoclavicular and temporomandibular joints present evidence of arthritis, and there may also be localized tenderness or pain under or behind the os calcis. (See Fig. 214.)

Constitutional symptoms are usually mild, being largely limited to fatigue and weight loss, although occasionally a patient comes to manifest general ill health, expressed, for instance, in low grade fever, anorexia, loss of weight, and widespread aching. The erythrocyte sedimentation rate is elevated in ankylosing spondylitis, in proportion to the activity of the disease process. Also, it is not unusual for a patient in whom the disease is pronounced and of long duration to show ocular abnormalities in the form of iritis or iridocyclitis, sometimes so severe as to lead to blindness. In a very small percentage of cases, ankylosing spondylitis is associated with cardiovascular changes, and specifically with aortitis (aortic insufficiency), myocarditis (resulting in angina, cardiac enlargement and insufficiency), and also evidence of left bundle branch block (caused by inflammatory damage which results in scarring of the bundle of His) (see Julkunen and Luomanmäki). In addition, the subject may have a pericarditis. Subcutaneous nodules are hardly ever (if ever) encountered in patients affected with ankylosing spondylitis, and the rheumatoid factor is not demonstrable in the serum. In a survey of the literature, Rosenthal et al. found that the presence of subcutaneous nodules was reported in 2 of 1,306 patients affected with ankylosing spondylitis. This extremely low incidence suggests to the present writer the possibility that these two cases actually represented instances of rheumatoid arthritis with advanced and extensive involvement of the vertebral column.

Early in the course of the disease, when the *physical signs* are minimal, one may find merely limitation of movement of the lumbar spine, especially in the lateral directions. Pain on forced movement of, or pressure against, the sacroiliac joints is a highly reliable sign of sacroiliitis, being almost as valuable as positive roentgenographic findings (see Mason). When, later in the course of the disease, the sacroiliac joints become fused, pain is no longer elicited by mild forced movement of, or pressure against, these joints. Ankylosis of the costovertebral and costotransverse articulations leads to restriction of respiratory excursion of the chest and a dorsal kyphosis with limitation of rotation of the dorsal spine. Involvement of the cervical spine naturally results in limitation of movement of the neck, and some degree of atlanto-axial subluxation may be present. With further progress of the spondylitis, peripheral joints become affected. Early or late involvement of the hip joints is a common and particularly disabling feature of the disorder. The rigidity of the hip joints, in conjunction with rigidity of the vertebral column, results in a serious functional handicap (see Hart and Robinson).

It should be evident from what has already been said that there is a wide range of variation in the clinical course of ankylosing spondylitis. In cases pursuing a mild course, in which the onset is insidious and there are minimal constitutional symptoms or none, and little or no elevation of the erythrocyte sedimentation rate, the disease process evolves slowly and may subside temporarily or permanently. However, even if it does subside without having advanced beyond involvement of the sacroiliac joints, the spondylitis may flare up again, perhaps after having remained dormant for some years. When the clinical manifestations of the disease are moderately severe from the beginning, the patient may come to present, within a period of some years, the full-fledged clinical picture of ankylosing spondylitis. This picture is characterized by a lumbodorsal stoop, a forward droop of the head, restricted mobility of the back, and diminished chest expansion. However, in the course of this general trend, there may have been periods of temporary improvement alternating with periods of exacerbation of the condition. When the disease is severe from the beginning, it is associated with constitutional manifestations, the evolution of the disability relating to the vertebral column is rapid, and within a few years the entire column becomes rigid and otherwise deformed.

With modern methods of treatment, the ultimate prognosis is not so doleful now as it was in the past. Indeed, only a small percentage of the afflicted subjects become permanently incapable of any work (see Blumberg and Ragan, and also Hart). However, in cases in which the disease continues and progresses in spite of treatment, amyloidosis sometimes develops, and involvement of the kidneys may result in uremia and the death of the patient.

ROENTGENOGRAPHIC AND PATHOLOGIC FINDINGS

The *roentgenographic findings* in relation to ankylosing spondylitis are rather distinctive and naturally reflect the *pathologic changes* characteristic of the condition. As already noted, the principal sites of these changes insofar as the vertebral column is concerned are the sacroiliac joints, the apophysial articulations, the intervertebral disks, and the paraspinal ligaments. In addition to the sacroiliac joints, other amphiarthroses, such as the manubriosternal articulation and the symphysis pubis, are particularly likely to present evidence of severe damage. Of the large diarthrodial joints, it is especially the hip joints and the shoulder joints that are likely to be involved first, and these may become severely affected and eventually even ankylosed. The knee joints and ankle joints, too, are often implicated and may likewise undergo bony ankylosis. A small percentage of the subjects show involvement of one or both temporomandibular joints (see Maes and Dihlmann).

The presence of *sacroiliitis* (almost always bilateral) is the earliest and most helpful finding in arriving at the roentgenographic diagnosis of ankylosing spondylitis (see Boland and Shebesta, and also Dilsen *et al.*). The details of the changes vary among the cases, in accordance with the duration and severity of the local disease process. At first, an affected sacroiliac joint will show blurring of the joint space (particularly in the lower part of the joint) due to loss of distinctness of the articular margin. Concomitantly, the sacrum and the parts of the iliac bones in the immediate vicinity of the sacroiliac joints come to show small patches of increased radiolucency (osteoporosis) intermingled with patches of radiopacity (osteosclerosis). Progression of the sacroilitis is manifested in a serrated appearance of the joint margins. In the course of time, the joint spaces narrow and then become obliterated, in part or throughout, in consequence of patchy or complete ankylosis of the sacrum with the iliac bones. After obliteration of the sacroiliac joints and fusion of the bones in question, the increased radiopacity presented by these bones recedes, and their radiodensity may now be normal or even somewhat less than normal.

The roentgenographic changes relating to the vertebrae are numerous, and in addition to the dorsal and lumbar portion of the spine, the cervical portion may also be affected (see Meijers *et al.*). Roentgenographs of normal vertebral bodies taken in lateral projection show a concave curve anteriorly. In cases of ankylosing spondylitis, the vertebral bodies often lose this curve and come to present a "squared-off" appearance in the lateral projection. As a result of ossification developing in the peripheral portion of the annulus fibrosus of some of the intervertebral disks, the roentgenographs will show slender, radiopaque bridges (often denoted as *syndesmophytes*) which arch across contiguous vertebral bodies. Eventually, chondroid metaplasia and ossification may also take place in the rest of the annulus and in the nucleus pulposus, and the disks as such may eventually be destroyed, in part or throughout. The replacement of many of the intervertebral disks by spongy bone, the bridging of vertebral bodies by bone formed in the outer part of the annulus fibrosus of the disks, and ossification of the anterior longitudinal ligament help to create the classic roentgenographic picture denoted as the "bamboo spine" of ankylosing spondylitis. (See Figs. 215 and 216.)

One may expect to find roentgenographic changes involving apophysial joints (the facet joints) if clear-cut evidence of sacroiliitis is already present, and if the above-mentioned changes relating to the vertebral bodies and the intervertebral disks are already evolving. In an individual case, only a few of the apophysial joints, here and there, may show clear-cut roentgenographic indications of abnormality. However, the intervening apophysial joints of normal appearance may already have undergone some pathologic changes, even though these are not yet apparent roentgenographically. The progress of the alterations in the apophysial joints is similar to that taking place in the sacroiliac joints. In particular, early in the course of the changes, the outline of the joint is likely to be indistinct, and this appearance is associated with the presence of spotty foci of radiolucency and radiopacity in the pertinent articulating vertebral facets. With further progress of the arthritis involving the facet joints, erosions and irregularities of the articular surfaces become apparent, and finally the severely affected facet joints become obliterated in consequence of bony ankylosis.

Rigidity of the vertebral column is the result of ankylosis of the facet joints and

Figure 215

A, Roentgenograph of the lumbar vertebrae, in anteroposterior projection, from the case of a man 57 years of age who died of myocardial infarction and had no difficulties relating to his vertebral column. This picture is presented as a normal control for the purpose of comparison with *B*. Note that the facet joints stand out clearly, the intervertebral disks show no evidences of ossification, and the interspinous ligaments are neither calcified nor ossified.

B, Roentgenograph of the lumbar vertebrae, in anteroposterior projection, from the case of a man 45 years of age who was affected with ankylosing spondylitis. On admission to the hospital, he stated that he had been in good health until the age of 30, at which time he began to have pain and difficulty relating to the sacroiliac region. Subsequently, he began to complain of difficulties involving his elbows, knees, and hip joints. Physical examination showed that he had complete ankylosis of the vertebral column, hips, knees, and ankles. There was also some evidence of arthritis involving the shoulder and elbow joints. Because both hip joints were ankylosed, an arthroplasty was carried out on the right hip joint. The patient died about 6 weeks after this surgical intervention. The autopsy revealed, in addition to the ankylosing spondylitis and ankylosis of various large diarthrodial joints, the presence of amyloidosis and also pulmonary infarction. In the roentgenograph the facet joints are no longer discernible, having undergone synostosis. The intervertebral disks show radiopacities representing the presence of osseous tissue in them. The spinous processes between the vertebrae are bridged by radiopaque shadows indicative of calcification and ossification of the interspinous ligaments. (Figure 216 also relates to this case.)

C, Roentgenograph of the lumbar vertebrae and part of the sacrum, in lateral projection, from the same case illustrated in *A*. As is normal, the contour of the anterior margin of the vertebral bodies shown is slightly concave. The facet joints are clearly visible.

D, Roentgenograph of part of the vertebral column, in lateral projection, from the same case of ankylosing spondylitis illustrated and described in *B*. Note that the facet joints are no longer discernible, having been obliterated by ossification. The spinous processes are bridged by osseous tissue resulting from ossification of the interspinous ligaments. The intervertebral disks show radiopacities representing the presence of osseous tissue in them. The contour of the anterior margin of the vertebral bodies shown is no longer clearly concave, and this is in accord with the "squaring off" of the bodies. Several of the intervertebral disks reveal that ossification has occurred in the annulus fibrosus and resulted in the formation of so-called syndesmophytes.

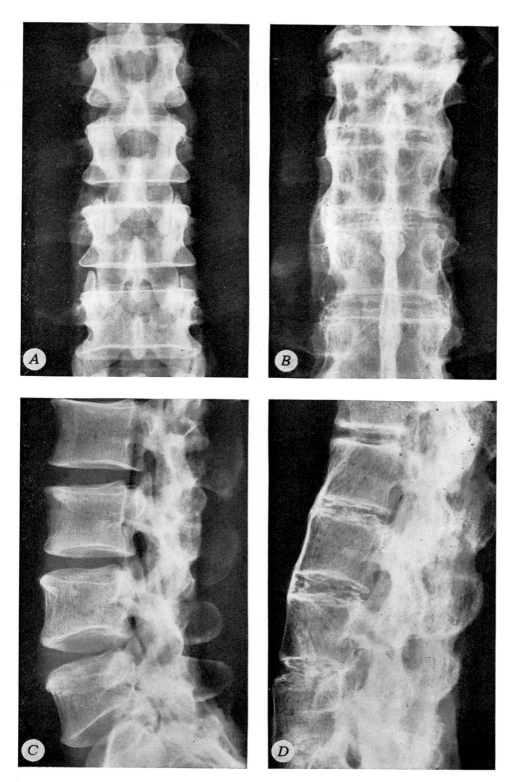

Figure 215

bony bridging of vertebral bodies occurring through ossification of the annulu-fibrosus of the intervertebral disks and also of the interior of the disks. The pathos logic changes relating to the disks result in partial or complete bony fusion of adjacent vertebral bodies. The rigidity of the column is increased by the development of ossifications in the interspinous ligaments and other posterior ligaments, such as the costovertebral ligaments and the ligamenta flava. Furthermore, a vertebral column which is already rigid not uncommonly becomes the site of a fracture or fracture-dislocation after a trauma (for instance, a fall or automobile accident), and the fracture is quite likely to be complicated by neural involvement due to associated injury of the spinal cord (see Grisolia *et al.*, and also Hansen *et al.*). An instance of nontraumatic fracture of the thoracic spine in a case of ankylosing spondylitis has been reported in which the fracture followed upon the minor stress of sitting up forcibly in bed (see Good).

The *pathologic changes* as they relate to the synovial (diarthrodial) joints of the extremities may be regarded as representing a nonspecific chronic arthritis. As already noted, the predilected diarthrodial joints are the hip joints, shoulder joints, and knee joints, and involvement of the small diarthrodial joints of the hands and feet is unusual. In its *early stage*, the inflammatory arthritis implicating the large joints of the extremities in ankylosing spondylitis has pathologic features in common with those of rheumatoid arthritis, but its *terminal stage* tends to be different from that of rheumatoid arthritis involving such joints.

The resemblance between the pathologic changes in affected diarthrodial joints in cases of ankylosing spondylitis and in cases of rheumatoid arthritis relates in particular to the synovial membrane. In both conditions, during their early stages the inflamed synovial membrane shows villous hyperplasia, proliferation of its lining cells, congestion and edema, and infiltration with lymphocytes, plasma cells, and histiocytes. The cells may have diffusely infiltrated the membrane; they may be present in focal collections (sometimes as large follicles having germinal centers); or they may present a perivascular distribution, especially in the deeper layers of the membrane. During the progress of the articular changes, the inflamed synovial membrane undergoes fibrosis, and eventually granulation tissue pannus (fibrovascular pannus) extends from the membrane onto the articular cartilages. The underlying cartilages are eroded and may finally be completely destroyed, and the granulation tissue may penetrate into the subchondral bone. After the articular cartilages have been eroded, union of the bone ends of the joint by cancellous osseous tissue tends to occur, resulting in bony ankylosis. In a knee joint, the intra-articular ligaments and menisci are also destroyed. Thus the difference between the pathologic changes in affected diarthrodial joints in ankylosing spondylitis as compared

Figure 216

A, Photograph of part of the acetabulum and the upper third of the left femur (sectioned in the frontal plane) from the case of the man who had ankylosing spondylitis and arthritis involving various large peripheral joints, and whose case history is given in Figure 215–*B*. Note that the femoral head and the acetabulum are no longer covered by articular cartilage, and that the articular cavity is obliterated because of bony ankylosis.

B, Roentgenograph of the specimen shown in *A* revealing more clearly the bony ankylosis of the hip joint. In several places, trabeculae of bone can be seen joining the femoral head with the acetabulum.

C, Photograph of the left knee joint area removed at autopsy in the same case. The patella is ankylosed to the femoral condyles in the region of the intercondylar groove. The femur is ankylosed to the tibia in a position of slight flexion.

D, Roentgenograph of the ankylosed area shown in *C* after the specimen had been sectioned in the frontal plane, the line of sectioning being deep to the patella.

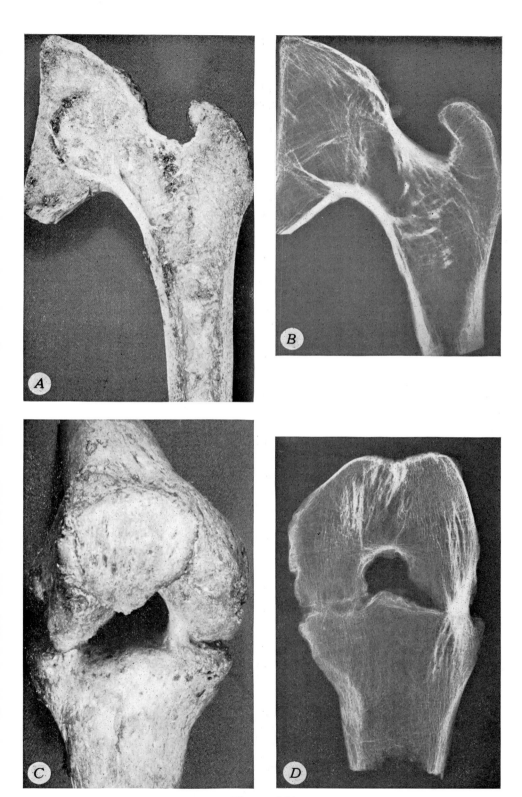

Figure 216

with rheumatoid arthritis, insofar as the ultimate status is concerned, is that in ankylosing spondylitis the joint often undergoes bony ankylosis, while in rheumatoid arthritis the terminal stage is usually a fibrous ankylosis associated with pronounced erosion of the articular bone ends (see Collins, Cruickshank, and also Rutishauser and Jacqueline). (See Fig. 217.)

TREATMENT

The primary objectives of treatment are the abolition of pain and the maintenance of mobility. In cases in which the pain is still mild, it may be overcome by the regular administration of adequate doses of aspirin or other salicylates. If the salicylates do not relieve the pain, the latter will almost certainly yield to the administration of phenylbutazone (Butazolidin). In view of the potential toxicity of the drug, the patient should have careful and continuous medical follow-up, and administration of the drug discontinued if the patient shows such toxic effects as peptic ulceration, skin rashes, and/or blood dyscrasias.

Overcoming or at least reducing the pain is highly important not only in increasing the patient's comfort but in encouraging participation in postural exercises and various other forms of physiotherapy. Normal activity should be encouraged, to facilitate the maintenance of mobility. Good breathing habits are important, and posture should be carefully supervised so that fixation of the spine in a position of forward flexion can be avoided.

The administration of *adrenal corticosteroids* is a treatment of last resort, to be used only if the disease is severe, active, and progressive, and is not controlled by any of the therapeutic measures mentioned above. At any rate, the long-term use of steroids is a hazard in cases of ankylosing spondylitis, since it is associated with

Figure 217

A and B, Photomicrographs ($\times$ 3) showing two intervertebral disks and parts of adjacent vertebral bodies from a case of ankylosing spondylitis. The subject was a middle-aged man whose vertebral column was found at autopsy to be rigidly fixed in a position of pronounced arcuate kyphosis. Some of the ribs were so firmly fused with the vertebral bodies that one could no longer recognize the pertinent intervening joint spaces. Likewise, many of the facet joints were completely synostosed. On sectioning the vertebral column, one could note that the peripheral part of the annulus fibrosus of some of the intervertebral disks had undergone ossification (syndesmophyte formation). In A, at the extreme left, syndesmophyte formation is clearly apparent, and toward the midportion of the disk, the nucleus pulposus is being replaced by spongy bone and marrow. It is also evident that the small portion of the vertebral body above the disk is very poor in spongy bone. In B, at the extreme left, the osseous tissue between the two adjacent vertebral bodies represents a syndesmophyte. Furthermore, it is clear that the annulus fibrosus and a part of the nucleus pulposus have been replaced by spongy bone containing fatty and myeloid marrow. Those portions of the vertebral bodies which are adjacent to the remaining part of the intervertebral disk show a definite sparsity of spongy trabeculae.

C and D, Photomicrographs ($\times$ 4) illustrating even more pronounced destruction of intervertebral disks and their replacement by spongy bone and marrow, resulting in bony synostosis between the adjacent vertebral bodies. The subject in this case was a woman 72 years of age who had clinical manifestations of ankylosing spondylitis for many years, as manifested by a pronounced arcuate kyphosis. In C a portion of the intervertebral disk is still clearly apparent on the right side of the picture, while on the left side, only small fragments of disk tissue are still discernible. In D, practically the entire disk has been destroyed and replaced by spongy bone, but a few small fragments are still discernible and mark its previous site.

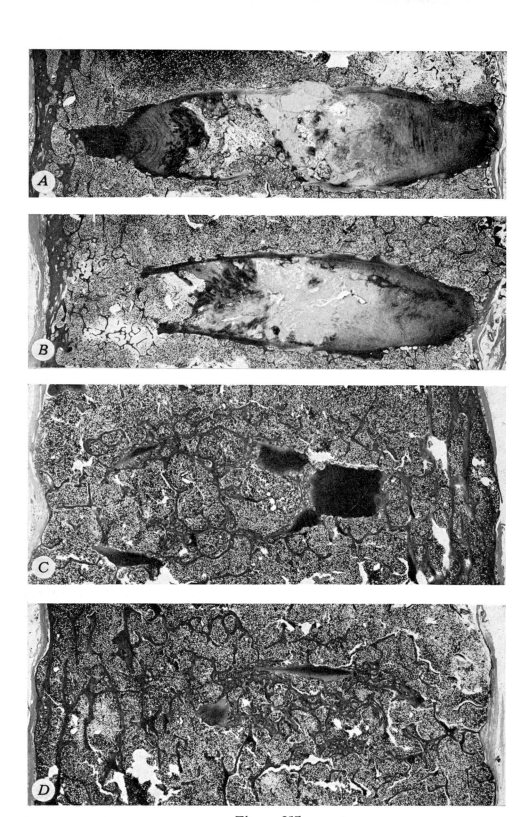

Figure 217

the same complications as those ensuing from their use in instances of classic rheumatoid arthritis.

The use of *radiation therapy* over areas of the spine which are tender, painful, and stiff usually results in relief from symptoms.   However, even when there is a fairly prompt favorable response to radiation therapy, relapses tend to occur, and the long-term course of the condition is not favorably influenced.   Moreover, radiation therapy seems to be fraught with definite hazards in cases of ankylosing spondylitis. In particular, it appears that patients affected with the condition who have been given repeated irradiation therapy show an almost tenfold increase in their chance of developing leukemia (especially myeloid leukemia) in comparison with non-irradiated patients or with the general population (see Court Brown and Abbatt, and also Abbatt and Lea).   It is also known that in the irradiated spondylitics the incidence of aplastic anemia is about 40 times as high as in the general population. Furthermore, one must consider the danger of radiation injury to the spinal cord (radiation-induced myelitis) if the total dose given is large and if the daily dose is much more than 100 *r*.

Surgical procedures, too, are sometimes used, mainly for the correction of advanced kyphosis and for relief of the disability caused by the pain, loss of mobility, and flexion deformity due to involvement of the hip joints.   *Osteotomy* of the laminae and articular facets is the surgical procedure appropriate for the correction of the kyphosis.   The purpose of vertebral osteotomy is not to restore mobility of the spine but to correct the deformity and achieve subsequent re-ankylosis in a better position (see Herbert, and also Goel).   *Arthroplasty* is the usual surgical procedure for difficulties relating to a hip joint or both hip joints.

REFERENCES

Abbatt, J. D. and Lea, A. J.: The Incidence of Leukaemia in Ankylosing Spondylitis Treated with X Rays, Lancet, *2*, 1317, 1956.

Abruzzo, J. L. and Christian, C. L.: Induction of a Rheumatoid Factor-Like Substance in Rabbits, Arthritis Rheum., *4*, 103, 1961.

Alexander, W. R. M. and McCarthy, D. D.: The Clinical Significance of the Rheumatoid Factor, in *Modern Trends in Rheumatology*, edited by A. G. S. Hill, New York, Appleton-Century-Crofts, 1966.

Ansell, B. M. and Bywaters, E. G. L.: Rheumatoid Arthritis (Still's Disease), Pediat. Clin. North America, *10*, 921, 1963.

Ansell, B. M. and Wigley, R. A. D.: Arthritic Manifestations in Regional Enteritis, Ann. Rheumat. Dis., *23*, 64, 1964.

Arapakis, G. and Tribe, C. R.: Amyloidosis in Rheumatoid Arthritis Investigated by Means of Rectal Biopsy, Ann. Rheumat. Dis., *22*, 256, 1963.

Astorga, G. and Bollet, A. J.: Diagnostic Specificity and Possible Pathogenetic Significance of Inclusions in Synovial Leucocytes, Arthritis Rheum., *8*, 511, 1965.

Avila, R., Pugh, D. G., Slocumb, C. H. and Winkelmann, R. K.: Psoriatic Arthritis: A Roentgenologic Study, Radiology, *75*, 691, 1960.

Baer, G. J.: Fractures in Chronic Arthritis, Ann. Rheumat. Dis., *2*, 269, 1941.

Baker, H., Golding, D. N. and Thompson, M.: Psoriasis and Arthritis, Ann. Int. Med., *58*, 909, 1963.

Barland, P., Novikoff, A. B. and Hamerman, D.: Lysosomes in the Synovial Membrane in Rheumatoid Arthritis: A Mechanism for Cartilage Erosion, Tr. A. Am. Physicians, *77*, 239, 1964.

————: Fine Structure and Cytochemistry of the Rheumatoid Synovial Membrane, with Special Reference to Lysosomes, Am. J. Path., *44*, 853, 1964.

Bauer, W. and Engleman, E. P.: A Syndrome of Unknown Etiology Characterized by Urethritis, Conjunctivitis, and Arthritis (So-called Reiter's Disease), Tr. A. Am. Physicans, *57*, 307, 1942.

Bennett, P. H. and Scott, J. T.: Autonomic Neuropathy in Rheumatoid Arthritis, Ann. Rheumat. Dis., *24*, 161, 1965.

Black, R. L. and O'Brien, W. M.: Observations on Psoriatic Arthritis, Arch. Interamerican Rheumatol., *7*, 44, 1964.

BLUHM, G. B., RIDDLE, J. M. and BARNHART, M. I.: Inflammatory Dynamics in the Rheumatoid Joint, J. Bone & Joint Surg., *49–A*, 1234, 1967.

BLUMBERG, B. and RAGAN, C.: The Natural History of Rheumatoid Spondylitis, Bull. Rheumat. Dis., *6*, 95, 1955.

BOLAND, E. W. and SHEBESTA, E. M.: Rheumatoid Spondylitis: Correlation of Clinical and Roentgenographic Features, Radiology, *47*, 551, 1946.

BRODIE, B. C.: *Pathological and Surgical Observations on Diseases of the Joints*, London, Longman, Hurst, Rees, Orme and Brown, 1818 (see p. 54).

BROWN, S. I. and GRAYSON, M.: Marginal Furrows. A Characteristic Corneal Lesion of Rheumatoid Arthritis, Arch. Ophth., *79*, 563, 1968.

BUCHAN, J. F.: Reiter's Disease: A Review of the Present Position, Proc. Roy. Soc. Med., *48*, 432, 1955.

BUNIM, J. J., BURCH, T. A. and O'BRIEN, W. M.: Influence of Genetic and Environmental Factors on the Occurrence of Rheumatoid Arthritis and Rheumatoid Factor in American Indians, Bull. Rheumat. Dis., *15*, 349, 1964.

BYWATERS, E. G. L.: The Relation between Heart and Joint Disease including "Rheumatoid Heart Disease" and Chronic Post-Rheumatic Arthritis (Type Jaccoud), Brit. Heart J., *12*, 101, 1950.

BYWATERS, E. G. L. and DIXON, A. St. J.: Paravertebral Ossification in Psoriatic Arthritis, Ann. Rheumat. Dis., *24*, 313, 1965.

BYWATERS, E. G. L., GLYNN, L. E. and ZELDIS, A.: Subcutaneous Nodules of Still's Disease, Ann. Rheumat. Dis., *17*, 278, 1958.

CAPLAN, A.: Certain Unusual Radiological Appearances in the Chest of Coal-miners Suffering from Rheumatoid Arthritis, Thorax, *8*, 29, 1953.

CAPLAN, A., PAYNE, R. B. and WITHEY, J. L.: A Broader Concept of Caplan's Syndrome Related to Rheumatoid Factors, Thorax, *17*, 205, 1962.

CARTER, M. E.: Sacro-Iliitis in Still's Disease, Ann. Rheumat. Dis., *21*, 105, 1962.

CARTER, M. E. and LOEWI, G.: Anatomical Changes in Normal Sacro-Iliac Joints during Childhood and Comparison with the Changes in Still's Disease, Ann. Rheumat. Dis., *21*, 121, 1962.

CASSIDY, J. T., and VALKENBURG, H. A.: A Five Year Prospective Study of Rheumatoid Factor Tests in Juvenile Rheumatoid Arthritis, Arthritis Rheum., *10*, 83, 1967.

CASSIDY, J. T., BRODY, G. L. and MARTEL, W.: Monarticular Juvenile Rheumatoid Arthritis, J. Pediat., *70*, 867, 1967.

CHARCOT, J. M.: Études pour servir a l'histoire de l'affection décrite sous les noms de goutte asthénique primitive, nodosités des jointures, rhumatisme articulaire chronique (forme primitive), etc., Paris Theses, No. 44, 1853.

CLAUS, G., McEWEN, C., BRUNNER, T. and TSAMPARLIS, G.: Microbiological Studies of Reiter's Disease, Brit. J. Ven. Dis., *40*, 170, 1964.

CLAWSON, B. J. and WETHERBY, M.: Subcutaneous Nodules in Chronic Arthritis, Am. J. Path., *8*, 283, 1932.

CLAWSON, B. J., NOBLE, J. F. and LUFKIN, N. H.: Nodular Inflammatory and Degenerative Lesions of Muscles from Four Hundred and Fifty Autopsies, Arch. Path., *43*, 579, 1947.

COATES, V. and COOMBS, C. F.: Observations on the Rheumatic Nodule, Arch. Dis. Childhood, *1*, 183, 1926.

COLLINS, D. H.: *The Pathology of Articular and Spinal Diseases*, Baltimore, The Williams & Wilkins Company, 1950 (p. 169).

COSTE, F. and SOLNICA, J.: La polyarthrite psoriasique, Rev. franç. d'études clin. et biol., *11*, 578, 1966.

COURT BROWN, W. M. and ABBATT, J. D.: The Incidence of Leukaemia in Ankylosing Spondylitis Treated with X Rays, Lancet, *1*, 1283, 1955.

COVENTRY, M. B., POLLEY, H. F. and WEINER, A. D.: Rheumatoid Synovial Cyst of the Hip, J. Bone & Joint Surg., *41–A*, 721, 1959.

CRUICKSHANK, B.: Histopathology of Diarthrodial Joints in Ankylosing Spondylitis, Ann. Rheumat. Dis., *10*, 393, 1951.

————: The Arteritis of Rheumatoid Arthritis, Ann. Rheumat. Dis., *13*, 136, 1954.

————: Lesions of Cartilaginous Joints in Ankylosing Spondylitis, J. Path. & Bact., *71*, 73, 1956.

————: Pathology of Ankylosing Spondylitis, Bull. Rheumat. Dis., *10*, 211, 1960.

DAMESHEK, W. and WELCH, C. S.: *Hypersplenism and Surgery of the Spleen*, New York, Grune & Stratton, Inc., 1953.

DAWSON, M. H.: A Comparative Study of Subcutaneous Nodules in Rheumatic Fever and Rheumatoid Arthritis, J. Exper. Med., *57*, 845, 1933.

DE FOREST, G. K., BUNTING, H. and KENNEY, W. E.: The Diagnostic Significance of Focal Cellular Accumulations in the Skeletal Muscles of Patients with Rheumatoid Arthritis, Ann. Rheumat. Dis., *6*, 86, 1947.

DE GRUCHY, G. C. and LANGLEY, G. R.: Felty's Syndrome, Australasian Ann. Med., *10*, 292, 1961.

DESMARAIS, M. H. L., GIBSON, H. J. and KERSLEY, G. D.: Muscle Histology in Rheumatic and Control Cases: A Study of One Hundred and Nineteen Biopsy Specimens, Ann. Rheumat. Dis., 7, 132, 1948.

DILSEN, N., McEWEN, C., POPPEL, M., GERSH, W. J., DiTATA, D. and CARMEL, P: A Comparative Roentgenologic Study of Rheumatoid Arthritis and Rheumatoid (Ankylosing) Spondylitis, Arthritis Rheum., 5, 341, 1962.

DINGLE, J. T.: Lysosomal Enzymes and the Degradation of Cartilage Matrix, Proc. Roy. Soc. Med., 55, 109, 1962.

DIXON, A. ST. J. and GRANT, C.: Acute Synovial Rupture in Rheumatoid Arthritis, Lancet, 1, 742, 1964.

DUTHIE, J. J. R., BROWN, P. E., KNOX, J. D. E. and THOMPSON, M.: Course and Prognosis in Rheumatoid Arthritis, Ann. Rheumat. Dis., 16, 411, 1957.

ENGLEMAN, E. P. and WEBER, H. M.: Reiter's Syndrome, Clin. Orthopaedics, 57, 19, 1968.

EPSTEIN, B. S.: Sternoclavicular Arthritis in Patients with Scleroderma and Rheumatoid Arthritis, Am. J. Roentgenol., 89, 1236, 1963.

FAHR, T.: Zur Frage des Rheumatismus nodosus, Centralbl. allg. Path., 29, 625, 1918.

FAVREAU, J. C. and LAURIN, C. A.: La maladie rhumatoïde de l'enfant, Union méd. Canada, 92, 848, 1963.

FEARNLEY, G. R. and LACKNER, R.: Amyloidosis in Rheumatoid Arthritis, and Significance of "Unexplained" Albuminuria, Brit. M. J., 1, 1129, 1955.

FELTY, A. R.: Chronic Arthritis in the Adult, Associated with Splenomegaly and Leucopenia, Bull. Johns Hopkins Hosp., 35, 16, 1924.

FERGUSON, R. H. and SLOCUMB, C. H.: Peripheral Neuropathy in Rheumatoid Arthritis, Bull. Rheumat. Dis., 11, 251, 1961.

FINGERMAN, D. L. and ANDRUS, F. C.: Visceral Lesions Associated with Rheumatoid Arthritis, Ann. Rheumat. Dis., 3, 168, 1942–43.

FORD, D. K.: Non-Gonococcal Urethritis and Reiter's Syndrome: Personal Experience with Etiological Studies During 15 Years, Canad. M. A. J., 99, 900, 1968.

FORD, D. K. and VALLIS, D. G.: The Clinical Course of Arthritis Associated with Ulcerative Colitis and Regional Ileitis, Arthritis Rheum., 2, 526, 1959.

FREUND, E.: Über rheumatische Knötchen bei chronischer Polyarthritis, Wien. Arch. inn. Med., 16, 73, 1928.

FREUND, H. A., STEINER, G., LEICHTENTRITT, B. and PRICE, A. E.: Peripheral Nerves in Chronic Atrophic Arthritis, Am. J. Path., 18, 865, 1942.

GARDNER, D. L. and ROY, L. M. H.: Tissue Iron and the Reticulo-endothelial System in Rheumatoid Arthritis, Ann. Rheumat. Dis., 20, 258, 1961.

GARROD, A. E.: A Treatise on Rheumatism and Rheumatoid Arthritis, Philadelphia, P. Blakiston, Son & Company, 1890.

GIBBERD, F. B., GILBERTSON, C. and JEPSON, E. M.: Felty's Syndrome: Radio-active Isotope Studies and Splenectomy, Ann. Rheumat. Dis., 24, 46, 1965.

GLAY, A. and RONA, G.: Nodular Rheumatoid Vertebral Lesions versus Ankylosing Spondylitis, Am. J. Roentgenol., 94, 631, 1965.

GOEL, M. K.: Vertebral Osteotomy for Correction of Fixed Flexion Deformity of the Spine, J. Bone & Joint Surg., 50-A, 287, 1968.

GOFTON, J. P.: Differential Diagnosis of Ankylosing Spondylitis and Rheumatoid Arthritis, M. Clin. North America, 52, 517, 1968.

GOOD, A. E.: Nontraumatic Fracture of the Thoracic Spine in Ankylosing Spondylitis, Arthritis Rheum., 10, 467, 1967.

GOODE, J. D.: Synovial Rupture of the Elbow Joint, Ann. Rheumat. Dis., 27, 604, 1968.

GREENBURY, C. L.: A Comparison of the Rose-Waaler, Latex Fixation, "RA-Test," and Bentonite Flocculation Tests, J. Clin. Path., 13, 325, 1960.

GRISOLIA, A., BELL, R. L. and PELTIER, L. F.: Fractures and Dislocations of the Spine Complicating Ankylosing Spondylitis, J. Bone & Joint Surg., 49-A, 339, 1967.

GRUENWALD, P.: Visceral Lesions in a Case of Rheumatoid Arthritis, Arch. Path., 46, 59, 1948.

HALL, A. P. and SCOTT, J. T.: Synovial Cysts and Rupture of the Knee Joint in Rheumatoid Arthritis, Ann. Rheumat. Dis., 25, 32, 1966.

HAMERMAN, D.: New Thoughts on the Pathogenesis of Rheumatoid Arthritis, Am. J. Med., 40, 1, 1966.

————: Views on the Pathogenesis of Rheumatoid Arthritis, M. Clin. North America, 52, 593, 1968.

HANSEN, S. T., Jr., TAYLOR, T. K. F., HONET, J. C. and LEWIS, F. R.: Fracture-Dislocations of the Ankylosed Thoracic Spine in Rheumatoid Spondylitis. Ankylosing Spondylitis, Marie-Strümpell Disease, J. Trauma, 7, 827, 1967.

HART, F. D.: Ankylosing Spondylitis, Brit. M. J., 2, 1082, 1958.

HART, F. D. and ROBINSON, K. C.: Ankylosing Spondylitis in Women, Ann. Rheumat. Dis., *18*, 15, 1959.

HERBERT, J.-J.: Vertebral Osteotomy for Kyphosis, Especially in Marie-Strümpell Arthritis, J. Bone & Joint Surg., *41–A*, 291, 1959.

HOLLANDER, J. L., REGINATO, A. and TORRALBA, T. P.: Examination of Synovial Fluid as a Diagnostic Aid in Arthritis, M. Clin. North America, *50*, 1281, 1966.

HUTCHISON, H. E. and ALEXANDER, W. D.: Splenic Neutropenia in the Felty Syndrome, Blood, *9*, 986, 1954.

HUTT, M. S. R., RICHARDSON, J. S. and STAFFURTH, J. S.: Felty's Syndrome. A Report of Four Cases Treated by Splenectomy, Quart. J. Med., *20*, 57, 1951.

JAJIĆ, I.: Radiological Changes in the Sacro-iliac Joints and Spine of Patients with Psoriatic Arthritis and Psoriasis, Ann. Rheumat. Dis., *27*, 1, 1968.

JAYSON, M. I. V. and BOUCHIER, I. A. D.: Ulcerative Colitis with Ankylosing Spondylitis, Ann. Rheumat. Dis., *27*, 219, 1968.

JEREMY, R., SCHALLER, J., ARKLESS, R., WEDGWOOD, R. J. and HEALEY, L. A.: Juvenile Rheumatoid Arthritis Persisting into Adulthood, Am. J. Med., *45*, 419, 1968.

JOHANSEN, P. E.: Synovial Lining Cells and Plasma Cells in the Synovial Membrane in Cases of Classic Rheumatoid Arthritis, Acta rheumat. scandinav., *11*, 4, 1965.

JOHNSON, R. L., SMYTH, C. J., HOLT, G. W., LUBCHENCO, A. and VALENTINE, E.: Steroid Therapy and Vascular Lesions in Rheumatoid Arthritis, Arthritis Rheum., *2*, 224, 1959.

JULKUNEN, H. and LUOMANMÄKI, K.: Complete Heart Block in Rheumatoid (Ankylosing) Spondylitis, Acta med. scandinav., *176*, 401, 1964.

KAPLAN, D., PLOTZ, C. M., NATHANSON, L. and FRANK, L.: Cervical Spine in Psoriasis and in Psoriatic Arthritis, Ann. Rheumat. Dis., *23*, 50, 1964.

KELLGREN, J. H., LAWRENCE, J. S. and AITKEN-SWAN, J.: Rheumatic Complaints in an Urban Population, Ann. Rheumat. Dis., *12*, 5, 1953.

KELLY, J. J., III, and WEISIGER, B. B.: The Arthritis of Whipple's Disease, Arthritis Rheum., *6*, 615, 1963.

KIMURA, S. J., HOGAN, M. J., O'CONNOR, G. R. and EPSTEIN, W. V.: Uveitis and Joint Diseases, Arch. Ophth., *77*, 309, 1967.

KNAGGS, R. L.: Report on the Strangeways Collection of Rheumatoid Joints in the Museum of the Royal College of Surgeons, Brit. J. Surg., *20*, 113, 309, 425, 1932–33.

KREBS, A.: Über Psoriasis arthropathica, Schweiz. med. Wchnschr., *92*, 29, 1962.

KULKA, J. P.: Vascular Derangement in Rheumatoid Arthritis, in *Modern Trends in Rheumatology*, edited by A. G. S. Hill, New York, Appleton-Century-Crofts, 1966.

LAAKSONEN, A.-L.: A Prognostic Study of Juvenile Rheumatoid Arthritis, Acta paediat. scandinav., Suppl. 166, 1, 1966.

LAINE, V. A. I.: Rheumatic Complaints in an Urban Population in Finland, Acta rheumat. scandinav., *8*, 81, 1962.

LASSUS, A., MUSTAKALLIO, K. K. and LAINE, V.: Psoriasis Arthropathy and Rheumatoid Arthritis, Acta rheumat. scandinav., *10*, 62, 1964.

LASSUS, A., MUSTAKALLIO, K. K., LAINE, V., and WAGER, O.: The Lack of Rheumatoid Factor in Psoriatic Arthritis, Acta rheumat. scandinav., *10*, 69, 1964.

LAWRENCE, J. S., LAINE, V. A. I. and de GRAAFF, R.: The Epidemiology of Rheumatoid Arthritis in Northern Europe, Proc. Roy. Soc. Med., *54*, 454, 1961.

LEHMAN, M. A., KREAM, J. and BROGNA, D.: Acid and Alkaline Phosphatase Activity in the Serum and Synovial Fluid of Patients with Arthritis, J. Bone & Joint Surg., *46–A*, 1732, 1964.

LINQUIST, P. R., and McDONNELL, D. E.: Rheumatoid Cyst Causing Extradural Compression, J. Bone & Joint Surg., *52-A*, 1235, 1970.

LUNDBERG, M. and ERICSON, S.: Changes in the Temporomandibular Joint in Psoriasis Arthropathica, Acta dermat.–venereol., *47*, 354, 1967.

MAES, H. J. and DIHLMANN, W.: Befall der Temporomandibulargelenke bei der Spondylitis ankylopoetica, Fortschr. Geb. Röntgenstrahlen, *109*, 513, 1968.

MARTEL, W. and DUFF, I. F.: Pelvo-Spondylitis in Rheumatoid Arthritis, Radiology, *77*, 744, 1961.

MARTEL, W., HOLT, J. F. and CASSIDY, J. T.: Roentgenologic Manifestations of Juvenile Rheumatoid Arthritis, Am. J. Roentgenol., *88*, 400, 1962.

MASON, D. T. and MORRIS, J. J., Jr.: The Variable Features of Felty's Syndrome. Review of the Literature, and Report of a Case with Massive Splenomegaly, Am. J. Med., *36*, 463, 1964.

MASON, R. M.: Ankylosing Spondylitis, Chap. XII in *Textbook of the Rheumatic Diseases*, edited by W. S. C. Copeman, 3rd ed., Edinburgh and London, E & S Livingstone Ltd., 1964.

MAUDSLEY, R. H. and ARDEN, G. P.: Rheumatoid Cysts of the Calf and Their Relation to Baker's Cysts of the Knee, J. Bone & Joint Surg., *43–B*, 87, 1961.

McEWEN, C., LINGG, C., KIRSNER, J. B. and SPENCER, J. A.: Arthritis Accompanying Ulcerative Colitis, Am. J. Med., *33*, 923, 1962.

MEIJERS, K. A. E., HEERMA VAN VOSS, S. F. C. and FRANÇOIS, R. J.: Radiological Changes in the Cervical Spine in Ankylosing Spondylitis, Ann. Rheumat. Dis., *27*, 333, 1968.

MELLORS, R. C., HEIMER, R., CORCOS, J. and KORNGOLD, L.: Cellular Origin of Rheumatoid Factor, J. Exper. Med., *110*, 875, 1959.

MÉNDEZ-BRYAN, R., GONZÁLEZ-ALCOVER, R. and ROGER, L.: Rheumatoid Arthritis: Prevalence in a Tropical Area, Arthritis Rheum., *7*, 171, 1964.

MESARA, B. W., BRODY, G. L. and OBERMAN, H. A.: "Pseudorheumatoid" Subcutaneous Nodules, Am. J. Clin. Path., *45*, 684, 1966.

MEYNET, P.: Rhumatisme articulaire subaigu avec production de tumeurs multiples dans les tissus fibreux périarticulaires et sur le périoste d'un grand nombre d'os, Lyon méd., *20*, 495, 1875.

MIALL, W. E.: Rheumatoid Arthritis in Males. An Epidemiological Study of a Welsh Mining Community, Ann. Rheumat. Dis., *14*, 150, 1955.

MILGROM, F. and WITEBSKY, E.: Studies on the Rheumatoid and Related Serum Factors. I. Autoimmunization of Rabbits with Gamma Globulin, J.A.M.A., *174*, 56, 1960.

MILGROM, F., WITEBSKY, E., GOLDSTEIN, R. and LOZA, U.: Studies on the Rheumatoid and Related Serum Factors. II. Relation of Anti-Human and Anti-Rabbit Gamma Globulin Factors in Rheumatoid Arthritis Serums, J.A.M.A., *181*, 476, 1962.

MILLER, B., MARKHEIM, H. R. and TOWBIN, M. N.: Multiple Stress Fractures in Rheumatoid Arthritis, J. Bone & Joint Surg., *49–A*, 1408, 1967.

MONGAN, E. S. and JACOX, R. F.: Erythrocyte Survival in Rheumatoid Arthritis, Arthritis Rheum., *7*, 481, 1964.

NATHAN, F. F. and BICKEL, W. H.: Spontaneous Axial Subluxation in a Child as the First Sign of Juvenile Rheumatoid Arthritis, J. Bone & Joint Surg., *50–A*, 1675, 1968.

NICHOLS, E. H. and RICHARDSON, F. L.: Arthritis Deformans, J. Med. Research, n.s. *16*, 149, 1909.

NOER, H. R.: An "Experimental" Epidemic of Reiter's Syndrome, J.A.M.A., *197*, 693, 1966.

NORTON, W. L. and STORZ, J.: Light and Electron Microscopic Studies of Synovium from Sheep Polyarthritis Caused by an Agent of the Psittacosis-lymphogranuloma Venereum-trachoma Group, Arthritis Rheum., *9*, 528, 1966.

OKA, M. and VAINIO, U.: Effect of Pregnancy on the Prognosis and Serology of Rheumatoid Arthritis, Acta rheumat. scandinav., *12*, 47, 1966.

PALMER, D. G.: Synovial Cysts in Rheumatoid Disease, Ann. Int. Med., *70*, 61, 1969.

PARONEN, I.: Reiter's Disease, Acta med. scandinav., *131*, Suppl. 212, 1948.

PEDEN, J. C., Jr.: Hypersplenism: Two Cases with Leg Ulcers Treated by Splenectomy, Ann. Int. Med., *30*, 1248, 1949.

PEKIN, T. J., Jr., MALININ, T. I. and ZVAIFLER, N. J.: Unusual Synovial Fluid Findings in Reiter's Syndrome, Ann. Int. Med., *66*, 677, 1967.

PERRI, J. A., RODNAN, G. P. and MANKIN, H. J.: Giant Synovial Cysts of the Calf in Patients with Rheumatoid Arthritis, J. Bone & Joint Surg., *50–A*, 709, 1968.

PETERS, J. H.: Reiter's Syndrome with Keratotic Dermatitis, Arch. Dermat. & Syph., *59*, 217, 1949.

PETERSON, C. C., Jr. and SILBIGER, M. L.: Reiter's Syndrome and Psoriatic Arthritis, Am. J. Roentgenol., *101*, 860, 1967.

PINALS, R. S.: Rheumatoid Arthritis Presenting with Laryngeal Obstruction, Brit. M. J., *1*, 842, 1966.

PIRANI, C. L. and BENNETT, G. A.: Rheumatoid Arthritis: A Report of Three Cases Progressing from Childhood and Emphasizing Certain Systemic Manifestations, Bull. Hosp. Joint Dis., *12*, 335, 1951.

PORTIS, R. B.: Pathology of Chronic Arthritis of Children (Still's Disease), Am. J. Dis. Child., *55*, 1000, 1938.

POTTER, T. A. and KUHNS, J. G.: Rheumatoid Tenosynovitis, J. Bone & Joint Surg., *40–A*, 1230, 1958.

REED, W. B.: Psoriatic Arthritis, Acta dermat.-venereol., *41*, 396, 1961.

REITER, H.: Ueber eine bisher unerkannte Spirochäteninfektion (Spirochaetosis arthritica), Deutsche med. Wchnschr., *42²*, 1535, 1916.

ROBINSON, H. S.: Rheumatoid Arthritis—Atlanto-Axial Subluxation and Its Clinical Presentation, Canad. M. A. J., *94*, 470, 1966.

ROSENTHAL, S. H., LIDSKY, M. D. and SHARP, J. T.: Arthritis With Nodules Following Ankylosing Spondylitis, J.A.M.A., *206*, 2893, 1968.

RUDERMAN, M., MILLER, L. M. and PINALS, R. S.: Clinical and Serologic Observations on 27 Patients with Felty's Syndrome, Arthritis Rheum., *11*, 377, 1968.

RUTISHAUSER, E. and JACQUELINE, F.: Involvement of the Hip in Ankylosing Spondylitis and Rheumatoid Arthritis, Documenta Geigy, Acta rheumatologica, No. 16, Basle, 1964.

SCHACHTER, J., BARNES, M. G., JONES, J. P., Jr., ENGLEMAN, E. P. and MEYER, K. F.: Isolation of Bedsoniae from the Joints of Patients with Reiter's Syndrome, Proc. Soc. Exper. Biol. & Med., *122*, 283, 1966.

SCHIERZ, G., STOEBER, E., MEIGEL, W., UNCKELL, F.-M., and KÖLLE, G.: Der Rheumafaktor bei juveniler rheumatoider Arthritis und bei Morbus Still, Munchen. med. Wchnschr., *46*, 2684, 1968.

SCHLESINGER, B.: Still's Disease, Chap. XI in *Textbook of the Rheumatic Diseases*, edited by W. S. C. Copeman, 3rd ed., Edinburgh and London, E & S Livingstone Ltd., 1964.

SCHMORL, G. and JUNGHANNS, H.: *Die gesunde und kranke Wirbelsäule im Röntgenbild*, Leipzig, Georg Thieme, 1932.

SCHWAB, J. H., CROMARTIE, W. J., OHANIAN, S. H. and CRADDOCK, J. G.: Association of Experimental Chronic Arthritis with the Persistence of Group A Streptococcal Cell Walls in the Articular Tissue, J. Bact., *94*, 1728, 1967.

SERRE, H., SIMON, L., GIVAUDAND, A. and BENAMARA, M.: La radiographie du pied dans le diagnostic de la polyarthrite chronique évolutive, J. radiol. et électrol., *43*, 728, 1962.

SHARP, J.: Ankylosing Spondylitis, Reports on Rheumatic Diseases, No. 12, Empire Rheumatism Council, London, 1962.

SHARP, J. and PURSER, D. W.: Spontaneous Atlanto-Axial Dislocation in Ankylosing Spondylitis and Rheumatoid Arthritis, Ann. Rheumat. Dis., *20*, 47, 1961.

SHERMAN, M. S.: Psoriatic Arthritis. Observations on the Clinical, Roentgenographic, and Pathological Changes, J. Bone & Joint Surg., *34–A*, 831, 1952.

SHERRY, M. G.: The Incidence of Positive RA Tests in Hodgkin's Disease and Leukemia, Am. J. Clin. Path., *50*, 398, 1968.

SHLIONSKY, H. and BLAKE, F. G.: Arthritis Psoriatica; Report of a Case, Ann. Int. Med., *10*, 537, 1936.

SHORT, C. L., BAUER, W. and REYNOLDS, W. E.: *Rheumatoid Arthritis*, Cambridge, Harvard University Press, 1957.

SINCLAIR, R. J. G. and CRUICKSHANK, B.: A Clinical and Pathological Study of Sixteen Cases of Rheumatoid Arthritis with Extensive Visceral Involvement ('Rheumatoid Disease'), Quart. J. Med., *25*, 313, 1956.

SMITH, R. J. and KAPLAN, E. B.: Rheumatoid Deformities at the Metacarpophalangeal Joints of the Fingers, J. Bone & Joint Surg., *49–A*, 31, 1967.

SOKOLOFF, L. and BUNIM, J.: Vascular Lesions in Rheumatoid Arthritis, J. Chronic Dis., *5*, 668, 1957.

SOREN, A.: Joint Affections in Regional Ileitis, Arch. Int. Med., *117*, 78, 1966.

STEINBERG, V. L. and PARRY, C. B. W.: Electromyographic Changes in Rheumatoid Arthritis, Brit. M. J., *1*, 630, 1961.

STILL, G. F.: On a Form of Chronic Joint Disease in Children, Med.-Chir. Tr., *80*, 47, 1897.

SWIFT, H. F.: Rheumatic Fever, J.A.M.A., *92*, 2071, 1929.

TEILUM, G. and LINDAHL, A.: Frequency and Significance of Amyloid Changes in Rheumatoid Arthritis, Acta med. scandinav., *149*, 449, 1954.

TOURAINE, A. and RUEL, A.: La pseudo-gonococcie entéritique, Ann. dermat. et syph., *6*, 61, 1946.

TRIBE, C. R.: Amyloidosis in Rheumatoid Arthritis, in *Modern Trends in Rheumatology*, edited by A. G. S. Hill, New York, Appleton-Century-Crofts, 1966.

VASSALLO, C. L.: Rheumatoid Arthritis of the Cricoarytenoid Joints, Arch. Int. Med., *117*, 273, 1966.

VAUGHAN, J. H. and BUTLER, V. P., Jr.: Current Status of the Rheumatoid Factor, Ann. Int. Med., *56*, 1, 1962.

WEBB, F. W. S., HICKMAN, J. A. and BREW, D. St. J.: Death from Vertebral Artery Thrombosis in Rheumatoid Arthritis, Brit. M. J., *2*, 537, 1968.

WEICHSELBAUM, A.: Über die senilen Veränderungen der Gelenke und deren Zusammenhang mit der Arthritis deformans, Sitzungsb. Kais. Akad. Wissensch. Math.-natur. Classe. Wien, *75–76*, 193, 1877.

WEINBERGER, H. W., ROPES, M. W., KULKA, J. P. and BAUER, W.: Reiter's Syndrome, Clinical and Pathologic Observations, Medicine, *41*, 35, 1962.

WELDON, W. V. and SCALETTAR, R.: Roentgen Changes in Reiter's Syndrome, Am. J. Roentgenol., *86*, 344, 1961.

WEST, H. F.: The Aetiology of Ankylosing Spondylitis, Ann. Rheumat. Dis., *8*, 143, 1949.

WHALEY, K. and DICK, W. C.: Fatal Subaxial Dislocation of Cervical Spine in Rheumatoid Arthritis, Brit. M. J., *2*, 31, 1968.

WISEMAN, B. K. and DOAN, C. A.: Primary Splenic Neutropenia; A Newly Recognized Syndrome, Closely Related to Congenital Hemolytic Icterus and Essential Thrombocytopenic Purpura, Ann. Int. Med., *16*, 1097, 1942.

WRIGHT, V.: Psoriatic Arthritis, Ann. Rheumat. Dis., *20*, 123, 1961.

WRIGHT, V., and REED, W. B.: The Link between Reiter's Syndrome and Psoriatic Arthritis, Ann. Rheumat. Dis., *23*, 12, 1964.

ZELLNER, E.: Arthropathia psoriatica und Arthritis bei Psoriatikern, Wien. Arch. inn. Med., *15*, 435, 1928.

ZIFF, M., BROWN, P., LOSPALLUTO, J., BADIN, J., and McEWEN, C.: Agglutination and Inhibition by Serum Globulin in the Sensitized Sheep Cell Agglutination Reaction in Rheumatoid Arthritis, Am. J. Med., *20*, 500, 1956.

Chapter

27

Neuropathic Arthropathies and Neuropathic
Fractures of Bone Shafts

CHARCOT, in 1868, directed attention to the fact that, in subjects affected with *tabes dorsalis*, the neural disorder may constitute the basis for the appearance of devastating articular lesions. Since then, it has become clear that these arthropathies are initiated and sustained mainly by painless fractures at the ends of the bones entering into the formation of the joint. The condition presented by a joint so altered is generally denoted as a "Charcot arthropathy." It has also been reported that paretics sometimes develop neuroarthropathies, but when the latter appear in such subjects they are ascribable to a concurrent tabes dorsalis rather than to the paresis *per se*. That entirely analogous articular lesions may occur in association with *syringomyelia* was demonstrated by Schlesinger in a monograph published in 1895.

Both tabes dorsalis and syringomyelia are also likely to be responsible for painless spontaneous fractures through the shafts of bones—that is, away from joints and independent of articular involvement. It has been claimed that general paresis, too, may favor the development of such fractures. However, if they do appear in a paretic, they (like neuroarthropathies developing in such subjects) can usually be attributed to a co-existing tabes dorsalis. More rarely, fractures in tabetics have their basis in an actual skeletal demineralization conditioned by the incidental development of a nutritional deficiency.

For a long time, tabes dorsalis and syringomyelia together were held to account for almost all cases of neuropathic arthropathy. However, in 1936, Jordan called attention to the fact that neuritic manifestations frequently appear in connection with *diabetes mellitus*. Since persons affected with diabetes are now surviving into middle life and old age, cases of *diabetic neuroarthropathy* are being encountered in increasing numbers. Neuropathic arthropathies (alone or with other skeletal lesions) have also been observed in cases of *congenital insensitivity to pain* (see Fanconi and Ferrazzini, Murray, Silverman and Gilden, van der Houwen, and also Siegelman *et al.*). In rare instances, a neuropathic arthropathy has been found to have its basis in still another neural disorder (see Shands). Thus a Charcot arthropathy occasionally appears in association with *transverse myelitis* from traumatic injury to the cord. A few cases have also been reported in which it appeared after *injury to, or inflammation of, peripheral nerves*.

In the present chapter we shall consider: (1) the skeletal manifestations conditioned by the pathologic changes occurring in the spinal cord in cases of tabes dorsalis and syringomyelia; (2) neuroarthropathy associated with diabetes mellitus and apparently representing the result of neuropathy due to the diabetes; and (3) the various skeletal aberrations observed in cases of congenital insensitivity to pain. However, we shall not discuss the soft-tissue ossifications which frequently appear (particularly in relation to the hip and knee joints) in cases of paraplegia caused by injuries to the spinal cord and resulting in transverse myelitis (see Dejerine and Ceillier, Voss, Heilbrun and Kuhn, Benassy *et al.*, and also Damanski). These ossifications will not be considered here for the following reasons: (1) In paraplegics, the para-articular and parosteal ossifications develop in the absence of neuropathy-induced alterations in the bone ends of the affected joint area; and (2) there have been instances in which pertinent tissue has become available for histologic examination and showed that the ossification (new bone formation) and erosion of the local bones are to be related to the presence of decubitus ulcers which result in chronic local infection of the soft tissues overlying the bones and extension of the infection to the bones themselves.

TABES DORSALIS AND SYRINGOMYELIA

CLINICAL CONSIDERATIONS

Incidence and Distribution of the Skeletal Lesions.—Most estimates of the incidence of *neuroarthropathy among tabetics* range between 5 and 10 per cent. Almost any joint may be involved, but about 75 per cent of the tabetic arthropathies occur in the lower extremities, and about 25 per cent occur in the upper extremities or in joints elsewhere in the skeleton. As to the specific distribution, it is clear that the knee joint is by far the one most often affected, accounting for almost half of all tabetic arthropathies. The hip, shoulder, ankle (including the midtarsal) and elbow joints, in order of descending frequency of involvement, together account for

Figure 218

A, Photograph showing the left knee joint area in the case of a woman 60 years of age who was affected with tabes dorsalis. The clinical history obtained when she was admitted to the hospital indicated that the joint had been swollen and unstable for about a year. About 4 years prior to admission, she had had similar complaints relating to her *right* knee joint, and that joint had been fused at another hospital. Because of the fusion of the right knee joint and the swelling of the left knee joint, she walked with great difficulty even with crutches, and could not walk at all without them. That she had tabes dorsalis was confirmed by the presence of Argyle-Robertson pupils, and neurological examination revealed absence of knee and ankle jerks. A synovectomy was carried out, and the synovial membrane was found thickened and roughened, and in some places showed villous hypertrophy. In other areas the membrane was somewhat gritty, as is revealed in the photomicrograph shown in Figure 224–*A*.

B, Photograph of a man 48 years of age presenting advanced articular changes of syringomyelia in the joints of both upper extremities. Neurological examination disclosed atrophy of the muscles of the hands, and disturbance in the perception of pain and temperature in the upper extremities, particularly in the right extremity. Abdominal reflexes were absent, while the knee and ankle reflexes were exaggerated. The huge swelling of the joints of the upper extremities, along with atrophy, sensory dissociation, and signs of involvement of the pyramidal tracts, finally led to the diagnosis of syringomyelia. While the neuroarthropathic changes were most striking in the upper extremities, there was also some evidence of arthropathy in the knee joints. (See also *C* and *D*.)

C, Roentgenograph of the right elbow joint disclosing extensive disintegration of the articular ends of all the bones entering into the formation of the joint. The capsule of the joint is greatly distended, and the region of the joint discloses a great number of small radiopacities representing fracture fragments from the articular bone ends. Some of these fragments probably lie free in the articular cavity, while others may be adherent to the synovial membrane and/or embedded in the capsule of the joint.

D, Roentgenograph of the left hand and wrist in the same case. Extensive destructive changes are manifest in the interphalangeal joints and in the intercarpal joints.

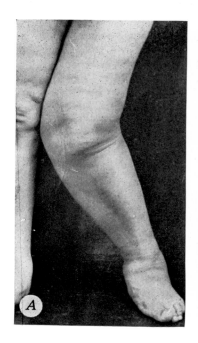

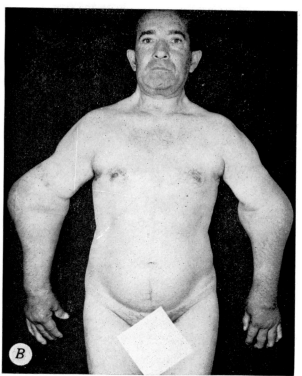

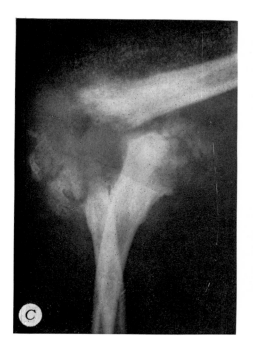

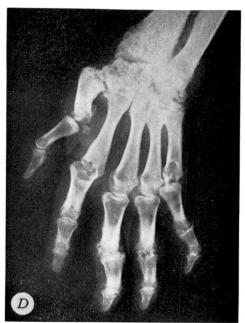

Figure 218

most of the rest of these arthropathies. The remaining small percentage is distributed among the other joints, including those of the vertebral column (especially in the lower thoracic and/or lumbar region), the temporomandibular and sternoclavicular joints, and those of the fingers and toes. (See Fig. 218–*A*.)

Tabes has definitely been established as a frequent cause of the so-called "malum perforans pedis" (see Scaglietti). In this condition, chronic analgic indurations and ulcerations of the soles of the feet are associated with extensive resorption of the articular ends of the phalanges and metatarsal bones and disruption of their joints. The severity of these lesions is exaggerated by a complicating osteomyelitis resulting from the presence of a suppurative inflammation in the local soft tissues.

In about half of the cases of tabes dorsalis with arthropathy, only one joint is affected. However, involvement of two joints is by no means uncommon, and cases have even been reported in which as many as six or seven joints were found implicated. When more than one joint is involved, the arthropathy is not infrequently symmetrical—notably in the knees or hips. Moreover, though rarely, two pairs of large joints are sometimes affected simultaneously—for instance, both knees and both hips or both knees and both ankles. In tabetics the *spontaneous shaft fractures*, too, involve mainly the bones of the lower limbs and are fairly often multiple.

The incidence of *neuroarthropathies and nonarticular fractures* is higher in *syringomyelia* than in tabes dorsalis. Indeed, it has been estimated that as many as 25 per cent, and perhaps even more, of the subjects affected with syringomyelia develop such skeletal lesions. In regard to the distribution of the arthropathies, it is of interest that about 80 per cent of them occur in the joints of the upper extremities and the rest of them mainly in those of the lower extremities. Thus the localization of the neuroarthropathies in syringomyelia is nearly the reverse of what it is in tabes dorsalis. The explanation for this seems to be that in syringomyelia the neural lesion is usually located in the cervical and upper dorsal part of the cord, while in tabes it is in the lower dorsal and lumbar region. Furthermore, bilateral and symmetrical articular involvement is much less common in syringomyelia than in tabes, probably because the cord involvement is not symmetrical in the former disease.

Within an upper extremity, the arthropathy in syringomyelics is observed most often in the shoulder joint. Next in order come the elbow and wrist joints and finally the other joints of the hand. (See Fig. 218.) In a lower extremity, the arthropathy seems to be distributed almost evenly among the knee, ankle, and hip joints. In syringomyelics with neuropathic skeletal lesions in the hands, the latter may come to show destructive perforating lesions of the soft tissues and extensive bone necrosis, analogous to the familiar "malum perforans pedis" of tabes dorsalis. *Diaphysial fractures* occur much less frequently in cases of syringomyelia than in cases of tabes dorsalis. When they do appear in syringomyelia, they are found most often in the bones of the upper extremities and particularly of the forearms.

Clinical Findings.—In *tabes dorsalis* a Charcot arthropathy or a spontaneous shaft fracture may be the feature first calling attention to the fact that a subject is affected with the disease. In such a case, neurologic examination may as yet give only slight or equivocal evidences of the neural disease, although the correct diagnosis can usually be established through serologic examination of the spinal fluid. The latent period between arthropathies and shaft fractures on the one hand and clear-cut clinical manifestations of the tabes dorsalis on the other is not one lasting for years, as some have supposed. However, Blencke and Blencke are probably right in maintaining that the majority of tabetic arthropathies and an even larger proportion of the spontaneous shaft fractures do appear at least before the tabetic subjects manifest ataxia. As to the time of appearance of the arthropathies and shaft fractures in *syringomyelia*, it has been observed, for instance by Schlesinger, that they usually occur during the late period of the underlying neurologic disorder. In some instances of syringomyelia, however, the arthropathy is the presenting clinical manifestation, despite the fact that the basic lesion of the spinal cord has already evolved. In a case of syringomyelia, it is not unusual to encounter an arthropathy involving a shoulder joint in which roentgenologic examination reveals that the head of the humerus has been substantially destroyed, the joint is subluxated, and radiopaque bodies are present in the articular cavity and also in the para-articular soft tissues. In such a case, the clinical and roentgenographic findings may lead to the erroneous interpretation of the articular lesion as a sarcoma (see Walbom-Jørgensen).

A Charcot arthropathy may make its appearance while the subject is in bed, during ordinary functional use of the joint, or after a misgauged movement of the joint during the day's activity. Even if there has been an immediately antecedent direct trauma to the joint, the trauma is rarely sufficient to account for the subsequent changes. Ordinarily, the first clinical manifestation of a tabetic (or syringomyelic) *neuroarthropathy* is rapid, painless, and resistant swelling of the affected articular region. More rarely, the commencement of the arthropathy is not abrupt and may be indicated by articular crepitation or by repeated dislocations, but these are usually followed in time by an episode of articular swelling. The swelling results in part from the accumulation of large amounts of fluid (frequently sanguineous) in the joint space, but to a greater extent from liberation and penetration of this fluid into the neighboring para-articular and subcutaneous tissues because of rupture of the capsule and tearing of the overlying soft parts. *Roentgenographs* of the region at this stage would usually demonstrate one or more fractures through the articular bone ends whose occurrence would seem to explain the joint effusion and swelling. Indeed, unless such fractures are observed (for they occur without the subject's knowledge and without adequate trauma), it may be difficult or impossible at this stage to know that one is dealing with a neuroarthropathy. (See Fig. 219.)

In startling contrast to the objective findings, the *complaints* are very mild, and there may be none at all. Thus, as noted, acute pain is absent, though a sensation of heaviness and fatigue in the affected extremity is common. There is almost never any increased local heat or any fever. Despite the considerable swelling, movement and function of the affected articulation may not be much restricted. The skin over the swollen joint is pale, but a network of engorged veins may be seen shimmering through it.

In most instances the affected joint never returns to the normal, although much of the swelling recedes, and very rapidly (usually in the course of some weeks or months) much more radical changes occur, conditioned mainly by additional fractures in the articular bone ends. In some cases, however, the initial manifestations regress so completely in the course of some weeks or months that clinically the joint appears normal again. Nevertheless, if it is palpated, one can often detect friction and crackling within the joint when it is moved. Recurrence of the effusion, with subsequent severe joint destruction, is not at all uncommon.

When the arthropathy is well advanced, the capsule and ligaments of the affected joint are quite loose, so that the occurrence of subluxations or even luxations is favored. Especially since there is little or no pain, this looseness, in conjunction with the recurrent fractures taking place in the joint, may finally distort the latter tremendously. Though free use of an affected joint certainly encourages its disruption, a neuropathic arthropathy may also become quite extreme even while the patient is resting in bed. Furthermore, it may not be until the joint is very badly broken up that the subject feels the need of medical attention.

As for *spontaneous shaft fractures* in tabetics, these too arise after relatively slight trauma, and are completely painless. It is possible to move the bone ends against each other without arousing protest. The type of fracture line may be any one of the various types to be observed in fractures of normal bones also. There is no particular likelihood of delayed union or nonunion. Hence, one may expect that under proper immobilization the healing of these fractures will proceed essentially like that of fractures in bones of normal persons. However, one does observe, in relation to the healing of shaft fractures in tabetics, an increased tendency toward luxuriant callus formation and toward pseudarthroses. Furthermore, after union, if the bone in question is subject to excessive functional punishment because of the analgia and possibly also ataxia, refracture is likely to occur. Finally, it should be realized that not all fractures in tabetics or syringomyelics are of the "spontaneous" type.

ROENTGENOGRAPHIC AND PATHOLOGIC FINDINGS

These aspects of neuropathic arthropathies will be discussed mainly in relation to tabes dorsalis rather than syringomyelia, since tabetic neuroarthropathies are encountered much more frequently than syringomyelic neuroarthropathies. Because

Figure 219

A, Roentgenograph of the right knee joint in the case of a man 53 years of age who, on admission to the hospital, presented clinical manifestations of tabes dorsalis and serological evidence of syphilis. Note the fragmented appearance of the medial condyle of the tibia, and also that the contour of the articular surface of the condyle is greatly depressed. About $2\frac{1}{2}$ years before coming under medical care at our hospital, the patient became aware that the knee was swollen and somewhat unstable. In the course of the physical examination at the time of admission, it was noted that he walked with a cane and wore a brace. Without a brace, he walked with a pronounced right-sided limp, associated with instability of the right knee joint. The knee was swollen and the patella was movable almost to the point of dislocation. Also, the knee could be hyperextended, striking lateral instability was apparent, and crepitation could be felt on movement of the joint. Deep tendon reflexes, notably of the knee and ankle joints, were absent. Surgery was carried out, the fragmented medial condyle being resected and replaced by a Vitallium mold. The *specimen* consisted of: (1) a substantial part of the upper end of the tibia, including all of the medial condyle; (2) the menisci of the knee joint, and a portion of the joint capsule, which showed thickening of the synovial membrane lining it; and (3) two small, somewhat flattened, oval-shaped osseous bodies covered in part by cartilage. The medial condyle was definitely enlarged, and its articular surface was deepened, being almost saucer-shaped. On palpation, the outer margin of the condyle was found irregular and nodular. The articular cartilage of the condyle did not appear normal anywhere, and in many places it had undergone substantial erosion. The impacted, comminuted fractures revealed in the clinical roentgenograph were not apparent on gross examination of the uncut specimen. Because of the fibrous ankylosis between the fracture fragments, practically no movement could be elicited on manipulation of the specimen. The resected medial condyle was sectioned serially in the longitudinal axis on a band saw, and the slices were then roentgenographed and photographed. Three sets of the pictures in question are illustrated below.

B and *C*, *D* and *E*, *F* and *G*, Alternating roentgenographs and photographs of 3 slices prepared from the medial condyle shown in *A* after it had been resected in the course of the surgical intervention. In all of these pictures, the photographs (which are on the right) are mirror images of the corresponding roentgenographs. The fracture fragments stand out clearly both in the roentgenographs and the photographs of the specimen slices. The fact that the fracture fragments are firmly held together by fibrous tissue can also be deduced from the photographs.

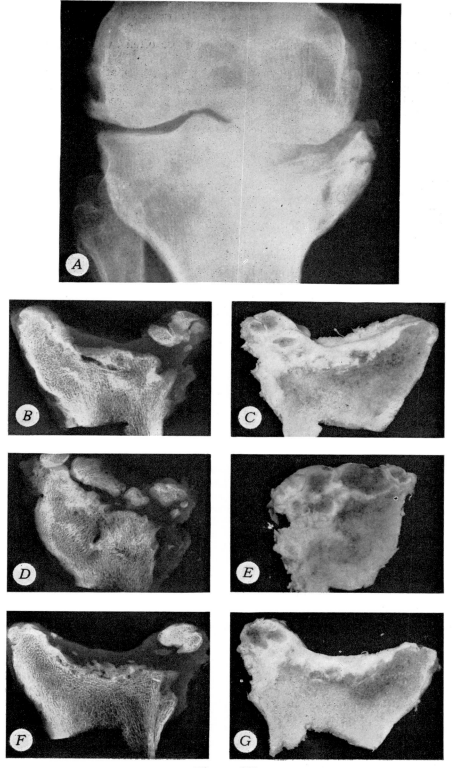

Figure 219

of this, tabetic neuroarthropathies have been more often available for anatomic study.

The *roentgenographic features* of a fully evolved neuropathic arthropathy are striking and are not likely to raise any diagnostic problems. (See Fig. 220.) On the other hand, the *early* roentgenographic changes displayed by a Charcot joint often raise problems of diagnosis, especially if the articular involvement is the presenting manifestation and the subject does not as yet show obvious indications of the neurological disease. In such a case the articular lesion might even be interpreted roentgenographically as representing merely a mild form of osteoarthritis. Somewhat later, but still relatively early, the changes visible roentgenographically include: persistent joint effusion; minimal subluxation; evidence of slight erosion and reactive sclerosis of the articular bone ends, suggestive of osteoarthritis; and occasionally even the presence of a clinically silent fracture (see Katz *et al.*).

The present writer has encountered a number of instances in which a synovectomy was carried out on a knee joint in a relevant case, on the assumption that the joint in question was the site of an osteoarthritis. On gross and microscopic examination of the synovial membrane, the finding of considerable amounts of cartilage and bone debris attached to, and incorporated in, the synovial membrane alerted the writer to the possibility that the joint was the site of an evolving tabetic arthropathy. Detailed clinical and laboratory examination of the patients in the cases in question supported that inference.*

* The cases were reported by Horwitz, who had worked as a Research Fellow in the laboratory of the Hospital for Joint Diseases.

Figure 220

A, Roentgenograph of the right knee joint of a man 50 years of age who was admitted to the hospital with a 5-month history of swelling of the joint. This was associated with a slight amount of pain on weight-bearing during the last 2 or 3 months of this period. The patient also stated that, once weekly for the 5 weeks preceding admission to the hospital, the knee joint was aspirated and large amounts of fluid were removed in the course of each aspiration. The clinical record revealed that he had contracted syphilis when he was 25 years of age. While in the hospital, tests of the blood and spinal fluid for syphilis gave positive results. Neurological examination indicated that the patient was affected with tabes dorsalis. Within a week after the patient's admission, a synovectomy was carried out on the knee joint, and the present writer made a gross and microscopic examination of the synovial membrane. Since he found considerable amounts of minute fragments of bone and cartilage adherent to the synovial membrane and embedded in it, he regarded the pathologic findings as indicative of an early stage of tabetic arthropathy of the knee.

B, Roentgenograph of the knee shown in *A* taken 14 months later. The articular bone ends have undergone pronounced disintegration, and one can see numerous small and some large radiopacities representing osteochondral fracture fragments. Most of these fragments are undoubtedly adherent to the synovial membrane, while others are actually incorporated in the synovium and the articular capsule. An above-knee amputation was carried out, and the articular ends of the knee joint are illustrated in Figure 225.

C, Roentgenograph of the left knee joint area in the case of a man 63 years of age affected with tabetic arthropathy. Note the striking disruption of the articular bone ends which has resulted from the occurrence of numerous fractures. The clinical record in this case indicates that the left knee became enlarged about 1 year before the patient's admission to the hospital. The knee joint was not very painful, but was unstable. It contained a considerable amount of fluid, but was not red and not tender on palpation. Because of the numerous fracture fragments within the joint, movement of the joint elicited very pronounced crepitation. An ophthalmologist found early signs of Argyle-Robertson pupils. Neurologic examination disclosed loss of deep pain sense and of vibratory sense. Furthermore, the knee and ankle joint reflexes could not be elicited.

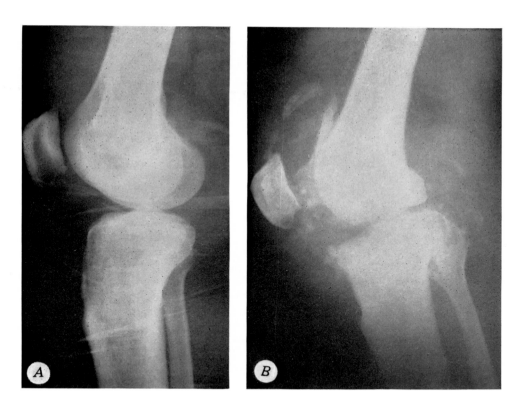

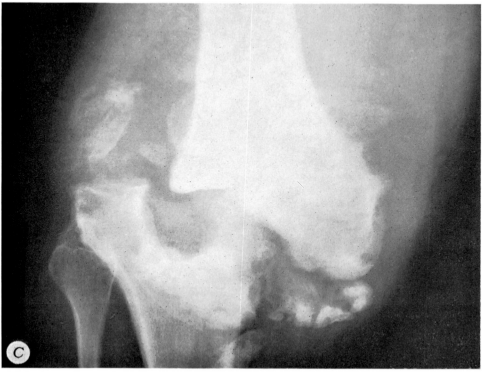

Figure 220

When a joint is the site of advanced changes, roentgenographs will disclose striking destructive and hypertrophic alterations. The bone ends of the joint will manifest fragmentation, absorption of subchondral bone, proliferation of new bone at the articular margins, and the presence of intra-articular fracture fragments. The joint area may acquire a bizarre configuration as a result of the fractures and the presence of intra-articular and para-articular masses of bone. (See Fig. 221.) A supervening infection, which is not uncommon in cases of Charcot arthropathy involving the ankle joint and/or joints of a foot, may exaggerate all these roentgenographic findings. (See Fig. 222.)

In respect to the *gross pathology*, it is to be noted that the great majority of tabetic Charcot joints of long duration are very much enlarged. Their increase in size results mainly from the healing of fracture fragments at the articular bone ends in malaligned positions, from the formation of marginal exostoses and extensive periosteal osteophytes, and from the incorporation of fracture fragments into the capsule, together with thickening and ossification of the capsule and para-articular tissues. On the other hand, one sometimes finds a tabetic Charcot joint in which the changes have tended mainly in the opposite direction, so that, despite some thickening of the capsule, the joint region is not enlarged. This is the case when, instead of being consolidated, the fracture fragments separated from the bone ends become resorbed and the ends themselves undergo erosive resorption.

If the arthropathy is far advanced, whether or not the joint region is enlarged, the capsule will be found irregularly thickened by fibrous tissue. The synovial lining is likewise thickened and usually shows considerable villous transformation, but

Figure 221

A and *B*, Roentgenographs of the left knee joint (in anteroposterior and lateral projections) of a man 55 years of age who had tabes dorsalis. He also presented evidence of neuroarthropathy involving the left ankle joint and the *right* knee. The difficulties relating to the knee joints were already of 6 years' duration when these roentgenographs were taken. Clinical examination disclosed a varus deformity of the left knee, which was also markedly swollen. There was pronounced hypermobility of that joint, and considerable crepitus was evident on flexion and extension. Knee and ankle jerks were absent bilaterally, and the patient also presented Argyle-Robertson pupils. Serological tests for syphilis yielded positive results in regard to the blood and spinal fluid. The articular ends of the femur and tibia are severely deformed, because numerous fracture fragments have broken away from the condyles of these bones. The alteration in the contour of these condyles is most pronounced in relation to the medial condyles. There is a large amount of fluid in the articular cavity, and in addition it is apparent that many of the fragments which have broken away from the femur and tibia have become adherent to, and/or incorporated in, the synovial membrane or the subsynovial layer of the capsule.

C, Photograph of the articular surface of the femur. The condyle on the right side of the picture appears flattened and even somewhat saucer-shaped, because the fractures have resulted in the loss of much of its substance. The surface is devoid of cartilage and is covered by fibrous tissue. The condyle on the left side of the picture appears ridged and nodular, likewise because of the breaking away of fracture fragments. Attached to the condyle on the left is a small piece of the articular capsule, and its inner surface discloses a number of small osteocartilaginous fracture fragments adherent to, or incorporated in, the synovial membrane. In the intercondylar area, a small piece of the posterior wall of the capsule is also apparent, and here, too, the synovial surface reveals a number of small adherent nodules representing osteochondral fracture fragments.

D, Photograph showing the synovial surface of most of the rest of the articular capsule. The surface is studded with numerous small and some large nodules consisting of fragments of cartilage and bone which are incorporated in the capsule or attached to it by short stalks. This illustration supplements and helps to explain the roentgenographic changes disclosed by *A* and *B* in relation to the joint capsule.

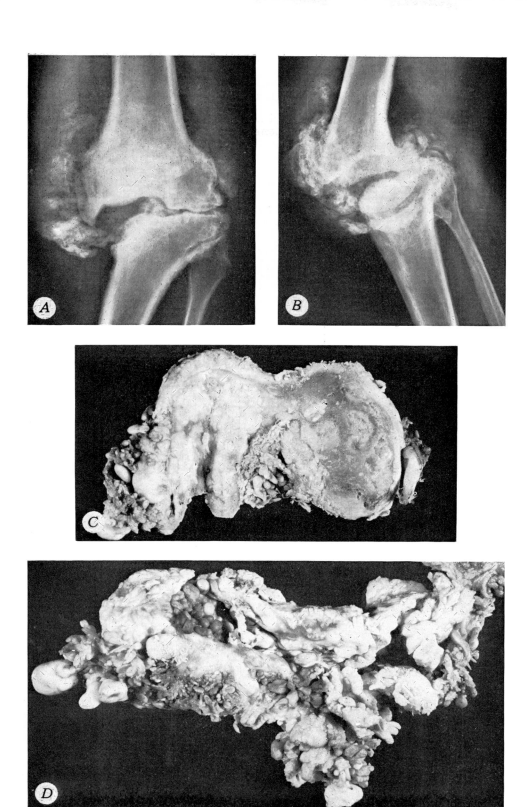

Figure 221

Figure 222

A, Roentgenograph showing the ankle region and part of the right foot in a case of tabes dorsalis in which, because of neurotrophic ulcers on the sole of the foot, infection had become superimposed upon the arthropathy. The affected limb was amputated at the level of the distal quarter of the femur. The patient, a man, was 58 years of age when the amputation was performed. During the preceding 10 years, he had had 3 admissions to the hospital. His case history revealed that he had contracted syphilis when he was 21 years of age. He was 48 years old at the time of his first admission to the hospital, and neurological examination at that time clearly indicated the presence of tabes dorsalis. In particular, the knee and ankle joint reflexes were absent, and the serological findings were positive for syphilitic infection. At the time of his second admission, when he was 56 years of age, his chief complaint was that the right foot had been swollen for 5 weeks, but there was no history of local trauma. Examination of the foot disclosed that the swelling extended distally from the midportion of the foot to the toes, and was chiefly on the dorsal and lateral aspects of the foot. The local skin had a dusky hue, and there was some local edema and heat. On his third admission, the destructive and inflammatory changes in the right foot and ankle had become so much more severe that he was no longer able to bear weight on the foot, and an above-knee amputation was therefore carried out.

B, Photograph of the cut surface of the amputated foot in question reveals extensive destructive changes involving the bones and joints of the ankle and midtarsal regions. In particular, the lower end of the tibia is fractured, the astragalus (talus) has been dislocated forward, and the upper surface of that bone is irregular. The upper surface of the os calcis has also been the site of a fracture, and the loosened fragment can be seen to be embedded in the soft tissues immediately above that bone. The cuboid, the navicular, and the cuneiform bones had been fractured and had undergone such pronounced disintegration that they can no longer be recognized as separate structures. Though the midtarsal bones and the joints between them are no longer identifiable, it was clear that the entire anatomic area in question had been the site of a chronic infection. The infection also extended up the muscle planes of the lower part of the leg, and, as can be seen in *A*, an osteoperiostitis is present on both the tibia and the fibula.

C, Roentgenograph of part of the right foot in another case of tabes dorsalis showing the destructive changes in the pertinent bones and joints. The patient was a man 52 years of age. On admission to the hospital he stated that, 2 years before, he had twisted his right ankle while at work. He did not consult a physician until a few weeks later, since he experienced no significant clinical difficulties during the interim, and the initial treatment by the patient's physician was strapping of the ankle. However, when the patient entered the hospital, the right foot and ankle were tremendously swollen. Examination now also disclosed pronounced redness and local heat and a small ulcer of the skin in the region of the external malleolus. Since it was evident from the roentgenograph, the clinical history, and the clinical findings that the condition represented a tabetic neuroarthropathy with a superimposed infection, and that conservative therapy would be of little value, an amputation through the middle of the leg was carried out. Examination of the amputation specimen disclosed that the ankle region was enlarged and puffy, and a small ulceration of the skin was present in the area of the external malleolus. The specimen was then cut in the sagittal plane with a band saw, through the web between the second and third toes. As the saw went through the ankle joint, about 200 cc. of yellowish creamy pus exuded from the articular cavity of that joint. Inspection of the cut surface of the foot and ankle region revealed extensive destructive changes in the bones and joints, and also evidence of infection. In particular, many small pieces of bone were seen to have broken off from the lower articular surface of the tibia, and a small wedge of bone had also become detached from the posterior surface. The talus was also strikingly modified. Its articular surface was pitted and irregular and covered by fibrocartilaginous tissue. The talus seemed likewise to be fractured in a number of places, the fracture fragments being held together by fibrous tissue. Not only was the bone fractured, but it was displaced anteriorly. The cuboid, too, was fractured in a number of sites.

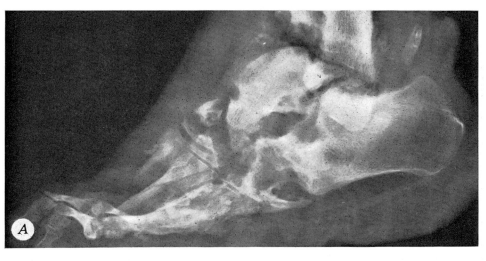

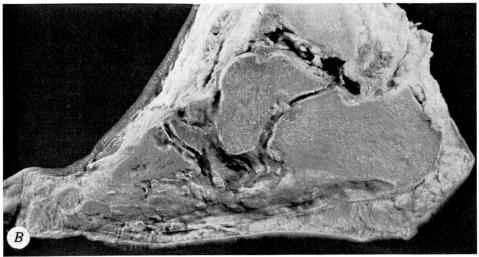

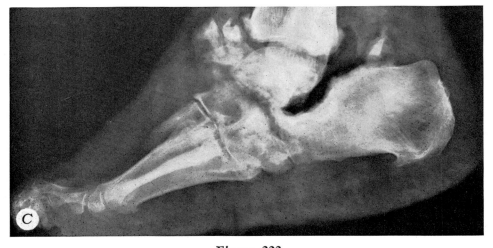

Figure 222

859

where this lining has recently been injured its surface will be covered with fibrin. Intra-articular connective tissue adhesions are also found, and it is likely that the joint cavity will contain some excess fluid. The synovial membrane may show numerous bits of cartilage and osseous tissue adherent to the surface or incorporated into it. The fragments of cartilage and bone in question have been derived from the bone ends of the joint in the course of abrasion of their articular surfaces. (See Figs. 223 and 224.) In time, the fragments of cartilage and bone which have become incorporated into the synovial membrane may take on some growth activity. Lying free in the articular space or adherent to the capsule (often in capsular recesses), there may be large and/or small fragments of bone. In addition, one may find some evidence of metaplastic ossification at sites of attachment of tendons and ligaments. Furthermore, the present writer's experience indicates (at least insofar as tabetic arthropathy is concerned) that intracapsular formation of cartilage and bone is rarely found as pronounced on dissection of the joint as roentgenographic appearances would lead one to think it would be. Actually, any large masses of supposedly metaplastic bone observed roentgenographically nearly always turn out to be fragments fractured from the articular bone ends and partly incorporated into the capsule and synovial membrane.

The articular bone ends ordinarily show little or none of the original covering cartilage. Where the latter is absent, it has usually been replaced, wholly or in part, by fibrous tissue and fibrocartilage. This new cartilage is rough, bulgy, and white, in contrast to any remnants of original cartilage, which are smooth and brownish yellow. Where the articulating surface has been worn down by friction, there will be no covering cartilage whatever, and the exposed underlying bone is eburnated, presenting a polished, or mirror-like, surface. The contours of the articular ends are generally distorted, because fractures have occurred and the fracture fragments have separated away completely or been reunited to the articular end in a malaligned position. The reunion may have been so complete that all signs of previous fracture lines have disappeared.

Figure 223

A, Photograph of the synovial membrane of the left knee joint, excised during the course of a synovectomy, in the case of a man 61 years of age affected with tabes dorsalis. On his admission to the hospital, he stated that the left knee joint had gradually swelled, and the swelling was now so pronounced that he was almost unable to bear weight on the leg. There was considerable fluid in the joint, and the circumference of that joint area was 19.5 cm., while that of the right knee joint area was only 14 cm. Though the patient denied having contracted syphilis, physical examination disclosed the presence of Argyle-Robertson pupils and also the absence, on neurological examination, of reflex responses of the knee and ankle regions. Study of the excised synovial membrane disclosed that it was thick and boggy. Furthermore, in some areas of the membrane (see left half of the picture), numerous tiny fragments of cartilage and/or bone were sprinkled over and adherent to the surface of the membrane and, in some places, even incorporated into it. In the right half of the picture, one can see large, discrete pieces of cartilage-covered bone adherent to the surface of the membrane in some sites and lying within the substance of it in others.

B, Roentgenograph of the excised synovial membrane shown in *A*. The oval or roundish discrete radiopacities represent the larger pieces of cartilage-covered bone which are attached to the membrane or incorporated into it.

C, Photomicrograph ($\times$ 18) of an area from the synovial membrane in the same case. On or immediately under the surface of the membrane, there are tiny fragments of cartilage and bone detritus. Deep in the membrane (on the left and on the right of the picture), there are two foci of cartilage and bone, apparently representing minute fragments which have become incorporated in the membrane, and which are viable and have evidently been enlarging in the manner of autoplastic transplants.

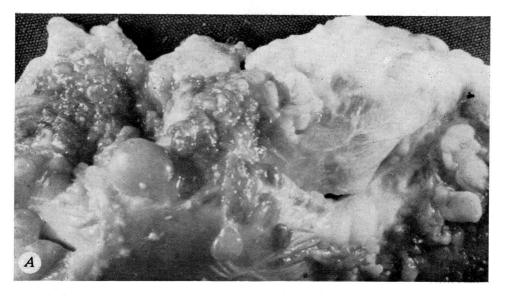

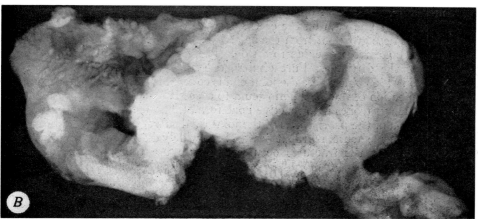

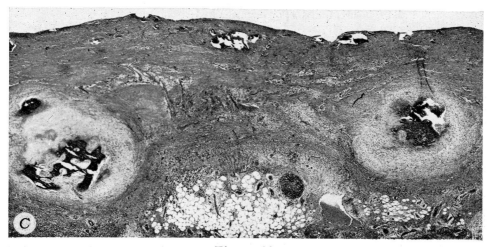

Figure 223

When a fracture line has extended obliquely through the diaphysis, and the periosteum has become separated from the diaphysial cortex, extensive deposits of subperiosteal new bone may be present. As pointed out by Moritz, these osteophytic deposits are often large enough to act as ledges, or brackets, which splint and hold together the comminuted bone ends. Instead of becoming reunited with the articular bone ends, some of the fracture fragments may, as already noted, become embedded in the capsule. Other fragments—especially in the shoulder and hip joints—may be ground up in the joint space as though in a mortar. In a Charcot hip joint, for instance, the rim of the acetabulum can become eroded, the flattened and irregular depression extending posteriorly and upwards onto the ilium. All of the head and most of the neck can become worn down. The femoral end of such a joint will be found covered with connective tissue and dislocated upward or even buried in the musculature.

Malalignments which develop in a Charcot joint lead to overloading of one side of the articulation and deloading of the other. In consequence, osteosclerosis appears in the overloaded bone ends and atrophy in the deloaded ends. Where the bones are dislocated and the joint dangles, its ends will generally show atrophy of the spongy trabeculae and thinning of the cortex, both from the periosteal and from the endosteal side. Such atrophies are ascribable to non-use of the part.

Exostoses may be found on the cartilage-covered articulating surfaces as bumpy elevations. These grow out from the spongiosa, and as they form, the cartilage is invaded by bone from the marrow side. There may also be exostoses at the periphery of the cartilage. Furthermore, one may find osteophytic outgrowths arising beyond the point where the joint end is covered by cartilage. These develop through subjection of the local periosteum to excessive friction from ligaments and tendons, which provokes it to reactive bone formation. (See Fig. 225.)

The question of the *pathogenesis* of the joint (and shaft) fractures in tabetics and the evolution of the neuroarthropathies has been widely discussed. The view held by Charcot was that the fractures occurred because the tabes dorsalis created a

Figure 224

A, Photomicrograph (× 12) of a tissue section prepared from the synovial membrane removed from the knee joint in the case illustrated in Figure 218–A. The synovial membrane was thickened and roughened, and showed villous hypertrophy in some places. In other areas the membrane was somewhat gritty, and this picture illustrates the histology of such an area. The great numbers of small dark spots toward the surface of the thickened synovial membrane represent minute fragments of bone which have been rubbed off from the articular bone ends of the Charcot joint in question.

B, Photomicrograph (× 35) again illustrating the incorporation of fragments of bone and also of cartilage into the synovial membrane of a knee joint which was the site of a Charcot arthropathy. The patient was a woman 49 years of age who, for about a year before admission to the hospital, complained of gradually increasing instability and intermittent swelling of her right knee joint. Roentgenographically the knee revealed the changes typical of a neuropathic joint. Neurological examination disclosed the absence, bilaterally, of knee and ankle reflexes. The patient also showed Argyle-Robertson pupils. Serological tests of the blood and spinal fluid yielded positive results in respect to syphilitic infection.

C, Photomicrograph (× 45) of a tissue section prepared from the synovial membrane which was removed from the right knee of a man 51 years of age whose blood and spinal fluid yielded positive findings in respect to syphilitic infection. Roentgenographic examination of the knee joint disclosed well-advanced tabetic arthropathy. Note the fragments of cartilage and bone debris on the surface of the synovial membrane and within it. Similar changes were widespread throughout all the histologic sections prepared from the excised synovial membrane.

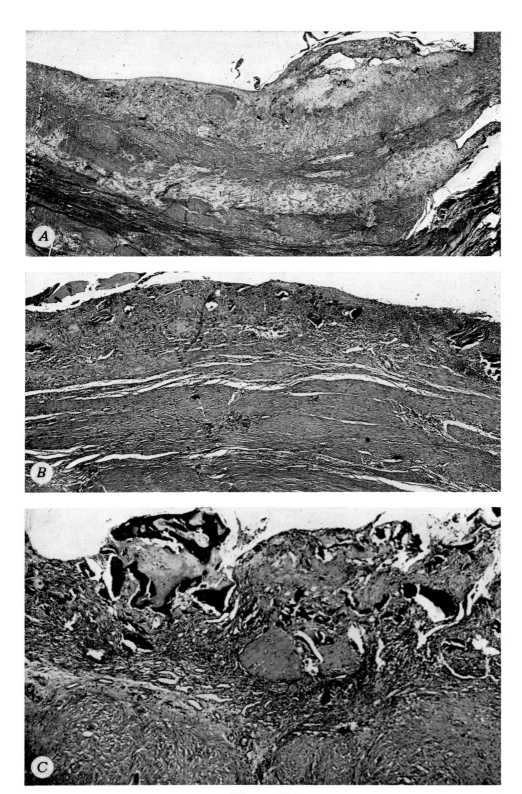

Figure 224

trophic disturbance, which he presumably thought made the bones porotic and/or brittle. Actually, however, the bones of such subjects are ordinarily not porotic before the occurrence of the fractures. Indeed, Corbin found that the sensory defect created by section of the dorsal roots in the lumbosacral region in cats was associated with thickening of the bones of the hind limbs in these animals if they continued to use the deafferentated extremities.

It is now generally agreed that neuroarthropathies result from trauma to the affected joints because of loss of the protective sense of pain and deep sensation. The loss of deep sensation leads to relaxation of the supporting structures and chronic instability of the joint, and when exposed to the stress of daily movement the joint is deprived of the normal protective reaction. As a consequence, the articulation becomes at least slightly malaligned, and the malalignment leads to excessive friction and abnormal loading, and to changes suggesting a mild degree of osteoarthritis. Cumulative injury causes synovial effusion and additional damage to the cartilage, and it is this that in turn leads to degeneration and disorganization of the joint. In support of this opinion, we have the fact that very many of the tabetic arthropathies develop in subjects who are not yet atactic. If, later on, the factor of ataxia is added, the liability to the occurrence and recurrence of fractures is, of course, greatly increased. Occasionally a case is encountered in which the joint becomes severely disorganized within a very short period of time—a few weeks or a month or two. The arthropathy in such cases has been denoted as "acute neuropathic arthropathy" (see Norman *et al.*).

TREATMENT

As Steindler pointed out, the early use of splints or other devices to protect the neuropathic joint from further damage is of supreme therapeutic importance. Unless such protection is given, distortions and subluxations will permit recurrent fractures and in general exacerbate the existing pathologic conditions. The patient should be cautioned to protect himself against trauma to, and overuse of, the affected joints. Johnson, on the basis of a large experience relating to the treatment of neuropathic fractures and joint injuries, stressed the idea that if an involved joint is inadequately protected, the immediate local changes (fractures, sprains, and/or intra-articular effusions) are likely to constitute the foundation for additional de-

Figure 225

A, Photograph of the articular end of the femur and the joint capsule of the knee joint shown in Figure 220–*B*, the photograph having been taken at the time of anatomic examination of the amputation specimen. Note that the articular surface is completely abnormal. Most of the femoral condyle on the left has been broken off, and the condyle on the right presents a bumpy appearance. In the region of the intercondylar area, the articular surface has been substantially eroded, and many tabs of fibrous tissue can be observed between the condyles and toward the upper end of the condyle on the right. There is massive thickening of the joint capsule, due to the presence of osteochondral fracture fragments which have become incorporated into the synovial membrane and the capsule.

B and *C*, Photographs of the lower end of the femur and upper end of the tibia and fibula from the case shown in *A* and Figure 220–*B*. The bones were cut in the frontal plane and then macerated to remove all the soft tissue. The photographs show strikingly the extent to which the contour of the femoral condyles has been distorted, and also reveal that much of the medial condyle of the tibia has been broken away. *C* represents a mirror image of the specimen shown in *B*, and reveals the posterior surface of the femur, tibia, and fibula.

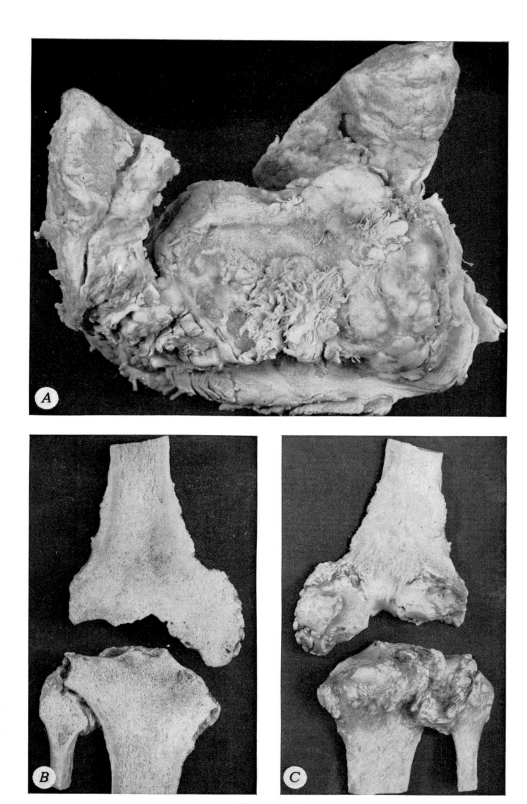

Figure 225

structive changes in the joint. Furthermore, he points out that, if adequate protective treatment is given early in the course of the evolution of a neuroarthropathy, healing of the lesion can often be expected. In a case in which the articular changes are already advanced when the subject comes under medical care, the joint may be massively swollen in consequence of effusion into it, and the enlarged joint may feel like a "bag of bones" because of the presence of numerous intra-articular fracture fragments. At this stage, the general objective of treatment is to prevent further damage to the joint by means of immobilization and repeated aspirations. Months may elapse before subsidence of the reactive inflammatory changes and resorption of the devitalized tissue in and about the joint is likely to occur.

If a surgical intervention (débridement) is proposed or carried out on a badly damaged joint, the danger of a postoperative infection and the possibility of failure of the procedure must be considered.

DIABETIC NEUROARTHROPATHY

It has long been known that, in cases of diabetes mellitus, *peripheral neuropathy* is not uncommon. The term "diabetic neuropathy" serves to denote the manifestations of impaired function of peripheral nerves—aberrations which are frequent and important accompaniments of the diabetic state. It has been reported that, among cases of diabetes of long duration, especially in middle-aged or elderly persons, neuropathy is present in about 30 to 50 per cent of the subjects (see Mulder *et al.*, and Dolman). Furthermore, neuropathy may also be found in some cases of latent diabetes mellitus—that is, in cases in which the presence of diabetes was established merely on the basis of an abnormal glucose tolerance test result (see Leffert). In consequence of the neuropathy, especially in those cases in which nerves of the lower extremities are affected, neuroarthropathies may develop, notably in the feet. In the great majority of cases of diabetic neuroarthropathy (sometimes also denoted as diabetic osteopathy), it is the bones and joints of the feet that are involved. Occasionally an ankle joint is implicated. Much less often diabetic neuroarthropathy is observed in a knee joint, rather rarely it appears in some part of the vertebral column, and exceptionally it involves joints of an upper extremity (see Feldman *et al.*).

CLINICAL CONSIDERATIONS

As already pointed out, the *neuropathy* developing in diabetics appears mainly in those who have passed middle age. It involves principally the nerves of the *lower extremities*, and its chief manifestations include: pain, paresthesia, hypoesthesia and hyperesthesia, diminution or absence of reflex responses, some muscular paresis, and tenderness of the nerves and muscles (see Jordan). When peripheral nerves of the *upper extremities* are affected, the neuropathy is likewise expressed in pain, paresthesias, and/or paresis. In brief, the clinical expressions of the neuropathy range from a mere loss of reflexes, loss of vibration sense, and loss of the proprioceptive sense of position of the legs, to severe pain involving the limbs or the trunk but not tending to be associated with clearly evident objective findings.

Arteriosclerosis (very common in diabetics) does not appear to play a direct role in the development of the neuropathy. In an occasional instance the neuropathy may be related to pressure on the nerves, focal infection, alcoholism, and/or an abnormal reaction to insulin. In the feet, the neuropathy may be the basis for perforating

ulcers or drop foot. Visceral manifestations of diabetic neuropathy include disordered functioning of the bowel and/or bladder. It has been pointed out that
neuropathic symptoms and signs indistinguishable from those presented by diabetics are also encountered in elderly nondiabetic persons. However, their frequency is lower among such persons than it is among diabetics (see Mayne). Although diabetic neuropathy is occasionally observed in a subject whose diabetes is
under good medical control, its incidence is much higher among diabetics who have
failed to follow instructions relating to diet or have not been under medical treatment
for their diabetes.

In consequence of the neuropathy, and especially because of impaired sensation
in the feet, destructive changes not uncommonly develop in the metatarsal bones
and phalanges, their related joints becoming affected secondarily. In regard to the
common involvement of the bones and joints of the foot, it is likely that the
arthropathy is instigated by slight but often-repeated local injury to the small bones
and joints of the foot, abetted by the comparative weakness of their capsules and
ligaments (see Degenhardt and Goodwin).

The first clinical indication that a foot is implicated is painless swelling of the
foot, associated with little heat or redness, if any. The fact that infection is a common complication in cases of diabetes raises the question of whether an infection
has contributed to the clinical and roentgenographic features of the diabetic neuroarthropathy in a particular case. However, there are unquestionable instances of
diabetic neuroarthropathy (or osteopathy) in which no evidence of infection is
present (see Rodnan *et al.*).

ROENTGENOGRAPHIC AND PATHOLOGIC FINDINGS

Roentgenographically the bones of the feet present a wide variety of abnormalities
(see Azerad *et al.*, Pogonowska *et al.*, and also Gondos). The mildest and least
characteristic change is osteoporosis, which may be present in bones of one foot or
both feet. In an individual case, the osteoporosis may be localized to one or another
of the bones of the affected foot, or may involve practically all of its bones. Another
early nonspecific alteration consists of the presence of small erosion defects located
in the juxta-articular area of the cortex of some of the phalanges or in corresponding
areas of the distal ends of the metatarsal bones. Further progression of the condition is associated with destruction (osteolysis) of the proximal ends of some of the
phalanges and the distal ends of some of the metatarsal bones. The progression of
the osteolysis may be rather rapid, and, in its course, the articular ends of the
affected phalanges and metatarsal bones come to present a ragged appearance.
Eventually, the altered bone ends become more or less smoothly tapered. These
alterations may occur in the absence of a local infection, but if an infection of the
overlying soft tissues does supervene, the progress of the osteolysis is accelerated.

When the adjacent bones of a metatarsophalangeal joint become tapered, the
altered bone ends undergo luxation. Approximation of the stumps of adjacent
phalanges which have been substantially resorbed produces a telescoping effect and
results in shortening of the toes. Another roentgenographic alteration presented
by the feet in diabetics affected with advanced neuroarthropathy is absence of the
tips of the terminal phalanges. A slight degree of periosteal new bone formation
may be observed in some cases, especially on the metatarsal bones, whether or not
there is evidence of infection involving the adjacent soft tissues. In the presence of
a soft-tissue infection, one or another of the phalanges may appear fragmented, or
its shadow may no longer be clearly apparent. A phalanx so altered may eventually
again cast a normal or almost normal shadow, but evidence of such restitution is

only rarely observed, because it is likely that a toe in which a phalanx has undergone such alterations will have been amputated. Roentgenographic indications of osteolysis similar to those observed in the phalanges and metatarsal bones are not commonly encountered in the bones constituting the distal portion of the tarsus.

The ankle joint sometimes presents roentgenographically the abnormalities characteristic of a Charcot arthropathy. In particular, an ankle so altered shows irregularity and fragmentation of the articular surfaces of the bones entering into the formation of the joint, and also some increased radiopacity of these bones, extending somewhat beyond the disrupted joint. As already noted, diabetic neuroarthropathies are rarely encountered in large diarthrodial joints other than the ankle joint. (See Fig. 226.)

In contrast to the roentgenographic findings, the gross and microscopic *pathologic findings* relating to diabetic neuroarthropathy *per se* are very meagerly represented in the literature. This is understandable in view of the fact that the pathologic changes in question center mainly in the bones of the feet, and an affected foot is not likely to be available for anatomic examination until the foot has been ablated because of a superimposed infection and/or gangrene. Under these circumstances, the basic changes which have taken place in the affected bones have been obscured by those due to the infection and gangrene. In a case in which: (1) a knee joint is the

Figure 226

A, Roentgenograph of the lower end of the left leg and ankle region from the case of a woman who had been aware for 17 years that she was a diabetic. She was 45 years of age at the time of admission to the hospital. For the first 10 years after the diagnosis of diabetes had been made, the treatment was limited to restriction of carbohydrate intake. Subsequently, the diabetes could no longer be controlled by careful attention to the diet, and antidiabetic drug therapy was instituted. At the time of her admission, the patient stated that her left ankle region had been more or less swollen for 2 years, and that the swelling was intermittent. She had difficulty in walking, and there was an ulcer on the lateral aspect of the ankle. Material was obtained from the site of the ulcer for bacteriological examination, and the microorganisms isolated were *Staphylococcus aureus* (coagulase positive) and *Klebsiella pneumoniae*. The illustration reveals striking abnormalities in the region of the ankle and foot. In particular, the talus has undergone complete dissolution, and there is fragmentation of the os calcis and complete disruption of the tarsus as well as of the ankle mortise. In addition, there is evidence of some periosteal new bone formation along the shaft of the tibia. These findings were interpreted as being characteristic of a diabetic neuroarthropathy complicated by an infection.

B, Roentgenograph of the right foot and ankle of a woman 54 years of age who, on admission to the hospital, gave a history of diabetes for 14 years. About 3 years before her hospitalization, she began to develop difficulties relating to the right leg and foot. The roentgenograph shows destruction of the ankle mortise, as well as fragmentation, sclerosis, and disruption of the subtalar joint. Additional pictures taken at this time revealed midtarsal subluxation and considerable soft-tissue swelling about the ankle. These changes, along with the clinical findings and the biochemical data relating to the serum (blood sugar values 164 to 430 mg. per cent), led to the diagnosis of diabetic neuroarthropathy. The patient also had hypertensive arteriosclerotic heart disease, congestive heart failure, and hypertensive retinopathy, and she died of uremia 2 years later.

C and *D*, Roentgenographs of the left foot and right foot, respectively, of a man 55 years of age who had been aware for 7 years that he had diabetes mellitus. From *C* it is evident that the bones of the midtarsus and the intertarsal joints are disrupted, as are most of the tarsometatarsal joints. In *D* the joints between the medial cuneiform, the intermediate cuneiform, and the lateral cuneiform are substantially obliterated. Also, the joint between the navicular and the three cuneiform bones is not well delineated. These changes, too, are indications of an evolving neuroarthropathy in the foot in question.

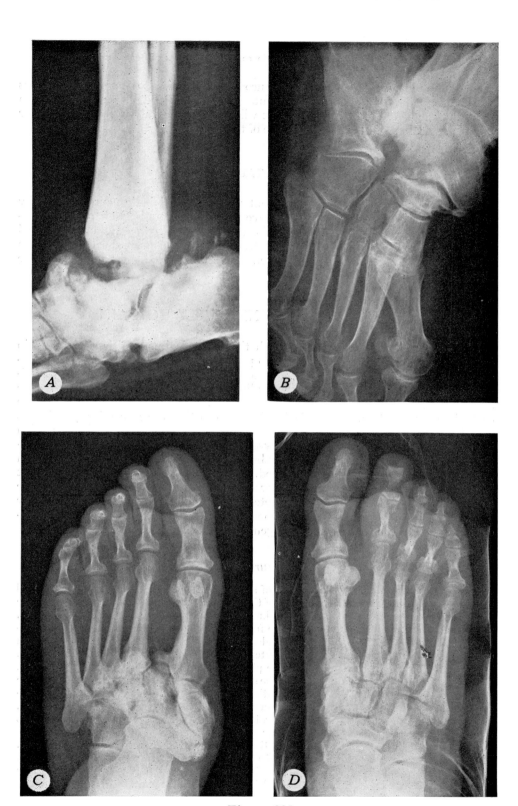

Figure 226

site of diabetic neuroarthropathy; (2) neuroarthropathy is also present in the bones of the feet; and (3) an above-knee amputation has been done because of infection and gangrene of the foot, the knee joint will reveal essentially the same anatomic changes as a Charcot knee joint in a case of tabes dorsalis.

TREATMENT

The appropriate treatment of a patient manifesting diabetic neuroarthropathy of a foot varies in accordance with the severity, location, and extent of the pathologic changes. In general, a *conservative (nonsurgical) approach* should be tried first and can occasionally be expected to lead to improvement and sometimes even to complete healing. Surgical treatment is recommended only if conservative treatment fails.

CONGENITAL INSENSITIVITY TO PAIN

In this section we are concerned with the skeletal abnormalities appearing in consequence of congenital indifference to pain. The subjects are usually still children at the time the neurological deficiency in question is discovered. In a pertinent case, Feindel found normal nerve endings in the skin and periosteum from the region of the right hip joint, and concluded that the abnormality was based in the central nervous system. In particular, it is known that the *perception of pain* is a function of the cerebral cortex, and it is supposed that the center for pain perception is in the parietal lobe. The affective evaluation of pain is likewise a cortical function. However, the precise anatomic aberrations in the brain area in question in these cases have not yet been determined. In the detailed discussion of the subject by Fanconi and Ferrazzini, these workers have analyzed the various aspects of the condition on the basis of 32 cases collected from the literature and 3 cases of their own. They denote the condition as "congenital analgia," but use that name interchangeably with the term "congenital generalized indifference to pain."

Figure 227

A, Roentgenograph of both knee joints of a girl 12 years of age affected with congenital indifference to pain. Clinical examination of the knees revealed pronounced instability of the joints. Note the enlargement of the *right* knee joint area (on the left side of the picture), due to intra-articular effusion, and also the fragmentation of the inferior and posterior surfaces of the lateral condyle of that femur, along with lateral dislocation of the patella. An infraction of the cortex is apparent on the outer surface of the distal metaphysis of the femur. The *left* knee joint (on the right side of the picture) shows only a slight degree of swelling. The patient's clinical record indicated that she sat up at 7 months of age, was able to take some steps at 12 months, and walked at 18 months. As a very young child, she would fall frequently, but she did not cry or complain when this happened. When she was somewhat older, she manifested corneal ulcerations on several occasions. When she was 7 years of age, it was necessary to suture the eyelids long enough to permit healing of the corneal ulcers.

B, Roentgenograph of the lower part of the right leg and ankle region in the same case. The distal epiphysis of the tibia is the site of a fracture.

C, Roentgenograph of the left foot, taken when the girl was about 10 years of age. At this time, she had suffered a fracture of the os calcis and of the first metatarsal bone. The shaft of the first metatarsal bone is greatly thickened, in consequence of subperiosteal new bone formation. The fracture site is just distal to the epiphysis of the bone, and it is clear that the fracture has not yet healed.

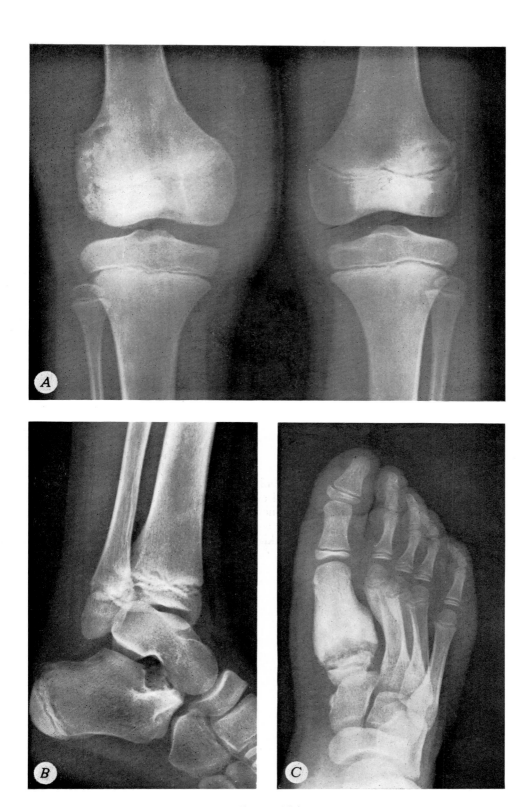

Figure 227

CLINICAL CONSIDERATIONS

To judge from the cases reported in the literature, slightly more than half of the subjects are males. In most of the cases the insensitivity to pain may be denoted as *absolute* on the basis of a completely negative case history in respect to perception of pain, and the complete absence of pain in the course of an objective physical examination. Those in whom the insensitivity to pain could be denoted as *relative* may have had only one episode in which they were aware of pain. As to intelligence, most of the subjects appear to be average or below average, but a few have superior intelligence. Aside from abnormalities relating to the skeleton, physical examination of a given subject may reveal scars on the tongue and fingers or elsewhere on the surface of the body.

In those cases in which the insensitivity to pain is already present during infancy, the parents or other members of the family may notice that, when the infant begins to crawl or walk, it fails to respond to stimuli which would normally arouse pain. However, in some cases, several years pass before medical advice is sought. Murray has presented succinctly the highlights of the clinical course and findings relating to the condition in such children. He notes that burns and lesions due to infection are particularly common among them, and that corneal opacities may develop as a result of unfelt trauma or the introduction of foreign bodies into one or both eyes. The affected child may also bite its tongue repeatedly. As Murray also points out, such children may appear to be aggressive in their relations with other children, since, because of their insensitivity to pain, they feel no necessity to yield in fights. In consequence, they may suffer much physical damage.

When the child comes under medical care, the presenting manifestation may be an uncontrolled but painless focus of infection or a frank deformity. At that time, a *roentgenographic survey* of the skeleton may already reveal obvious abnormalities. (See Fig. 227.) In particular, the survey may disclose the presence of neuro-arthropathies, fractures, and/or one or more foci of osteomyelitis (see Silverman and Gilden). Once in a while, a case of congenital indifference to pain first comes to be recognized when the subject has reached adult life, and, in these cases, lesions involving bones and/or joints may or may not be present.

In cases of congenital insensitivity to pain, the most common sites for the neuro-arthropathies (Charcot joints) are the ankle joint and the joints of the tarsus. Van der Houwen has described a case in which both knee joints, one elbow joint, and the lumbosacral part of the spine were sites of neuroarthropathy. Aside from fractures of the articular ends of the bones entering into the formation of a joint which is the site of a neuroarthropathy, a fracture of the shaft of one or another bone may be encountered. Since the shaft fractures in these cases are practically painless and tend to undergo union in malposition, they may reveal themselves clinically only because of the resultant deformity. If the fracture is a compound fracture and the associated open wound has not received appropriate medical attention, the fracture area often becomes the site of an osteomyelitis. If a plaster cast is applied to a joint where a Charcot arthropathy is present, or if a cast has been applied in the treatment of a shaft fracture (irrespective of whether it is a compound fracture), the lack of sensitivity to pain may delay the recognition of the osteomyelitis for a long time and permit its progression. Even in the absence of a fracture, a bone area may be the site of a local abscess which may likewise go unrecognized for a long time.

In the *treatment* of the syndrome as a whole, the primary requisite is to impress upon the subject or (if the patient is a young child) upon the parents and others involved in the child's care the need for caution directed toward avoidance of injuries whose presence might be unrecognized because of the sensory deficiency. As the subject grows older, he may become aware of these dangers, partly because other qualities of sensation, and especially intellectual functions, take over as substitutes for the missing sensitivity to pain. Consequently, normal duration of life can be expected for most of the subjects, even though they never develop a true sense of pain. If a knee joint is the site of an advanced neuroarthropathy, an arthrodesis may be indicated (see Abell and Hayes).

REFERENCES

ABELL, J. M., Jr. and HAYES, J. T.: Charcot Knee due to Congenital Insensitivity to Pain, J. Bone & Joint Surg., *46–A*, 1287, 1964.

AZERAD, E., STUHL, L., LUBETZKI, J. and SLOTINE, M.: Étude radiologique des ostéopathies du diabète sucré. "Le pied diabétique," Ann. radiol., *6*, 421, 1963.

BENASSY, J., BOISSIER, J.–R., PATTE, D., and DIVERRES, J.–C.: Ostéomes des paraplégiques (Contribution à l'étude de l'ossification neurogène), Presse méd., *68*, 811, 1960.

BLENCKE, A. and BLENCKE, B.: Die neuropathischen Knochen- und Gelenkaffektionen, Deutsche Orthopädie, *8*, 1931.

CHARCOT, J. M.: Sur quelques arthropathies qui paraissent dépendre d'une lésion du cerveau ou de la moelle épinière, Arch. physiol. norm. et path., *1*, 161 and 379, 1868.

CORBIN, K. B.: Alterations in the Hip Joint After Deafferentation, Arch. Surg., *35*, 1145, 1937.

DAMANSKI, M.: Heterotopic Ossification in Paraplegia, J. Bone & Joint Surg., *43–B*, 286, 1961.

DEGENHARDT, D. P. and GOODWIN, M. A.: Neuropathic Joints in Diabetes, J. Bone & Joint Surg., *42–B*, 769, 1960.

DEJERINE and CEILLIER, A.: Para-ostéo-arthropathies des paraplégiques par lésion médullaire (étude clinique et radiographique), Ann. méd., *5*, 497, 1918.

DOLMAN, C. L.: The Morbid Anatomy of Diabetic Neuropathy, Neurology, *13*, 135, 1963.

FANCONI, G. and FERRAZZINI, F.: Kongenitale Analgie (kongenitale generalisierte Schmerzindifferenz), Helvet. paediat. acta, *12*, 79, 1957.

FEINDEL, W.: Note on the Nerve Endings in a Subject with Arthropathy and Congenital Absence of Pain, J. Bone & Joint Surg., *35–B*, 402, 1953.

FELDMAN, M. J., BECKER, K. L., REEFE, W. E. and LONGO, A.: Multiple Neuropathic Joints, Including the Wrist, in a Patient With Diabetes Mellitus, J.A.M.A., *209*, 1690, 1969.

GONDOS, B.: Roentgen Observations in Diabetic Osteopathy, Radiology, *91*, 6, 1968.

HEILBRUN, N. and KUHN, W. G., Jr.: Erosive Bone Lesions and Soft-Tissue Ossifications Associated with Spinal Cord Injuries (Paraplegia), Radiology, *48*, 579, 1947.

HORWITZ, T.: Bone and Cartilage Debris in the Synovial Membrane. Its Significance in the Early Diagnosis of Neuro-Arthropathy, J. Bone & Joint Surg., *30–A*, 579, 1948.

JOHNSON, J. T. H.: Neuropathic Fractures and Joint Injuries. Pathogenesis and Rationale of Prevention and Treatment, J. Bone & Joint Surg., *49–A*, 1, 1967.

JORDAN, W. R.: Neuritic Manifestations in Diabetes Mellitus, Arch. Int. Med., *57*, 307, 1936.

KATZ, I., RABINOWITZ, J. G. and DZIADIW, R.: Early Changes in Charcot's Joints, Am. J. Roentgenol., *86*, 965, 1961.

LEFFERT, R. D.: Diabetes Mellitus Initially Presenting as Peripheral Neuropathy in the Upper Limb, J. Bone & Joint Surg., *51–A*, 1005, 1969.

MAYNE, N.: Neuropathy in the Diabetic and Non-diabetic Populations, Lancet, *2*, 1313, 1965.

MORITZ, A. R.: Tabische Arthropathie. Histologische Studie, Virchows Arch. path. Anat., *267*, 746, 1928.

MULDER, D. W., LAMBERT, E. H., BASTRON, J. A. and SPRAGUE, R. G.: The Neuropathies Associated with Diabetes Mellitus, Neurology, *11*, 275, 1961.

MURRAY, R. O.: Congenital Indifference to Pain, with Special Reference to Skeletal Changes, Brit. J. Radiol., *30*, 2, 1957.

NORMAN, A., ROBBINS, H. and MILGRAM, J. E.: The Acute Neuropathic Arthropathy—A Rapid, Severely Disorganizing Form of Arthritis, Radiology, *90*, 1159, 1968.

POGONOWSKA, M. J., COLLINS, L. C. and DOBSON, H. L.: Diabetic Osteopathy, Radiology, *89*, 265, 1967.

RODNAN, G. P., MACLACHLAN, M. J. and BROWER, T. D.: Neuropathic Joint Disease (Charcot Joints), Bull. Rheumat. Dis., *9*, 183, 1959.

SCAGLIETTI, O.: Klinik und Pathologie des Malum perforans mit besonderer Berücksichtigung der Skeletveränderungen, Arch. orthop. u. Unfall-Chir., *30*, 392, 1931.

SCHLESINGER, H.: *Die Syringomyelie*, Leipzig and Vienna, F. Deuticke, 1895.

SHANDS, A. R., Jr.: Neuropathies of the Bones and Joints: Report of a Case of an Arthropathy of the Ankle Due to a Peripheral Nerve Lesion, Arch. Surg., *20*, 614, 1930.

SIEGELMAN, S. S., HEIMANN, W. G. and MANIN, M. C.: Congenital Indifference to Pain, Am. J. Roentgenol., *97*, 242, 1966.

SILVERMAN, F. N. and GILDEN, J. J.: Congenital Insensitivity to Pain: A Neurologic Syndrome with Bizarre Skeletal Lesions, Radiology, *72*, 176, 1959.

STEINDLER, A.: The Tabetic Arthropathies, J.A.M.A., *96*, 250, 1931.

VAN DER HOUWEN, H.: A Case of Neuropathic Arthritis Caused by Indifference to Pain, J. Bone & Joint Surg., *43–B*, 314, 1961.

VOSS, H.: Über die parostalen und paraartikulären Knochenneubildungen bei organischen Nervenkrankheiten, Fortschr. Geb. Röntgenstrahlen, *55*, 423, 1937.

WALBOM-JØRGENSEN, S.: Neuropathy of the Shoulder Joint Primarily Diagnosed as Sarcoma, Clin. Radiol., *17*, 365, 1966.

Chapter

28

Idiopathic Inflammatory Histiocytosis

In this chapter, we shall consider: (1) eosinophilic granuloma of bone; (2) Letterer-Siwe disease; and (3) Schüller-Christian disease. These three conditions, while differing in their clinical manifestations, appear to be interrelated in their basic pathology, and it is hence to be inferred that they share a common though still-unestablished etiology. On this assumption, despite the existence of transition forms among these three conditions: (1) Eosinophilic granuloma of bone would represent the limited expression of the disorder (the mildest form); (2) Letterer-Siwe disease the acute disseminated expression (the most serious form); and (3) Schüller-Christian disease the chronic disseminated and most widely varied expression of idiopathic inflammatory histiocytosis (see Jaffe and Lichtenstein). The conception that Letterer-Siwe disease and Schüller-Christian disease are anatomically interrelated was not new, having previously been proposed by Flori and Parenti, Glanzmann, and also Wallgren, among others. However, our idea of interrelating eosinophilic granuloma of bone with Letterer-Siwe disease and Schüller-Christian disease was new, and constituted what is now generally recognized as a forward step toward the understanding of these three clinical and pathologic expressions of inflammatory histiocytosis. The concept that eosinophilic granuloma of bone (in solitary or multiple foci) and Schüller-Christian disease and Letterer-Siwe disease have a common underlying process and represent different phases of the same disease has won the support of a number of investigators, including Avery *et al.*, Oberman, Arcomano *et al.*, and also Uehlinger. However, this opinion has been rejected by others, including McGavran and Spady, and also Lieberman *et al.* One reason for the rejection, cited by the latter authors, is the contention that the expression "Letterer-Siwe disease" is a clinical term which has been used to characterize various histiocytic lymphomas and occasional infectious processes, and should therefore not be linked with eosinophilic granuloma and Schüller-Christian disease. This opinion was controverted by Richter in his discussion of the article by Mermann and Dargeon. Those authors maintained that Letterer-Siwe disease is to be regarded as a neoplastic process presenting a histologic similarity to monocytic leukemia. In refuting this view, Richter, a specialist in hematologic pathology, stated: "On the basis of present knowledge I am unwilling to classify it [Letterer-Siwe disease] among the neoplastic diseases."

The term "histiocytosis X" was introduced by Lichtenstein in 1953 and is now also frequently used by others as a comprehensive designation for the three conditions. His reason for advocating the term "histiocytosis X" was that use of this term would do away with "slavish adherence to the eponyms of Letterer-Siwe disease and Schüller-Christian disease, at least as primary designations." In other words, he advocated that the eponyms be used only as qualifying terms in conjunction with the designation "histiocytosis X." In particular, "histiocytosis X localized in bone" would represent eosinophilic granuloma of bone, "acute or subacute disseminated histiocytosis X" would denote Letterer-Siwe disease, and "chronic disseminated histiocytosis X" would refer to Schüller-Christian disease. Actually, there is nothing significant in regard to the concept of histiocytosis X which distinguishes it from the view already expressed in 1944 in the article by Jaffe and Lichtenstein in which the three clinical manifestations of idiopathic inflammatory histiocytosis were discussed under the descriptive title: "Eosinophilic Granuloma of Bone: A Condition Affecting One, Several or Many Bones, But Apparently Limited to the Skeleton, and Representing the Mildest Clinical Expression of the Peculiar Inflammatory Histiocytosis Also Underlying Letterer-Siwe Disease and Schüller-Christian Disease."

EOSINOPHILIC GRANULOMA OF BONE

In 1940, Lichtenstein and Jaffe described 3 cases presenting a solitary destructive bone lesion which the present writer had already recognized as being inflammatory in nature, and whose peculiarities seemed to him to be economically expressed in the name "eosinophilic granuloma of bone." Independently but at the same time, Otani and Ehrlich described under the name of "solitary granuloma of bone" 4 cases showing the same type of lesion, and they favored the idea that trauma might be the initiating cause of it.

In the cases which we reported, the lesion was found to be characterized histologically by conspicuous sheetlike collections of histiocytes (including some revealing phagocytic activity), interspersed among which there were more or less prominent accumulations of eosinophilic cells and especially eosinophilic leukocytes. In addition, however, there were usually some fields of hemorrhage and necrosis, and, particularly in relation to these latter fields, one could note larger or smaller numbers of multinuclear giant cells, some of which likewise showed phagocytic activity. The modifications which may be superimposed on this histologic picture—for instance, by the scarring effects of a fracture at the site of the lesion—will be brought out later. In any event, the name "eosinophilic granuloma of bone" was applied to the lesion because of the imprint which the eosinophils give it, though it was recognized and stressed that its basic cells are the histiocytes.

Not long after the appearance of the article published in 1940, the writer became aware that one may also encounter cases showing multiple bone lesions presenting the same histologic picture as the solitary eosinophilic granuloma. The case which first brought about this realization showed lesions in a number of bones roentgenographically, though only one of the lesions was giving rise to clinical complaints when the patient was first admitted to our hospital. It thus also became clear that, even in cases in which supposedly there is only a solitary lesion, lesions may be present in other bones too, though clinically silent, and should be searched for roentgenographically.

In 1941, Farber confirmed the occurrence of cases of eosinophilic granuloma both with solitary and with multiple skeletal lesions. In the subsequent fuller report by Green and Farber, the clinical peculiarity of these cases was stressed, and, on the pathologic side, the peculiar granulomatous character of the lesion's tissue was emphasized. Indeed, Green and Farber, too, pointed out the necessity for singling out these cases on the basis of their special character. Others concurred in our designation of the lesion as "eosinophilic granuloma of bone" (see Hatcher, Mallory, Held and Rutishauser, and also Hunter).

CLINICAL CONSIDERATIONS

In respect to *age incidence*, it is to be noted that eosinophilic granuloma of bone is seen mainly in children, though sometimes in young adults. If tissue from a bone lesion of a middle-aged or elderly adult suggests on histologic examination that one might be dealing with an eosinophilic granuloma, there is considerable likelihood that the lesion actually represents a focus of Hodgkin's disease. In regard to the *number of bones involved* in a particular case, our original article, as already noted, concerned itself with instances in which only one bone seemed to be affected. That cases may be encountered in which several or even many bones are involved is now also clear. Of the 10 cases reported by Green and Farber, 4 showed single and 6 showed multiple lesions, and none of their patients was more than 11 years old, though it should be pointed out that these cases were reported from The Children's Hospital in Boston.

In respect to *localization*, it is to be noted that apparently almost any bone, with the possible exception of the bones of the hands and feet, may be the site of a lesion in a case of eosinophilic granuloma, whether the skeletal involvement is single or multiple. In the cases in which more than a few bones are affected, those implicated are likely to include one or more bones of the cranial vault, the mandible, some of the ribs, one or more of the vertebrae, and several of the long bones—especially the femur and humerus. In a long tubular bone, the lesion nearly always appears in the shaft of the bone. In the total experience of the present writer, there was only one instance in which the eosinophilic granuloma developed in an epiphysis of a long tubular bone. A case in which an eosinophilic granuloma appeared in the distal epiphysis of a femur is included among the 20 cases reported by Ochsner.

In one instance of eosinophilic granuloma with multiple involvement which was followed by the writer, 8 bones were affected, but those of the skull were spared. At the time of her first admission, the patient in question, a girl 8 years of age, presented a lesion in each of the following bones: right femur, left femur, ninth and eleventh right ribs, and also the second and ninth left ribs. On a subsequent admission, the additional bones found implicated were the eighth left rib and the seventh cervical vertebra.

The purely *visceral forms* of eosinophilic granuloma will not be discussed in this book. They are most commonly observed in the lungs (see Williams *et al.*, Knudson *et al.*, Cruthirds and Johnson, and Weber *et al.*), and have also been encountered in lymph nodes, in the absence of skeletal lesions (see Traissac *et al.*).

The *clinical difficulties* are usually limited to such local complaints as may arise from the skeletal lesions, systemic manifestations being entirely absent as a rule, even in the cases presenting involvement of several or many bones. However, as already stated, when a number of bones are affected in a given instance, it may be only one lesion that gives rise to local complaints, all the other lesions being clinically silent, at first or even for some time. Thus, in the case mentioned in the foregoing paragraph, in which there were lesions in 8 different bones, only one—the one in the neck of the right femur—was causing difficulties at the time of the patient's original admission. Subsequently, involvement of the seventh cervical vertebra led to collapse of the body of that vertebra, thus becoming an additional source of complaints. The fact that in a given case there can be so many silent lesions definitely suggests that occasional cases, even those in which a number of bones are involved and, *a fortiori*, cases in which only one bone is affected, may entirely escape clinical detection.

When there are complaints referable to an affected bone, local tenderness and pain are the most common. Other findings will depend on the part involved. For instance, if the part affected is rather superficial—a rib or the calvarium, for example—a local swelling without heat may be palpable. A lesion in the neck of a femur will usually be associated with a limp. The presence of an eosinophilic granuloma in a *vertebral body* is very likely to lead to wedging collapse of that body and to suggest vertebra plana (so-called Calvé's disease) roentgenographically (see Compere *et al.*, Fripp, Yabsley and Harris, Kieffer *et al.*, and also Nesbit *et al.*).

Figure 228

A, Roentgenograph of the left shoulder region of a child about 3 years of age. The radiolucent lesion in the scapula was established to be an eosinophilic granuloma on the basis of the histologic findings presented by tissue curetted from the lesional area. For several weeks prior to the time this roentgenograph was taken, there was clinical evidence that movement of the shoulder was somewhat limited, and some tenderness was present on deep palpation of the axillary area.

B, Roentgenograph showing a large area of radiolucency in the interior of the lateral end of the right clavicle, and also the deposition of subperiosteal new bone on the cortex of the affected portion of the clavicle. The patient was a child 2 years of age whose principal difficulty was pain of 3 weeks' duration, and curettage of the lesional area revealed that it was an eosinophilic granuloma. Two roentgenographic surveys of the skeleton, done about $2\frac{1}{2}$ months after the lesion in the clavicle was recognized, showed several areas of decreased radiodensity in the left frontal and parietal regions of the calvarium. In addition, lesions were noted in the right femur, left acetabulum, right pubic bone, right ilium, the left fourth and fifth ribs, the right sixth rib, and the fourth thoracic vertebral body. The child was treated with nitrogen mustard and then with methotrexate. After the methotrexate had been given for about 4 months, examination of the blood showed that the treatment had not resulted in any hematopoietic depression. After another 6 months, a roentgenographic skeletal survey revealed filling in of the radiolucent areas in the frontal and parietal bones and considerable healing of the lesion in the clavicle, but the body of the fourth thoracic vertebra was still flattened. Furthermore, this survey failed to reveal any new areas of disease. The child finally made a complete clinical recovery.

C, Roentgenograph showing wedging collapse of the body of the seventh thoracic vertebra in a case of eosinophilic granuloma in which the calvarium was also the site of a lesion. The patient was a girl 12 years of age whose chief complaint was of increasing pain in the thoracic region of the back. Tissue curetted from the lesional area in the calvarium revealed indubitable evidence of eosinophilic granuloma. The calvarial lesion healed in after the curettage, but follow-up information is lacking in regard to the collapsed vertebral body.

D, Roentgenograph showing, in the femoral head, a round, radiolucent area abutting on the epiphysial cartilage plate. The patient was a boy 7 years of age. A needle biopsy established that the lesion was an eosinophilic granuloma, and the lesional area subsequently healed in.

E, Roentgenograph of the left femur, which is the site of a large eosinophilic granuloma involving the upper portion of the shaft, including part of the intertrochanteric area. The patient was a girl 4 years of age who, 3 weeks before admission to the hospital, complained of discomfort and pain in the left thigh. At the same time, the mother noted that the child limped. About a week after the onset of these complaints, there was some swelling of the left thigh, and that led to the child's admission to the hospital. The picture discloses a somewhat fusiform area of intramedullary rarefaction, and also periosteal new bone formation which extends downward below the site of the lesion to the junction of the proximal and middle thirds of the femur. The cortex in the region of the lesion is thinned in consequence of erosion from the medullary surface. At surgery, the area in question was found to contain 10 to 15 cc. of bloody fluid, and soft, yellowish tissue was curetted from the interior of the bone. Histologic examination of the tissue led to designation of the lesion as an eosinophilic granuloma of bone. Postoperatively, the child was given some roentgen therapy, and the lesional area filled in. One year after the surgery, the child appeared well and active and was symptom-free. See Figure 229 for the histologic pattern of the lesional tissue.

F, Roentgenograph illustrating the alterations caused by an eosinophilic granuloma in the shaft of the left femur of a girl 10 years of age. For about one month prior to admission to the hospital, she experienced pain in the thigh and limped slightly. Note the extensive destruction of the medullary area of the midportion of the shaft, erosion of the cortex from the medullary side, and some subperiosteal new bone formation. The lesional area was curetted, and the diagnosis of eosinophilic granuloma was established on the basis of the histologic findings. After surgery, the lesional area began to heal in, and the general health of the child also improved.

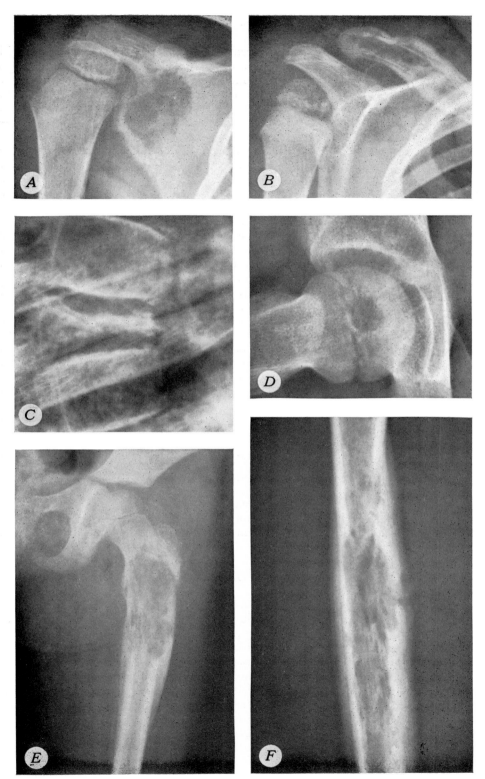

Figure 228

Wedging collapse of the ossification center of a vertebral body of a young child was long held to be due to aseptic necrosis of the center, and was denoted as Calvé's disease. In recent years it has become increasingly clear that wedging collapse of a vertebral body in a child usually results from an eosinophilic granuloma. Indeed, one may doubt whether Calvé's disease in the original sense actually exists. When an eosinophilic granuloma involving a vertebral body has resulted in collapse of the body, the presence of the lesion may be associated with severe local pain and perhaps even with paraplegia. Occasionally one encounters an instance of eosinophilic granuloma of a vertebra which has not resulted in wedging collapse of the body. In these cases the absence of vertebra plana is ascribable to the fact that the eosinophilic granuloma involved only the posterior aspect of the vertebral body, the neural arches, and/or the appendages (see Kaye and Freiberger).

In relation to bone sites other than vertebrae, the duration of the patient's complaints may vary from a few days to several weeks. In an occasional case, inquiry may reveal that the onset of the complaints was associated with slight fever for a few days. In one of our cases the disease seemed to have been ushered in by an attack of moderate but generalized abdominal pain.

In an occasional instance, *leukocytosis*, of moderate severity but not associated with any change in the differential count, is found. In some cases, also, whether or not there is leukocytosis, the differential count shows a slight increase of the *eosinophilic leukocytes* in the blood smears. In one of our patients presenting a solitary lesion, it was not until $1\frac{1}{2}$ years after the lesion had been curetted and had healed that the eosinophil count (4 per cent on admission) dropped to normal. Furthermore, although the peripheral blood may fail to reveal an abnormally high eosinophil count in a particular case, it is very likely that bone marrow obtained from a bone remote from the one which is the site of the eosinophilic granuloma will yield an unusually high eosinophil count (see Marcove, and also Casuccio and Melanotte). The erythrocyte sedimentation rate is often increased (see Fowles and Bobechko).

In the cases in which *chemical estimations* were made, including those of blood cholesterol, cholesterol esters, and total lipid, they yielded normal findings. In the few instances in which tissue from lesions was *cultured for bacteria and viruses*, the results were negative. In a further search for evidences of virus infection, material from two lesions was inoculated into mice, rabbits, and guinea pigs by various routes (including the intracerebral and intratesticular), again with negative results.

ROENTGENOGRAPHIC AND PATHOLOGIC FINDINGS

Roentgenographically the individual bone lesion generally presents as a small or large radiolucent focus. In the calvarium, the lesional area tends to be more or less circular and rather sharply delimited, the focus of radiolucency even appearing punched out. Extensive resorption of the tables, particularly the outer table, will generally be found associated with swelling of the overlying soft parts. In a scapula or an innominate bone, too, the lesion tends to reveal itself in the roentgenograph as an oval or rather circular, sharply delimited area of rarefaction. In a rib, the affected region, in addition to being rarefied, may be expanded and also fractured in one place or another, and if a fracture is present there may even be evidence of subperiosteal deposition of new bone and thickening of the overlying soft tissue. In regard to long bones, too, it can be noted that the lesion begins to evolve in the interior of the bone shaft and that, as it enlarges to implicate the regional cortex, the latter becomes eroded from the medullary side. Furthermore, the cortex may undergo expansion and even be perforated, and, where perforation has taken place, deposition of subperiosteal new bone usually becomes evident. In relation to long tubular bones, it is only very rarely, as already noted, that an eosinophilic granuloma makes its appearance in an epiphysis, and the writer's total experience has included only one case in which the lesion had this location. (See Fig. 228.)

Altogether, there is nothing distinctive about the roentgenographic appearance of an individual lesion. For that reason, one can readily understand why, in cases in which eosinophilic granuloma is limited to a single bone (especially a long tubular bone), the focus of bone destruction as seen in the roentgenograph may even suggest, in the light of the clinical picture as a whole, that the lesion is a sarcoma, and in particular a Ewing sarcoma. At the time the concept of the Ewing sarcoma was first delineated, and even somewhat later, it was customary to make the diagnosis on the basis of the roentgenographic findings, without histologic examination of a biopsy specimen. Under these circumstances, in cases in which a cure of a supposed Ewing sarcoma was obtained by means of radiation therapy, the great likelihood is that the lesion in question was an eosinophilic granuloma rather than a Ewing sarcoma. In the cases in which several or many bones are involved, the roentgenographic appearances may again suggest a cancerous growth—specifically a malignant lymphoma or a tumor metastatic to the skeleton. Furthermore, and more logically, the roentgenographic picture in these cases (particularly in the presence of lesions in the skull) may suggest Schüller-Christian disease.

In regard to details of the *pathologic anatomy* of eosinophilic granuloma of bone, one is confronted by a wide range of histologic findings varying with the duration of the lesion and also with the presence or absence of superimposed secondary changes, such as reparative scarring in response to perforation or fracture of the bone at the site of the lesion. If an unmodified eosinophilic granuloma is exposed surgically when it is still in its early phase (a few weeks or at most a few months after its appearance), it is likely that the lesional area will be found more or less hemorrhagic and cystic, and will show a relatively small amount of soft, brownish tissue which may be streaked with yellow. Microscopic examination may reveal that some or much of this tissue is necrotic.

Characteristically, the non-necrotic tissue presents on *microscopic examination*, as already noted, conspicuous sheetlike collections of large phagocytic cells of the nature of histiocytes, interspersed among which are more or less conspicuous numbers of eosinophilic cells and especially of eosinophilic leukocytes. Furthermore, one finds actively phagocytic multinuclear giant cells, especially in the vicinity of fields of hemorrhage and necrosis. It is the *histiocytes* that constitute the basic component of the lesion. Most of them contain a single nucleus, but a small number have two nuclei or even more. The nuclei are large and usually roundish, although some are oval, kidney-shaped, or otherwise modified in contour. In the cytoplasm of the uninuclear or multinuclear cells, one often observes phagocytosed erythrocytes and granulocytes (usually eosinophils) in various stages of disintegration, as well as brownish hemosiderin granules. The leukocytes and hemosiderin particles are readily discernible in preparations stained with hematoxylin and eosin. The red blood cells, though refractile, are not always easy to detect in such preparations, but can be seen reasonably well in sections stained with eosin and methylene blue. Particularly in the vicinity of fields of necrosis, some of the unicellular and many of the multicellular or giant histiocytes may be found to contain sudanophilic droplets. These are not doubly refractile, as a rule, and apparently represent phagocytosed particles of the neutral fat normally present in the invaded interior of the affected bone. (See Fig. 229.)

As already noted, the eosinophils, though not the basic cellular constituent of the lesion, yet give it a striking imprint, especially when present in large numbers. For the most part, these cells present irregular or bilobed nuclei, though in some lesions or in some places in a given lesion the nuclei of the eosinophilic cells are found to be roundish and not indented.   Incidentally, the small size of these uninuclear eosinophils militates against the idea that they might be eosinophilic myelocytes.   In connection with the finding of the eosinophilic leukocytes in the lesions, it should be pointed out that it may be difficult to demonstrate these cells in tissue which has been left too long in decalcifying fluid (for instance, nitric acid). In some lesions or parts of lesions, one may also find small numbers of lymphocytes, plasma cells, and even neutrophilic polymorphonuclear leukocytes.   In appropriately processed tissue, Charcot-Leyden crystals derived from the nuclei of eosinophils are very often demonstrable in areas where the tissue is necrotic (see Ayres and Silliphant).

If a fracture through the site of the lesion has been followed by a reparative reaction to it, the interior of the bone at that site may be found filled in more or less completely by a cellular tissue which is reddish gray-white on the whole and even tinged with yellow.   On histologic examination, however, it will be found that, though the lesion as a whole has undergone connective tissue scarring in many places, it has nevertheless not lost its characteristic histologic features.   That is, one can still see large fields or even delineated foci of tissue dominated by histiocytes which are intermingled with eosinophils and especially with eosinophilic leukocytes. Though the lesion as a whole may be traversed in an irregular way by strands and patches of connective tissue, the latter tissue can be traced to the fracture because of its association with parosteal scarring, periosteal new bone formation, and callus formation.   Hence, the presence of scarring under these circumstances should not be taken as indicating that scarring represents a phase in the healing of the eosinophilic granuloma *per se*.   (See Fig. 230.)

It seems pertinent at this point to consider the question of the histologic changes undergone by an eosinophilic granuloma which had not been treated (by surgery or radiation) and has had a chance to pursue its natural course.   Green and Farber have stated that when the lesion first passes from the early to the older stage, eosinophils are no longer to be found in it, large vacuolated mononuclear cells are seen predominating, and the ingrowth of connective tissue is evident.   They went on to say that further along in the evolution of the lesion the large mononuclear cells become lipophages and take on the typical appearance of "foam cells." They maintained that, still later, connective tissue crowds out the mononuclear cells and lipophages and in turn is transformed into bone.   The present writer interprets the description given by Green and Farber of the progression of the pathologic changes as indicating that the lesion passes from the early stage of a histiocytic granuloma

Figure 229

A, Photomicrograph ($\times$ 150) prepared from tissue curetted from the femoral lesion shown in Figure 228-*E*.   The small, deeply stained cells are eosinophilic leukocytes which, in this picture, are present mainly in large focal collections.   The larger cells, which are not deeply stained, are the histiocytes, and some eosinophilic leukocytes are interspersed among them.

B, Photomicrograph ($\times$ 475) showing a tissue field in which some eosinophilic polymorphonuclear leukocytes are dispersed among the histiocytes.   Especially in the upper part of the picture, the bilobed nuclei of the eosinophils are clearly apparent, and granules (which take the eosin stain) can be seen plainly in the cytoplasm of most of these cells.

C, Photomicrograph ($\times$ 700) showing a compacted, tumor-like aggregation of histiocytes. Note that some of the latter have more than one nucleus, as does, for instance, the large cell near the lower right-hand corner of the picture.   Furthermore, some of the histiocytes contain phagocytosed eosinophils and erythrocytes, as well as eosinophilic granules and iron-containing particles.

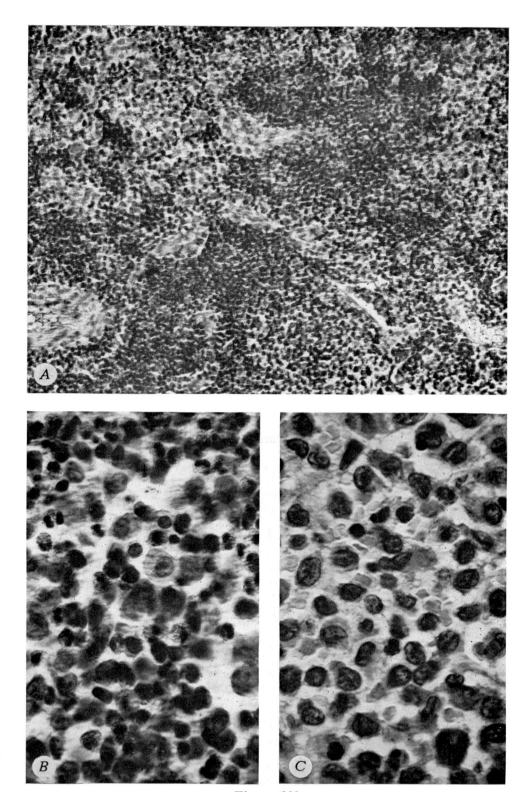

Figure 229

dominated by eosinophils to a stage in which the picture becomes interpretable as that of lipogranuloma (reminiscent of the lesion of Schüller-Christian disease).

The present writer has studied histologically 2 untreated lesions in a case of eosinophilic granuloma of bone which would appear to indicate that *such lesions may heal through resolution* instead of through the mediacy of lipidization and connective tissue scarring. The 2 lesions in question were located in ribs and were from the same patient mentioned previously—a girl 8 years of age in whom 8 lesions, in all, were demonstrable roentgenographically. Of these 8 lesions, only 2 (the one in the right femoral neck and the one in the body of the seventh cervical vertebra) had given rise to clinical difficulties. The other lesions (including the one in the upper portion of the shaft of the left femur) were entirely silent clinically. At the time of the patient's first admission to the hospital, the lesion in the neck of the right femur and the one in the upper portion of the shaft of the left femur were treated surgically by curettage. Serial roentgenographic examinations undertaken in the course of the next 9 months demonstrated that, in the 2 curetted femoral sites, healing through ossification was taking place. Furthermore, the roentgenographs ultimately revealed that the ninth and eleventh ribs, which were also sites of eosinophilic granuloma and which were untreated, likewise presented evidence of healing. Consent was obtained for resection of the involved areas of the ribs in question, so that it was possible to ascertain directly what had happened in the course of spontaneous healing of these rib lesions.

Both rib segments were sectioned transversely into small blocks for embedding in paraffin. Then almost all of these tissue blocks were serially sectioned and studied microscopically. Surprisingly, the stained tissue slides revealed but little evidence of previous disease in the interior of these ribs. It was clear from all the sections

Figure 230

A, Roentgenograph of the sixth right rib, which is the site of an eosinophilic granuloma. The patient was a boy 11 years of age who had become aware of pain in the area of the involved rib about 2 months before he was hospitalized. Several weeks before admission, he had noted that one of the ribs in that area was swollen. The pertinent roentgenographs were seen by numerous radiologists and were interpreted by all of them as indicative of the presence of a malignant tumor—probably a Ewing sarcoma. This evaluation of the lesion is entirely understandable in view of the fact that the roentgenographs which were studied were taken during July or August 1939—that is, at a time when the concept of eosinophilic granuloma as a disease entity was still quite new. The expanded portion of the rib was resected, and histologic examination of pertinent tissue revealed that the lesion was indeed an eosinophilic granuloma. The present writer saw the case in consultation at the time the surgery was carried out at The Mount Sinai Hospital in New York City, and arrived at the diagnosis of eosinophilic granuloma on the basis of examination of a frozen section of tissue from the resected rib. This case was one of the cases reported by Otani and Ehrlich in 1940. Reference was also made to it in the article by Lichtenstein and Jaffe (1940) and in the article by Jaffe and Lichtenstein (1944). The patient made a prompt and complete recovery after the surgery, and no additional lesions developed.

B, Photomicrograph (× 20) of a tissue section prepared from the resected rib. Note that there is a defect in the cortex, and that the diseased tissue in the interior of the rib appears partitioned off into fields. Study of the slide under higher magnification revealed that the delimited areas consisted mainly of histiocytes intermingled with larger or smaller numbers of eosinophils. The delimiting strands and tracks are composed of vascular connective tissue permeated by eosinophils.

C, Photomicrograph (× 265) revealing the eosinophils (small, darkly stained cells) which are concentrated in some places in the lower part of the picture, and are intermingled with the histiocytes in the upper part of the picture.

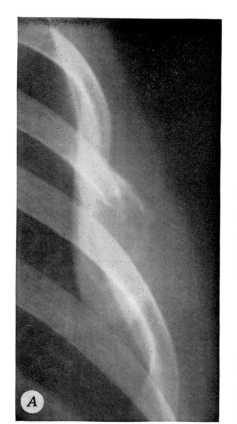

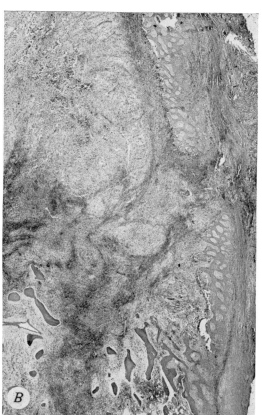

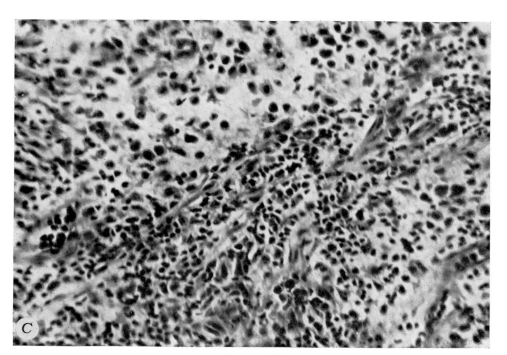

Figure 230

that the interior of the ribs now contained a substantial amount of hematopoietic and fatty marrow between reconstituted spongy trabeculae. However, this hematopoietic marrow showed an excess of leukocytes, especially of eosinophilic leukocytes, and in some places the excess of the eosinophils was even pronounced. Furthermore, one could still see in the marrow, here and there, some macrophages containing blood pigment and even phagocytosed red blood cells. The section which was prepared from a transverse slice through the widest portion of the ninth rib showed the clearest evidence of residual disease. However, even this consisted merely of one small field in which there were many histiocytes containing blood pigment and fragmented red blood cells, supported in a loose and somewhat vascular edematous meshwork. The latter was rather heavily infiltrated with small cells having dark-staining nuclei and appearing to be young marrow cells.

Altogether, then, such traces of residual disease as we could still find in the great number of tissue slides prepared from all parts of the two rib segments were at most reminiscent of the original inflammatory histiocytic and eosinophilic lesion. Even though one now found, somewhere in these healed lesions, a few nests of foam cells, this finding itself would not be significant as pointing in the direction of lipogranuloma. Indeed, a few small nests of foam cells would have little specific meaning, since they are frequently seen even in inflammatory granulation tissue curetted from lesions in cases of chronic pyogenic osteomyelitis. Nevertheless, it may be countered that a lipogranulomatous process had replaced the histiocytic-eosinophilic process in the ribs in question but had already disappeared by the time the ribs were examined microscopically. As noted, Green and Farber held that this is indeed the chronology of the natural healing of the eosinophilic granulomatous lesion. This may be so, but the two rib specimens just described failed to yield any evidence in that direction, and furthermore suggested instead that the lesion of eosinophilic granuloma of bone can heal by resolution without passing through a lipogranulomatous stage. (See Fig. 231.)

In this connection it should be noted that, in the healing phases of a fibrous corti-

Figure 231

A, Roentgenograph showing an eosinophilic granuloma lesion in the right ninth rib in the case of a girl 8 years of age who, in the course of her illness, developed lesions in 8 bone sites, only 2 of which gave rise to clinical difficulties. The patient was admitted to the hospital for treatment of a lesion in the neck of the right femur. Subsequently (about 9 months after her first admission) a roentgenographic skeletal survey revealed involvement of the right ninth and eleventh ribs. In particular, the contour of the ninth rib is expanded, and the diseased area presents as a focus of radiolucency. The rib lesion was not treated either surgically or by radiation, but healed spontaneously (see B).

B, Roentgenograph showing the appearance of the affected ninth rib, 7 months after the picture shown in A was taken. Though the contour of the rib is still expanded, the area of radiolucency is no longer evident, spontaneous healing having occurred.

C, Photomicrograph (× 15) of a tissue slide prepared from the resected healed ninth rib in question. The slide was prepared from a block of tissue taken through the widest part of that rib. The interior of the rib (that is, the medullary cavity) reveals fatty and myeloid marrow and numerous dilated blood vessels. No obvious scarring is present, and residual tissue ascribable to the pathologic process is minimal. Such tissue is apparent, however, in the area delimited by the arrows.

D, Photomicrograph (× 475) showing in detail the cellular composition of the small residual area of disease marked out by the arrows in C. The large histiocytes, which are supported in a loose, edematous meshwork, contain pigment granules in their cytoplasm. The dark-staining nuclei are mainly the nuclei of eosinophilic leukocytes. (The fingerprints visible in the right side of the picture could not be eliminated from the negative.)

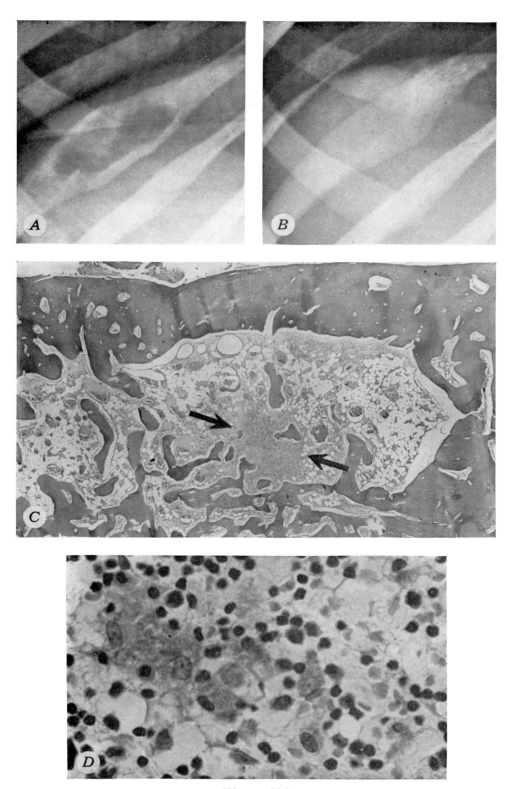

Figure 231

cal defect or a nonossifying fibroma, many of the stromal cells in certain of the tissue fields may become lipidized and converted into foam cells. On this account, one finds occasional instances in the literature in which a lipidized fibrous cortical defect or a nonossifying fibroma is described as a xanthoma, xanthofibroma, or xanthogranuloma, often with the specific implication (an erroneous one) that the lesion represents a healed, lipidized focus of eosinophilic granuloma. However, the writer has yet to encounter an indubitable solitary focus of eosinophilic granuloma which, even in part, has become so lipidized as to present the pattern of the lipidized tissue fields sometimes seen in a nonossifying fibroma (see Jaffe).

TREATMENT

Patients affected with eosinophilic granuloma involving a *single bone* enter the hospital only because of local complaints referable to the affected area of the bone and usually come under surgical treatment rather promptly, with one diagnosis or another. Since the definitive diagnosis is ordinarily made only after histologic study of tissue obtained from the lesion, one cannot know what would regularly happen to any solitary eosinophilic granuloma lesion if it were left undisturbed. We do know, however, that solitary lesions which are curetted show gradual repair of the affected area after this procedure alone. More often, curettage and supplementary radiation therapy (with employment of relatively small doses—400 to 500 r) have been used, but it is not certain that the roentgen therapy accelerates the healing process. However, if healing is delayed and the local complaints do not subside, one should be alert to the possibility that lesions may appear in other bone sites.

Roentgen therapy alone has also been used against one or another remaining lesion in cases of *multiple involvement* of bones after the diagnosis has been made on the basis of curettings from one of the lesions. For a large lesion in a surgically inaccessible site, Green and Farber have advocated giving a total dose of 1,500 r through two fields, in small divided doses, over a period of 6 days. Under such treatment, while some lesions heal within a few months, others do not, requiring a year or more. Nevertheless, as mentioned above, some of the lesions may undergo spontaneous healing.

Corticosteroids (notably in the form of Prednisone) have been used in some cases of eosinophilic granuloma involving a number of bones, despite the fact that prolonged administration of cortisone may induce clinical features of the Cushing syndrome. The use of corticosteroids may be prompted by the fact that: (1) In cases presenting multiple lesions, it often happens that some of the symptomatic lesions are in sites not readily accessible for curettage; and (2) it is obviously necessary to avoid the overexposure of the subject to irradiation of many individual lesions. However, if one or more of the lesions involve bone sites where their progression could create a serious clinical complication, irradiation of these lesional sites is indicated in addition to the use of corticosteroids. In a case in which there are multiple lesions and in which, despite the use of the foregoing therapeutic measures, clinical progress toward healing has not been made, Marcove advocates the cautious use of methotrexate.

LETTERER-SIWE DISEASE

As already noted, it appears that eosinophilic granuloma of bone (conceived in a clinico-anatomic sense), Schüller-Christian disease, and Letterer-Siwe disease constitute different expressions of the same basic disorder. Certainly, on clinical grounds alone one would not suspect that there were any points of correspondence between eosinophilic granuloma of bone and Letterer-Siwe disease. Indeed, from all that has already been said about eosinophilic granuloma of bone, it is clear that the latter is clinically a mild disorder ordinarily limited to the skeleton and often involving only a single bone. Letterer-Siwe disease, on the other hand, is clinically a serious disorder in which lesions are widely distributed through the body, including the skin and the bones.

Especially in the older literature, cases which would now be classed as instances of Letterer-Siwe disease have been described under a variety of names, such as "aleukemic reticulosis," "acute (or infectious) aleukemic reticulosis," "reticuloendotheliosis," "infectious granulomatous (or nonlipoid) reticuloendotheliosis," and "nonlipoid histiocytosis." Also in the older literature, some cases of Letterer-Siwe disease are to be found reported as instances of Schüller-Christian disease. If, in the light of our present knowledge, one studies the case reported by Hand which has linked his name with the names of Schüller and Christian, it seems more than likely that Hand's case would now be classed as an instance of Letterer-Siwe disease *per se* rather than as one of Hand-Schüller-Christian disease.

The designation "Letterer-Siwe disease" was applied by Abt and Denenholz in 1936 to give credit to Letterer for his description of a case from the standpoint of the pathologic anatomy, and to Siwe for his presentation of the clinical observations in a case of his own, and compilation of the clinical findings relating to a number of cases already reported by others. It should be noted, however, that Letterer held at first that the pathologic changes underlying the disorder have a tumorous basis, while the common current opinion is that they represent an inflammatory reaction of unknown cause. Furthermore, the clinical picture delineated by Siwe has been found to require supplementation and even amendment. Be that as it may, valuable contributions to the understanding of the clinical and pathologic aspects of Letterer-Siwe disease soon began to accumulate (see Guizetti, Podvinec and Terplan, Roussy and Oberling, Foot and Olcott, Paige, van Creveld and ter Poorten, Flori and Parenti, Glanzmann, and also Wallgren).

CLINICAL CONSIDERATIONS

Letterer-Siwe disease has its *onset* mainly in infants and in children below the age of 2 (rarely appearing after the age of 4). A case has also been reported in which a full term but stillborn infant manifested Letterer-Siwe disease in fully evolved form at birth (see Ahnquist and Holyoke). This case of congenital Letterer-Siwe disease represents a rare instance (apparently the first one reported) in which the disease completed the full course *in utero*. A case of fully evolved Letterer-Siwe disease has also been described in which the subject was a somewhat premature infant who died immediately after delivery and on whom an autopsy was performed which established the diagnosis (see Cohen *et al.*). Furthermore, a few cases have been recorded in which only one feature of Letterer-Siwe disease (such as skin lesions or abdominal enlargement) had been noted at birth but in which the full-fledged clinical picture evolved in the course of the next few weeks or months and the infant died not long thereafter (see Batson *et al.*). Even if the infant shows no manifestations of the disease at birth, the condition ordinarily runs an acute or subacute course, the infant dying some weeks or months later. In an occasional instance, however, the course is semichronic, being protracted over a year or two or even a somewhat longer period. Indeed, the condition sometimes passes over into what may already be called Schüller-Christian disease, as will be made clear presently. A clinico-anatomic complex denoted as "familial reticuloendotheliosis with eosinophilia" has been described which should be differentiated from Letterer-Siwe disease even though the infants in question do present severe skin eruptions, hepato- and splenomegaly, and generalized lymphadenopathy (see Omenn).

The principal *clinical findings* to be noted in cases of Letterer-Siwe disease as a whole are: (1) a febrile course; (2) enlargement of the spleen, of the liver, and of superficial lymph nodes; (3) a cutaneous eruption, generally purpuric in character and often particularly pronounced shortly before death; (4) hypochromic secondary anemia, often profound terminally; and (5) one or more destructive lesions in bones, particularly in the skull bones (specifically the calvarium, the mandible, and the base of the skull in the region of the sphenoid). Less regularly, the cases present: (1) leukocytosis of moderate severity; (2) evidence of secondary bacterial infection in the form of purulent otitis media and mastoiditis, ulcerative or even necrotizing angina, or acute lymphadenitis; (3) mottling or honeycombing and even emphysema of the lungs, evident roentgenographically; and (4) terminally, pleural and abdominal effusion and subcutaneous edema.

PATHOLOGIC AND ROENTGENOGRAPHIC FINDINGS

Anatomically, Letterer-Siwe disease is characterized by wide dispersion of histiocytes through the tissues of the body, in the form of either *nodular foci* or *diffuse collections*. Histologic examination reveals that the histiocytes occur (as more or less conspicuous nodular collections) particularly in the lymph nodes, the tonsils, the thymus, the spleen, the bone marrow, the liver, the lymphoid tissue of the alimentary tract, and the skin. Diffusely distributed histiocytes are found in the lungs, the dura, the periosteum overlying the affected bone areas, the interstitial or fatty connective tissue of the heart, the pancreas and the renal pelves, and even in some of the endocrine glands (pituitary, parathyroid, and adrenal). Interspersed among the histiocytes there may be small numbers of lymphocytes and plasma cells and sometimes also a sprinkling of eosinophils.

A basis of relationship between Letterer-Siwe disease and eosinophilic granuloma of bone is afforded by the gross and histologic character of the destructive skeletal

Figure 232

A, Roentgenograph showing a large, destructive lesion involving the distal half of the shaft of the left radius of a female infant 10 months of age. When this picture was taken, the left wrist and forearm had been swollen for about 2 months. A biopsy was carried out on the lesion in the forearm, and the histologic pattern of the tissue removed conformed to that of an eosinophilic granuloma (see *B*). In the course of the subsequent 2 months, this infant manifested petechial hemorrhages and superficial ulcerations of the skin, including the scalp. Furthermore, enlargement of the liver, spleen, and superficial lymph nodes became evident clinically. The child died about 4 months after the onset of her clinical difficulties, and an autopsy confirmed the diagnosis of Letterer-Siwe disease.

B, Photomicrograph ($\times$ 150) of tissue curetted from the lesion in the radius illustrated in *A*. The lighter cells are histiocytes, and the small, dark ones are eosinophils. In respect to cytologic appearance, the curettings from this lesion in a case of Letterer-Siwe disease are interchangeable with those from a case of eosinophilic granuloma in which the latter condition is limited even to one bone.

C, Photomicrograph ($\times$ 60) of a lymph node removed at autopsy in the case of the infant who died of Letterer-Siwe disease and about whom some clinical information is given in *A*. The lymphoid cells have been substantially replaced by histiocytes (see *D*).

D, Photomicrograph ($\times$ 165) showing a nodular focus of histiocytes in the lymph node illustrated in *C*, where the area in question is more or less indicated by the arrows.

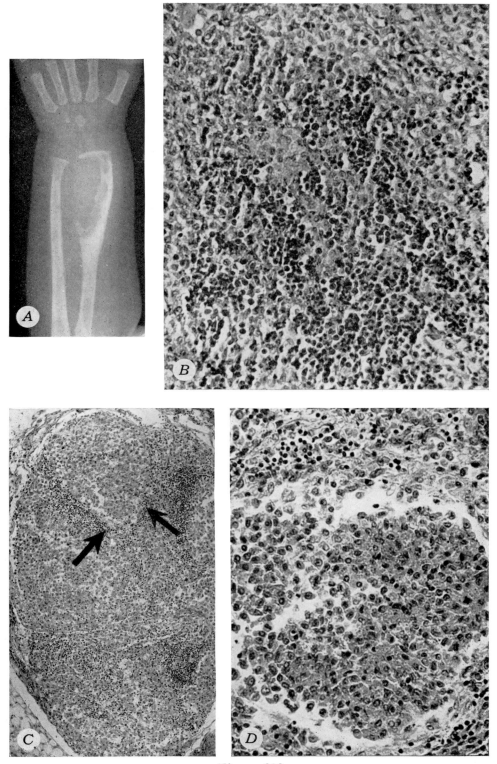

Figure 232

lesions encountered in the former. Specifically, the granulation tissue present in the destructive skeletal lesions of Letterer-Siwe disease in an early stage of their evolution may be indistinguishable microscopically from such tissue in corresponding lesions of eosinophilic granuloma of bone. This statement is supported by the findings in one of the cases of Letterer-Siwe disease which was studied by the writer at the time the full concept of eosinophilic granuloma of bone was being formulated. The case described by Falk and Brown represents another pertinent instance.

The subject in the case studied by the writer was a female infant 10 months of age who came under medical care because of pain and swelling (of 3 weeks' duration) in the area of the left wrist and forearm. There was no history of antecedent trauma to the region in question. A roentgenographic skeletal survey revealed a destructive lesion involving almost the entire distal half of the shaft of the left radius, but no lesions in any other bones. However, the clinical condition of the infant became rapidly worse in the course of the subsequent 2 months. She was febrile, and enlargement of the liver, spleen, and superficial lymph nodes became evident. The skin, including the scalp, presented superficial ulcerations and innumerable petechial hemorrhages. Thus there was clinical evidence that the infant was suffering from Letterer-Siwe disease, and she died about 4 months after the onset of the swelling in the area of the left wrist and forearm. An autopsy confirmed the clinical diagnosis. Indeed, both the clinical and the anatomic findings in this case were in line with those already reported in the literature under the headings of Letterer-Siwe disease, reticulosis (or reticuloendotheliosis) and nonlipoid histiocytosis. Furthermore, the evaluation of the histologic changes in the case was greatly aided by the opportunity of reviewing, for comparison with it, the histologic slides in the relevant cases reported by Abt and Denenholz, Paige, and Foot and Olcott. (See Fig. 232.)

Sections prepared from the various organs and tissues removed at autopsy in the case described here showed, on microscopic examination, a wide distribution of histiocytes through the various tissues of the body—specifically in lymph nodes (both peripheral and internal) and in the spleen, the liver, the bone marrow, the lungs, the skin, the lymphoid tissue of the large intestine and the appendix, the periappendiceal fat, the interstitial tissue of the pancreas, the peripancreatic (subperitoneal) connective tissue, the adrenal medulla, the periadrenal fat, and the hili of the kidneys. Other changes included areas of focal necrosis in the spleen, severe degeneration and fatty change of the hepatic parenchyma, degeneration of the renal epithelium and of the myocardium, and the presence of foci of extramedullary hematopoiesis in the liver and kidneys.

The collections of histiocytes in the lymph nodes, the intestinal lymphoid tissue, and the spleen were particularly large, and focal nodular groups of them even

Figure 233

A, Photomicrograph (× 130) showing a pulmonary field containing numerous histiocytes in the instance of Letterer-Siwe disease to which Figure 232 likewise pertains. At the pleural surface of the lung (represented in the upper margin of the picture), there are many large histiocytes, some of which have double nuclei. In consequence of the accumulation of histiocytes in the interstitium between the alveoli, the alveolar spaces are compressed. Histiocytes are also to be observed within the alveoli.

B, Photomicrograph (× 100) of a tissue section prepared from the colon in the same case. Histiocytes have substantially replaced the submucosal lymphoid nodule.

C, Photomicrograph (× 100) showing a small part of an intra-abdominal lymph node removed at autopsy in this case. Note that most of the lymphoid cells have been replaced by histiocytes.

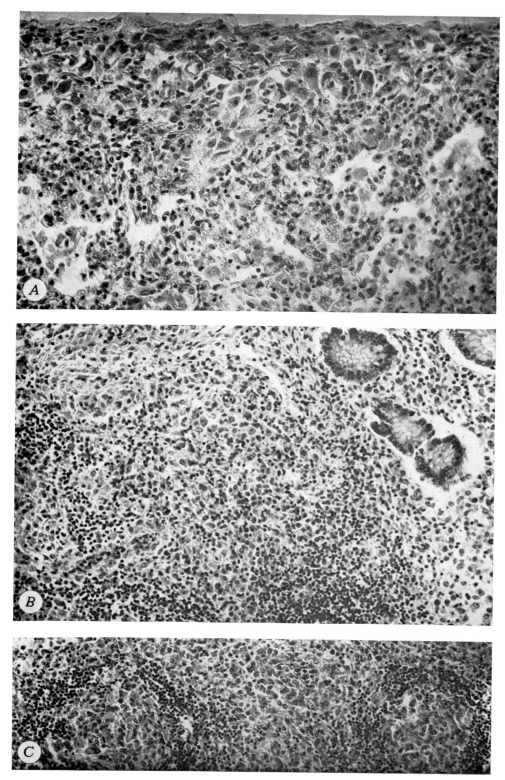

Figure 233

tended to be confluent. In the other tissues, the nests were relatively small and tended to be well separated, or the histiocytes were diffusely distributed. The histiocytes presented, on the whole, faintly acidophilic cytoplasm and rather large, pale, rounded or oval nuclei. Some of the cells were binuclear, and some rather large ones were even multinuclear. Many of the histiocytes contained phagocytosed red blood cells and brownish pigment granules in their cytoplasm. Some of the larger nodular collections presented evidence of hemorrhage and of degeneration or necrobiosis of their component cells and even some fibroblastic scarring. Furthermore, in some sites the focal collections of macrophages were interspersed with a few plasma cells, lymphocytes, and polymorphonuclear leukocytes.

Thus the case of the infant in question made it possible to recognize a connection between Letterer-Siwe disease and eosinophilic granuloma of bone.* This connection resides in the anatomic character of the lesion in the radius of the patient. As noted, when this lesion was examined, it presented a histologic picture identical with that seen in characteristic lesions of eosinophilic granuloma of bone. That is, one saw hemorrhage and necrosis in the inflammatory tissue, and large fields of histiocytes intermingled with fields of eosinophils—a picture which, when once seen, is sufficiently striking to remain firmly in one's mind. (See Fig. 233.)

On the other hand, in relatively old or more chronic skeletal lesions—that is, lesions in cases of Letterer-Siwe disease in which the disorder has run for more than a year—one is likely to find considerable fibrous scarring of the lesional tissue and transformation of some or many of the histiocytes into lipophagic foam cells, in conformity with the picture of so-called lipogranulomatosis supposedly characteristic of Schüller-Christian disease. One finds this fibrous scarring and secondary lipidization (through the conversion of histiocytes into lipophagic foam cells) not only in the lesions of bones and their coverings but also in the granulomatous lesions developing in the thymus and the lungs.

Thus, at one stage or another, a case of Letterer-Siwe disease (reticulosis, reticuloendotheliosis, nonlipoid histiocytosis) may show interrelations through some of its lesions not only with eosinophilic granuloma of bone but also with Schüller-Christian disease. Anatomic support for this idea was given by Flori and Parenti in 1937 in their paper on hyperplastic infectious reticuloendotheliosis with granulo-

* The writer is indebted to Dr. Herman Bolker, who placed at his disposal the roentgenographs showing the destructive lesion in the shaft of the left radius of the infant, and also some of the tissue obtained at the surgical intervention, in the course of which the affected site in the radius was curetted. He is also indebted to Dr. Caspar Burn, who made available to him a clinical abstract, the autopsy protocol, and sections prepared from tissue removed at autopsy in this particularly instructive case.

Figure 234

A, Roentgenograph of the skull of a child 21 months of age who died within a few months after this picture was taken. A diagnosis of Letterer-Siwe disease was established on the basis of both the clinical findings and the autopsy findings. Note the roundish areas of radiolucency in the frontal, parietal, and temporal bones. The child presented a purplish red petechial eruption on the neck, trunk, and extremities, and also petechiae on the gums, tongue, and buccal mucosa. Splenomegaly and hepatomegaly were evident clinically. A roentgenographic skeletal survey showed osteolytic lesions in many bones elsewhere than in the skull.

B, Roentgenograph illustrating lesions in both clavicles and also in both scapulae in this case. Many of the ribs were also sites of lesions, but those ribs were mainly below the ones shown in this illustration.

C, Roentgenograph revealing large osteolytic lesions in both iliac bones in this case of Letterer-Siwe disease.

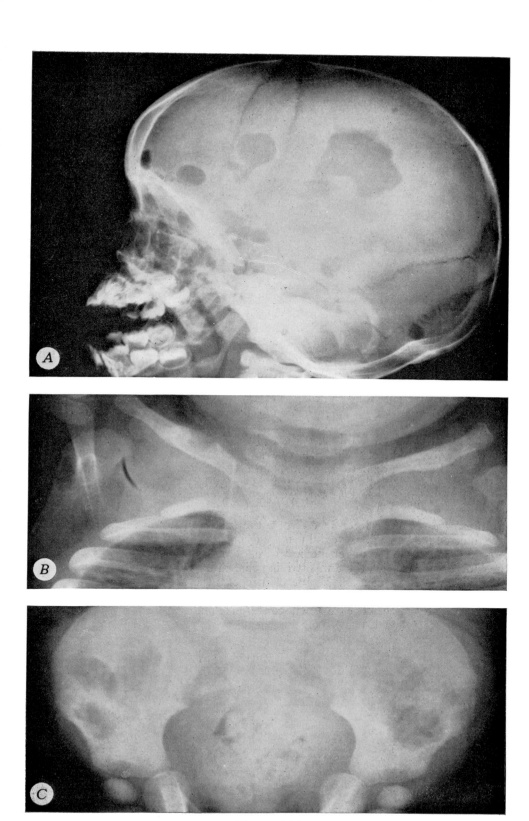

Figure 234

xanthomatous evolution (of the type observed in Schüller-Christian disease). It was also maintained by Glanzmann, who held that cases of so-called reticuloendotheliosis (Letterer-Siwe disease) may pass over into Schüller-Christian disease. More specifically, he held that Letterer-Siwe disease apparently represents the acute septic expression of the pathologic process which in more chronic form is represented by Schüller-Christian disease. A similar point of view was taken by Wallgren, who stressed the importance of the time factor in the transition from one disease state into the other. Additional exponents of the anatomic kinship between the two disorders include Gross and Jacox, and also Mallory.

In connection with the question of the mergence of Letterer-Siwe disease in its chronic stage into what may already be called Schüller-Christian disease, a few additional remarks on the skeletal lesions in the former may be in order. As already noted, skeletal lesions evident clinically or at least *roentgenographically* in Letterer-Siwe disease are particularly likely to include lesions in skull bones. Specifically, it is the calvarium that tends most strongly to show one or more lesions in one or several of its component bones. However, involvement of the base of the skull is by no means uncommon, and occasionally one or another of the facial bones has been found affected. When lesions are present in bones of the skull, one is likely to find them elsewhere in the skeleton also, in one or even many bones, with apparent exception of the bones of the hands and feet. In the cases described by Gerstel and by Flori and Parenti, implication of the skeleton was particularly widespread.

Even when a number of bones (including bones of the skull) are involved, all of the skeletal lesions may be clinically silent. On the other hand, one of them may instigate a search for additional skeletal lesions, so that others are then discovered roentgenographically. In connection with involvement of the sphenoid bone and of the bones delimiting the orbits, diabetes insipidus and exophthalmos have been noted. Indeed, some of the cases have even presented the complete Christian triad of calvarial defects, diabetes insipidus, and exophthalmos. (See Fig. 234.)

TREATMENT

In most cases of Letterer-Siwe disease the condition runs a fulminating course, the affected infant or young child usually dying within a few months or possibly a year after first coming under medical care. However, an occasional instance has been observed in which there was striking clinical improvement or even cure under antibiotic therapy (see Fisher). Bierman reports the 17-year survival of identical twins who, at 8 months of age, had been found (through tissue examination) to have Letterer-Siwe disease. The treatment consisted of multiple antibiotic chemotherapy (the drugs employed being penicillin, chlortetracycline, streptomycin, and/or chloramphenicol), and one of the two patients also received small doses of irradiation limited to the skull. Furthermore, Bierman lists 6 other reported cases which were treated with various antibiotics, along with radiation in 2 of them and cortisone in another. Corticotropin (ACTH) and cortisone have been used with good results in the treatment of some cases of Letterer-Siwe disease, when the dosage of these steroids was adequate. Prouty has described a case of Letterer-Siwe disease in which the patient showed improvement when treated with Prednisone. In particular, the lesions present in bone and soft tissue healed, the hepatomegaly and lymphadenopathy regressed, the anemia was corrected, and the fever disappeared. In an occasional case, methotrexate has also been found to be of therapeutic value. A case of Letterer-Siwe disease has also been reported which set in when the subject was 4 months of age and in which the disease process underwent spontaneous resolution, the child being free of relevant signs and symptoms 2 years later (see Meenan and Cahalane).

SCHÜLLER-CHRISTIAN DISEASE

As is well recognized, the clinical category of Schüller-Christian disease (lipogranulomatosis) is a miscellaneous one. This is true even apart from the fact, now clearly established, that the presence or the absence of the Christian triad (calvarial defects, exophthalmos, and diabetes insipidus) is not by itself an adequate basis for a decision as to whether or not a particular case belongs in the category of Schüller-Christian disease. As to the Christian triad, its presence depends solely on extensive involvement of the bones at the base of the skull, and is neither essential in the diagnosis nor specific for the disease. In any series of cases, it is much more likely to be absent than present (see Takahashi *et al.*).

CLINICAL CONSIDERATIONS

There is wide variety among the cases which have been assigned to the category of Schüller-Christian disease. This is already evident from some of the previous remarks relating to Letterer-Siwe disease. In that connection, it was stated that cases of Letterer-Siwe disease pursuing an exceptionally protracted course of a year or several years may eventually cross the border into the domain of Schüller-Christian disease. The cases reported by Merritt and Paige and also by Green and Flaherty seem to represent excellent examples of progression of the basic pathologic changes from those of Letterer-Siwe to those of Schüller-Christian disease. Such cases, with their coloring of Letterer-Siwe disease, relatively rapid course, and appearance in very young children, contrast with the classic cases of Schüller-Christian disease. In the latter cases (of which the one reported by Chiari is a good example), even though the subjects come to present the full Christian triad, the course of the illness is more protracted, sometimes extending over a period of 10 or even 15 years. Furthermore, while the illness is often found to have set in at some time between the ages of 5 and 10, there are many cases in which the onset dates from some time in the second or third decade or even later.

It may be one or more phenomena of the Christian triad that first direct attention to the disease. Or instead, especially in young subjects, it may be stunting of growth (due to damage to the pituitary gland) that alerts one to it. In still other cases, the first abnormality observed may be a lesion in a jaw bone, in a long tubular bone, or even in some other bone. It has been demonstrated that lesions of the oral mucous membrane resulting in detachment of the gingiva from the underlying structure may precede involvement of the contiguous area of one or both jaw bones (see Lyon and Meyer, Ross *et al.*, and Takahashi *et al.*). The appearance of such gingival lesions, along with implication of the maxilla or mandible, may lead to loosening of the regional teeth and the roentgenographic picture of so-called "floating teeth." (See Fig. 235.)

In association with the various skeletal lesions and some or all of the features of the Christian triad, one may find pulmonary fibrosis, adiposity, and even hypogenitalism. In the case reported by Chiari, the autopsy findings included lipogranulomata in the central nervous system. Altogether, it is clear that the classic cases of Schüller-Christian disease present a wide variety of clinical findings. As to the ultimate *prognosis*, this is poor if, because of lesions in the base of the skull, there has been damage to the hypothalamus, the infundibulum, and the pituitary gland. Other influences tending to make the prognosis unfavorable include scarring of the lungs, ultimately leading to right ventricular heart failure. In addition, the heart itself and even the brain and cord or their coverings may be the site of lipogranulomata, and such lesions likewise have a deleterious effect on the prognosis.

PATHOLOGIC AND ROENTGENOGRAPHIC FINDINGS

It appears that any case which is placed in the category of Schüller-Christian disease should be expected to show, as the *anatomic prerequisite*, collagenized and lipidized lesions classifiable as lipogranulomata. Nevertheless, one can often demonstrate in the lipogranulomatous lesions of a given case (much more easily in certain cases than in others) that the collagenization and lipidization have been engrafted on lesions which originally were dominated by the presence of compacted histiocytes still free of lipid. In other words, it seems to be fairly clear that the fibroblastic scarring and collagenization, and the varying amounts of cholesterol (free or in the cytoplasm of lipophagic foam cells) which give the characteristic lipogranuloma imprint to the lesions of Schüller-Christian disease, represent secondary engraftments on a lesion which was originally neither scarred nor lipidized.

The question which now arises is: In Schüller-Christian disease, what is the cytologic character of the skeletal lesions in particular before they undergo scarring and lipidization? That is, do they show, before that, a granulation tissue dominated

Figure 235

A, Roentgenograph of a large, destructive lesion involving the left scapula of a boy 14 years of age who came to manifest the features of Schüller-Christian disease. Seven months before this picture was taken, he noticed difficulty in abducting the left shoulder, but at that time there was no pain or any history of relevant trauma. About 4 months after the onset of his complaint relating to the shoulder, a hemorrhagic, ecchymotic area appeared on the posterior axillary fold. About 6 weeks later, his left arm suddenly became very painful and he was unable to move it. Concomitantly, an ecchymotic area appeared on the lateral aspect of the upper third of the arm. A roentgenographic skeletal survey made at this time failed to reveal any other bone lesions, but such lesions did become manifest later. A biopsy of the scapular lesion was carried out, and microscopic examination of the tissue revealed the histologic pattern of an eosinophilic granuloma. In contrast to the histologic pattern which one observes in a case of eosinophilic granuloma which has not eventually taken on the features of Schüller-Christian disease, the histologic pattern of the biopsy specimen in this case showed in particular that: The lesional tissue was rather cellular; more histiocytes were present in proportion to the eosinophils; and there was hardly any evidence of necrosis, such as one would encounter in a large eosinophilic granuloma *per se*. These histologic details emphasize the difference between an intrinsic eosinophilic granuloma and a lesion presenting the histologic pattern of an eosinophilic granuloma destined to take on the histologic pattern of a lipogranuloma, such as would be characteristic of Schüller-Christian disease. After the diagnosis was established, 500 *r* of radiation were given to the affected scapula, and substantial healing occurred within a period of a few months.

B, Roentgenograph revealing involvement of the left innominate bone (ilium and the acetabular area) and the head of the left femur 2 years after the roentgenograph shown in *A* was taken. Permission for removal of a biopsy specimen from the innominate bone was refused, but radiation therapy was given and these lesions also healed in.

C, Roentgenograph showing a lytic lesion in the frontal region of the skull in the same patient. This lesion was discovered at about the same time that the lesions portrayed in *B* were uncovered. This skull lesion, too, was treated with radiation therapy and healed in.

D, Roentgenograph disclosing involvement of the mandible in this case. Because of the alterations in the mandible, several of the regional teeth have become loosened, and the picture illustrates the so-called "floating teeth" not infrequently observed in cases of Schüller-Christian disease. The jaw lesion, too, was irradiated and healed in. In the course of the 6 years during which the various bone lesions in this patient were treated with radiation therapy, he received a total of about 12,000 *r*. The latest follow-up information available is that, 20 years after the onset of his disease, he is well, has no complaints, and is working regularly. The patient's recovery was favored by the fact that no lesions developed at the base of the skull or in the lungs, heart, brain, or spinal cord.

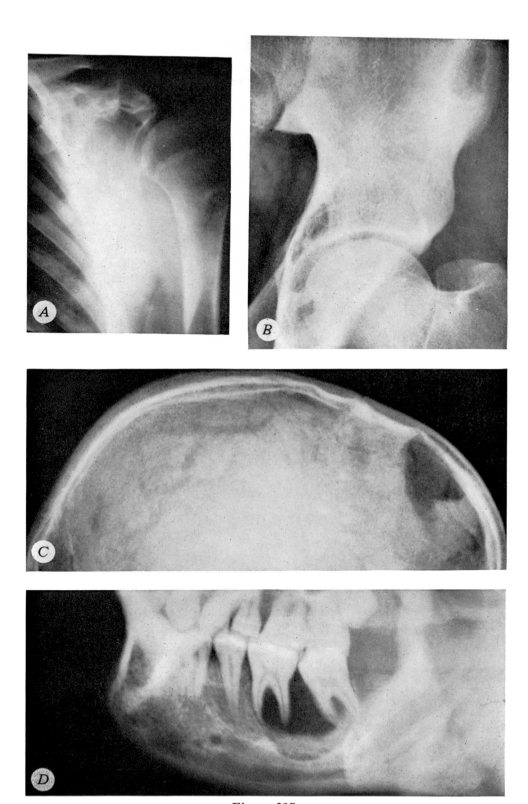

Figure 235

by the presence of histiocytes or of histiocytes and eosinophils—a picture such as one sees in the lesions of eosinophilic granuloma of bone? In 2 cases in which the writer examined tissue from the presenting osteolytic bone lesions, the histologic pattern was that of eosinophilic granuloma, but the subsequent course in these cases was that of Schüller-Christian disease characterized by the presence of lipogranulomata in the bone lesions and viscera. This finding is supported by Uehlinger on the basis of anatomic material he studied in 2 cases which he reported. It is also corroborated by the 5 cases reported by Engelbreth-Holm *et al.* In these 5 cases, in which the subjects were children 2 to 9 years of age, histologic examination revealed a gradual transition, in various lesions, from lipid-free eosinophilic granuloma to the presence of histiocytes containing lipid and finally histologic changes in the direction of fibrous scarring and lipogranuloma formation. Two pertinent cases have also been described by Dumermuth.

One of the problems in establishing this temporal relationship between the lesion presenting the characteristic histologic features of an eosinophilic granuloma and the lesion presenting the histologic features of a lipogranuloma is that the pertinent tissue may not have been examined microscopically until the lesion had already passed into a late stage in its evolution—that is, into the lipogranulomatous stage. Further support for the concept that this represents the sequence of events is furnished by 2 additional facts: (1) In the early stages of evolution of Letterer-Siwe disease, one may find destructive skeletal lesions resembling cytologically those of eosinophilic granuloma of bone; and (2) in its chronic stages, Letterer-Siwe disease takes on some of the anatomic aspects of Schüller-Christian disease, the skeletal and even certain visceral lesions undergoing lipogranulomatous transformation.

Figure 236

A, Roentgenograph showing the left sacroiliac region in the case of a woman 29 years of age who, shortly after giving birth to a somewhat premature infant, began to experience pain in the lower part of the back on the left side, and was aware that the pain was aggravated by walking. In addition to the osteolytic changes in the left ilium and on the left side of the sacrum, lesions in various ribs were found.

B, Roentgenograph revealing osteolytic lesions in the seventh and eighth ribs on the right side in the same case. There was no involvement of the skull bones. The radiologist concluded that the lesions in the ribs and the left sacroiliac region represented foci of metastatic carcinoma. However, the orthopaedic surgeon (Dr. Harry Sonnenschein) was unwilling to accept that diagnosis and decided to resect a small portion of the right seventh rib to obtain a definitive diagnosis based on tissue examination. The present writer examined that rib specimen, which measured 1.5 cm. in length. The periosteal surface was rough and irregular, and one area showed a nodular protrusion. On sectioning the specimen in its long axis, the marrow cavity was found to be filled with homogeneous grayish yellow tissue. Microscopic examination of this tissue led to the diagnosis of lipoid granulomatosis (Schüller-Christian disease), and the histologic appearance of the tissue is shown in Figure 237.

C, Roentgenograph of the left sacroiliac region showing sclerosis and healing after radiation therapy (1,200 *r*) had been given to the area in this case. There was an almost immediate cessation of pain when the therapy was instituted.

D, Roentgenograph of the left hip joint area revealing extensive osteolytic changes in the ilium, and faint evidence of involvement of the neck of the femur. The patient was a boy 17 years of age who came under hospital care with a history of intermittent sharp pain in the region of the left hip, the pain radiating down the medial aspect of the thigh to the knee. The pain was noted only when the patient was sitting, and was not aggravated by activity. A biopsy specimen was obtained from the ilium, and tissue slides were submitted to the present writer for his opinion. These slides were evaluated as showing an inflammatory histiocytosis, which, in this case, is probably best characterized as Schüller-Christian disease. Radiation therapy was advised, but no follow-up information is available.

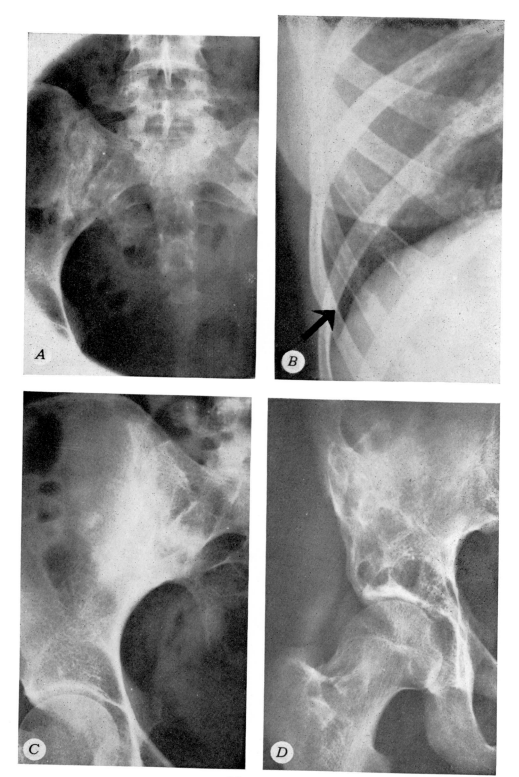

Figure 236

However, in the writer's opinion, no case, irrespective of the clinical picture it presents, should be designated as one of Schüller-Christian disease unless or until at least some of its lesions (visceral or skeletal) already have the cytologic character of lipogranulomata.

Occasionally one encounters a case in which a number of bone lesions are present whose tissue, on histologic examination, presents the pattern of a lipogranuloma but in which the clinical picture is not compatible with a diagnosis of Schüller-Christian disease. In one pertinent case studied by the writer, the patient was a woman 29 years of age who, a few weeks after delivery of a $7\frac{1}{2}$-month fetus, noticed pain across the lower part of the back and particularly in the left sacroiliac region. Roentgenographs of the skeleton taken some weeks after the appearance of this pain showed a large area of osteolysis about the left sacroiliac articulation and also destructive changes involving the right seventh and eighth ribs. The skull bones presented nothing abnormal. (See Fig. 236.) The nature of the clinical picture and the roentgenographic findings in this case suggested that the skeletal abnormalities were manifestations of carcinoma metastatic to the bones from an undetermined focus. In a desire to obtain further information, a biopsy specimen was removed from the affected right seventh rib. Examination of the specimen by the writer showed that the lesion was clearly a lipogranuloma. (See Fig. 237.) The patient received 1,200 r to the affected sacroiliac region and ribs. The lesions healed rapidly, and the patient had no further difficulties in the ensuing 7 years (see Sonnenschein).

In connection with such clinically ambiguous cases, one may mention the two reported by Chester. * One subject was a woman 44 years of age and the other a man 69 years of age, and in neither case was lipogranulomatosis suspected clinically, though in both cases the presence of xanthelasmic patches on the eyelids was noted at autopsy. Both subjects were free of skeletal complaints during life, but the presence of skeletal lipogranulomatosis (particularly in the diaphyses of the long tubular bones) was discovered when bones routinely removed at autopsy were cut open. Furthermore, in the case of the woman, lipogranulomatous lesions were found in the lungs, in the heart, and to an insignificant degree in the liver. The scarring of the lungs in this case was so extensive that it had led to cardiac hypertrophy and right ventricular failure. Indeed, in some pulmonary fields, the fibrous replacement was so thorough that the damaged parenchyma could scarcely be recognized as pulmonary tissue at all. In addition, the lipogranulomatous lesions in the bones had provoked an osteoplastic reaction there which was so pronounced that the af-

* The pathologic material from these two cases became available to the present writer for restudy. This happened because Chester's report emanated from the laboratory of the late Viennese pathologist, Jakob Erdheim, and much of the latter's personal collection of interesting pathologic material was willed to Dr. Ernst Freund (a long-time associate of Professor Erdheim), who in turn willed it to the present writer, with whom Freund was subsequently associated.

Figure 237

A, Photomicrograph ($\times$ 16) of a slide prepared from part of the resected rib to which reference was made in the legend of Figure 236–B. It is clear that the cortex of the rib has been fractured. Subperiosteal new bone can be observed on the atrophic cortex seen in the upper part of the picture and also on the cortex near the lower part of the picture. The marrow cavity of the rib shows the presence of dense fibrous tissue, some endosteal new bone formation, and also focal collections of lipophages. The collections of lipophages are walled off and separated from each other by fibrous tissue.

B, Photomicrograph ($\times$ 225) of the blocked-out area shown in A. The lipoid content of the foam cells was found to stain orange-red with sudan, and this finding indicates that the lipid is mainly cholesterol. The fibrous tissue characterizing the lesion as a lipoid granuloma can be seen near the bottom of the picture.

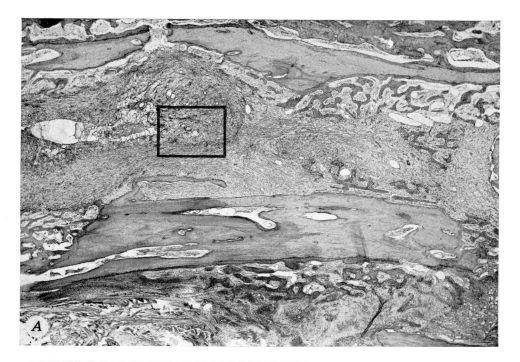

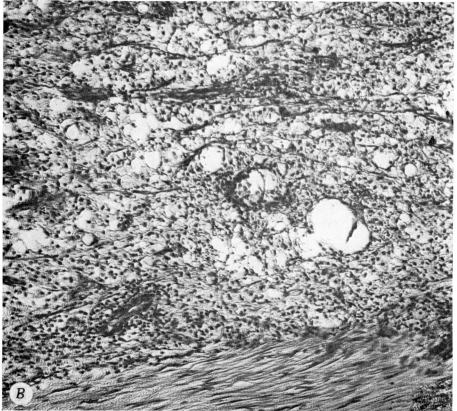

Figure 237

fected areas were extremely sclerotic. Such cases should be held distinct from cases of Schüller-Christian disease, and have also been discussed and illustrated in Chapter 18 under the title of "Lipid (Cholesterol) Granulomatosis" (p. 535).

TREATMENT

The generally advocated treatment for the bone lesions of Schüller-Christian disease is radiation therapy given in small repeated doses over a long period of time. The total amount of irradiation administered to any particular lesional area should not exceed 1,000 r, and doses as low as 600 or 700 r have been found effective (see Jørgsholm).

REFERENCES

ABT, A. F. and DENENHOLZ, E. J.: Letterer-Siwe's Disease: Splenohepatomegaly Associated with Widespread Hyperplasia of Nonlipoid-Storing Macrophages; Discussion of the So-Called Reticulo-Endothelioses, Am. J. Dis. Child., *51*, 499, 1936.

AHNQUIST, G. and HOLYOKE, J. B.: Congenital Letterer-Siwe Disease (Reticuloendotheliosis) in a Term Stillborn Infant, J. Pediat., *57*, 897, 1960.

ARCOMANO, J. P., BARNETT, J. C. and WUNDERLICH, H. O.: Histiocytosis X, Am. J. Roentgenol., *85*, 663, 1961.

AVERY, M. E., MCAFEE, J. G. and GUILD, H. G.: The Course and Prognosis of Reticuloendotheliosis (Eosinophilic Granuloma, Schüller-Christian Disease and Letterer-Siwe Disease), Am. J. Med., *22*, 636, 1957.

AYRES, W. W. and SILLIPHANT, W. M.: Charcot-Leyden Crystals in Eosinophilic Granuloma of Bone, Am. J. Clin. Path., *30*, 323, 1958.

BATSON, R., SHAPIRO, J., CHRISTIE, A. and RILEY, H. D., JR.: Acute Nonlipid Disseminated Reticuloendotheliosis, Am. J. Dis. Child., *90*, 323, 1955.

BIERMAN, H. R.: Apparent Cure of Letterer-Siwe Disease. Seventeen-Year Survival of Identical Twins with Nonlipoid Reticuloendotheliosis, J.A.M.A., *196*, 368, 1966.

Case Records of the Massachusetts General Hospital (Cabot Case #26302), New England J. Med., *223*, 149, 1940.

CASUCCIO, C. and MELANOTTE, P. L.: Eosinophilic Granuloma of Bone, Acta med. belg., p. 715, 1960.

CHESTER, W.: Über Lipoidgranulomatose, Virchows Arch. path. Anat., *279*, 561, 1930.

CHIARI, H.: Die generalisierte Xanthomatose vom Typus Schüller-Christian, Ergebn. allg. Path. u. path. Anat., *24*, 396, 1931.

————: Über Veränderungen im Zentralnervensystem bei generalisierter Xanthomatose vom Typus Schüller-Christian, Virchows Arch. path. Anat., *288*, 527, 1933.

CHRISTIAN, H. A.: Defects in Membranous Bones, Exophthalmos and Diabetes Insipidus; An Unusual Syndrome of Dyspituitarism, M. Clin. North America, *3*, 849, 1920.

COHEN, D. M., MITCHELL, C. B. and ALEXANDER, J. W.: Letterer-Siwe Disease in a Newborn, Arch. Path., *81*, 347, 1966.

COMPERE, E. L., JOHNSON, W. E. and COVENTRY, M. B.: Vertebra Plana (Calvé's Disease) Due to Eosinophilic Granuloma, J. Bone & Joint Surg., *36–A*, 969, 1954.

CRUTHIRDS, T. P. and JOHNSON, H. R.: Solitary Primary Eosinophilic Granuloma of Lung, J.A.M.A., *196*, 295, 1966.

DUMERMUTH, G.: Reticulogranulomatose: Zwei Fälle von eosinophilem Granulom mit Übergang in Hand-Schüller-Christiansche Krankheit, Helvet. paediat. acta, *13*, 15, 1958.

ENGELBRETH-HOLM, J., TEILUM, G. and CHRISTENSEN, E.: Eosinophil granuloma of Bone—Schüller-Christian's disease, Acta med. scandinav., *118*, 292, 1944.

FALK, A. G. and BROWN, A. F.: Acute Disseminated Histiocytosis-X, with Destructive Skeletal Lesions in Rib and Mandible, Arch. Path., *81*, 90, 1966.

FARBER, S.: The Nature of "Solitary or Eosinophilic Granuloma" of Bone, Am. J. Path., *17*, 625, 1941.

FISHER, R. H.: Multiple Lesions of Bone in Letterer-Siwe Disease, J. Bone & Joint Surg., *35-A*, 445, 1953.

FLORI, A. G. and PARENTI, G. C.: Reticuloendoteliosi iperplasica infettiva ad evoluzione granuloxantomatosa (tipo Hand-Schüller-Christian), Riv. clin. pediat., *35*, 193, 1937.

FOOT, N. C. and OLCOTT, C. T.: Report of a Case of Non-Lipoid Histiocytosis (Reticuloendotheliosis) with Autopsy, Am. J. Path., *10*, 81, 1934.

FOWLES, J. V., and BOBECHKO, W. P.: Solitary Eosinophilic Granuloma in Bone, J. Bone & Joint Surg., *52-B*, 238, 1970.

FRIPP, A. T.: Vertebra Plana, J. Bone & Joint Surg., *40-B*, 378, 1958.

GERSTEL, G.: Über die Hand-Schüller-Christiansche Krankheit auf Grund gänzlicher Durchuntersuchung des Knochengerüstes, Virchows Arch. path. Anat., *294*, 278, 1934.

GLANZMANN, E.: Infektiöse Retikuloendotheliose (Abt-Letterer-Siwe'sche Krankheit) und ihre Beziehungen zum Morbus Schüller-Christian, Ann. paediat., *155*, 1, 1940.

GREEN, A. E., JR. and FLAHERTY, R. A.: Histiocytosis X. Report of a Case of Hand-Schüller-Christian Disease, Radiology, *75*, 572, 1960.

GREEN, W. T. and FARBER, S.: "Eosinophilic or Solitary Granuloma" of Bone, J. Bone & Joint Surg., *24*, 499, 1942.

GROSS, P. and JACOX, H. W.: Eosinophilic Granuloma and Certain Other Reticulo-endothelial Hyperplasias of Bone. A Comparison of Clinical, Radiologic, and Pathologic Features, Am. J. M. Sc., *203*, 673, 1942.

GUIZETTI, H.-U.: Zur Frage der infektiös bedingten Systemerkrankungen des reticuloendothelialen Apparates im Kindesalter, Virchows Arch. path. Anat., *282*, 194, 1931.

HAND, A.: Defects of Membranous Bones, Exophthalmos and Polyuria in Childhood: Is It Dyspituitarism? Am. J. M. Sc., *162*, 509, 1921.

HATCHER, C. H.: Eosinophilic Granuloma of Bone, Arch. Path., *30*, 828, 1940.

HELD, A.-J. and RUTISHAUSER, E.: L'histiocyto-réticulose dite granulomatose éosinophile des maxillaires, Bull. Acad. suisse sc. méd., *4*, 415, 1948.

HUNTER, T.: Solitary Eosinophilic Granuloma of Bone, J. Bone & Joint Surg., *38-B*, 545, 1956.

JAFFE, H. L.: *Tumors and Tumorous Conditions of the Bones and Joints*, Philadelphia, Lea & Febiger, 1958 (p. 88).

JAFFE, H. L. and LICHTENSTEIN, L.: Eosinophilic Granuloma of Bone: A Condition Affecting One, Several or Many Bones, But Apparently Limited to the Skeleton, and Representing the Mildest Clinical Expression of the Peculiar Inflammatory Histiocytosis Also Underlying Letterer-Siwe Disease and Schüller-Christian Disease, Arch. Path., *37*, 99, 1944.

JØRGSHOLM, B.: Roentgen Therapy in Hand-Schüller-Christian and Related Diseases, Acta radiol., *50*, 468, 1958.

KAYE, J. J. and FREIBERGER, R. H.: Eosinophilic Granuloma of the Spine Without Vertebra Plana, Radiology, *92*, 1188, 1969.

KIEFFER, S. A., NESBIT, M. E. and D'ANGIO, G. J.: Vertebra Plana Due to Histiocytosis X: Serial Studies, Acta radiol. (diagn.), *8*, 241, 1969.

KNUDSON, R. J., BADGER, T. L. and GAENSLER, E. A.: Eosinophilic Granuloma of the Lung, Med. Thorac., *23*, 248, 1966.

LETTERER, E.: Aleukämische Retikulose. (Ein Beitrag zu den proliferativen Erkrankungen des Retikuloendothelialapparates.) Frankfurt. Ztschr. Path., *30*, 377, 1924.

LICHTENSTEIN, L.: Histiocytosis X. Integration of Eosinophilic Granuloma of Bone, "Letterer-Siwe Disease," and "Schüller-Christian Disease" as Related Manifestations of a Single Nosologic Entity, Arch. Path., *56*, 84, 1953.

LICHTENSTEIN, L. and JAFFE, H. L.: Eosinophilic Granuloma of Bone, Am. J. Path., *16*, 595, 1940.

LIEBERMAN, P. H., JONES, C. R., DARGEON, H. W. K. and BEGG, C. F.: A Reappraisal of Eosinophilic Granuloma of Bone, Hand-Schüller-Christian Syndrome and Letterer-Siwe Syndrome, Medicine, *48*, 375, 1969.

LYON, E. and MEYER, H.: Krankheitserscheinungen in der Mundhöhle bei der Schüller-Christianschen Krankheit, Ztschr. Kinderh., *49*, 768, 1930.

MALLORY, T. B.: Pathology: Diseases of Bone, New England J. Med., *227*, 955, 1942.

MARCOVE, R. C.: Bone-marrow Eosinophilia with Solitary Eosinophilic Granuloma of Bone, J. Bone & Joint Surg., *41-A*, 1521, 1959.

————: Personal communication.

MCGAVRAN, M. H. and SPADY, H. A.: Eosinophilic Granuloma of Bone, J. Bone & Joint Surg., *42-A*, 979, 1960.

MEENAN, F. O. and CAHALANE, S. F.: Spontaneous Resolution of Histiocytosis X, Arch. Derm., *96*, 532, 1967.

MERMANN, A. C. and DARGEON, H. W.: The Management of Certain Nonlipid Reticulo-endothelioses, Cancer, *8*, 112, 1955.

MERRITT, K. K. and PAIGE, B. H.: Xanthomatosis (Schüller-Christian Syndrome): Report of a Case with Necropsy, Am. J. Dis. Child., *46*, 1368, 1933.

NESBIT, M. E., KIEFFER, S. and D'ANGIO, G. J.: Reconstitution of Vertebral Height in Histiocytosis X: A Long-Term Follow-up, J. Bone & Joint Surg., *51-A*, 1360, 1969.

OBERMAN, H. A.: Idiopathic Histiocytosis. A Clinicopathologic Study of 40 Cases and Review of the Literature on Eosinophilic Granuloma of Bone, Hand-Schüller-Christian Disease and Letterer-Siwe Disease, Pediatrics, *28*, 307, 1961.

OCHSNER, S. F.: Eosinophilic Granuloma of Bone, Am. J. Roentgenol., *97*, 719, 1966.

OMENN, G. S.: Familial Reticuloendotheliosis with Eosinophilia, New England J. Med., *273*, 427, 1965.

OTANI, S. and EHRLICH, J. C.: Solitary Granuloma of Bone Simulating Primary Neoplasm, Am. J. Path., *16*, 479, 1940.

PAIGE, B. H.: A Case of Reticulosis, Am. J. Dis. Child., *49*, 266, 1935.

PODVINEC, E. and TERPLAN, K.: Zur Frage der sogenannten akuten aleukämischen Retikulose, Arch. Kinderh., *93*, 40, 1931.

PROUTY, M.: Remission of Letter-Siwe Disease After Prednisone Therapy, J.A.M.A., *169*, 1877, 1959.

RICHTER, M. N.: See article by Mermann and Dargeon, p. 121.

ROSS, I. F., BROWN, G. N. and CONRAD, S. C.: Chronic Disseminated Histiocytosis X (Hand-Schüller-Christian Type) with Oral Mucosal Lesions, Oral Surg., *9*, 529, 1956.

ROUSSY, G. and OBERLING, C.: Akute, wahrscheinlich infektiöse aleukämische Retikulose bei einem Säugling, Wien. med. Wchnschr., *84*, 407, 1934.

SCHÜLLER, A.: Über eigenartige Schädeldefekte im Jugendalter, Fortsch. Geb. Röntgenstrahlen, *23*, 12, 1915.

SIWE, S. A.: Die Reticuloendotheliose—ein neues Krankheitsbild unter den Hepatospleno-megalien, Ztschr. Kinderh., *55*, 212, 1933.

SONNENSCHEIN, H. D.: Disseminated Lipoid Granulomatosis without the Schüller-Christian Syndrome, Bull. Hosp. Joint Dis., *2*, 63, 1941.

TAKAHASHI, M., MARTEL, W., and OBERMAN, H. A.: The Variable Roentgenographic Appearance of Idiopathic Histiocytosis, Clin. Radiol., *17*, 48, 1966.

TRAISSAC, M., MARTIN, C. and MORTUREUX: Forme macropolyadénopathique sans lésions osseuses du granulome éosinophile chez un nourrisson, Arch. franç. pédiat., *17*, 559, 1960.

UEHLINGER, E.: Das eosinophile Knochengranulom, in *Handbuch der gesamten Hämatologie*, Munich, Urban & Schwarzenberg, 1963 (see *IV*, p. 56).

VAN CREVELD, S. and TER POORTEN, F. H.: Infective Reticulo-endotheliosis Chiefly Localized in Lungs, Bone Marrow and Thymus, Arch. Dis. Childhood, *10*, 125, 1935.

WALLGREN, A.: Systemic Reticuloendothelial Granuloma: Nonlipoid Reticuloendotheliosis and Schüller-Christian Disease, Am. J. Dis. Child., *60*, 471, 1940.

WEBER, W. N., MARGOLIN, F. R. and NIELSEN, S. L.: Pulmonary Histiocytosis X, Am. J. Roentgenol., *107*, 280, 1969.

WILLIAMS, A. W., DUNNINGTON, W. G. and BERTE, S. J.: Pulmonary Eosinophilic Granuloma: A Clinical and Pathologic Discussion, Ann. Int. Med., *54*, 30, 1961.

YABSLEY, R. H. and HARRIS, W. R.: Solitary Eosinophilic Granuloma of a Vertebral Body Causing Paraplegia, J. Bone & Joint Surg., *48-A*, 1570, 1966.

Chapter

29

Syphilis of Bones and Joints

In this chapter, consideration will be given to: (1) the historical aspects of syphilis, and (2) the skeletal manifestations of congenital and acquired syphilis. The skeletal lesions of syphilis, both congenital and acquired, are certainly much less often encountered now than they were 50 to 100 years ago. Because of its previous high prevalence, and because the earlier anatomic pathologists were very much interested in the skeletal lesions of syphilis, they made careful studies of these lesions, and wrote detailed reports based on their findings. Hence one must consult the older literature to obtain the most complete accounts of the skeletal aspects of syphilis. It is for these reasons that many of the references to the literature in this chapter relate to articles written many years ago by pathologists, surgeons, dermatologists, and clinicians who had devoted a great deal of attention to the various aspects of syphilitic infection. Since there has recently been a resurgence of syphilitic infection (both congenital and acquired), a detailed presentation of the pertinent skeletal lesions seems appropriate.

ANTIQUITY OF SYPHILIS

At the end of the fifteenth century, an epidemic of what was later called syphilis spread throughout southern Europe. The earliest descriptions of the pestilence ascribed its introduction into Europe to the sailors who returned from America with Columbus. Since syphilis may leave permanent traces in the bones, skeletons antedating the fifteenth century, from many scattered parts of the globe, have been carefully examined to test the correctness of this assumption. The possibility that syphilis may have existed in the Old World prior to Columbus's discovery of America received strong support from the evidence presented by Sudhoff, Cripps and Curtis, and also Hudson. However, the trend of the results of some archaeological investigations is against this hypothesis. In particular, Smith and Dawson have reported that the bones of Egyptian mummies yielded no indications of syphilis. Of all who have studied Egyptian remains in this connection, Michaëlis alone (on the basis of comparatively limited material) considers it probable that syphilis—or some disease resembling it—was extant in Egypt before the return of Columbus from America. Against its existence in Europe previous to that time, Bloch (another medical historian) stated that no presenting evidence of syphilis has ever been found in any old Slavic or prehistoric German mound, or in any European burial site of the Middle Ages.

On the other hand, Jones directed attention to definite indications of syphilis in ancient bones excavated in the state of Tennessee (in the United States), although he did not claim that these bones were surely pre-Columbian. Since then, corroborative evidence appears to have established the syphilitic character of certain pre-Columbian bones excavated at points in the Americas as widely separated as the

United States, Peru, and possibly Argentina (see Hooton, and also Tello and Williams). The skeletal remains of Pueblo Indians which were studied by Hooton, and which other American anthropologists agree are definitely pre-Columbian, include three skulls diagnosed by Williams as almost certainly syphilitic. As Williams states, there seems to be no difference of opinion among experts as to what constitutes a typical specimen of a dried syphilitic skull in which the changes are those due to gummatous erosion. Therefore, most reliance has been placed upon calvarial changes, and in particular upon calvarial erosion by gummata. On the whole, the weight of present evidence favors the view that syphilis was brought to Europe from America. This evidence was summarized by Pusey and more recently by Jarcho. This conclusion is somewhat qualified by Jarcho as follows: "Hence it is inferred that syphilis was conveyed from America to Europe in virulent form, and probably by the companions of Columbus. This does not deny the possibility that a mild form of the disease may have existed in Europe previously, at a low level of prevalence."

CONGENITAL SYPHILIS

The skeletal changes to be discussed here are those that result from syphilitic infection of the fetus during its intra-uterine development. Bone involvement in congenital syphilis, to the extent to which it was understood at all, was considered rare before 1870. At that time, Wegner, from studies made principally on the long tubular bones of fetuses, gave the first gross and microscopic descriptions of the hitherto unrecognized luetic lesion—syphilitic osteochondritis. Soon afterward, Parrot, studying bones of young syphilitic infants, confirmed and supplemented Wegner's findings. He demonstrated that syphilitic osteochondritis appears in flat bones and in short tubular as well as in long tubular bones. Furthermore, advanced stages of syphilitic osteochondritis were established by Parrot as the precursors of epiphysial separation. This placed Ranvier's earlier observation of the occurrence of epiphysial separation in congenitally syphilitic infants on a firm anatomic basis. Taylor's monograph, published in 1875, critically discussed the contributions mentioned above, and made available many practical clinical observations on congenital lues in infants which are still valid today. He was one of the first to make a definite clinical distinction between the bone changes of congenital syphilis and those of rickets.

These early investigations led to further important progress in the understanding of congenital syphilis. First came the correlation of abnormalities noted roentgenographically with the gross and microscopic pathologic findings in the bones. This was supplemented by the discovery that the *Treponema pallidum* could be demonstrated, by means of staining techniques, in the bones of congenitally syphilitic stillborn fetuses and also neonates dying shortly after birth. Finally, of great help in both prophylaxis and scientific knowledge was the use of serologic reactions diagnostic of lues. Since 1900, there have appeared a number of comprehensive reports and outstanding reviews relating to osseous involvement in congenital syphilis. Prominent among them are those of Schmidt, Hochsinger, Herxheimer, Wieland, Thomsen, Schneider, Pick, McLean, and also Wechselberg and Schneider.

Incidence of Congenital Syphilis.—The incidence of congenital syphilis is difficult to estimate, since it varies in accordance with the countries evaluated, their population, and race (see Cole). Herxheimer in 1928, on the basis of estimates from several different sources, placed this incidence in developed countries at 2 to 4 per cent. The prophylactic and therapeutic work of the modern prenatal clinics has greatly facilitated the recognition of syphilis in pregnant women, and has thus led to a striking reduction in the incidence of congenital syphilis in all such countries. It has now been definitely established that adequate antepartum treatment of pregnant syphilitic women strikingly lowers the percentage of fetal stillbirths due to syphilis and also the percentage of full term neonates born with syphilis. McCord stated that sufficient antepartum treatment practically assures the syphilitic woman that her baby will be born free of the disease. On the basis of his total experience, he states that 95 per cent of the neonates of adequately treated mothers are free of syphilis. The longer and more intensive the treatment, the better the results, but even a few treatments in the last weeks of pregnancy will definitely increase the likelihood that the newborn infant will be free of syphilis (see Philipp and Richter, McKelvey and Turner, and also Eastman and Dippel).

As a result of appropriate therapy, congenital syphilis became almost a rarity in the United States, at least in large urban areas, whereas before the introduction of the measures in question about 60,000 syphilitic neonates were born annually in this country. Furthermore, the concomitant Public Health campaign against syphilitic infection in general brought about a reduction in the incidence of syphilis in adults which was maintained for many years. In recent years, however, a resurgence of syphilis among adolescents and young adults has led to a rise in the incidence of congenital syphilis in areas of the country where routine serologic testing of pregnant women and prompt treatment of those found infected is not being carried out.

When the fetus does become infected, *syphilitic osteochondritis* is probably a constant manifestation of the disease. If this lesion can be demonstrated roentgenographically during the first two weeks of extra-uterine life, one can be certain of the presence of syphilitic infection even if the infant appears normal on external examination. Shipley *et al.* examined white fetuses listed as normal in the catalogue of the Carnegie Institute of Embryology, and found that, in 25 per cent of the first 100 studied, the bones presented roentgenographic evidence of congenital syphilis. Even if the osteochondritis cannot be demonstrated roentgenographically at this time, however, it may nevertheless be present and would be apparent on microscopic examination. Drucker and Mankin urge that orthopaedists become fully cognizant of the early skeletal manifestations of congenital syphilis.

Pathogenesis.—In regard to pathogenesis, it is established that after the third or fourth month of gestation the *Treponema pallidum* invades the fetus from the placenta, and the spirochetes are then distributed to the bones by way of the fetal blood stream. The spirochetes multiply perivascularly (forming pericapillary webs) and then intercellularly and interstitially (see Schneider). The spirochetes are then to be found in the actively proliferating areas of the perichondrium and periosteum, in the cartilage vessel canals, in the bone marrow itself, and particularly at the sites of active endochondral ossification, especially in the metaphysial regions of long tubular bones and at the periphery of any secondary centers of ossification which may already have developed. The osteoblasts in these sites take up the spirochetes, and in consequence their osteogenetic function is inhibited and the osteoblasts may even degenerate.

At autopsies of syphilitic stillborn fetuses and neonates dying shortly after birth, spirochetes can easily be demonstrated in the bones. They may be discerned by means of dark field examination of fresh scrapings from the metaphyses, or in decalcified and undecalcified paraffin sections appropriately stained (see Turnbull, and also Bertarelli). Because of the strong tendency of the spirochetes to disintegrate, it is essential that the material on which the search for them is carried out be as fresh as possible. The question has been raised whether the great numbers of spirochetes found in stillborn fetuses that have undergone severe maceration develop by multiplication after death of the fetus. Some think that they do, but others firmly believe that the excessive numbers of spirochetes in such stillborn fetuses are independent of maceration.

After birth, the spirochetes tend to disappear rapidly from the bones. When antisyphilitic treatment has been begun (even in very young infants), it is well-nigh impossible to demonstrate the spirochetes by staining methods. Healing of the syphilitic lesions is associated with regression in the numbers of spirochetes. A few remaining ones may be retained within the bone cells, particularly in those areas where the spirochetes had previously been most numerous. Such spirochetes are apparently the means of rekindling the infection and are the basis for the recurrence of syphilitic lesions in childhood and later life.

SKELETAL LESIONS OCCURRING EARLY IN CONGENITAL SYPHILIS

The osseous lesions of congenital syphilis as they appear in the fetus, the neonate, and the very young infant (in the first few months of life) are: *osteochondritis, diaphysial osteomyelitis*, and *periostitis*. These pathologic changes as a group represent the bone lesions developing *early* in the course of congenital syphilis (see Bandirali and Pratesi).

Syphilitic Osteochondritis.—According to the findings of Thomsen and others, this lesion does not appear before the end of the fifth month of fetal life. Most investigators emphatically deny that syphilitic osteochondritis as described by Wegner can make a first appearance extra-uterinely, or that it occurs with lues acquired early in infancy. In macerated syphilitic fetuses or other stillborn syphilitics beyond the fifth month of fetal life, however, osteochondritis may be the only

Figure 238

A, Roentgenograph of the femur and humerus of a somewhat premature male syphilitic neonate who died 3 days after birth. Note the widened and somewhat serrated radiopaque shadows at the metaphysial-epiphysial junctions of these bones. These shadows reflect the presence of the calcified cartilage lattice characteristic of congenital syphilis, and are likely to be most prominent at sites where endochondral ossification is normally most active. (See *F*.)

B and *C*, Photographs showing the appearance of the epiphysial-metaphysial junctions at the upper and lower ends of a sectioned femur from a 6 week old male infant born somewhat prematurely. In addition to presenting syphilitic osteochondritis, he had gummata in both lungs. The clearly delineated and somewhat irregular whitish zones at the metaphysial-epiphysial junctions of the femur reflect the presence of the wide lattice of cartilage matrix, which suggests the diagnosis of syphilitic osteochondritis.

D, Photograph of the cut surface of the lower end of a femur from the case of a $2\frac{1}{2}$ month old female infant affected with congenital syphilis. The clearly visible white zone at the epiphysial-metaphysial junction is indicative of the presence of syphilitic osteochondritis. The presence of syphilitic osteochondritis is not clearly evident grossly at the periphery of the epiphysial center of ossification.

E, Photomicrograph ($\times$ 30) showing the histologic appearance presented by the epiphysial-metaphysial junction at the lower end of a femur of a full term (nonsyphilitic) neonate. Note the cartilage cells lined up in columns at the upper part of the picture. Shaftward, trabeculae of spongy bone extend into the metaphysis, and myeloid marrow is prominent in the intertrabecular marrow spaces.

F, Photomicrograph ($\times$ 40) illustrating the histologic findings of the syphilitic osteochondritis at the lower end of the femur shown in *A*. The proliferating cartilage cells are lined up in columns. The cores of calcified cartilage matrix that extend downward represent the cartilage lattice characteristic of syphilitic osteochondritis. Note that practically no osseous tissue is deposited on these cores of cartilage matrix. The intertrabecular marrow spaces are devoid of myeloid marrow, and contain vascularized inflammatory granulation tissue in which spirochetes could have been demonstrated by appropriate staining techniques.

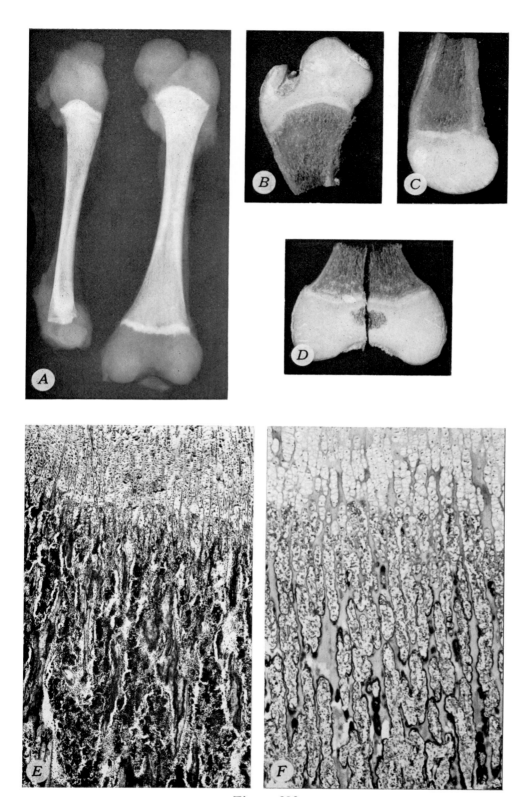

Figure 238

definitive luetic lesion. If not discernible grossly or roentgenographically, its presence, as already noted, may be demonstrable microscopically.

When syphilitic osteochondritis develops, it is likely to involve all regions of endochondral ossification. The lesions are more or less symmetrically disposed, but different bones of the same skeleton may manifest different degrees of involvement. The earlier the osteochondritis has begun intra-uterinely, and the longer the fetus survives, the more apparent are the changes. When the extent of the osteochondritis is not pronounced, the more rapidly growing regions (epiphysial-metaphysial junctions of long tubular bones and costochondral junctions) are the only ones measurably affected. In severe cases, the flat bones, the short tubular bones, the centers of ossification of the vertebrae and sternum, etc. are affected just as frequently as the long tubular bones and the ribs. A fair estimate of the severity of the osteochondritic involvement can, however, be gained by examination of the costochondral junctions alone.

Abnormalities in the provisional calcification zone constitute the earliest manifestations of the osteochondritis. In *normal neonates* the provisional calcification zone of a long tubular bone presents as a very delicate, yellow-whitish line immediately beneath the proliferating epiphysial cartilage. This yellowish white line is often rather difficult to discern grossly. Its depth is almost invariably less than 0.5 mm. In *syphilitic neonates,* widening of the provisional calcification zone, to as much as 2 mm., can occur in the earlier stages of syphilitic osteochondritis. Simultaneously, a slight yellowing of this line and an accentuation of its serrations toward the proliferating epiphysial cartilage become evident. Greater widening, irregularity, and serration of the provisional calcification zone are marks of a more advanced osteochondritis. The zone now acquires a striking yellow color and takes on a chalky, crumbly texture. During the development of the osteochondritis, the proliferating cartilage may remain entirely normal in color and width. On the other hand, it may widen somewhat and even become injected. (See Fig. 238.)

Histologic examination of a region showing syphilitic osteochondritis will disclose that there is diminished osteoblastic activity in the area. This interference with normal endochondral ossification permits the overgrowth of the ordinarily narrow provisional calcification zone. The yellow, widened layer of provisional calcification thus formed—the calcium latticework—appears microscopically as a network of densely calcified cartilage pillars, free of deposits of new bone. This latticework extends into the diaphysis and replaces most of the normal subchondral trabeculae of spongy bone, which, in turn, recede further into the diaphysis. The few spongy trabeculae remaining in the vicinity of the epiphysial-metaphysial junction are observed to be extremely thin. In the earlier stages of the syphilitic osteochondritis, myeloid marrow is still interspersed between the calcified columns of cartilage matrix. Furthermore, calcium deposits, in finger-like protrusions, may extend even into the resting cartilaginous epiphyses, particularly in the neighborhood of the larger cartilage vessel canals. As noted above, the proliferating cartilage zone may remain apparently unchanged or appear widened. It has even been demonstrated that it may be underdeveloped and atrophied, especially in the presence of large numbers of spirochetes.

In the fullest development of the osteochondritis (the last stage), soft and gray granulation tissue appears in the metaphyses. The granulation tissue may vary in amount, color, and consistency. When extensive, it causes a loosening of the connection between the epiphysis and metaphysis, thus creating a likelihood of *epiphysial separation.* The presence of granulation tissue is of the greatest assistance in the gross and microscopic recognition of syphilitic osteochondritis. To obtain specimens for study without disrupting the bone-cartilage junctions, Fraenkel suggested freezing formalin-fixed specimens and then cutting them with an electric saw. The granulation tissue in the metaphysis usually, though not always, occupies an intermediary position in the zone of abnormal calcification. It may show penetration into the shaft or toward the epiphysis, or may even send processes into the resting cartilage. While the granulation tissue tends to extend completely across the metaphysis, more limited localization is also to be observed. At first it consists of simple connective tissue containing numerous blood vessels which are free of endangiitic changes. There may likewise be lymphoid cells in perivascular accumulations, while polymorphonuclear leukocytes are less prominent. Minute foci of fatty degeneration and necrosis may appear, and other more purely leukocytic or granulomatous foci may also ultimately develop. Apparently, necroses are induced by the toxic effects of degeneration of the spirochetes. However, the necrotic lesions do not seem to be gummata, for, as Pick points out, true coagulation necrosis and endangiitic changes are absent. Some trabeculae of bone may appear in the granulation tissue, and it is held that they are formed in it by metaplasia. The growth of the granulation tissue is also associated with erosion of the calcified lattice and existing trabeculae of spongy bone. Osteoclasts make their appearance in such regions.

In regard to the *pathogenesis* of syphilitic osteochondritis, it is to be noted that the first two of Wegner's stages have been designated by Schneider as "passive or degenerative" osteochondritis, while he interpreted the granulation-forming third stage as "active" osteochondritis. In stillborn fetuses and premature syphilitic neonates, "passive" osteochondritis is characteristic. The "active" osteochondritis is a more usual finding in young infants, and its development is an expression of early syphilitic inflammation of the mesenchymal tissues of bones (as of other organs). Thus the evolution of the osteochondritis is conditioned by diminution or cessation of normal osteoblastic activity, as well as by inflammatory changes in regions of endochondral bone growth. The toxic products of spirochetal activity induce disturbances of the physiologic relations existing between: (1) normal cartilage proliferation and (2) the deposition of osseous tissue on the calcified trabeculae of cartilage matrix at the provisional calcification zone, which occurs normally in the course of endochondral ossification.

The role of the chondral-perichondrial tissues in the formation of the diaphysial granulation tissue has not been clarified. Schmidt and most others contend that the granulation tissue appearing in the cartilage vessel canals of the epiphyses is the essential basis for the diaphysial granulations, while Thomsen lays greater stress on the periosteal tissues as the foundation for these granulations. The perichondrium of the epiphyses, with its extensions into the cartilage vessel canals, assuredly participates in the tissue reaction to the syphilitic infection. At first, there is active hyperemia of the blood vessels in these canals. With advance of the osteochondritic process, the cartilage vessel canals become filled with granulation tissue, and metaplastic fiber bone may appear in the granulations or on the walls of the vessel canals. Finally, widening of the canals, with dissolution of the bordering cartilage, may occur. It is striking that, under these circumstances, the cartilage lining the joint space wholly escapes involvement.

In older fetuses, neonates, and in infants up to 3 months of age, *epiphysial separation* occurs. This is observed only in the long tubular bones. It is generally conceived as a culmination of the granulation-forming stage of osteochondritis. Its incidence has been variously estimated. McLean, in a survey of osseous lesions in young infants affected with congenital syphilis, observed it in 24 of 102 cases. Generally, more than one separation occurs in the same patient. In McLean's 24 cases, epiphysial separation was seen in a total of 100 sites. Many of the separations which he observed were impacted. It is not wholly established whether the occurrence is more frequent in the upper extremity than the lower, but statistics seem to favor the upper. Here, separation of the lower epiphysis of the humerus is undoubtedly the most frequent.

The line of cleavage usually runs through the metaphysis, but the fracture line is not necessarily exactly transverse. The final separation is due to disruption (usually mechanical) of the fragile connections which exist between the epiphysis and the diaphysis because of the growth of the granulation tissue. Ordinarily, the dislocation is not pronounced, since the periosteum remains intact. Sometimes the separation is only partial. As opposed to the usual form of separation (through the metaphysis), separation of the epiphysis may take place through the proliferating cartilage zone because of necrosis of the cartilage.

In all pronounced cases of syphilitic osteochondritis with epiphysial separation, the inflammatory reaction to the syphilitic infection may spread to the surrounding tendons and muscle bellies, amalgamating them into a uniformly inflamed mass. Thus, the added participation of the parosteal inflammation in the so-called syphilitic *pseudoparalysis of Parrot* is clear. Some hold that the epiphysial separation need not be confined to the granulation stage, but sometimes takes place through disintegration or fracture of the calcified cartilage lattice on a mechanical basis— either intra-uterine or during birth. Others contend that epiphysial separation before the granulation stage is always an artifact.

On *roentgenographic examination* the ends of the shafts (diaphysial ends) of the long tubular bones of a *normal fetus or newborn infant* appear sharply outlined, while the epiphyses of these bones are not apparent unless a secondary center of ossification is already present. These diaphysial lines are straight or somewhat curved, but in any case delicate and clear-cut. On the other hand, *syphilitic osteochondritis* is reflected in the appearance of abnormal shadows, particularly at the ends of the diaphyses of long tubular bones. For this reason, roentgenographic

Figure 239

A, Roentgenographs of both hands, one forearm, and one foot of a 7 month old fetus who died 3 days after delivery. Wassermann tests done on both the mother and the infant gave definitely positive results. However, the father's blood was seronegative for syphilis. The mother had not received antiluetic therapy before or during the course of the pregnancy. The indications of syphilitic osteochondritis are best represented at the distal ends of the radius and ulna by a somewhat irregular radiopaque zone in each of these bones. Immediately proximal to these radiopacities, one can observe an area of relative radiolucency which is the result of the inflammatory changes caused by the *Treponema pallidum* in the local intertrabecular marrow spaces. To a lesser degree, similar changes are to be observed in the metacarpal and metatarsal bones.

B and C, Roentgenographs of a femur and tibia from a case of congenital syphilis. The subject was an infant 7 months of age at the time of death. Both parents had syphilis, but the infant had not received any antiluetic treatment. The metaphysial-epiphysial junction at the lower end of the femur (B) shows two relatively radiolucent zones delimited by three relatively radiopaque borders. The radiolucent zones represent sites occupied by syphilitic granulation tissue, and these changes are the basis for a subepiphysial fracture or infraction. The lower end of the tibia (C) also shows a narrow transverse radiolucent zone just proximal to the epiphysis. In this region the cortex (on the left side of the picture) shows a small defect, and this defect may be considered the basis for an epiphysial separation. In relation to both the femur and the tibia, some periosteal new bone formation is apparent, and this probably represents what is designated as "specific ossifying periostitis."

D, Photomicrograph (× 2.5) showing the distal half or so of the humerus in the case referred to in B and C. There had been a separation of the epiphysis at the epiphysial-metaphysial junction, and the epiphysis is slightly dislodged to the left. The cortex of the shaft is very much thickened as a result of the deposition of periosteal new bone.

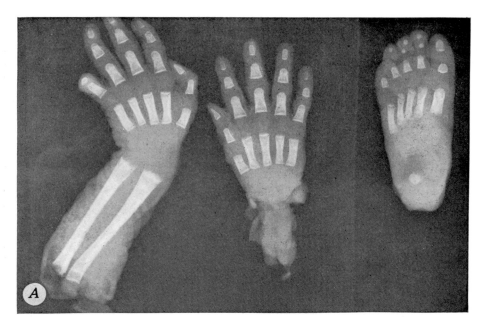

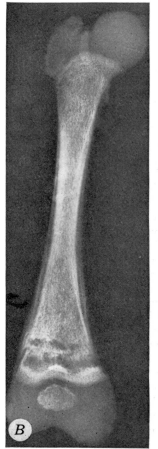

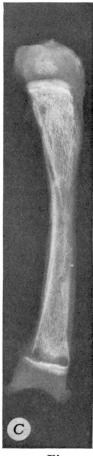

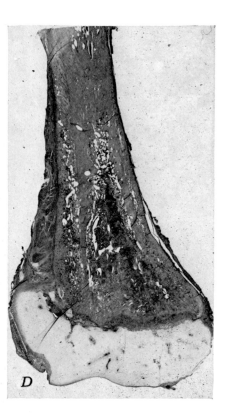

Figure 239

examination, since the pioneer work of Fraenkel, has come to occupy a very prominent place in the diagnosis of the bone lesions of congenital syphilis in stillborn
fetuses, neonates, and very young infants. In the latter, *clinical manifestations*
of congenital syphilis may be entirely lacking during the first weeks of life, and the
diagnostic advantage of roentgenographic study under such circumstances is obvious. As Pick emphatically stated, however, osteochondritis in its earliest stages
of development may be below the threshold of roentgenographic recognition. Therefore, in the pathologic examination of fetuses for evidences of skeletal syphilis,
roentgenographic studies cannot entirely substitute for microscopic examination.
When the increase in the depth of the zone of provisional calcification is not great,
and when it constitutes the only deviation from the normal, even microscopic
diagnosis may be inconclusive unless the presence of spirochetes can be demonstrated. (See Fig. 239.)

In the first stages of syphilitic osteochondritis, the roentgenographs of tubular
bones show radiopaque shadows at the epiphysial-diaphysial junctions. These
shadows are exaggerations of those normally cast. They represent the widened
provisional calcification zone. The shadows cap the ends of the trabeculae of the
spongiosa. The shadows vary in thickness, in accordance with the stage to which
the osteochondritis has progressed. It is very likely that the radiopaque shadow
will show serrations projecting toward the epiphyses; toward the diaphysis, the
shadow is delimited by a straight or slightly wavy line.

When the osteochondritis advances to the stage of granulation tissue formation,
roentgenographs may exhibit, near the ends of the metaphyses, a narrow, transverse, relatively radiolucent zone between two darker shadows. This relatively
radiolucent zone represents the granulation tissue. Less often, one may observe
two narrow radiolucent zones delineated by three relatively radiopaque borders.
Eventually the end of the diaphysis may have a quite irregularly notched, or serrated, appearance (see Maggi and Grassi). In such instances, the basis is being
laid for a subepiphysial fracture or infraction.

If the syphilitic osteochondritis is very widespread, it may also be observed
roentgenographically in the short tubular bones, where the lesions may likewise
show symmetrical distribution and be of uniform extent. Roentgenographic indications of syphilitic osteochondritis are also to be seen in flat bones. In cases of
severe syphilitic infection, indications of osteochondritis may also be observed
around any secondary centers of ossification present. The nuclei of such centers
are outlined peripherally by dense shadows, reflecting wide zones of provisional
calcification. In these regions the lighter and denser roentgenographic zones may
also be demonstrated. Of course, it is always necessary (as McLean points out) to
exercise great caution in interpreting roentgenographic appearances, especially
when they are not clearly diagnostic. A slight widening and more definite density
of the lines marking the ends of the diaphyses may mislead the observer to a diagnosis of congenital syphilis if these are the only roentgenographic abnormalities
present. The associated presence of a periostitis or syphilitic osteomyelitis would
dispel all doubts. It should be borne in mind that the epiphysial-diaphysial junctions and costochondral junctions are sites which register many pathologic changes
in bones, such as lead lines, phosphorus bands, rickets, scurvy, etc. While these
conditions can very often be promptly excluded, they suggest the need for constant
alertness in the interpretation of borderline lesions. In recent years, because of the
tendency toward active treatment of pregnant syphilitic women, the roentgenographic signs of syphilis in the infants of treated mothers are likely to be meager
and mild, so that the pertinent findings in the neonate must be viewed in the light
of this fact. In the presence of such mild indications of congenital syphilis, there is
a strong probability that, if the infant in question is not appropriately treated,

additional skeletal evidence of the disease will become manifest fairly soon (see Grävinghoff).

Furthermore, Caffey points out that the lesions visible roentgenographically in the bones in congenital syphilitics may, if not pronounced, be simulated by a wide variety of conditions affecting nonsyphilitic young infants. He lists the causes of these other conditions as follows: (1) bacteremia (due to staphylococcus, pneumococcus, and tubercle bacillus); (2) erythroblastosis fetalis; (3) septic hemolytic anemia; (4) familial hemolytic anemia; (5) multiple birth injuries; (6) congenital atresia of the biliary apparatus; (7) severe malnutrition; (8) unexplained hemiparesis; (9) protozoan encephalitis; and (10) maternal bismuth therapy. Others, too, have emphasized the possible sources of diagnostic confusion in the roentgenographic evaluation of the skeletal changes of congenital syphilis (see Evans, and also Müller).

In any event, if a syphilitic infant survives, the *osteochondritis heals*, even without treatment. In fact, all manifestations of congenital syphilis in early infancy decrease after the sixth month. The healing of the osteochondritis may be so complete as to leave no trace, even when epiphysial separation has previously taken place. Under antiluetic treatment, the healing is particularly rapid. With healing, numerous osteoblasts reappear and deposit bone on the calcified cartilage lattice. This lattice is resorbed, and a narrow provisional calcification zone reappears. The granulation tissue is also obliterated, as is any new bone in it. Thus, normal endochondral ossification is restored. If healing occurs after epiphysial separation, continuity is reestablished by a reparative proliferation of callus. Altogether, there exists an inclination toward establishing normal anatomic appearances, but the details of the healing process have not been very well studied. After healing of the osteochondritis, the bones continue to grow normally. It is said that growth may sometimes be rather stimulated. At any rate, bone growth rarely appears to be retarded in consequence of the osteochondritis.

Diaphysial Osteomyelitis Early in Congenital Syphilis.—This rather distinctive type of lesion may be clearly present in the diaphyses of long tubular bones during the first months of infancy. (See Fig. 240.) As Pick indicates, such foci are even more evident roentgenographically than grossly, and microscopic examination discloses the lesion with even greater clarity. Degrees of osteomyelitic involvement not sufficiently advanced to be recognizable roentgenographically will also be evident on microscopic examination. The osteomyelitic foci vary in size and location. They may be rather diffuse or more circumscribed. If they are located near the epiphyses and are wedge-shaped, the base of the wedge usually lies against the periosteum.

The foci apparently arise in one of two ways. The subchondral granulation tissue (formed in the late stages of osteochondritis) may extend and grow deep into the diaphysis, or foci of connective tissue may be generated independently of the osteochondritic granulation tissue. Microscopically, the osteomyelitic foci show themselves to be composed of cellular connective tissue, not infrequently delimited from the normal marrow. While the trabeculae of bone originally present may be resorbed, metaplastic new bone may make its appearance in the connective tissue. Necroses, of microscopic size, may be encountered, and numerous spirochetes have been demonstrated in the necrotic areas. The overlying periosteum may thicken. With rarefaction of the bone, there may even be expansion of the cortex.

Wimberger made a special study of the radiographic appearances of various osteomyelitic foci in the shafts of long tubular bones early in congenital syphilis. Particular attention was directed to the presence of the rather characteristic symmetrically disposed osteomyelitic foci in the upper quarters of the medial aspects of the tibiae. The roentgenographic demonstration of these tibial lesions during

59

the first months of infancy, even in the absence of other evidences of syphilis, seems to warrant a diagnosis of congenital lues. In the later months of infancy, too, when differential diagnosis becomes more difficult, the presence of symmetrically distributed osteomyelitic foci likewise suggests congenital syphilis, as Péhu *et al.* also noted.

Periostitis Early in Congenital Syphilis.—A clear understanding of the periosteal changes was slow in evolving. Frank periostitis appears much less frequently than osteochondritis, and there have been relatively few systematic pathologic studies of it. Outstanding among these are those by Fraenkel, which contributed extensively to the subject. It is maintained that three types of periosteal changes can be distinguished early in congenital syphilis: One of these, *specific ossifying periostitis*, is apparently directly due to syphilis; the other two, *reactive periostitis* and *late reparative periostitis*, are nonspecific.

Specific ossifying periostitis, though originating independently of other bone lesions of syphilis, may be seen in combination with them. While this form of periostitis can sometimes be observed (even well developed) in fetuses, it is more usually a syphilitic manifestation to be observed in surviving infants. The combination with osteochondritis is exceptional, since it usually develops after the subsidence of the osteochondritis. Association with a diaphysial lesion is more common. While relatively few congenitally syphilitic infants show this form of periostitis, it may be widely and symmetrically distributed when it does occur.

The subperiosteal bone deposits may be found on the shafts of long tubular bones and also on one or both surfaces of such flat bones as the ilia and scapulae. These deposits may cloak the shafts of the long tubular bones completely or partially. The layer of subperiosteal new bone in such cases usually reaches its maximum thickness in the midportion of the shaft and tapers down toward the ends of the shaft. The underlying original cortex either retains its normal thickness or becomes porotic. The cortex has been described as being "boxed in" by the newly deposited subperiosteal bone. Usually this bone is clearly composed of several layers of new bone—sometimes as many as four layers. Interposed between these layers are fissure-like spongy spaces containing red marrow. At first, the new layers are composed of fiber bone. Later, the fiber bone is transformed into lamellar bone, which may become very dense. Schneider described the presence of spirochetes in the cambium layer of the overlying periosteum. The subperiosteal de-

Figure 240

A, Photograph showing the cut surface of the lower part of a femur, the knee joint, and the entire tibia sectioned in the longitudinal plane. The subject, an infant affected with congenital syphilis, was 3 months of age at the time of death. Some, but not adequate, antiluetic treatment had been administered. In the upper third of the shaft of the tibia, a focus of syphilitic diaphysial osteomyelitis is visible (see arrows). In addition, the cortex of the shaft, especially in its midregion, is greatly thickened as a result of subperiosteal new bone deposition (see *B*).

B, Photomicrograph ($\times$ 3) showing the focus of syphilitic osteomyelitis delineated by the arrows in *A*, and also the thickening of the cortex due to subperiosteal new bone formation in the general region of the osteomyelitic focus.

C, Photomicrograph ($\times$ 13) detailing the histologic pattern of a cross section of the tibia shown in *B* at the level of the thickest part of the periosteal new bone. From above down, the thick layer of subperiosteal new bone stands out clearly from the original cortical bone, which is undergoing rarefaction. On the inner surface of the original cortical bone, a small area of the focus of syphilitic osteomyelitis is apparent.

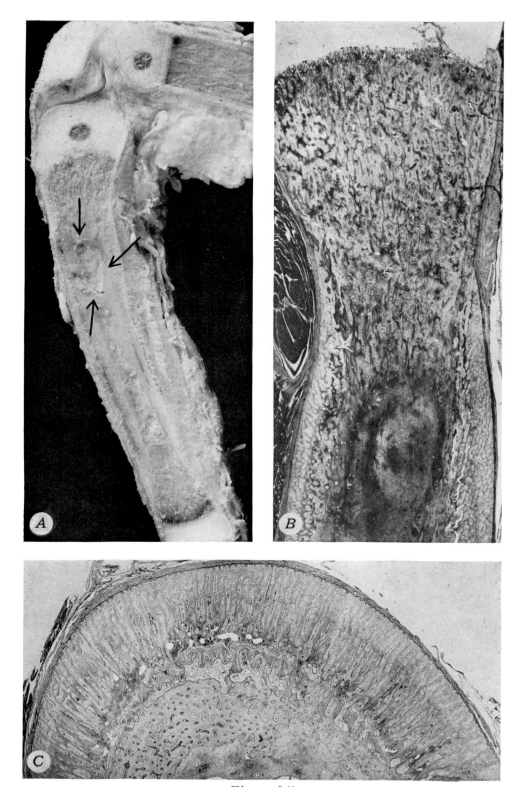

Figure 240

posit is clearly evident roentgenographically in relation to long tubular bones, and strata formation is definitely manifest in some cases. However, the early specific ossifying periostitis is not demonstrable roentgenographically on the ilia and scapulae, and barely so on the ribs. The periostitis subsides under treatment, but rather slowly.

In respect to *reactive periostitis*, it should be stressed that this is not an independent manifestation of congenital syphilis, but is simply a healing response, involving the formation of callus containing cartilage. This type of periosteal proliferation takes place in association with the healing of partially detached epiphyses, or as a reparative response occurring wherever the cortex has been destroyed in the wake of syphilitic osteomyelitis. The callus periostitis reaches its fullest extent at the site of the fracture or cortical defect. It is particularly characterized by the sparsity of spirochetes in the reparative tissues.

The frequency of occurrence of *late reparative periostitis* is not known, because both anatomic and roentgenographic material bearing upon it has been scarce. Its recognition is based essentially on roentgenographic findings. Fraenkel states that late reparative periostitis appears with the regression of the osteochondritis (under the influence of antiluetic treatment). It intensifies as the osteochondritic healing progresses. It is characteristic that, before the initiation of treatment, roentgenographs show a complete absence of periosteal thickening or only the faintest indications of it. The periosteal thickening may persist for months after the osteochondritis is completely healed. As with the specific ossifying periostitis described above, layers of new bone are found deposited on the cortex of the shaft. These may finally merge with the original cortex, and a very thick, dense compacta may result. It is obvious that it may be difficult, without some previous knowledge of the case, to differentiate between the late reparative periosteal response and the early specific ossifying periostitis.

Other Skeletal Changes Early in Congenital Syphilis.—Alterations in the *skull* are now relatively infrequent and unimportant for the diagnosis and understanding of the skeletal aspects observed early in the course of congenital syphilis. Descriptions of cranial bone involvement in very young congenital syphilitics are to be found particularly in the older literature, such as the articles by Parrot, Fournier, and also Hochsinger. Circumscribed erosions have been noted on both the outer and inner surfaces of the calvarium, but in contrast to caries sicca (of acquired lues), the pronounced "worm-eaten" aspect of the calvarium is exceptional. Very large single lesions of rarefying osteitis and osteomyelitis have also occasionally been seen. Circumscribed osteophytic deposits on, or diffuse sclerotic thickenings of, the calvarial bones have likewise been recorded. The development of hydrocephalus, attributable to the extension of luetic periostitis from the skull bones to the meninges, is possible. In addition, caput natiforme (commonly a rachitic manifestation) may have its origin in congenital syphilis.

In tubular bones, *gummata* ranging from a few millimeters to 2 cm. in diameter have been reported, in notably rare instances, as occurring early in congenital syphilis. Gummata of the calvarium have also been described, although rarely. Most authors, however, have regarded these lesions merely as large areas of necrosis in syphilitic granulation tissue rather than as genuine gummata.

Early in congenital syphilis (usually within the first 3 months of the infant's life), epiphysial dissolution or separation may take place, culminating in so-called pseudoparalysis. As a consequence of such changes, *intra-articular effusion* may occur, and the fluid may give a very strongly positive test reaction for syphilis. Unless pus accumulates in the joint, the articular cartilages are not destroyed. However, since a pyogenic infection is often engrafted upon the affected joint, such suppuration is not at all uncommon.

SKELETAL LESIONS OCCURRING LATE IN CONGENITAL SYPHILIS

When the syphilis of the newborn infant remains untreated or is inadequately treated, the early skeletal changes nevertheless regress. They may even completely disappear in the course of the first year or two of life. The syphilitic infection is still latent, however, and very often flares up again. This is especially likely to happen in subjects in whom the syphilitic infection in early infancy has run a mild course and hence been unrecognized (see Smith). The later bone lesions begin to appear from about the fourth year of life onward. (See Fig. 241.) Unlike the lesions appearing early in congenital syphilis, they tend to resemble those of acquired syphilis in their appearance, their distribution, and their entire nature. In exceptional instances, however, the juxta-epiphysial areas of the metaphyses of some of the long tubular bones of older children reveal lesions simulating those of syphilitic osteochondritis of neonates, and such lesions have been denoted as representing "osteochondritis syphilitica tarda" (see Pick). Furthermore, should the skeletal lesions of congenital syphilis become manifest during adult life, as they sometimes do, they may erroneously be regarded as expressions of acquired syphilis.

The bone lesions developing late in congenital syphilis are of two main types: *gummatous* and *nongummatous (hyperplastic)* osteomyelitis or periostitis (pp. 926 and 929). While almost any bone may be affected, the skull bones and such tubular bones as the radius, tibia, and ulna are the ones chiefly involved. Their special susceptibility has been ascribed to the particular exposure of these parts to trauma. It must also be borne in mind, however, as Schneider has indicated, that it is precisely in these bones that the spirochetes may remain dormant for a long time, directly favoring the appearance of lesions in these localizations. While the lesions may be widespread, the predominating clinical manifestations are those resulting from involvement of the skull bones and tibiae (see Pendergrass *et al.*). Several instances of syphilitic osteomyelitis of the mandible have been reported (see Heslop, and also Olmstead).

Saber tibia is a significant finding late in congenital syphilis (see Fournier). It is held that stimulated longitudinal growth of the bone is a factor in the production of this striking abnormality. The acceleration of tibial growth results from epiphysial irritation. Since the fibula is not affected in the same manner, the diseased tibia usually grows at an increased rate between two fixed points. It becomes bent forward and flattened laterally, and the marrow canal also becomes bent. Thus, we may find a true bowing. The idea that this deformity arises not on the basis of weight-bearing but rather on that of the abnormally increased growth is supported by the fact that it also occurs, though only rarely, in the radius and ulna. In rickets, the tibia is bent laterally instead of forward. Bowing deformity of the tibia also occurs in association with acquired syphilis, and this finding has led to much discussion of the differential diagnosis between monostotic Paget's disease of the tibia and the saber tibia of syphilis.

The provoking lesion may be either a gummatous or a nongummatous osteomyelitis or periostitis. New bone is deposited by the periosteum. This subperiosteal new bone tends to remain distinct from the original cortex. The underlying cortex may become porous, and the initial porous state is followed by one of sclerosis involving periosteally and endosteally formed new bone. In the final stages, examination discloses a diffuse hyperostosis with a narrowed major cavity, which may also be filled with spongy bone (see Wilhelm). In time, often after many years, as Pick points out, all the subperiosteal new bone fuses with the cortex.

Another skeletal feature appearing late in congenital syphilis is *dactylitis*, which involves the short tubular bones of the fingers much more often than those of the toes. The dactylitis may appear in several phalanges, but the distribution is not symmetrical. Most frequently it develops in the proximal phalanx of the index finger. The joints and overlying soft tissues are not affected at first. Roentgenographically, the affected bone shows a strongly increased radiolucency of the expanded diaphysis. The cortical shadow is very thin. Healing is associated with the appearance of periostitis and hyperostosis. These lesions have not been very adequately investigated anatomically.

The involvement of the *bones of the skull* has been discussed by a number of investigators (see Parrot, Fournier, and also Hochsinger). Destruction of the osseous and cartilaginous nasal framework may lead to the chronic and often symptomless "saddle," "bulldog pug," "goat," or "terrace-shaped" nose. Destruction of the calvarium by gummata taking their departure in the pericranium was found, along with other syphilitic lesions, in 2 of 100 cases of congenital syphilis analyzed by Dunham.

The significance of the changes occurring in the *teeth* have been the subject of much discussion in relation to the differential diagnosis of congenital syphilis. The general consensus appears to be that the dental changes supposedly characteristic of syphilis should be regarded as syphilitic only if they are concomitant with other changes in the skeleton that are unquestionably luetic. Quite similar dental changes have been found in the teeth of nonluetic children (see Kranz). The dental changes (in permanent teeth) most frequently stressed as being due to syphilis are those that were found in the incisors by Hutchinson and in the molars by Moon. The so-called "Hutchinson's teeth" are notched and narrowed incisors, especially the permanent central incisors of the upper jaw, brought about by arrest in development of the central denticles of these teeth. Moon described the changes occurring in the 6-year molars in congenital syphilis. These so-called "Moon's molars" are dome-shaped and reduced in size through dwarfing of the central denticles of each cusp. It should be borne in mind that these changes in the molars may occur without changes in the incisors (see Lucas). In any event, the alterations occurring in the teeth in cases of congenital syphilis do not regress under antiluetic therapy as do the changes in the bones (see Sarnat *et al.*).

The *pathogenesis* of the dental changes has been explained in various ways. Some investigators inculpate the direct action of spirochetes on the tooth germ,

Figure 241

A, Photograph of the forearms and wrists of a 9 year old boy in whom a diagnosis of congenital syphilis was made shortly after birth. He had received some antiluetic treatment in infancy, but treatment had not been continued. On his admission to our hospital at the age of 9, his history indicated that he had had swelling in the region of both wrists for about 2 months.

B, Roentgenograph of the left forearm in the same case at the time of his admission to the hospital. The epiphysial-metaphysial junctions at the lower end of both the radius and the ulna show areas of radiolucency which, in all probability, reflect the presence of foci of syphilitic osteomyelitis or of gumma formation. The ulna in particular is the site of periostitis which involves practically the entire shaft. Under antiluetic treatment, there was rapid regression and healing of the lesions involving the upper extremities. A follow-up roentgenograph taken 3 years later showed that there was no recurrence of these bone lesions.

C, Roentgenograph showing the left knee joint area in the case of a 12 year old boy who was admitted to the hospital because of swelling of both knees. Clinical and roentgenographic examinations revealed that both joints were swollen and contained fluid. The father's blood was seropositive for syphilis, and the patient's blood was also seropositive. The picture is characteristic of a "Clutton joint." A deposit of some periosteal new bone on the cortex of the tibial shaft is evident, and has caused slight bowing of the contour of the bone. Under antiluetic treatment, his clinical complaints subsided.

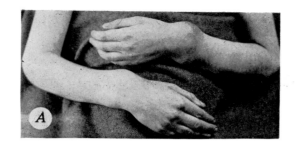

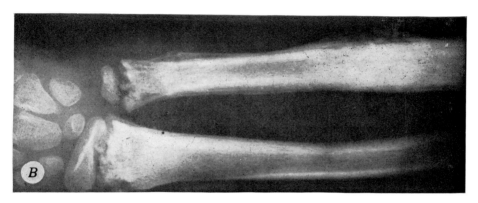

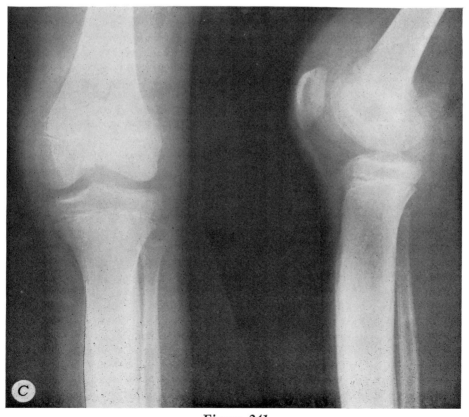

Figure 241

especially on the odontoblasts and ameloblasts (see Del Guasta). Others hold that disturbance in function of the parathyroid and other endocrine glands is a causal factor (see Kranz). Still others relate the changes to a luetic process in the jaw bones, and particularly in the intermaxillary portion of the upper jaw. Hypoplasia of the milk teeth in congenital luetics has been familiar from the time of the first studies of the dental changes in congenital syphilis. In this connection it is interesting to note that a number of observers have found spirochetes in the jaws and teeth of syphilitic fetuses (see Schneider). In a macerated fetus, Bauer demonstrated great numbers of spirochetes in the upper and lower jaw bones. The incisor and canine teeth within these bones were found deluged with the *Treponema pallidum*. The spirochetes were seen in the tooth germ, the pulp, the uncalcified dentine, the calcified dentine, the dental follicle, the enamel pulp, and the enamel epithelium. There were changes in the odontoblasts, ameloblasts, and dental follicles. Bauer held that the hypoplasia of the enamel in the deciduous and permanent teeth of congenital syphilitics is probably to be ascribed to injury to the ameloblasts. Similar findings relating to the dental stigmata of prenatal syphilis have also been reported by Bradlaw.

Particularly in older children (usually 8 to 15 years of age), and especially in the knee joints, bilateral chronic hydrops associated with little or moderate pain and perhaps a low grade fever is by no means an unusual finding late in congenital syphilis. These articular manifestations of syphilis (which may simulate those of tuberculosis) are usually denoted as *Clutton's joints*. The correct etiologic diagnosis of bilateral chronic syphilitic hydrops in children is important (see Borella *et al.*). In the first place, bilateral knee joint effusion is often a warning of the possible approach of a syphilitic interstitial keratitis. Secondly, immobilization of such diseased joints is contraindicated, since it may lead to irremediable chronic changes.

Aside from the skeletal lesions occurring late in congenital syphilis, it should be pointed out that occasionally an adolescent or a young adult affected with congenital syphilis may come to manifest either tabes dorsalis or paresis. Such cases are now rare, but were seen not infrequently in the pre-penicillin era (see Carruthers *et al.*). The present writer had seen at least 3 cases of tabes dorsalis in congenital syphilitics during the 1920s and 1930s, and 2 of these subjects also presented tabetic neuroarthropathies.

ACQUIRED SYPHILIS

Whatever the historical facts relating to the antiquity of syphilis may be, it is clear that the skeletal lesions resulting from acquired syphilis were already known and recognized by the end of the sixteenth century. However, it was only a little more than a hundred years ago that the modern conception of the chronologic evolution of these lesions made it possible to categorize them in detail. This conception was developed through the work of Ricord, which included a study of the relation which certain bone lesions bear to the course of the disease. In his time, bone lesions of acquired syphilis were encountered fairly often, both on clinical examination of affected subjects and in the course of autopsies on such subjects. Now clinicians observe them only occasionally and pathologists see them very rarely indeed (see King and Catterall). For instance, one revelatory lesion with which the older pathologic-anatomists were thoroughly familiar—calvarial erosion due to gummata—is now practically unseen. The relative rarity of osseous lesions of acquired syphilis today in developed countries may be largely attributed to the institution of early systematic and intensive antiluetic treatment. Whether, in addition, the virulence of the *Treponema pallidum* has become attenuated in certain parts of the globe is still an unsettled question. Certainly, the incidence of acquired syphilis in its so-called malignant form has decreased considerably in recent years.

Since the institution of modern methods of treatment, *skeletal lesions occurring early in the course of acquired syphilis* (primary and secondary stages of syphilis) have been almost entirely eliminated in adequately treated subjects. The older literature, however, contains descriptions of such early complaints. Transitory drawing or boring pains in the bones (osteocopic pains), not aggravated by pressure, were formerly prominent in the primary stage of the disease, particularly in those subjects who had fever. The sites of predilection were the upper ends of the tibiae and humeri and the frontal region of the skull. No objective changes in the bones have been recorded to account for these pains.

Periosteal swellings accompanied by violent nocturnal and often radiating pains sometimes appeared during the second stage. These were localized especially to superficial bones, and particularly to the frontal region of the calvarium and the upper portions of the anterior surfaces of the tibiae. Mild degrees of periosteal inflammation, sometimes associated with moderate amounts of subperiosteal new bone formation, were the cause of these swellings. Effusion into the knee joint sometimes accompanied them (p. 943). Complete spontaneous subsidence or disappearance of both the symptoms and the swellings under antiluetic treatment was the usual event.

SKELETAL LESIONS OCCURRING LATE IN ACQUIRED SYPHILIS

Skeletal lesions occurring late in the course of acquired syphilis may be due to the formation of gummata or may represent nongummatous syphilitic inflammation, or even both. It is principally the superficially located bones, or portions of such bones, that are subject to these changes. Such localizations are generally attributed to trauma, to which exposed bones are, of course, more prone. However, it is not usually a solitary injury that induces the localization of a syphilitic lesion, but apparently persistent low grade irritation, as, for instance, from continued pressure or mild friction. Nevertheless, a syphilitic lesion may localize, though rarely, at the site of a single severe injury (see Lanyar). It must not be forgotten, however, that syphilitic lesions sometimes also appear at bone sites in the absence of trauma.

The presence of a gumma, whether in the periosteum, in the substance of the bone, or in the medullary cavity, is conclusive evidence of the syphilitic nature of the process. Gummata in bones generally do not appear until years or even decades after the acquisition of the disease, although instances are recorded of gummatous bone lesions manifesting themselves less than one year after the subject became infected. In addition to the gumma, the affected bone may present more or less severe nongummatous periostitis or osteomyelitis. However, such nongummatous lesions may also appear even though no gumma has developed in the bone. Thus, both gummatous and nongummatous lesions may contribute toward the production of a syphilitic bone condition in a particular case. For example, there may be a gummatous lesion in the medullary cavity of a bone with a nongummatous periosteal lesion overlying it.

From the clinical as well as the anatomic point of view, bone lesions appearing late in acquired syphilis are of two main types. There is the more common clinical form, which is distinguished by the presence of gummata, and the rarer clinical form, in which parts of one bone, an entire bone, or several bones become diffusely diseased and apparently do not develop circumscribed gummatous lesions (see Axhausen). The tendency of the diseased bone to soften and to involve concurrently the adjacent soft tissues, in which ulcers are likely to develop, is found with the gummatous type of lesion. This tendency is entirely absent if the affected bone shows only nongummatous periostitis or osteomyelitis. (See Fig. 242.)

PATHOLOGIC FINDINGS

Gumma Formation.—*Grossly*, gummata appearing in bones coincide in most respects with gummatous nodules occurring in other tissues. Furthermore, whether the gummata evolve in the medullary cavity or in the periosteum, they have much in common. When fully developed, however, those arising in the periosteum are usually much smaller than those occurring in the marrow cavity. The so-called "syphilitic tophus" results from the elevation of the periosteum by a gumma. Gummata are generally discrete, but may become confluent. They may be barely visible grossly, or range up to such a size that they entirely fill the marrow cavity. Grossly, the caseous necrotic material of gummata (which is more or less centrally placed) is yellowish in color and has a dry, pulpy, rather crumbly consistency. The gummata may manifest, from the beginning, an inclination to regress and even to heal, though sometimes they show a considerable tendency to enlarge. Encapsulation of the caseous area by fibrous tissue is evidence of healing. In regressing, the caseous material may rest within the fibrous capsule for a long time. Gradually the dense capsule tends to cut off the caseated area from the neighboring tissues. If the gumma is bordered by spongy bone, the intertrabecular marrow of the latter is quite hyperemic. The osseous tissue in the immediate vicinity of a fully developed gumma tends to undergo sclerosis.

Microscopically, early in its evolution the gumma is represented by granulation tissue abundantly interspersed with engorged capillaries and densely infiltrated with lymphoid cells. Benda claims that, in the formation of gummata, the granulation tissue is preceded by accumulations of polymorphonuclear leukocytes. As the lesion advances at its periphery, caseation appears at the center. The histologic details vary with the stage of evolution of the gumma. Thus, for example, smaller gummata may strongly suggest tubercles in their microscopic appearance. This suggestion is largely due to the presence in them of central caseation, of a few epithelioid and Langhans' giant cells at the periphery of the caseous zone, and of a peripheral lymphoid cell layer. In larger gummata, however, epithelioid and giant cells may be scant or even absent.

Figure 242

A, Roentgenograph of part of the skull showing radiolucent areas in the frontal portion of the calvarium which are the result of gummatous erosions of the outer table. The subject was a woman 45 years of age who had acquired syphilis about 15 years before this picture was taken. She had not been adequately treated prior to her admission to the hospital, at which time a skeletal survey showed lesions also in several of her ribs and in the upper part of her left radius. Serologic tests for syphilis were positive, and she was given antiluetic therapy, particularly large doses of penicillin.

B and C, Roentgenographs showing the left elbow region in the patient referred to in A. In B it is evident that there is some periosteal new bone deposition on the cortex of the upper end of the shaft of the radius, and the radiolucencies reflect the presence of syphilitic osteomyelitis and/or gummatous inflammation involving not only the shaft but also the epiphysial end of the bone. C shows the roentgenographic appearance of the same area 18 days after antiluetic therapy had been started. The picture reveals that there has been substantial healing in this relatively short interval.

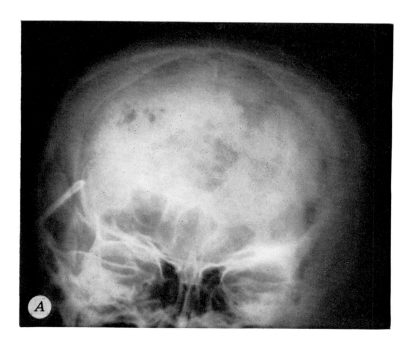

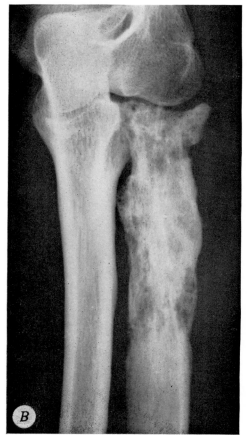

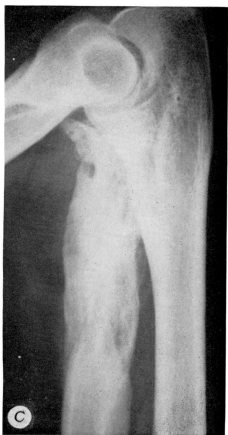

Figure 242

Within the caseating area, necrosis eventually occurs in all the local tissues (vascular, cellular, and supportive). When the caseation is complete, staining of the cell nuclei is generally lacking, and the necrotic amorphous mass appears deep pink when stained with eosin. In areas of fresh necrosis, blood vessels filled with red blood cells may be temporarily retained. The framework of certain structures (particularly the basic tissue of thrombosed blood vessels) may be preserved for a time. Osseous tissue within the gumma likewise undergoes necrosis. The central caseous mass, in gummata of long standing, may also contain cholesterol crystals in rather large numbers, and small scattered spaces, which presumably had contained fat, may appear. The border regions of gummata, as long as they have not succumbed to caseation, are extremely rich in engorged blood vessels, and hyperemia also often extends far beyond the periphery of the gumma. The capsule about the caseous tissue is formed from the surrounding, rather cellular granulation tissue, which becomes poorer in cells as the gumma matures.

Circumscribed lymphoid collections about capillaries, only microscopically discernible, are exceedingly common in syphilitic bones. They are frequently found in the neighborhood of larger gummata, but are seen independently as well. Whether these lymphoid collections are to be regarded as microscopic gummata is still dubious (see Benda). Nevertheless, Freund contends that such sharply circumscribed lymphoid collections should be held to represent the early developmental stages of gummata, since he claims to have observed all stages of transition of such local lymph cell accumulations into definite, small gummata. He states, however, that they do not necessarily develop to any larger size, and that it is quite possible for them to recede entirely.

In regard to the *genesis of the caseous necrosis,* most observers believe that gummatous caseation is due to the effect of the toxic products of spirochete degeneration, although it must be conceded that spirochetes are not readily found in such bone lesions. The inability to demonstrate spirochetes does not exclude the possibility of their presence. In addition, various observers have considered it plausible that the generally recognized form of *Treponema pallidum* may be only one stage in the evolutionary cycle of the syphilitic organism, and that infravisible (ultramicroscopic) forms may exist (see Levaditi *et al.*). While necrosis is probably initiated through the action of toxic products, thrombosis of blood vessels within the granulation tissue may contribute to its progression.

The toxic theory is supported by the similarity of the bone lesions of acquired syphilis to those occurring late in congenital syphilis. Schneider reports that, in congenitally syphilitic infants, resting spirochetes may be found in the bone cell lacunae, between the cell protoplasm and the bone ground substance. Liberation of these spirochetes in any considerable number (during bone reconstruction) creates opportunities for the fresh development, in childhood, of a local syphilitic lesion. When such a lesion does develop, the spirochetes can no longer be demonstrated, because they have disintegrated. Since, as just stated, the lesions of acquired syphilis and those appearing late in congenital syphilis are entirely analogous, the idea is favored that the bone lesions of acquired syphilis in the tertiary stage (and particularly the gummata) are likewise the result of the local growth and degeneration of spirochetes.

In regard to the *healing of a gumma,* it is to be noted that, after encapsulation of the gumma, resorption of the caseous matter may finally take place in the course of the healing process. This resorption occurs through the agency of leukocytes and histiocytes, which invade the necrotic area by way of the capsule around the gumma. Eventually the caseous material may be completely replaced by a dense connective tissue scar. Such scars are poor in cells (even at their borders) and also poor in blood vessels. The scars may become impregnated with calcium, especially at their borders. If the caseous material is incompletely removed, calcium deposits may be found within the residuum. If bone is included within the gumma, such scars retain whatever bone had been incorporated within the caseous material. In the calvarium, such scars fill out the erosive defects produced by the gumma and are intimately attached to the pericranium and the base of the area of bone erosion. Gumma healing may sometimes—though very rarely—be so complete that even an indurated calcified scar may eventually be entirely resorbed. Thus, in exceptional instances, all traces of a gumma even in the marrow cavity may be completely effaced and replaced by new spongy bone and normal fatty marrow (see Freund).

Nongummatous Syphilitic Periostitis.—This type of lesion occurs very frequently late in the course of acquired syphilis and is clinically very important. Here, we shall limit ourselves to a discussion of its anatomic aspects, leaving the clinical aspects for subsequent presentation. The periosteal reaction may be limited and circumscribed, but occasionally it is so extensive that it implicates the entire periosteum of a bone. Under such circumstances it may be associated with extensive nongummatous medullary inflammation, and as a result, in rare instances the bone may become very much thickened and even deformed. This is especially likely to be the case in long tubular bones, such as the tibia, radius, and ulna. (Such thick bones found among ancient skeletal remains have been interpreted, in conjunction with calvarial lesions, as evidence of syphilis.)

As already noted, nongummatous syphilitic periostitis may occur independently of, or in association with, gummata in the marrow cavity. Before periosteal new bone formation advances to any considerable degree, the inflamed periosteum shows a greatly thickened fibrous layer and a cambium layer which is usually well developed. If the periosteum is incised at this stage, it will be found swollen and gelatinous. Larger or smaller accumulations of lymphoid cells, often surrounding vessels or nerves, may be found in it. The medium-sized arteries in the cellular portion of the periosteum may manifest intimal thickening and narrowed lumina.

This early stage of inflammation is followed by one of osteophyte formation. In the course of this process, new bone is deposited on the original cortex but only loosely connected with it. The spaces between the osseous trabeculae are filled with cellular fiber marrow, and the trabeculae are lined by osteoblasts, sometimes several layers thick. As the osteophyte grows in thickness, the coarse-fibered osseous tissue constituting its trabeculae comes to be replaced by lamellar osseous tissue. When the subperiosteal new bone is completely replaced by lamellar osseous tissue, the newly deposited osseous tissue may merge completely with the underlying cortex. Eventually it may even become functionally important. If thick, it may substitute for the original cortex, which may gradually be resorbed. Under these circumstances the outermost layers of the periosteal osteophyte become condensed into a new compacta, while the deeper layers and original cortex are resorbed. The newly formed periosteal bone may act in the same manner, if gummata of the marrow cavity destroy the cortex. In that case, the new subperiosteal bone may encircle the necrotic cortex of a tubular bone, just as an involucrum does in suppurative osteomyelitis. However, gummata sometimes invade the subperiosteal new bone and even destroy it.

Nongummatous Syphilitic Osteomyelitis.—Some degree of nongummatous syphilitic osteomyelitis is frequently found in the close neighborhood of intramedullary gummata. This type of osteomyelitis is usually of limited extent, whether or not it borders on gummata. The intertrabecular marrow spaces of the spongiosa of a long tubular bone which is the site of nongummatous syphilitic osteomyelitis will be found filled with moderately cellular connective tissue in which blood vessels are abundant. In its earliest stages, the connective tissue is rather cellular and contains lymphoid cells which are usually sparse and tend to be diffusely distributed, but occasionally the lymphoid cells are aggregated into sharply delimited foci. The spongy trabeculae within a small area of syphilitic osteomyelitis are usually atrophic. Only infrequently does osteomyelitis spread out over an area wide enough to involve the cellular tissue of the entire marrow cavity and its ramifications. Such an occurrence in tubular bones, in association with the formation of large amounts of subperiosteal new bone, results in pronounced thickening of the affected bone.

Syphilitic Caries.—As already noted, it is well known that gummatous lesions may lead to destruction of adjacent or encircled bone. The term *"caries sicca"* has been applied to indicate resorption of cortical bone in the vicinity of an area of gummatous inflammation (see Virchow). In this process, bone destruction is conditioned by the presence of the gumma. It is not the gumma itself, however, that erodes the bone, but rather the inflammatory process *per se*. In caries sicca, the bone resorption takes place slowly, and necrosis is therefore not clearly evident as a rule, either grossly or microscopically.

On the other hand, the gummatous inflammation may be associated with obvious bone destruction, in which the bone becomes manifestly necrotic. The *"caries necrotica"* results from the rapid spread of the gummatous tissue. It leads to necrosis of the affected area of bone and usually to its delimitation from the rest of the osseous tissue. The necrotic and separated bone (sequestrum) may become included in the caseous portion of the gumma. The rapidity with which the sequestrum is incorporated within the substance of the gumma determines whether this bone shall retain its original compactness or become porotic. The rapid progression of a gumma may cause caries necrotica to appear where caries sicca had at first been present. When gummata spread rapidly, there seems to be a predisposition to a superimposed pyogenic infection. Such an occurrence adds to the severity and extent of the bone necrosis.

MANIFESTATIONS OF ACQUIRED SYPHILIS IN INDIVIDUAL SKELETAL AREAS

In the *skull, erosion of the calvarium by gummata* has long been regarded as especially characteristic of acquired syphilis. The frontal and parietal bones are predilected. More rarely, the temporal bones become diseased, and only in exceptional cases do the syphilitic changes extend into the occipital region. While either the inner or the outer surface of the calvarium may be the first to become eroded, it is very unusual for this erosion to begin on the inner surface. In fact, Erdheim maintained that initial involvement of the outer table was a significant

Figure 243

A, Photograph of a middle-aged man who had acquired syphilis while he was still young. The forehead shows a large area of ulceration as a result of gummatous involvement, a characteristic finding in cases of syphilis of long duration in which the subject has not been adequately treated. A small area of the calvarium is exposed, and to the right of it, gummatous granulation tissue is apparent. The calvarium beneath the gumma is ulcerated. Death was caused by renal insufficiency due to gummatous involvement of the kidneys.

B, Photomicrograph ($\times$ 50) showing gummatous erosion of the outer surface of the calvarium in the case of the man shown in *A*. On higher magnification the histologic structure of the tissue eroding the calvarium is found to be composed of some connective tissue heavily infiltrated with lymphocytes, and in tissue fields beyond that illustrated, there is evidence of caseous necrosis of the gumma.

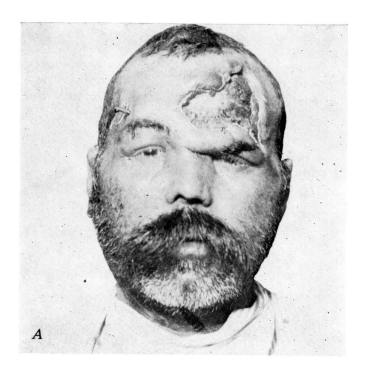

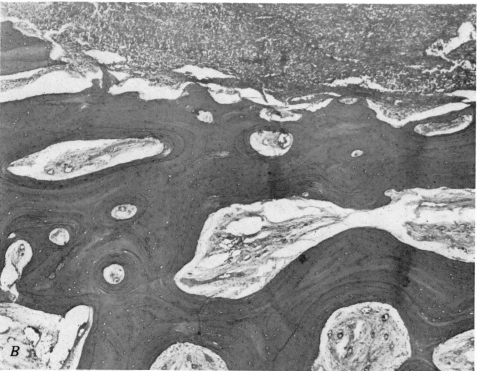

Figure 243

gross finding which differentiated syphilitic from tuberculous calvarial erosion. However, Soloweitschik held that the gumma formation sometimes begins within the substance of the calvarium, without causing much erosion of either table.

Typically, the outer surface of the calvarium becomes eroded by extension of the gummatous inflammation from the pericranium. Clinically, the gummatous lesions in the pericranium take the form of more or less circumscribed hemispherical or flat swellings which are usually somewhat firm on palpation but occasionally rather soft (pseudofluctuant). From the site of the gumma in the pericranium, the syphilitic inflammatory process may reach the interior of the calvarium by way of the walls of the blood vessels which extend from the pericranium through the outer table. The actual disintegration of the outer table of the calvarium by the gumma is brought about by a number of influences: active vascularization of the diseased area, pressure from the gumma, and destruction of fragments of bone in the gummatous area. (See Fig 243.) Sometimes only one small area of calvarial erosion appears, while in other instances the erosions are numerous and even confluent, so that the calvarium may be extensively implicated (see von Eicken, and also Gregory and Karpas).

Virchow maintained that two apparently opposed processes are demonstrable in each area of calvarial erosion. In its center, a rarefying (atrophic-regressive) process occurs, while peripherally a condensing (hypertrophic-progressive) process takes place. He described the rarefaction as beginning with widening and confluence of the vessel canal spaces in the diseased portion of the calvarial table, resulting in a funnel-shaped and stellate depression in the table. Further progression of the erosion increases the extent and depth of the depression. The excavation is deepest in the central part of the eroded area. Gradually, the table is perforated, and the base of the excavation extends into the diploic area of the calvarium. As the erosion deepens, new bone is deposited peripherally around the edge of the excavation, and the borders acquire a somewhat split-up, sinused, folded or wrinkled appearance. This new bone merges with the surface of the table and may finally become very sclerotic and even ivory-like. When the destruction is pronounced, the newly deposited bone may form an irregular wall about the border of the depression. Eventually, a thin film of new bone is also deposited on the base of the erosion, so that the marrow spaces of the exposed diploë become obliterated.

The eroded area is finally filled in by somewhat dense, poorly vascular connective tissue scars which are adherent to the overlying scalp and/or underlying dura, and they remain after the gummatous inflammation has healed. Complete restoration of the bone is quite unlikely. Hence, when the depressions are already present on the outer surface of the calvarium, they are evident on palpation. When multiple calvarial gummata heal, the surface of the cranial vault acquires bumps and hollows. Visible changes in the scalp overlying such calvarial erosions may be absent. Loss of hair is said to ensue eventually.

When the calvarial erosion is very deep and extensive, the inflammatory changes may penetrate to the dura mater. The latter then becomes detached from the inner table, so that any residual bone lying between the pericranium and the dura mater tends to be cut off from its blood supply. Necrosis of bone is favored by the rapid progress of the gummatous inflammation in all directions and the frequent occurrence of a superimposed pyogenic infection. Thus more or less extensive bone necrosis comes to be added to the erosive changes. The large necrotic masses of bone may remain *in situ* for long periods of time. Ultimately they become delimited, tending to separate themselves as sequestra from the rest of the calvarium. The continued suppuration can result in destruction of the overlying scalp, after which such sequestra become visible. Finally, loosening or even expulsion of a massive sequestrum can result (see Frangenheim). Although surgical intervention for the removal of such sequestra is poorly tolerated by the patient, it can sometimes greatly abridge the clinical course and may be carried out when the sequestra have definitely been delineated and loosened (see Adson).

Perforation of the entire thickness of the calvarium so that the dura is exposed is infrequent, but if it does occur, it is apparently more often associated with lesions that originate between the dura and the inner table than with those between the pericranium and the outer table. Large exostoses present on the inner table may give rise to manifestations resulting from pressure on the brain. Calvarial necrosis advancing to the dura may favor the extension to the brain of a super-imposed pyogenic infection.

Even mild degrees of calvarial erosion are now very infrequently observed in cases of acquired syphilis. If pronounced, however, the pathologic manifestations induced in a calvarium by the erosion are so striking and typical that their recognition at autopsy is a simple matter. It should also be noted, however, as Williams has indicated, that some ancient skulls with symmetrical osteoporosis of the calvarium have been mistakenly regarded as syphilitic. Symmetrical osteoporosis was apparently common among some ancient races. Furthermore, it has been suggested that leprosy may have produced, in some ancient skulls, changes similar to those of syphilis, but little information is available on this point (see Williams).

Gummatous lesions in *skull bones other than the calvarium* are now rarely encountered. Formerly, however, syphilitic involvement of these other bones of the skull was rather common. In particular, *nasal cartilages and bones* were frequently the site of gummatous erosion and necrosis. Usually, such lesions were the consequence of extension of syphilitic ulcers from the nasal mucosa. However, primary gummatous involvement of these bones, independent of mucosal disease, was also encountered. Destruction of the nasal bones and cartilages through the growth of the gummata often led to the formation of sequestra. When appearing in these sites, the gummatous involvement was likely to be most severe in the posterior and upper portions of the nasal cavity, and to spread from there. As a result, the cartilaginous portion of the nose, the vomer, the nasal bones, and the thin lamellae of the ethmoid, as well as the nasal processes of the upper jaw, sometimes underwent necrosis. Involvement of the ethmoid and vomer tended to destroy the nasal root and lead to the so-called "saddle nose," even if the nasal bones themselves were not implicated. The anatomic alterations due to lesions affecting the nasal bones in acquired syphilis are the same as those encountered late in congenital syphilis, and have been particularly well described in conjunction with the latter (see Parrot, Fournier, and also Hochsinger).

In the *upper jaw*, the hard palate, especially in its central region, is most susceptible to destruction. This begins by extension of gummata from the floor of the nose or from the roof of the mouth. Perforation of the palate and the ejection of small sequestra are thus brought about. The deformations resulting from destruction of parts of the facial portion of the skull may persist even after the syphilitic infection has received thorough treatment. Before any abnormal dried skulls in which the nasal region is the principal part involved are interpreted as syphilitic, one should consider the possibility that the changes observed may have resulted from lupus, leprosy, yaws, or tropical leishmaniasis—conditions which, in relation to the skull, chiefly attack the nasal parts (see Williams). In this connection, some believe that, on the basis of present knowledge, there are no clear criteria permitting differentiation between syphilis and yaws in affected dried skulls (see Blacklock, and also Butler).

The *lower jaw*, which is less frequently affected, may show circumscribed gummata, diffuse gummata, or subperiosteal new bone formation. Among untreated cases of advanced syphilis reported by Downes, there were 6 cases in which the lower jaw showed extensive necrosis. When there is gummatous involvement, there may also be evidence of suppuration. Disease of the *malar bones* may accompany syphilis of the cranial vault.

In the *skull, diffuse nongummatous syphilitic lesions* have also been observed. These are due to subperiosteal new bone formation, affecting particularly the calvarium, and the changes in question are not so characteristic of syphilitic involvement of the skull as are the erosions of the calvarium by gummata. Such nongummatous periostitis produces thickening of the outer surface of the calvarium, which may either become roughened or remain smooth. Axhausen mentions examining one such skull, the calvarium of which had the thickness of a thumb. The thickening of the skull bones may even be so pronounced that the skull as a whole presents the appearance characteristic of leontiasis ossea (p. 276). The thickening makes the skull abnormally heavy. Furthermore, it may be difficult to distinguish the thickening in such skulls from that produced by other causes of chronic periostitis, such as osteomyelitis.

In relation to *long tubular bones, gummatous involvement* is observed much more often in the interior of an affected bone than on the surface. In the medullary cavity of a long tubular bone, which is most likely to be a femur or a tibia, the gummata may be limited to the diaphysial portion of the shaft, but they are also quite commonly situated in the spongy ends (metaphysial ends) of the bone, or in both places simultaneously. When present in the interior of a long tubular bone, the gumma or gummata may be clinically latent, and encapsulated anatomically. Under such circumstances, their presence may be revealed by means of detailed roentgenographic examination of the bone. If the subject comes to autopsy and the affected bone is removed from the body and sawed open in its long axis, the gummata will be apparent. Among 27 cases of syphilis of long duration which came to autopsy, Chiari observed 9 cases in which central medullary gummata had been clinically latent. If the gummatous focus is small, if the periostitic reaction which it has provoked is not very intense, and if the bone is surrounded by voluminous muscle masses, a gummatous lesion, even if not actually dormant anatomically, may nonetheless be inconspicuous clinically. On the other hand, gummata in long tubular bones may give pronounced clinical evidence of their presence by pain, swelling, deformity, or a change obvious roentgenographically. They become especially conspicuous clinically if they break into joints or if they destroy considerable areas of the overlying cortex, provoking changes in the periosteum and surrounding muscles.

Figure 244

A, Photograph showing ulcerations on the medial and lateral aspects of the left leg resulting from gummatous involvement of the soft tissues. The patient was a woman, 47 years of age at the time of her admission to the hospital, whose difficulties relating to this leg set in 10 years before this picture was taken. At the onset, she developed one small ulcer on the leg, and in the course of the next 3 or 4 years a few more appeared, which subsequently healed. The demonstrated ulcerations began to appear about 3 years before this picture was taken. The individual ulcers enlarged and merged, and their presence was associated with a foul-smelling discharge. There was also a considerable amount of pain during the 6 months preceding her admission to the hospital. Roentgenographic examination revealed the presence of an osteoperiostitis on the shafts of the fibula and tibia. Examination of the blood showed that she was seropositive for syphilis.

B, Photomicrograph (× 125) of a tissue section prepared from a nodular swelling in the soft tissues of the thigh at a site well above the ulcerated area in the leg shown in *A*. The tissue is heavily infiltrated with lymphocytes and plasma cells, and a few Langhans' giant cells are seen. The histologic pattern represents the early stage of gumma formation.

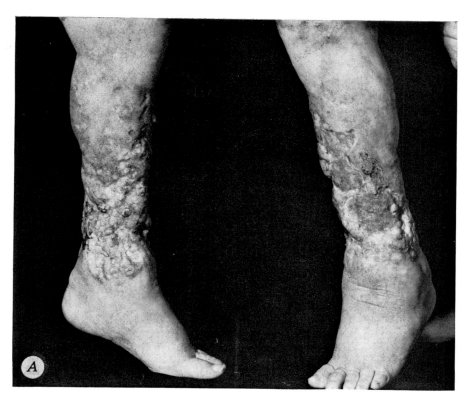

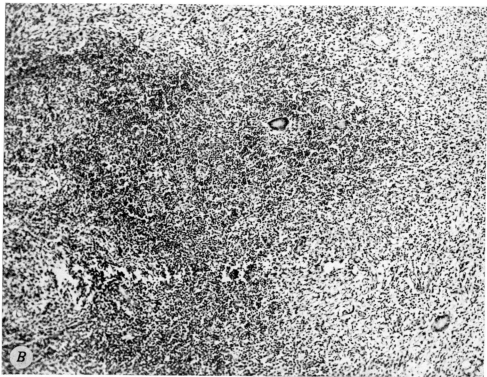

Figure 244

Those gummata which spread through a considerable portion of the major marrow cavity have been designated as diffuse syphilomata (see Gangolphe). These diffuse lesions show no tendency to remain dormant, as there is almost always periosteal thickening due to associated gummatous or nongummatous periostitis. The resulting periosteal new bone formation may double or treble the circumference of the diaphysis of a bone thus involved. The muscles are implicated in the syphilitic inflammation and become merged with the neighboring bone and fascia. Carious erosion and necrosis of the cortical bone result from the spread of the gummatous process. Pyogenic infection tends to supervene. This increases the extent of the necrosis, and large and small cortical perforations may appear. Finally, the skin may be perforated in various places, and fistulae with winding passages from which pus exudes may lead to the interior of such a bone. (See Fig. 244.)

In relation to a long tubular bone, as already indicated, the initial site of a gumma may even be at the surface of the bone, the gumma starting its development in the periosteum. In that site the gummata appear singly or in groups as circumscribed hemispherical or flat swellings, which are more or less firm and show pseudofluctuation. The inflammatory process often extends into the underlying cortical bone and erodes it. In consequence of the reaction caused by the presence of the gumma in the periosteum, a reparative process takes place at the periphery of the focus. This process is characterized by the formation of periosteal new bone. Roentgenographically, therefore, the erosion defect may ultimately be outlined by a radiopaque shadow of dense bone. Periosteal gummata may regress or may extend toward the surface and perforate the skin. Or, instead, gummatous lesions of the periosteum may extend into the interior of the bone and cause extensive caries and necrosis.

The *periosteum* of long tubular bones may also be the site of inflammatory changes on a nongummatous basis. *Rather limited (localized) periosteal inflammations* are much more common than those which are diffuse. When the periosteal inflammation is of limited extent, it originates within the inner surface of the periosteum. The overlying skin may be reddened and edematously swollen, and the involved region may be painful to pressure. Sometimes the periostitis is accompanied by severe pain. Periostitis is very likely to occur if treatment of the syphilitic subject is neglected (see Jordan). Clinically, one or more swellings may be evident on roentgenographic examination, and these are found to be lying on the bone but not attached to it. The development of periosteal new bone leads to the formation of an osteophyte. Such new bone is often to be recognized roentgenographically as enveloping the original cortical bone in a circular sheath. Furthermore, a certain degree of stratification of the subperiosteal new bone is to be demonstrated roentgenographically. Ultimately, the deposited periosteal new bone may become entirely ossified and intimately amalgamated with the underlying cortex (see Hahn and Deycke-Pascha).

The *diffuse periosteal inflammations* may be striking, and are of interest historically. They may affect part of a bone, an entire bone, or several bones. This type of syphilitic bone involvement is most familiar in relation to the tibia, where it can lead to distorting thickenings and deformities (see Axhausen). If a bone thus affected is sawed longitudinally, radical structural abnormalities may be noted. The original cortex in the affected area may be found replaced by porous osseous tissue, and the marrow cavity partially obliterated by close-meshed spongy bone. On the other hand, the cortex may be found abnormally thick and sclerotic, parts being of ivory-like consistency. The surface of such a bone may be smooth or rough; many openings for the admission of blood vessels may be seen and, often, longitudinal grooves. Such radical departure from the original structure is the result of periosteal and intramedullary new bone formation, and is the significant characteristic of syphilis involving a long bone diffusely. Sometimes, only a portion of a bone may be thus involved, and in such instances, especially in young persons, the impression may be created that one is dealing with a sarcoma of bone. If there is a massive deposit of periosteal new bone, the differential diagnosis between syphilis and a periosteum-oriented sarcoma may be particularly difficult. A serological reaction indicative of syphilis may be the first clue to the real nature of the disease process, which rapidly subsides under antiluetic treatment.

Diffuse syphilitic disease of a tibia may induce lengthening and deformity of the bone, resulting in the so-called *"saber tibia."* Such a deformed tibia might be confused with the saber tibia of monostotic Paget's disease, since in both of these conditions the affected tibia shows curvature, thickening, and lengthening of the bone. The saber tibia appearing in the course of acquired syphilis is more often due to pseudobowing than to true bowing. With pseudobowing, the vertical direction of the major marrow cavity remains essentially normal, the outward deformity of the bone being due to voluminous arched thickening of the anterior surface of the tibia. The fibula, if involved, may be lengthened but remains straight. True bowing of the tibia, with actual curvature of the major marrow cavity, does occur in association with congenital syphilis (see Fournier).

Wilhelm described features permitting differentiation between these two types of saber tibia on the basis of gross anatomic and roentgenographic study of macerated specimens. He stressed the roentgenographic finding of clearly defined layers (or mantles) of subperiosteal new bone on the shaft cortex of a syphilitic saber tibia. Comparative study of tibiae from cases of monostotic Paget's disease failed to reveal such mantles of new bone on the cortex of the bone shaft. Others, too, have stressed the significance of the subperiosteal new bone as a roentgenographic and anatomic feature of syphilitic saber tibia (see Weber). However, Weber was unable to discern, in ground disk preparations, any anatomic feature characteristic of syphilitic periostitis. In syphilis the periosteally formed new bone at first tends to remain distinct from the cortex, but in cases of diffuse syphilitic inflammation of long duration, it has been shown that the division between periosteal new bone and the original cortex may eventually become indistinct and even completely disappear (see Axhausen).

It is clear that cortical thickening in Paget's disease, as in syphilis, is the result of periosteal new bone formation (see Schmorl). In Paget's disease, however, the newly formed periosteal bone is almost always rapidly merged with the underlying cortical bone, and hence there may be no roentgenographic evidence of it. Rarely, even in Paget's disease, a very prominent deposit of periosteal new bone can be recognized grossly and roentgenographically (see Freund, and also Jaffe). More certain criteria for differentiating between the two diseases in a tibia are: the lamellation of the cortex, the widened and uneven medullary cavity, and the presence of the mosaic architecture (histologically) in a bone transformed by Paget's disease. The value of the mosaic pattern as a differential criterion is further demonstrated by histologic examination of macerated and/or unmacerated syphilitic tibiae (see Nestmann). In only one of the syphilitic tibiae which Nestmann studied could any semblance of mosaic architecture be seen. Even in this case it was not so widely distributed through the osseous tissue as it is in a tibia which is the site of Paget's disease. Furthermore, on a clinical basis, an increase in the serum alkaline phosphatase value in Paget's disease presents another finding which helps in the differentiation between the two conditions (see Bodansky and Jaffe).

One of the rarer lesions of acquired syphilis is *syphilitic dactylitis.* This is observed very much less often in acquired syphilis than in congenital syphilis. In any event, the involvement of the phalanges or the metacarpal and/or metatarsal bones in the dactylitis is to be attributed to gummatous periostitis or gummatous osteomyelitis or both. Occasionally, as Eschle points out, it seems to be caused by the extension of gummatous lesions from the soft parts to the regional bone or bones. (See Fig. 245.) In acquired syphilis the dactylitis is apparently more often the result of gummatous periostitis than of gummatous osteomyelitis, while late in congenital syphilis the primary lesion is more often a gummatous osteomyelitis. However, the presence of a gummatous osteomyelitis *per se* may be obscured by an overlying periosteal reaction. The fingers are implicated much more frequently than the toes. It is characteristic of the condition that the diseased fingers present externally the appearance of spina ventosa. Therefore, confusion with tuberculous spina ventosa is possible, particularly if the condition is limited to one or a few fingers. Such diseased fingers are first broadened and lengthened. The back of the hand becomes swollen and thickened, eventually presenting a cushion-like appearance. The skin is glistening, taut, and livid in color. Though the movement of the fingers may be impeded by swellings, the joints remain uninvolved for some time. The implicated bone or bones may eventually be completely destroyed, so that local shortening and deformity appear.

Syphilitic lesions involving the *vertebral column* are most likely to occur in conjunction with syphilitic lesions of other bones. Vertebral bodies are implicated much more commonly than the arches and processes. Usually, only a single vertebra is affected, but the disease may progress to neighboring vertebrae, and, if it does, the local intervertebral disks are destroyed. In any event, involvement of more than four vertebrae in a series is uncommon. The upper cervical vertebrae are much more frequently affected than any of the other vertebrae. The anatomic changes range from periostitis of a mild degree to advanced gummatous changes resulting in necrosis of bone and the formation of sequestra (see Ziesché). Usually it is only when the pathologic changes are advanced that they give rise to clinical manifestations and roentgenographic findings. The presence of small gummata scattered throughout the vertebral column is rare. The finding of syphilitic lesions in two different portions of the spine may be of clinical value in the differential diagnosis between syphilis and tuberculosis.

Clinical complaints resulting from vertebral syphilis depend upon the site of the lesion and the degree of destruction of the neighboring tissues. In gummatous disease of the *cervical spine*, a mass in the posterior pharynx may cause painful

Figure 245

A, Roentgenograph of the left foot in the case of a woman 44 years of age who was admitted to the hospital because of a soft-tissue swelling in the region of the first metatarsal bone. In addition, the picture shows erosion of that bone. She gave a history that, 7 months before admission, she noted some swelling of the ankle, and the swelling gradually included the medial aspect of the left foot. In the course of the evolution of these changes, the skin became discolored (dark red) and somewhat roughened. Physical examination disclosed swelling of the foot, the swelling extending from the medial and plantar aspect of the first metatarsal bone to the fourth metatarsal, and also from the region of the metatarsophalangeal joints to the region of the midtarsus. Serologic examination yielded positive findings for syphilis.

B, Photomicrograph ($\times$ 85) of one of the tissue fragments removed at surgery from the lesion shown in *A.* Note that the marrow is replaced by granulation tissue which in some places is heavily permeated by small cells. On higher power, these were found to be mainly lymphocytes and some were plasma cells. In addition to fragments of bone, a number of irregular fragments of soft, gray-yellow, necrotic-appearing nonosseous tissue were submitted for histologic examination. Sections prepared from the soft tissue showed almost complete necrosis. Apparently these tissue fragments represented gummatous areas which had undergone extensive necrosis.

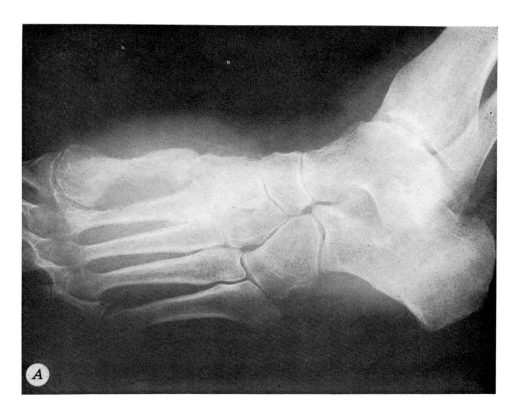

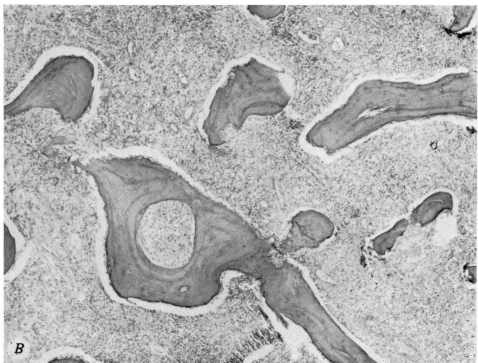

Figure 245

939

swallowing, with trismus, stiffness, and eventually even gibbus formation. In the breaking down of the tissues, the anterior arch of the atlas (as well as other portions of the cervical vertebrae) has been described as having been "sequestrated" through the ulcerated tissues of the posterior part of the pharynx. Collapse of the vertebral column at the cervical level has been known to cause sudden death. However, in the cases collected by Ziesché, healing, sometimes with astonishingly good functional result, was noted quite often, even after the sequestration of necrotic bone. In *other areas of the vertebral column*, similar if less pronounced conditions are manifested. However, the pain and the rigidity so evident with gummatous lesions in the cervical region are not apparent when other parts of the column are affected. Nevertheless, syphilitic spondylitis, wherever situated in the spinal column, may lead to involvement of the spinal cord and its meninges, with such serious sequelae as meningitis, myelitis, and compression phenomena. Final healing is almost always associated with stiffness of the involved portion of the vertebral column.

In syphilitic bones, *fractures* are not the result of brittleness or osteoporosis of the bones but rather of the presence of gummata in them (see Freund). So completely can a portion of bone be permeated and weakened by a gumma that a pathologic fracture may easily appear through the diseased region. The humerus, femur, and clavicle are the more usual sites of such so-called "spontaneous" fractures, occurring most frequently in the vicinity of an articular end of the bone. Multiple fractures have been observed (see Gangolphe). The fractures often heal rather rapidly, in the course of which abundant callus is formed. However, delayed healing is not infrequent. Major fractures are often bound together by indurated scar tissue, but the latter does not show caseation. A high degree of mobility at the fracture site may result in the formation of a pseudarthrosis.

The spongy trabeculae may undergo *thickening* or *sclerosis*, not necessarily in the immediate vicinity of a gumma. Furthermore, newly formed trabeculae appearing about the connective tissue capsule of a gumma and consisting mainly of primitive fiber bone may become concentrically compacted about the gumma. Subsequently, this encircling layer of osseous tissue may be converted into a dense sclerotic wall which comes to frame the gumma. This may be clearly apparent roentgenographically, and is of considerable value in the diagnosis of intramedullary gummata. However, as roentgenographic and pathologic examinations have shown, gummata may be present without a surrounding wall of condensed osseous tissue. The subperiosteal new bone deposited on a bone cortex in the wake of syphilitic inflammation of the periosteum also commonly undergoes densification.

In regard to the *roentgenographic differential diagnosis* between syphilis and tuberculosis of bone, the presence of osteoporosis and the absence of osteosclerosis are usually held to be indications in favor of tuberculosis. Nevertheless, although this is the general rule, the absence of sclerosis roentgenographically and even the presence of rather severe degrees of bone atrophy or osteoporosis do not necessarily eliminate the possibility of syphilis. Sometimes, even when gummatous lesions are present, atrophy and osteoporosis may supersede the sclerosis either partly or wholly. Occasionally the osteoporosis and atrophy develop without being preceded by sclerosis, their occurrence being instigated by inactivity, or being the direct result of the presence of the syphilitic inflammation in the bone.

A considerable degree of *repair and reconstruction* is possible in a bone altered by syphilitic infection. If the cortex has been extensively diseased, it may be replaced by new bone. This new bone may finally be reconstructed so as to appear and function as a new cortex. Microscopically the restored cortex presents a picture which may simulate, to some degree, the mosaic architecture presented by the osseous tissue of Paget's disease (see Freund). Reconstruction of the interior of an affected bone is also possible though less likely. In rare instances, an indurated medullary scar, the residue of a previous gumma, may finally be resorbed and replaced by fatty marrow containing spongy trabeculae.

The *muscles* in the vicinity of gummatous bone lesions often manifest pronounced but not uniform atrophy. The atrophic muscles show narrowing of their fibers and a reduction in the number of fibers. Eventually the atrophic muscles may be replaced by fatty tissue containing some lymphocytes. The connective tissue septa between the muscle bundles are often very much thickened, as is the internal perimysium. In addition, gummatous lesions may extend directly into the muscle, and after healing has occurred, one may find connective tissue scars containing lymphoid cells. Thus the muscle atrophy may be the direct result of extension of inflammation from the bone, or it may be due to inactivity. The *tendons* lying apposed to a bone area which is the site of a syphilitic lesion may become involved by extension of the inflammation to them, and in time, such tendons may be partially destroyed.

SYPHILIS OF JOINTS

In either congenital or acquired syphilis, joints may come to be involved. The anatomic features characterizing the pertinent abnormalities in the articular tissues were not fully understood for a long time. The underlying reasons for this delay are the following: (1) The stage in the course of the disease at which time joints become involved varies widely, since implication of joints may not become evident for years or even decades after the syphilitic infection has been acquired, although sometimes articular manifestations appear shortly after the onset of the infection; (2) frequently the syphilitic nature of the arthritis is clinically quite obscure; and (3) sometimes severe arthritis with deformity evolves before the syphilitic basis for the arthritis is recognized.

CLINICAL CONSIDERATIONS

The statistics relating to the *incidence of articular involvement* in syphilis as recorded in the older literature are not now generally applicable. Currently, in evaluating the incidence, a number of factors must be considered, including: the prevalence of syphilis in the geographical area under consideration; the efficiency of the methods used in the treatment of the syphilitic infection; and the probable skill of the local physicians in the detection of joint syphilis. Articular involvement is undoubtedly not frequent with either congenital or acquired syphilis. However, it is interesting to note that: (1) Brünauer and Hass reported in 1924 that about 2 per cent of all joint disease is due to syphilis; (2) Strauss, in evaluating 100 cases of chronic arthritis in 1926, stated that in 6 of them the arthritis had a luetic basis; and (3) von Hippel noted in 1903 that syphilitic arthritis was present in 56 per cent of a series of 77 congenitally syphilitic children with keratitis. Von Hippel's findings must, of course, be considered in relation to the time of his report and the methods of treatment prevalent at that time.

In regard to the *distribution of syphilitic arthritides*, it is particularly the large joints that are likely to be involved. Of these, the knee joint is most frequently affected. Next in order comes the elbow joint; much less often affected are the ankle, shoulder, and wrist joints. Furthermore, the involvement is quite commonly bilateral and symmetrical. Thus, in both congenital and acquired syphilis, both knee joints may be simultaneously diseased, although in one of them the lesion may be very slight and even difficult to detect clinically. It was Clutton who first emphasized the diagnostic significance of bilateral painless hydrops of the knee in children and adolescents as evidence of congenital syphilis. Of the smaller joints, the sternoclavicular is rather often the site of the luetic involvement.

In congenital syphilis, the *time of onset* of articular involvement varies. While joints are hardly ever implicated *early in congenital syphilis*, they are, by contrast, frequently involved *late in congenital syphilis*. In *acquired syphilis*, one or several joints may become inflamed in the *secondary stage* of the infection—that is, during or near the time of the skin eruption. Much more often, it is in the *tertiary stage* of acquired syphilis that the joint involvement shows itself. The *site of departure* of the syphilitic articular inflammation may actually be the soft tissues of the joint (for example, the synovial or parasynovial tissues); or, instead, the inflammation may reach the joint secondarily from a focus of syphilis in the articular end of a bone entering into the formation of a joint. Late in *acquired syphilis*, the origin of the joint affection is as likely to be primarily osseous as primarily synovial. Late in *congenital syphilis*, it is more often primarily synovial.

Clinical Complaints and Findings.—There are very few arthritides that may not be simulated by some type of syphilitic joint involvement. Procedures available for the *diagnosis* of joint syphilis include: roentgenographic examination of the joint region; testing of both the blood and the synovial fluid for evidence of syphilitic infection; the recovery of *Treponema pallidum* from the synovial fluid in early cases of syphilis; and the clinical improvement represented by antisyphilitic treatment. Even with all of these aids, the diagnosis often requires critical evaluation. Cases remain in which, after all factors have been considered, the luetic etiology of the arthritis is still not definitely established. Nevertheless, the possibility of lues must always be borne in mind when one is confronted with articular disease of obscure origin. Furthermore, it is important to remember that even if a patient is luetic, the pathologic process in his joints need not necessarily be due to syphilis.

The *clinical history* may or may not point toward the correct diagnosis. Clinical factors in favor of a diagnosis of joint syphilis—though certainly not establishing it definitely—are: periodic exacerbations of the arthritic condition; frequently the mild character of the pain and the tendency of the pain to become worse at night; the retention, for a long time, of good active and passive mobility, and delay in the appearance of muscle atrophy. Roentgenographically, the joint region may fail to demonstrate findings suggestive of syphilis; however, in some cases the articular ends of the bones do show syphilitic periostitis or syphilitic lesions (gummata) in the epiphysial ends of the bones.

Aspiration of fluid from the joint, if possible, may aid further in arriving at the diagnosis. The physical character and cytology of this fluid are not in themselves distinctive. In rare cases, apparently, the synovial fluid yields a positive test result for syphilis while the blood serum of the patient does not. In such isolated instances, it is reasonably certain that the articular condition is luetic. Conversely, if the test result from the joint punctate is negative when the test result from the blood is positive, the articular condition is probably *not* syphilitic. Almost invariably, if the synovial fluid yields a positive test result, the blood also will yield a positive result. In considering the diagnosis of syphilitic arthritis, one must always exclude the possibility of tuberculosis. This is accomplished by inoculating some of the synovial fluid subcutaneously or intraperitoneally into a guinea pig, or by culturing the fluid in an attempt to grow the tubercle bacillus.

Chesney *et al.* were able to recover *Treponema pallidum* from the knee joint fluid in 3 of 10 cases of syphilis with articular involvement. Two to 4 cc. of freshly drawn synovial fluid were inoculated into one or both testes of rabbits. Subsequently, treponema were found by dark field examination of scrapings from the inflamed testes. In these 3 cases the syphilitic infection was of recent origin. In one of the cases from which the spirochetes were recovered, the arthritis preceded the exanthem, while in another the arthritis appeared less than 3 months after the subject was infected. These findings have been confirmed by other investigators (see Gerškowič and Brenner). It is of interest that treponema can be found in synovial fluid not long after the syphilitic infection was acquired. In contrast, Chesney et al. were unable to recover spirochetes from cases of arthritis occurring late in the course of syphilis.

The frequent dramatic success of antisyphilitic therapy is the most nearly conclusive, as well as the most practical, evidence of the syphilitic nature of a joint affection. Such success is greatest before the occurrence of severe destructive changes and the consequent appearance of articular deformity. Even in the presence of such changes, antisyphilitic treatment is likely to have some therapeutic value, however, since it arrests the progress of the inflammatory process.

Syphilis as it relates to joints presents a wide range of both clinical and anatomic manifestations. Mention has already been made of intra-articular effusion occurring early in the course of *congenital syphilis* (p. 920), and the occurrence of bilateral painless hydrops (so-called Clutton's joints) late in the course of congenital syphilis (p. 924). In this section of the chapter, our attention will be focused mainly upon the articular aspects of *acquired syphilis*. During the secondary stage of acquired syphilis—that is, at the time of the appearance of the multiform skin eruptions (or shortly before or after)—there may be pains referred to bones and joints, and even swelling of some joints. Since early and energetic treatment of syphilis is now common, the swelling of joints relating to the secondary stage of acquired syphilis has become relatively infrequent.

Simple *arthralgia* is the more usual manifestation during the secondary stage of acquired syphilis, the pain being referred to a single joint or, less frequently, to several joints. It is the large joints (knee, ankle, or shoulder) that are the most common sites of the pain. However, clinical examination of the painful joint reveals no limitation of motion, no crepitus, and no intra-articular effusion. In this respect, these arthralgias appear to be analogous to those which occur in other acute infectious diseases. The pains, of widely varying intensity, are so undistinctive that in themselves they would not suggest the presence of syphilis. The arthralgia tends to increase during repose, and to decrease after exercise of the joint. Nothing exact is known about the anatomic condition in such joints. Furthermore, it is not possible to state whether or not the localization of spirochetes in the soft tissues of the joint is a factor in the causation of the pain. Hydrarthrosis is much less likely to occur with the exanthem than is simple arthralgia. When effusion is found, the knee is the most common site. As a rule, only one joint is affected, functional difficulty is not pronounced, and persisting pain is not present. However, the pain is ordinarily more severe at night. The synovial effusion, which is often scant, sets in rather abruptly and apparently spontaneously. The fluid gives a positive test reaction for syphilis, and disappears rapidly under antiluetic treatment.

An even more serious form of joint involvement with secondary syphilis simulates rheumatic fever (see Fournier). This articular manifestation is rather rare and is likely to present diagnostic problems (see Hoffmann). One or several large joints become painful, limited in mobility, and moderately swollen. In addition, the body temperature may be slightly elevated, but there is no sweating. If the condition is neglected, actual joint changes are likely to ensue. In the absence of other signs of syphilis, such cases might be treated for acute rheumatism and the syphilis itself escape attention and treatment. Chesney et al. have described one such case with eosinophilia and enlarged and tender lymph nodes. They recovered *Treponema pallidum* from the knee fluid of this patient.

PATHOLOGIC FINDINGS

Pathogenesis.—Syphilis of joints may take its departure from: (1) syphilitic inflammation developing in the synovial membrane, or (2) the extension of a syphilitic lesion into the joint from a focus of syphilis in an articular end of a bone. (See Fig. 246.)

Late in either congenital or acquired syphilis, a joint may become affected by a luetic process originating in the synovial or parasynovial tissues. The instigating factor of the synovial inflammation is sometimes a gumma. In only a very few instances, however, have gummata in the synovial or parasynovial tissues been demonstrated histologically by tissue examination. The clinical appearance and course do not necessarily give any indication of the presence of gummata in the synovial membrane. Joints so involved show principally intra-articular effusion and thickening of the capsule. Borchard described a surgically extirpated synovial membrane containing gummata. This membrane was very much thickened and velvety and showed villus formation with miliary gummata in the villi. There was one large stalked gumma attached to the capsule and hanging into the joint. The articular cartilages were not eroded. Lancereaux's case at autopsy showed the gummatous synovial membrane in both knees to be thickened and injected. The surface of the synovium was covered in places by pseudomembranous deposits. The articular cartilage of one of the femoral condyles was ulcerated and eroded. Hoffmann examined a biopsy specimen from a knee joint which revealed gummata, and described the remaining synovium as red and granulating. In connection with gummatous synovial inflammation, Virchow stressed the diagnostic significance of radiating scars in the articular cartilages resulting from the erosive action of gummata.

More often, gummata are not to be observed with luetic inflammations originating in the synovial or parasynovial tissues. In such joints, thickening of these tissues

Figure 246

A, Roentgenograph of a knee joint which was the site of syphilitic inflammation in a case of acquired syphilis. The subject was a man 33 years of age who, when admitted to the hospital, gave a history of pain and swelling of the right knee of 1 year's duration. He had acquired syphilis about 13 years before—that is, at the age of 20. Examination revealed marked enlargement of the knee. There was local heat, fluid in the joint, and thickening of the capsule. The knee joint had been aspirated several times prior to admission to the hospital. On palpation of the knee, the region of the internal condyle of the femur was found to be somewhat tender, as was the tibia. A synovectomy was performed, in the course of which it was found that in the supracondylar region, immediately above the articular cartilage, there was a defect in the cortex of the bone. In the region of the defect there was granulation tissue, indicating that the involvement of the joint was the result of extension into it of the syphilitic inflammation from the medullary cavity of the femur. Involvement of the end of the shaft of that bone is apparent in the picture.

B, Photograph of the resected synovial membrane from the involved knee joint shown in *A*. The membrane is enormously thickened. The surface is very irregular, presenting smooth and roughened areas, white and deeply discolored ones, as well as a few fibrinous deposits. Sectioning showed that, within the substance of the thickened synovial membrane, there were areas which appeared to be necrotic.

C, Photomicrograph ($\times$ 35) of one of the tissue sections prepared from the synovial membrane shown in *B*. On the left side of the picture, thick villi are apparent which contain collections of round cells, mainly lymphocytes. Some lymphocytes are present even deeper in the membrane. On the right side of the picture, a gumma is present, and only a small amount of caseous material is apparent. The periphery of the gumma is heavily infiltrated with lymphocytes.

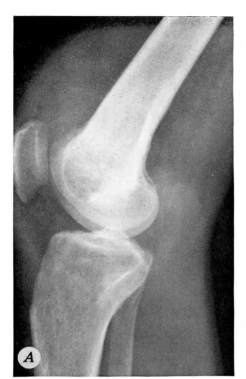

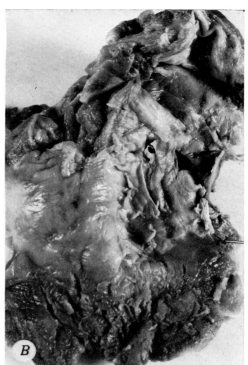

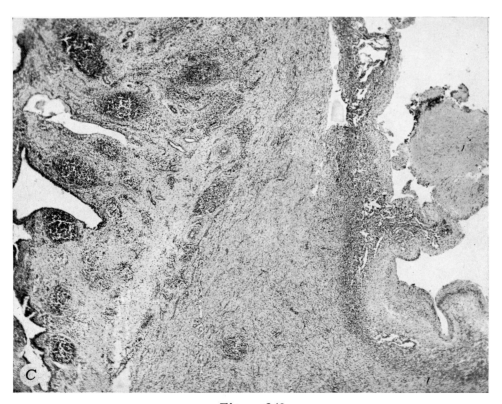

Figure 246

occurs; villus formation and effusion may also be part of the pathologic picture. It may indeed be difficult, if not impossible, to differentiate the inflammatory changes under such circumstances from those provoked by nonsyphilitic agents. The villi may contain numerous lymphoid cells and large numbers of blood vessels, but the characteristic indications of syphilis may be entirely lacking. In such joints, pannus may appear and lead to the destruction of the articular cartilages. If the types of syphilitic joint involvement described so far are promptly treated, however, the syphilitic changes may rapidly regress. This is especially the case if no erosion or secondary changes have yet appeared in the articular cartilages or the underlying bone.

Late in *either* congenital or acquired lues, syphilitic inflammation in the articular end of a bone may come to implicate the soft tissues of the joint. Under these circumstances, the joint involvement is usually the result of the extension of a gumma from the bone into the joint. The penetration occurs most often where the synovial membrane is attached to, and reflects from, the bone. As the gumma in the bone may be clinically latent, only a roentgenograph may reveal its presence and its relation to the arthritis. On the whole, the arthritis due to the extension of syphilitic inflammation from bones into joints is more severe than that resulting from inflammation originating primarily in the synovial or parasynovial tissues.

When it is possible to establish the fact that a gumma has broken through from a bone into the adjacent joint, the syphilitic nature of the condition of the joint is established *a priori*. The active inflammation that is set up in the joint results from the degenerated gummatous matter which has entered the joint from the bone, but the inflammatory process which ensues is not at all likely to be gummatous. Furthermore, it is known that joints may be inflamed sympathetically—that is, without the direct penetration of a gumma into the joint. In these cases the joint inflammation may be due to a syphilitic periostitis at the end of the bone or a syphilitic lesion in the substance of the bone not far from the joint. Gangolphe and also Chiari are among those who have made anatomic studies of syphilitic articular affections which have resulted from the invasion of gummata from one or another articular bone end into the joint. An important contribution to our knowledge of this subject is represented by Freund's detailed report emphasizing the microscopic changes.

Progression of the Pathologic Changes.—As noted above, luetic arthritis may either originate in the synovial membrane or extend to the joint from an adjacent bone. In either case, the degree of the *ultimate pathologic changes* to be observed is determined by the severity of the inflammation, the time that has elapsed since its onset, and various secondary factors. Supervening nonsyphilitic processes, partly mechanical, may be added to the syphilitic joint changes *per se*. In other words, arthritic changes of nonluetic character may be engrafted upon the original syphilitic lesion. In consequence, a severe deforming arthritis may ensue. Freund has made practically the only detailed histologic study of syphilitic joints showing advanced pathologic changes. His work is therefore an essential source of reference on this aspect of the subject.

The *synovial membrane* may be made up of loose connective tissue lined by one or several layers of cells. In some places the connective tissue may be quite vascular and contain foci of lymphoid and plasma cells. Lymphoid cells are also to be found in the more superficial lining layer. Varying degrees of villus hypertrophy may be noted. Furthermore, under certain conditions, portions of the synovium may show fibrinoid deposits on its surface, raveling, and desquamation. Where inflammation has been of long duration, thickening of the joint capsule may be prominent. On histologic examination, the latter will be found to be composed of dense and poorly cellular connective tissue. Such a capsule may eventually become contracted.

In time, *erosion of the articular cartilage* becomes manifest. This is due to the destructive action of pannus formed in the active stage of the synovial inflammation. The pannus, composed of connective tissue, grows out from the synovium. As it forms, the pannus tends to spread over the articular surface, continually destroying the cartilage. In the course of this destruction, shallow or deep erosive hollows appear. These become filled with cellular connective tissue. The destruction of cartilage may go so deep that the connective tissue may come to lie directly on the subchondral bony end plate. Any cartilaginous residue on this plate is subject to further destruction from below by invading blood vessels from the marrow. Between areas of erosion, there may, however, be areas in which the original cartilage still remains. Because of changed mechanical conditions in such joints, rests of original cartilage are subject to cell proliferation, swelling, fibrillation, abrasion, degeneration, and even necrosis.

In some places where the articular cartilage has been destroyed by pannus, regeneration of the cartilage may take place. The new cartilage is formed from the connective tissue which has filled in the erosion defects in the cartilage. Early in the regenerative stage, such new cartilage, if examined histologically, presents the usual histologic characteristics of regenerating hyaline cartilage. In particular, it has a more or less basophilic ground substance, it is fibrillar on the whole, and it has numerous small separate cells lying close together. Even this regenerated cartilage may be destroyed by pannus erosion from the surface, or by blood vessels from the marrow cavity. If the regeneration of the cartilage continues, calcification of its deepest layer may take place. In young subjects, this new cartilage thus acquires a provisional calcification zone and may hence participate in a revival of local endochondral ossification.

Where the arthritis has progressed even further, *sievelike perforations* may be found on the articular surface of syphilitically inflamed joints. These surface perforations lead into the spongiosa, sometimes by a narrow bottle-like neck. Such pouchlike cavities in the spongiosa are lined by a wall of dense connective tissue, which may be covered by a modified synovium. The perforations may represent openings left after the irruption of a gumma from the subchondral spongiosa into the joint, or they may be the result of minute fractures which extend through the provisional calcification zone and which have forced the subchondral spongiosa apart.

In a syphilitic joint which has undergone such extensive changes, mobility may eventually be very much limited. This limitation may result from irregularities of the articulating surfaces or, more definitely, from the formation of dense intra-articular connective tissue adhesions. The appearance of such adhesions is favored by very extensive destruction in, and by lack of use of, the joint. Rarely, the adhesions may become cartilaginous or bony and result in ankylosis of the joint. Thickening and shriveling of the capsule may also contribute to the ankylosis. In the subchondral spongiosa, atrophy and sclerosis in varying degrees is demonstrable grossly and roentgenographically. The tendency to osteosclerosis may be increased by changed mechanical conditions in the joint which result from abnormal friction of the bone ends against each other. The supervention of atrophy, even in some of these sclerotic trabeculae, is favored by immobility.

REFERENCES

ADSON, A. W.: The Surgical Treatment of Gummatous Osteitis of the Skull, J.A.M.A., *74*, 385, 1920.

AXHAUSEN, G.: Beiträge zur] Knochen- und Gelenksyphilis, Berl. klin. Wchnschr., *50*, 2361, 1913.

BANDIRALI, G. R., and PRATESI, A. C.: Su alcuni casi di sifilide ossea congenita precoce di recente osservazione, Ann. radiol. diag., *36*, 349, 1963.

BAUER, W.: Ueber Befunde am Zahnkeim und Kieferknochen bei angeborener Syphilis, Wien. klin. Wchnschr., *44*, 879, 1931.

BAUER, W. H.: Tooth Buds and Jaws in Patients with Congenital Syphilis. Correlation between Distribution of Treponema pallidum and Tissue Reaction, Am. J. Path., *20*, 297, 1944.

BENDA, C.: Allgemeine pathologische Anatomie der Syphilis, *Handbuch der Haut- und Geschlechtskrankheiten, 15(2),* 225, 1929.

BERTARELLI, E.: "Spirochaete pallida" und Osteochondritis, Centralbl. Bakt., *41* (pt. 1), 639, 1906.

BLACKLOCK, D. B.: Relationship of Syphilis and Yaws, Brit. M. J., *1*, 97, 1933.

BLOCH, I.: *Der Ursprung der Syphilis. Eine medizinische und kulturgeschichtliche Untersprung.* 1. *Der Ursprung der Syphilis,* Jena, Gustav Fischer, 1901.

————: *Der Ursprung der Syphilis.* 2. *Kritik der Lehre von der Altertumssyphilis,* Jena, Gustav Fischer, 1911.

————: The History of Syphilis, in: *A System of Syphilis,* edited by D'Arcy Power and J. Keogh Murphy, 2nd ed., London, Oxford University Press, 1914.

BODANSKY, A., and JAFFE, H. L.: Phosphatase Studies. III. Serum Phosphatase in Diseases of the Bone: Interpretation and Significance, Arch. Int. Med., *54*, 88, 1934.

BORCHARD: Ueber luetische Gelenkentzündungen, Deutsche Ztschr. Chir., *61*, 110, 1901.

BORELLA, L., GOOBAR, J. E., and CLARK, G. M.: Synovitis of the Knee Joints in Late Congenital Syphilis. Clutton's Joints, J.A.M.A., *180*, 190, 1962.

BRADLAW, R. V.: The Dental Stigmata of Prenatal Syphilis, Oral Surg., *6*, 147, 1953.

BRÜNAUER, S. R., and HASS, J.: Über syphilitische Gelenksaffektionen und deren Erkennung, Med. Klinik, *20*, 1453 and 1490, 1924.

BUTLER, C. S.: Yaws and Syphilis, J.A.M.A., *102*, 148, 1934.

CAFFEY, J.: Some Roentgenologic and Anatomic Changes in the Growing Skeleton After the Administration of Bismuth and Arsenic, Am. J. Dis. Child., *49*, 264, 1935.

————: Syphilis of the Skeleton in Early Infancy: The Nonspecificity of Many of the Roentgenographic Changes, Am. J. Roentgenol., *42*, 637, 1939.

CARRUTHERS, M. M., AKBARI-FARD, M., and LERNER, A. M.: A Case of Congenital Paresis in 1966, Ann. Int. Med., *66*, 1204, 1967.

CHESNEY, A. M., KEMP, J. E., and RESNIK, W. H.: Syphilitic Arthritis with Eosinophilia: Recovery of T. Pallidum from the Synovial Fluid, Johns Hopkins Hosp. Bull., *35*, 235, 1924.

CHESNEY, A. M., KEMP, J. E., and BAETJER, F. H.: An Experimental Study of the Synovial Fluid of Patients with Arthritis and Syphilis, J. Clin. Invest., *3*, 131, 1926-27.

CHIARI, H.: Zur Kenntniss der gummösen Osteomyelitis in den langen Röhrenknochen, Vrtljschr. Dermat. u. Syph., *9*, 389, 1882.

CLUTTON, H. H.: Symmetrical Synovitis of the Knee in Hereditary Syphilis, Lancet, *1*, 391, 1886.

————: Symmetrical Synovitis of the Knee in Hereditary Syphilis, Clin. Orthop., *57*, 5, 1968. (This is a reprint of the 1886 article.)

COLE, H. N.: Congenital and Prenatal Syphilis, J.A.M.A., *109*, 580, 1937.

CRIPPS, D. J., and CURTIS, A. C.: Syphilis Maligna Praecox. Syphilis of the Great Epidemic? An Historical Review, Arch. Int. Med., *119*, 411, 1967.

DEL GUASTA, F.: Sulla patogenesi delle alterazioni dentarie nella sifilide congenita, Nuova rass. odontoiatria, *9*, 2, 1928.

DOWNES, E.: Six Cases of Syphilitic Necrosis of the Jaw; Removal of Sequestra, in Three Cases by Incision from Without, and in Three by Operation Inside the Mouth; Recovery, Lancet, *2*, 870, 1881.

DRUCKER, M. G., and MANKIN, H. J.: Congenital Syphilis in 1970: A Case Report, Bull. Hosp. Joint Dis., *31*, 132, 1970.

DUNHAM, E. C.: Gummatous Osteoperiostitis of the Skull in Congenital Syphilis, Am. J. Dis. Child., *30*, 690, 1925.

EASTMAN, N. J., and DIPPEL, A. L.: The Passage of Arsenic through the Human Placenta Following Arsphenamine Therapy, Bull. Johns Hopkins Hosp., *53*, 288, 1933.

VON EICKEN: Tertiär-luetische Veränderungen des Schädeldaches, Sitzungsb. oto-laryng. Gesellsch. zu Berlin, p. 20, 1932.

ERDHEIM, J.: Über Tuberkulose des Knochens im allgemeinen und die des Schädeldaches im besonderen, Virchows Arch. path. Anat., *283*, 354, 1932.

ESCHLE, F.: Beiträge zu Casuistik der syphilitischen Dactylitis, Arch. klin. Chir., *36*, 356, 1887.

EVANS, W. A., JR.: Syphilis of the Bones in Infancy. Some Possible Errors in the Roentgen Diagnosis, J.A.M.A., *115*, 197, 1940.

FOURNIER, A.: *La Syphilis héréditaire tardive,* Paris, G. Masson, 1886.

————: *Traité de la syphilis,* Paris, J. Rueff, 1899.

FRAENKEL, E.: Die kongenitale Knochensyphilis im Röntgenbilde, Fortschr. Geb. Röntgenstrahlen, Suppl. *26*, 1911.

————: Über die angeborene Syphilis platter Knochen und ihre röntgenologische Erkennung, Fortschr. Geb. Röntgenstrahlen, *19*, 422, 1912–13.

FRANGENHEIM, P.: Die Syphilis der Knochen, *Handbuch der Haut- und Geschlechtskrankheiten, 17(3)*, 168, 1928.

FREUND, E.: Zur Frage der Ostitis deformans Paget, Virchows Arch. path. Anat., *274*, 1, 1929.

————: Über Knochensyphilis, Virchows Arch. path. Anat., *288*, 146, 1933.

————: Über Syphilis der Gelenke, Virchows Arch. path. Anat., *289*, 575, 1933.

GANGOLPHE, M.: Contribution a l'étude des localisations articulaires de la syphilis tertiaire. De l'ostéoarthrite syphilitique, Ann. dermat. et syph., *6*, 449, 1885.

————: *Maladies infectieuses et parasitaires des os*, Paris, G. Masson, 1894.

GERŠKOWIČ, Z., and BRENNER, M.: Zur Frage der Diagnostik der Gelenksyphilis, Arch. klin. Med., *175*, 637, 1933.

GRÄVINGHOFF, W.: Über die Schwachzeichen der angeborenen Lues am Knochen, Jahrb. Kinderh., *133*, 189, 1931.

GREGORY, M. S., and KARPAS, M. J.: Syphilitic Bone Disease of the Skull, J. Nerv. & Ment. Dis., *40*, 651, 1913.

HAHN, R., and DEYCKE-PASCHA: Knochensyphilis im Röntgenbild, Fortschr. Geb. Röntgenstrahlen, Suppl. *14*, 1907.

HERXHEIMER, G.: Zur pathologischen Anatomie der kongenitalen Syphilis, Ergebn. allg. Path., *12*, 499, 1908.

————: Die pathologische Anatomie der angeborenen Syphilis. Allgemeine Gesichtspunkte, Verhandl. deutsch. path. Gesellsch., *23*, 144, 1928.

HESLOP, I. H.: Syphilitic Osteomyelitis of the Mandible, Brit. J. Oral Surg., *6*, 59, 1968.

VON HIPPEL, E.: Ueber die Häufigkeit von Gelenkerkrankungen bei hereditär Syphilitischen, München. med. Wchnschr., *50(2)*, 1321, 1903.

HOCHSINGER, C.: *Studien über die hereditäre Syphilis. II. Knochenerkrankungen und Bewegungsstörungen bei der angeborenen Frühsyphilis*, Leipzig, Franz Deuticke, 1904.

————: Die Besonderheiten der kongenital-syphilitischen Erkrankungen der inneren Organe (einschliesslich des Zentralnervensystems) und des Bewegungsapparates, *Handbuch der Haut- und Geschlechtskrankheiten, 19*, 116, 1927.

HOFFMANN, E.: Zur Frage der Lues articularis praecox unter dem Bilde der Polyarthritis rheumatica, Klin. Wchnschr., *12*, 1837, 1933.

HOFFMANN, V.: Befunde zur Kenntnis der Gelenksyphilis, Arch. klin. Chir., *171*, 635, 1932.

HOOTON, E. A.: *The Indians of Pecos Pueblo: A Study of their Skeletal Remains*, New Haven, Yale University Press (Chap. 10. Pathology), 1930.

HUDSON, E. H.: Christopher Columbus and the History of Syphilis, Acta trop., *25*, 1, 1968.

HUTCHINSON, J.: *Syphilis*, London, Cassell & Co., 1887.

JAFFE, H. L.: Paget's Disease of Bone, Arch. Path., *15*, 83, 1933.

JARCHO, S.: Some Observations on Disease in Prehistoric North America, Bull. Hist. Med., *38*, 1, 1964.

JONES, J.: Explorations of the Aboriginal Remains of Tennessee, Smithsonian Contributions to Knowledge, Washington, *22*, No. 259, 1876.

JORDAN, A.: Zur Statistik der syphilitischen Osteoperiostosis, Dermat. Wchnschr., *81*, 1737, 1925.

KING, A. J., and CATTERALL, R. D.: Syphilis of Bones, Brit. J. Ven. Dis., *35*, 116, 1959.

KRANZ, P.: Über Zahnanomalien bei kongenitaler Lues, Sammlung Meusser: No. 8, 1920.

————: Zahndeformitäten bei angelborener Syphilis, *Handbuch der Haut- und Geschlechtskrankheiten, 19*, 240, 1927.

LANCEREAUX, E.: *Traité historique et pratique de la Syphilis*, Paris, J. B. Baillière et Fils, 1866.

LANYAR, F.: Ein Beitrag zur Frage der traumatischen Auslösung luetischer Knochenerkrankungen, Arch. Dermat. u. Syph., *163*, 326, 1931.

LEVADITI, C., VAISMAN, A., SCHOEN, R., and MEZGER, J. G.: Nouvelles recherches expérimentales sur la syphilis, Ann. Inst. Pasteur, *50*, 222, 1933.

LUCAS, R. C.: "Inherited Syphilis," Rep. Soc. Study Dis. Child., *8*, 62, 1908.

MAGGI, G. C., and GRASSI, E.: Aspetti radiologici delle localizzazioni scheletriche dell'eredolue precoce, Minerva pediat., *15*, 938, 1963.

McCORD, J. R.: Syphilis and Pregnancy. A Clinical Study of 2,150 Cases, J.A.M.A., *105*, 89, 1935.

McKELVEY, J. L., and TURNER, T. B.: Syphilis and Pregnancy. An Analysis of the Outcome of Pregnancy in Relation to Treatment in 943 Cases, J.A.M.A., *102*, 503, 1934.

McLEAN, S.: The Roentgenographic and Pathologic Aspects of Congenital Osseous Syphilis, Am. J. Dis. Child., *41*, 130, 1931.

————: The Correlation of the Roentgenographic and Pathologic Aspects of Congenital Osseous Syphilis, with Particular Reference to the First Months of Life, Am. J. Dis. Child., *41*, 363, 1931.

61

————: Correlation of the Roentgenologic Picture with the Gross and the Microscopic Examination of Pathologic Material in Congenital Osseous Syphilis, Am. J. Dis. Child., *41*, 607, 1931.

————: The Correlation of the Clinical Picture with the Osseous Lesions of Congenital Syphilis as shown by the X-Rays, Am. J. Dis. Child., *41*, 887 and 1128, 1931.

————: The Osseous Lesions of Congenital Syphilis. Summary and Conclusions in One Hundred and Two Cases, Am. J. Dis. Child., *41*, 1411, 1931.

MICHAËLIS, L.: Vergleichende mikroskopische Untersuchungen an rezenten, historischen und fossilen menschlichen Knochen. Zugleich ein Beitrag zur Geschichte der Syphilis, Veröffentl. Kriegs- u. Konstitutions Path., *6(2)*, No. 24, 1930.

MOON, H.: Quoted by Lucas.

MÜLLER, G.: Epiphysäre Entkalkungszonen bei kongenitaler Viruspneumonie. Über die Beobachtung von luesähnlichen Röntgenbefunden an den Knochen einer Frühgeburt, Ann. paediat., *193*, 33, 1959.

NESTMANN, F.: Histologische Untersuchungen an syphilitisch veränderten Tibien, Arch. orthop. u. Unfall-Chir., *26*, 237, 1928.

OLMSTEAD, E. G.: Gummatous Osteomyelitis with Pathologic Fracture Complicating General Paresis, Am. J. Syph., *32*, 243, 1948.

PARROT, M. J.: Sur une pseudo-paralysie causée par une altération du système osseux chez les nouveau-nés atteints de syphilis héréditaire, Arch. physiol. norm. et path., *4*, 319, 470, 612, 1871–72.

————: The Osseous Lesions of Hereditary Syphilis, Lancet, *1*, 696, 1879.

PÉHU, CHASSARD, and ENSELME, J.: Étude radiologique de la syphilis congénitale des os longs envisagée dans la première enfance, J. radiol. et électrol., *10*, 54, 1926.

PENDERGRASS, E. P., GILMAN, R. L., and CASTLETON, K. B.: Bone Lesions in Tardive Heredo-syphilis, Am. J. Roentgenol., *24*, 234, 1930.

PHILIPP, E., and RICHTER, W.: Lues und Geburtshilfe. Aufgaben des Geburtshelfers bei der Bekämpfung der kongenitalen Lues, München. med. Wchnschr., *80*, 1540, 1933.

PICK, L.: Zur Röntgendiagnose der angeborenen Knochensyphilis, Deutsche med. Wchnschr., *45*, 953, 1919.

————: Neuere Forschungen über die kongenitale Knochensyphilis, Dermat. Wchnschr., *74*, 540, 1922.

————: Über die Röntgenuntersuchung als Hilfsmittel für die Diagnose der congenitalen Frühsyphilis des Skelettsystems, insbesondere bei Veränderungen an der Diaphyse der grossen Röhrenknochen, Deutsche Ztschr. ges. gerichtl. Med., *12*, 159, 1928.

————: Über Osteochondritis syphilitica im Kindesalter (Osteochondritis syphilitica tarda), Verhandl. deutsch. path. Gesellsch., *23*, 248, 1928.

————: Angeborene Knochensyphilis. In *Handbuch der speziellen pathologischen Anatomie und Histologie*, edited by F. Henke and O. Lubarsch, Berlin, Julius Springer, 1929 (*9*(part 1), see p. 240).

PUSEY, W. A.: *The History and Epidemiology of Syphilis*, Springfield, Charles C Thomas, 1933.

RANVIER: Syphilis congénitale; péri-hépatite syphilitique; gommes du foie et décollement des épiphyses, Gaz. méd. Paris, *19*, 596, 1864.

RICORD, P.: *Lectures on Venereal and Other Diseases Arising from Sexual Intercourse.* (Reported and Translated by Victor de Meric), Philadelphia, E. Barrington and G. D. Haswell, 1849.

————: *Traité complet des maladies vénériennes*, Paris, J. Rouvier, 1851.

————: *A Practical Treatise on Venereal Diseases; or, Critical and Experimental Researches on Inoculation, Applied to the Study of these Affections, with a Therapeutical Summary and Special Formulary.* (English Translation by A. S. Doane), 13th ed., New York, Redfield, 1854.

SARNAT, B. G., SCHOUR, I., and HEUPEL, R.: Roentgenographic Diagnosis of Congenital Syphilis in Unerupted Permanent Teeth, J.A.M.A., *116*, 2745, 1941.

SCHMIDT, M. B.: Allgemeine Pathologie und pathologische Anatomie der Knochen, Ergebn. allg. Path., *7*, 221, 1900–01.

SCHMORL, G.: Über Ostitis deformans Paget, Virchows Arch. path. Anat., *283*, 694, 1932.

SCHNEIDER, P.: Anatomie, Röntgenologie und Bakteriologie der angeborenen Frühsyphilis de s Knochensystems, Ergebn. allg. Path., *20(2)*, 185, 1923–24.

————: Über die Organveränderungen bei der angeborenen Frühsyphilis, Verhandl. deutsch. path. Gesellsch., *23*, 177, 1928.

SHIPLEY, P. G., PEARSON, J. W., WEECH, A. A., and GREENE, C. H.: X-Ray Pictures of the Bones in the Diagnosis of Syphilis in the Fetus and in Young Infants, Johns Hopkins Hosp. Bull., *32*, 75, 1921.

SMITH, F. R., JR.: Late Congenital Syphilis. A Study of the Results of Treatment in 267 Patients, Bull. Johns Hopkins Hosp., *53*, 231, 1933.

SMITH, G. E., and DAWSON, W. R.: *Egyptian Mummies*, London, Allen & Unwin, 1924.

SOLOWEITSCHIK, E.: Beiträge zur Lehre von der syphilitischen Schädelaffection, Arch. path. Anat., *48*, 55 and 193, 1869.

STRAUSS, H.: Über Gelenkerkrankungen bei Spätlues, Ther. Gegenw., *67*, 107, 1926.

SUDHOFF, K.: *Graphische und typographische Erstlinge der Syphilisliteratur*, Munich, C. Kuhn, 1912.

————: *Aus der Frühgeschichte der Syphilis*, Leipzig, J. A. Barth, 1912.

————: *Der Ursprung der Syphilis*, Leipzig, F. C. W. Vogel, 1913.

TAYLOR, R. W.: *Syphilitic Lesions of the Osseous System in Infants and Young Children*, New York, Wm. Wood & Co., 1875.

————: Bone Syphilis, Hereditary and Acquired. I. Early and Late Hereditary Bone Syphilis, New York M. J., *85*, 1, 1907.

————: Bone Syphilis, Hereditary and Acquired. II. Early and Late Acquired Bone Syphilis, New York M. J., *85*, 57, 1907.

TELLO, J. C., and WILLIAMS, H. U.: An Ancient Syphilitic Skull from Paracas in Peru, Ann. M. Hist., *2*, 515, 1930.

THOMSEN, O.: *Pathologisch-anatomische Veränderungen über die congenitale Syphilis bei dem Foetus und dem neugeborenen Kind*, Copenhagen, Levin & Munksgaard, 1928.

TURNBULL, H. M.: Recognition of Congenital Syphilitic Inflammation of the Long Bones, Lancet, *1*, 1239, 1922.

VIRCHOW, R.: Ueber die Natur der constitutionell-syphilitischen Affectionen, Arch. path. Anat., *15*, 217, 1858.

————: Ueber syphilitische Gelenkaffectionen, Berl. klin. Wchnschr., *21*, 534, 1884.

WEBER, M.: Schliffe von mazerierten Röhrenknochen und ihre Bedeutung für die Unterscheidung der Syphilis und Osteomyelitis von der Osteodystrophia fibrosa sowie für die Untersuchung fraglich syphilitischer, prähistorischer Knochen, Beitr. path. Anat., *78*, 441, 1927.

WECHSELBERG, K., and SCHNEIDER, J. D.: Morbidität und klinische Symptomatik der konnatalen Lues im Säuglingsalter, Deutsche med. Wchnschr., *95*, 1976, 1970.

WEGNER, G.: Ueber hereditäre Knochensyphilis bei jungen Kindern, Arch. path. Anat., *50*, 305, 1870.

WIELAND, E.: Spezielle Pathologie des Bewegungsapparates (Stützapparates) im Kindesalter. In *Handb. allg. Path. u. path. Anat. d. Kindesalters*, edited by H. Brüning and E. Schwalbe, Wiesbaden, J. F. Bergmann, 1913 (*2*, page 148).

WILHELM, S. F.: Osteitis Fibrosa and the Hyperostotic Form of Bone Syphilis. A Comparative Anatomical and Roentgenological Study, Surg. Gynec. & Obst., *41*, 624, 1925.

WILLIAMS, H. U.: Human Paleopathology, with Some Original Observations on Symmetrical Osteoporosis of the Skull, Arch. Path., *7*, 839, 1929.

————: The Origin and Antiquity of Syphilis: the Evidence from Diseased Bones. A Review, with Some New Material from America, Arch. Path., *13*, 779 and 931, 1932.

WIMBERGER, H.: Klinisch-radiologische Diagnostik von Rachitis, Skorbut und Lues congenita im Kindesalter, Ergebn. inn. Med. u. Kinderh., *28*, 264, 1925.

ZIESCHÉ, H.: Ueber die syphilitische Wirbelentzündung, Mitt. Grenzgeb. Med. u. Chir., *22*, 357, 1910–11.

Chapter

30

Tuberculosis and Sarcoidosis of Bones and Joints

There can be no doubt that what we now call *skeletal tuberculosis* has been a familiar and common condition for thousands of years. This fact is attested by illuminating descriptions of the condition in the earliest known medical writings. It is also corroborated by the results of archaeological excavations, which have quite frequently unearthed ancient human bones presenting abnormalities indicative of tuberculous involvement, especially of the thoracolumbar portion of the vertebral column (see Lichtor and Lichtor). The references to skeletal tuberculosis in the early medical literature became increasingly precise in the course of years. Thus Wiseman in 1686, in discussing the King's Evil (scrofula), described instances of "white swelling," especially in children, and it is apparent from his text that many were cases of tuberculosis of bones and joints.

As the specialty of pathology developed, skeletal tuberculosis came to be clearly delimited and differentiated from skeletal lesions due to other causes. One of the first modern contributions to the understanding of tuberculosis of bones and joints was made in 1826 by Margot. His work was important because of his recognition of tubercles on anatomic examination of articular lesions diagnosed clinically as "tumor albus." Rokitansky, advancing pertinent knowledge a step further, stressed the similarity of the basic pathology of skeletal tuberculosis and visceral tuberculosis.

In connection with the diagnosis of tuberculosis, it is worth pointing out that, even before Koch identified the tubercle bacillus in 1882, guinea pig inoculation had been used as an aid in the diagnosis of tuberculosis. That is, although the tubercle bacillus had not yet been discovered, it was known that if fluid or pus obtained from a human, and in particular from a lesion thought to be tuberculous, was injected into a guinea pig, the pathologic changes induced in the animal would justify a clinical diagnosis of tuberculosis. From these beginnings, knowledge regarding skeletal tuberculosis accumulated as our understanding of tuberculous infection in general increased. Among the important early contributions subsequent to Koch's crucial discovery were those of Volkmann, König, Krause, Cheyne, and Nichols.

Sarcoidosis is being considered in this chapter because the lesional granulation tissue, which consists of quasi-tuberculous nodules, may be confused, on a histologic basis, with the tubercles of tuberculosis. However, a distinction is possible because of the fact that the tubercles of sarcoidosis, even when agglomerated, do not undergo caseation.

TUBERCULOSIS

In *tuberculosis* the lesions of the skeleton, as well as those of tendon sheaths and bursae, may be induced by either the *human* or the *bovine* type of the tubercle bacillus. Clinically, the changes induced by the bovine type are indistinguishable from those induced by the human type. The bovine bacilli are at least as virulent for man as are the human bacilli. Griffith clearly established the importance of the bovine type in the causation of skeletal tuberculosis. The bovine tubercle bacillus is ordinarily conveyed to the human body by cow's milk and enters it by way of the intestinal tract. There are no reports of human skeletal lesions arising from avian or reptilian tubercle bacilli.

The question of whether, and to what extent, there is a relationship between *trauma* and skeletal tuberculosis has aroused a good deal of discussion in the past. The problem is a very complex one, partly because of confusion regarding the various possible roles of trauma. Certainly in many cases of skeletal tuberculosis there is a history of preceding trauma, but careful analysis of all factors will usually show that the trauma merely called attention to an already existing tuberculous skeletal lesion. It is probably only in about 1 per cent of cases of skeletal tuberculosis that trauma acts as an initiating or even as a localizing agent (see Schuberth and Mayr-Weber). Von Meyenburg maintained that the only cases in which one can be absolutely certain that trauma is to be inculpated are those in which the trauma coincided with the actual introduction of tubercle bacilli into the wound. Confusion and disagreement as to the importance of trauma are also created by differences of opinion regarding: (1) the degree of severity of the trauma, (2) the time elapsing between the trauma and the onset of the tuberculous lesion, and (3) the relationship of the site of the trauma to the site of the tuberculous lesion. However, if, within 2 to 6 months after a definite injury to a particular skeletal part, tuberculosis develops precisely in the injured area, it would certainly seem reasonable to suppose that the trauma had some connection with the tuberculous skeletal lesion. In regard to the role of trauma, it should be pointed out that in 1944 Meyer reported that in Denmark only one new case of skeletal tuberculosis was noted per 30,000 of the general population. He discussed the relation of trauma to tuberculosis of bones and joints, but stated that, with an incidence as small as it was in Denmark, the statistical evaluation of the role of trauma in skeletal tuberculosis was not possible.

Incidence.—Even when pulmonary tuberculosis was a rather common disease, skeletal tuberculosis was, by comparison, infrequently encountered. In regard to the over-all incidence of skeletal tuberculosis at that time, there were few data available. In 1913, de Quervain and Hunziker estimated that in the canton of Basel in Switzerland there were, on the average, 12.8 cases per 10,000 of population. Johansson reported that in the city of Gothenburg, Sweden, between 1909 and 1922, an average of 5.65 new cases of skeletal tuberculosis were diagnosed each year among 10,000 children under 15 years of age, and 1.62 new cases among 10,000 subjects over 15 years of age. Other statistical evaluations at about that time placed the incidence of skeletal tuberculosis (new and chronic) in children under 15 years of age at about 10 cases per 10,000 subjects; the incidence of *new cases per year* was apparently about 3 or 4 per 10,000.

In any event, it seems worth pointing out that, between 1938 and 1957, various evaluations of the occurrence of skeletal tuberculosis among cases of tuberculosis in general was approximately 3 to 5 per cent. However, on the basis of mortality statistics relating to persons dying of *extrapulmonary* tuberculosis, the proportion of those affected with *skeletal* tuberculosis in particular was relatively high, ranging approximately between 25 and 35 per cent (see Kastert and Uehlinger).

No general or permanent validity should, of course, be assigned to these statistical data. They applied specifically to the time and the country in which they were calculated. It is well known that, in underdeveloped countries, poverty (as manifested in undernutrition and overcrowding) shows a pronounced statistical association with morbidity from tuberculosis in general (see Percy-Lancaster, and also

Dickson). Skeletal tuberculosis is no exception to this rule, in spite of the fact that milk (the carrier of bovine tubercle bacilli) is likely to be scarce where there is poverty. In addition, overcrowding ensures intimate and prolonged contact with open cases of tuberculosis. The frequent occurrence of tuberculosis (usually pulmonary) in the immediate family or among relatives of persons suffering from skeletal tuberculosis is generally recognized. Estimates of this frequency have been as high as 50 per cent, but 10 to 20 per cent would seem to be more accurate.

PATHOGENESIS OF SKELETAL TUBERCULOSIS

The course of tuberculous infection in man is usually subdivided into three stages. The first of these stages, commonly referred to as the *primary complex*, is the one in which the initial tuberculous focus is established, and is often not associated with clinical manifestations, though in some cases there is fever, cough, and/or loss of weight. There can be no doubt that, in the past, a large percentage of persons developed a primary tuberculous complex during childhood or adolescence. To judge from the older reports, practically everyone, especially in cities, acquired a primary focus of infection before reaching adult life. In fact, in the older statistics, young children up to 5 years of age (except during the first year of life) showed a very high incidence of such a primary infection. However, recent roentgenographic and pathologic studies have revealed that the primary complex is being acquired later and later in life (early and middle adult life). Now, even in cities, the proportion of children who go through adolescence without acquiring a primary tuberculous complex is larger than it used to be. When fresh primary complexes are acquired as late as middle life, the condition is often asymptomatic (see Uehlinger).

The *primary complex* consists of a tuberculous lesion at the site of the initial infection, and of spread of the tubercle bacilli from there to the regional lymph nodes. In its fresh state, the lesion is rather exudative and caseous. While the site of most primary foci is in the lungs, the primary lesion may appear elsewhere, particularly in the cervical lymph nodes, or in the intestine and its regional lymph nodes. In the lungs, as Parrot, Küss, and also Ghon have shown, the lesion, which is about 1 cm. in diameter, is usually situated near the surface of one of the lobes, and in addition the regional (hilar) lymph nodes are involved. In the intestinal tract, the small intestine and its regional lymph nodes are more often affected than is the large intestine (see Ghon and Pototschnig). The tubercle bacilli initiating *intrathoracic* primary foci are air-borne in most cases and are nearly always of the human type. The bacilli initiating *intra-abdominal* primary lesions are usually of the bovine type and are ordinarily milk-borne.

In the large majority of the cases, the primary lesion eventually heals, within a year or several years, and the healing tends to follow a rather characteristic course (see Weber *et al.*). The tuberculous focus, which is caseous and calcareous, becomes encapsulated by fibrous connective tissue. It may ultimately be transformed into a hyalinized fibrous nodule, often containing large amounts of calcareous material and frequently bone. Virulent tubercle bacilli may remain in the primary lesion for a long time (see Puhl).

In a study of the incidence of primary complexes in *childhood*, Blacklock reported findings based on autopsies carried out on 1,800 children whose ages ranged from a few hours to 13 years, and of these, 1,439 were under 2 years of age. He found that 283 of the subjects showed evidences of tuberculous infection. The primary lesion was in the chest in about 61 per cent of those infected, in the abdomen in 35 per cent, in the cervical lymph glands in 2 per cent, and could not be located in 2 per cent. In only about one fifth of the cases in which the primary complex was in the abdomen was there gross evidence of intestinal ulceration. In more than half of this last group of cases, the subjects were less than 1 year of age. Opie, supplementing the pathologic findings with roentgenographic examination of the lungs, found evidence of the primary lesion in the lungs in 92 per cent of *adults* investigated by him. It is also known that more than one primary complex may develop in an organ, and especially the lung.

Ranke pointed out that the primary stage was likely to be followed by a *secondary stage*, also denoted as "postprimary reinfection." The first stage, he thought, may merge directly into the second, or the second stage may appear after an interval, not infrequently a number of years, during which the primary lesion may have been healing or even had healed. Postprimary reinfection may be an exogenous reinfection (through the inhalation of tubercle bacilli), or it may be an endogenous reinfection (caused by organisms which were present in the primary lesion and survived). The reinfection may result in rapidly fatal generalized miliary tuberculosis, or may proceed so inconspicuously that it entirely escapes clinical recognition.

It is maintained that in the course of spread of the infection, tubercle bacilli are discharged into the blood or lymph stream from the primary focus or (apparently more often) from the tuberculous lymph nodes draining the focus. It has been contended that the bone marrow, the suprarenal glands, and the brain are among the tissues particularly likely to be the sites of localization of the tubercle bacilli during the spread (dissemination stage) of the infection. It is thought that these bacilli may remain dormant or, sooner or later, incite the development of metastatic tuberculous lesions. Aschoff regarded the rapidly fatal generalized miliary tuberculosis of childhood as a manifestation of dissemination of the tubercle bacilli during the secondary stage. He held that this occurs in those cases in which a tuberculous lesion that has involved the intima of a large blood vessel or lymph channel has broken into the lumen of the structure, thus permitting tubercle bacilli to gain access to the circulating blood and/or lymph. Even Ranke conceded that not all persons who acquired tuberculous infection are subject to a secondary stage. Others have maintained that in most cases the lesion of the primary complex shows early healing, and that the infection does not pass into the so-called second stage. Even in regard to generalized miliary tuberculosis as an evidence of secondary dissemination, many (including Opie) believe that it is an indication of an overwhelming primary infection in a susceptible subject who had not developed any immunity to the disease.

Involvement of one or another organ is a manifestation of the *tertiary stage* of tuberculosis. The most frequent form of tuberculosis affecting a single organ is pulmonary tuberculosis (phthisis). It is believed that pulmonary tuberculosis, as observed mainly in adults, results from aerogenous or exogenous reinfection or superinfection rather than from reactivation of a dormant tuberculous infection which has passed through the primary and secondary stages. Tuberculosis of an organ is peculiar in that metastasis from the diseased area is uncommon. If tubercles obviously of hematogenous origin do appear in distant tissues or organs, they only infrequently show a tendency to develop into disease foci, since the miliary foci of metastases tend to become obliterated by focal scarring (see Uehlinger). Thus there is clearly a considerable degree of immunity in the distant tissues and organs. However, local spread of the tuberculous process is possible. The peculiarities of the anatomic character of organ tuberculosis are explicable on the basis of an immunologic state induced by the primary infection.

In attempting to determine the proper pathogenetic relation of skeletal tuberculosis (including that of tendon sheaths and bursae) to the total concept of human tuberculous infection, one must consider the three-stage interpretation discussed above, even if only as a point of departure. A primary focus of tuberculous infec-

tion is not known to appear in the skeletal system, although theoretically this might
be possible. One way in which, conceivably, a primary lesion might develop in a
skeletal area is by the direct introduction (through the agency of trauma) of
tubercle bacilli into the area. Ordinarily, a tuberculous infection in a skeletal part
reaches that area by the blood stream from an already existing extraskeletal
tuberculous disease focus.

In regard to the possible relation of clinical skeletal tuberculosis to the so-called
secondary stage (postprimary reinfection), most of the investigators who believe in
the existence of that stage maintain that tubercle bacilli are deposited in the bones
and synovial membranes. This seeding occurs in the course of blood-borne dissemination of the bacilli, following postprimary reinfection. Certainly in *children*,
the nidus for the development of tuberculosis in a bone or joint is brought to the
area through hematogenous dissemination, whether or not this process is regarded
as the secondary stage. Indeed, in children there is a strong tendency for the localization (through hematogenous spread) of all types of bacteria in the skeletal tissues.
As to *adults*, it is unlikely that tubercle bacilli remaining from a dissemination
during childhood would lead to skeletal tuberculosis years later. It is more probable
that the bacilli were entirely destroyed or that the tubercles which they induced had
healed completely. It is entirely conceivable that in adults the reactivation of a
dormant primary complex might lead to a late hematogenous invasion of the skeletal
tissues by tubercle bacilli. While this would explain the occurrence of skeletal
tuberculosis as the result of late endogenous reinfection from a primary complex,
it is difficult to be certain that this actually is a common basis for the skeletal
lesions in adults.

Certainly, skeletal tuberculosis seems often to belong to the category of tuberculosis affecting a specific body area. Consequently, skeletal tuberculosis, like chronic
pulmonary tuberculosis, must be regarded as developing, frequently at least, on the
basis of an exogenous reinfection. Evidence that the tubercle bacilli of the reinfection are of exogenous origin is of interest not only in connection with pulmonary
tuberculosis, but also in relation to skeletal tuberculosis. Thus, in attempts to reduce the incidence of skeletal tuberculosis, continued careful attention should be
given to prevention of the spread of tubercle bacilli from exogenous sources (such as
milk) or from contact with cases of active pulmonary tuberculosis.

CLINICAL CONSIDERATIONS

Age and Sex Incidence.—Though skeletal tuberculosis may appear at any age, it
rarely sets in during the first year of life. In regard to *age incidence*, statistical
studies relating to the first half of the twentieth century have shown that, in about
50 per cent of all cases, the subjects were between 3 and 15 years of age. It should
be remembered, however, that such data necessarily vary with the institutions
from which they are derived. Whitman, in 1927, stated that, of a group of 5,461
persons treated for skeletal tuberculosis, about 87 per cent were less than 14 years
of age. In our institution, for example, the proportion of adults among the patients
with skeletal tuberculosis was fairly high. Formerly (as is shown by the older data,
especially from Europe), of the cases appearing in subjects up to 15 years of age,
more than a third were under 5 years of age; about a third were between the ages
of 5 and 10; and in somewhat less than a third, between the ages of 10 and 15.
However, both the number and the proportion of cases in which the subjects were
below 5 years of age, and especially below 3 years of age (when the prognosis of the
disease is gravest), have been diminishing. Current statistical evaluations have
indicated a drop in the incidence of skeletal tuberculosis during childhood and early

adult life, and an increase in the incidence of the condition in adults past middle age (see Kastert and Uehlinger, and also Hald).

As to *sex incidence*, skeletal tuberculosis does not seem to predilect either sex. Such differences as have been reported in various studies tend to cancel each other, and at best they are probably too small to be statistically significant.

Localization.—With few exceptions, statistical compilations indicate that the three anatomic areas most frequently affected are, in descending order, the vertebral column, the hip, and the knee. In approximately 25 to 40 per cent of *all cases of skeletal tuberculosis*, the disease is located in the vertebral column, and more specifically, in about three fourths of these cases, in some part of the column between the sixth dorsal and the third lumbar vertebrae (see Sevastikoglou and Wernerheim). In about 25 per cent of all cases of skeletal tuberculosis, the hip joint is affected, and in about 20 per cent the knee. The region of the ankle is generally considered to be the next most important site after the aforementioned three, and is much more often affected in adults than in children. Data based on large numbers of cases indicate that involvement of the joints of the lower extremities exceeds by far the joints of the upper extremities. Moreover, in relation to the upper extremities, tuberculosis occurs more frequently in adults than in children.

On the whole, the simultaneous tuberculous implication of two or more different skeletal areas is rather uncommon, especially in cases in which the spine, hip, or knee is affected. If concomitantly another skeletal lesion does develop, it is one of the other two members of this trio that is most likely to be affected. For instance, if the spine is involved and a second lesion appears at another skeletal site, that site will probably be a hip or a knee joint. Of these three locations, tuberculosis involving a knee seems least likely to be complicated by another skeletal tuberculous focus. Tuberculosis of one of these three regions may, however, be complicated by tuberculous spina ventosa. Spina ventosa itself generally affects more than one finger or toe. In an affected vertebral column, it is not unusual, as has been supposed, to observe areas of tuberculous involvement separated by uninvolved areas of the column.

If multiple lesions develop, they may become clinically apparent within a few weeks or months of each other. This finding has led to the general belief that such multiple lesions are initiated at the same time, but manifest themselves clinically at different times. It has been maintained by various authors that the presence of multiple foci of involvement has an unfavorable prognostic significance (see Broca). It was stressed by Ménard that cases of spondylitis and/or coxitis complicated by spina ventosa also have a poor prognosis. In children, skeletal tuberculosis is sometimes observed in which multiple lesions seem to be the outstanding characteristic of the pathologic condition. Such cases have been denoted as instances of disseminated bone tuberculosis (see McTammany *et al.*, Seedat and Wolpert, and also O'Malley and Zeft).

As has already been stated, the *vertebral column* is the most common site of skeletal tuberculosis, most of the spondylitides being located in the region of the column between the lower thoracic and the lumbar vertebrae. The disease is relatively infrequent in the cervical vertebrae and also in the sacrum *per se*, although tuberculosis of the sacroiliac joint is not rare. Its presence may be associated with the formation of an intrapelvic or extrapelvic abscess. It is only exceptionally that the lesion remains confined to a single vertebra. About as often as not, two or more adjacent vertebrae become implicated, usually by rapid extension of the disease from one vertebra to a neighboring one. Sometimes as many as 8 or 10 may ultimately be involved. (See Fig. 247.)

Multiple lesions in the vertebral column—that is, two or more separate diseased areas with uninvolved vertebrae in between—had been considered rather uncommon. Peabody and others pointed out, however, that careful search for multiple foci by roentgenographic examination has shown them to be more frequent than they were formerly thought to be. Moreover, multiple foci are often revealed at autopsy even when detailed roentgenographic examination had disclosed only a single focus. The separate foci apparently arise independently, through infection carried by the blood stream to the different sites rather than through contact infection from burrowing abscesses (see Thrap-Meyer, and also Kastert and Uehlinger).

Of skeletal tuberculosis in general, *tuberculous spondylitis* has the longest period

Figure 247

A, Photograph showing the cut surface of part of a spine, sectioned in the sagittal plane, from a case of vertebral tuberculosis. The kyphotic angulation is the result of tuberculous involvement and caseation leading to destruction of the vertebral bodies of T_8 through T_{12}. Some of the affected thoracic vertebral bodies bulge toward the spinal canal, and made pressure upon the regional part of the spinal cord. The subject was a woman who was 34 years of age when she was admitted to our hospital. Her clinical history indicates that a focus of vertebral tuberculosis was already present when she was 3 years old. From then until the age of 7, she was in a plaster-of-Paris cast, and after that she continued to wear braces. When she was 9 years old, her lower extremities became paralyzed for a short period of time. On admission to our hospital because of dyspnea, palpitation on exertion, and increasing general weakness and difficulty in walking, physical examination revealed cardiac murmurs (indicating the presence of an endocarditis) and a markedly deformed vertebral column. The apex of the kyphosis was in the lower dorsal region. Four days after her admission, the patient died. The autopsy revealed not only the illustrated changes in the vertebral column, but also mitral endocarditis, hydrothorax on the right side of the chest, healed hilar tuberculosis, and chronic passive congestion of the lungs, liver, and kidneys.

B, Roentgenograph of the part of the vertebral column shown in *A*. Note that the intervertebral disks have been destroyed in the affected portion of the spine. The focal radiopacities within the diseased vertebrae reflect calcium deposition in the caseous areas.

C, Photograph of part of a vertebral column (from another case) sectioned in the sagittal plane. The illustration demonstrates in particular the cut surface of the bodies of the fifth through the eleventh thoracic vertebrae. Note that the intervertebral disk between the bodies of the eighth and ninth vertebrae has been destroyed, and that both of these bodies are completely affected. Bulging of the posterior surfaces of these vertebral bodies is obvious, and this bulging has led to narrowing of the spinal canal and compression of the cord. The anterior surfaces of these bodies have become expanded by pathologic tissue pressing forward under the anterior longitudinal ligament. In addition to the tuberculous changes already noted, a focus of tuberculosis is evident in the anterior part of the body of the tenth thoracic vertebra and also in the posterior part of the body of the seventh thoracic vertebra. The clinical history of this 58 year old woman indicated that she had experienced pain in the lower thoracic area for almost a year. About 6 months before admission to the hospital, she became aware of progressive weakness of both lower extremities, and during the month before admission she was unable to move either limb. Neurological examination disclosed complete paraplegia with bilateral pyramidal signs—manifestations ascribed to compression of the cord by an epidural abscess. A laminectomy was carried out in an effort to decompress the cord, but the patient died the following day as a result of cardiac failure. The autopsy revealed cardiac hypertrophy and dilatation, and healed pulmonary tuberculosis in the apices of both lungs.

D, Roentgenograph of the portion of the specimen shown in *C*. The destruction of the intervertebral disk between the eighth and ninth thoracic vertebral bodies is clearly apparent, as is the bulging of the tuberculous tissue under the anterior longitudinal ligament. In addition, one can note that there is clear-cut lytic destruction of the anterior part of the eighth thoracic body, and also some destruction of the ninth body anteriorly. The focus of tuberculosis in the anterior part of the tenth vertebral body, visible in *C*, is also evident in the roentgenograph as an area of relative radiolucency.

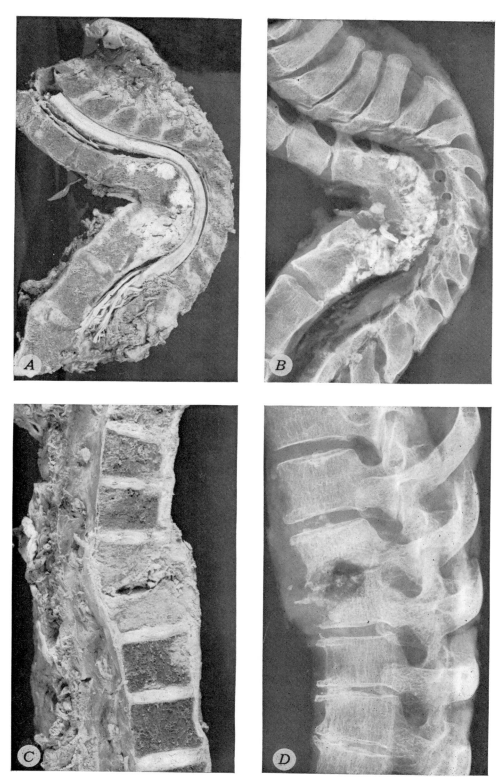

Figure 247

of morbidity and the highest mortality rate. The mortality rate for tuberculous spondylitis as reported by Johansson was 26 per cent, by Valtancoli 16.5 per cent, by Wullstein 27 per cent, and by Seemann 31 per cent. It may be well to mention, also, that of all the forms of skeletal tuberculosis, Pott's disease is the one most frequently associated with pulmonary tuberculosis. Among the 100 cases of Pott's disease reported by Adams, there were 22 in which the subjects showed pulmonary tuberculosis.

Diagnosis.—The clinical diagnosis of skeletal tuberculosis often presents problems, especially if the pathologic changes are not advanced. However, in about half to two thirds of the cases admitted to hospital services, the lesions have progressed sufficiently to permit a reasonably accurate clinical diagnosis, provided that pertinent roentgenographic findings are available. The other cases present diagnostic difficulties, largely because of their ambiguous clinical course and features, and also because the possibility of tuberculous infection is often not considered now. Such cases require keen clinical judgment, the use of diagnostic laboratory procedures, repeated roentgenographic examinations, and sometimes (when large joints are involved), an exploratory biopsy. In even more obscure cases, the correct diagnosis is often made only after histologic examination of tissue obtained during a surgical intervention undertaken because of an erroneous clinical diagnosis. Such instances include those in which the tuberculosis has an unusual location (as, for example, in the diaphysis of a long tubular bone) or presents in a very atypical form.

There are several factors which may create diagnostic difficulties even when the disease is in an advanced stage: (1) Certain joints which are predilected by skeletal tuberculosis are also predilected by other pathologic conditions. Thus, when it occurs in the hip of a child, skeletal tuberculosis may be confused with Legg-Perthes disease. (2) The clinical features may be misleading because they simulate those appearing in other conditions. For instance, syphilitic arthritis of the knee in children (Clutton's joints) may be mistaken for tuberculous gonitis, and *vice versa*. (3) Another diagnostic difficulty may arise from the false conclusion that, because a patient presents definite evidence of tuberculosis elsewhere, the skeletal lesion under evaluation is also tuberculous. For example, it is well known that adults with pulmonary tuberculosis often complain of pain and swelling in one or more joints. These joints are by no means necessarily tuberculous, however. Many of the sources of confusion in the differential diagnosis of skeletal tuberculosis have been emphasized by Milgram.

There are, of course, certain features that favor a diagnosis of skeletal tuberculosis: (1) Skeletal tuberculosis is not uncommon in children, although it is by no means so common in them now as it was in the past; (2) the clinical manifestations usually develop slowly and insidiously; (3) the infection is particularly likely to appear in the spine, hip, or knee; (4) in relation to large joints, the involvement is usually monarticular; (5) if more than one joint is affected, the contralateral joint is almost never affected (except in cases of spina ventosa).

As has already been mentioned, the *clinical evolution* of skeletal tuberculosis tends to be gradual. Thus, it may be months or even a year or more before the clinical manifestations are sufficiently advanced to enable one to evaluate the condition and arrive at a diagnosis with the usual clinical, roentgenographic, and laboratory aids. Nevertheless, there are also many cases in which these manifestations develop abruptly or at least very rapidly.

The principal *complaints* and *findings* are: (1) pain, which is usually mild, but in some locations (especially the hip) is sometimes severe, and in a few regions (cervical spine) is always severe; (2) swelling due to joint effusion and to thickening of the periarticular tissues; (3) local heat, without redness of the skin; (4) muscle spasm and/or local muscle atrophy; (5) limitation of movement of the joint, especially if the articular cartilages are eroded; (6) a limp, particularly in association with tuberculous coxitis; (7) local tenderness, especially pronounced in diaphysial tuberculosis; (8) local and burrowing cold abscesses; (9) contractures and subluxations of large joints; and (10) gibbus of the vertebral column.

These clinical features vary in character, number, and severity from case to case and are related to the particular site of the lesion. Thus, in tuberculous spondylitis a more or less angular deformity is the most common clinical evidence of the disease. Furthermore, there may be referred pain. Characteristically, with disease of the hip joint, the pain is referred to the region of the knee.

Shortly after undergoing a primary infection by the tubercle bacillus, almost all of the infected persons react positively to a *tuberculin test*. As a diagnostic test, a negative tuberculin reaction is more significant than a positive one. In interpreting the tuberculin test result, it must always be borne in mind that a positive test result does not prove that a given lesion is tuberculous, although it does prove that the individual has been previously infected by tubercle bacilli. Under proper safeguards, the tuberculin test may, however, yield valuable information. A positive tuberculin response in infancy (below 2 years) more than at any other age is of considerable diagnostic value. It suggests, as Hart, among others, pointed out, that the tuberculous infection present is developing into a focus of clinical tuberculosis or will soon develop into it. A negative reaction, if the dose of tuberculin has been adequate, is more illuminating, and is of diagnostic value at all ages. A negative reaction is most likely to be obtained in young children who have not yet become tuberculin-sensitized through the acquisition of a tuberculous infection. As pointed out in the section on pathogenesis (p. 954), the primary tuberculous infection is now being acquired later and later in life, even in large cities. Therefore, the presence of a negative tuberculin reaction in childhood or adolescence is becoming more and more significant diagnostically.

A negative tuberculin reaction need not, however, necessarily mean that a tuberculous infection is not present. Thus it is well known that a small percentage of frankly tuberculous patients also give a negative tuberculin reaction. This is found especially in those patients who are moribund with pulmonary, generalized miliary, or meningeal tuberculosis, and who are tested a few days or weeks before death. Also, if there is substantial healing of the tuberculous infection, the skin reaction may occasionally become weak or even negative (see Cummins). Nevertheless, a negative tuberculin test result has a special significance and applicability in the diagnosis of skeletal lesions of the sarcoid type (p. 1006). Where it is suspected that the lesion is related to sarcoidosis, a positive tuberculin reaction is evidence against that diagnosis, while a negative reaction strongly supports it.

The induction of tuberculosis in guinea pigs through the *inoculation* of material suspected of being tuberculous (usually fluid or pus obtained from affected bones and joints or draining sinuses) remains the best single laboratory procedure for the diagnosis of a local tuberculous infection. (As already noted, this was a well-known diagnostic method in relation to tuberculosis even before the discovery of the tubercle bacillus.) Thus, for example, of a group of 44 specimens (from cases later proved to represent tuberculosis of bones or joints), only 3 failed to induce tuberculosis in guinea pigs (see Blair and Hallman). Perhaps the tubercle bacilli were lacking in these 3 particular specimens. The material may be inoculated subcutaneously and/or intraperitoneally. In our experience, the subcutaneous tissues of the axilla constitute the most satisfactory site for inoculation. By utilizing this site, it is possible to reduce to a minimum the loss of animals through infection by contaminating microorganisms.

One of the disadvantages of guinea pig inoculation is that 6 to 8 weeks and sometimes more must elapse before the result of the test is clear. Many methods have been devised in an effort to shorten this time. One of the most valuable of these methods is to test the inoculated animal with tuberculin. Magath, among others, found that the test period could usually thus be shortened to about 4 weeks. If the guinea pig has really been infected by the tuberculous material, it usually dies within 48 hours after subcutaneous injection of 0.5 cc. of old tuberculin. Nontuberculous guinea pigs are not killed by this amount of tuberculin. Our own experience confirms the value of this procedure.

The alternative to guinea pig inoculation is the *bacteriologic culture* of suspected material. This procedure often permits the demonstration of the presence of tubercle bacilli earlier than through the inoculation of guinea pigs. However, the culture method does not yield as high a percentage of correct results as does the method of guinea pig inoculation. This statement applies particularly to material from cases of bone and joint tuberculosis.

In the study from our institution reported in 1933 by Blair and Hallman, 44 specimens taken from lesions subsequently proved to be tuberculous yielded only 34 positive cultures of tubercle bacilli. On the other hand, as previously noted, the presence of tubercle bacilli was revealed in 41 of these specimens by guinea pig inoculation. On the basis of that experience, Blair and Hallman maintained that the culture method for diagnosing tuberculous infection could not at that time replace the method of guinea pig inoculation. Although methods for culturing tubercle bacilli have now been greatly improved, this procedure is not yet replacing guinea pig inoculation.

Effort should be made to establish the diagnosis *without resorting to biopsy of the synovial membrane*, as arthrotomy creates some danger of local spread of the infection and also the possibility of introducing a superimposed infection. Frequently, the information yielded by the biopsy is inadequate or even misleading. Too often, the specimen removed is not characteristic of the suspected tuberculous lesion. Furthermore, frozen sections of synovial tissue are difficult to interpret. In fact, the present writer has long regarded as tentative any diagnosis reached on the basis of tissue slides of synovial membrane prepared by the frozen section method. If a biopsy is carried out, some of the tissue should be submitted for bacteriologic culture and should also be inoculated into a guinea pig. It should be pointed out that granulomata quite similar microscopically to those of tuberculosis or brucellosis may be caused by acid-fast bacilli other than tubercle bacilli—organisms sometimes denoted as *anonymous* (or unclassified) *mycobacteria*. These bacteria are culturally

Figure 248

A, Photomicrograph (× 38) of a lymph node removed from the left elbow region (the supratrochlear area) in the case of a female child 16 months of age. The child was admitted to our hospital because of pain and swelling of that elbow for 4 days. A roentgenograph showed some destructive changes at the upper end of the ulna. Since the clinical diagnosis was not clear, a surgical exploration of the left elbow region was undertaken. A lymph node measuring 1 cm. in length and 0.7 cm. in width and thickness was excised, and histologic examination established the diagnosis of tuberculosis. Note the agglomerated tubercles, some of which, as indicated by the arrows, reveal the presence of caseous necrosis.

B, Photomicrograph (× 38) of a lymph node removed from the supraclavicular area of the neck (right side) in the case of a woman 25 years of age who was admitted to our hospital because of the mistaken impression that the palpable lymph node and the roentgenographic pulmonary findings were related to Hodgkin's disease. The excised lymph node measured 4 × 1.5 × 1 cm. Its capsule was intact and smooth. The cut surface of the node appeared slightly lobulated and somewhat yellow, and the tissue had a fleshy consistency. Note the numerous tubercles, many of which are agglomerated. Despite the agglomeration of the tubercles, no evidence of caseous necrosis is apparent. This negative finding clearly differentiates the histologic picture of sarcoidosis from that of tuberculosis, as shown in *A*.

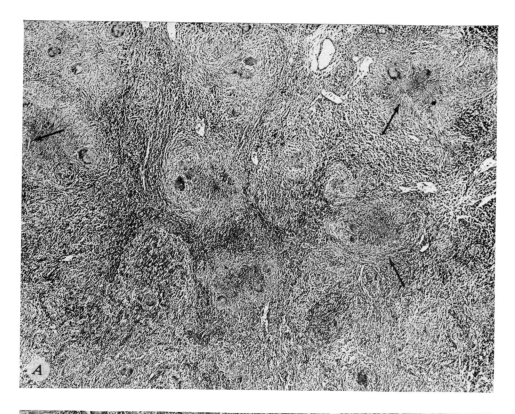

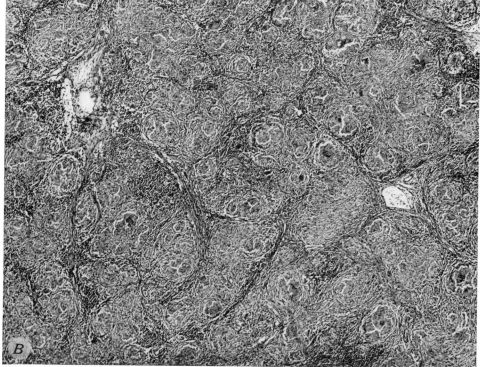

Figure 248

different from the tubercle bacillus. They are not susceptible to the chemothera-
peutic agents which are effective against tubercle bacilli, and are not virulent for
guinea pigs (see Kelly *et al.*, and Heitzman *et al.*).

Biopsy of lymph glands draining the region of a supposedly tuberculous lesion is
often of diagnostic value. The lymph glands in question should be prepared for
microscopic examination, and some of the lymphoid tissue should also be inoculated
into a guinea pig. Girdlestone and also Seddon have emphasized the clinical significance of enlargement of the regional glands in the groin as an aid in the diagnosis
of tuberculous gonitis. The present writer has also seen an adult (a man) in
whom a monarticular gonitis was established as tuberculous through the histologic examination of enlarged glands present in the groin. Ottolenghi, studying 19
cases of skeletal tuberculosis, found that in all but 4 the diagnosis could be confirmed by biopsy and histologic examination of regional lymph nodes. (See Fig.
248.)

ROENTGENOGRAPHIC FINDINGS

During the early stage of the evolution of a tuberculous bone or joint lesion, it is
often difficult to arrive at a diagnosis on the basis of *roentgenographic examination.*
In cases of suspected tuberculous spondylitis, especially in children, roentgenographs
may fail to reveal changes in the vertebral column for some time after significant
clinical complaints have appeared. In advanced cases of skeletal tuberculosis, the
roentgenographic changes may be pronounced and yield pertinent diagnostic information. However, it should be pointed out that certain tuberculous lesions are
difficult to distinguish roentgenographically from nontuberculous lesions. Thus,
for example, tuberculosis of the shaft of a tubular bone can scarcely be differentiated
from nontuberculous pyogenic osteomyelitis of the shaft of a bone. Again, tuberculous dactylitis is almost indistinguishable roentgenographically from syphilitic
dactylitis. In still other instances, even when the lesion is in a large joint, the
roentgenographic picture is occasionally so atypical that it not only does not suggest
tuberculosis but does suggest an entirely different condition. Phemister and
Hatcher gave particular consideration to the temporal sequence of some of the
alterations appearing in large joints. It should be borne in mind that most of the
significant roentgenographic alterations relating to skeletal tuberculosis are those to
be observed in the large joints and the vertebral column.

The *principal roentgenographic findings* suggestive of skeletal tuberculosis may be
summarized as follows: (1) In relation to diarthrodial joints, swelling of the periarticular soft tissues is frequently noted. There may be narrowing of the joint space
in consequence of destruction of the articular bone ends. In tuberculous arthritis
the narrowing of the joint space usually develops gradually and late in the course of
the disease. This is particularly true in those large diarthrodial joints in which the
articular surfaces are normally in close contact and subjected to weight-bearing.
On the other hand, in such joints a tuberculous effusion may at first even widen the
joint space. As a result of partial or complete resorption of the subchondral bony
end plate and its adjacent trabeculae by granulation tissue, there is evidence of
osteoporosis manifested by reduction or loss in radiodensity of the normally sharp
shadow of the articular ends of the bones entering into the formation of the joint.
(2) As the tuberculous process advances, gouged-out areas of reduced radiodensity
(erosions) appear on the surface of the bone ends adjacent to the periphery of the
articular cartilages. (3) Wedge- or cone-shaped areas of destruction or clearly
delimited sequestra are found if there is extensive involvement of the epiphysial
ends of the bones. The sequestra border on the articular surfaces of the joint, and

their shadows are more radiopaque than those representing the perifocal bone, and are delimited wholly or partially by narrow radiolucent shadows. Sequestra on both sides of the joint space constitute the so-called "kissing sequestra." (See Fig. 249.) (4) In the vertebral column, there is paravertebral soft-tissue swelling at the involved area, and narrowing of the regional intervertebral disk spaces usually occurs. The roentgenographic diagnosis of tuberculous spondylitis is generally regarded as dependent upon narrowing of the intervertebral disk spaces and deformation of vertebral bodies. This finding is held by many to be the earliest and most constant roentgenographic indication of tuberculosis of the spine (see Doub and Badgley). It is known, however, that tuberculous spondylitis occasionally is present without such roentgenographic evidence. In fact, tuberculous foci may be present in several neighboring vertebral bodies without their collapse and/or narrowing of the intervertebral disks. Sclerosis about such foci sometimes leads to misinterpretation of these changes as indicative of metastatic carcinoma (see Petter and Medelman). In this connection it should be pointed out that vertebral tuberculosis may sometimes be unrecognized clinically despite careful roentgenologic examination, and be found only at autopsy. Furthermore, where the vertebral column is known to be the site of tuberculosis, additional tuberculous lesions in the column may be found at autopsy which were not revealed roentgenographically. (5) Increased radiopacity due to sclerotic osseous tissue may be observed, particularly about an abscess within the bone. In vertebral tuberculosis this finding is especially frequent. However, osteosclerosis appearing early in association with disease of a large joint may be regarded as evidence that the lesion is not tuberculous. (6) Another suggestive finding is the presence of periosteal osteophyte formation near the edge of the articular cartilage, sometimes extending slightly up the shaft. (7) Also of help in arriving at the diagnosis is the finding of burrowing abscesses, which produce dissecting opacities in the soft tissues and eventually may lead to the formation of sinuses. Extension of a paravertebral density equally above and below a focus of vertebral tuberculosis may signify that the bulk of the lesional tissue is granulation tissue (see Freund). The presence of large fusiform or saccular shadows is probably indicative of the fact that the content of the abscess cavity is largely seropurulent fluid. In the lumbar region, the earliest indication of an abscess may be an outward bulge in the shadow of the psoas muscle. (8) The finding of deformities (gibbus, contractures, and subluxations) is important for the roentgenographic diagnosis. (See Fig. 250.)

In summary, the roentgenographic changes which afford the strongest evidence in favor of tuberculosis in the large joints are: the presence of wedge- or cone-shaped lesions, "kissing sequestra," and late narrowing of the joint space; in the vertebral column: the presence of cold or burrowing abscesses.

PATHOLOGIC CONSIDERATIONS

In this section of the chapter we shall consider, in the following order: (1) the histopathology of tuberculous inflammation in general; (2) the various anatomic aspects of skeletal tuberculosis; (3) skeletal tuberculosis as manifested in individual skeletal sites; (4) tuberculosis of tendon sheaths and bursae; (5) extraskeletal tuberculous lesions with concomitant skeletal lesions; and (6) the progress of the disease in respect to morbidity and mortality.

Histopathology of Tuberculous Inflammation.—The specific response to tuberculous infection of the skeletal tissues is influenced by the anatomic structure of the particular skeletal part affected. In most respects, however, the changes induced in the skeletal tissues by the localization of tubercle bacilli are of the same general type as those induced in other tissues or organs.

62

The formation of *tubercles* is the most characteristic response of the tissues to the localization of tubercle bacilli. Single tubercles can barely be seen with the naked eye. However, they tend to coalesce and cluster. Groups of tubercles thus combine to form the minute, translucent, grayish nodules observed in tuberculous lesions and generally designated as "miliary tubercles." *Histologically*, mature tubercles appear more or less sharply demarcated from the surrounding tissue. They are composed of cells which are clustered around a central zone. These cells are sometimes arranged in laminae, but usually the arrangement is less orderly, and the cells are attached to one another. The characteristic cell (the epithelioid cell) has an elongated, vesicular nucleus with little chromatin. Its faintly outlined irregular cell body has processes which connect with processes of neighboring cells. In the central part of the tubercle, there may be one or more multinuclear giant cells. Each of these is a mass of protoplasm containing many nuclei which are usually arranged at the periphery or at opposite poles of the cell. Giant cells also give off processes which mingle with those of the neighboring epithelioid cells. A mantle of lymphocytes may be observed at the periphery of the tubercle. When clusters of tubercles undergo central necrosis, they present yellowish centers (see MacCallum, Miller, and also Foot).

Tubercles have no independent blood supply. However, because of their small size, they can absorb nourishment from the surrounding tissue and thus stave off necrosis for some time. Hence it is not necessarily the lack of blood supply that

Figure 249

A, Roentgenograph of the left knee area, which is the site of a tuberculous infection. The subject was a man who was 32 years of age when he was admitted to our hospital. The clinical record indicates that he had had pain in the left knee for about $2\frac{1}{2}$ months. Physical examination revealed some swelling of the joint area, obliteration of the normal local depressions, slight local heat, and some restriction of extension and flexion of the knee. The articular ends of the femur and tibia show numerous small roundish and/or oval areas of rarefaction, probably representing local foci of osteoporosis due to inactivity. Note also the transverse linear rarefactions in the condyles of the femur (particularly the lateral condyle). These rarefactions apparently reflect the presence, beneath the articular cartilage, of a narrow zone of tuberculous granulation tissue separating the cartilage from the subchondral bone (see Fig. 254-*A*). On the medial aspect of the tibial plateau, there is a similar, though smaller and less well-delineated, linear rarefaction. In the course of the surgical intervention, a piece of synovial membrane was removed, and pathologic examination established the diagnosis of tuberculosis (see Fig. 253-*B*).

B, Roentgenograph of a knee joint demonstrating sequestra oriented to the condyle of the femur and the upper end of the tibia, respectively. Since the sequestra are apposed to each other, they may be designated as "kissing sequestra." In addition, the lower end of the femur and the upper end of the tibia present evidence of advanced osteoporosis. Moreover, the articular cavity is distended, apparently by the accumulation of fluid in the joint space, and the synovial membrane appears to be thickened. The patient, a man, was 23 years of age at the time of his admission to our hospital. His clinical record indicates that for the preceding 5 years he had had pain and some swelling of the right knee. In the course of time, the pain increased, so that it became difficult for him to walk without the aid of a cane, and even with it he was able to walk for only short distances. Physical examination of the right lower extremity revealed pronounced atrophy of the thigh muscles and considerable thickening of the soft tissues in the popliteal space. Some enlarged lymph nodes were palpable in the right inguinal region. An arthrodesis was carried out.

C, Photomicrograph ($\times$ 5) illustrating the histologic architecture of part of one of the sequestra shown in *B*. The sequestrum consists of necrotic bone whose articular surface is devoid of cartilage. The sequestrum is clearly delimited from the neighboring osseous tissue, which is porotic.

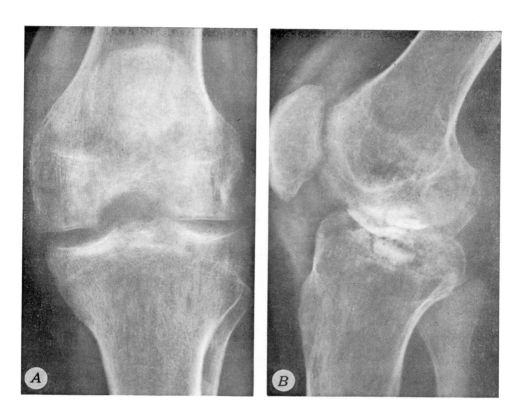

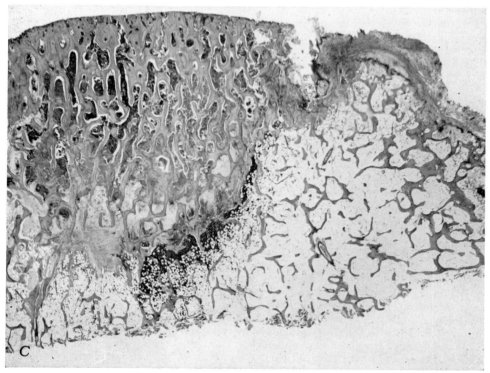

Figure 249

induces the central caseous necrosis to which they are subject; instead, the degeneration is incited by the tuberculin produced by the bacilli in the tubercles. Fatty droplets in the epithelioid cells are doubtless evidence of beginning degeneration. In the course of necrosis, degenerating and disintegrating epithelioid cells become agglomerated into a central amorphous mass.

There are variations in the details relating to the histologic structure of tuberculous lesions among different species and even within a particular species. If one studies the tissues of large numbers of guinea pigs which had been inoculated with tuberculous material from humans, one becomes aware of the wide range of differences in the histologic detail presented by various tissues of the infected guinea pigs.

Many reports have centered about the problem of the *genesis of the tubercle*, particularly with respect to its epithelioid cells (see Sabin, Opie, Sabin *et al.*, and

Figure 250

A, Roentgenograph of part of a vertebral column from a case in which there was tuberculous involvement of the tenth and eleventh dorsal vertebrae, and in which the intervening disk had been destroyed. The picture shows, though only faintly, a paravertebral soft-tissue swelling at the level in question. The patient was a woman 47 years of age whose clinical history indicated that she had had pain across the back for about 1 year prior to her admission to the hospital. The pain, mild at first, became severe after a few months, and was aggravated by coughing and sneezing. In addition, there was some pain localized to the lateral aspects of both calves. The patient was placed on antibiotic therapy, and this treatment was followed by a surgical intervention which consisted of fusion of the area.

B, Roentgenograph of part of a vertebral column from a case in which a diagnosis of tuberculosis involving the eleventh and twelfth thoracic vertebrae was established. The patient, a girl, was $11\frac{1}{2}$ years of age when she was first admitted to our hospital. About 9 months before admission, back pain and fever were noted. The fever subsided after several days, but the back pain persisted, though it was not severe and did not radiate. In time, she had difficulty in standing, and as her condition worsened, she could not walk, and she even had to support her trunk with her arms while sitting. Her back muscles were in spasm and did not relax in any position. A costal transversectomy was performed on the eleventh rib on the right side. Pus was encountered, the area was curetted, and the evacuated material was submitted for bacteriologic and pathologic examinations, which confirmed the clinical impression of a tuberculous infection.

C, Photograph of part of the vertebral column and contiguous ribs from a case of tuberculosis involving some of the lower thoracic vertebrae. The subject, a male, was 16 years of age when he was first admitted to our hospital and the diagnosis of vertebral tuberculosis was made. Subsequently, for about a year, he was a patient in the hospital's extended care unit for skeletal tuberculosis. On readmission to the hospital, physical and roentgenographic examinations disclosed the presence of a huge posterior mediastinal abscess and also erosion of the anterior surfaces of several of the thoracic vertebrae. He died a few months later and an autopsy was performed. The vertebral column from D_5 to S_1 was removed, and it showed the presence of a large paravertebral abscess, located mainly between D_5 and D_{10}. The abscess was opened, and the abscess cavity contained a large quantity of pus, amounting to several hundred cubic centimeters. Anteriorly the pus was walled off by the anterior longitudinal ligament, and laterally on each side it was walled off by the parietal pleura over the head and neck regions of the local ribs. As is evident in the illustration, the anterior surfaces of the regional vertebral bodies were covered by tuberculous granulation tissue.

D, Photograph revealing the cut surface of the vertebrae shown on the right in *C*. A considerable part of the body of the eighth dorsal vertebra has been destroyed. Moreover, the intervertebral disk between the eighth and ninth vertebral bodies has undergone almost complete destruction. Small areas of tuberculous involvement can be observed in the ninth vertebral body and in the proximal part of the tenth body. The intervening disk is also affected. The spinal canal is not narrowed, since there is no tuberculous granulation tissue or pus making pressure against the posterior longitudinal ligament.

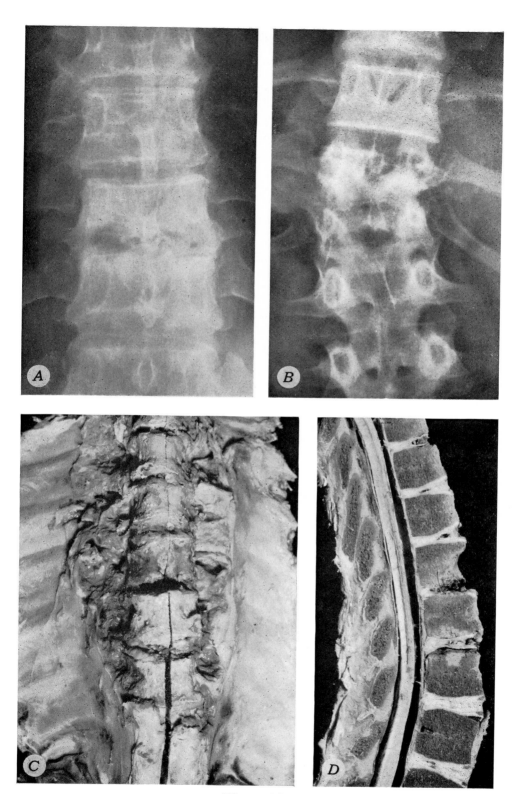

Figure 250

969

Long). Experimental studies have shown that, where tubercle bacilli localize in a tissue, they first induce a scant exudation of fluid and an active, though transient, immigration into the area of polymorphonuclear leukocytes (see Vorwald). According to others, tubercle formation is actually preceded by "primary tissue damage," which is held to be necrosis induced by the tubercle bacilli at the site of their localization before the tubercles form (see Huebschmann). Others deny the occurrence of such immediate local degenerative changes (see Tschistowitsch and Winogradow, and also Mandelstamm). However, most other investigators do not stress the temporal sequence between the supposed primary tissue damage and the subsequent changes.

At the site of localization of tubercle bacilli, a tubercle evolves by the accumulation of mononuclear cells which mature to form epithelioid cells. Collections of these cells constitute the essential element of the specific reaction—the formation of the tubercle. There is still disagreement as to whether the epithelioid cells are derived solely from the phagocytes of fixed tissues, such as the connective tissues, or also from mononuclear leukocytes in the circulating blood. The opinion most widely favored is that the epithelioid cells are derived mainly from the phagocytes in the fixed tissues. It is also recognized, however, that circulating mononuclear leukocytes may enter an area of tuberculous inflammation and be converted into epithelioid cells. In regard to the Langhans giant cells, it is generally accepted that they are derived from the epithelioid cells by fusion of several of the latter or by their inordinate growth with division of the nucleus only.

In the course of the development of the tubercle, new mononuclear cells appear about the original epithelioid cells, and these monocytes also mature into epithelioid cells. It is probable that this process continues from the periphery inward as long as tubercle bacilli remain alive in the area in question. It seems likely, however, that disintegrating and/or dead bacilli also play an important role in inducing the formation of tubercles. The experimental work of Sabin and her co-workers demonstrated the significance of the insoluble fat or wax content of such dead bacilli in provoking the formation of tubercles. Notably, they showed that tubercles can be produced experimentally by dead bacilli as well as by live ones, and that the histologic response of the tissues to tubercle bacilli is similar to the response provoked by the insoluble fat or wax extracted from tubercle bacilli.

It is generally recognized that, at any stage in the evolution of a tuberculous lesion, *caseation* may be prominent among the pathologic changes and may even dominate them. This aspect of the inflammatory changes of tuberculosis has been investigated experimentally, and various conclusions have been drawn. The necrosis of the lesional tissue is usually rapid, and the caseous material consists of the necrotic tissue intermingled with coagulated exudate. Polymorphonuclear leukocytes may be distributed sparsely or diffusely through the necrotic tissue, or they may form a wall around the caseous focus. Tubercle bacilli may be preserved in the caseous material. Areas of caseation tend to undergo secondary transformation, such as softening and liquefaction. The softening apparently occurs through the action of proteolytic enzymes present in the leukocytes. The softened material is inspissated or resorbed, or tends to be eliminated in other ways.

In the course of time, evidence of *healing* may be seen in an area of tuberculous inflammation. For instance, young miliary tubercles frequently heal into hyaline fibrous nodules. Large caseous foci generally become encapsulated, the encapsulation occurring mainly through the formation of nonspecific connective tissue at the periphery of the focus. The encapsulating tissue may be highly collagenous and hyaline, although within the capsule the formation of epithelioid cell tubercles is also sometimes observed. Ultimately, the whole caseous area may be replaced by a connective tissue scar developing from the capsule surrounding the caseous focus.

A caseous area may also be the site of *calcium deposition* resulting from diffusion and precipitation into the caseous focus of calcium carbonate and phosphates. Even in a calcified focus, virulent tubercle bacilli may still be retained. In time, a calcified caseous area may become the site of bone deposition, and bone marrow may also be present. A tuberculous focus is often surrounded by a zone of non-specific inflammation, which has been variously designated as a *collateral* or a *perifocal inflammation*. It has been attributed, on the one hand, directly to the toxins of the tubercle bacillus and, on the other hand, to the degenerative products of tissue catabolism originating in the tuberculous focus. Anatomically, such a perifocal zone of inflammation consists of granulation tissue with varying quantities of tissue fluid and infiltrated cells.

The Various Anatomic Aspects of Skeletal Tuberculosis.—The tubercle bacilli inciting tuberculous inflammation in a *bone or synovial membrane* are almost always carried to the region by the blood stream. Only on rare occasions does a bone or a synovial membrane become affected by extension from an extraskeletal focus of tuberculosis, particularly a bursa or tendon sheath, which in turn was infected by way of the blood stream. In very exceptional instances, tubercle bacilli may be introduced into a skeletal area directly, through a break in the skin. For example, Preiser observed a man with pulmonary tuberculosis who, in a state of alcoholic delirium, had bitten himself in the region of the wrist and subsequently developed tuberculosis in that area.

Furthermore, it seems established beyond doubt, in connection with *tuberculosis of joints*, that the disease may begin in the articular end of a bone, break into the joint, and then involve the synovial membrane. (See Fig. 251.) On the other hand, at least half of the cases in which the tuberculosis is predominantly in the synovial membrane are *not* the result of spread of the infection from a bone adjacent to, or entering into, the formation of the affected joint. In these cases the synovial membrane becomes infected directly by way of the blood stream. Even while the primary bone lesion is still very small, infectious matter from it may penetrate the articular cartilage and reach the synovial membrane. The changes consequently appearing in this membrane are difficult to distinguish from, if not identical with, those of tuberculosis originating there.

Tissue available for pathologico-anatomic study of skeletal tuberculosis in an active state is mainly tissue removed in the course of surgical procedures. Such material is only moderately satisfactory for this purpose, as it is often difficult for the pathologist to visualize correctly the relations of the various bits of tissue to the disease focus as a whole. However, correlation of the roentgenographic appearance of the involved area with the pathologic material is very helpful and may give a clue to the site of origin of the infection. Nevertheless, in many instances it is indeed difficult to determine, at the time of observation in the clinic or in the laboratory (and even under the most favorable circumstances), whether the disease process began in the bone or in the synovial membrane.

Almost any bone may be the site of tuberculous infection. In a long tubular bone the tuberculous process usually takes its departure in one of the epiphysial ends, particularly near its articular surface. From there, the infection soon tends to spread to the synovial membrane. The diaphysis (or shaft) of a *long tubular bone* is occasionally the site of a tuberculous infection, though the diaphysis of a *short tubular bone* is more frequently affected. When the pathologic process originates in a *vertebra*, it usually starts in the body of the vertebra. Of the *short bones*, it is especially those of the tarsus and sometimes those of the carpus that are the sites of tuberculous infection. As the individual bones of the carpus and tarsus ordinarily articulate with several others, it is very likely that the disease process will spread to neighboring bones and joints.

When tubercle bacilli localize in a bone, the pathologic process is initiated by tubercle formation in the marrow, the trabeculae of spongy bone becoming affected subsequently. It is held that the bacilli tend to predilect the myeloid marrow (see Huebschmann). The trabeculae of bone which are bordered by newly formed tubercles undergo progressive resorption. The focus of disease enlarges and spreads as a result of the formation of additional tubercles in the marrow. At this early stage, histologic examination will disclose that the lesion still consists of tuberculous granulation tissue interspersed with spongy trabeculae in various stages of resorption. When caseation sets in, the tuberculous focus increases in size. Extensive caseation may already be manifest even when the lesion has existed for only a short time. It should be noted that most large tuberculous foci in bone eventually become predominantly caseous.

In those rare instances in which an osseous tuberculous focus of long duration fails to show any special tendency toward caseous necrosis or liquefaction, the pathologic process is likely to remain circumscribed and limited to the bone. It is mainly in superficially located areas of epiphyses and epicondyles that such lesions are to be encountered. Roentgenographically they suggest cystic or fibrocystic *non*tuberculous lesions (see Kienböck). So-called cystic tuberculosis of bone may affect a single bone, and the part of the bone involved may be the metaphysial area or a metaphysial-epiphysial area. In other instances there are *multiple* cystlike lesions, and such cases have been denoted as "*multiple* pseudocystic tuberculosis of bone." The affected subjects are much more often children than adults (see Murray, Karlén, and also Hayes).

Figure 251

A, Roentgenograph of part of the pelvis and both hip joints in the case of a 3 year old male child whose right hip joint was the site of a tuberculous infection. The presence of the large multiloculated area in the acetabulum on the left side of the picture is in harmony with the idea that the infection spread from there to the articular cavity of the hip joint and subsequently involved the articular surface of the head of the femur. The case history of the child indicates that there had been complaints relating to the right hip for about 6 months before he was admitted to our hospital. In particular, the affected joint was painful, there was some local tenderness and fullness, movement of the joint was limited, and the child limped. He died 5 months later, and an autopsy was performed. The affected right hip joint area was removed *in toto*. The autopsy also disclosed the presence of: tuberculous meningitis, internal hydrocephalus, disseminated miliary tuberculosis, and a calcifying focus of primary tuberculous infection in the upper lobe of the right lung.

B, Photograph of the right hip area which had been removed at autopsy and sectioned in the longitudinal plane. The articular cartilage of the head of the femur has been eroded, and the femoral head is covered by a pannus of tuberculous granulation tissue. The head of the femur is somewhat flattened, and the articular surface of the acetabulum is covered by a thick layer of compacted fibrin containing granulation tissue. Near the fovea, a large tuberculoma is present which measures about 2 cm. across the thickness of the acetabulum. That is, it extends from the articular surface across the entire thickness of the structure. In the transverse direction, the tuberculoma measures at least 3 cm. There can be little doubt that the involvement of the hip joint took its departure from the tuberculous focus in the acetabulum. The tuberculous tissue then entered the joint and infected the lining of the joint capsule, with the result that the articular cartilage of the femoral head was destroyed, and the subchondral spongiosa also became implicated.

C, Photomicrograph ($\times$ 35) of part of the articular surface of the femoral head. The surface is completely devoid of cartilage. In the upper half of the picture it can be noted that much of the subchondral spongiosa has been destroyed, and that the enlarged marrow spaces are filled with agglomerated tubercles. In the lower half of the picture one can observe that the intertrabecular marrow spaces still show fatty and myeloid marrow.

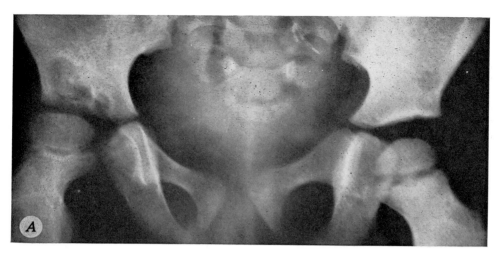

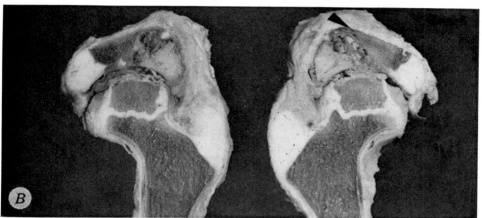

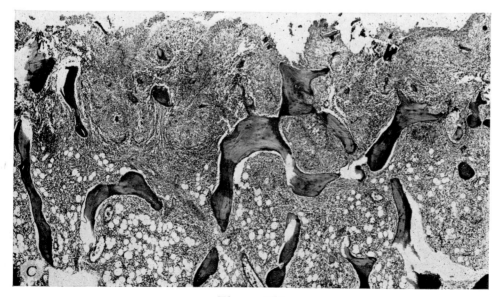

Figure 251

If *caseous bone foci* have not yet liquefied, they appear yellowish and may be rather firm. The degree of firmness depends in part upon the length of time during which the tuberculous lesion had existed before necrosis took place. If necrosis supervenes early or rapidly, it implicates the regional bone that has not yet become extensively resorbed despite the presence of granulation tissue between the spongy trabeculae. Under such circumstances, many of the necrotic trabeculae within the caseous focus retain their original size, form, and arrangement.

The firmness may be only relative, however; that is, the pathologic focus may be firm only in comparison with the atrophic nontuberculous bone neighboring upon the diseased area. Under these conditions, microscopic examination will disclose that many of the trabeculae give evidence of having been more or less extensively eroded. Apart from the considerations already mentioned, coagulation of the inter-trabecular granulations *per se* contributes some degree of firmness to the caseous area.

Sites of more recent caseation are likely to be bordered by tuberculous granulation tissue containing epithelioid cells and some giant cells. What appears to be fibrin-like material may be admixed with the necrotic tissue at the periphery of the caseous focus. As the caseous region softens, a more definite encapsulating zone becomes delimited around it.

Figure 252

A, Roentgenograph showing, in lateral projection, a knee joint of a 21-month-old child. The oval-shaped radiolucent area in the metaphysis at the lower end of the femur is a focus of so-called cystic tuberculosis. The periosteal new bone formation represents a reaction to the involvement of the cortex just above the epiphysial cartilage plate. The articular cavity of the joint is distended as a result of implication of the synovial membrane. The child died of miliary tuberculosis 6 or 8 weeks after this picture was taken.

B, Roentgenograph of a knee joint, in the anteroposterior projection, which presents a large area of radiolucency in the upper metaphysis of the left tibia and concomitant involvement of the adjacent epiphysis. The subject was a girl 3 years of age, and the difficulties relating to the lesion in question had begun 3 months before the patient was admitted to our hospital. At that time, the child fell, injured her left knee, and complained of pain. On clinical examination, it was found that the knee area was slightly swollen, painful to pressure, and motion was somewhat limited. The lesional area was curetted, and tissue was processed for histologic examination. Some tissue was also injected into a guinea pig. The laboratory findings confirmed the preoperative diagnosis of tuberculosis.

C, Photomicrograph ($\times$ 5) of a section prepared from a vertebral body presenting a tuberculoma (see the upper left-hand part of the picture). The subject was a woman 28 years of age who was admitted to our hospital because of pain, of about 6 months' duration, in the right ankle. There was fluctuant swelling on the external surface of that ankle, and aspiration yielded some purulent fluid which, on bacteriologic examination, revealed the presence of tubercle bacilli. An ankle fusion was carried out. Pertinent tissue was examined histologically, and the fact that the ankle was the site of a tuberculous infection was confirmed. Several weeks after the ankle fusion, the patient began to complain of pain in the lower part of the back. Roentgenographs of the spine showed lesions in the bodies of the first and second lumbar vertebrae which were interpreted as tuberculous. A spinal fusion was performed and was apparently successful. Two years after the patient's first admission to our hospital, she was readmitted for additional surgery on the spine, since the vertebral lesion was progressing, and a second spinal fusion was carried out. The patient died 4 days later. An autopsy disclosed the presence of miliary tuberculosis, tuberculous meningitis, and tuberculous empyema on the left side. The affected pleural cavity contained about 1,000 cc. of thick, creamy pus, which showed the presence of tubercle bacilli when smears were prepared from it and stained. The vertebral column from the eighth thoracic to the fourth lumbar vertebrae was removed. The vertebral body illustrated was one of several vertebral bodies presenting tuberculous involvement.

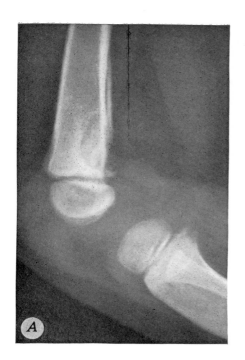
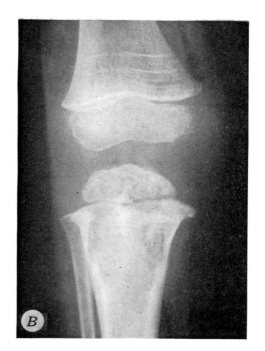
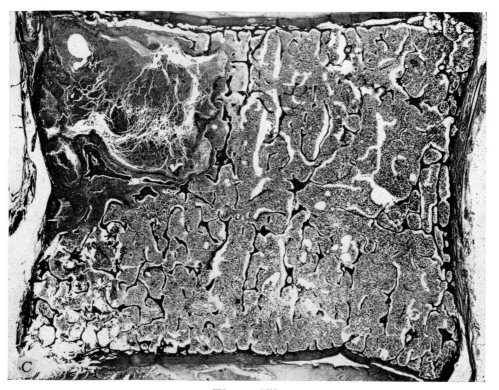

Figure 252

As a result of liquefaction of a caseous focus in the bone, an *abscess cavity* may develop. Contained within it is pus in which there may be floating fragments of bone and even fine granules—the so-called "bone sand." An abscess cavity is usually bordered by a wide perifocal zone whose intertrabecular marrow is mainly nonspecific granulation tissue. Immediately surrounding the cavity, there is ordinarily a narrow layer of connective tissue containing variable quantities of lymphocytes, polymorphonuclear leukocytes, and some fibrin. Fully formed epithelioid cell tubercles are generally not seen in the delimiting connective tissue layer. The bone trabeculae in the perifocal zone about an abscess are often sclerotic. Thus an abscess cavity frequently comes to be surrounded by a wall of sclerotic bone and fibrous intertrabecular tissue. This encapsulating wall may be interpreted as evidence of a reparative process. (See Fig. 252.)

The chemical processes by which the dissolution of the osseous tissue in the necrotic focus takes place are not clear. Some have stated that it occurs through the medium of proteolytic enzymes derived from leukocytes. The dissolution of the bone trabeculae probably takes place concomitantly with the softening of the rest of the caseous tissue. Liquefaction is especially conspicuous in foci of caseous tuberculosis in the vertebrae, and the softening may finally extend to the cortical bone and may favor the formation of subligamentous pus and burrowing abscesses.

The bone defect or abscess cavity almost never comes to be filled in by bone, and only rarely is it filled in by tuberculous or nontuberculous granulation tissue. Thus, the perifocal reactive healing process, including the osteosclerosis, remains limited to the immediate vicinity of the abscess. As a rule, the contents of an old bone cavity consist of inspissated pus or caseous calcareous matter. Eventually, even the perifocal osteosclerosis may recede to a considerable degree.

Roentgenographically, the necrotic bone (*sequestrum*) within a caseous focus may appear sharply demarcated from the surrounding bone and may persist in this delimited form for some time. In an end of a long bone, such as the femur, the sequestrum may appear as a cone-shaped area in a zone of destruction bordering upon the articular surface (see Phemister and Hatcher). Occasionally one encounters tuberculous sequestra which are located in the articular ends of the bones on opposite sides of the joint and which have been denoted as "kissing sequestra." Infarction of the bone, occurring as a result of vascular occlusion, was long regarded as the basis for the formation of such sequestra. Anatomic studies have failed, however, to corroborate this opinion.

It should be pointed out that the *synovial membrane* of the *knee joint* is the one that best lends itself to gross examination upon removal because of the large amount of tissue provided by the quadriceps bursa. It is for this reason that descriptions relating to the pathologic findings in a tuberculous synovial membrane are based primarily upon the alterations presented by the synovial membranes of affected knee joints.

All other things being equal, the pathologic changes in a synovial membrane are likely to be more severe if the inflammation follows the penetration of a caseous bone focus into the joint space than if it starts *de novo* in the synovial membrane. Tuberculous involvement of a synovial membrane is associated with inflammatory thickening of the periarticular connective tissue and fat. This thickening contributes to the enlargement of the joint area, which is often already swollen by effusion. At first, the periarticular soft-tissue swelling is of a nontuberculous perifocal character. Biopsy of such tissue at this stage will not show evidence of tuberculosis, and therefore does not aid in arriving at a diagnosis. Subsequently, the inflammatory changes very often do penetrate the joint capsule and extend into the periarticular tissues.

When a synovial membrane is severely inflamed, it appears extremely thickened.

Heavy layers of fibrin may be spread irregularly over its surface. It is likely that the articular cavity will contain a considerable amount of purulent fluid or liquefied caseous matter, though sometimes its contents consist largely of coagulated pus. Microscopic examination of such a thickened membrane shows the presence of richly vascular tuberculous granulation tissue, upon which necrotic and fibrin-like material may be found deposited. In addition, within the granulation tissue there are necrotic and caseous areas, fibrin masses, collections of leukocytes, and large numbers of dispersed mononuclear phagocytes. Epithelioid cells and full-fledged epithelioid tubercles are also present, especially in the vicinity of areas of caseation. In some specimens, even if considerable caseation is present, few, if any, clearly differentiated tubercles or nests of epithelioid cells are to be found.

When the inflammatory changes are less florid, the thickened synovial membrane is gray-red in color. Even in these milder cases there is often a thin deposit of fibrin on the surface of the membrane. Contained within the latter, and sometimes extending into the subsynovial connective tissue, small areas discolored brownish red by blood pigment may be observed. On gross inspection, some miliary tubercles are often clearly visible on the surface of such a membrane. Their differentiation from miliary lymphoid collections is not very difficult. Any fluid present in the joint space is likely to be cloudy and to contain shreds of fibrin. In these less florid cases the microscopic appearance of the synovial membrane varies. The outer surface of the membrane has usually lost its lining layer of cells. Within the substance of the thickened membrane, there are often myriads of typically developed epithelioid tubercles, some or many of which may show central necrosis. In other instances, the histologic evidence of the tuberculous nature of the inflammation may not be so apparent, for the inflammatory granulation tissue may contain few epithelioid cells. Nevertheless, some scattered tubercles are always present, even though other evidence of tuberculosis may be slight. In any case, however, no large areas of caseation are found. (See Fig. 253.)

Sometimes the tuberculous changes in the synovial membrane are even less striking than those described above. In these instances the membrane is only moderately thickened, somewhat injected, and succulent. There may be no deposit of fibrin on its surface, the joint space having been filled with thin yellow fluid. Various degrees of villus formation may be observed at the reflections of the synovial membrane. Close inspection of the surface of such a membrane will usually reveal, even grossly, some miliary tubercles in its substance. In such cases the tuberculous inflammation may remain limited to the synovial membrane. The clinical and roentgenographic evidence may then in no way suggest a diagnosis of tuberculosis, and under these conditions the nature of the lesion can be clarified only by microscopic examination of the synovial membrane removed in the course of surgery.

With tuberculous involvement (whether primary or secondary) of a synovial membrane, partial or complete erosion and destruction of the *articular cartilages* is likely to take place. The erosion starts with the spread of granulation tissue from the inflamed synovial membrane onto the free surface of the cartilage. The granulation tissue advances insidiously from the border of the cartilage, progressing centripetally across its surface. Through the action of its vascular and phagocytic elements, portions of the cartilage are eroded, and leukocytes in the joint exudate may also participate in the process. The erosion does not pursue an even course. In some joints it may be the midportion of the cartilage, for instance, that ultimately becomes most severely ulcerated. In others, multiple ulcerations with islands of somewhat changed intervening cartilage produce a highly bizarre appearance. The erosion may continue for a long time, but the surface destruction may be arrested, even very early, if the eroding granulation tissue becomes necrotic.

The course of the surface erosion also varies in accordance with intra-articular conditions. Where the articular cartilages are in contact, compression and motion seem capable of checking the advance of the granulation tissue (see Phemister and Hatcher). Furthermore, since the articular cartilage is much thicker in growing children than in adults, complete destruction of this cartilage is less likely to occur in children.

Frequently it is the subchondral granulation tissue that separates the cartilage from the bone and is the basis for the destruction of the articular cartilage. This granulation tissue inserts itself at the periphery, and as it advances under the articular cartilage, it loosens and even detaches it from the subchondral bony end plate. The detached cartilages may become extensively necrotic, and sometimes disappear completely. Their destruction may be hastened by a superimposed pyogenic infection brought to the joint by way of regional sinuses or the blood stream. The subchondral bone trabeculae become atrophic. Many of the trabeculae, especially in the vicinity of the granulation tissue, are resorbed, along with portions of the bony end plate.

Where the articular cartilages are in close contact (as in the hip joint and ankle joint), subchondral destruction may be more severe than that on the surface of the articular bone ends. Even before the subchondral inflammation has progressed very far, portions of subchondral bone at the periphery of the joint may become necrotic. Such necrotic foci are likely to be somewhat wedge-shaped, and are referred to as *sequestra*, because they become more or less delimited from the surrounding bone. Corresponding necrotic areas may appear in the bone ends on opposite sides of a joint, giving rise to the so-called "kissing sequestra." (See Fig. 254 and also Fig. 249-A.)

As happens in relation to other articular inflammations, an intra-articular *effusion* almost always accompanies tuberculous infection of the synovial membrane. In fact, there may already be considerable effusion while the synovial inflammation is still in an early stage. Even if the tuberculous lesion is limited to a bone, the synovial membrane not yet being affected, a sympathetic effusion may be induced if the disease focus borders on a joint.

Figure 253

A, Photomicrograph ($\times$ 38) showing a villously proliferated synovial membrane of a knee joint and the presence of many tubercles within the villi. The patient was a girl 11 years of age who had first been admitted to our hospital when she was 6 years old. Her clinical record indicates that, at about the time of her first admission, her father died of pulmonary tuberculosis, and one of her brothers was under treatment for pulmonary tuberculosis. Difficulties relating to her left knee joint had already been present for about 2 months before her first admission, and physical examination revealed definite swelling of the knee area, increased local heat, and some limitation of extension and flexion. A roentgenograph of the affected knee joint disclosed periarticular swelling and definite thickening of the synovial membrane, but failed to reveal any abnormalities relating to the bones of that joint. Though the tuberculin test was strongly positive, it was decided to treat the child conservatively. She was transferred to the country home branch of the hospital, where she remained for 4 years before being sent back to the hospital. About 6 months after readmission, an arthrodesis was carried out, and the excised tissue, which consisted of fragments of synovial membrane and osteoarticular shavings, was submitted for histologic examination, which clearly established the diagnosis of tuberculosis of the knee joint.

B, Photomicrograph ($\times$ 50) revealing the histologic pattern of the synovial membrane removed in the course of the surgical intervention on the knee joint illustrated in Figure 249-A. The synovial membrane is greatly thickened, and on the surface of the membrane there is fibrin, which is rather closely compacted. The thickened synovial membrane is inflamed and permeated by numerous tubercles, some of which are agglomerated.

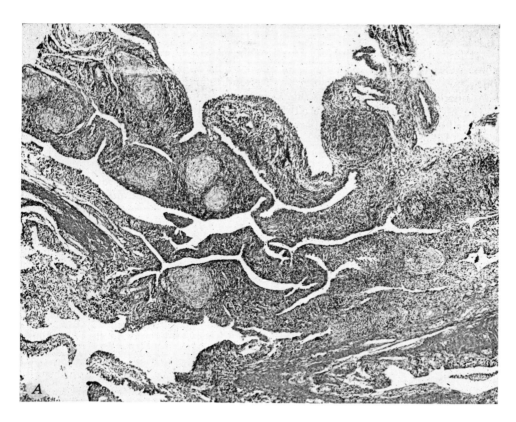

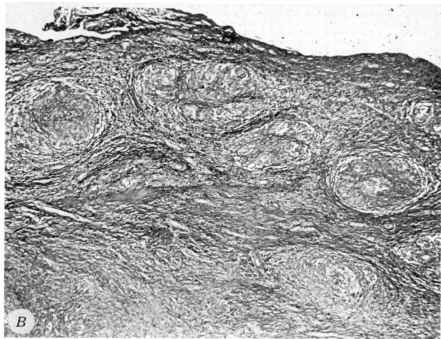

Figure 253

At first, the synovial fluid is usually thin, straw-colored, and fairly clear. In some cases it remains so, while in others it soon becomes thick and more or less purulent. The ultimate character of the exudate is determined by the severity of the tuberculous inflammation. The thickest and most purulent exudates are seen in the most advanced cases, where the purulent matter is thickened by fibrin and by liquefied caseous and necrotic tissue. However, even in the absence of a sinus or sinuses, tuberculous joints may become secondarily infected by pyogenic bacteria, which can also modify the character of the exudate. If the pathologic process in the joint is active but aspiration elicits no fluid, the intra-articular fluid is probably coagulated. Eventually, with spontaneous regression and the formation of intra-articular adhesions, much of the fluid becomes resorbed, and under these circumstances, aspiration may also fail to yield fluid.

Tubercle bacilli virulent for guinea pigs are to be found in joint exudates even when the inflammation is subsiding spontaneously and even if the effusion has existed for a long time. If, at the time of removal of the fluid, the synovial membrane has not yet been invaded by tubercle bacilli, the fluid will not, of course, induce tuberculosis in guinea pigs. This may be one of the reasons why a small percentage of exudates from joints subsequently proved to be tuberculous are likely to yield negative results from this important diagnostic procedure. If this happens, the guinea pig inoculation test should be repeated.

The thickened synovial membrane of some actively tuberculous joints (especially knees) may be studded with irregular, *knobby projections* whose stalks vary in length and thickness. These pedunculated masses result mainly from fibrinous transformation of the inflamed synovial tissue. They show a strong tendency to be molded by intra-articular pressure. On microscopic examination, they are found to consist largely of fibrinoid material in which collagen fibrils are still recognizable. As the result of the action of intra-articular mechanical forces, the roundish knobs often become separated from the stalks and may lodge in recesses of the synovial membrane.

Figure 254

A, Photomicrograph ($\times$ 12) illustrating tuberculous granulation tissue which has extended beneath the articular cartilage of the head of the radius and has separated the articular cartilage from the subchondral bone, which is somewhat atrophic. The articular surface of the cartilage has a thin layer of granulation tissue extending partly over it. The subject was a girl 19 years of age who was admitted to our hospital because of pain, swelling, and limitation of motion of the right elbow joint for about 1 year. Roentgenographic examination disclosed that the articular ends of the bones entering into the formation of the elbow joint were distinctly atrophic, and there were also other changes suggestive of tuberculosis. A surgical intervention was carried out, and the tissue removed from the elbow joint was submitted for anatomic examination. The material consisted of several pieces of bone and soft tissue. One of the osseous fragments was the head of the radius, whose articular surface was covered by granulation tissue. The head of the radius was extremely soft and compressible, thus indicating that the subchondral bone was highly atrophic.

B, Photomicrograph ($\times$ 30) showing tuberculous granulation tissue which has penetrated the articular cartilage of a tibia, and presents as a small mass protruding into the articular cavity. Residual fragments of articular cartilage are visible on both sides of the mass. On the right side of the picture, a subchondral tubercle is apparent (see arrow). The clinical record of the patient, a man 64 years of age at the time of his admission to our hospital, indicates that for about 3 years prior to admission he had complaints relating to the left knee joint. The joint was painful and swollen, and there was also limitation of motion and difficulty in walking. Smears of fluid aspirated from the knee joint showed the presence of tubercle bacilli. A fusion of the knee joint was carried out, and anatomic examination of the excised tissue confirmed the diagnosis of tuberculosis.

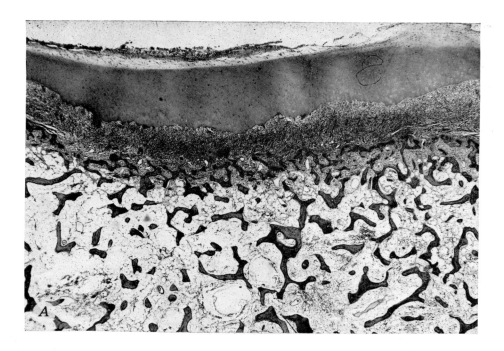

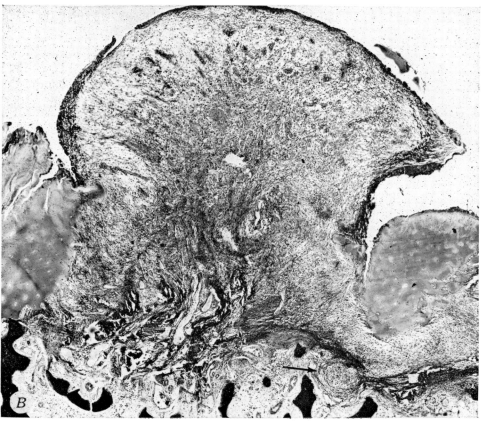

Figure 254

Bodies of rice-grain size (so-called *rice bodies*) are more common and more abundant in tuberculous joints or tendon sheaths than are the larger bodies. They occur especially in cases in which the inflammation is milder and the condition has run a chronic course. In general, these rice bodies likewise arise from fibrinous transformation of the synovial tissue, but they are not always composed entirely of fibrin. Sometimes they still contain remnants of epithelioid tubercles and of swollen collagen fibers. It must be remembered that rice bodies, even in as large numbers as may be encountered in tuberculous tenosynovitis, may also be encountered in some cases of nontuberculous synovial inflammation. Therefore, one should not attach too much diagnostic significance to the mere finding of rice bodies at the surgical intervention.

The so-called *cold abscess* is a highly characteristic manifestation of skeletal tuberculosis. In general, it is only in cases of tuberculous spondylitis that the burrowing properties of such abscesses are likely to be prominent. The cold abscesses, after burrowing for a long time and over a considerable distance, may perforate the skin or penetrate into a body cavity or organ. If an abscess forms in a pelvic bone or in the region of the hip joint, it may also burrow, but if it does, the abscess tract is ordinarily not very long.

The mechanism underlying the formation and progress of burrowing abscesses has been a subject of keen interest. It seems fairly well established that the direction of the burrowing is not determined by gravity alone. It also seems clear that the pus within the abscess is not derived solely from the purulent bone focus (see Tschistowitsch and Winogradow), but is continually being supplemented by material arising from the caseous necrosis and suppurative liquefaction of tuberculous granulation tissue which is steadily being formed along the abscess tract. As the abscess burrows, the new tuberculous granulation tissue lying in the vicinity of its head or directly in its path is being cleared away by caseation and liquefaction. Factors contributing to the ultimate size of the abscess are: (1) the amount of the tuberculous granulation tissue formed, (2) the extent of its caseation, and (3) the degree of its suppurative liquefaction. These factors vary from case to case.

A burrowing abscess of long duration may develop a delimiting wall consisting of connective tissue, and the older the abscess, the denser the wall. Ultimate calcification of the wall is by no means uncommon and may greatly facilitate roentgenographic demonstration of the abscess. The inner surface of the delimiting wall of the capsule may be lined by tuberculous granulation tissue. While the burrowing abscess is enlarging, its inner wall may show a deposit of irregular masses of crumby caseous material. Histologic examination of the tuberculous granulation tissue usually shows a striking scarcity of mature epithelioid cell tubercles. The tissues, particularly the muscles, compressed or penetrated by the burrowing abscesses undergo extensive degeneration and atrophy and fibrous replacement.

The contents of a cold abscess vary. In the early stages, the pus is rather thin and of a light green-yellow color, and it may contain crumby masses. In older abscesses, the pus is more fluid and brownish. If the lesion in connection with which the abscess has developed is healing spontaneously, much of the abscess content may be resorbed. Closed tuberculous abscesses rarely contain any bacteria other than tubercle bacilli, and even these may be scarce. That is, the pus is likely to be "sterile" so far as nontuberculous elements are concerned. This is particularly the case in burrowing abscesses confined to the thorax. Burrowing psoas abscesses become secondarily infected somewhat more frequently.

Skeletal Tuberculosis as Manifested in Individual Skeletal Sites.—In *tuberculous spondylitis* the pathologic process usually begins in the body of the affected vertebra, close to an intervertebral disk. The lower thoracic and lumbar vertebrae are predilected. The cervical vertebrae are seldom involved. The tuberculous tissue first develops in the marrow, the osseous tissue becoming affected only secondarily. The disease focus, as a result of enlargement and caseation, frequently extends beneath the anterior and/or posterior longitudinal ligaments to the periphery of one or two regional intervertebral disks. However, postmortem findings indicate that tuberculosis almost never starts in an intervertebral disk. Before the age of 25, initial involvement of a disk is theoretically possible, because up to this age there may still be blood vessels nourishing the disks, but after this age the intervertebral disk is apparently not nourished in this way. Therefore in adults, vertebral tuberculosis is not likely to start in the intervertebral disk. It is only very rarely that the tuberculous lesion spreads from the vertebral body to the lamina, the spinous process, or the transverse processes of the affected vertebra.

The *postmortem findings* relating to tuberculous spondylitis differ in accordance with the severity and duration of the condition. However, the bodies of tuberculous vertebrae nearly always reveal lesions which have already advanced at least to the stage of caseation. The caseous lesions may be small, or so large as to involve one or several entire vertebral bodies. Although the bodies may have retained their shape during the early clinical course, postmortem examination usually shows them collapsed to some extent.

In an involved area, the intervertebral disks may be found destroyed totally or in part. The loose structure of the nucleus pulposus favors the extension of the infection when once the cartilage-bone border between the vertebral body and the adjacent disk or disks has been broken through. On the whole, a disk is most vulnerable at the point where the nucleus pulposus lies closest to the vertebral body. In the lower part of the spinal column, the extension of the disease into the intervertebral disk tends to take place in the posterior part of the disk. In adults, the disk will be penetrated, especially where such a disk has undergone regressive changes.

Collapse of vertebral bodies in the course of tuberculous spondylitis tends to give rise to severe *deformities*. In particular, the collapse is likely to create an angular posterior projection at the site of maximum involvement of the column. The angle of the projection is most acute when only one or two vertebrae have been destroyed. It is naturally less sharp when three or more vertebrae are involved. If the diseased bodies collapse sooner or more extensively on one side than on the other, there may be lateral as well as posterior angulation. The degree of angulation is least with collapse in the cervical or lumbar regions of the spine. In the mid-dorsal region, of course, the deformity may be severe and striking, often taking the form of the traditional hunchback. However, the diameter of the spinal canal is not usually significantly narrowed by such angular distortions of the column. (See Fig. 247.)

Paravertebral thickening or enlargement is very frequently—in fact, almost always—present at some stage in the evolution of a tuberculous spondylitis. This thickening results from the accumulation of tuberculous granulation tissue and/or pus between the involved vertebrae and the anterior longitudinal ligament. In exceedingly rare instances, there may be an extension of the paravertebral abscess to the wall of the aorta. This can lead either to the formation of an aneurysm or to the development of miliary tuberculosis (see Fossel). As has been known for a long time, penetration of a lung by a paravertebral abscess is by no means rare. In particular, it was noted in a pertinent report that penetration of a lung by a paravertebral abscess occurred in 32 of 327 cases of tuberculous spondylitis of the thoracic spine (see Yau and Hodgson).

Temporary or permanent paresis or even complete paralysis, through pressure on the spinal cord, is certainly a fairly frequent complication, although there is considerable variation in the figures relating to its incidence. The pressure on the cord is usually due to the accumulation of tuberculous granulation tissue and/or pus in the epidural space which results from penetration of the posterior longitudinal ligament by the inflammatory tissue. When the spondylitis is located in the upper and/or middle thoracic part of the column, paresis or paralysis is most likely to develop. Matsumoto, among others, held that the reason for this is that the spinal canal is narrower in the upper and middle thoracic area than in the cervical region. He maintained that the size of the spinal canal in a given region of the vertebral column stands in inverse relation to the frequency of Pott's paralysis in that region. Sometimes, apparently, cord symptoms are due rather to irritation from adhesions between the dura and the pia-arachnoid than to an epidural bulge. *Regional herpes zoster* has also been described as occurring in connection with tuberculous spondylitis (see Kobro). Estimates of the frequency of paresis or paralysis differ widely: Seemann reported 36 per cent; Wullstein, on the basis of many cases, reported 12.7 per cent. Data from various sources, summarized and analyzed by Whitman, indicate that paralysis occurs in about 5.6 per cent of children and 13 per cent of adults under treatment for tuberculous spondylitis. In his opinion, the percentage of neglected cases developing paralysis is still higher, though just how high is not known.

In at least half of the cases of tuberculous spondylitis, *burrowing abscesses* develop. These abscesses tend to come to the surface of the body, sometimes above the thorax (as, for instance, in the posterior part of the pharynx or in the suboccipital triangle) but usually below the diaphragm, where they point along one of several definite anatomic paths. As already stated, the direction of the burrowing is not determined solely by gravity but also by the site of the vertebral lesion. The course pursued and the site at which the abscess comes to the surface are useful indications of its site of origin. Willis noted that abscesses may be found subdivided into successive pockets, which, although effectively shut off from the thoracic and abdominal cavities, may open dorsally between the transverse processes and ribs.

The various courses which the abscess may take have been described in detail by Boeminghaus. Abscesses may burrow along both sides of the spine without communicating with each other. Sometimes a burrowing abscess is directed toward the surface of the body before the vertebral tuberculosis is clearly evident roentgenographically. In such cases it may be difficult to recognize the true cause of a bulge produced by the abscess. Burrowing abscesses may open on one or another body surface and thus form fistulae which often drain indefinitely. These distinctly increase the unfavorableness of the prognosis of tuberculous spondylitis.

In relation to tuberculosis involving *cervical vertebrae*, abscesses developing in the atlanto-occipital region may localize below the occiput, in the suboccipital triangle. They may then pass forward to the region behind the ear. Abscesses associated with other upper cervical vertebrae usually present as retropharyngeal accumulations of pus. In contrast to most burrowing abscesses, those in the retropharyngeal region interfere with vital functions—namely, swallowing and breathing—and consequently, of all tuberculous burrowing abscesses, have the most unfavorable prognosis. Especially in children, they sometimes perforate into the oral cavity and thus may cause death through suffocation or aspiration pneumonia. Even if the perforation does not lead rather promptly to death, there still remains the grave danger of the formation of fistulae and the occurrence of mixed infections in this region. Abscesses forming in the lower cervical region may extend along the course of the regional arteries. For instance, they may appear anteriorly at the inner border of the sternocleidomastoid attachments. The abscesses may finally extend into the mediastinum, or they may burrow along the subclavian vessels and reach the axilla.

Abscess formation resulting from tuberculosis of *thoracic vertebrae* may be difficult to detect, even in cases in which the abscess has extended down to the attachment of the diaphragm. The soft-tissue swelling brought about by abscesses oriented to thoracic vertebrae is very gradual. Not infrequently, an abscess developing in relation to thoracic vertebrae perforates through the pleura or into the lung. Bilateral abscesses are usually prevented from uniting by the strong anterior longitudinal ligament. Occasionally, instead of descending, an abscess resulting from tuberculosis of upper thoracic vertebrae may burrow upward in the direction of the cranium.

The *lumbar vertebrae* are particularly common locations for tuberculosis, and hence are especially likely to be the sites of origin of burrowing abscesses. As a rule, these abscesses develop bilaterally, although only one may become clinically prominent. Pus collecting from tuberculous lesions of the first and second lumbar vertebrae is often blocked by the tough mesh of the medial crura of the diaphragm. It is for this reason that the abscesses associated with these vertebrae burrow only a little way down, and tend to spread laterally. Pus accumulating above the diaphragm can burrow caudally only where the psoas muscle penetrates the lumbo-costal arch. In tuberculosis of the lower lumbar vertebrae, the pus may burrow into the sacral excavation. Such retroperitoneally located abscesses may compress the rectum. If they are sufficiently large, they may be palpated on rectal examination.

Pus collecting beneath the fascia of the psoas muscle produces the so-called *psoas abscess*. The pus burrows subfascially and very frequently penetrates below Poupart's ligament. It is then most likely to appear under the skin of the thigh at a point medial to the large femoral vessels. A psoas abscess may continue to develop below Poupart's ligament and appear in the space between the adductors and the rectus femoris. If it does not extend to the surface or is not surgically evacuated, the abscess may continue to develop further in various ways, under the influence of increasing pressure. In doing this, it may follow the course of the circumflex femoral artery, approach the femur, and subsequently break through to the posterior or lateral surface of the thigh. More rarely, the abscess develops in the musculature of the adductors, showing itself in a corresponding swelling and enlargement on the medial surface of the thigh. (See Fig. 255.)

Instead of burrowing anteriorly below Poupart's ligament, the abscess may follow the course of the sciatic nerve through the *sciatic foramen*. In its subsequent extension, it may either: (1) reach the surface at the lower border of the gluteus maximus (in the region between the tuberosity of the ischium and the greater trochanter) or (2) continue its descent along the sciatic nerve and even finally extend to the region of the popliteal fossa.

The pus sometimes extends below the fascia of the iliac muscle. An iliac abscess may advance below Poupart's ligament and thus reach the thigh. If the sac is constricted in the region of Poupart's ligament, communicating collections of pus are present above and below this ligament. Occasionally an abscess points under the skin of the back. This happens when pus bores below the fascia of the quadratus muscle of the back and advances along the path of the lowest intercostal vessels. If these abscesses burrow somewhat further down, they may present in the so-called lumbar triangle.

One of the aforementioned abscesses may perforate its sac, and the pus may then spread along the retroperitoneal pelvic cellular tissue. This pus, in continuing its descent, may compress the bladder or parts of the intestinal tract. The retroperitoneal suppuration may reach the anterior abdominal wall and, on further increase of the internal pressure, extend upward between the wall and the peritoneum.

At one time, *tuberculous coxitis* probably comprised more than half of all cases of hip disease in childhood, and was exceeded in frequency only by tuberculosis of the spine. Tuberculous coxitis may appear at any age. In the past, the vast majority of the affected persons were under 15 years of age, the condition was common between the ages of 3 and 6 years, and the mortality rate was high. Smith reported that among 150 subjects treated conservatively and followed for 3 years or more, 24 per cent died in the course of this period.

In the hip, as in the other joints, tuberculosis may start in the synovial membrane or in one of the bones entering into the formation of the joint. The point of departure for the coxitis is more commonly in one of the bones than in the synovial membrane. Various sites of predilection have been reported for the initial disease focus when it starts in a bone. Waldenström, evaluating 83 cases of tuberculous coxitis (nearly all in children), reported that the lesion started as often in the femur as in the acetabulum. On the other hand, others have reported that the disease process

Figure 255

A, Photograph of the first three lumbar vertebrae and part of the fourth lumbar vertebra removed at autopsy in a case of vertebral tuberculosis and sectioned in the sagittal plane. The upper and posterior portion of the third lumbar vertebra shows a focus of tuberculosis which has bulged the posterior longitudinal ligament somewhat and also the dura mater, and extended upward to implicate a small portion of the posterior surface of the second lumbar vertebra. Tuberculous tissue is present beneath the anterior longitudinal ligament in the region of the second lumbar vertebra. The patient was a 25-year-old man who, 1 year before his death, slipped on the sidewalk and fell on his back. One month later, he went to a clinic for treatment, and his record there indicates that he had sharp pain in the lumbar part of the spine and that the pain radiated around his hips to the front. He also complained of occasional dizziness and headaches. He was admitted to our hospital 2 weeks before his death. He was febrile, and neurological examination revealed generalized hyperesthesia and muscle tenderness. The fundi showed bilateral papilledema. The deep reflexes were hyperactive, and the clinical findings suggested the diagnosis of tuberculous meningitis. The course was progressively downhill, and he died. The autopsy revealed, in addition to the pathologic findings mentioned above concerning the second and third lumbar vertebrae: (1) disseminated miliary tuberculosis with involvement of the lungs, liver, spleen, kidneys, heart, aorta, pancreas, and adrenals; (2) tuberculomata in the brain; and (3) miliary tubercles in the meninges.

B, Roentgenograph of the portion of the vertebral column shown in *A*. The focus of tuberculosis in the third lumbar vertebra stands out clearly, but the small focus of tuberculosis which is extending under the posterior ligament to involve the second lumbar vertebra has not produced a significant defect in the posterior contour of that body. Anteriorly, the second lumbar vertebra shows a crescent-like area of radiolucency reflecting the pressure erosion caused by the tuberculous tissue beneath the local part of the anterior longitudinal ligament.

C and *D*, Photographs of cross sections of vertebrae and overlying soft tissues at the level of L_2 (*C*) and L_3 (*D*) in the case of a woman who had tuberculosis of the vertebral column. A spine fusion was carried out, and she died about $1\frac{1}{2}$ months later. The patient was 30 years of age at the time of her admission to our hospital, and her clinical history indicates that she had had pain in the lower part of her back for 2 years. Physical examination revealed pronounced restriction of motion in the spine, and tenderness at the level of L_1 and L_2. Subsequently she began to complain of pain in the back of her head, and all movements of the neck were restricted and painful. The neck became rigid, and abdominal reflexes were absent. A spinal tap, which established the presence of tuberculous meningitis, was carried out. The patient became confused, and also lost the use of her lower extremities. An autopsy revealed tuberculous meningitis, disseminated miliary tuberculosis, and bilateral psoas abscesses. In *C* (L_2), it is clear that the body of the vertebra has foci of tuberculosis, and that the spinal canal has been narrowed because the tuberculous tissue has penetrated the posterior longitudinal ligament and is making pressure against the dura mater. On each side of the vertebral body there is a psoas abscess. In *D* (L_3), at the level of this cross section, no involvement of the vertebral body is recognizable, but above this level the body was involved. The bilateral psoas abscesses are clearly apparent, and the abscess on the left side of the picture is very large.

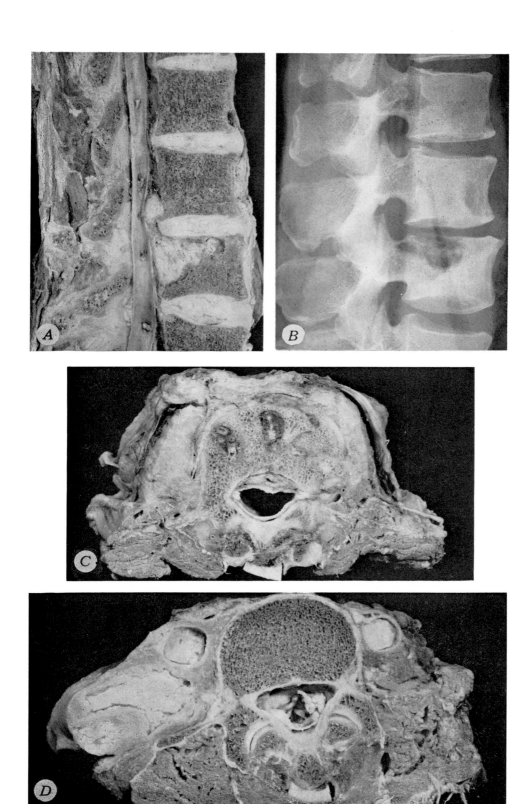

Figure 255

begins more frequently in the pelvic bone than in the femur (see Bankart). In this connection, it is held that the lesion starts in the interior of the ilium, immediately above the acetabulum, and that it spreads from that area to the acetabulum and through the ligamentum teres to the head of the femur. In this way the joint space becomes affected. When the acetabulum is extensively destroyed, the head of the femur may migrate upward. (See Fig. 251.)

Other workers, however, hold the opposite view—that tuberculous coxitis of osseous origin begins much more often on the femoral side of the joint. As to the specific localization of the initial lesion within the femur, there have also been different opinions, the most common being that the lesion begins in the capital femoral epiphysis, not far from the articular cartilage. However, Phemister and Hatcher reported that in children, particularly young ones, the tuberculous process takes its departure more frequently in the femoral neck or metaphysis than in the capital epiphysis. Within the neck the lesion is more often at the lower border than at the upper. Roentgenographically it presents as an area of radiolucency (see Ratliff, and also Ahern). From the femoral head or neck, the disease usually spreads to the joint space. The synovial membrane and the adjoining surface of the acetabulum become implicated. However, if the presenting lesion is still limited to the femoral neck, and if antibiotic therapy is given and the lesional area is evacuated surgically, the likelihood of a cure is strong. With advanced tuberculous coxitis, necrotic and purulent matter may find an exit from the joint space through the capsule and burrow for a short distance between the muscles of the thigh.

Rather infrequently, tuberculosis may spread to the hip joint from the *greater trochanter*. Meyerding and Mroz made a study of a number of cases of tuberculosis of the greater trochanter and the trochanteric bursa beneath the gluteus maximus muscle. The pathologic condition was usually limited to this region and ordinarily caused local tenderness and a cold fluctuating swelling. In a few cases, motion of the hip joint was impaired, notably when the lesion spread to the neck of the femur. Involvement of the hip joint is likely to follow surgical excision of the affected greater trochanter, since the intervention makes it possible for tubercle bacilli to enter the joint and infect the synovial membrane (see McNeur and Pritchard).

Tuberculosis of the *knee joint* is exceeded in frequency and clinical importance only by tuberculosis of the spine and of the hip. However, it is definitely less serious prognostically, since it is more accessible and amenable to treatment than is tuberculosis of the vertebral column or hip joint. Although tuberculosis of the knee joint is frequently observed in childhood and puberty, it is less strictly limited to these age groups than is tuberculous spondylitis and coxitis. Simultaneous involvement of both knees is extremely rare. In this respect, tuberculous gonitis contrasts with syphilitic gonitis, but resembles the latter in its frequently insidious onset. A persisting monarticular gonitis should be suspected of being tuberculous until some other basis for it has been definitely established.

The tuberculous inflammation often begins in the synovial membrane of the joint, and in some cases it shows a strong tendency to remain limited to the membrane. Under such circumstances there is a delay in the appearance of abscesses in the epiphyses or extensive destruction of the articular cartilages of the bone ends of the affected joint. Nevertheless, roentgenographic examination may disclose pitlike excavations at the margins of the articular cartilages, due to erosion of the local bone cortex.

More often, the pathologic process begins in one of the bones entering into the formation of the joint—particularly in the *distal* epiphysis or epiphysial end of the femur or the *proximal* epiphysis or epiphysial end of the tibia, but sometimes in the patella. When located in the patella, the lesional area may appear roentgenographically as a focus of radiolucency (see Hartofilakidis-Garofalidis). Rarely, tuberculous gonitis may develop from a disease focus in the head of the fibula. Occasionally a focus starting in one of the bones shows a tendency to remain limited to that bone. In most cases, however, the infection spreads to the joint cavity, because the infected bone area undergoes caseous necrosis and some of the caseous material is subsequently discharged into the articular cavity. Both clinically and anatomically, tuberculosis of a knee joint taking its departure in an articular bone end is more severe than when the inflammatory process begins in the synovial membrane. (See Fig. 256.)

In the *tarsal* and *carpal* areas, also, the tuberculous process may start in a bone or in the synovial membrane of a joint. Because of the relative smallness of the tarsal and carpal bones and the multiplicity of the local articulations (due to the irregular shape of the bones in question), it is not at all likely that the tuberculosis will remain limited to one bone or one joint in these regions. Moreover, bilateral involvement of the tarsal or carpal bones is very rare. It is in adults that most instances of tuberculosis in these regions are observed.

The incidence of tuberculosis of the *tarsal region* (including also the ankle joint and the lower end of the tibia and fibula) stands next in frequency to tuberculosis of the spine, hip, and knee, respectively. Nevertheless, it is encountered much less often in the tarsal region than in these other sites. In more than half of the cases of tuberculosis of the tarsal region, the talus (astragalus) or the calcaneus will be found involved, the talus being more often affected than the calcaneus. Spread from the talus to the ankle joint and secondarily to the tibia and/or fibula, or from the calcaneus to the talocalcaneal joint, is not at all uncommon. (See Fig. 257.) In the midtarsal region it is the navicular and the cuboid that are most likely to be affected. Tuberculosis of the navicular may remain localized to that bone, but more frequently the talonavicular joint is concomitantly involved (see Pouzet).

Tuberculosis of the *carpal region* is definitely rare, especially in persons below 15 years of age. When it appears in this area, the bones of the distal row are more likely to be the site of origin than the bones of the proximal row. In the carpal region, tuberculosis tends to spread and involve several bones and joints more often than it does in the tarsal region. That is, tuberculosis limited to a single carpal bone is very unusual. Particularly in adults, the prognosis of tuberculosis of the carpal region is generally held to be unfavorable, especially because the subjects frequently are also afflicted with active pulmonary tuberculosis (see Satta).

The *elbow region* is more often involved than the shoulder or even the wrist. Among the three bones entering into the formation of the elbow joint, the frequency of involvement, in descending order, is: the olecranon process of the ulna, the lower end of the humerus (especially the external condyle), and the head of the radius. Tuberculosis of the bones of the *pelvis* (excluding the immediate vicinity of the hip joint) is observed especially in young adults. It predilects the sacroiliac joints, but it may be limited to the sacrum, the ilium or (less frequently) the os pubis (see Madlener, Fares and Pagani, and also Nicholson). Involvement of the sacroiliac joints is the most common localization in relation to the pelvis *per se*. (See Fig. 258.) If the lesion in one or both of the sacroiliac joints is associated with sinus formation and the presence of foci of tuberculosis in other bone sites, the prognosis is unfavorable, and the mortality rate in these cases has been reported to be as high as 58.6 per cent (see Strange).

Tuberculosis is less often encountered in the *shoulder joint* than in the elbow or wrist, and, of course, rare by comparison with the spine, hip, knee, or ankle. When it does involve the shoulder joint, the site of its onset is most often the head of the humerus, and the lesion spreads from there to the articular cavity. Very *infrequently*, it begins in the scapula. As in other articular regions, the infection may also arise in the synovial membrane. The *clavicle* seems to be affected very rarely, if ever. In this respect, skeletal tuberculosis again contrasts with skeletal syphilis, in which the clavicle is rather frequently involved.

As is natural, in view of their closer proximity to the lungs, the *ribs* are more frequently affected by tuberculosis than is the *sternum*. Most often the infection spreads to these bones directly from the pleura or lungs. In some cases, however, especially in children, the involvement of the ribs is independent of inflammation of the lungs or pleura. It is these latter cases that are amenable to treatment by resection (see Rechtman, and also Johnson and Rothstein).

The *shafts of long tubular bones* (and especially their diaphyses) are only exceptionally an initial site of tuberculous inflammation, at least in occidental countries. In fact, most data indicate that tuberculosis starting anywhere in the shaft of a long tubular bone constitutes less than 1 per cent of all cases of skeletal tuberculosis in

Figure 256

A, Photograph of a tuberculous right knee joint, dissected to disclose the pathologic changes in the articular capsule, the patella, and the femoral condyles. The synovial lining of the capsule is thickened and covered by fibrin, and in the region of the quadriceps pouch the synovial membrane has undergone villous proliferation. The articular cartilage of the patella is eroded at its periphery. The lateral condyle of the femur (on the left side of the picture) is completely denuded of articular cartilage, and is covered by granulation tissue which had been situated subchondrally and had led to detachment of the articular cartilage. Above the condyle, a small, roundish fragment of articular cartilage is visible (see arrows), and this piece of cartilage may be a residual fragment of the cartilage which had been separated from the lateral femoral condyle. The articular cartilage over the medial condyle (on the right side of the picture) shows an area where the cartilage has been separated from the underlying bone. The patient in this case, a boy, was 10 years of age when he was admitted to our hospital. His clinical history indicated that he had had difficulties (limp and swelling) relating to his right knee for a number of years. About 2 years after admission, he died of miliary tuberculosis. An autopsy was performed, in the course of which the knee joint was opened and photographed.

B, Photograph of the right elbow joint removed at autopsy in the case of a 69-year-old man who died 6 months after he was admitted to our hospital. The cause of death was generalized miliary tuberculosis. In the course of the autopsy, the right elbow joint was removed *in toto*, along with 3 inches of the distal end of the humerus and 2 inches of the proximal end of the radius and of the ulna. The capsule of the joint was opened, and that part of the capsule which encircles the head of the radius was found thickened, as was the synovial membrane. The synovial membrane lining the posterior part of the elbow joint was also affected. Note that the articular cartilage of the head of the radius, as well as the cartilage of the contiguous part of the humerus, present evidence of erosion. Much of the regional cartilage of the humerus was found loosened from the subchondral bone, as a result of granulation tissue on the deep surface of the cartilage. The articular cartilage lining the trochlea of the ulna also showed evidences of erosion. Histologic study of tissue removed from various areas of the joint established the presence of tuberculous inflammation.

C and *D*, Photographs of the cut surface of the patella shown in *E*. The lesional area is a tuberculoma which had broken out of the bone and infected the synovial membrane of the knee joint.

E, Roentgenograph of the left knee joint in the case to which reference was made in *C* and *D*. The clinical record of the patient, a man who was 36 years of age at the time of his admission to our hospital, indicates that he had pain and swelling of the knee, and that the complaints had set in spontaneously. The knee was aspirated, and about 80 cc. of turbid yellowish fluid were removed. About 6 weeks later, the patella and some of the capsule of the joint were excised. An arthrodesis of the joint, through the use of a sliding bone graft placed across the joint anteriorly, was carried out. Histologic examination of the tissue established the diagnosis of tuberculosis of the knee joint. Two years after the surgical intervention, roentgenographic examination revealed complete bony fusion of the knee joint.

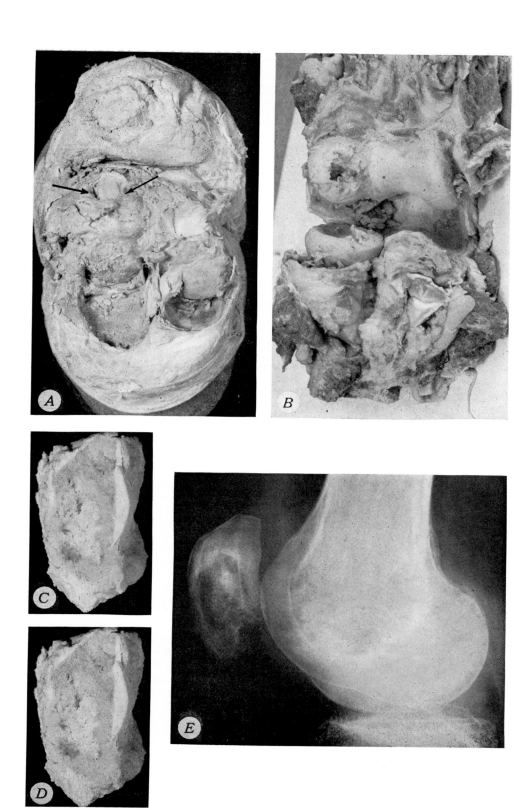

Figure 256

these countries. On the other hand, among Chinese, as stated by Hsieh *et al.*, tuberculosis of bone shafts is encountered more frequently, and comprised 4.8 per cent of 786 cases of skeletal tuberculosis treated between 1921 and 1932 at their hospital in Peiping.

A tuberculous lesion taking its departure in the shaft of a long bone may show close similarity (clinically and roentgenographically) to the inflammatory lesions induced in bones by pyogenic bacteria. For this reason, errors in differential clinical diagnosis may easily arise. It is often only by histologic and/or bacteriologic examination of tissue or pus from the lesion in question that its tuberculous basis is established. Destructive tuberculous diaphysial lesions have also been described which, because of their acuteness and extensiveness, were at first thought to be the result of pyogenic infection (see Drevermann, and also Gralka).

Figure 257

A, Photograph showing the cut surface of the *right* foot and ankle region of a boy who was 11 years of age at the time of an amputation through the lower third of the leg. The amputation was carried out during his fourth admission to our hospital. On his first admission, 21 months before the amputation of the right foot, he had had swelling of the *left* ankle joint and of the *left* big toe (metatarsophalangeal joint area), and both of these areas were aspirated. The aspirated material was inoculated into 2 guinea pigs, and both of them developed tuberculosis. During that first admission, there was already some clinical indication that a lesion was also present in the *right* foot, and the subsequent amputation was done because the ankle area had become enlarged to about twice the normal size. Immediately over the internal malleolus there was a granulating ulcer measuring about 1½ inches in diameter; below and behind that malleolus was another granulating ulcer about 1 inch in diameter. Clinical examination revealed a draining sinus on the outer aspect of the ankle, immediately above and behind the external malleolus, and also a draining sinus immediately below the external malleolus. The specimen was cut in the sagittal plane, through the web between the second and third toes, and showed that practically the entire calcaneus was involved. In some places this bone was sclerotic, and in other places it was softened and cystified. The cystic areas were filled with pus and granulation tissue. The infection extended into the posterior tubercle of the talus and also into the posterior part of the tibiotalar joint. Liberal sectioning of half of the foot showed that the inflammatory changes had extended into the fascial planes and tendon spaces about the ankle region. The clinically evident ulcerations were the result of spread of the tuberculous infection from the bone and joint regions and from the other foci of soft-tissue involvement.

B, Roentgenograph of part of the right foot taken 11 months before that foot (shown in *A*) was amputated. The focus of tuberculosis in the calcaneus presents as a large area of somewhat loculated radiolucency. The soft-tissue mass oriented to the superior surface of the os calcis reflects the spread of the tuberculous lesion from the calcaneus to the soft tissues around the Achilles tendon and to the local subcutaneous tissues, as is also evident in *A*.

C, Roentgenograph showing the distal end of the radius and the ulna, the carpal bones, and the proximal ends of the metacarpal bones of the left upper extremity. The abnormalities apparent in the picture were proved to have their basis in a tuberculous infection. The patient, a man, was 30 years of age at the time of admission to our hospital. When he was 25 years old, he was hospitalized at another institution for treatment of chronic pulmonary tuberculosis. About a year later he was discharged, because it was thought that his pulmonary tuberculosis was arrested. His clinical record at our hospital indicates that, about 1 year before admission, he had struck his left wrist with a hammer, but that, even before the injury, he already had some difficulty relating to that wrist area. After the injury, a swelling developed which slowly increased in size and eventually interfered with the use of the wrist. A surgical intervention was undertaken which consisted of resection of the flexor tendons of the palm and fingers. Lesional tissue was curetted from the affected part of the lower end of the radius. On gross examination, the tissues revealed the presence of minute tubercles, and histologic examination confirmed the diagnosis of tuberculosis.

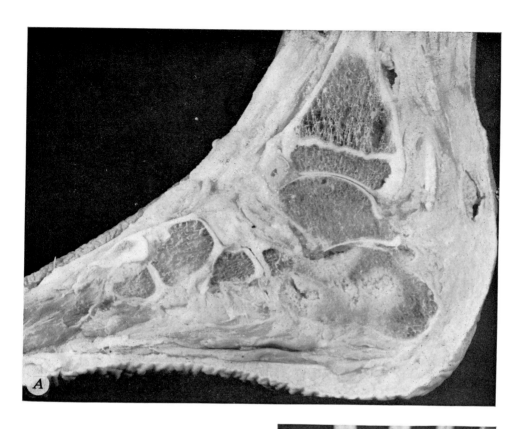

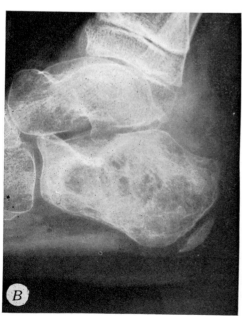

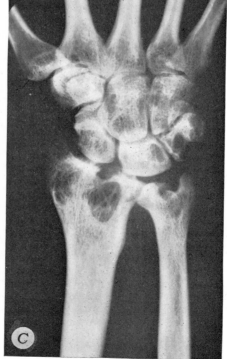

Figure 257

Most cases of tuberculosis starting in a bone shaft take one of the two following pathologic forms: (1) They may present as solitary metaphysial foci which are more or less circumscribed, destructive lesions, usually located centrally in or near the metaphysis, and simulating a pyogenic osteomyelitic abscess; or (2) diaphysial tuberculosis may take the form of diffuse lesions involving the medulla and cortex of one fourth to one half of the shaft of the bone. When the diaphysis is involved, scattered areas of bone destruction and periosteal new bone formation are present,

Figure 258

A, Roentgenograph showing a tuberculous lytic lesion in the region of the right sacroiliac joint. The patient, a woman 45 years of age, was admitted to the hospital with a 6-month history of pain in the buttock, and the pain also radiated down the right thigh and leg. Note that the joint space is narrowed, and that the margin of the iliac bone entering into the formation of the sacroiliac joint is moderately eburnated. The roentgenograph was interpreted as reflecting either tuberculosis of the sacroiliac joint or (less probably) a focus of metastatic carcinoma. The patient died about 1 year after this picture was taken, but an autopsy was not performed.

B, Roentgenograph of the left hip joint showing an area of radiolucency in the region of the greater trochanter of the femur. The patient was a man 36 years of age whose clinical record indicates that when he was 19 years old he contracted pulmonary tuberculosis, and that when he was 31 years old the pulmonary tuberculosis was considered cured. A few days after his admission to our hospital, a surgical intervention was carried out. This consisted of excision of a sinus tract and abscess cavity in the soft tissues in the region of the greater trochanter, and also of removal of some bone from the trochanter itself. Histologic examination of the excised tissue revealed the presence of a tuberculous abscess in the greater trochanter and also tubercles in the skin around the opening of the sinus tract.

C, Roentgenograph of the right elbow joint region in the case of a man 39 years of age. His clinical record shows that, 7 months before, he twisted his right upper extremity while bowling, struck his elbow against the side of a table, and the elbow became very painful. The severe pain subsided, but mild, aching pain persisted, and the elbow region swelled. The roentgenograph, taken the day after the patient was admitted to our hospital, discloses the presence of an active process which had destroyed the articular surface of the ulna, caused irregular erosion of the subchondral cortex of the humerus, and destruction of the proximal end of the radius. An arthrotomy, carried out a week after admission, revealed inflammatory tissue within the joint space. This tissue was excised and the upper end of the radius was removed. The specimen consisted of some fragments of scarred and inflamed noncaseous tissue, and a number of fragments of obviously inflamed cortical and spongy bone. These latter fragments included the head of the radius, whose articular cartilage had been completely eroded and whose spongiosa had clearly been infected. Microscopic examination of sections prepared from the excised nonosseous tissue revealed the presence of numerous tubercles. The fragments of bone also showed evidence of tuberculosis.

D, Roentgenograph of part of a right hand and forearm in the lateral projection. On the dorsal surface of the hand, in the region of the carpal bones, there is a large oval shadow representing a tuberculous tenosynovitis. The clinical record of the patient, a woman 30 years of age at the time of her admission to our hospital, indicates that for 3 years a painful swelling had been present on the dorsum of her right hand, and the swelling had gradually increased during the third year. The patient was also unable to extend her fingers completely. Physical examination showed the presence of small, nontender lymph nodes in each axilla. The skin over the mass on the dorsum of the wrist was freely movable. Palpation of the mass revealed that it was circumscribed, multilocular, and fluctuant. The lesional area was explored surgically and when the mass was incised a large number of rice bodies were removed. It was also noted that the common digital extensor tendons were frayed, and in the further course of the surgery the distended tendon sheath was excised. The surgical specimen consisted of several pieces of tissue, all of which, when fitted together, formed a structure about as big as a large egg. Histologic examination disclosed the presence of caseous and noncaseous tubercles, and the diagnosis was clearly tuberculous tenosynovitis.

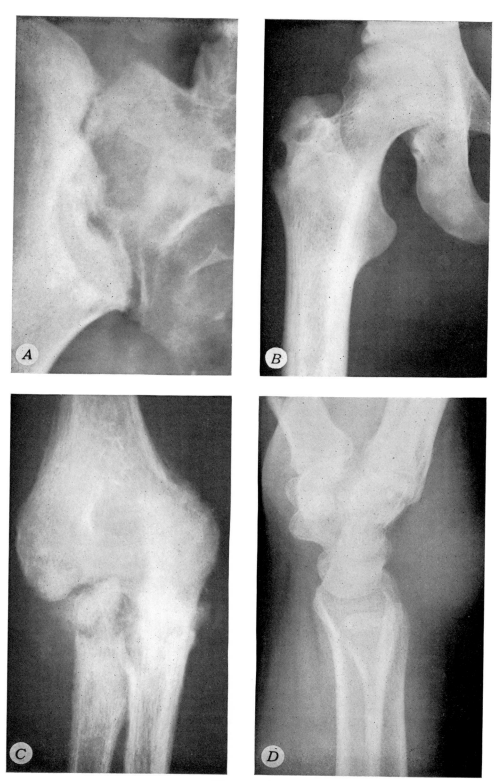

Figure 258

and the changes resemble chronic pyogenic osteomyelitis without circumscribed abscess formation. Some of the cases falling within these two groups represent transition forms between the two. This was shown by Hsieh *et al.*, who attempted to classify the various types of shaft tuberculosis on the basis of roentgenographic appearances.

More rarely, as described by Van Gorder, diaphysial tuberculosis induces swelling and cyst formation in the shaft of a long tubular bone. The cases of multiple cystic tuberculosis of long tubular bones reported by Van Alstyne and Gowen, and also by Sanes and Smith, seem to belong in this category. In the cases showing swelling and cysts, the cortex becomes thickened as a result of periosteal new bone formation, but it is also rarefied. One or more large abscesses containing sequestra may occupy the central portion of the diaphysis of a bone so diseased. Endosteal new bone formation frequently obliterates the medullary cavity about the abscesses. When the condition is in an advanced stage, the soft tissues adjacent to the bone

Figure 259

A, Roentgenograph showing a tuberculous lesion in the distal half of the shaft of the left ulna. The picture reveals rarefaction of the cortex in the involved area of the ulna, and the presence of a thin layer of periosteal new bone on the modified cortex. The patient, a boy 4 years of age, had had swollen glands on the right side of the neck for about $2\frac{1}{2}$ years before his admission to our hospital. The difficulties relating to his left arm set in about 1 week prior to admission. At that time his arm had been twisted by a playmate. Since then, he had had pain in the region of the wrist, and slight swelling, local heat, and tenderness of the affected area of the forearm. The child also had some fever and appeared acutely ill. Since aspiration of the implicated part of the forearm yielded no fluid, a decision was made to carry out a biopsy on the ulna. The specimen submitted for anatomic examination consisted of several slivers of cortical bone. Adherent to the inner surface of the fragments of bone were tiny bits of yellowish tissue. All of the tissue was processed for histologic examination, and some of the tissue slides showed tubercles oriented to the bone. About 2 weeks after the surgery, the child was transferred to another hospital, where he soon showed signs of cerebral irritation and stiffness of the neck. He became delirious, went into coma, and died. An autopsy was not performed, but it seems highly probable that the cause of death was disseminated miliary tuberculosis.

B, Roentgenograph of part of the right fibula and tibia showing abnormalities relating to the fibula. The cortex of part of the shaft of the fibula is thickened and somewhat rarefied, and also presents a layer of subperiosteal new bone on the modified cortex. The patient was a woman 22 years of age who was admitted to our hospital because of pain and swelling in the right leg of 2 months' duration. Her complaints began about a week after she had injured the leg, and became aggravated by a subsequent minor injury. She walked with a right-leg limp and, in the course of walking, tended to rotate that leg externally. Her clinical record also indicates that, for about 1 year before admission, she had night sweats and bronchitis, representing evidence of a pre-existing tuberculous infection. About 1 week after her admission, a surgical intervention was carried out, and approximately 6 inches of the fibular shaft were resected. In the midportion of the specimen, the shaft was found somewhat expanded. The specimen was cut in its long axis. The cut surface revealed thickening of the cortex as a result of deposition of a moderate amount of subperiosteal new bone. In the medullary cavity the tissue was glistening and of whitish color, and tended to be slightly mucoid in consistency. Histologic examination established the diagnosis of tuberculosis (see *C*).

C, Photomicrograph ($\times$ 30) illustrating the histologic pattern of the pathologic changes in the fibula. The cortical bone in the upper part of the picture shows enlargement of some of the haversian canals, which are filled with inflammatory tissue faintly suggesting the pattern of tubercles. In the medullary cavity, and especially on the left side of the picture, there are numerous discrete and agglomerated tubercles. The cortical bone in the lower part of the picture discloses tubercles extending from the medullary cavity and perforating the cortex. Significant follow-up information concerning this patient is not available.

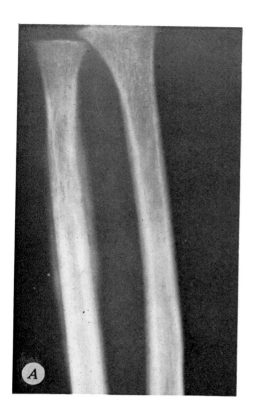

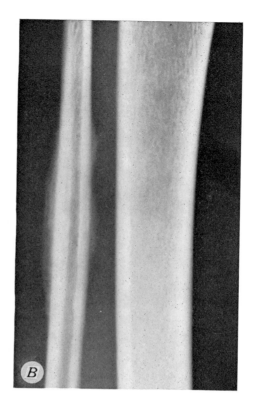

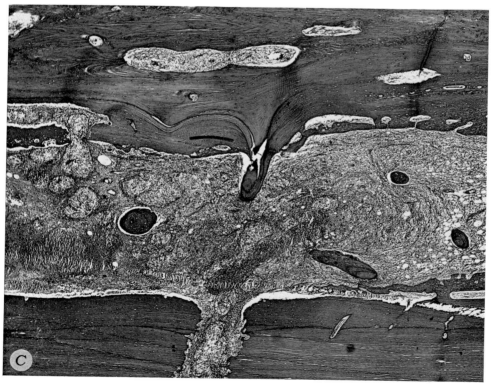

Figure 259

may become involved. In 5 of the 6 cases reported by Van Gorder, radical excision of the diseased bone area was followed by complete cure. In an instance of cystic tuberculosis of several long bones in an infant 1 year of age, the tuberculous lesions gradually underwent spontaneous resolution (see Schwentker).

Very exceptionally, tuberculosis of a bone shaft may be manifested merely by a periostitis, as pointed out by Allison, among others. Roentgenographically, such tuberculous lesions may closely resemble those of bone syphilis or possibly even osteogenic sarcoma. The differential diagnosis in such cases can be established only by histologic examination of tissue. (See Fig. 259.)

Tuberculosis of the bones of the fingers and toes, resulting in *spina ventosa*, seems to appear almost solely in early childhood, and the condition is observed about 5 times as often in the hands as in the feet (see Bailleul). From half to two thirds of the cases in which spina ventosa is present also show other foci of skeletal tuberculosis. An affected *phalanx* usually reveals a thin and expanded cortex, which may even be perforated in places. Some periosteal new bone formation may also be evident. The marrow cavity of such a bone usually contains considerable tuberculous granulation tissue. Varying amounts of nonspecific granulation tissue may also be present, however. The tuberculous tissue often extends through and beyond the cortex and periosteum, appearing in the neighboring soft tissues and fascia. Furthermore, the tuberculous granulation tissue may pierce the articular cartilage and enter the joint. Not infrequently, pyogenic infection supervenes to complicate the clinical and pathologic findings. Even when this happens, resolution of the lesions sometimes takes place in the course of several years.

Data concerning the frequency of spina ventosa show variations, and many of the larger statistical compilations omit the condition entirely. However, Johansson reported that spina ventosa was present in about one fifth of the cases of skeletal tuberculosis appearing before the age of 15. This extremely high proportion is due in part to the fact that he included as a separate case each finger or toe that showed tuberculous dactylitis, and in part to the peculiarities relating to localization of skeletal tuberculosis in the geographical area from which his report emanated.

In most of the cases recorded in the older literature, the subjects presenting spina ventosa were almost always very young children. Possibly its occurrence at this age was related to the early dissemination of the tuberculous infection. In the United States, the tendency to very early primary infection, and hence to its early generalized spread, has become less and less pronounced. This fact may help to explain the discrepancies in different reports concerning the incidence of spina ventosa in relation to tuberculosis in other skeletal sites. Certainly, in the United States, spina ventosa was not observed often. In our hospital, it comprised a very small percentage of all the cases of skeletal tuberculosis.

Tuberculosis involves the *metacarpals* more frequently than the *metatarsals*, but neither of these sites is implicated so often as are the phalanges. (See Fig. 260.) The clinical diagnosis of tuberculosis of the metacarpal and metatarsal bones is difficult, and can often be made only by means of histologic examination of a tissue specimen from the affected bone (see McMaster and King).

Though the *skull* is not one of the common sites, tuberculosis in that area is not rare in geographical regions where tuberculosis is common (see Barton). It is particularly the *calvarium* that is likely to be affected. Calvarial tuberculosis is much more often observed in children between the ages of 1 and 10 than in infants, adults, or elderly people. The predominance of children among the patients is generally ascribed to the frequency of trauma to the head in this age group. The tuberculosis of the flat bones of the calvarium often leads to serious complications. Erdheim pointed out that, in adults, the lesions of calvarial tuberculosis, in contrast to those of calvarial syphilis, are more extensive on the inner than on the outer surface of the cranial vault. Thus a relatively small defect on the outer surface of the calvarium may be associated with very extensive erosions on the inner surface. Large erosion cavities may contain sequestra, and a tuberculous pachymeningitis may spread the infection to the brain. If, on the other hand, the tuberculosis is localized in the *infra-orbital margin*, for instance, the condition may be without pronounced clinical manifestations, and may never require hospitalization. In relation to the *upper jaw*, tumor-like swellings of tuberculous origin have been described (see Bronner and Krumbein). In such cases the diagnosis is often first made on the basis of histologic examination of a biopsy specimen. Instances of tuberculosis of the *mastoid bone* have also been described (see Battaglia).

As to *healing*, it is often difficult to decide clinically whether a focus of skeletal tuberculosis is merely in a latent stage or has healed. It may be years before the lesion reaches either stage, but spontaneous recurrence is nevertheless possible. Recurrence may be defined as the local reactivation of a focus which had become latent or had apparently healed. The presence of necrotic foci or sequestra tends to delay and interfere with healing, and a secondary pyogenic infection may also hinder healing. Under particularly favorable conditions, however, virtually complete spontaneous healing can occur. This is especially likely to take place if the tuberculosis is limited to the synovial membrane or at least has not destroyed much bone.

In joints in which the articular ends have been involved, healing proceeds mainly through the development of fibrous ankylosis, and fibrous adhesions come to bind the articular surfaces. The eroded articular cartilages are not regenerated, and ultimately some degree of bony ankylosis may take place. The tendency to healing is greater in children than in adults. In the presence of ankylosis, the infection enters a quiescent stage rather than a state of healing. This was illustrated in an instance of tuberculous coxitis observed by the present writer. In that case the infection was latent for many years, during which the only clinical complaint was stiffness of the hip. Surgical correction of the difficulty was attempted. This led to reactivation and subsequent dissemination of the tuberculous infection, and death from miliary tuberculosis ensued within a few months.

The clearest examples of healing in skeletal tuberculosis are observed in cases of tuberculous spondylitis. The intervertebral disks never regenerate, but healing by actual bony fusion of adjacent diseased bodies may ultimately take place. Thus, it is possible to encounter healed tuberculous spondylitides in which several vertebral bodies are solidly fused into a single large block. The anatomic divisions between the original bodies are completely obliterated or are indicated only by remnants of intervertebral disk tissue. However, the repair and healing of the tuberculous process are usually not complete. Under these circumstances, some residua of the disease (in the form of caseous-calcareous foci) are often to be found in the fused vertebral bodies. The perifocal osteosclerosis that was originally present about the abscesses recedes or disappears in the course of healing of the spondylitis.

It may be worthy of note that, in vertebral columns showing a lumbar lordosis secondary to a thoracic kyphosis, the lumbar vertebrae are likely to be distinctly taller than they would normally be. This increased height appears to be a compensation for the kyphosis. It can occur only in the vertebral columns of young subjects, since, in them, longitudinal growth of the vertebral bodies is still possible. Such lengthening of the lumbar bodies is found not only with tuberculous spondylitis but with kyphotic deformity of the thoracic region caused by other conditions.

Tendon Sheaths and Bursae. — *Tuberculous tenosynovitis* is not frequently encountered. As to *age incidence*, most of the affected subjects are between 20 and 50 years of age. In respect to *localization*, it has been reported that in the *hand* the volar tendon sheaths at the wrist are as likely to be affected as the dorsal tendon sheaths. In addition, especially if the volar sheaths are involved, the tendon sheaths of one or more fingers may also be implicated. In regard to *sex incidence*, tuberculous tenosynovitis occurs in both males and females, but the specific sex ratio seems to vary somewhat from institution to institution. In Felländer's experience, the condition was somewhat more common among females, while others have observed it somewhat more frequently in males (see Bickel *et al.*). In females, the volar sheaths are more often affected, while in males it is the dorsal sheaths that are more often implicated. (See Fig. 258-*D*.)

Furthermore, even in the absence of involvement of the volar or dorsal tendon sheaths at the wrist, tuberculous tenosynovitis limited to the sheaths of one or more flexor tendons of the fingers may be encountered. In the region of the *foot*, an occasional instance of tuberculous tenosynovitis is observed in which the dorsiflexor sheath at the ankle is affected (see Pimm and Waugh). In a large percentage of the cases of tuberculous tenosynovitis, the subjects have had tuberculosis in some other site—most often the lungs. However, the temporal relationship between the development of the tuberculous tenosynovitis and the associated tuberculous infection at some other site is not clearly established. The *treatment* of the tenosynovitis in any site should consist of thorough surgical resection and complete removal of the infected tendon sheath. Appropriate chemotherapy is also imperative. Indeed, the chemotherapy should be started even before the surgery is undertaken, and continued for several months thereafter (see Pitzler).

Tuberculous bursitis may occur even without involvement of a regional bone or joint. In relation to the hip area, the occurrence of tuberculosis involving the trochanteric bursa, without implication of the underlying bone, is well established. The writer has seen several cases of this type. He has also examined tissue from an instance of tuberculosis of the subdeltoid bursa. In that case, too, there was no evidence of involvement of the regional bone or bones.

Extraskeletal Tuberculous Lesions with Concomitant Skeletal Lesions.—It is known that when a focus of skeletal tuberculosis appears, other tuberculous lesions are usually present elsewhere in the body. Most often, the lesion already existing

Figure 260

A and *B*, Roentgenographs of the hands of a child about 10 years of age who was affected with tuberculous dactylitis. In each hand the first metacarpal bone is expanded and presents focal areas of rarefaction. The distal phalanx of the thumb of the right hand is also implicated, and the proximal phalanx of the index finger discloses involvement not only of its shaft but also of its epiphysis. The shaft of the middle phalanx of the fifth finger of the left hand is apparently also implicated. As is usual in tuberculous dactylitis in children, many of the short tubular bones have become affected. The clinical record in this case indicates that the tuberculous dactylitis had already been present for about 1 year. The diagnosis was established by examination of tissue obtained by a needle biopsy of the proximal phalanx of the right index finger.

C, Photograph of an amputated finger (the third finger of the right hand), cut in the sagittal plane, from another case of tuberculous dactylitis. The subject was a boy 15 years of age. The proximal phalanx has been almost completely replaced by tuberculous granulation tissue, and the inflammatory process has broken out of the bone into the overlying soft tissues and made pressure on the flexor tendon of the finger.

D, Photograph of the cut surface of the costal cartilage of the third *left* rib and the articulating part of the sternum (upper picture). The costosternal articulation of the third *right* rib is shown in the lower picture. Both costosternal junctions were the sites of cold abscesses, as is evident from the distention of the local articular cavities. The subject was a man 32 years of age who died of advanced pulmonary tuberculosis.

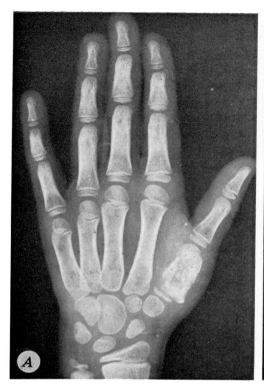
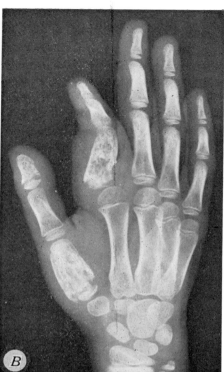
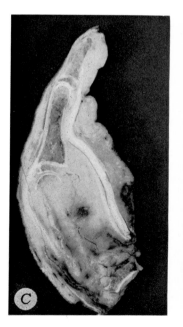
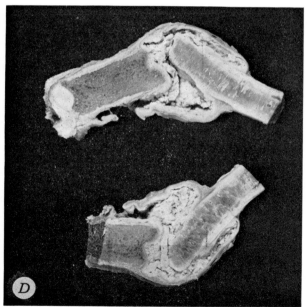

Figure 260

is merely the nonclinical so-called *primary complex*. Thus, if death should occur from accident or intercurrent infection in a case of skeletal tuberculosis, especially in childhood, postmortem examination will ordinarily not reveal two fully evolved clinical forms of tuberculosis. Instead, one will find, as a rule, only the lesions of a primary complex (most often within the thorax), in addition to the principal tuberculous lesion in the skeleton. In children, a healed intrathoracic primary complex is often demonstrable roentgenographically. In nonmoribund adult patients with skeletal tuberculosis, *chronic pulmonary tuberculosis* is sometimes present. The actual frequency of this combination of involved sites is somewhat difficult to evaluate. Certainly the two conditions (pulmonary and skeletal tuberculosis) are not found together so often as are skeletal tuberculosis and an intrathoracic primary complex.

Among subjects with skeletal tuberculosis admitted to an orthopaedic service, those also affected with *chronic* pulmonary tuberculosis are relatively few. On the other hand, it is striking that, despite the previous widespread occurrence of tuberculosis of the lungs, skeletal tuberculosis was infrequent among those patients affected with pulmonary tuberculosis. However, the pulmonary specialist may be inclined to overestimate the frequency of lung tuberculosis among patients with skeletal tuberculosis, since he, of course, sees instances of skeletal tuberculosis which are complicated by pulmonary tuberculosis. In contrast, the orthopaedic surgeon tends rather to underestimate the frequency of the association, since patients with skeletal tuberculosis who are also suffering from *active* pulmonary tuberculosis are not likely to come to his attention.

In any group of patients in whom the two conditions are associated, it will be found that, more often than not, the skeletal tuberculosis has preceded the pulmonary involvement. Pulmonary tuberculosis complicating skeletal tuberculosis is observed more frequently in adults than in children, and the pulmonary lesions are more often in a state of fibrosis or healing than in an active state. Where the pulmonary disease is florid, it is important to determine whether it antedated or followed the onset of the skeletal lesion. Jacquemin regarded the development of a tuberculous skeletal lesion in the course of pulmonary tuberculosis as a favorable factor, and he considered the prognosis unfavorable if the pulmonary lesion followed the osseous lesion. Furthermore, as has been recognized for a long time and especially stressed by Fishberg, in patients in whom the pulmonary tuberculosis shows a strong tendency toward healing, dormant skeletal lesions sometimes flare up. Conversely, the observation has been made that when the skeletal lesion heals, a fibrotic pulmonary focus is likely to be reactivated.

There are many *statistical studies* bearing upon the pulmonary findings in patients with skeletal tuberculosis. Thus, in analyzing 27 cases of skeletal involvement in children, Dietl found that 21 had no clinical evidence of pulmonary tuberculosis. Of the other 6 cases, only 2 showed a coexistence of florid pulmonary and florid skeletal lesions. Schaafhausen, investigating roentgenographically 100 cases of skeletal tuberculosis in children and adolescents, found no intrathoracic lesions in 24, only a primary pulmonary complex in 46, a healed (fibrotic) pulmonary process of some extent in 24, and florid pulmonary changes in only 6.

Progress of the Disease with Respect to Morbidity and Mortality.—The highest degree of morbidity and the highest mortality rates occur in association with tuberculous spondylitis, coxitis, and gonitis. Tuberculous spondylitis has the gravest prognosis because of the burrowing abscesses and long-standing suppuration often encountered in this condition. In relation to the mortality statistics, it is also important to consider the different methods of treatment (surgery, conservative treatment, chemotherapy, heliotherapy, etc.).

Years ago, Johansson reported a mortality rate of 22 per cent for skeletal tuberculosis in children under 15 years of age. That relatively high death rate was probably related to the fact that a large proportion of the affected subjects were below the age of 5. The mortality rate for skeletal tuberculosis at ages below 3 years was notoriously high everywhere. It was lowest when the skeletal tuberculosis was acquired late in childhood, in adolescence, or in early adult life; later in adult life, the rate rose again, more or less steadily.

It may be very difficult to evaluate the role of the skeletal lesion *per se* in the fatal outcome in a given case. Often all that can be concluded, even after careful postmortem examination, is that the skeletal lesion appears to be directly or indirectly a factor in the death. By far the most common causes of death in cases of skeletal tuberculosis are tuberculous meningitis, miliary tuberculosis, amyloid degeneration of the internal organs, and chronic pulmonary tuberculosis. Very often, generalized miliary tuberculosis and tuberculous meningitis occur together. Thus the immediate cause of death is frequently an extraskeletal tuberculous lesion, or some other complicating factor.

Of the causes of death mentioned above, *tuberculous meningitis* is the most frequent. As a rule, it sets in within a year after the onset of the skeletal lesion. As a complication, it occurs particularly in young children. Generalized *miliary tuberculosis*, too, tends to occur especially in young children, not very long after the skeletal lesion has become evident. As to *amyloid infiltration* of the internal organs, this was, in the past, often a complication, and not infrequently was the immediate cause of death. Many years may intervene, however, between the onset of the skeletal tuberculosis and death from amyloidosis, which is directly related to long-standing suppuration. Infection with other bacteria may be superimposed, and the presence of fistulae permits continued drainage of the pus. In cases of skeletal tuberculosis with a fatal outcome, *chronic pulmonary tuberculosis* is also not at all infrequent, and is observed more often in adults than in children. The time relationship between the two lesions is often difficult to establish. One should bear in mind, however, that the chronic pulmonary tuberculosis may appear concurrently with the skeletal tuberculosis, or even antedate it.

In cases of generalized miliary tuberculosis, especially in *infants* and *young children*, tubercles in various quantities are almost always present in the *myeloid portions of the bone marrow*, particularly in the vertebrae, the ribs, the sternum, and the epiphyses of long tubular bones. Not infrequently, they can also be located in the synovial membranes, especially of large joints. In *adults*, however, tubercles are not so widely disseminated and are found mainly in the marrow of the vertebral bodies and ribs. The basis for the great susceptibility of the myeloid marrow to tubercle formation is not yet clearly known. Because of the rapidly fatal outcome in cases of generalized miliary tuberculosis, there are no distinctive clinical manifestations so far as the skeleton is concerned.

Such tubercles as are formed are rarely recognizable with the naked eye. So far as their microscopic features are concerned, Huebschmann states that the lesions range from tiny circumscribed areas of marrow necrosis (areas of "primary tissue damage") to the completely typical epithelioid cell tubercles showing central necrosis. Tschistowitsch and Winogradow and others, however, have been unable to find areas of necrosis or primary tissue damage preceding the formation of tubercles. The tubercles are usually separated from the neighboring bone trabeculae by unmodified marrow. The spongy trabeculae do not show erosion or necrosis unless the tubercles abut against them.

In fatal cases of *extra-osseous tuberculosis* (especially pulmonary tuberculosis), miliary tubercles are sometimes present in the myeloid marrow of the bones. However, if such tubercles are formed at all, they are demonstrable only microscopically, and are usually scant and scattered. As stressed by Randerath, it may be necessary to examine the marrow of many bones to find the tubercles, which tend to be discrete and composed mainly of epithelioid cells. Ordinarily, their presence is not associated with significant changes in the neighboring spongy trabeculae. Randerath reported that he observed tubercles in the bone marrow in 18 of 22 cases of chronic extraskeletal tuberculosis, mainly pulmonary.

Gelatinous degeneration of the fatty marrow is a frequent accompaniment of chronic organ tuberculosis, especially pulmonary, although its exact incidence is not known (see Michael). However, it is not specific for tuberculosis, since it occurs with other conditions, such as cirrhosis of the liver. Droplet degeneration of the fat cells of the marrow, sometimes to the point of complete destruction of these cells, has also been observed in patients dying of chronic pulmonary tuberculosis (see Ponfick).

TREATMENT

Perhaps the most important single factor in determining appropriate therapeutic procedure in an individual case is the location of the tuberculous lesion. Tuberculous spina ventosa is ordinarily treated conservatively; tuberculosis of the shaft of a long tubular bone may warrant radical excision of the diseased area. In tuberculous spondylitis, the treatment may be: (1) conservative (bed rest, immobilization, and chemotherapy) and/or (2) surgical (decompression, grafting, or fusion), along with pre- and postoperative chemotherapy. In either case, the treatment is directed toward the prevention or reduction of deformities and the supporting of the diseased area to stimulate healing (see Friedman, Brackett *et al.*, Freund, Bakalim, Cleveland *et al.*, Arct, Kohli, Goel, and also Funk *et al.*).

SARCOIDOSIS

Sarcoidosis is a disease of unknown etiology, characterized pathologically by the presence of epithelioid tubercles which do not tend to undergo necrosis even if they agglomerate. The tubercles may appear in any organ or tissue, and not infrequently their giant cells reveal the presence of laminated and apparently calcified bodies. Roentgenographic examination of the chest is likely to show the presence of striated and/or spotty shadows radiating from the hilus of the lungs. In cases of Boeck's sarcoid (also designated as lupus pernio), lesions are frequently present in the bones, the phalanges in particular being affected. The skeletal lesions may be well developed even when the cutaneous manifestations are so slight as to escape notice except under careful observation. Thus it is that we sometimes encounter, as stressed by Jüngling, cases in which the skeletal lesions precede the cutaneous lesions or develop entirely without accompanying cutaneous lesions.

The possibility of the existence of skeletal lesions of the sarcoid type without a related condition in the skin is corroborated in an instance observed by the present writer. The subject was a girl 8 years old who suffered from a chronic multiple joint affection. Several tendon sheaths and synovial membranes were removed at different times. Histologically these tissues showed changes characteristic of sarcoidosis. The unusual feature of the case was the fact that neither the skin nor the bones were involved. Sundelin described a pertinent case in which the subject was 14 years of age. Roentgenographic examination of the lungs revealed the nodular mottling typical of sarcoidosis. In addition, the patient presented chronic swelling of the parotid glands and of the submandibular lymph glands. Examination of the blood revealed the presence of eosinophilia and monocytosis. In that case, too, lesions in the skin and bones were entirely lacking.

CLINICAL CONSIDERATIONS

Incidence.—Sarcoidosis is by no means a rare disease in the United States. The highest concentration of cases in this country is in the eastern part, and particularly in the southeast. Statistical findings relating to age, sex, and race indicate that: (1) More than half of the subjects are young adults; (2) males are more often affected than females; (3) Negroes definitely predominate among the subjects; and (4) the disease seems to be rare among the Chinese.

Clinical Complaints and Findings.—Despite the fact that sarcoidosis was originally delineated as a disease complex on the basis of its dermal manifestations, it is now accepted that, in many cases, lesions in the skin are absent at the time the presence of the disease is discovered. By far the most common complaints relate to the respiratory tract. In particular, they are cough, pain in the chest, and dyspnea, and result from the presence of sarcoid granulomata involving the hilar lymph nodes and the pulmonary parenchyma. Moreover, there are subjects affected with the disease who are asymptomatic but in whom roentgenographic examination of the chest already reveals abnormalities characteristic of sarcoidosis (see Bacharach). The nonrespiratory manifestations of the disease include: malaise, loss of weight, spindle-shaped enlargement of the fingers and/or toes, ocular abnormalities (such as painless iritis and/or iridocyclitis), and, of course, dermal lesions. When dermal lesions are present they appear as discrete or agglomerated, flat or only slightly raised, reddish brown nodules. The lesions in the skin are usually asymptomatic, develop slowly, do not ulcerate, and often heal spontaneously. Their presence is generally associated with regional lymphadenopathy.

The initial involvement of the bones of the fingers and toes is usually ushered in by reddening of the skin, rather rapid swelling, and aching pains. There may also be slight fever. These initial acute changes regress to some degree, but the attacks recur from time to time. Eventually the affected fingers or toes show pronounced chronic swelling. The skin of these swollen parts manifests clear signs of lupus pernio (the sarcoid of Boeck). Trophic disturbances may also appear in the affected parts. In rare instances, mutilation (due to destruction especially of terminal phalanges) may be observed. In milder cases, however, swelling and thickening of fingers or toes sets in gradually and painlessly. When bones are involved, the periphalangeal soft tissues are very likely to be swollen and diseased, even if the skin does not become affected. (See Fig. 261.)

In sarcoidosis, the bones of the hands appear to be more severely, if not more often, affected than those of the feet. The distribution of the lesions tends to be more or less symmetrical. The proximal and middle phalanges of the fingers and toes are most likely to be involved. Next, in descending order of frequency, come the metacarpal bones, the terminal phalanges, and the metatarsal bones. Sometimes, though rather rarely, the carpal, tarsal, and nasal bones are affected. Very exceptionally, lesions of the sarcoid type have been reported to involve a long tubular bone. However, extreme caution is necessary before including in this category tubercle-like lesions in the long tubular bones. Such cases may represent merely instances of atypical diaphysial tuberculosis.

Clinical Laboratory Findings.—As to the *hematological findings*, it is to be noted that the hemoglobin level is occasionally below normal, and that the sedimentation rate of the blood is often elevated. The leukocyte count is likely to be within normal limits, but if the subject has fever, the count may be elevated—that is, there may be leukocytosis. A more frequent finding (representing a manifestation of hypersplenism) is leukopenia. In respect to the differential leukocyte count, a relative lymphocytosis is common, but has no diagnostic significance. On the other hand, the frequent finding of eosinophilia does have diagnostic significance (see Singer *et al.*, and also Bacharach).

In regard to the *blood chemistry findings* (and in particular the plasma protein values), a reduction in the serum albumin and an increase in the serum globulin can often be noted. Normally, the albumin value is higher than the globulin value. In sarcoidosis, the reduction in the serum albumin and the increase in the serum globulin results in a reversal of the normal albumin-globulin ratio of the serum.

In approximately 20 to 25 per cent of cases of sarcoidosis, hypercalcemia is present. Ordinarily the serum calcium values in these cases are only slightly or moderately above the normal figure, which is 10.0 ± 0.5 mg. per cent for adults and 11.0 ± 0.5 mg. per cent for children. In association with the hypercalcemia, there may be hypercalciuria. The serum phosphorus value is usually normal and, if elevated at all, is only slightly above the normal figure, which is 3.5 ± 0.5 mg. per cent for adults and 5.0 ± 0.5 mg. per cent for children. Even if a hypercalcemia is present, the normal or perhaps slightly elevated serum phosphorus value serves to negate the possibility that one is dealing with a case of hyperparathyroidism. The latter diagnosis is also controverted by the fact that, in sarcoidosis, the administration of cortisone reduces the hypercalcemia.

If the presence of hypercalcemia is not promptly recognized and the condition is not appropriately treated, the kidneys may undergo irreversible impairment, and/or the eyes may become severely and irreversibly damaged (see Goetz). In addition to the hypercalcemia, mineral balance studies have shown significant abnormalities relating to the metabolism of magnesium and phosphorus. Vitamin D depletion significantly improves the hypercalcemia, hypercalciuria, and negative calcium balance, while vitamin D in normal or excessive amounts aggravates the negative mineral balance (see Hendrix).

Biologic Skin Tests.—In sarcoidosis, the skin usually shows no reaction to the intracutaneous injection of *tuberculin* in the amounts used to ascertain the presence of a tuberculous infection. Tuberculin sensitivity testing by O.T. (old tuberculin) has been replaced by P.P.D. (purified protein derivative). P.P.D. is used in 3 dilutions: .00002 mg.; .0002 mg.; and .005 mg. In using P.P.D., 0.1 cc. of the weakest solution is injected intracutaneously, and the test is read in 48 hours. If the test result is negative, a retest is made with the strongest solution. A *negative tuberculin reaction* is important in arriving at the diagnosis of sarcoidosis. The skin is usually *hyposensitive* to tuberculin, even in high concentration. This anergy is considered as evidence of desensitization to tuberculin (see Sulzberger). Skin lesions should be searched for, but, as previously stated, they need not necessarily be present. Guinea pigs inoculated with lesional tissue from cases of sarcoidosis yield negative findings.

The *Kveim test* for sarcoidosis has proved to have a definite diagnostic value, though it presents certain difficulties and disadvantages. Wells and Halsted describe the Kveim test as follows: "The antigen is an aqueous Merthiolate suspen-

Figure 261

A and *B*, Roentgenographs of the hands and feet of a young woman who was admitted to our hospital because of pain and swelling of several fingers of both hands and the toes of both feet. The roentgenographic findings, the fact that the patient was a Negro, and the negative result of a test made with 3 dilutions of P.P.D. tuberculin led to the clinical conclusion that the changes in the hands and feet were ascribable to sarcoidosis. This diagnosis was supported by the presence of a number of small reddish papules on the woman's face, in accordance with what is commonly seen in cases of sarcoidosis. One of the papules on the face was excised, and some tissue was removed from the proximal phalanx of the index finger of the left hand. Microscopic examination of these tissue specimens confirmed the diagnosis of sarcoidosis. (See Fig. 262 and also Fig. 248-*B*.)

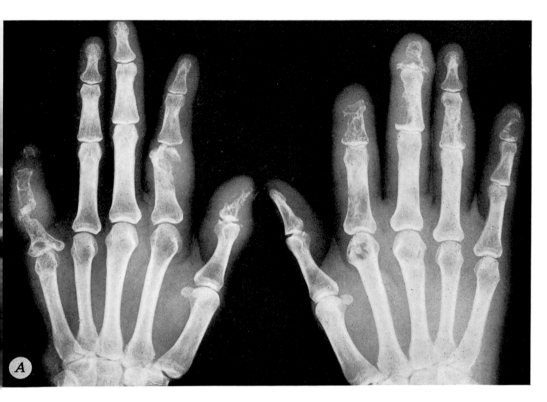

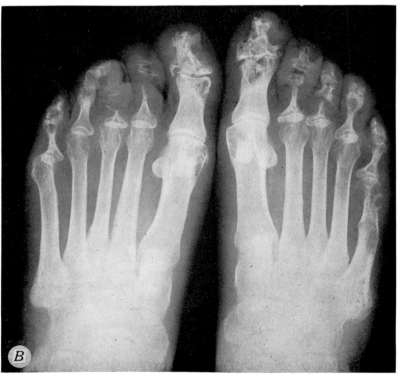

Figure 261

1007

sion of ground lymph node tissue known to contain the lesions of sarcoidosis. This material is checked for sterility and made up as a 10 per cent suspension for use in the test. An intradermal inoculation of 0.1 ml. is made in the same manner as for the tuberculin test. Patients are asked to return in six weeks, at which time the test site is excised for histologic examination. With a positive test, a characteristic papule develops which lasts for months and usually disappears in about a year. The gross appearance of the papule alone is probably not sufficient evidence of a positive reaction. Microscopic examination showing a tuberculoid lesion similar to that of cutaneous sarcoidosis is a more reliable criterion."

PATHOLOGIC AND ROENTGENOGRAPHIC FINDINGS

The *pathologic changes* in the bones are the result of the growth of granulomatous tissue, which is rather characteristic histologically. It is composed of discrete hyperplastic tubercles consisting mainly of epithelioid cells. Such quasi-tuberculous nodules may be bordered by lymphocytes and may even contain a few Langhans giant cells. However, it is distinctive of these tubercles that they do not show caseation. This type of tubercle, whether located in skin, bone, subcutaneous connective tissue, synovial membrane, bursae, tendon sheaths, or even internal organs (such as the lung), is diagnostically characteristic of sarcoidosis. (See Fig. 262.) In the case of lupus pernio with bone lesions which was described by Schürer-Waldheim, the histologic findings in the bone lesions were the same as those in the skin lesions. Rieder seems to have been the first to give a *roentgenographic description* of the bone lesions seen in lupus pernio. Jüngling later developed the subject further and designated the condition in the bones as *"ostitis tuberculosa multiplex cystica."*

Since phalanges are almost invariably affected, the *roentgenographic appearances* will be described as observed in these bones. The essential condition revealed by the roentgenograph is the presence of radiolucent areas within the involved bones. These areas of increased radiolucency may be distributed throughout the affected bone or may appear as discrete, circumscribed foci of rarefaction, especially in the phalangeal heads. Periosteal new bone formation does not occur, and the growth of the affected bones is not disturbed. Jüngling reported that the skeletal lesions, as revealed roentgenographically, are of two basic types—the *diffuse* and the *circumscribed*. Frequently, however, cases are seen in which the roentgenographic changes take an intermediate form. In the *diffuse* form the phalanges are likely to lose their normal dumbbell shape by becoming widened in their midportions. The cortex is diminished to a paper-thin shell. The demarcation between compacta and marrow space becomes obliterated. The head and diaphysis of the affected phalanx acquire a coarse, honeycomb appearance, the spaces being largest in the head of the bone, and the walls of the spaces are not delimited by perifocal sclerosis. There also

Figure 262

A, Photomicrograph ($\times$ 38) of tissue removed from the region of the proximal phalanx of the index finger of the left hand illustrated in Figure 261-*A*. Note the tubercles, many of which are agglomerated, and the absence of caseous necrosis. These findings support the diagnosis of sarcoidosis.

B, Photomicrograph ($\times$ 24) of tissue removed from the face of the woman referred to in *A* and in Figure 261. Note that the epithelium in the region of the papule is somewhat thinned. In the corium there is a granulomatous lesion which is composed of numerous round cells, epithelioid cells, other mononuclear elements, and an occasional multinuclear giant cell. The histologic pattern of this papule likewise supports the diagnosis of sarcoidosis.

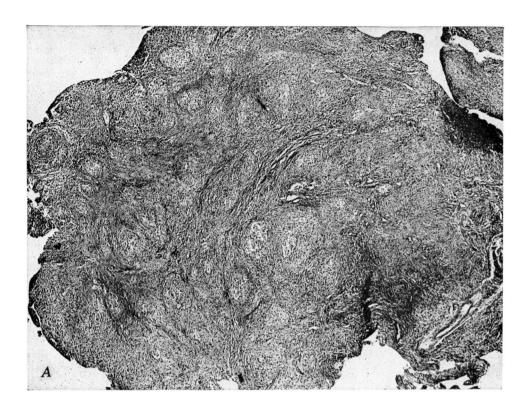

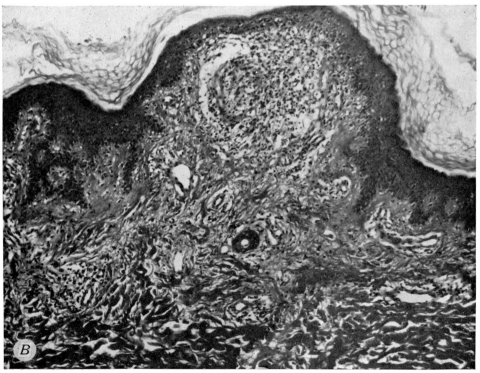

Figure 262

exists a variant of this diffuse form, characterized roentgenographically by diffuse, small, and spotty rarefactions. As in the diffuse form first described, there is obliteration of the normal architecture of the phalanx. In the *circumscribed* form the heads of the phalanges in particular show the areas of rarefaction. These areas present a "punched-out" appearance, and tend to be circular or nearly so. The spongiosa about these spotty rarefactions may still appear normal, and the shafts of the phalanges are frequently free of pathologic changes.

When the changes in the bone have been present for some time, osteophytic overgrowth may appear about the joints. In phalanges showing the coarse rarefactions, areas of mutilation may eventually develop. However, sequestra do not form. Extension of the disease process into the joints is rare, except where the pathologic changes are very advanced. The presence of large areas of coarse rarefaction, as described in relation to the diffuse form, seems to indicate a more florid form of the disease process. The small, spotty, diffuse form, on the other hand, seems to be the expression, in Jüngling's opinion, of an extremely torpid form of sarcoidosis.

The *differentiation* of sarcoidosis involving the small bones of the hands and feet from tuberculous spina ventosa is usually easy, but may present some problems. The roentgenographic appearance of the bone lesions is of great value in the differential diagnosis, but problem cases may be clarified by roentgenographic examination of the lungs, which may reveal the rather characteristic nodular mottling not infrequently present in sarcoidosis.

Several instances of sarcoidosis which involved vertebrae and in which the diagnosis was established ante mortem by biopsy have been reported (see Zener *et al.*, and also Berk and Brower). Pain referred to the back and local tenderness were consistently the chief presenting clinical complaints. In all these cases, roentgenographs of the chest revealed the changes in the lungs which are characteristic of sarcoidosis. In the affected vertebrae, the lesions involved one or more vertebral bodies and presented as roundish areas of radiolucency with sclerotic margins. The intervertebral disk spaces were usually not narrowed, and the vertebral bodies themselves were not compressed.

In a bone, the lesion tends to pursue a chronic course. *Spontaneous complete healing* of an individual bone lesion takes place only rarely, while the skin lesions of sarcoidosis heal relatively often. Radiation therapy has much less effect on the bone lesion than on the skin lesion. Lomholt reported that typical cases of sarcoid of Boeck responded well to intravenous injections of chaulmoogra oil, formerly used in the treatment of leprosy.

REFERENCES

ADAMS, Z. B.: Tuberculosis of the Spine, J. Bone & Joint Surg., *16*, 200, 1934.
AHERN, R. T.: Tuberculosis of the Femoral Neck and Greater Trochanter, J. Bone & Joint Surg., *40-B*, 406, 1958.
ALLISON, N.: Tuberculosis of Bone, Arch. Surg., *2*, 593, 1921.
ARCT, W.: Operative Treatment of Tuberculosis of the Spine in Old People, J. Bone & Joint Surg., *50-A*, 255, 1968.
ASCHOFF, L.: *Lectures on Pathology*, New York, Paul B. Hoeber Inc., 1924.
BACHARACH, T.: Sarcoidosis, Am. Rev. Resp. Dis., *84*, 12, 1961.
BAILLEUL, L.: *Des ostéites tuberculeuses des petits os longs de la main et du pied (spina-ventosa) et des difformités qui peuvent leur succéder au niveau des doigts chez l'enfant*, Paris Thèses, No. 192, G. Steinheil, 1911.
BAKALIM, G.: Tuberculous Spondylitis. A Clinical Study with Special Reference to the Significance of Spinal Fusion and Chemotherapy, Acta orthop. scandinav., Suppl. *47*, 1960.
BANKART, A. S. B.: The Treatment of Tuberculous Disease of the Hip-joint, Brit. J. Surg., *20*, 551, 1933.
BARTON, C. J.: Tuberculosis of the Vault of the Skull, Brit. J. Radiol., *34*, 286, 1961.
BATTAGLIA, B.: Tuberculosis of the Mastoid, Am. Rev. Resp. Dis., *84*, 431, 1961.

BERK, R. N., and BROWER, T. D.: Vertebral Sarcoidosis, Radiology, *82*, 660, 1964.

BICKEL, W. H., KIMBROUGH, R. F., and DAHLIN, D. C.: Tuberculous Tenosynovitis, J.A.M.A., *151*, 31, 1953.

BLACKLOCK, J. W. S.: *Tuberculous Disease in Children: Its Pathology and Bacteriology*, Medical Research Council, Special Report Series, No. 172, London, His Majesty's Stationery Office, 1932.

BLAIR, J. E., and HALLMAN, F. A.: Diagnosis of Surgical Tuberculosis: Comparison of Diagnosis by Inoculation of Guinea-Pigs and by Culture, Arch. Surg., *27*, 178, 1933.

BOEMINGHAUS, H.: Senkungsabszesse, Deutsche med. Wchnschr., *59*, 1559, 1933.

BRACKETT, E. G., BAER, W. S., and RUGH, J. T.: Report of the Commission Appointed to Investigate the Results of Ankylosing Operations of the Spine, J. Orthop. Surg., *3*, 507, 1921.

BROCA, A.: Ostéites tuberculeuses multiples du nourrisson, Nourrisson, *10*, 209, 1922.

BRONNER, H., and KRUMBEIN, C.: Über tumorartige Kiefertuberkulose, Bruns' Beitr. klin. Chir., *137*, 346, 1926.

CHEYNE, W. W.: *Tuberculous Diseases of Bones and Joints. Their Pathology, Symptoms, and Treatment*, 2nd ed., London, Henry Frowde, 1911.

CLEVELAND, M., BOSWORTH, D. M., FIELDING, J. W., and SMYRNIS, P.: Fusion of the Spine for Tuberculosis in Children, J. Bone & Joint Surg., *40-A*, 91, 1958.

CUMMINS, S. L.: The Significance of Intradermal Tuberculin Tests, Brit. M. J., *1*, 336, 1929.

DICKSON, J. A. S.: Spinal Tuberculosis in Nigerian Children, J. Bone & Joint Surg., *49-B*, 682, 1967.

DIETL, K.: Über Lungenbefunde bei Kindern mit extrapulmonaler Tuberkulose, Med. Klinik, *19*, 1192, 1923.

DOUB, H. P., and BADGLEY, C. E.: The Roentgen Signs of Tuberculosis of the Vertebral Body, Am. J. Roentgenol., *27*, 827, 1932.

DREVERMANN, P.: Über Osteomyelitis tuberculosa, Deutsche Ztschr. Chir., *220*, 166, 1929.

ERDHEIM, J.: Vorlesung ueber Tuberkulose des Schaedeldaches, in *Libman Anniversary Volumes*, *1*, 375, 1932.

————: Über Tuberkulose des Knochens im allgemeinen und die des Schädeldaches im besonderen, Virchows Arch. path. Anat., *283*, 354, 1932.

FARES, G., and PAGANI, A.: La osteite tubercolare del pube, Minerva ortop., *17*, 459, 1966.

FELLÄNDER, M.: Tuberculous Tenosynovitis of the Hand Treated by Combined Surgery and Chemotherapy, Acta chir. scandinav., *111*, 142, 1956.

FISHBERG, M.: *Pulmonary Tuberculosis*, 4th ed., Philadelphia, Lea & Febiger, 1932.

FOOT, N. C.: Studies on Endothelial Reactions. IX. The Formation of Reticulum in the Lesions of Experimental Tuberculosis in Rabbits, Am. J. Path., *1*, 341, 1925.

FOSSEL, M.: Allgemeine Miliartuberkulose durch Einbruch einer Wirbelkaries in die Aorta, Zentralbl. allg. Path., *56*, 328, 1932–33.

FREUND, E.: Zur Klinik und Radiographie der Spondylitis tuberculosa, Arch. klin. Chir., *159*, 434, 1930.

————: Zur Klinik der Hüftgelenkstuberkulose, insbesonders über deren moderne chirurgische Behandlung, Ztschr. orthop. Chir., *59*, 19, 1933.

FRIEDMAN, B.: Chemotherapy of Tuberculosis of the Spine, J. Bone & Joint Surg., *48-A*, 451, 1966.

FUNK, F. J., JR., WELLS, R. E., and GOLDING, J. R.: Pott's Disease in Children, J. Bone & Joint Surg., *50-A*, 839, 1968.

GHON, A.: *Der primäre Lungenherd bei der Tuberkulose der Kinder*, Berlin, Urban & Schwarzenberg, 1912.

GHON, A., and POTOTSCHNIG, G.: Über den Unterschied im pathologisch-anatomischen Bilde primärer Lungen- und primärer Darminfektion bei der Tuberkulose der Kinder, Beitr. Klin. Tuberk., *40*, 87, 1918–19.

GIRDLESTONE, G. R.: The Pathology and Treatment of Tuberculosis of the Knee-joint, Brit. J. Surg., *19*, 488, 1932.

————: *Tuberculosis of Bone and Joint*, Revised by E. W. Somerville and M. C. Wilkinson, 3rd ed., London, Oxford University Press, 1965.

GOEL, M. K.: Treatment of Pott's Paraplegia by Operation, J. Bone & Joint Surg., *49-B*, 674, 1967.

GOETZ, A. A.: Effect of Cortisone on Hypercalcemia in Sarcoidosis, J.A.M.A., *174*, 380, 1960.

GRALKA, R.: Akute tuberkulöse eitrige Osteomyelitis, Monatsschr. Kinderh., *32*, 153, 1926.

GRIFFITH, A. S.: The Types of Tubercle Bacilli in Human Bone and Joint Tuberculosis, J. Path. & Bact., *31*, 875, 1928.

————: Observations on the Bovine Tubercle Bacillus in Human Tuberculosis, Brit. M. J., *2*, 501, 1932.

HALD, J., JR.: The Value of Histological and Bacteriological Examination in Tuberculosis of Bones and Joints, Acta orthop. scandinav., *35*, 91, 1964.

HART, P. D'A.: *The Value of Tuberculin Tests in Man with Special Reference to the Intracutaneous Test*, Medical Research Council, Special Report Series, No. 164, London, His Majesty's Stationery Office, 1932.

HARTOFILAKIDIS-GAROFALIDIS, G.: Cystic Tuberculosis of the Patella, J. Bone & Joint Surg., *51-A*, 582, 1969.

HAYES, J. T.: Cystic Tuberculosis of the Proximal Tibial Metaphysis with Associated Involvement of the Epiphysis and Epiphyseal Plate, J. Bone & Joint Surg., *43-A*, 560, 1961.

HEITZMAN, E. R., BORNHURST, R. A., and RUSSELL, J. P.: Disease Due to Anonymous Mycobacteria, Am. J. Roentgenol., *103*, 533, 1968.

HENDRIX, J. Z.: Abnormal Skeletal Mineral Metabolism in Sarcoidosis, Ann. Int. Med., *64*, 797, 1966.

HSIEH, C. K., MILTNER, L. J., and CHANG, C. P.: Tuberculosis of the Shaft of the Large Long Bones of the Extremities, J. Bone & Joint Surg., *16*, 545, 1934.

HUEBSCHMANN, P.: Pathologische Anatomie der Tuberkulose, in: *Die Tuberkulose und ihre Grenzgebiete in Einzeldarstellungen*, Berlin, J. Springer, *5*, 1928.

JACQUEMIN, A.: Tuberculose pulmonaire et génitalité, Bull. Acad. méd., Paris, *91*, 517, 1924.

JOHANSSON, S.: *Über die Knochen- und Gelenk-Tuberkulose im Kindesalter*, Jena, Gustav Fischer, 1926.

JOHNSON, M. P., and ROTHSTEIN, E.: Tuberculosis of the Rib, J. Bone & Joint Surg., *34-A*, 878, 1952.

JÜNGLING, O.: Ostitis tuberculosa multiplex cystica (eine eigenartige Form der Knochentuberkulose), Fortschr. Geb. Röntgenstrahlen, *27*, 375, 1919–21.

————: Über Ostitis tuberculosa multiplex cystoides, zugleich ein Beitrag zur Lehre von den Tuberkuliden des Knochens, Bruns' Beitr. klin. Chir., *143*, 401, 1928.

KARLÉN, A.: On Cystic Tuberculosis of Bone, Acta orthop. scandinav., *31*, 163, 1961.

KASTERT, J., and UEHLINGER, E.: Skelettuberkulose, in *Handbuch der Tuberkulose*, Vol. IV, Stuttgart, Georg Thieme, 1964 (p. 443).

KELLY, P. J., WEED, L. A., and LIPSCOMB, P. R.: Infection of Tendon Sheaths, Bursae, Joints, and Soft Tissues by Acid-Fast Bacilli Other than Tubercle Bacilli, J. Bone & Joint Surg., *45-A*, 327, 1963.

KIENBÖCK, R.: Über tuberkulöse Epiphysenfugen-Cysten und Abscesse, Arch. orthop. u. Unfall-Chir., *29*, 67, 1930 and *30*, 204, 1931.

KOBRO, M.: Zoster and Tuberculosis of the Spine, Acta med. scandinav., *82*, 300, 1934.

KOHLI, S. B.: Radical Surgical Approach to Spinal Tuberculosis, J. Bone & Joint Surg., *49-B*, 668, 1967.

KÖNIG, F.: Die Tuberculose der menschlichen Gelenke sowie der Brustwand und des Schädels, Berlin, August Hirschwald, 1906.

KRAUSE, F.: Die Tuberkulose der Knochen und Gelenke, Deutsche Chir., Lief. 28a, p. 106, 1899.

KÜSS, G.: *De l'hérédité parasitaire de la tuberculose humaine*, Paris, Asselin et Houzeau, 1898.

LICHTOR, J., and LICHTOR, A.: Paleopathological Evidence Suggesting Pre-Columbian Tuberculosis of the Spine, J. Bone & Joint Surg., *39-A*, 1398, 1957.

LOMHOLT, S.: Tolv Tilfaelde af Boecks Sarkoid behandlet med et spedalskhedsmiddel (Antileprol), Hospitalstid., *77*, 187, 1934.

LONG, E. R.: The Inflammatory Reaction in Tuberculosis, Am. J. M. Sc., *185*, 749, 1933.

MACCALLUM, W. G.: *A Text-Book of Pathology*, 5th ed., Philadelphia, W. B. Saunders Co., 1932.

MADLENER, M.: Die Tuberkulose des Schambeins, Deutsche Ztschr. Chir., *196*, 329, 1926.

MAGATH, T. B.: Large Doses of Tuberculin in Testing Guinea Pigs Inoculated for Diagnostic Purposes, Am. J. M. Sc., *188*, 403, 1934.

MANDELSTAMM, M.: Experimentelle Beiträge zum Studium der Knochentuberkulose, Beitr. Klin. Tuberk., *82*, 98, 1933.

MARGOT, E.: Mémoire sur les tumeurs blanches des articulations, Arch. gén. méd., Series 1, *11*, 5, 1826.

MATSUMOTO, N.: Ueber die Pathogenese der sogenannten Kompressionsmyelitis, Fukuoka-Ikwadaigaku-Zasshi, *20*, 62, 1927.

McMASTER, P. E., and KING, R. W.: Tuberculosis of Metatarsal Bones, J. Bone & Joint Surg., *16*, 202, 1934.

McNEUR, J. C., and PRITCHARD, A. E.: Tuberculosis of the Greater Trochanter, J. Bone & Joint Surg., *37-B*, 246, 1955.

McTAMMANY, J. R., MOSER, K. M., and HOUK, V. N.: Disseminated Bone Tuberculosis. Review of the Literature and Presentation of an Unusual Case, Am. Rev. Resp. Dis., *87*, 889, 1963.

MÉNARD, V.: *Étude sur la coxalgie*, Paris, Masson et Cie, 1907.

VON MEYENBURG, H.: Beiträge zur traumatischen Tuberkulose, Schweiz. med. Wchnschr., *64*, 589, 1934.

MEYER, J.: Trauma and Tuberculosis, Acta path. et microbiol. scandinav., *21*, 571, 1944.

MEYERDING, H. W., and MROZ, R. J.: Tuberculosis of the Greater Trochanter, J.A.M.A., *101*, 1308, 1933.

MICHAEL, P.: Gelatinous Degeneration of the Bone Marrow, J. Path. & Bact., *33*, 533, 1930.

MILGRAM, J. E.: Diagnostic Inaccuracy in Tuberculosis of Bone, Joint and Bursa, J.A.M.A., *97*, 232, 1931.

MILLER, W. S.: The Reticulum of the Lung. IV. Its Presence in the Reparative Process of the Tuberculous Lesion with and without Caseation, Am. J. Path., *3*, 217, 1927.

MURRAY, R. O.: Observations on Cystic Tuberculosis of Bone, with a Report on Two Cases, Proc. Roy. Soc. Med., *47*, 133, 1954.

NICHOLS, E. H.: Tuberculosis of Bones and Joints, Tr. Am. Orthop. A., *11*, 353, 1898.

NICHOLSON, O. R.: Tuberculosis of the Pubis, J. Bone & Joint Surg., *40-B*, 6, 1958.

O'MALLEY, B. W., and ZEFT, H. J.: Disseminated Bone Tuberculosis Without Pulmonary Manifestations, Am. J. Med., *38*, 932, 1965.

OPIE, E. L.: The Focal Pulmonary Tuberculosis of Children and Adults, J. Exper. Med., *25*, 855, 1917.

————: The Relation of Apical Tuberculosis of Adults to the Focal Tuberculosis of Children, J. Exper. Med., *26*, 263, 1917.

————: Cellular Reactions of Tuberculosis and Their Relation to Immunity and Sensitization, Arch. Path., *14*, 706, 1932.

OTTOLENGHI, C. E.: Diagnóstico de la tuberculosis ósteoarticular por la biopsia ganglionar, Rev. ortop. y traumatol., *3*, 1, 1933.

PARROT, J. M. J.: Compt. rend. Soc. de biol., Series 6, *3*, 308, 1876.

PEABODY, C. W.: Secondary Foci of Tuberculosis in the Spine in Pott's Disease, Ann. Surg., *75*, 95, 1922.

PERCY-LANCASTER, R.: The Problems of Tuberculosis in the Bantu as Seen by an Orthopaedic Surgeon, J. Bone & Joint Surg., *42-B*, 861, 1960.

PETTER, C. K., and MEDELMAN, J. P.: An Atypical Case of Tuberculosis of the Spine, J.A.M.A., *102*, 1378, 1934.

PHEMISTER, D. B., and HATCHER, C. H.: Correlation of Pathological and Roentgenological Findings in the Diagnosis of Tuberculous Arthritis, Am. J. Roentgenol., *29*, 736, 1933.

PIMM, L. H., and WAUGH, W.: Tuberculous Tenosynovitis, J. Bone & Joint Surg., *39-B*, 91, 1957.

PITZLER, K.: Über die tuberkulöse Tendovaginitis an der Hand und ihre Behandlung, Zentralbl. Chir., *85*, 529, 1960.

PONFICK, E.: Ueber die sympathischen Erkrankungen des Knochenmarkes bei inneren Krankheiten, Arch. path. Anat., *56*, 534, 1872.

POUZET, F.: La tuberculose astragalo-scapho-cunéenne chez l'enfant, Rev. d'orthop., *15*, 308, 1928.

PREISER, R. A.: Selbstverletzung eines Geisteskranken mit nicht alltäglichem Verlauf (Bisswunde, Knochentuberkulose), Psychiat.-neurol. Wchnschr., *35*, 331, 1933.

PUHL: Ueber Primär-und Reïnfekte der Lungenphthise, Deutsche med. Wchnschr., *48*, 278, 1922.

DE QUERVAIN, F., and HUNZIKER, H.: Die Statistik der chirurgischen Tuberkulosen in Basel für das Jahr 1913, Cor.-Bl. schweiz. Ärzte, *49*, 761, 1919.

RANDERATH, E.: Pathologisch-anatomische Untersuchungen über die Tuberkulose des Knochensystems, Beitr. Klin. Tuberk., *79*, 201, 1932.

RANKE, K. E.: Primäre, sekundäre und tertiäre Tuberkulose des Menschen, München. med. Wchnschr., *64*, 305, 1917.

RATLIFF, A. H. C.: Tuberculosis of the Femoral Neck in Childhood, J. Bone & Joint Surg., *39-A*, 1365, 1957.

RECHTMAN, A. M.: Tuberculous Osteitis with Pathologic Resection of Seventh Rib, J. Bone & Joint Surg., *11*, 557, 1929.

RIEDER, H.: Über Kombination von chronischer Osteomyelitis (Spina ventosa) mit Lupus Pernio, Fortschr. Geb. Röntgenstrahlen, *15*, 125, 1910.

VON ROKITANSKY, C.: In *Handbuch der pathologischen Anatomie*, (*Handbuch der speciellen pathologischen Anatomie*), *2*, 91, 1844.

SABIN, F. R.: Cellular Studies in Tuberculosis, Am. Rev. Tuberc., *25*, 153, 1932.

SABIN, F. R., DOAN, C. A., and FORKNER, C. E.: Studies on Tuberculosis, J. Exper. Med., *52*, Suppl. 3, 1930.

SANES, S., and SMITH, W. S.: Osteitis Tuberculosa Multiplex Cystica of Fibula and Tibia, J.A.M.A., *102*, 1206, 1934.

SATTA, F.: La tuberculose du poignet, Rev. d'orthop., *19*, 609, 1932.

SCHAAFHAUSEN, R.: Die Knochen- und Gelenktuberkulose in ihrer Beziehung zur Lungentuberkulose, Ztschr. Tuberk., *59*, 111, 1930–31.

SCHUBERTH, K., and MAYR-WEBER, V.: Besteht ein Zusammenhang zwischen Trauma und Knochentuberkulose?, Beitr. Klin. Tuberk., *74*, 668, 1930.

65

Schürer-Waldheim, F.: Beitrag zur Klinik, Morphologie und Ätiologie der Ostitis tuberculosa multiplex cystoides, Arch. klin. Chir., *160*, 680, 1930.

Schwentker, F. F.: Cystic Tuberculosis of the Bone, Am. J. Dis. Child., *42*, 102, 1931.

Seddon, H. J.: Inguinal Lymph Gland Biopsy in the Diagnosis of Tuberculous Disease of the Knee, Brit. M. J., *1*, 105, 1939.

Seedat, Y. K., and Wolpert, S. M.: Disseminated Tuberculosis of Bone: Report of Two Cases, Brit. M. J., *1*, 1291, 1965.

Seemann, O.: Ueber Verlauf und Ausgang der Tuberkulose der Wirbelsäule, Beitr. klin. Chir., *87*, 146, 1913.

Sevastikoglou, J., and Wernerheim, B.: Some Views on Skeletal Tuberculosis, Acta orthop. scandinav., *23*, 67, 1953.

Singer, E. P., Hensler, N. M., and Flynn, P. F.: Sarcoidosis, Am. J. Med., *26*, 364, 1959.

Smith, T.: *Parasitism and Disease*, Princeton, Princeton University Press, 1934.

Strange, F. G. St. C.: The Prognosis in Sacro-iliac Tuberculosis, Brit. J. Surg., *50*, 561, 1963.

Sulzberger, M. B.: Sarcoid of Boeck (Benign Miliary Lupoid) and Tuberculin Anergy, Am. Rev. Tuberc., *28*, 734, 1933.

Sundelin, F.: Fall av benign miliarlupoid (Boeck), Hygiea, *95*, 481, 1933.

Thrap-Meyer, H.: Spondylitis tuberculosa multiplex, Acta orthop. scandinav., *4*, 154, 1933.

Tschistowitsch, A. N., and Winogradow, I. S.: Über die pathologische Histologie der Knochentuberkulose, Beitr. path. Anat., *91*, 236, 1933.

————: Über die Histologie der Senkungsabscesse, Beitr. Klin. Tuberk., *82*, 765, 1933.

Uehlinger, E.: Die tuberkulöse Spät-Erstinfektion und ihre Frühevolution, Schweiz. med. Wchnschr., *72*, 701, 1942.

————: Pathogenese und allgemeine pathologische Anatomie der hämatogenen Tuberkulose, Ztschr. Tuberk., *125*, 365, 1966.

————: Die pathologische Anatomie der hämatogenen Tuberkulose, Schweiz. med. Wchnschr., *97*, 1523, 1967.

Valtancoli, G.: La tubercolosi della colonna vertebrale. In *Ricerche statistiche sulla tubercolosi ossea ed articolare*, by Cicconardi, G., Sacco, R., Vacchelli, S., and Valtancoli, G., Bologna, L. Cappelli, 1922.

Van Alstyne, G. S., and Gowen, G. H.: Osteitis Tuberculosa Multiplex Cystica (Jüngling). Report of a Case Involving the Larger Long Bones With Complete Proof of Its Tuberculous Etiology, J. Bone & Joint Surg., *15*, 193, 1933.

Van Gorder, G. W.: Tuberculosis of the Shaft of Long Bones, J. Bone & Joint Surg., *16*, 269, 1934.

Volkmann, R.: Die chronischen fungösen und purulenten Gelenkentzündungen. Tumor albus and Arthrocace, in *Handbuch der allgemeinen und speciellen Chirurgie*, *2(2)*, Chapt. XLII, 1882.

Vorwald, A. J.: The Early Cellular Reactions in the Lungs of Rabbits Injected Intravenously with Human Tubercle Bacilli, Am. Rev. Tuberc., *25*, 74, 1932.

Waldenström, H.: *Die Tuberkulose des Collum Femoris im Kindesalter und ihre Beziehungen zur Hüftgelenkentzündung*, Stockholm, P. A. Norstedt & Söner, 1910.

Weber, A. L., Bird, K. T., and Janower, M. L.: Primary Tuberculosis in Childhood with Particular Emphasis on Changes Affecting the Tracheobronchial Tree, Am. J. Roentgenol., *103*, 123, 1968.

Wells, B. B., and Halsted, J. A.: *Clinical Pathology*, 4th ed., Philadelphia, W. B. Saunders Co., 1967 (p. 502).

Whitman, R.: *A Treatise on Orthopaedic Surgery*, 8th ed., Philadelphia, Lea & Febiger, 1927.

Willis, T. A.: Pott's Abscess, Surg. Gynec. & Obst., *43*, 285, 1926.

Wiseman, R.: *Several Chirurgical Treatises*, 2nd ed., London, R. Norton and J. Macock for R. Royston and B. Took, 1686.

Wullstein, L.: Die Wirbelentzündungen, in *Handbuch der orthopädischen Chirurgie*, *1*, 1225, 1905–1907.

Yau, A. C. M. C., and Hodgson, A. R.: Penetration of the Lung by the Paravertebral Abscess in Tuberculosis of the Spine, J. Bone & Joint Surg., *50-A*, 243, 1968.

Zener, J. C., Alpert, M., and Klainer, L. M.: Vertebral Sarcoidosis, Arch. Int. Med., *111*, 696, 1963.

Chapter

31

Skeletal Lesions Caused by Certain Other Infectious Agents

As is common knowledge, the term *"pyogenic osteomyelitis"* is generally understood to signify a bone infection in which the causative agent is a *Staphylococcus*. Indeed, one or another strain of staphylococci is the pathogenic agent in about 90 per cent of cases of so-called pyogenic osteomyelitis. Infection by *Streptococcus* (usually a hemolytic *Streptococcus* but occasionally a nonhemolytic variety) accounts for about 3 per cent of cases of osteomyelitis. Infection by other bacteria, such as the pneumococcus, *Brucella*, the colon bacillus, and bacilli of the *Salmonella* group, together account for only 1 or 2 per cent. Only an occasional instance of osteomyelitis (at least in the United States) is due to an infection by a fungus or a virus.

STAPHYLOCOCCAL OSTEOMYELITIS

As noted, the causative agent of pyogenic osteomyelitis is usually a *Staphylococcus*, and more specifically the *Staphylococcus aureus*. Furthermore, when considering pyogenic osteomyelitis, one has in mind those cases in which the staphylococcal infection is blood-borne (hematogenous) rather than those in which it reaches the bone by contamination from the surface (as, for instance, with compound fractures, war wounds, and a surgical intervention). A *hematogenous pyogenic osteomyelitis* develops as a result of the lodgment, in a bone site, of bacteria from some other focus of infection (skin, ear, throat, etc.). More often than not, however, the extraskeletal focus of infection is not clinically evident when the osteomyelitis is first recognized. At any rate, the bacteria are carried to the affected skeletal area by the blood stream, and when a tubular bone is implicated, the bacteria reach it by way of the nutrient artery. Ultimately, they enter the capillaries in the spongiosa of the juxta-epiphysial and/or metaphysial region of the bone. Even when the bacteria are lodged in a bone area, an osteomyelitis does not always set in promptly, because, as a result of the original extra-osseous infection, there are pertinent antibodies in the blood, and consequently the bacteria which had localized in the bone marrow are either destroyed or become dormant and inactive. Under these circumstances it may not be until some months later that the bacteria become reactivated and a focus of osteomyelitis is established. Various aspects of the pathogenesis of pyogenic osteomyelitis in man have been confirmed through the experiments of Thompson and Dubos, who induced osteomyelitis in rabbits by the intravenous injection of staphylococci which were grown on culture media. These investigators concluded that the inflammatory osteomyelitis produced in the rabbits bears a close resemblance to hematogenous staphylococcal osteomyelitis occurring in man.

CLINICAL CONSIDERATIONS

Incidence.—As is generally known, the incidence and also the clinical and pathologic aspects of pyogenic (staphylococcal) osteomyelitis have undergone a striking change since the introduction of the antibiotic drugs. Before that time, the over-all mortality rate was 20 to 30 per cent (see Pyrah and Pain, and also Crossan). It has been established that the antibiotics can largely avert the development of acute osteomyelitis by curing the infection in the primary site (in the throat, upper respiratory tract, genitourinary tract, skin, etc.).

With regard to *age incidence*, it is known that the disease sets in most often between the ages of 3 and 15 years—that is, during the period of most active skeletal growth. An instance of acute osteomyelitis is occasionally observed in a neonate or in an infant up to the age of 1 year (see Madgwick). In a neonate the bacterial infection may take its departure from the umbilicus (see Trueta), and in neonates and older infants the osteomyelitis is often the result of an infection by *Streptococcus*, and particularly by *beta*-hemolytic *Streptococcus*. Hematogenous staphylococcal osteomyelitis of long tubular bones does not often set in during middle or late adult life; instead, the likelihood is that the condition is chronic (that is, of long duration) and had set in at some time during childhood. When it does start during adult life, acute hematogenous osteomyelitis tends to involve short bones, particularly vertebrae, the infection spreading to these bones from the pelvis (see Wiley and Trueta).

In relation to *sex incidence*, it should be noted that, among the cases of staphylococcal osteomyelitis becoming manifest during childhood, the proportion of males to females affected is about 3 or 4 to 1. This fact is in harmony with the greater frequency of injuries, along with infection of parosteal or other soft tissues, among male children. In *infants* the incidence of osteomyelitis is about the same in males as in females (see Green and Shannon). Among *adults*, males predominate over

Figure 263

A, B, C, D, and *E,* Roentgenographs from the same case of pyogenic staphylococcal osteomyelitis, the time interval between *A* and *E* being 5 months. The subject, a boy 13 years of age when he was admitted to our hospital, had twisted his right ankle 3 days earlier. He complained of pain and swelling, and was febrile. There was no past history of pain in any joint. Physical examination revealed that the boy was acutely ill, with a temperature of 104.4° F. The right ankle was somewhat swollen, and an area of redness, swelling, local heat, and localized tenderness was present on the medial aspect of the lower portion of the leg.

A, The roentgenograph taken on the day of admission shows that the area outlined by the arrows is vaguely radiolucent, indicating that the infection is already brewing in the distal metaphysis of the tibia.

B, Roentgenograph taken 11 days later clearly reveals that the medial surface of the cortex in that part of the tibia has been substantially resorbed, and the rest of the metaphysis shows mottled radiolucency.

C, Roentgenograph taken 16 days after the one shown in *B* discloses that the infection has provoked subperiosteal new bone formation, which is evident in the interosseous space and also on the medial aspect of the lower part of the shaft of the tibia.

D, Roentgenograph of the involved area taken 6 weeks after the one shown in *C.* The pathologic changes revealed here are very much more advanced. The subperiosteal new bone formation on the medial side is definitely more pronounced. As indicated by the arrows, there are three areas of radiolucency, and these appear to be the sites of abscesses.

E, Roentgenograph taken 10 weeks after the one shown in *D* discloses that the radiolucent areas now stand out even more clearly, and their presence is associated with a considerable amount of new bone formation in the interosseous space.

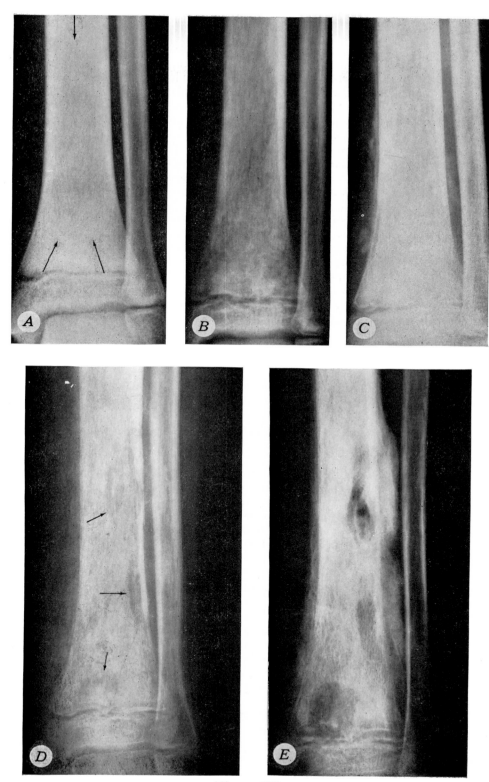

Figure 263

females in a ratio of about 6 or 7 to 1. Rather frequently, the osteomyelitis is preceded by a traumatic incident, such as a contusion, twist, sprain, or other injury to the area in question (see Hanzawa and Suda).

Localization.—Almost any bone may become the presenting site of an acute staphylococcal osteomyelitis. However, it is well established that those of the *lower limbs* are more frequently affected than are those of the upper limbs (see Harris, and also Gilmour). It is clear that the femur and the tibia are most often implicated, the two most common sites of involvement being the proximal and distal ends of their shafts, in the general vicinity of the pertinent epiphysial cartilage plates. (See Fig. 263.) Occasionally, however, the focus of osteomyelitis develops in the midportion of the shaft. From the metaphysis, the infection may spread to the neighboring articular end of the bone and even to the regional joint, inducing a pyogenic arthritis. In the *upper extremities* the humerus is most often implicated, and in that bone, too, the lesion tends to appear in the upper or lower metaphysis rather than in the midportion of the shaft. The other long tubular bones of the extremities (that is, the fibula, radius, and ulna) are affected much less frequently than are the femur, tibia, and humerus.

Septic arthritis of the *hip joint* frequently occurs in those infants and young children in whom the upper end of the femur is the site of pyogenic osteomyelitis. Unless its presence is recognized early (by means of roentgenographic examination or the aspiration of pus from the joint) and appropriate therapy is instituted, the pyogenic arthritis may endanger the life of the patient. Moreover, if the subject is still a child or an adolescent, it is likely that the future growth of one or both bones entering into the formation of the joint will be disturbed, and the function of the joint may undergo restriction (see Roberts, Eyre-Brook, Brantschen, Jones and Roberts, Borella *et al.*, Louw and Shandling, and also MacEwan and Dunbar). Septic arthritis of the hip joint in adults is rather uncommon, and its diagnosis may be difficult unless the presence of the infection is established by aspiration of the joint (see Bulmer, and also Kelly *et al.*). Pyogenic osteomyelitis of the *patella* is uncommon (see Evans).

A focus of pyogenic osteomyelitis in a *phalanx* of a hand or foot sometimes represents an individual localization of a multifocal infection. More often, osteomyelitis of phalanges (especially those of the fingers) occurs when an infection involving the overlying soft tissues spreads to one or more of those bones, or is the result of fracture of a phalanx with laceration and infection of the overlying soft tissues. As a rule, the entire bone becomes infected and the phalanx (especially if it is a terminal phalanx) undergoes destruction. Osteomyelitis of the *sesamoid bones* of the first metatarsophalangeal joint has been reported, but is definitely of rare occurrence (see Colwill, and also Torgerson and Hammond).

Of the bones of the *trunk*, those of the pelvis and of the vertebral column are most often affected, while ribs are only rarely implicated. When an area of the *vertebral column* is the site of a hematogenous pyogenic osteomyelitis, the lesion is most likely to be at the lumbar level. The vertebral sites next in order of frequency of involvement are the thoracic, thoracolumbar, and cervical areas (see Garcia and Grantham). In a vertebra, the body is involved much more frequently than the arch. When a vertebral body is affected, a paravertebral abscess may develop (see Klages).

With regard to the bones of the *skull*, osteomyelitis is most often observed in the *jaw bones*, particularly the mandible. In that bone the infection tends to be chronic, and is usually located in the body and/or the junction of the body and a ramus. The most common basis for involvement of the mandible is an infection originating about an impacted lower third molar tooth, or ensuing upon extraction of one or more teeth which were already the site of dental caries (see Bauer, Baranoff, Kinnman and Lee, and also Razim and Friedberg). An instance of osteomyelitis of the upper jaw in an infant 2 weeks of age was reported as having taken its departure in a tooth germ of the upper jaw (see Remky). Osteomyelitis of the *nasal septum* is of rare occurrence, but several cases have been described in which the infection spread from the nasal septum to the local region of the calvarium (see Benjamins). An instance of circumscribed osteomyelitis of the *calvarium* has been reported in which the condition developed during intra-uterine life (see Ladewig). The vault of the skull may also become infected from the nasal sinuses, or following a trauma to the calvarium, or may even appear after a surgical intervention on the skull (see Cohen, Adelstein and Courville, Wilensky, and also Marek).

Clinical Complaints and Findings.—Discussion of these aspects of staphylococcal osteomyelitis necessitates consideration of the site of the presenting lesion, the duration of the infection, and the question of whether the subject had already received treatment with antibiotics. Ordinarily, especially in *children*, the clinical onset of *acute* osteomyelitis is rather abrupt. Its principal manifestations consist of pain in the affected skeletal area, fever, and tachycardia. If a *long tubular bone* is involved, severe localized tenderness will be evoked on palpation, even in the absence of swelling or redness. Local swelling, if present, results from the accumulation of pus under the periosteum. (See Fig. 264.) Under these circumstances, aspiration of the fluctuant area will yield some purulent material which, on bacteriologic examination, will reveal another bacterium, if the infecting organism is not *Staphylococcus aureus*. Moreover, hematologic examination will very likely disclose a neutrophilic leukocytosis and an increased sedimentation rate.

In *adults* the clinical onset of pyogenic osteomyelitis tends to be subacute, and the progress of the disease will be slow and insidious (see Zadek). Such cases have been denoted as instances of *primary subacute pyogenic osteomyelitis*. Roentgenographically the lesional area is usually apparent in the shaft of the affected long bone—most often a tibia (see Harris and Kirkaldy-Willis). Specifically, the focus of infection may be a localized abscess, either small (a so-called Brodie's abscess) or much larger. The larger abscesses tend to develop in the metaphysis (particularly in the lower metaphysis) of the tibia. In an occasional instance of so-called primary subacute pyogenic osteomyelitis, there may be *multiple* abscess cavities in the shaft of the affected bone.

A focus of pyogenic osteomyelitis in the *vertebral column* is characterized clinically by persistent and progressive backache. In accordance with the particular site of the lesion within the column, the pain may radiate into the chest or abdomen, or even into one of the lower limbs. Early in the course of the vertebral involvement, roentgenographs may fail to disclose the lesion. On this account, serial roentgenographs should be taken, and these will ultimately demonstrate changes in the affected vertebral body or bodies and in the regional intervertebral disks (see Pritchard and Thompson, Bruno *et al.*, Klein, and Ambrose *et al.*).

Lateral displacement of the linear thoracic paraspinal shadow of Brailsford is held to be an early roentgenographic sign of osteomyelitis of the thoracic spine (see Millard). This shadow, which is a slender vertical line usually detectable in an anteroposterior view, normally extends downward from the fourth thoracic vertebra to the site of reflection of the pleura onto the diaphragm, and is usually observed on the left side, though it may also be present on the right side. With pyogenic osteomyelitis of the upper thoracic vertebral bodies, a large paraspinal vertebral abscess may develop and present as a posterior mediastinal mass, which may even displace the trachea forward (see de Lorimier *et al.*).

Furthermore, a focus of hematogenous osteomyelitis in a vertebra occasionally results in the development of a paraplegia, which is due to narrowing of the spinal canal and pressure on the spinal cord. This pressure is caused by bulging of the posterior longitudinal ligament and consequent collapse of one or more of the affected vertebrae, leading to gibbus formation (see Kulowski, and Freehafer *et al.*). (See Fig. 265.)

PATHOLOGIC FINDINGS

The discussion of the pathologic findings relating to staphylococcal osteomyelitis will center mainly on the condition in long tubular bones. In addition, pyogenic arthritis will be discussed.

Histology of Acute Hematogenous Osteomyelitis of Long Tubular Bones.—The histologic details concerning the initial changes at the site of localization of the bacteria in human bones have not been extensively studied, since pertinent material is not ordinarily available. On the basis of such relevant data as we have, however, it is known that the bacteria, on entering a long bone, lodge in the marrow spaces of the metaphysis, not far from the epiphysial cartilage plate in a young subject or the epiphysial end of the bone if the epiphysis has already fused with the shaft. In the marrow spaces of the spongiosa, the bacteria (in the course of a week or so) give rise to one or several small abscesses. The periphery of such an abscess may be heavily infiltrated with viable polymorphonuclear leukocytes, but in the more central part of the abscess the leukocytes are largely necrotic. In time, the inflammatory process makes its way to the adjacent part of the cortex, enters the cortex by way of its haversian canals, and then spreads through the cortex along its haversian canals, which become enlarged.

The porosity of the bone cortex is usually induced by lacunar resorption, associated with the formation of numerous osteoclasts, but is apparently also sometimes caused by so-called "smooth resorption." In particular, in some places one finds that the widened haversian canals have smooth borders—a finding which cannot be related to lacunar resorption. The porosity is evident not only where the suppuration has spread to the bone cortex, but also in adjacent parts, often over a wide area. The blood supply to portions of the cortex may be obstructed, and where this happens the formation of cortical sequestra is favored. In the course of time, the

Figure 264

A, *B*, *C*, and *D*, Roentgenographs of the distal end of the right femur showing the progression of a pyogenic osteomyelitis during a period of 6½ weeks. The patient was a boy 14 years of age when he was first admitted to our hospital.

A, Roentgenograph taken on admission shows that the anterior surface of the distal end of the shaft cortex appears rarefied, and the trabecular markings at the end of the shaft are not clear.

B, Roentgenograph taken 3 weeks later shows progression of the osteomyelitis. In addition to more pronounced rarefaction of the cortex anteriorly, there is a thin layer of subperiosteal new bone formation. Some rarefaction of the shaft cortex posteriorly is also apparent, and a distinct deposit of periosteal new bone can also be seen near the upper end of the picture.

C, Roentgenograph taken 6½ weeks after admission even more clearly delineates the subperiosteal new bone formation present anteriorly, and also the subperiosteal deposit of bone on the posterior surface of the cortex. It can also be noted that a part of the cortex has become delimited as a sequestrum *in situ* (see arrows).

D, Roentgenograph taken in the anteroposterior projection at the same time as the one shown in *C*. One can observe changes which are not clearly evident in the lateral projection. In particular, it is apparent here that the infection has broken out of the shaft, just above the epiphysial cartilage plate. The plate is substantially obliterated.

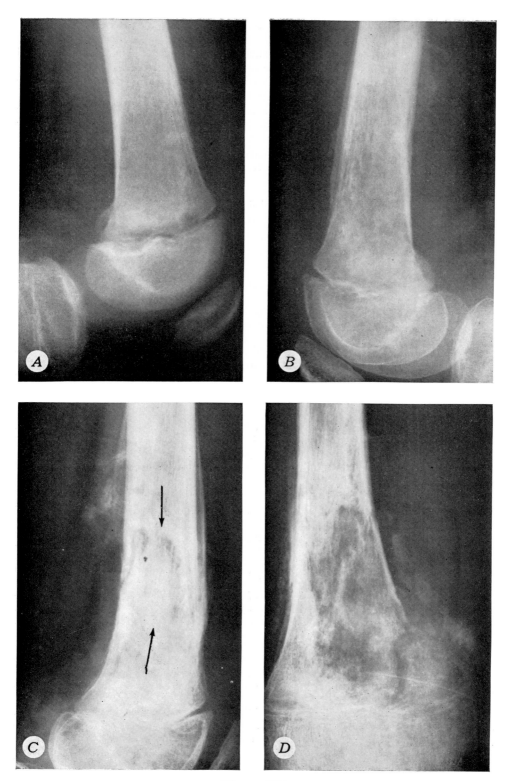

Figure 264

inflammatory process reaches the outer surface of the cortex, inducing subperiosteal new bone formation and even giving rise to a subperiosteal abscess. The abscess in the marrow cavity comes to be surrounded by a thick, feltlike zone of connective tissue fibers. Small foci of hemorrhage result not from trauma but from toxic damage to the regional blood vessels. If the cortex of an affected long tubular bone is thickened, and if the medullary cavity is likewise the site of reparative new bone formation, the roentgenographic appearance may raise diagnostic problems, and one may misinterpret the picture as indicating the presence of a tumor, and particularly of an osteogenic sarcoma (see Elliott, Stewart, and also Cohn).

Figure 265

A, Roentgenograph showing in lateral projection a lesion involving the bodies of the fourth and fifth lumbar vertebrae. There is also destruction of the intervertebral disk between these two bodies. The basis for these abnormalities was a pyogenic infection caused by *Staphylococcus aureus*, *Streptococcus*, and *Escherichia coli*. The subject was a 37-year-old man who was admitted to our hospital with a 1-year history of pain in his back. A surgical intervention was carried out. The incision was in the midline and extended from the second lumbar vertebra to the ilium. When the fascia was incised, there was a gush of foul-smelling, very fluid pus mixed with blood. A large abscess cavity was opened which extended to the vertebrae in the midline and downward toward the psoas muscles. A second incision, made at the same level as the first, but to the right of the midline, led into another pus-filled cavity, which was also found to extend toward the vertebrae and downward along the psoas muscle. The patient died 2 days after the surgical intervention, and an autopsy revealed: (1) osteomyelitis of the fourth and fifth lumbar vertebrae, with complete destruction of the intervening disk; (2) bilateral psoas abscesses; and (3) acute generalized peritonitis.

B, Photograph of the cut surface of the part of the vertebral column referred to in *A*. The picture shows that the intervertebral disk between the fourth and fifth lumbar vertebrae is completely destroyed, and in the general vicinity of the disk, the posterior longitudinal ligament bulges somewhat toward the spinal canal and makes pressure against the dura mater. Sclerosis of the spongiosa in the lower portion of the fourth lumbar vertebra and the upper portion of the fifth is evident, and is consistent with the appearances presented by these vertebral bodies in *A*.

C, Roentgenograph, from another case, showing in lateral projection the lower third of the thoracic part of the vertebral column. The intervertebral disk between the tenth and eleventh bodies has undergone destruction, and these bodies are bridged anteriorly by bony projections. The patient was a woman 62 years of age who, for 5 months before her admission to our hospital, had been under treatment (at another hospital) for the same complaints. A biopsy performed at that institution established the diagnosis of chronic osteomyelitis. The clinical and laboratory findings recorded at our hospital were: (1) a healing lumbodorsal scar in the midline, with some drainage at the lower end, and (2) the presence of *Staphylococcus aureus*, coagulase-positive, in some of the pus from the draining sinus. A costotransversectomy on the left side of the involved area was performed, but paraplegia, which developed shortly afterward, necessitated a decompression laminectomy at the level of D_{10}–D_{11}. Despite this intervention, the paraplegia persisted, and several weeks later the woman died. An autopsy revealed a *Staphylococcus aureus* osteomyelitis involving D_{10} and D_{11}, destruction of the intervertebral disk, compression collapse of the bodies, and also compression of the spinal cord. There was also evidence of pyelonephritis, septic splenic infarcts, and bronchopneumonia, all of which were related to the *Staphylococcus aureus* septicemia, which was established by blood cultures.

D, Photograph of the cut surface of part of the vertebral column removed at the autopsy, and specifically the lesional area shown in *C*. The intervertebral disk has undergone complete destruction, and it can be seen that the two vertebral bodies are bridged anteriorly by projections of bone.

E, Roentgenograph of the specimen shown in *D*. The picture exemplifies with special clarity the writer's view that the roentgenograph represents an important aspect of the gross pathologic findings.

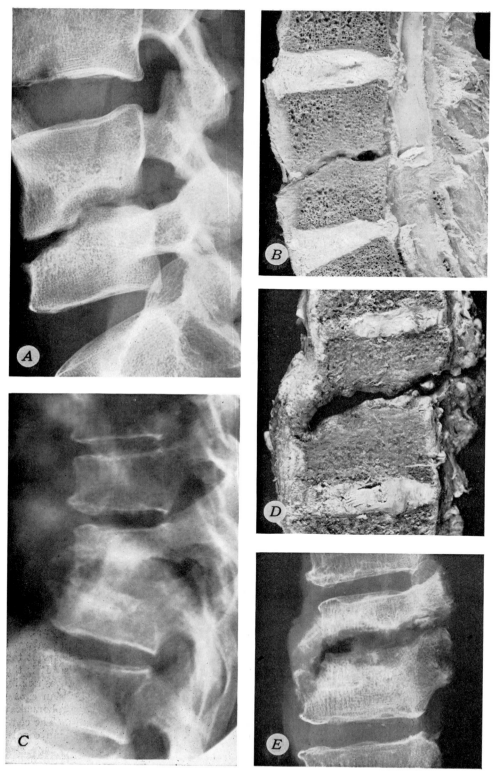

Figure 265

Figure 266

A, Photograph of the lower part of the left tibia (cut in the frontal plane) from a case of pyogenic osteomyelitis in which the subject died of staphylococcemia, and the tibia was removed during an autopsy. The picture shows that the epiphysis is separated from the shaft, the separation having occurred in the course of removal of the bone. Note that the spongiosa in the shaft of the bone presents small, spotty, whitish areas and one large roundish area in the metaphysis just proximal to the plate. Some similar discolored areas can be seen in the epiphysis, and a large one can be noted in the lower left side of the epiphysis, where the inflammatory focus abuts on the articular cartilage. These whitish areas are sites in which the intertrabecular marrow spaces are crowded with inflammatory cells, which on microscopic examination were found to be mainly polymorphonuclear leukocytes. The subject in this case was a 13-year-old girl who had had pain and swelling in the region of the left ankle for 1 day before admission to our hospital. When she entered the hospital, her temperature was 104.4° F. A blood culture revealed the presence of *Staphylococcus aureus*. Aspiration of the left ankle region yielded pus, and an incision and drainage was carried out. On the following day, another surgical intervention revealed that the tissues overlying the lower third of the tibia were red and fluctuant. The periosteum was found thickened, and some of it was stripped from the underlying cortex. Histologic examination disclosed the presence of an infection. The patient's condition became worse, and she died 1 week later. One day before her death, another blood culture revealed the presence of numerous colonies of *Staphylococcus aureus*. In addition to the presence of acute osteomyelitis of the left tibia, the autopsy disclosed that: (1) the left ankle was the site of pyarthrosis, and (2) there were abscesses in the kidneys and lungs and also under the parietal pleura, associated with osteomyelitis of the thoracic ends of some of the ribs.

B, Photomicrograph (× 6) disclosing the presence of an osteomyelitic infection in the intertrabecular marrow spaces of the distal end of the shaft of a femur from an analogous case. The subject was 2 years and 4 months old when she was admitted to our hospital. Four or 5 months prior to admission, she had contracted a "cold," which had lasted about 2 weeks, and then developed some difficulties relating to the kidneys. Pyelitis was revealed by the cloudiness of the urine and the numerous pus cells found in it. Subsequently, a painful area ("sore") appeared on the back of the lower part of the left thigh. About 3 days prior to admission, the child fell on the left knee, and the next day there was pain in, and slight swelling of, that knee. One day before admission, she had convulsions and became cyanotic. Physical examination on admission revealed a temperature of 104.4° F., a somewhat congested pharynx, and slight rigidity of the neck. The left lower extremity was red and swollen, felt warmer than the right, and was tender to pressure. An incision was made over the lateral aspect of the thigh, about 2 inches above the knee. When the periosteum was incised, seropurulent material gushed out, apparently from the area in the vicinity of the condyle. The next day, her temperature rose to 108.6° F., and she died. The autopsy revealed acute osteomyelitis and periostitis of the distal end of the femoral shaft. The tissue section from which this photograph was made revealed that the intertrabecular marrow spaces contained numerous microabscesses composed of polymorphonuclear leukocytes.

C, Photomicrograph (× 30) showing the histologic architecture of an area of cortical bone from a case of chronic osteomyelitis of a tibia. The cortex had become somewhat porotified. The illustration shows, in cross section, many haversian canals which are still not enlarged or otherwise modified (see arrows). The large, irregularly contoured spaces represent the result of enlargement and fusion of neighboring and adjacent haversian canals. It is the fusion of such enlarged canals that accounts for the bizarre histologic appearance, especially at the left and upper part of the picture. The spaces of these enlarged haversian canals are filled with inflammatory granulation tissue containing numerous polymorphonuclear leukocytes. Osteoclasts are also present on the surfaces of many of the canals. The communicating passages between the haversian canals represent so-called Volkmann canals.

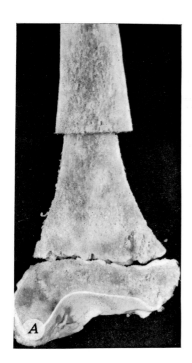
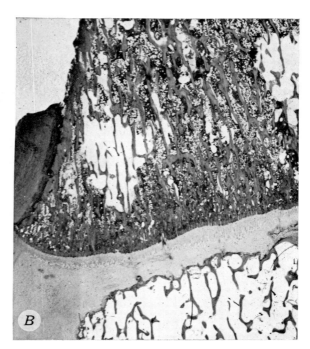
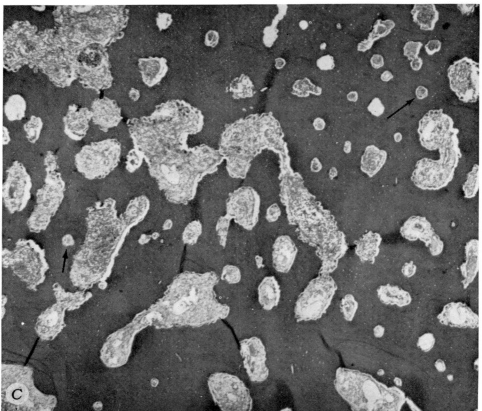

Figure 266

The eruption of the pus outward (spontaneously or in the course of a surgical intervention) is followed by a remission of the hyperemia and, in cases running a favorable course, also soon by cessation of the bone resorption and the beginning of repair through apposition of new bone on the walls of the widened haversian canals. The apposition of new bone lamellae may even lead to a densification (eburnation) of the cortex. In sites where the suppuration has rapidly and completely destroyed the content of the haversian canals, the bone becomes necrotic before resorption has begun. A fragment of necrotic cortical bone can, of course, become detached only from neighboring bone which has remained viable. The separation of the necrotic osseous tissue takes place because of osteoclastic activity, and occurs at a site somewhat away from the bone area which is still viable. The areas of necrotic bone cortex which are in immediate contact with viable cortex are likely to be resorbed and replaced by new bone, rather than undergo sequestration. The porosity of the bone cortex is conditioned not only by the widening of the haversian canals but, in addition, by the formation of perforating canals—so-called Volkmann canals (see Volkmann, and also Jaffe). (See Figs. 15 and also 266.)

Course of Healing in Acute Suppurative Osteomyelitis.—In a bone in which the osteomyelitic process is rather advanced, the progress of the healing is slow, but the pertinent literature contains few reports on the anatomic details relating to the healing. The reason for the paucity of such information is that bones in which the disease process is still active ordinarily do not become available for gross and microscopic examination unless the subject dies and the bones in question are removed at autopsy. A case in point was described in detail by Freund: The subject was a man 23 years of age who, in the preceding 6 years, had developed osteomyelitis in various bones. He died of generalized amyloidosis, and an autopsy was performed. After examining many of the affected bones, Freund reported the course of the healing process as follows: When the acute inflammation has subsided, the suppuration (formation of pus) gradually diminishes. After disintegration and resorption of the leukocytes, the marrow cavity is filled in by granulation tissue, which is replaced by fibrous tissue. In the course of these changes, one may note (here and there) persisting minute abscesses surrounded by capsules of connective tissue. At the periphery of these connective tissue capsules, there may be some lipoid-bearing phagocytes and sometimes also a few foreign body giant cells oriented to tiny fragments of bone. More rarely, fine spongy trabeculae are formed around the abscesses. The neighboring spongy trabeculae are often thickened and, on more detailed examination, present a "striated appearance," due to the numerous newly formed layers of osseous tissue separated by conspicuous cement lines.

Advancing from the vicinity of healing foci, the bone marrow may slowly press forward against the fibrous wall of the abscess and replace the scar tissue by either cellular or fatty marrow. However, large abscesses are transformed into cystic cavities, since a large abscess cavity, like a pleural empyema, does not undergo complete replacement by granulation tissue. Furthermore, because of its rigid environment (bone formation around the abscess), the bone abscess cannot collapse. The resorption of large collections of pus takes place so slowly that meanwhile the connective tissue capsule becomes firm because of its richness in collagenous fibers. In consequence, no additional granulation tissue can be formed on its inner surface. Also, after the interior of the abscess has become completely liquefied, organizing connective tissue can no longer be deposited on its wall. The densification of the scar tissue in the vicinity of healed foci occasionally leads to angioma-like dilatation of the vessels, which, in such cases, are surrounded by gelatinous, edematous marrow poor in cells. In the case of a suppurative osteomyelitis which has run a rather protracted course, *amyloid* is sometimes deposited in the vessel walls of the bone marrow, as it is in the liver, kidneys, spleen, intestines, and other organs.

Transition from Acute to Chronic Osteomyelitis.—In all cases of *acute* osteomyelitis in which large sequestra develop, the progress of healing is protracted unless the sequestra are removed surgically. If large sequestra are present, spontaneous healing is possible only rarely, for usually the fistulae which form are not adequate for expulsion of the necrotic bone fragment or fragments. Sequestra sometimes continue to lie in the marrow cavity for decades, and are the basis for a persistent suppuration. In such cases, death is often caused by generalized amyloidosis.

In other instances, *chronic* osteomyelitis develops, because the bacteria giving rise to the inflammatory changes have not been completely eliminated. The infectious agents may remain viable in small abscesses and probably also in fragments of necrotic bone (small sequestra). At intervals of months or years, the residual viable bacteria may cause recurrent flare-ups of the osteomyelitis. The subjects then suffer from repeated bouts of fever, the development of new fistulae, and the elimination of sequestra through these fistulae if the sequestra are very small. If the osteomyelitis comes under control, there may be evidence of substantial repair, in the form of reappearance of large amounts of spongiosa (interspersed with some small abscesses) in the marrow cavity of the affected bones, and the deposition of subperiosteal new bone on the already altered cortex. If a bone which has undergone such changes is macerated, the appearance of the altered bone fits into the general category of so-called "sclerosing osteomyelitis." On the other hand, if resorption predominates for a long time in a given bone, that bone may become the site of a *fracture*. However, such fractures tend to heal under appropriate treatment with splints or other support to the area (see Capener and Pierce). (See Fig. 267.)

Osteomyelitis Chronic from the Beginning.—These cases stand out clinically in sharp contrast to cases of acute suppurative osteomyelitis in which, in the past, the infection often led to death of the subject. Death resulted from complications, such as the development of numerous metastatic abscesses in the lungs, kidneys, and other organs, and/or purulent inflammation of the pleura, pericardium, peritoneum, or meninges. In the instances pursuing a chronic course from the beginning, sequestrum formation is meager or entirely lacking, and there is almost no formation of pockets of pus. For these reasons, such lesions have also been denoted as "dry osteomyelitis" or "atypical osteomyelitis" (see Freund, and also Melchior). This form of the disease tends to occur at a somewhat more advanced age than the acute form, the majority of the persons affected being more than 30 years old. The clinical manifestations of so-called "dry osteomyelitis" are often vague and usually offer little help in establishing the diagnosis. The condition may have been present for many years, and occasionally its anatomic basis consists of inflammatory foci taking the form of small bone abscesses. Rarely do these abscesses reach the periosteum or become oriented to it. They are located within the substance of the bone, and their presence therefore may be revealed only by roentgenographic examination or in the course of an autopsy. Since a bone site containing a number of small abscesses may appear roentgenographically as a focus of radiopacity, the condition in such cases has sometimes been denoted as "chronic sclerosing nonsuppurative osteomyelitis of Garrè." This designation is inaccurate, since Garrè was actually referring to instances of conventional acute osteomyelitis pursuing a course which, in the early phase of its evolution, did not result in the formation of an abscess, fistula, or sequestrum (see Jaffe and Lichtenstein). Furthermore, cases of "dry" or "atypical" osteomyelitis do not fit into the category of so-called "Brodie abscess."

Chronic Bone Abscess (Brodie Abscess).—A so-called Brodie abscess is a sharply delimited focus of infection usually present in only one bone site but sometimes also at more or less the same site in the corresponding opposite bone. The affected subjects are predominantly young people whose skeletal growth is not yet complete. The abscess may have been *in situ* for years before it was discovered, and during this time may have failed to give rise to any serious clinical complaints, those present consisting of intermittent bouts of pain, often more severe at night. In such a case, it can no longer be established that the abscess represents merely a local manifestation of an acute suppurative osteomyelitis.

The most common site of a Brodie abscess is the tibia, where it is located more often in the distal than in the proximal metaphysis. Other sites are the distal metaphyses of the radius and femur. (See Fig. 268.) Less often, an abscess develops in other tubular bones, and it is not unusual, when a long tubular bone is affected, for the abscess to be located more or less in the midportion of the shaft (see Wehner, and also Kasakow and Pokrowski). Rarely are such bones as a vertebra, patella, or calcaneus affected. Occasionally the presence of the abscess is discovered in the course of roentgenographic examination of a bone site which is painful, although the cause of the pain is not clear. The abscess may be only 1 cm. or as much as 3 or 4 cm. in diameter. Its wall is lined by inflammatory granulation tissue, and around its periphery, the spongy bone is likely to present areas of sclerosis. (See Fig. 269.)

Figure 267

A, B, C, D, and *E,* Photographs of various bones from different cases. These bones were the sites of pyogenic osteomyelitis. The overlying soft tissues have been removed. Unfortunately, the clinical details are not available except in regard to the femur illustrated in *C.*

A, The upper end of a femur showing irregularity in the contour of the femoral head, a large depression in the region of the fovea, and periosteal new bone deposition on the cortex of the intertrochanteric area of the shaft. There is some new bone deposition in the region of the lesser trochanter. There are erosions, lacunae, and new bone deposition in relation to the greater trochanter. An oblique fracture line can be seen extending downward from the junction of the upper and middle thirds of the shaft.

B, There is a clear-cut fracture line at the junction of the upper and middle thirds of this specimen (a femur). Especially below the fracture site, but also above, one can note deposits of new bone on the cortex. A large sequestrum *in situ* is apparent below the fracture.

C, The cut surface of a right femur is shown sectioned in the sagittal plane. The interior of the lower third of the shaft was the site of an abscess, as is evident from the lack of spongy trabeculae in that area. The epiphysial end of the bone shows two small cavities in the spongiosa, one of which contains a fragment of bone. The subject, 50 years of age when he was admitted to our hospital, had developed an osteomyelitis of the right femur in childhood, and after about 3 years of treatment, his local complaints subsided temporarily. Subsequently he had numerous recurrent complaints relating to the osteomyelitis, and a number of discharging sinuses appeared. Several days after his admission to our hospital, surgery disclosed a large abscess cavity in the lower third of the femoral shaft, and the tissue lining the wall of the cavity was curetted. Histologic examination revealed that the bone was the site of a chronic osteomyelitis. Bacteriologic examination of direct smears disclosed the presence of pus cells and gram-positive cocci, and culture of the specimen revealed that the infecting organism was *Staphylococcus aureus*. The man died about 1 week after the surgery. An autopsy was performed, in the course of which the femur was removed for anatomic examination. The cause of death was renal insufficiency, and the kidneys showed advanced chronic glomerular nephritis.

D, Part of a fibula showing thickening of the bone due to subperiosteal new bone deposition. Toward the right, one can see three openings leading from the surface of the cortex into the medullary cavity, and also some spicules of bone, representing sequestra, which are more clearly evident in *E.*

E, The fibula shown in *D,* sectioned in the longitudinal plane. The bone cortex has been thickened as the result of the deposition of subperiosteal new bone. The sequestra in the medullary cavity stand out clearly.

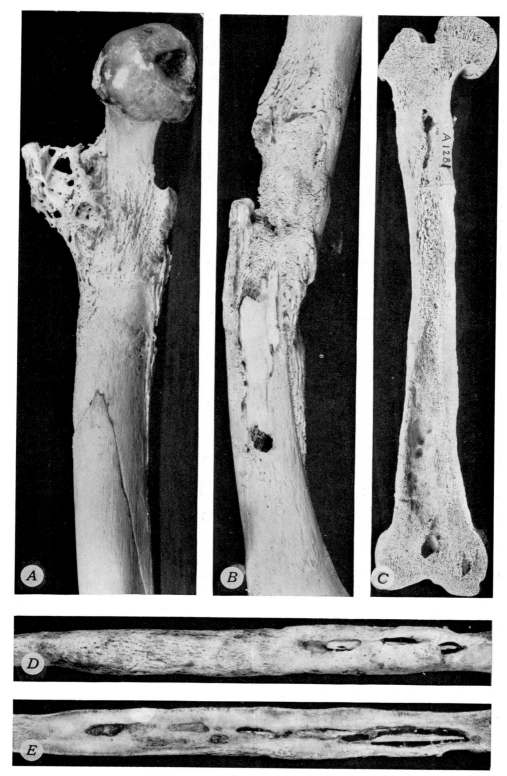

Figure 267

The fluid content of the abscess cavity is not the same in all cases. It may be purulent or oil-like or even mucoid or slimy. The infectious agent is also not always the same, and in an occasional instance, bacteriologic examination fails to reveal any organisms at all. If the abscess cavity is not sterile, bacteriologic examination will disclose the presence of staphylococci or streptococci and sometimes even both of them in the same abscess. In some cases the bacterial agent giving rise to the abscess is the typhoid bacillus.

Anatomically the inner surface of the abscess cavity is lined by a layer of granulation tissue which is infiltrated by leukocytes and sometimes even covered by a layer of fibrin. Toward the outer surface, the granulation tissue merges with a layer of connective tissue of varying thickness and density. This connective tissue represents the capsule of the abscess cavity, delimiting it from the neighboring osseous tissue. The spongy bone bordering on the abscess is somewhat compacted, though the densification is more conspicuous in some places than in others. The marrow spaces of the spongy bone neighboring on the abscess cavity contain myeloid and fatty marrow and a relatively small amount of connective tissue cells.

Figure 268

A, Roentgenograph showing a roundish area of radiolucency in the distal end of the shaft of the left radius of a 5-year-old boy. The boy was well until he fell off a bicycle and injured his left hand about 5 months before his admission to the hospital. Since the injury, he had pain in the wrist, with gradual swelling at the distal end of the forearm. He tended to spare the left wrist, and the pain occasionally kept him awake at night. Clinical examination disclosed a fluctuant swelling on the dorsoradial aspect of the left wrist. In addition, a chain of lymph glands was palpable in the left arm, from above the medial epicondyle, and a few shotty nodes were also palpable in the axilla. At the surgical intervention, the lesional area was found filled with granulation tissue and pus. Bacteriologic examination revealed the presence of a nonhemolytic coagulase-positive *Staphylococcus aureus.* The curettings from the wall of the lesion showed, on histologic examination, a loose, vascular granulation tissue heavily permeated with polymorphonuclear leukocytes and also mononuclear cells, most of which were macrophages.

B, Roentgenograph of the distal end of the left tibia, in which there are two adjacent foci of radiolucency, one of which extends to the epiphysial cartilage plate and into the medial aspect of the epiphysis. The patient was a boy 11 years of age who, about 1½ years before his admission to our hospital, developed some pain and swelling in the region of the left ankle. The pain subsided after several months, but the swelling persisted. Four months before the patient was admitted, the ankle again became painful, and a roentgenograph revealed the lesion in question. A surgical intervention was carried out, and several small bits of white and brownishly discolored tissue were curetted from the lesional area. Microscopically, this tissue was found to be highly vascular granulation tissue which was heavily permeated with polymorphonuclear leukocytes. Bacteriologic examination revealed the presence of coagulase-positive *Staphylococcus aureus,* and a diagnosis of staphylococcal osteomyelitis (localized bone abscess) was made.

C and *D,* Roentgenographs of a knee area, in anteroposterior and lateral projections, showing a bone abscess in the lateral condyle of a femur. The patient was a woman 31 years of age who was admitted to our hospital because of fever associated with pain and swelling of the left knee. These difficulties had been present for several weeks but had become definitely worse 1 week before admission. Physical examination revealed tenderness in the region of the knee, which was also swollen because of an intra-articular effusion. A surgical intervention was carried out, and the lesional area was saucerized. Histologic examination of the curettings revealed spongy bone manifesting inflammatory changes in the intertrabecular marrow spaces, and in some places there was a thick layer of inflammatory cells (mainly leukocytes) in a connective tissue substratum. Such areas represented the wall of the bone abscess. Staphylococci were cultured from the pus and tissue submitted for bacteriologic examination.

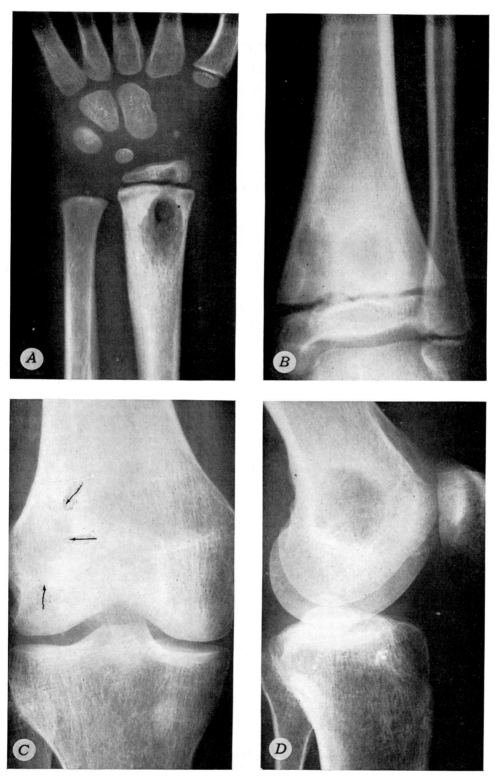

Figure 268

Suppurative Periostitis.—This is the result of an accumulation of pus in the loose layers of the periosteum—in particular, that part of the periosteum which is in immediate contact with the underlying bone. As the pus accumulates, the outer and more fibrous portion of the periosteum is elevated, and the blood supply which it brings to the bone is reduced, because the lumina of the periosteal blood vessels are narrowed as a result of compression and stretching of the vessels. Some of the blood vessels are also destroyed. Consequently, the nutrition of the cortical bone is disturbed, so that, if there is a large accumulation of pus, some small fragments of the outer portion of the cortical bone may become necrotic. If the subperiosteal pus enters the haversian canals and thus comes to obstruct the blood supply to deeper portions of the cortex, larger areas of the cortical bone become necrotic.

The accumulation of large amounts of pus under the periosteum also tends to stretch and destroy its outer coat. The pus may then make its way into the soft tissues overlying the bone (particularly into the muscle), and an abscess may form which sometimes eventually breaks through the skin and leads to the formation of a fistula. If the periosteum is not destroyed, the outer layer of the cortex often reveals

Figure 269

A, Roentgenograph of the right tibia and fibula which shows thickening of part of the medial aspect of the tibial cortex. Note that (as indicated by the arrows) the central part of the thickened cortex has a small area of relative radiolucency, which was found to represent an intracortical abscess. Though the roentgenograph might suggest that the lesion was an osteoid-osteoma, neither the clinical findings nor the clinical history supported that diagnosis. The patient was a 42 year old woman who was admitted to our hospital because of episodes of recurrent pain in her right leg of about 2 years' duration. The pain, which usually set in during the night and disappeared by morning, was associated with localized tenderness over the midportion of the tibia. Resection of the affected part of the tibial cortex was carried out. The specimen consisted of a block of cortical bone which measured 3.5 cm. in length, 2 cm. across, and 1.5 cm. in depth. The resected block of bone was cut longitudinally, and in the midportion of its cut surface a small focus of granulation tissue completely filled a defect in the cortex (see *B*).

B, Photomicrograph ($\times$ 8) disclosing a full cross section of the abscess which is located in the interior of the affected part of the tibial cortex shown in *A*. The thickening of the cortex is due to the apposition of subperiosteal new bone on the original cortical bone. Histologic examination clearly revealed that the lesion was a bone abscess. The granulation tissue was permeated with lymphocytes, plasma cells, and histiocytes. In the central part of the abscess, numerous polymorphonuclear leukocytes were still present.

C, Roentgenograph of a fibula (right) which is the site of an abscess. The patient was a boy 10 years of age who had fallen and injured his right leg about 4 months before his admission to our hospital. At the time of the accident he began to experience pain in the leg, his calf was swollen, and subsequently he became febrile. This roentgenograph, taken on the day after the patient's admission, shows thickening of the fibula due to the deposition of subperiosteal new bone. The arrows point out a small, faintly radiolucent, roundish area at the junction of the original cortex and the deposited subperiosteal new bone. This area was subsequently established as the site of a small cortical abscess at the border between the original cortical bone and the subperiosteal new bone. Surgery was carried out, about 8.5 cm. of the shaft of the fibula being resected. The bone was found somewhat thickened, particularly in the central portion of the specimen, which, when sawed open, disclosed a small, somewhat rounded defect at the junction of the cortex with the overlying subperiosteal new bone (see *D*).

D, Photomicrograph ($\times$ 8) of a tissue section from the lesional area of the fibula shown in *C*. It is clear that the abscess is located mainly near the outer surface of the original cortex, which has a thick layer of subperiosteal new bone deposited on it. The defect contained some soft, slightly granular inflammatory tissue.

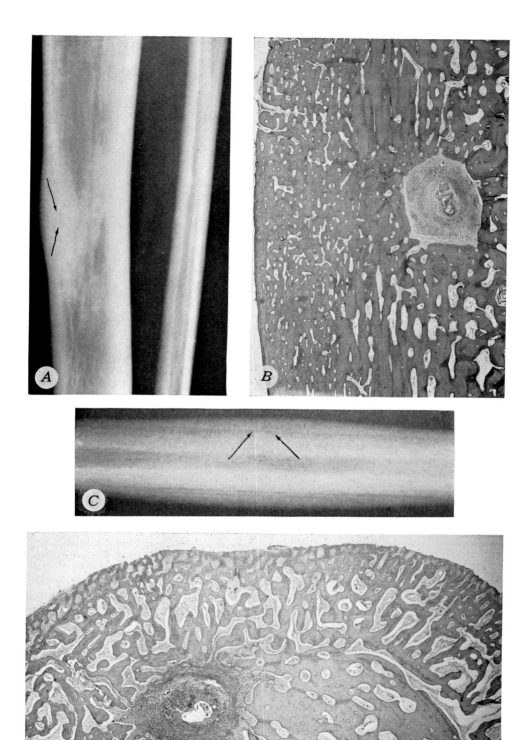

Figure 269

a considerable amount of subperiosteal new bone, which may present as irregular, flat and/or spiked osteophytes. If the affected bone is a tibia or a radius, there may be a bridge of new bone (osteophyte) which fuses the bone in question with its neighboring bone (tibia with fibula, radius with ulna). (See Fig. 270 and also Fig. 271–A and B.)

Pyogenic Arthritis.—This is one of the most common complications of pyogenic osteomyelitis, and is observed much more frequently in infants and young children than in adults. With osteomyelitis of bones of the carpus or tarsus (bones which are only infrequently involved), spread of the infection to adjacent joints is almost the rule. In accordance with the fact that the articular ends of long tubular bones are predilected sites of pyogenic osteomyelitis, the infection frequently spreads from such an affected bone to a neighboring joint. The joints most often involved are the knee and the hip (see Klemm, Heberling, and also Soeur). In large diarthrodial joints, the infection often spreads from the bone cortex to the periosteum and then into the joint at the site of attachment of the capsule.

However, a joint may become the site of a pyogenic arthritis in consequence of direct infection of the synovial membrane, the bacteria reaching it by way of the blood stream. From the articular cavity, the infection may spread to one or another of the bones entering into the formation of the joint. An acute purulent infection of a hip joint (especially in children) not infrequently leads to an intra-

Figure 270

A, Roentgenograph of the knee joint area and upper half of the tibia and fibula in the case of a man 65 years of age. Ten years before his admission to our hospital, he developed a draining abscess in the region of the left thigh. Chemotherapy was administered, and in a few months there was some clinical improvement. However, the knee became stiff, and about 10 months later, pus began to drain from the medial side of the knee. Further clinical study and roentgenographic examination of the limb disclosed that the left femur was the site of a chronic osteomyelitis, and that infection also implicated the tibia and fibula. Note that the patella is fused to the condylar area of the femur as a result of bony ankylosis. There are some small spikelike outgrowths of bone projecting from the proximal end of the patella, and a very large bony spike protrudes from the posterior surface of the femur. Similar but smaller projections are apparent at the proximal end of the tibia and of the fibula. A midthigh amputation was performed. On the medial aspect of the knee, the skin showed an area of ulceration measuring about 3 × 4 cm. The soft-tissue defect extended inward to the bone, the entire area was filled with granulation tissue, and pus was draining from the area. Further examination of the amputated extremity disclosed that the knee joint was rigid and could be moved only a few millimeters. Dissection of the knee area revealed that the rigidity of the joint was due to fibrous ankylosis of the articular capsule from the patellar ligament to the tibia, and was also due to fibrous adhesions between the articular ends of the femur and tibia. The remaining illustrations on this plate are from the same case.

B, Photograph of the tibia and fibula after their overlying soft tissues were removed. The upper end of the fibula is thickened, and its surface is irregular because of subperiosteal new bone deposition. The spikelike projections (osteophytes) from the tibia, visible on the right side of the picture, represent foci of periosteal bone formation, resulting from traction periostitis.

C, Photograph of the lower half of the femur after all the overlying soft tissues had been removed. Note that the patella is ankylosed to the condylar region of the femur. This finding conforms to the roentgenographic appearance shown in *A*. At the proximal end of the intercondylar region, an oval opening in the cortex is apparent. This opening led to an abscess cavity in the interior of the femur, and that abscess was the source of the pus.

D, Photograph showing the lower part of the shaft of the femur cut in the frontal plane. The cortex is very thick, and the medullary cavity is the site of an abscess containing, in some places, coagulated pus.

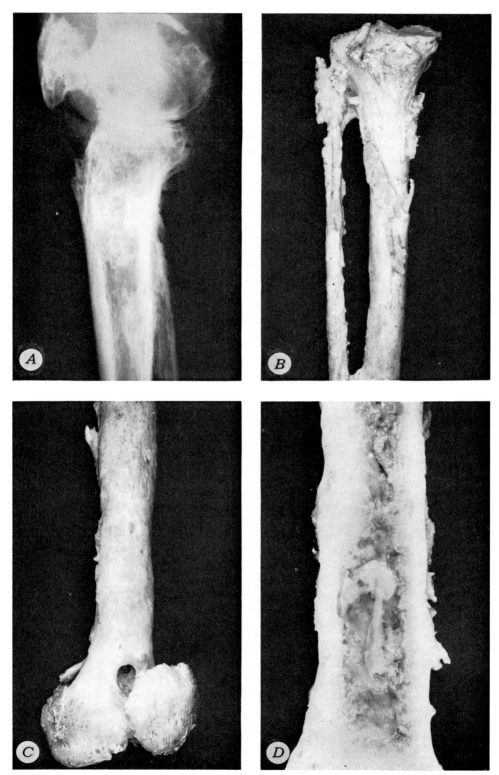

Figure 270

Figure 271

A, Photograph of the lower part of the left femur, cut in the frontal plane, in the case of a 54 year old woman whose left femur had been the site of osteomyelitis for 37 years. She was 38 years old at the time of her first admission to our hospital, and at that time she had a persistent sinus on the lateral aspect of the lower third of the left thigh. She also had increasing stiffness of the knee joint, and more frequent bouts of pain in the thigh. (Prior to her first admission here, she had had two surgical interventions for the osteomyelitis.) A saucerization was carried out, and tissue examination showed chronic osteomyelitis and sequestrum formation. The bacteriologic examination disclosed that the infectious agent was a coagulase-positive *Staphylococcus aureus*. During the next 5 years, she underwent two additional saucerizations. Bacteriologically, it was found that there was now a mixed bacterial infection, since (in addition to staphylococci) streptococci and diphtheroid bacilli were cultured. Two years after the last saucerization, the patient was readmitted because of fever and severe continuous pain in the region of the thigh, and a midthigh amputation was done. Note the large abscess in the interior of the lower end of the femoral shaft. The abscess is surrounded by a thick layer of dense white tissue (fibrous tissue) which extends into the epiphysial end of the bone. On the right, the fibrous tissue extends down to about an inch from the articular cartilage. However, though the encapsulating fibrous tissue extends to the subchondral spongiosa, it has not broken into the joint. At the distal end of the abscess cavity, there is a small, round fragment of bone, which is a sequestrum.

B, Roentgenograph of the specimen shown in *A*. The sequestrum in the abscess cavity is clearly evident. The fibrous tissue is relatively radiolucent, and where that tissue is not very dense it is even more radiolucent. The cortex in the vicinity of the abscess is definitely thickened.

C, Photograph of the lower end of the right femur and upper end of the tibia and of the fibula in the case of a man 63 years of age whose lower extremity had been amputated because of an osteomyelitis of 30 years' duration. The infection had begun in the knee joint. About 15 years before the patient was first admitted to our hospital, an arthrodesis had been carried out on the right knee joint, and that joint showed solid fusion at an angle of about 150°. Anteriorly the general area of the previous arthrodesis was found reddened, swollen, and sensitive to pressure. There was markedly increased local heat, and slight enlargement of the inguinal lymph nodes on the right side. Several months after his discharge, he was readmitted because of an acute exacerbation of the osteomyelitis at the distal end of the femur and proximal end of the tibia. A saucerization was carried out. When the superficial fascia was incised, a large amount of yellowish, thick, creamy pus gushed from the wound. Histologic examination revealed chronic osteomyelitis of the tibia, and *Staphylococcus aureus* was cultured from the material. The patient was discharged about a month after this surgical intervention, and was readmitted 15 years later. The right knee was found fused in complete extension, and there was a large area (about 3 inches) in the region of the knee joint anteriorly where the skin and subcutaneous tissues were absent. An amputation was carried out 14 cm. above the knee. On dissection, the knee joint was found fused. In the course of removal of the soft tissues from the region of the knee joint, the femoral and popliteal arteries were found thrombosed. A purulent exudate was present in the intermuscular spaces both superiorly and inferiorly. The periosteum of the lower part of the femur and upper part of the tibia was thickened, but stripped easily from the cortex. Note that, because of ankylosis of the knee joint, the articular cavity is no longer visible in this view. Part of the intercondylar area of the femur has been eroded, and inflammatory granulation tissue protrudes from it. Moreover, several inches of the anterior surface of the tibial cortex have been destroyed, and inflammatory granulation tissue extends to the surface of the tibia and fills its medullary cavity.

D, Posterior view of the specimen shown in *C*. The lateral condyle of the femur and the lateral plateau of the tibia are completely ankylosed, as is the tibiofibular joint. While some articular space still remains between the medial condyle of the femur and the medial plateau of the tibia, it is clear that, at a deeper level, there is some bony ankylosis of that part of the knee joint.

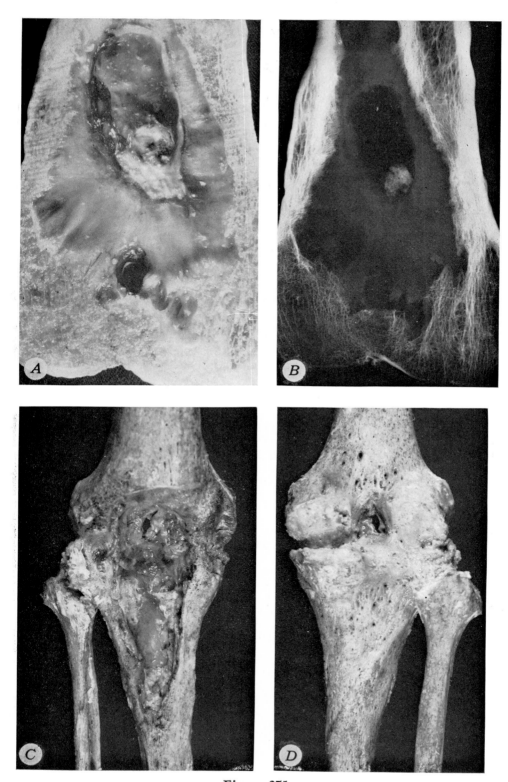

Figure 271

Figure 272

A, Roentgenograph of the right hip region in a case of acute osteomyelitis of the ilium and pyarthrosis of the hip joint. The patient, a boy, was 13 years of age when he was admitted to our hospital. He had fallen while playing basketball and injured his right hip region, but did not suffer any serious disability at that time. About a week later, however, he began to have pain in his right hip, and he also began to limp. In addition, he had some fever. At that time he was hospitalized at another institution. There, the right lower extremity was placed in traction, and a plaster-of-Paris cast was applied. About a week later, the cast was removed and the boy was discharged from the hospital. At home, he was in bed for about 2 weeks, after which he was admitted to our hospital. Physical examination at that time revealed the presence of a mass over the lateral aspect of the thigh between the greater trochanter of the femur and the crest of the ilium. The skin over the mass was movable, but the mass itself was adherent to the underlying structures. There was pronounced limitation of internal and external rotation of the hip joint. In the region of the acetabulum, it is evident that the ilium is eroded, and the hip joint is distended by fluid, which casts a somewhat radiopaque shadow, indicating that the fluid is thick inspissated pus. Immediately above the greater trochanter, there is a somewhat delimited shadow which may represent a fragment of bone that has separated from the eroded area of the ilium. A surgical intervention was carried out. The capsule of the joint was exposed and was found thick, tense, and bulging. The capsule was incised and a large amount of yellowish, turbid fluid was evacuated. The head of the femur appeared normal, but the upper rim of the acetabulum and the external surface of the ilium above the acetabulum were found slightly eroded. A few fragments of bone were removed. The histologic examination of the tissue disclosed the presence of a chronic osteomyelitis. The bacteriologic examination of the pus from the joint revealed that the infectious agent was the *Staphylococcus aureus*.

B, Roentgenograph from the case of a man 52 years of age in whom the right ischium and ascending ramus of the pubis were the site of a low grade osteomyelitis. A few months before the patient's admission to our hospital, he began to have some intermittent discomfort in the right buttock, the lateral aspect of the right thigh, and also the right knee joint. The lesion in the ischium and the affected part of the pubic bone discloses many small areas of relative radiolucency. At the site of junction between the ischium and the pubic bone, there is a perpendicular zone of radiolucency, vaguely suggestive of a fracture. A surgical intervention was carried out. The tissue sections prepared from the specimen revealed thickening of the osseous trabeculae, extensive scarring of the intertrabecular marrow, and evidence of chronic inflammation of the marrow spaces, as indicated by the presence of numerous lymphocytes and other inflammatory cells. These histologic changes were interpreted as representing a low grade chronic osteomyelitis (osteitis) of the ischium and pubis. Unfortunately, however, none of the tissue was submitted for bacteriologic examination.

C, Photograph of part of the right scapula and upper end of the humerus from a case of pyogenic arthritis. The patient was an 88 year old man. About 4 months before he was admitted to our hospital, he complained of pain in the right shoulder. The shoulder area became greatly swollen, and all the local landmarks were obliterated. Examination showed that the shoulder area was warm to touch and semifluctuant, and that the entire right upper extremity was enlarged. There was cyanosis of the hand, and the nails were also cyanotic. The skin was shiny and tense. The roentgenographs revealed definite soft-tissue swelling about the shoulder and an area of rarefaction in the medial half of the humeral head. One of the roentgenographs showed that the humeral head was not in proper relationship to the glenoid of the scapula. About 70 cc. of thick, whitish pus were aspirated from the joint anteriorly and laterally, and the infecting organism was found to be *Escherichia coli*. The man died and an autopsy was performed, in the course of which the affected shoulder region was removed. Note that the articular cartilage of the head of the humerus is completely eroded, as is the cartilage of the glenoid of the scapula. The autopsy also disclosed the presence of chronic pyelonephritis, cystitis, and urethritis. Additional findings included bronchopneumonia, a myocardial scar on the wall of the left ventricle, and a recently formed area of ischemic necrosis of the cardiac musculature.

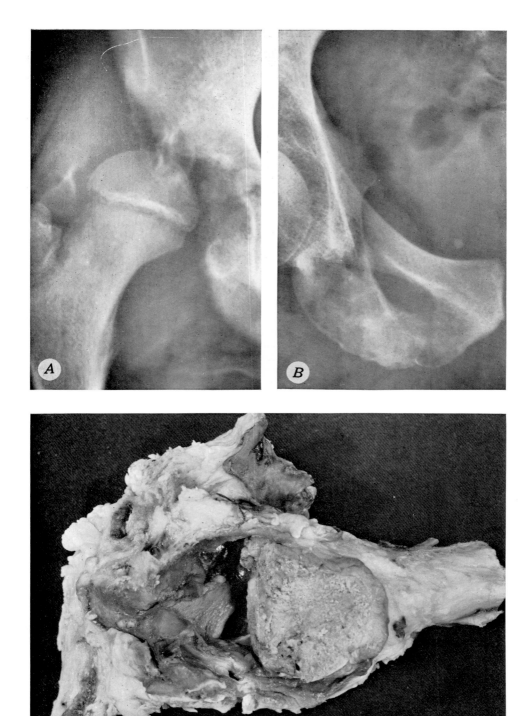

Figure 272

pelvic abscess, which results from extension of the infection to the retroperitoneal lymph nodes by way of the local lymphatic channels (see Freiberg and Perlman). (See Fig. 272.)

The establishment of the infection in the joint leads to purulent inflammation of the synovial membrane and destruction of the articular cartilages. In consequence, the marrow of the subchondral spongy bone becomes infected, and small abscesses are formed. The infection may then spread to the rest of the articular bone end, and large abscesses may develop there. Small or large areas of the articular bone end may become necrotic and appear as sequestra in roentgenographs. Extensive involvement of the articular bone ends of a joint and destruction of the

Figure 273

A, Roentgenograph illustrating bony ankylosis of the left hip joint in the case of a man who died at the age of 25. When the subject was 15 years of age, he developed *Staphylococcus aureus* septicemia and a pyogenic arthritis of the left hip joint, for which he was treated at another institution. Subsequently he was transferred to our hospital. He had a definite fluctuant area in the midportion of the left thigh, and this abnormal finding extended up toward the pelvis. There was ankylosis of the left hip joint, associated with slight adduction deformity. At the surgical intervention, an incision was made over the outer aspect of the left thigh, and a large amount of greenish pus was encountered. Bacteriologic examination of some of the pus revealed the presence of *Staphylococcus aureus*. About 1½ years after his first admission, he was readmitted because additional foci of osteomyelitis had appeared. One of these was located in the left radius, and another involved the external malleolus of the right tibia. Subsequently there were several additional admissions to our hospital. At the time of his death the patient had a 10-year history of osteomyelitis in multiple foci and also a 7-year history of drainage from a sinus in the region of the left ischium. An autopsy was performed and revealed chronic osteomyelitis of the sacrum, left innominate bone, and proximal end of the left femur; and ankylosis of the left hip joint (see *C*). Extensive amyloidosis of the liver, spleen, adrenals, pancreas, and kidneys was also present, the amyloidosis being the basic cause of his death.

B, Roentgenograph showing part of the right ilium and the upper part of the femur in the case of a man 64 years of age in whom this ilium was the site of an osteomyelitis. There was a concomitant pyogenic arthritis in the right hip joint. A surgical intervention was carried out, and inflammatory tissue was found on the outer surface of the ilium and in the medullary cavity of the affected part of that bone. Histologic examination established the presence of an osteomyelitis. The tissue sections showed subacute and chronic inflammatory changes in the bone marrow and in the extra-osseous soft tissues (the local fat and muscle).

C, Photograph of the pelvis, including the fifth lumbar vertebra and the upper end of the left femur, from the case whose clinical history is given in *A*. After these bones had been removed at autopsy, all the overlying soft tissues were removed, and hence the macerated specimen presents a clear picture of the sites of the osteomyelitis. Note that, in addition to the bony ankylosis of the left hip joint, there is erosion of the left side of the lower end of the sacrum. In the area above the acetabulum, the ilium is expanded and was apparently also a site of infection, as was the superior ramus of the pubis and also the upper end of the ischium on the left side.

D, Photomicrograph ($\times$ 7) of a slide prepared from the articular end of a femoral head in a case of pyogenic infection of the hip joint. It is clear that the articular cartilage has undergone complete destruction, which usually occurs with a pyogenic infection of a joint. The patient, a boy, was 13 years of age when he was first admitted to our hospital. He was transferred from another hospital whose clinical record indicated that there was a pyogenic infection of the upper end of the left femur and a concomitant infection of the hip joint. A surgical intervention was done at our hospital, during which a major portion of the capital epiphysis of the femur was removed, and pus was submitted for bacteriologic examination. The infecting organism was *beta*-hemolytic *Streptococcus*, and the histologic findings were consistent with a diagnosis of pyogenic arthritis.

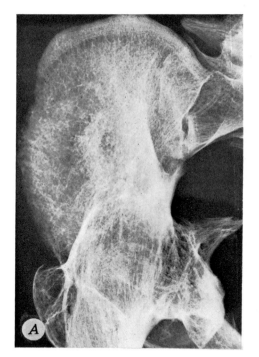
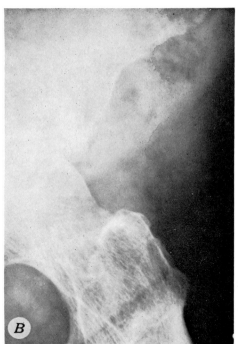
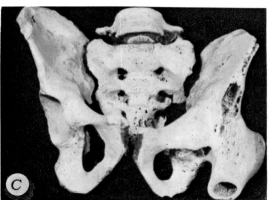
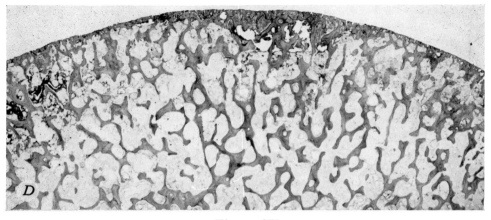

Figure 273

articular cartilages often lead to immobilization of the joint by fibrous adhesions or even by bony ankylosis. (See Fig. 271–C and D, and also Fig. 273.) It has been advocated by Paterson that these sequelae of acute suppurative arthritis can be avoided, especially in children, if: (1) an arthrotomy of the affected joint is done promptly; (2) the wound is closed without drainage; (3) adequate treatment with antibiotics is given; and (4) concurrently, the joint is immobilized for about 6 weeks.

Fistula Formation and its Sequelae.—Fistulae of long duration may have various unfavorable sequelae. Rather often, there is some bleeding from the granulation tissue lining the fistula, and if the bleeding continues for a long time, a severe anemia may ensue. The wall of a fistula frequently becomes epithelialized, the epithelium growing in from the skin around the external opening of the fistula. The epithelium lining the deep part of the fistula is likely to undergo repeated degeneration because of the presence of pus within the fistula. (See Fig. 274.) The epithelial lining of a fistula of long duration occasionally undergoes malignant transformation into a *squamous cell carcinoma* (see Jaffe). In the past, cancer developed in about 0.25 to 0.5 per cent of cases of protracted chronic osteomyelitis (see Benedict). It was usually only among those instances in which the bone infection had persisted for at least 20 or 30 years and in which sinuses were still present that this complication was likely to appear. The site of the tumor was most often a tibia. (See Fig. 275.) The writer has even observed an instance in which a sarcoma developed at the site of a chronic osteomyelitis. Cancer as a

Figure 274

A, Roentgenograph of the lower end of the right femur, which was the site of a chronic osteomyelitis and a draining sinus of long duration. The patient, a man 54 years of age when he was admitted to our hospital, sustained a football injury when he was 19 years of age. In the course of that injury, the distal epiphysis of the femur became separated from the shaft. (As indicated on p. 37, fusion of the distal femoral epiphysis with the shaft of the bone has already taken place by the age of 19 in at least 50 per cent of normal male subjects.) After the injury, an open reduction was carried out, but an infection developed. Over a period of many years, the man had a discharging sinus on the lateral surface of the lower part of the right thigh (see arrow). For a week or two prior to admission to our hospital, he was aware of increasing swelling of the lower part of the thigh and increasing discharge from the sinus. A midthigh amputation was done. On the lateral aspect of the leg, near the level of the knee joint, there was a healed scar about 19 cm. in length. This scar was apparently related to the site of the surgical intervention which was done when the subject was 19 years of age. In the region of the upper third of the scar, there was a sinus which measured up to 1 cm. in diameter. In the course of further dissection of the specimen, the knee joint was opened. The articular cartilages in the region of both femoral condyles showed slight pitting erosion and slight fibrillation.

B, Photograph of the cut surface of the femur, sectioned in the frontal plane. It should be noted that this photograph of the specimen is a mirror image of the roentgenograph shown in A. The opening of the sinus, indicated by the arrow on the left side in A, corresponds to the arrow on the right side in B. A large part of the interior of the femur was filled with very foul-smelling, white, inspissated, greasy, keratin-like material, similar in all respects to the contents of a large sebaceous or epidermoid cyst lined by stratified squamous epithelium. The material which filled the cystic area represents stratum corneum which had been shed by the squamous epithelium lining the cyst, and had accumulated within it.

C, Photomicrograph ($\times$ 5) of one of the tissue sections prepared from the region of the cyst in the femur illustrated in B. The section reveals in particular that the osseous wall of the cyst is lined by heavily keratinized squamous epithelium. The adjacent osseous tissue shows new bone formation, scarring of the marrow, and chronic inflammation. In processing the tissue for preparation of the sections, practically all of the greasy, keratin-like material was separated away from the underlying stratified squamous epithelium.

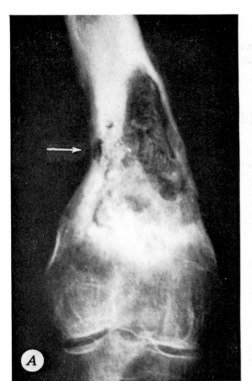

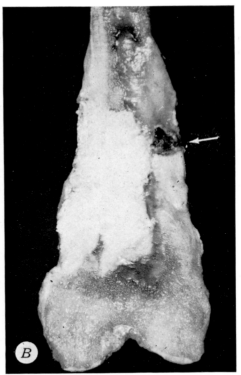

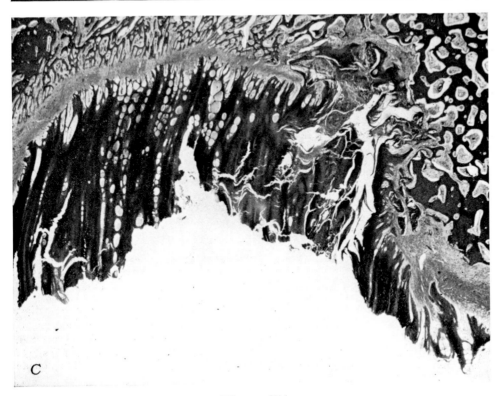

Figure 274

complication will probably be observed even less frequently in the future because of the modern management of such cases by aggressive surgery and antibiotic therapy.

SKELETAL INFECTIONS CAUSED BY OTHER BACTERIA

Salmonella Osteomyelitis.—*Salmonella* are gram-negative nonspore-forming bacilli. There are several species of *Salmonella*, but all are related with respect to their antigenic qualities. With one exception, they are pathogenic both for man and animals, the exception being *Salmonella typhosa* (the cause of typhoid fever), which is pathogenic for man but not for animals. An infection with *Salmonella typhosa* produces an acute fever due to intestinal inflammation, and as a complication of typhoid fever, a *Salmonella typhi* osteomyelitis was occasionally observed in the past (see Marbury and Peckham, and also Harris).

Salmonella osteomyelitis is a fairly frequent complication in cases of sickle cell anemia (p. 703). However, instances of *Salmonella* osteomyelitis have been observed in infants whose red blood cells do not sickle (see Ebrahim and Grech, and also Westerlund and Bierman). The present writer has also encountered two cases without sickle cell anemia: In one of them, the infecting bacillus was the *Salmonella oranienburg;* in the other, culture of the pus yielded a *Salmonella* bacillus, but the precise strain was not identified. The lower end of a tibia was affected in one of these instances, and the proximal half of the shaft of a radius in the other. (See Fig. 276.) Clinically, neither of the subjects appeared acutely ill. They had some intermittent pain in the affected region of the bone and some local swelling of the limb. Surgical exploration in both of these cases revealed thick yellow pus. Hematogenous osteomyelitis and pyarthrosis due to *Salmonella suipestifer* (the hog cholera bacillus) have also been encountered in infants, children, and young adults. The age of the subjects listed in the article by Weaver and Sherwood ranged from 5 weeks to 19 months. Harvey referred to 46 previously reported cases, and presented 21 additional instances. The clinical findings (aside from osteomyelitis) may include pneumonia, meningitis, endocarditis, and/or infection of the urinary tract. Harvey also pointed out that the majority of the cases of *Salmonella suipestifer* bacteremia occur during the first decade of life. However, the mortality statistics showed that

Figure 275

A, Roentgenograph showing a focus of chronic osteomyelitis in the lower part of the shaft of a tibia, at which site a squamous cell carcinoma appeared (see *C*). The patient was a man 66 years of age whose osteomyelitis dated back to late childhood. The lower part of the leg had been the site of several sinuses which had been draining more or less constantly for 26 years before the affected limb was amputated because of the complicating cancer.

B, Photograph showing a tibia which had been the site of a chronic osteomyelitis associated with the presence of a draining sinus. In this case a squamous cell carcinoma developed from the epithelium lining the sinus. The patient was a 64-year-old man who had suffered a shrapnel wound of the leg 38 years prior to admission, and developed a focus of osteomyelitis in the tibia. The carcinoma began to evolve about 1 year prior to amputation of the affected limb. At the time of the amputation, the regional inguinal lymph nodes were found enlarged. A subsequent radical lymph node resection revealed that the enlarged nodes were the site of metastases. The patient died of massive pulmonary embolism subsequent to the lymph node dissection.

C, Photomicrograph ($\times$ 75) illustrating the cytologic pattern of the squamous cell carcinoma from the case illustrated in *A*.

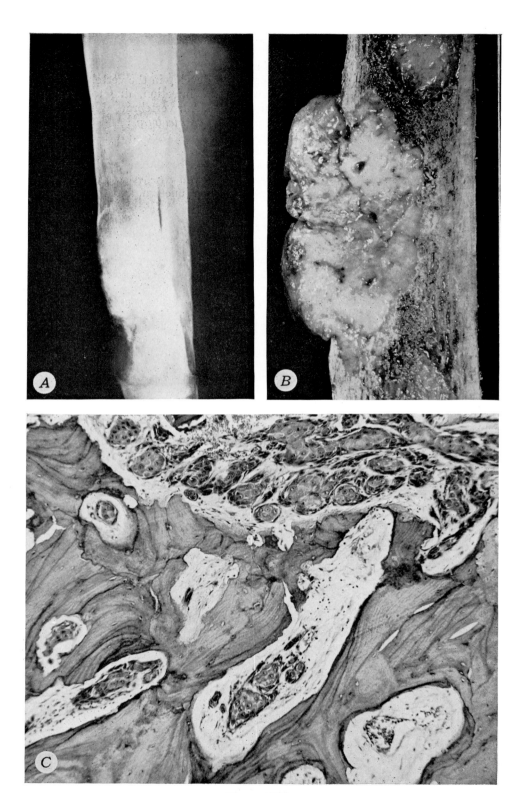

Figure 275

19 per cent of subjects under 25 years of age and 58 per cent over 25 years of age died. Only rarely does a salmonella osteomyelitis develop in the vertebral column. However, Ralston described a case in which the infection, due to *Salmonella cholerae suis*, was localized to the fourth and fifth lumbar vertebrae. Hunt reported a case of cervical spondylitis caused by *Salmonella oranienburg*.

Brucellosis.—*Brucella* are gram-negative coccobacilli which are nonmotile and nonsporulating. Brucellosis (also known as undulant fever, Bang's disease, Malta fever, etc.) is caused by an infection with any of the three known strains of *Brucella* organisms: *Brucella abortus*, *Brucella suis*, and *Brucella melitensis*. The pertinent bacteria infect man and animals via the skin, the conjunctiva, and the alimentary

Figure 276

A, Roentgenograph from a case in which the lower end of the right tibia was the site of *Salmonella* osteomyelitis. The patient, a 20-year-old man, was admitted to our hospital because of pain in the region of the right ankle. The pain had set in 5 years earlier, and during the intervening period it was mild and intermittent, the recurrent pain usually coming on after exertion. About 2 years before admission, the right ankle region swelled, a subcutaneous abscess became apparent, and some pus was evacuated from the abscess. Shortly before admission to the hospital, another episode of painful swelling of the ankle occurred. The clinical history does not make any reference to any intestinal disturbance or fever associated with the onset of the local difficulties. The temperature, pulse rate, and blood count were within normal limits. A surgical exploration of the affected part of the tibia and curettage of the area was performed. Some pus from within the lesional area was cultured and revealed a gram-negative bacillus of the *Salmonella* group which was subsequently identified as *Salmonella oranienburg*. Histologic examination of the tissue showed evidence of chronic osteomyelitis of a rather nondescript pattern. There were fields heavily permeated with polymorphonuclear leukocytes interspersed with macrophages, some of which were filled with lipid. In other fields the inflammatory cells in the marrow spaces were mainly lympho-cytes and macrophages. About 14 years later, swelling and a draining sinus in the region of the right ankle, representing a recurrence of the osteomyelitis of the lower end of the tibia, necessitated readmission to the hospital. Culture again revealed the presence of *Salmonella oranienburg*. Antibiotics were administered, the draining subsequently ceased, and the wound was healing well when the patient was discharged. About 9 months later, however, there was another recurrence of the osteomyelitis. The affected end of the tibia was again saucerized, antibiotic therapy was instituted, the wound closed, and he was finally discharged 2 months later as cured.

B, Roentgenograph of the upper part of the right forearm in a case in which the radius was the site of a *Salmonella* infection. Note the thinning of the cortex from the medullary side and the radiolucent appearance of the interior of the bone in the lesional area. The patient, a man 52 years of age, had had pain and swelling of the right forearm for 2 months prior to his admission to our hospital. Examination revealed that his temperature and pulse rate were within normal limits. The upper part of the affected forearm was moderately swollen and sensitive to touch; there was a slight increase in local heat and some restriction of motion at the elbow joint. The sedimentation rate was somewhat increased, as was the leukocyte count. During the surgical intervention on the radius, thick pus was encountered in the subcutaneous tissue, and an abscess was also found within the radius. A *Salmonella* organism was cultured from the pus. The tissue submitted for histologic examination con-sisted of a number of bone shavings which, for the most part, represented fragments of modified cortical bone. The details of the inflammatory changes are revealed in *C*.

C, Photomicrograph ($\times$ 120) prepared from a tissue section of the modified cortex of the affected radius. The cortex is rarefied, and the enlarged haversian canals contain inflamma-tory cells. In the upper part of the picture, the inflammatory disease process is character-ized by the presence of granulation tissue containing leukocytes and epithelioid cells. In some places the epithelioid cells were found agglomerated. The presence of these collec-tions of epithelioid cells is consistent with an infection by an organism of the *Salmonella* group.

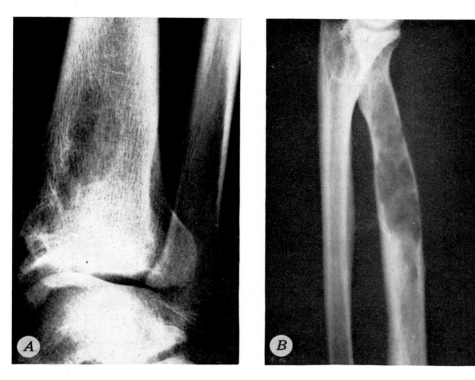

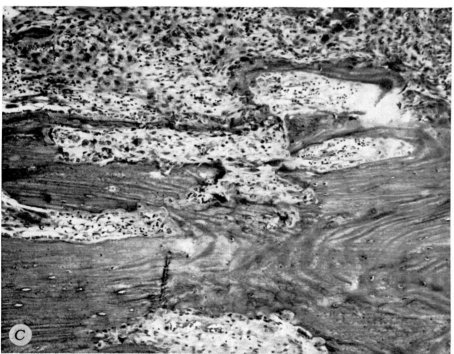

Figure 276

tract. Experiments on animals also indicate that under certain environmental conditions the respiratory tract is an important site of entry for the bacteria. Growth of the bacteria at the various portals of entry, and invasion of the regional lymph channels, leads to introduction of the bacteria into the blood stream. Consequently, they may localize in the spleen, liver, lymph nodes, bone marrow, joints, and/or kidneys.

The disease may take one of three clinical forms: It may start as an acute febrile disease with a strong tendency to become recurrent and chronic; it may start insidiously and pursue a chronic course, which may be interrupted by bouts of fever; or it may be present in a subclinical form (see Lowbeer). A focus of brucellotic osteomyelitis usually does not become manifest clinically for a few weeks or months after the onset of the infection. An instance has also been described in which a vertebral lesion appeared 1 year after the initial infection (see Bishop). When brucellosis is established in a bone or joint, pain is noted in the implicated part. If the infection is in the vertebral column, its most common site is the lumbosacral region. Another articulation frequently involved is the sacroiliac joint (see Serre *et al.*).

In regard to the *pathologic findings*, it is to be noted that when the brucella organisms leave the blood stream and enter one or another tissue site, the local reaction is characterized by the accumulation of large numbers of mononuclear cells (macrophages) rather than polymorphonuclear leukocytes. Instead of microabscesses, such as develop with staphylococcal infections, granulomas are formed. Microscopically the granulomas, in addition to the macrophages, show the presence of some lymphocytes, plasma cells, and perhaps a few multinuclear giant cells of the foreign body type. The brucella organisms are phagocytized by the macrophages, and those which survive and multiply in the macrophages may be transported by the latter to other body sites.

The reported *incidence of skeletal involvement* in brucella infections ranges from 2 per cent to 70 per cent, the highest incidence being observed in *Brucella melitensis* infections. Bursae and tendon sheaths, too, may become the site of a brucella infection. The bones most frequently affected are the vertebrae, but localization in various long and/or flat bones has also been reported. Within the vertebral column, a part of the lumbar or dorsolumbar area is most often implicated. When a vertebra becomes diseased, its body, especially the part nearest the disk, is usually affected. Under these circumstances, two adjacent vertebral bodies may be found involved. In particular, wedging of vertebrae and angulation or tilting of the spine are not uncommon. Extradural compression of the cord as a result of the spondylitis may be the cause of myelopathy in cases of brucellosis (see Ganado and Craig). An instance has been reported in which the infection took its departure in an intervertebral disk rather than in a vertebral body (see Aguilar and Elvidge). When the brucella organisms become localized in the marrow of a bone, minute granulomas are formed, and for a short time the osseous tissue itself is not modified. Eventually, however, the granulomas may undergo necrosis, and a caseous focus of brucellotic osteomyelitis may then develop. The caseous necrotic area is sometimes encapsulated by a thick layer of connective tissue.

With brucellosis melitensis, large diarthrodial joints (and occasionally only a single large joint) are frequently involved (see Makin *et al.*). More often than not, the only articular manifestation is a hydrarthrosis. Septic arthritis has also been noted, a pertinent instance resulting in solid ankylosis of the hip joint having been reported by O'Donoghue. A case of brucellosis of the sacroiliac joint, in which the condition led to ankylosis of that joint, was described by Steinberg, who also made reference to other cases reported in the literature.

Hemophilus influenzae.—These bacteria are capable of producing pyogenic infections. In children, the prognosis is frequently grave, while adults are less often affected and the disease pursues a milder form. Farrand *et al.* have described two instances of hemophilus infection in infants. In one, the lesion was in the neck of a femur, and in the other it presented as a suppurative arthritis of a knee joint. In these cases an infection of the respiratory tract preceded the hematogenous spread of the hemophilus bacteria to the skeletal areas. Other authors have also described instances in infants and young children of acute hematogenous pyarthrosis due to *Hemophilus influenzae* (see Wall and Hunt). As already stated, *Hemophilus influenzae* infection is not so common in adults as in children. A pertinent case of pyarthrosis involving an ankle joint in an adult was reported by Patterson and Levine, who point out that, in adults, septic arthritis caused by the *Hemophilus influenzae* might be associated with a concomitant meningitis.

Clostridium welchii.—*Clostridium welchii* is one of many species of bacteria belonging to the clostridia group, and is ordinarily classified as *Clostridium perfringens*. It is the most common etiologic agent of gas gangrene, and occasionally is the cause of an acute septic arthritis, the knee joint being the site of predilection. Clinically the complaints and findings in joints infected with *Clostridium welchii* are similar to those caused by other bacteria. With respect to treatment and prognosis, it is of interest that in the case of *Clostridium welchii* infection of a knee joint reported by McNae, and in the two cases reported by Torg and Lammot, excellent functional recovery followed upon surgical exploration of the affected joint, evacuation of the pus, and the administration of large doses of antibiotics—especially penicillin.

Meningococcus.—Articular inflammation caused by a meningococcal infection was already discussed in 1899 by Gwyn, who recovered meningococci from an involved joint and from the blood and spinal fluid in a case of cerebrospinal fever. Osler described the clinical characteristics of meningococcal arthritis. In 1919, Herrick and Parkhurst presented in detail the articular manifestations of meningococcal infection. Schein reported 23 cases of meningococcal infection in which there was involvement of joints: in 14, more than one joint was implicated; in 11, a knee joint was affected, either alone or in conjunction with other joints. It appears that in some of the cases the articular difficulties set in before the meningitis became clinically evident; in others, the arthritis did not become manifest for several days or even several weeks after the onset of the meningitis; and in still other cases the articular difficulties were apparently related to serum sickness. In any event, the affected joints were painful.

As described by Keefer *et al.*, the meningococcal infection of a joint pursues the following course: The bacteria usually reach the articular capsule by way of the blood stream, and become localized in the connective tissue beneath the synovial membrane. The infected tissue soon becomes infiltrated by polymorphonuclear leukocytes, lymphocytes, and plasma cells, many of which surround the local blood vessels. As the infection progresses and the inflammatory changes increase, the synovial lining cells are destroyed, and the inner lining of the capsule is covered by a layer of granulation tissue heavily infiltrated with polymorphonuclear leukocytes. The prognosis for meningococcal arthritis seems to be much better for children than adults. Only very infrequently, because of the high mortality rate, are the pathologic changes so advanced that the affected joints become ankylosed following destruction of the articular cartilages and infection of the articular ends of the bones entering into the formation of the joint.

Pneumococcus.—The over-all incidence of articular involvement in cases of pneumonia is only about 0.3 per cent, the arthritis becoming manifest sometimes before and sometimes after the pulmonary infection. Occasionally, pneumococcal arthritis appears as a result of an extrapulmonary infection: an infection of the skin in the region of the joint, or by extension of the pneumococcal infection from a bone directly into the neighboring joint. Even more rarely, the arthritis may set in without a pneumococcal infection elsewhere in the body, thus representing a "primary" or "cryptogenic" arthritis (see Boger, and also Keefer *et al.*).

Gonococcus.—As to skeletal infection by gonococci, it is to be noted that joints are usually involved, and that the arthritis is ordinarily associated with gonococcal infection of the urethra or some other part of the genitourinary tract. The arthritis is much more often polyarticular than monarticular. In descending order, the joints most frequently involved are the knees, ankles, and wrists, although almost any joint may be implicated. Concomitantly there may be tenosynovitis (especially if it is the wrist and ankle joints that are the sites of the arthritis), and Keefer and Spink emphasize the diagnostic significance of tenosynovitis.

The inflammatory process in a joint may be relatively mild. If it is, the lining cells of the synovial membrane are intact, but, deep to the lining cells, the membrane may be heavily infiltrated by polymorphonuclear leukocytes, lymphocytes, and plasma cells. If the inflammatory process is more pronounced, the synovial lining may be destroyed, and the inner surface of the articular capsule is then covered by granulation tissue containing polymorphonuclear leukocytes, macrophages, and also plasma cells. As the inflammation progresses, the articular cartilages may be destroyed and the infection may even come to involve the subchondral bone. On the other hand, a hematogenous gonococcal infection may localize first in an articular bone end of a joint, and may spread from there to the joint and involve the synovial membrane.

LEPROSY

Leprosy (Hansen's Disease).—Leprosy is a chronic infectious disease, long familiar and by no means rare. It is still a common disease in tropical and subtropical regions and in the Orient, and is rather prevalent in Central Africa and Central and South America. It is probably present more or less sparsely in most other regions of the world, but appears to be definitely rare in the Arctic and Antarctic zones. The historical aspects and the geographic distribution of leprosy have been presented in detail by Riordan.

The etiologic agent of leprosy is *Mycobacterium leprae* (the Hansen bacillus). The *Mycobacterium leprae* differs from all other bacteria in its propensity for invading peripheral nerves. The tiny dermal nerves are regularly involved in the skin lesions, and in many patients, large peripheral nerves are affected. The histopathologic reaction in nerves reflects the type of leprosy present. In the lepromatous type, as delineated by Binford, there are many bacilli in affected nerves but there is very little cellular reaction, while in the tuberculoid type, although there are few bacilli, the severe cellular reaction may completely destroy the nerve.

Leprosy is evidently at least mildly contagious, for it has been established that, through prolonged and intimate contact, it can be transmitted from a leper to a healthy person. Experimental attempts to transmit leprosy to humans or animals by inoculation have not yet yielded entirely conclusive results. However, Rees *et al.* have reported that, when the footpads of mice were injected with *Mycobacterium leprae*, local lepromatous lesions could be demonstrated after a 2-year period.

The condition is distinguished *pathologically* by a specific granulation tissue which may develop in almost any part of the body and which contains the acid-fast bacillus discovered by Hansen in 1874. The disease involves principally: the skin, certain peripheral nerves, the mucous membranes of the respiratory tract, the anterior part of the eye, and the testes. It is most likely that the nasal passage is the usual portal of entry, as the lepra bacilli tend to localize early in the nasal mucosa. The incubation period is very long, having been estimated as 3 to 6 years by a number of investigators.

Clinical Considerations.—With respect to *age incidence,* statistics indicate that the disease becomes clinically manifest when the subjects are under 20 or over 30 years of age. However, there is considerable variation in regard to the age of the subjects, and this variation is related to differences in the geographic distribution of the cases. For instance, in the United States, about 24 per cent of the patients are under 20 years of age, while in the Philippines about 65 per cent are in that age group. When the disease sets in after 30 years of age, 51 per cent are in this age category in the United States, while in the Philippines, only about 17 per cent are older than 30 (see Badger). That leprosy is encountered *more often in males* than in females is definitely established, the preponderance of males over females being almost 2 to 1. Irrespective of geographic distribution of the cases, if one spouse has leprosy, the incidence of leprosy in the other spouse is only 5 or 6 per cent.

The disease has traditionally been divided into two main types—*nodular leprosy* and the *neural form of leprosy*—although both types may be present in the same subject. In the *nodular type* the clinical picture is dominated by the presence of firm nodules (lepromata) located mainly in the skin of the face, hands, and feet, and in the mucous membranes of the nasal and oral cavities. In the *neural type,* because of the development of lepromatous granulation tissue in and around nerves, the clinical picture is dominated by neurologic phenomena. When the peripheral nerve trunks are affected, striking sensory and neurotrophic disturbances appear, especially in the hands and feet.

Leprosy is often ushered in by rather prolonged prodromal symptoms. Among these, malaise, drowsiness, profuse sweating, and slight continuous or intermittent fever are prominent, and rhinitis is also often present. In the neural form of the disease, the presenting complaints may be superficial sensory disturbances (pruritus, hyperesthesia, anesthesia) or lancinating pains, exacerbated by pressure, along the course of certain peripheral nerves. The principal clinical manifestations are: (1) the development of granulomatous nodules in the skin (characterizing lepromatous leprosy) and (2) involvement of peripheral nerves (characterizing the neural, or anesthetic, form of leprosy).

In the cases of *nodular leprosy* showing prominent superficial lesions, the skin of the face and of the extremities (especially the back of the hands and the fore part of the feet), and the mucous membrane of the cheeks, nose, fauces, and tongue are the sites where the leprous nodules are most likely to form. As the lepromata on the face grow larger, they raise the skin in folds and create the typical leonine countenance and characteristic bumps. The infiltrated patches may eventually become anesthetic merely through the direct effect of the inflammatory tissue upon local nerves. The leprous lesions in the skin and mucous membrane tend to soften and break down, turning into discharging phagedenic ulcers. The lepra bacilli are recoverable from the discharge. The erosive action of these ulcers is sometimes so severe that large areas of bone and cartilage, especially of the face, may be destroyed. Some of the ulcers may heal, leaving scars, while lepromata elsewhere ulcerate. If left to run their natural course, such cases often go on for decades before the patient dies.

In the *neural form of leprosy,* the clinical picture, as already stated, is dominated by neurologic abnormalities—especially sensory and neurotrophic changes. The skin of the back and of the extremities first shows a more or less symmetrical distribution of circular, oval, or irregularly shaped, brown, reddish, or purplish macules, or plaques. Not long thereafter, muscle atrophy may become clearly evident—for instance, in the hands. By this time, the affected large nerves of the extremities can sometimes be felt as thick, stiff cords. After a year or two, the plaques begin to enlarge, their edges become raised, and their centers yellowishly discolored. The affected skin areas (which may at first have been hyperesthetic) become definitely anesthetic. Muscular power also suffers progressive disturbance and loss, parts may become paralyzed, and the hands and feet finally distorted into clawlike positions. However, the sensory changes are already far advanced before motor disturbances become prominent. Finally, extensive mutilations on a neurotrophic basis, aggravated by mixed infection, may make their appearance.

Pathologic Findings.—As already stated, it is clear that lesions may evolve in almost any tissue or organ. Here, of course, we are interested primarily in the skeletal lesions. It may well be said at once that the initial leprous skeletal lesions are relatively unimportant as compared with those bone and joint changes which follow upon neural damage and secondary infection.

The formation of lepromata begins around blood vessels. The tissue constituting these lesions, wherever situated, is rather characteristic microscopically. Its foundation is a loose-meshed connective tissue which is cellular and contains an abundance of vascular channels and dilated lymphatic channels. It is distinguished by the presence of great numbers of cells which are loaded with globules of fat. These cells are mainly mononuclear, although a few multinuclear giant cells may also be seen. Some of the cells become so distended by fat globules that their cellular structure is greatly modified. They then appear vacuolated and foamy when the fat has been dissolved out in the course of processing the tissue for histologic examination. Often the lepromata contain acid-fast lepra bacilli, sometimes in great numbers. Sawtschenko and also MacCallum noted that numerous bacilli are usually observable in the vascular endothelial cells also. Only where the leprous granulation tissue has become necrotic or secondarily infected is more than an occasional polymorphonuclear leukocyte likely to be found in it.

Binford points out that, "On the basis of clinical and histopathologic examinations, the disease falls into two distinct reaction types: (1) the *lepromatous*, in which there is evidently poor host resistance (because the bacilli grow prolifically in host macrophages and Schwann cells), and (2) the *tuberculoid*, in which a small number of bacilli excite a severe granulomatous reaction similar to that seen in sarcoidosis or proliferative tuberculosis. In addition, a group of cases called *'borderline'* or *'dimorphous'* occurs, in which clinical and histopathologic features of each type are present. A fourth group, designated as *'indeterminate,'* is comprised of cases in which clinical and histopathologic changes are so mild that definite classification cannot be made." In the *neural form of leprosy* the sensory nerves in particular become implicated, and the areas served by these nerves are thus subject to damage due to loss of local sensation. In the neural lesions the bacilli which are present in the perineural and epineural tissues incite the formation of granulation tissue. In consequence the neural fibrils degenerate, and the resultant loss of motor function and sensory perception leads to atrophy of the implicated hands and feet. As a result, the parts in question are likely to be subjected to repeated injuries and may ultimately become severely damaged.

The ratio of the lepromatous to the nonlepromatous (tuberculoid) type of leprosy varies from area to area of the world. In particular, Skinsnes reported, on the basis of a survey of the literature, that in Japan 63.5 per cent of the affected subjects had the lepromatous form and 36.5 per cent the nonlepromatous (tuberculoid) form. In India, on the other hand, only 12 per cent of affected subjects were found to have the lepromatous form of the disease, while 88 per cent had the nonlepromatous form. In Uganda the proportion of lepromatous to nonlepromatous leprosy in 1958 was found to be 18.4 to 81.6 per cent. In the United States (Texas, in particular) in 1957, the proportion was 79.3 to 20.7 per cent. In Brazil, it was 60.7 to 39.3 per cent.

The *skeletal changes* of leprosy have their basis in: (1) actual local inflammatory leprous lesions, and (2) neural abnormalities leading indirectly to skeletal changes. The specific leprous alterations in the skeletal tissues appear mainly, if not solely, when the leprosy is characterized by the presence of nodular lesions on the surface of the body. (See Fig. 277.) In these cases, bone involvement usually takes place by *extension* of the infection from dermal or mucosal areas to directly underlying skeletal parts. It is for this reason that the phalanges and the skull bones are the skeletal tissues most frequently affected when the disease spreads in this way. Accordingly, also, *leprous periostitis* is the commonest and sometimes the sole resulting lesion. The underlying bone may, however, be penetrated and somewhat eroded by the periosteal leproma. Ordinarily there is very little periosteal new bone formation if there is no superimposed mixed infection. If a secondary infection is present, the periosteal reaction may be extensive and much new bone may be deposited. The underlying bone is likewise subject to the aggravating effects of secondary infection, which may induce necrosis of bone and the formation of sequestra.

Sometimes the bacilli reach the skeletal tissues by the *hematogenous route* instead of penetrating to them directly from overlying dermal lesions. Under these conditions, not only can periostitides develop, but also intra-osseous (intramedullary) foci. Ordinarily the periosteal lesions originating in this way are very small. They are encountered most often on the bones of the hands and feet, and on the tibia, radius, ulna, and ribs. Such leprous periostitides often evolve synchronously with spurts of new dermal eruption. They do not usually cause important changes in the underlying bones. In fact, they may fail to give any clinical evidence of their existence and may be apparent only roentgenographically.

The *intra-osseous foci* are most commonly situated in the ends of the bones affected. Less commonly involved are the diaphyses of short tubular bones and the small bones of the carpus and tarsus. In rare instances there is diffuse infiltration of the entire marrow cavity of a bone. Sawtschenko carefully traced the evolution of leprous osteomyelitic foci from the first changes in the bone marrow. Histologically the established lesions in the bone marrow resemble the leprous lesions in other types of tissue. The foci are usually of mustard seed to pea size. They are yellow and rather firm. The spongy trabeculae within them are more or less extensively resorbed, but ordinarily are not necrotic. If the focus grows, the neighboring cortical bone may be perforated. It is penetrated by the specific granulation tissue which enters the haversian canals, eroding and enlarging the canals. However, the destruction of the osseous tissue is very slow in leprous osteomyelitis. In this respect, the latter contrasts with most other osteomyelitides, including the tuberculous. Furthermore, the leprous infection *per se* does not seem to provoke much reactive proliferation of new bone. Altogether, the disease process in the bone is not very active when there is no complicating secondary infection. (See Fig. 278.)

Specific leprous arthritis seems to be rare, and no adequate pathologic studies have been made of it. The arthritis, too, occurs particularly with nodular leprosy. As described by Hirschberg and Biehler, the arthritis may manifest itself clinically (if a large joint is affected) in pain and swelling, with extreme hydrops. The effusion may distend the joint to such an extent that both active and passive motion are arrested, but this effusion usually eventually regresses. In specific leprous arthritis, the joints most often implicated, in order of decreasing frequency of involvement, are the ankle, knee, wrist, finger, and elbow. Articular involvement is usually the result of extension of a disease focus in the bone or periarticular tissues to the synovial membrane. Occasionally it seems to evolve in consequence of hematogenous infection of the synovial membrane.

The skeletal changes occurring on a *neurotrophic basis* are much more severe than those caused by actual leprous lesions. The clinical aspects of such cases were discussed by Hillis in 1881, and his monograph also contains some information on the pathologic basis for the clinical manifestations. Subsequently, Harbitz emphasized their neural origin. Hopkins and also Chamberlain *et al.* described in detail the roentgenographic aspects of the neurotrophic changes occurring in cases of leprosy of long duration.

It is mainly in the *bones of the hands and feet* that these alterations develop to the fullest extent. An instance of anesthetic leprosy in an early stage came to the attention of the writer. There was some numbness of both hands, and distinct dermal macules were present. The roentgenograph disclosed very early changes of bone atrophy, especially in the terminal phalanges of the fifth fingers and in the cortex of the proximal phalanx of one thumb. Such atrophic changes, which usually advance slowly in a proximal direction, arise through irregular, progressive, vascular resorption of the affected bones from their outer surfaces. This centripetal erosion may become so pronounced that the phalanges are finally sharpened to points or even entirely resorbed. Rows of phalanges may disappear and the affected fingers and toes become mere stubby, grotesque stumps. In bones affected by the neurotrophic atrophy but still retaining their original shape, the cortex will be strikingly thinned and show deep resorption lacunae, while the spongy trabeculae will have disappeared almost completely. Such bones contain very gelatinous fatty marrow. The surrounding soft parts, including the skin and nails, also show the effects of the sensory and trophic disturbance. The muscles are atrophied, but, on the whole, when not complicated by secondary infection, there is less damage in the soft parts than in the bone. If, in the course of its rarefaction, a bone undergoes a fracture, callus formation and healing do not take place and the fragments may ultimately be resorbed.

Figure 277

A, Photograph of a young man affected with leprosy whose difficulties relating to the disease were of about 5 years' duration. The slightly leonine appearance is due to lepromatous lesions in the skin of the face. The extensor surfaces of both thighs present more or less symmetrical, irregularly shaped, brownish areas of discoloration. A similar, though small, patch of discoloration is apparent on the abdominal wall, and there is also one on the anterior surface of the midportion of the right leg.

B, Photograph of part of the back and the posterior aspect of both thighs of the subject shown in *A*. The brownish discoloration of the skin is even more clearly apparent in this photograph.

C, Photograph of the dorsal aspect of both hands from another case of leprosy. The patient was a man 31 years of age who had been affected with leprosy for almost 7 years. At the onset of his illness, an eruption was noticed on the skin of one leg. Within a month, it also became evident elsewhere on his body, with the exception of the palms of his hands, the soles of his feet, and the flexor surfaces of the upper and lower extremities. Shortly thereafter, there was loss of mobility of the left hand, starting with the fifth finger and successively involving the rest of the fingers of that hand. There was also atrophy of the fifth finger and the palmar surface of the hand. The hand was numb, and he could not differentiate between warmth and heat. Six years later the fingers of the right hand lost their mobility in the same successive fashion as that of the left hand, and the numbness and loss of temperature differentiation were noted. Three weeks prior to admission, he attempted to light a stove, not knowing that the stove was already hot. Having touched the stove, he felt no sensation, retired to bed, and awoke the next morning with the burn blisters apparent in the picture. Physical examination showed clawlike hands, with marked atrophy of the fifth fingers. In the course of his hospitalization, a piece of skin and a nodule were removed for histologic examination, and the microscopic findings revealed the pathologic changes of leprosy.

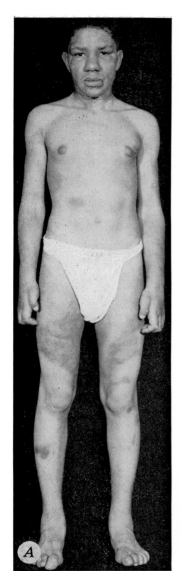

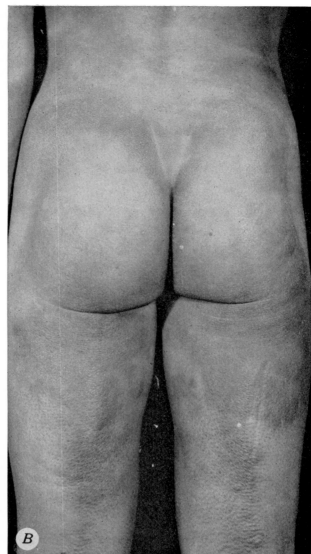

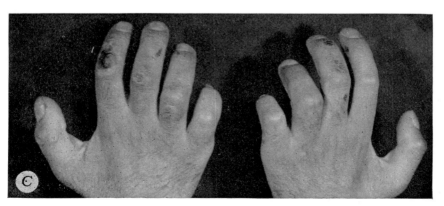

Figure 277

Because of the anesthesia resulting from the neural lesions, the leper is particularly prone to injuries, especially of exposed parts. The neurotrophic defect delays the healing of these injuries and makes them more liable to pyogenic infection. Consequently, ulcerations develop which may extend down to the bone (see Srinivasan and Desikan). Thus, sooner or later, the skeletal changes developing on a neurotrophic basis are very likely to be aggravated or even superseded by the far more devastating changes due to secondary pyogenic infection. In accordance with the severity of the suppurative inflammation, reactive periostitis or osteitis may ensue, or even necrosis and sequestration of the affected bone may take place (see Harris and Brand). Thrombosis of blood vessels and gangrene of soft parts may complete the picture. Parts of limbs so affected may slough off or, being anesthetic, be amputated by the patient himself. In this way arose many of the horrible mutilations which were so common in lepers and which were discussed in 1848 by Danielssen and Boeck.

Not only the bones but also the *joints* of an affected part register damage due to the anesthesia and the neurotrophic defect. The neuroarthropathies are most pronounced in the joints of the feet and ankles. Certain articulations, especially those of the ankles, show serous effusion, villous proliferation of the synovial membrane, erosion and (in other places) compensating proliferation of the articular cartilage, sclerosis and eburnation of exposed bone, formation of marginal exostoses, and even fragmentation of the articular ends. In short, one finds many of the changes characteristic of hypertrophic arthritis. Joints may also become subluxated or ankylosed. Harbitz held that much of the articular damage is ascribable to chronic trauma arising from altered conditions of weight-bearing. When all the influences described have been at work upon an articulation, it may come to resemble a Charcot joint or a syringomyelic joint; or, instead, it may merely be distorted through deformation of the constituent bones. Other types of articular change may be induced by pyogenic bacteria, which may enter a hitherto normal joint or a joint modified in any of these ways and cause suppurative arthritis with its well-known sequelae.

Autopsy Findings.—Powell and Swan have described the gross and microscopic *pathologic changes* observed in 50 consecutive cases coming to autopsy at the National Leprosarium (United States Public Health Service) at Carville, Louisiana. The average duration of life after the onset of obvious signs and symptoms in these cases was 20 years, and the average age at the time of death was just under 59 years. While leprosy is seldom a rapidly fatal disease, it is one often resulting in pronounced disability. In particular, its continued presence is frequently associated with con-

Figure 278

A, Photomicrograph ($\times$ 100) prepared from a tissue slide of skin from a hand in a case of leprosy. The picture shows the characteristic folding of the skin seen in well-developed cases of leprosy. The arrows point to a few of the subcutaneous lepromata which are the cause of the folding.

B, Roentgenograph of a hand of a man affected with leprosy. Note that the terminal phalanges are strikingly eroded, that several of the phalanges have been worn down to sharp points, and that the terminal phalanx of the middle finger has been completely resorbed. The indicated changes have a neurotrophic basis. (I wish to credit the Armed Forces Institute of Pathology for this illustration, made from their negative #69–3310–4, and also for the one shown as *C*, made from negative #69–3310–3. The case was submitted to the Armed Forces Institute of Pathology from the Ryder Hospital of Puerto Rico.)

C, Roentgenograph of the right foot of the same subject, revealing that the phalanges of the middle toe have disappeared—that is, have been resorbed. The terminal phalanx of the fifth toe has also been obliterated.

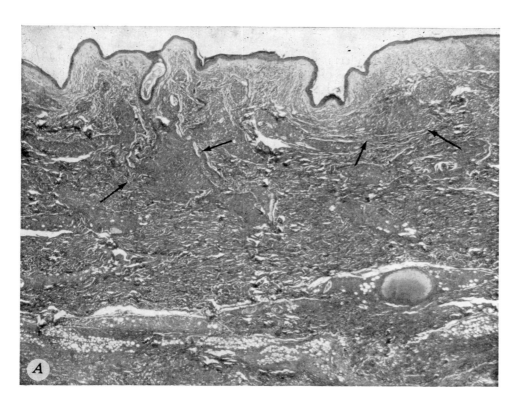

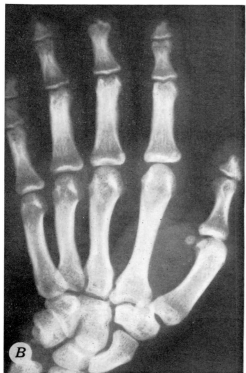

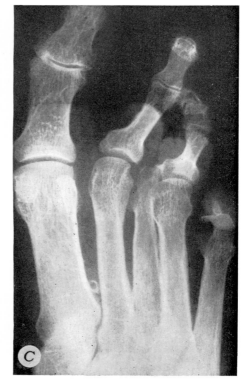

Figure 278

tractures, neurotrophic ulcers, renal insufficiency, and also blindness. In 48 of the 50 cases, the leprosy was of the lepromatous type. In one third of these cases, the spleen, liver, and adrenal glands also contained lepromatous lesions. In 23 cases, secondary amyloid deposits were noted in one or more tissues, the kidney being the organ most frequently involved. Renal insufficiency secondary to the deposition of amyloid was the most common cause of death. As reported by Hopkins and Faget, another important cause of death in cases of leprosy is tuberculosis.

Diagnosis.—In all cases in which it is suspected on a clinical basis that one is dealing with leprosy in an early stage, a search should be made for the acid-fast Hansen bacillus. It should be sought in the nasal secretions and in sections and smears from suspected lesions. The bacteriologic evidence in favor of a diagnosis of leprosy may be regarded as very strong if: (1) the bacilli found are acid-fast by the Ziehl-Neelsen staining method; (2) they are seen to be clumped; and (3) tissue containing them does not produce tuberculosis when injected into a guinea pig. Unfortunately, attempts to culture the lepra bacillus have not yielded unequivocal results, and altogether there are no conclusive bacteriologic, immunologic, or serologic tests for leprosy. In an advanced stage of the disease, the clinical manifestations, of course, speak for themselves.

SKELETAL INFECTIONS CAUSED BY FUNGI AND VIRUSES

Involvement of bones and/or joints in consequence of infections by fungi or viruses is not common, and the cases in question are usually difficult to diagnose on a clinical basis. A rare instance of histoplasmosis involving a knee joint was described by Key and Large.

Mycetoma.—This condition is a chronic granulomatous fungal disease which most often affects the feet (mycetoma pedis). The terms *Madura foot* and *maduromycosis* emphasize the particularly high prevalence of the condition in southern India. It should be pointed out, however, that mycetoma has been observed not only in India but in practically every part of the world except the Arctic regions. Furthermore, the disease is by no means limited to the feet, having also been recorded as occurring in the hand and/or arm, for instance (see Josefiak and Kokiko, Symmers and Sporer, and also Cockshott and Rankin). A case of infection of the skin and soft tissues of a leg, associated with a destructive lesion in the proximal

Figure 279

A, Roentgenograph of a foot which is the site of an infection by the mycetoma fungus— the cause of Madura foot. The subject was a middle-aged Nigerian man. The metatarsal bones in particular disclose the presence of the infection. In addition, there are indications that the infection may also involve several of the metatarsophalangeal joints, as well as some of the midtarsal bones. (I wish to credit the Armed Forces Institute of Pathology for this illustration, which was made from their negative #70–5282–2. The case was sent to the Institute by Dr. Stanley Bohrer of the University College of Ibadan, Nigeria.)

B, Photomicrograph ($\times$ 50) of tissue from a Madura foot revealing the presence of mycetoma fungi. The latter are clumped into small, irregular masses, and the small cells which surround the clumps of fungi are mainly polymorphonuclear leukocytes and epithelioid cells. At this low magnification the hyphae and chlamydospores which characterize the architecture of the mycetoma grains cannot be seen. (This photomicrograph was made from slide #17 of the Armed Forces Institute of Pathology collection of slides dealing with mycotic diseases.)

C, Photomicrograph ($\times$ 400) made from the same slide shown in B and illustrating the hyphae.

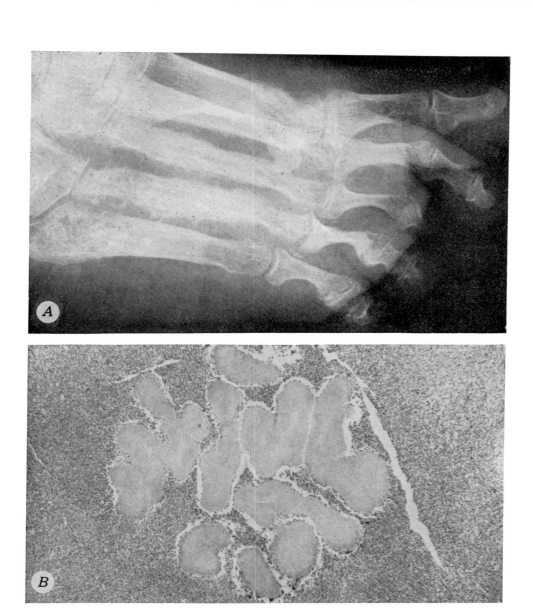

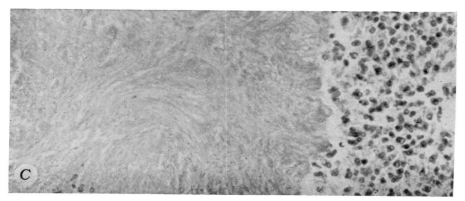

Figure 279

end of the tibia and also with involvement of the knee joint, has been reported by Hogshead and Stein. A case of maduromycosis in which the presenting lesion was in the shaft of a tibia was reported by Kulowski and Stovall. Furthermore, a case of primary mycetoma of a patella has also been reported (see Majid *et al.*).

The infection is acquired from fungi present in the soil. The relatively high incidence of mycetoma infection in the feet is due to the fact that, in the regions where the disease is endemic, the feet are not protected against the fungus, since the subjects do not wear shoes or sandals. A foot or hand in which the disease is present is painful, strikingly enlarged, and usually shows numerous sinuses with raised margins. As a consequence of the sinus formation, secondary infection by pyogenic microorganisms is not unusual as a complication. When a secondary pyogenic infection does occur, there is fever, and, as the infection advances, roentgenographic examination of the enlarged foot or hand reveals extensive destruction of bones in the affected part (see Oyston). (See Fig. 279.)

Cryptococcosis (Torulosis).—*Cryptococcus neoformans* is a yeastlike fungus which has a pronounced predilection for the central nervous system but may also infect the skin, the lungs, other organs, and even bones and/or joints. In man, the most common manifestation of cryptococcosis is chronic meningoencephalitis, which is consistently fatal. Infection of skeletal tissues by this fungus is uncommon, and if the infection is localized to a bone and/or joint and remains so, the prognosis is favorable. Almost any bone may be the site of an infection by cryptococci. As recorded in the literature, the pelvis, femur, spine, and tibia were among the most common sites of skeletal cryptococcosis (see Gosling and Gilmer). More often than not, skeletal involvement occurs in cases in which the cryptococcosis is generalized and implicates the central nervous system.

In a case of cryptococcosis with involvement of the skeleton, the initial symptom relating to a given bone (a limb bone in particular) is usually swelling and tenderness of the soft tissues adjacent to that affected part. This is likely to be associated with pain, particularly in relation to weight-bearing bones. Roentgenographically the lesional area in a bone presents as a focus of radiolucency, with or without evidences of local subperiosteal new bone formation (see Durie and MacDonald, and also Allcock). In the course of healing of the lesion, the affected bone area regains a normal roentgenographic appearance.

Histologic examination of tissue from a well-advanced bone lesion reveals the

Figure 280

A, Roentgenograph of the right hand of a man 59 years of age who had sustained an injury to the index finger. The picture reveals that the middle phalanx of that finger is the site of a cystlike lesion which was interpreted in Puerto Rico as an enchondroma. Subsequently the man developed a draining sinus in the vicinity of the affected phalanx. Several months later, the finger was amputated, and tissue examination revealed a granulomatous inflammation characteristic of *Cryptococcus neoformans*. (I wish to credit the Armed Forces Institute of Pathology for this illustration, which was made from their negative #53–18539.)

B, Photomicrograph (× 50) prepared from a tissue slide from a case of cryptococcosis. Note the torula-like organisms (encapsulated yeastlike bodies) particularly prominent in the left and upper part of the picture. The tissue (lung) came from the case of a 62 year old man who had had fever, malaise, and dyspnea. He died, and an autopsy revealed involvement of the lungs and brain by the fungus. The illustration shows that the alveoli are filled with the fungi, which are large and encapsulated. (This photomicrograph was made from slide #7 of the Armed Forces Institute of Pathology collection of slides dealing with mycotic diseases.)

C, Photomicrograph (× 320) prepared from the same slide illustrated in *B*. The encapsulated fungi (*Cryptococcus neoformans*) are clearly evident at this magnification.

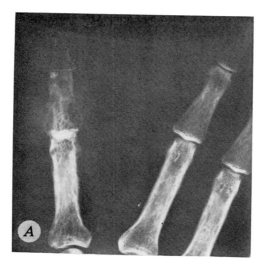

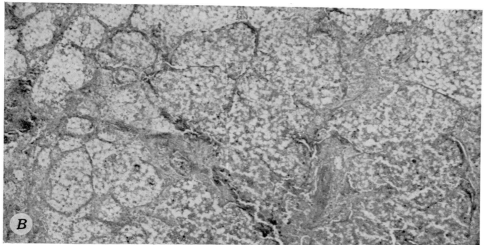

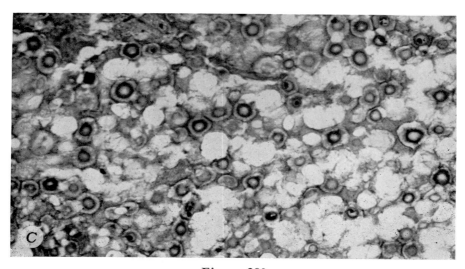

Figure 280

presence of granulation tissue containing multinuclear giant cells, lymphocytes, and histiocytes. If the biopsy tissue is properly stained, the presence of cryptococci in it can be demonstrated. Torula-like organisms (encapsulated yeastlike bodies) are found in tissue curetted from the bone lesion. They can also be demonstrated in smears of pus obtained from such a lesion. (See Fig. 280.)

Coccidioidomycosis.—The causative agent for this condition is the fungus *Coccidioides immitis*, which is a spherical, thick-walled, endospore-filled organism. In the United States, the incidence of the disease is highest in the arid southwestern part of the country (see Fiese). In the series of 95 cases of the disseminated type which was analyzed and discussed by Forbus and Bestebreurtje, 37 of the subjects were white Americans, 48 were colored Americans, 2 were Mexicans, 1 was a Filipino, 1 was an American Indian, 1 an oriental (Chinese), and 5 were of unknown race. In regard to the clinico-anatomic features of the disease, no racial differences were noted.

The *clinical manifestations* vary in accordance with the distribution of the lesions, which may be limited (localized) or disseminated throughout the body (widespread). The disease is primarily and predominantly a pulmonary affection, and may be roentgenographically indistinguishable from chronic pulmonary histoplasmosis or chronic pulmonary tuberculosis (see Sarosi *et al.*), and when it remains localized to the lungs, the mortality rate is low (see Klein and Griffin). The lungs become infected through the inhalation of dust containing the chlamydospores, which represent the vegetative stage of the fungus growing outside of the body (see Dickson and Gifford). On the other hand, when the disease is widely disseminated, the mortality rate is high.

With respect to the *histopathology*, coccidioidomycosis is an inflammatory granu-

Figure 281

A, Roentgenograph of a knee joint area disclosing a lesion in the upper half of the patella which (on the basis of tissue examination) had been found to be due to coccidioidomycosis. The subject was a man 33 years of age who had complained of pain in the knee for several months before the lesional area was subjected to surgery. (I wish to credit the Armed Forces Institute of Pathology for this illustration, which was made from their negative #117171–82170.)

B, Roentgenograph showing a destructive lesion involving the bodies of the twelfth thoracic and first lumbar vertebrae from another case of coccidioidomycosis. The subject was a 62 year old ranch worker in California. Two months prior to his hospitalization, he had developed small ulcerations on the medial surface of the right ankle from which there was a discharge of yellowish purulent material. One month before his admission, the lower thoracic part of his spine became painful. Purulent material from the ulcers in the region of the right ankle revealed spherules representing an infection by *Coccidioides immitis*. Approximately 3 months after the onset of his complaints, the man died. (I wish to thank the Armed Forces Institute of Pathology for permitting the use of their negative #498629 for this illustration.)

C, Photomicrograph ($\times$ 75) illustrating the histologic pattern presented by the synovial membrane of a knee joint from another case of coccidioidomycosis. The subject was a middle-aged man who lived and worked in southern California. He developed pain and swelling of one of his knees. Even after a few months, however, there was no destruction of the articular ends of the bones relating to the affected knee joint. A synovectomy was done, and the granulomatously inflamed synovial membrane was found to be thickened and fibrotic. Histologically the tubercle-like structures represent the characteristic spherules (sporangia) of coccidioidomycosis. Some of the sporangia contain endospores, and some are empty.

D, Photomicrograph ($\times$ 320) showing one of the sporangia characteristic of coccidioidomycosis. The endospore is clearly evident.

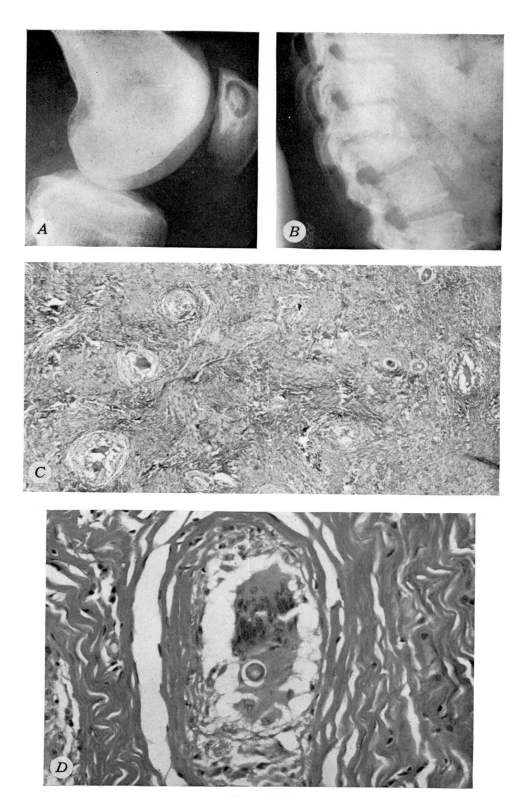

Figure 281

lomatous disease presenting histologic appearances resembling those of tubercles. If the presence of the fungi is not apparent in the stained tissue sections, the histologic pattern may lead to misdiagnosis of the condition as tuberculosis. When the skeleton is implicated, usually a number of bones are involved. Although the infection may occur in any part of the bone, it develops most often at the articular end or ends of the bone. Under these circumstances the infection not infrequently spreads to the articular cavity, involves the synovial membrane, and may ultimately lead to destruction of the articular cartilages. Cases of recurrent synovitis leading to swelling of the joint (most often the knee) have also been noted in which the point of departure for the coccidioidal synovitis was hematogenous infection of the synovial membrane by the fungi (see Pollock *et al.*). A case of coccidioidal synovitis of a knee joint and its rapid cure by means of the intra-articular injection of amphotericin B was reported by Aidem. (See Fig. 281.)

Blastomycosis.—*Blastomyces dermatitidis* is a spherical, thick-walled, budding yeastlike fungus. It induces a granulomatous infection involving the skin, internal organs (especially the lungs), and also bones and joints. Sometimes the inflammatory reaction induced by the fungus is dominated by suppuration, and in other cases there is a mixture of granulomatous and suppurative inflammation. The highest incidence of skeletal involvement is observed in cases in which the skin and lungs are also implicated. On rare occasions, skeletal blastomycosis has been observed in the absence of cutaneous and pulmonary manifestations, and under these circumstances the establishment of the diagnosis may present a problem (see Cushard *et al.*).

As to the *geographic distribution* of blastomycosis in the United States, its incidence is highest in the Ohio Valley, the Mississippi Valley, and the Middle Atlantic States (see Wilson and Plunkett). The disease has appeared in persons of all ages, but the majority are between 20 and 50 years of age. There is no racial predilection, but with respect to sex distribution, males are more often affected than females. Epidemiologic studies have consistently indicated that the infection is usually acquired by inhalation of the spores from the soil, in analogy with what occurs in relation to histoplasmosis, coccidioidomycosis, and other fungus infections (see Gehweiler *et al.*).

After acquiring the disease by inhalation of the spores, the subject may develop cough, fever, dyspnea, and chest pains. When the pulmonary infection is established, the blastomycotic fungi may be disseminated to other sites by way of the blood stream. Various organs may become involved, and lesions may develop in one or several bones, sometimes as many as 6 or 7 being affected. While almost any bone may be implicated, the most common sites are vertebrae, ribs, the tibia, and the bones of the tarsus and carpus. Anatomically the bone area may show evidence of necrosis and/or be the site of an abscess. Such viable tissue as remains in the implicated area may present the histologic pattern of a tubercle-like granuloma. If a joint becomes involved, the synovial membrane may be found heavily infected, and the articular cartilages undergo degeneration. If the joint is one in which there are intra-articular ligaments, they also degenerate.

Roentgenographically the bone lesions of blastomycosis have nothing distinctive about their appearance. If vertebrae are involved, the findings resemble those of tuberculous spondylitis. In both of these conditions, the vertebral bodies are eroded anteriorly, and, as the inflammatory process advances, the anterior longitudinal ligament is penetrated and a paraspinal mass (unilateral or bilateral), representing paravertebral abscess formation, becomes evident. In long tubular bones, small focal areas of radiolucency may be present in the subchondral or metaphysial-epiphysial region. These radiolucent areas, which are usually delimited by a sclerotic border, represent abscess formations. In addition, the shafts of some of the long tubular bones may reveal a fairly large area of radiolucency corresponding to an abscess-like focus of osteomyelitis. In the presence of such a lesion, the bone cortex may be thinned and perforated, and the infection may spread to the neighboring soft tissues and/or joint (see Schenken and Palik). If a large part of the shaft of a bone is involved, subperiosteal new bone formation may be conspicuous. Under these circumstances, soft-tissue swelling over the site of infection may be prominent, and draining sinuses may develop because of the presence of subcutaneous abscesses.

In summary, then, it can be stated, in regard to the *diagnosis*, that in the case of a patient with a chronic draining abscess who exhibits roentgenographic evidence of periostitis and/or a destructive lesion involving a regional bone, blastomycosis should be one of the conditions considered in the differential diagnosis, especially if the lungs and skin also show lesions (see Boswell). If it is suspected that a pathologic condition is the result of blastomycosis, a positive culture of the fungus will, of course, permit a definitive diagnosis (see Liggett and Silberman). If the case is one of blastomycosis, *microscopic examination* of a stained smear of pus, sputum, or pleural fluid will reveal the characteristic thick-walled yeast cells, which appear singly or in budding form. (See Fig. 282.)

Actinomycosis.—This fungal disease occurs in man, cattle, and other animals. It is a low grade, slowly progressive, chronic infection which gradually induces: (1) the formation of indurated granulomatous swellings occurring chiefly in the connective tissues; (2) some degree of suppuration; and (3) the presence of *Actinomyces* in the pus and/or lesional tissue. After the infection has been acquired, a few weeks or a number of months may elapse before it spreads locally from the site of entry of the fungi or becomes disseminated by way of the blood stream. Local spread of the infection may result in the formation of subcutaneous abscesses and in perforation of the skin, leading to the development of fistulae. In addition to being disseminated by way of the blood stream, the fungi may spread through the lungs by way of the bronchi. The roentgenographic manifestations of thoracic actinomycosis were described in detail by Flynn and Felson.

Actinomycotic involvement of the skeleton is by no means common in man. When such an infection becomes localized in the skull, the particular sites affected are the mandible and/or the maxilla, along with some other bones of the skull (see Everts). Involvement of one of the jaw bones most often follows in the wake of extraction of a tooth (see Nathan *et al.*).

Actinomycosis involving the soft tissues and one or more bones of a finger has been described. In such cases the infection usually sets in as the result of laceration of a finger which has been bitten by an adversary of the subject in the course of a fight. Burrows referred to such cases as "actinomycosis from punch injuries" (see Burrows, and also Wearne). (See Fig. 283.) Actinomycosis of a metacarpal bone, resulting from a punch injury to the hand sustained in the course of a fight, has also been described (see Mendelsohn). An instance of actinomycosis implicating the left humerus, radius, and ulna which was the result of spread of the infection from the skin and soft tissues overlying the bones in question has been described by Varadarajan. Actinomycosis involving the soft tissues and bones of the left upper extremity in a woman whose case had been followed for many years was described by Martinelli and Tagliapietra. In that case an amputation at the shoulder joint was carried out, but subsequently the scapula and overlying soft tissues came to show evidences of actinomycotic infection.

Actinomycotic infection of the vertebral column has also been encountered. Its clinical diagnosis presents problems, because it is likely that the lesion will be misinterpreted as tuberculous spondylitis (see Simpson and McIntosh). On roentgenographic examination of the affected part of the column, the characteristic finding is erosion of the cortex of the involved vertebra. The erosion is caused by a paravertebral abscess, the pus coming from a focus of actinomycotic infection in the lungs or in the intestinal tract—notably in the appendix. Along with the vertebral body itself, its transverse processes, the pedicles, laminae, and spinous processes may be implicated. If thoracic vertebrae are involved, the vertebral ends of the corresponding ribs are almost invariably also affected (see Young). In respect to the roentgenographic and anatomic differences between actinomycotic and tuberculous infection of the vertebral column, it is to be noted that in tuberculous spondylitis the lesion develops within the body of one or more vertebrae, and as the focus of disease enlarges, the affected vertebral body or bodies collapse, and an angular deformity of the column results. In actinomycotic spondylitis, on the other hand, central disruption of the vertebral body or bodies, resultant collapse of the affected vertebrae, and angulation of the column do not occur.

Smallpox.—Skeletal lesions ascribable to smallpox (variola) are by no means rare in areas of the world where the disease is still fairly prevalent. It has been reported that in former years 2 to 5 per cent of young children affected with smallpox developed *osteomyelitis variolosa* (see Cockshott and MacGregor). Rarely, instances of *vaccinia osteomyelitis* have been observed in children who had been vaccinated against smallpox by the inoculation of smallpox virus grown in laboratories.

In relation to *osteomyelitis variolosa*, Chiari reported that in subjects who had died of smallpox and been autopsied, foci of necrosis were very often found widely distributed through the marrow of the long bones and occasionally also in the marrow of the sternum and vertebrae. The pertinent lesions were noted as early as 2 days and as late as 2 months after the appearance of the eruption on the skin. Instances have also been recorded in which adults who had been affected with smallpox during childhood showed stunted long bones. The stunted growth was ascribed to pathologic changes in the epiphyses or at the epiphysial-metaphysial junctions of the affected bones (see Musgrave and Sison). Huenekens and Rigler have reported a case of nonsuppurative osteomyelitis variolosa which was characterized by destructive lesions in the vicinity of the epiphysial cartilage plates of the long bones. In the course of roentgenographic follow-up of the case, they found that the subsequent stunted growth of these bones could be explained on the basis of premature closure of the pertinent epiphysial cartilage plates. Three similar cases of osteomyelitis variolosa have been reported by Eikenbary and LeCocq. These subjects had contracted smallpox in childhood. In these instances, too, there were deformities of the limbs (inequality of growth of the long bones) in consequence of damage to the epiphysial cartilage plates and premature fusion of the epiphyses and relevant shafts.

Figure 282

A, Roentgenograph of the left knee joint area of a 24 year old woman who had had discomfort and mild pain in the area for about 10 months. The patella was excised and, when sectioned, revealed a circumscribed, grayish white, homogeneous mass measuring about 1.5 × 1 cm. Histologic examination of that tissue revealed the presence of *Blastomyces dermatitidis*. (I wish to credit the Armed Forces Institute of Pathology for this illustration, which was made from their negative #483904–14112.)

B, Photomicrograph (× 320) prepared from tissue removed in a case of blastomycosis. The subject was a South American woman 27 years of age. She died, and an autopsy revealed involvement of cervical, mesenteric, retroperitoneal, and para-aortic lymph nodes. There was also evidence of blastomycotic infection of the spleen and the pancreas. The pertinent fungi are surrounded by clumps of nuclei, and the fungi have the shape of tear drops. The other cellular elements in this picture are mainly lymphocytes, plasma cells, and polymorphonuclear leukocytes. (This picture was prepared from slide #13 of the Armed Forces Institute of Pathology collection of slides relating to mycotic diseases.)

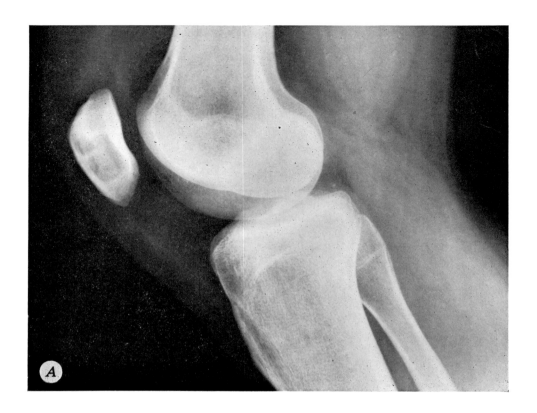

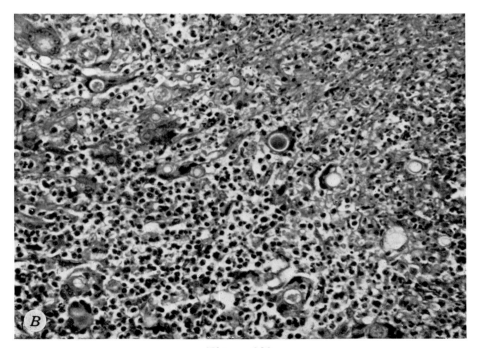

Figure 282

Other expressions of osteomyelitis variolosa are fairly common and even more serious. Within a week or a number of weeks after the smallpox becomes clinically evident, the onset of skeletal involvement may be indicated by swelling in the vicinity of one or more joints, especially the elbows, hips, and knees (see Bery and Chawla, and also Srivastava). However, occasionally it sets in with thickening of the shafts of one or more bones, which is the result of subperiosteal new bone formation. Roentgenographically, such changes resemble those of pyogenic osteomyelitis. In osteomyelitis variolosa, the changes in the bones are often bilateral and symmetrical. Implication of the three bones of an affected elbow joint (or both elbow joints) is rather common (see Davidson and Palmer). Bilateral involvement of the tibia and fibula can also frequently be observed, this involvement taking the form of a pronounced osteoperiostitis implicating the shafts of these bones. In the bones of the carpus and tarsus and also the tubular bones of the hands and feet, small foci of increased radiodensity may also become apparent. Such roentgenographic findings and the lack of response of the skeletal changes to antibiotics and chemotherapy in general are of value in differentiating osteomyelitis variolosa from bacterial osteomyelitis.

Vaccinia Osteomyelitis.—This condition is a very rare complication following vaccination against smallpox. Even though an osteomyelitis develops in an infant or child who has been so vaccinated, it should not be assumed that the lesion has been caused by the vaccinia virus unless it is established that the virus is present in tissue removed from the focus (or one of the foci) of osteomyelitis. The present writer has studied such a case, which was reported by Sewall. Figure 284 relates to that case, and the history is given in the pertinent legend.

The rarity of vaccinia osteomyelitis was emphasized by Cochran *et al.* who, in 1963, reported a case, and stated that it was the first instance observed in the British Isles in which the diagnosis was confirmed by isolation of the virus from

Figure 283

A, Roentgenograph of a mandible which was the site of actinomycosis. The patient was a 54 year old man who had developed a "pocket" behind the second molar tooth on the right side of the lower jaw. Food tended to accumulate in this site, and subsequently the tooth was extracted. An abscess developed at the site of the extraction, but this lesion healed. Four months later, pus began to drain intermittently from the site of the previous abscess. The area was again explored surgically, and the presence of actinomycosis was established. The so-called "sulfur granules" characteristic of an actinomycotic infection can be seen in the lesional area. (I wish to credit the Armed Forces Institute of Pathology for this illustration, which was made from their negative #126250–85065.)

B, Roentgenograph of the left thumb of a 54 year old man who developed an actinomycotic infection as a result of a bite inflicted on his thumb by another person 3 weeks before the subject was admitted to our hospital. The thumb reveals swelling of the soft tissues, most pronounced in the region of the distal phalanx. The roentgenograph also discloses considerable destruction of the distal phalanx. The surgical intervention consisted of incision, drainage, and saucerization. The bacteriologic examination of the tissue disclosed the presence of *Actinomyces bovis*, anaerobic streptococci, and fusiform bacilli. Histologic examination of tissue revealed that the osteomyelitis was the result of infection by *Actinomyces*.

C, Photomicrograph ($\times$ 200) revealing, in the upper left-hand part of the picture, the so-called "sulfur granules" (ray fungus). However, even under this magnification, the details of the typical granules are not distinguishable. In addition to the sulfur granules, one can note the presence of numerous polymorphonuclear leukocytes neighboring upon the collections of *Actinomyces*. In the right half of the picture there is granulation tissue, likewise interspersed with polymorphonuclear leukocytes.

D, Photomicrograph ($\times$ 320) prepared from the same slide shown in *C*. The ray fungi are clearly evident at the upper edge of the midportion of the agglomerated *Actinomyces*.

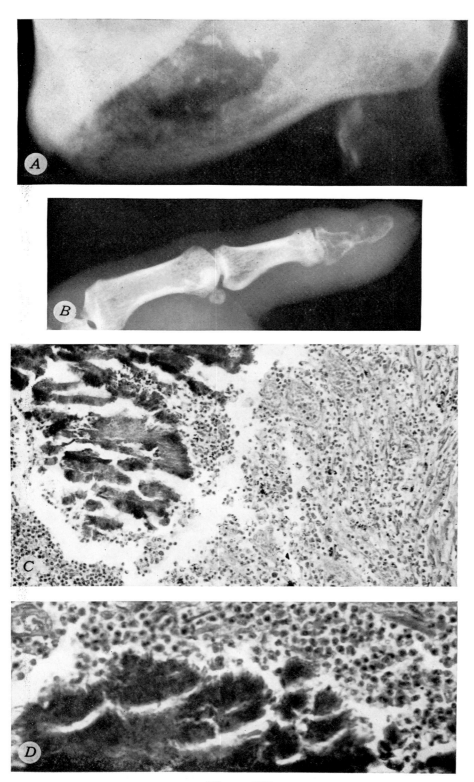

Figure 283

one of the bone lesions. The subject was a male infant who was vaccinated against smallpox when he was $3\frac{1}{2}$ weeks old. Four weeks after the vaccination, the patient developed a tender, diffuse swelling over the left scapula. Roentgenographic examination revealed considerable subperiosteal new bone formation on the costal and dorsal surfaces of the scapula. Seventy days postvaccination, the patient presented pallor, sniffles, fever, and conjunctivitis. Within 12 hours, the left side of the mandible was swollen and tender. Six days later, periosteal new bone formation was evident in that area of the lower jaw. A similar sequence of events occurred at 95 and 115 days after vaccination, the ribs and the entire mandible coming to show subperiosteal new bone formation. Treatment included repeated administration of human antivaccinial gamma globulin. After approximately one year, all of the involved bones (except the left scapula) had remodeled and were normal.

Rubella (German Measles).—It has long been known that a fetus developing in a mother who had acquired rubella in the early stages of her pregnancy (especially the first trimester) may present various abnormalities, including nonskeletal and skeletal aberrations. Specifically, the congenital rubella syndrome (also denoted as rubella embryopathy) includes: cardiac anomalies, cataract, chorioretinitis, deafness, intra-uterine retardation of growth, and roentgenographically evident skeletal changes (see Highman, Rabinowitz *et al.*, Singleton *et al.*, and Williams and Carey). The skeletal changes are localized mainly in the metaphysial regions of

Figure 284

A, Roentgenograph of the bones of the left forearm of a female child who was 17 months of age when she was admitted to our hospital. About 5 months earlier, she had been vaccinated in the left arm, and shortly thereafter there was evidence of a severe local reaction to the vaccine. The skin of the left forearm became discolored, and the forearm underwent progressive swelling. The roentgenograph shows destructive changes involving the distal two thirds of the shaft of the ulna and also extensive periosteal new bone formation. It is evident that there is a deformity of the ulna, and also a fracture of that bone. About 2 weeks after the patient's admission, a biopsy was carried out on the dorsomedial aspect of the left ulna. Part of the specimen was sent to the Public Health Research Institute of the City of New York for bacteriologic evaluation, and they reported: "The material sent us contained vaccinia virus which produced typical lesions on the chorioallantoic membrane as well as typical intracytoplasmic inclusions. It also produced skin lesions in rabbits and was neutralized by anti-vaccinia antiserum. The antiserum we used was not as potent as desirable but in view of all the other evidence, we have no doubt as to the identity of this strain." After $2\frac{1}{2}$ months, the child was discharged and was to be treated in our Out-Patient Department. Instead, however, the family admitted her to another hospital, where she died 5 months later. No autopsy was performed. The other pictures on this plate relate to the same case.

B, Roentgenograph of the anterior part of the skull. Three weeks prior to the child's admission to our hospital, the skin and underlying soft tissues of the forehead became discolored. The roentgenograph reveals a large area of radiolucency on the left side of the frontal bone. No biopsy specimen was taken from the skull.

C, Photomicrograph ($\times$ 50) showing the histologic architecture of one of the fragments of bone curetted from the shaft of the affected ulna shown in *A*. The osseous tissue is necrotic, as indicated by the empty bone cell lacunae. Under a higher magnification, one could observe that any osteocytes still present in the bone cell lacunae had undergone partial or complete degeneration. The bone itself is porous in consequence of enlargement of the haversian canals, and the very large irregular spaces represent the result of agglomeration of neighboring modified haversian canals. The tissue within these canals is strikingly devoid of polymorphonuclear leukocytes. It consists mainly of red blood cells, most of which have degenerated, and also contains sparse connective tissue cells, some fibrin, and an occasional macrophage.

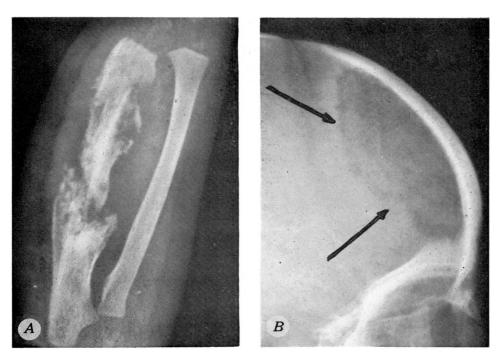

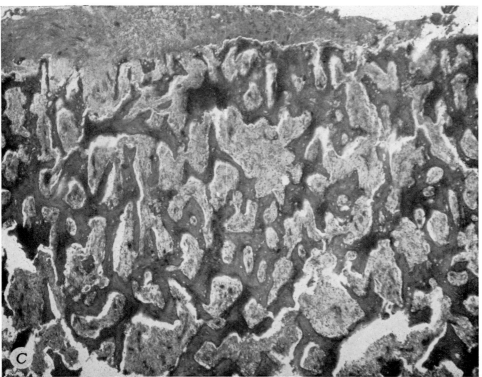

Figure 284

long tubular bones, and especially in the distal part of the femoral metaphysis and the proximal part of the tibial metaphysis. Roentgenographically the affected metaphyses show disorganization of their architecture. In particular, the metaphyses present linear and ovoid areas of radiolucency alternating with zones of coarse trabeculae. These deviations from the normal architecture tend to disappear within a month or two after birth. However, the nonskeletal aberrations characterizing the rubella syndrome may persist into adult life. Instances of rubella synovitis have also been described. In these cases the subjects were mainly adult females and, when hospitalized, presented evidence of acute polyarthritis and tenosynovitis affecting particularly the wrists, knee joints, and small joints of the hands (see Chambers and Bywaters).

Varicella (Chickenpox).—Chickenpox is a common disease caused by a virus, and ordinarily runs a mild course. The affected subjects are principally young children. The disease is characterized by a vesicular eruption of the skin and the mucous membranes, and the individual dermal lesions are surrounded by erythema. Despite the fact that chickenpox is a common disease, involvement of bones and/or joints has only rarely been recorded. An instance of arthritis developing in a knee of a 5-year-old girl affected with chickenpox was reported by Ward and Bishop. Attempts to isolate the virus from the involved joint in that case were not successful. Nevertheless, the fact that the arthritis subsided simultaneously with the chickenpox seemed to justify the assumption that the varicella virus was the cause of the arthritis. A case of dry gangrene appearing in connection with chickenpox and necessitating amputation of both lower extremities was reported by Bogumill, who also gives details on additional reported cases of varicella gangrenosa. Cheatham *et al.* have described in detail 2 cases of varicella in which the subjects died and were autopsied. In addition to the postmortem findings, these authors discuss the isolation of the virus, its identification, and also its propagation.

ECHINOCOCCOSIS

Echinococcosis is the most important of the infections caused by a larval tapeworm. The ova of the worm are ingested with contaminated food or water, and hatch in the intestine. The onchosphere penetrates the intestinal wall, enters the lymph or blood, and is carried to one or another part of the body, where the hydatid larvae develop. Although infection with *Echinococcus granulosus* is the most frequent basis for the destructive skeletal lesions caused by helminths, involvement of the skeleton is uncommon. It is estimated as occurring in about 2 per cent of cases of this disease. It is only in certain parts of the world—notably sheep-raising countries—that echinococcosis is encountered at all. It is therefore only in these regions that there is a reasonably good chance of observing cases in which human bones are implicated (see Alldred, and also Hogg *et al.*).

In soft tissue, such as the *liver*, a *larval hydatid echinococcus* is characterized by: (1) its distinct delimiting wall with a nuclear germinative inner lining and a chitinous outer lining; (2) a unilocular cystic structure determined by this wall; and (3) a fluid content in which brood capsules, daughter cysts, scolices and/or immature worms may be floating. A case of primary intramuscular hydatidosis is sometimes encountered, and in such instances, too, the lesion is found encapsulated (see Rask and Lattig). It should be noted that when hydatid echinococcosis is developing *intra-osseously* and while it is still confined within the bone, the lesion does not assume this conventional appearance. That is, within a bone there is not formed the classic thick-walled unilocular cyst mentioned above. Instead, the affected portion of the bone (usually the spongiosa) will be found permeated by minute though grossly visible separate thin-walled cysts. However, such a lesion, even while still completely intra-osseous, is easily identifiable at autopsy or in the course of surgery as representing hydatid echinococcosis (see Hutchison *et al.*). If the cyst erupts from the bone, as it frequently does, the erupted portion shows the development of large cysts, such as are found in connection with the classic unilocular hydatid of soft tissue. The *alveolar echinococcus* appears in *soft tissues* as a ramifying, porous, usually necrotic mass which is not definitely delimited from the host tissue by a wall, as is the hydatid echinococcus. The identification of the alveolar lesion in *bone* is extremely difficult at autopsy or during surgery, since, in a bone, it is not only rare but rather nondescript. Because of the associated necrosis and liquefaction, an alveolar echinococcal bone lesion is usually misinterpreted as tuberculous osteitis until the tissue is studied microscopically.

In regard to the localization of skeletal echinococcosis, Gangolphe in 1886 had already stressed the idea that, when a bone is affected, the lesion nearly always starts its development within the bone, and the disease does not reach the bone secondarily from the neighboring soft tissues. As in other skeletal infections dependent upon hematogenous dissemination, the lesions are initiated mainly in the spongiosa. It has been a common observation that the osseous involvement is usually limited to one bone, a few adjacent bones, or at least to one skeletal region. When several bones are implicated, it is often by direct invasion of one bone from another, as, for instance, of a femur from the pelvis, of a rib from a vertebra, or of one vertebra from another. Echinococcosis of an articulation without the presence of a disease focus in a neighboring bone is definitely rare.

As to the frequency of involvement of individual bones or skeletal parts, the data collected by Pasquali are representative. Altogether, they cover 406 cases of echinococcosis with bone lesions: (1) The vertebral column was found affected in 41.6 per cent; (2) the pelvis in 22.1 per cent, the sacral and iliac portions being those most frequently implicated; (3) the humerus in 9.4 per cent; (4) the tibia and fibula in 8.9; (5) the femur in 8.1; and (6) the skull in 5.2 per cent. Implication of certain bones, such as the sternum, scapula, and phalanges, was found to be relatively rare, while involvement of the bones of the tarsus, the carpus, and the forearm was not found at all. The ribs are frequently affected in connection with involvement of thoracic vertebrae.

As to the *pathologic findings*, in bones, as elsewhere, echinococcosis is usually of the hydatid variety. As already stated, however, the latter, while it is developing intra-osseously, assumes an atypical form. This fact has been stressed by numerous observers, including Gangolphe, Dévé, Yamato, and also Altmann, who have studied the pathologic anatomy of this condition.

Especially if the lesion is in the spongiosa, great numbers of small but usually grossly recognizable cysts will be present. As a rule, these are of approximately pinhead size, though they may become as large as cherries after they have succeeded in pushing aside the resistant spongy trabeculae. If the disease extends to the major medullary cavity, the cysts there, being less restricted, will develop even beyond cherry size. Thus, in hydatid echinococcosis of bone, no mother cyst with typical wall is to be found. The smaller cysts which are permeating the spongiosa have, however, developed from the germinative lining of a larva whose growth had been distorted from the start. Because of the resistance offered by the osseous tissue, this larva did not develop in the manner usual in soft tissues (endogenous growth) but instead by the process of exogenous budding or heterotrophic growth. Thus, osseous hydatid echinococcosis is associated with the presence of numerous small cysts growing outside the original focus of implantation of the larva. Furthermore, scolices only rarely develop in these cysts, and the latter are therefore usually sterile. The multiplicity of cysts appearing when bone is involved by hydatid echinococcosis has often led to erroneous classification of the lesion as one of the distinctly rare alveolar type.

The presence of the cysts between the trabeculae provokes the proliferation of connective tissue in the intertrabecular marrow. This tissue, which is heavily infiltrated with lymphocytes and eosinophils, encircles some of the cysts. Between the latter, giant cells, hemosiderin pigment, and cholesterol crystals will also appear. Many of the bone trabeculae in the vicinity are eroded and resorbed. As the lesion grows, the overlying bone cortex becomes thinned. Yielding of the weakened cortex results in expansion of the diameter of the bone. It is worth noting also that the periosteum does not ordinarily respond with new bone formation. (See Fig. 285.)

Extension of the disease into the parosteal tissues is frequent, and occurs most often with vertebral echinococcosis. Dévé has devoted considerable attention to the subject. When once liberated from the bone, the extra-osseous portion of the echinococcal lesion begins to approximate that of a hydatid which has been in soft tissue from the start. Large daughter cysts with scolices are formed. Since, when it becomes freed from bone, the lesion thus assumes the character of an ordinary hydatid, this character had evidently merely been distorted while the lesion was still intra-osseous. The parosteal echinococcal lesion sometimes attains tremendous proportions. It is delimited by a thick fibrous membrane resulting from reactive proliferation of the host tissue. It may contain seropurulent fluid and detritus, and has been designated as an "ossifluent hydatid abscess." With involvement of thoracic vertebrae, the extra-osseous cyst may spread beneath the parietal pleura into the intercostal spaces, along the vertebrae, and even into the spinal canal. If the pelvic bones are involved, the cysts may extend for a considerable distance in front of, or behind, the sacrum.

Occasionally a bone lesion takes the form of an *alveolar echinococcosis*, with or without involvement of regional soft parts, and may be misinterpreted as tuberculosis until it is examined microscopically. Such cases have been described in

Figure 285

A, B, C, and D, Roentgenographs of several bones from a case of echinococcosis. The subject, a South African man, was 34 years of age when he was admitted to a hospital in his country for treatment. Dr. Golda Selzer of Capetown gave the writer the clinical data and the material from which these illustrations were made. Ten years prior to hospitalization, the man had sustained a fracture of the right femur. He was confined to bed for a month and then was ambulatory on crutches. About 3 years after the fracture, he noticed a gradually increasing swelling of his right thigh. The affected extremity had wasted, and the entire right lower limb had become shorter than the left, mainly in consequence of shortening of the right thigh.

A, Roentgenograph of the upper half of the right tibia and fibula. One can note a large area of radiolucency in the shaft of the tibia, and thinning of the cortex from the medullary side. This picture was taken at the time of the fracture of the right femur.

B, Roentgenograph of the upper half of the right tibia, which, in the course of several years, had undergone expansion and appears multiloculated. This roentgenograph was taken about 7 years after the one shown in A.

C, Roentgenograph showing a multilocular lesion involving the right ischium, pubis, and acetabulum.

D, Roentgenograph of the right femur and part of the corresponding side of the pelvis. There is extensive destruction of the femur, which had been the site of the fracture 10 years before. The illustration shows a great number of cysts spread throughout the femur and the right side of the pelvis. A biopsy was carried out, and a large amount of gelatinous material and several small daughter cysts were removed. These findings, along with examination of the pertinent pathologic tissue, established the diagnosis of echinococcosis.

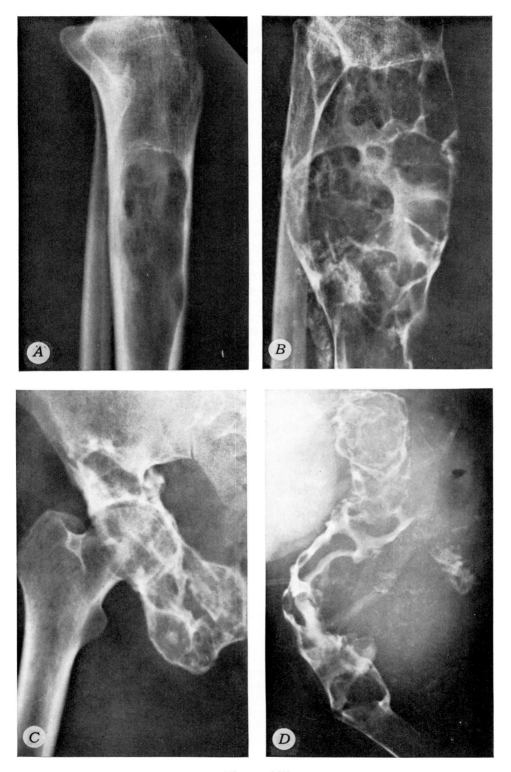

Figure 285

studies by Elenevsky, Brentano and Benda, and also Klages. In the latter two articles, instances are recorded in which the disease apparently began in the bone and only later invaded other tissues and organs.

On *microscopic examination* of tissue from the affected bone, the minute cystic parasitic structures (individual ones never quite filling out a mesh of spongiosa) can be observed between the trabeculae, which are in various stages of resorption and necrosis. The intertrabecular marrow in the affected region is necrotic and in some places shows proliferation of fibrous tissue. The necrosis so prevalent in lesions of alveolar echinococcosis is ascribable to toxins produced in the course of the growth of the larvae. The newly formed inflammatory granulation tissue is heavily infiltrated with leukocytes and tends to surround the parasites and may fill in cortical defects. Klages states that, not far from the disease focus, the periosteum may be stimulated to new bone formation. Elenevsky already showed that, when an alveolar echinococcus breaks out from bone into surrounding soft tissues, its pathologic anatomic features do not change.

It is doubtful whether echinococcosis starts in a joint without associated involvement of regional bone. If joints do become implicated, it is usually because the disease had broken into the joint from a neighboring bone. Among 50 cases of skeletal echinococcosis, Fischer collected 10 instances in which the disease broke into a joint. The hip joint is the large articulation most often thus invaded, in accordance with the relatively high frequency of involvement of the pelvis. With involvement of the pelvis, the acetabulum is often disrupted, and the head of the femur prolapses into the pelvic cavity. Except in the case of the hip joint, transition of the infection from one bone to another by way of a large joint is apparently also infrequent. On the other hand, penetration and extension of the disease by way of synchondroses or small joints (such as the costovertebral) are frequent. If the infection extends from one vertebra to another, this is likely to occur by contact with a paravertebral hydatid abscess rather than through an intervertebral disk.

As to the *clinical features* and *diagnosis* of skeletal echinococcosis, it has been established that the disease progresses very slowly. Dull, boring bone pains, particularly at night, may for years be its only clinical manifestation unless the pathologic process is also active in the liver, lungs, or some other soft tissue. There may be no other signs or symptoms until the bone is expanded or until the cortex is perforated. Then, as a result of compression of adjacent organs or tissues, pressure phenomena may appear and may even dominate the clinical picture. However, because of loss of bone substance, pathologic fractures occur with such frequency as to constitute one of the common clinical manifestations of skeletal involvement. In fact, especially if the disease is in a long tubular bone, it may be a fracture (spontaneous or precipitated by slight trauma) that first calls attention to its presence. If vertebrae are affected, they may collapse and a gibbus develop. In some instances, paravertebral burrowing abscesses and, in others, compression of the spinal cord have been noted as complications (see Mills, and also Murray and Haddad). Furthermore, the diseased area may become secondarily infected (with suppuration and fistula formation), and the patient may then be febrile.

When echinococcosis is suspected, *roentgenographic examination* may help to clarify the diagnosis. This aid lends itself much better to some regions (for instance, the pelvis) than to others (for instance, the thoracic vertebrae). In any event, as Hsieh indicated, roentgenographic examination is ordinarily insufficient in itself to establish the diagnosis, early or small lesions almost invariably being misdiagnosed as representing foci of osteomyelitis or tuberculous osteitis. If one of the bones of the pelvis presents a large unilateral lesion associated with pronounced expansion and thinning of the cortex, echinococcosis should be suspected. In a long tubular bone, the diseased area will likewise appear radiolucent and meshy and show a thin cortex. In the *differential diagnosis* of skeletal echinococcosis, one must consider a large focus of fibrous dysplasia, a giant-cell tumor, an enchondroma, metastatic carcinoma, or multiple myeloma. The roentgenographic diagnosis of echinococcus infection involving vertebrae and/or the skull often presents special difficulties. In the vertebrae and in the skull, such a lesion may easily be confused with one representing metastatic carcinoma or other lesions producing radiolucent areas.

Among other valuable *clinical diagnostic aids* in cases suspected of being echinococcosis are: (1) eosinophilia, present in about one fourth of the cases; (2) a positive complement fixation test (obtainable in most cases with the patient's blood serum when hydatid fluid is used as the antigen); and (3) a positive reaction to intradermal injection of hydatid fluid—a highly specific test devised by Dew *et al.* Apt and Knierim evaluated these diagnostic aids on 208 patients and found the indirect hemagglutination test had both the highest sensitivity and specificity. However, especially if the pathologic changes of the disease are limited to a small bone, the results of all these tests may be negative. Nevertheless, it should be noted that immunoelectrophoresis is the most valuable immunologic test for the presence of the disease (see Capron *et al.*).

In regard to *prognosis*, it is conceivable that in some cases the bone lesions due to hydatid echinococcus infection may become arrested and/or heal spontaneously. The only definitive *treatment*, however, is the complete surgical excision of all the affected tissue. This is, of course, by no means always possible. In the pelvis and in the vertebral column—precisely the regions most often involved—radical excision is always difficult and frequently impossible. In addition, these crucial areas offer poor prospects for healing, because surgical intervention permits further dissemination of the disease and even secondary infection. The ultimate prognosis depends not only upon the accessibility of the lesion to excision, but on the presence or absence of echinococcosis elsewhere in the body. The mortality rate for skeletal echinococcosis in general is very high. Indeed, the alveolar form, whether present in the skeleton or elsewhere, is almost always fatal.

REFERENCES

ADELSTEIN, L. J., and COURVILLE, C. B.: Traumatic Osteomyelitis of the Cranial Vault, Arch. Surg., *26*, 539, 1933.

AGUILAR, J. A., and ELVIDGE, A. R.: Intervertebral Disk Disease Caused by the *Brucella* Organism, J. Neurosurg., *18*, 27, 1961.

AIDEM, H. P.: Intra-Articular Amphotericin B in the Treatment of Coccidioidal Synovitis of the Knee, J. Bone & Joint Surg., *50-A*, 1663, 1968.

ALLCOCK E.: Torulosis, J. Bone & Joint Surg., *43-B*, 71, 1961.

ALLDRED, A. J.: Hydatid Disease of Bone in Australasia, J. Bone & Joint Surg., *52-B*, 787, 1970.

ALTMANN, F.: Über die Echinokokkenerkrankung der Beckenknochen, Virchows Arch. path. Anat., *272*, 662, 1929.

AMBROSE, G. B., ALPERT, M., and NEER, C. S.: Vertebral Osteomyelitis, J.A.M.A., *197*, 619, 1966.

APT, W., and KNIERIM, F.: An Evaluation of Diagnostic Tests for Hydatid Disease, Am. J. Trop. Med., *19*, 943, 1970.

BADGER, L. F.: Epidemiology, in *Leprosy in Theory and Practice*, 2nd ed., edited by R. G. Cochrane and T. F. Davey, Bristol, John Wright & Sons Ltd., 1964. (See p. 69.)

BARANOFF, A. F.: The Incidence of Osteomyelitis of the Jaw Bones Among the Chinese, Chinese M. J., *48*, 637, 1934.

BAUER, W. H.: The Importance of the Histologic Picture of Osteomyelitis of the Jaws Following the Extraction of Teeth for Treatment, Am. J. Orthodontics, *26*, 150, 1940.

BENEDICT, E. B.: Carcinoma in Osteomyelitis, Surg. Gynec. & Obst., *53*, 1, 1931.

BENJAMINS, C. E.: Osteomyelitis der Schädelknochen bei entzündlicher Erkrankung der Nasenscheidewand, Arch. Ohren- Nasen- u. Kehlkopfh., *126*, 133, 1930.

BERY, K., and CHAWLA, S.: Radiological Features in Small Pox Osteomyelitis, Indian J. Radiol., *23*, 11, 1969.

BINFORD, C. H.: Leprosy—A Model in Geographic Pathology, Internat. Path., *7*, 6, 1966.

BISHOP, W. A., JR.: Vertebral Lesions in Undulant Fever, J. Bone & Joint Surg., *21*, 665, 1939.

BOGER, W. P.: Pneumococcic Arthritis, J.A.M.A., *126*, 1062, 1944.

BOGUMILL, G. P.: Bilateral Above-the-Knee Amputations: A Complication of Chickenpox, J. Bone & Joint Surg., *47–A*, 371, 1965.

BORELLA, L., GOOBAR, J. E., SUMMITT, R. L., and CLARK, G. M.: Septic Arthritis in Childhood, J. Pediat., *62*, 742, 1963.

BOSWELL, W. L.: Roentgen Aspects of Blastomycosis, Am. J. Roentgenol., *81*, 224, 1959.

BRANTSCHEN, G.: Ostéomyélite du col fémoral, Radiol. clin., *27*, 351, 1958.

BRENTANO, and BENDA, C.: Ein Fall von multiloculärem Echinococcus, Deutsche Ztschr. Chir., *52*, 206, 1899.

BRODIE, B. C.: An Account of Some Cases of Chronic Abscess of the Tibia, Med.-Chir. Tr., *17*, 239, 1832.

————: Lecture on Abscess of the Tibia, London Med. Gaz., *36*, 1399, 1845.

BRUNO, M. S., SILVERBERG, T. N., and GOLDSTEIN, D. H.: Embolic Osteomyelitis of the Spine as a Complication of Infection of the Urinary Tract, Am. J. Med., *29*, 865, 1960.

BULMER, J. H.: Septic Arthritis of the Hip in Adults, J. Bone & Joint Surg., *48–B*, 289, 1966.

BURROWS, H. J.: Actinomycosis from Punch Injuries, with a Report of a Case Affecting a Metacarpal Bone, Brit. J. Surg., *32*, 506, 1945.

CAPENER, N., and PIERCE, K. C.: Pathological Fractures in Osteomyelitis, J. Bone & Joint Surg., *14*, 501, 1932.

CAPRON, A., YARZABAL, L., VERNES, A., and FRUIT, J.: Le diagnostic immunologique de l'échinococcose humaine, Path. Biol., *18*, 357, 1970.

CHAMBERLAIN, W. E., WAYSON, N. E., and GARLAND, L. H.: The Bone and Joint Changes of Leprosy: A Roentgenologic Study, Radiology, *17*, 930, 1931.

CHAMBERS, R. J., and BYWATERS, E. G. L.: Rubella Synovitis, Ann. Rheumat. Dis., *22*, 263, 1963.

CHEATHAM, W. J., WELLER, T. H., DOLAN, T. F., JR., and DOWER, J. C.: Varicella: Report of Two Fatal Cases with Necropsy, Virus Isolation, and Serologic Studies, Am. J. Path., *32*, 1015, 1956.

CHIARI, H.: Ueber Osteomyelitis variolosa, Beitr. path. Anat., *13*, 13, 1893.

COCHRAN, W., CONNOLLY, J. H., and THOMPSON, I. D.: Bone Involvement After Vaccination Against Smallpox, Brit. M. J., *2*, 285, 1963.

COCKSHOTT, P., and MACGREGOR, M.: Osteomyelitis Variolosa, Quart. J. Med., *27*, 369, 1958.

————: The Natural History of Osteomyelitis Variolosa, J. Fac. Radiologists, *10*, 57, 1959.

COCKSHOTT, W. P., and RANKIN, A. M.: Medical Treatment of Mycetoma, Lancet, *2*, 1112, 1960.

COHEN, I.: Osteomyelitis of the Skull, Ann. Surg., *97*, 733, 1933.

COHN, L. C.: Non-Suppurative Osteomyelitis, Radiology, *16*, 187, 1931.

COLWILL, M.: Osteomyelitis of the Metatarsal Sesamoids, J. Bone & Joint Surg., *51–B*, 464, 1969.

CROSSAN, E. T.: Hematogenous Osteomyelitis, Internat. Abstr. Surg., *66*, 176, 1938.

CUSHARD, W. G., JR., KOHANIM, M., and LANTIS, L. R.: Blastomycosis of Bone, J. Bone & Joint Surg., *51–A*, 704, 1969.

DANIELSSEN, D.C., and BOECK, W.: *Traité de la Spédalskhed ou éléphantiasis des Grecs*, Paris, J.-B. Baillière, 1848.

DAVIDSON, J. C., and PALMER, P. E. S.: Osteomyelitis Variolosa, J. Bone & Joint Surg., *45–B*, 687, 1963.

DE LORIMIER, A. A., HASKIN, D., and MASSIE, F. S.: Mediastinal Mass Caused by Vertebral Osteomyelitis, Am. J. Dis. Child., *111*, 639, 1966.

DÉVÉ, F.: L'échinococcose vertébrale, Ann. d'anat. path., *5*, 841, 1928.

DEW, H. R., KELLAWAY, C. H., and WILLIAMS, F. E.: The Intradermal Reaction in Hydatid Disease and its Clinical Value, M. J. Australia, *12*, 471, 1925.

DICKSON, E. C., and GIFFORD, M. A.: Coccidioides Infection (Coccidioidomycosis). II. The Primary Type of Infection, Arch. Int. Med., *62*, 853, 1938.

DURIE, E. B., and MACDONALD, W. L.: Cryptococcosis (Torulosis) of Bone, J. Bone & Joint Surg., *43–B*, 68, 1961.

EBRAHIM, G. J., and GRECH, P.: Salmonella Osteomyelitis in Infants, J. Bone & Joint Surg., *48–B*, 350, 1966.

EIKENBARY, C. F., and LECOCQ, J. F.: Osteomyelitis Variolosa, J.A.M.A., *96*, 584, 1931.

ELENEVSKY, K.: Zur pathologischen Anatomie des multiloculären Echinococcus beim Menschen, Arch. klin. Chir., *82*, 393, 1907.

ELLIOTT, G. R.: Chronic Osteomyelitis Presenting Distinct Tumor Formation Simulating Clinically True Osteogenic Sarcoma, J. Bone & Joint Surg., *16*, 137, 1934.

EVANS, D. K.: Osteomyelitis of the Patella, J. Bone & Joint Surg., *44–B*, 319, 1962.

EVERTS, E. C.: Cervicofacial Actinomycosis, Arch. Otolaryng., *92*, 468, 1970.

EYRE-BROOK, A. L.: Septic Arthritis of the Hip and Osteomyelitis of the Upper End of the Femur in Infants, J. Bone & Joint Surg., *42–B*, 11, 1960.

FARRAND, R. J., JOHNSTONE, J. M. S., and MACCABE, A. F.: Haemophilus Osteomyelitis and Arthritis, Brit. M. J., *2*, 334, 1968.

FIESE, M. J.: *Coccidioidomycosis*, Springfield, Illinois, Charles C Thomas, 1958.

FISCHER, G.: Ueber Echinococcus in Gelenken, Deutsche Ztschr. Chir., *32*, 205, 1891.

FLYNN, M. W., and FELSON, B.: The Roentgen Manifestations of Thoracic Actinomycosis, Am. J. Roentgenol., *110*, 707, 1970.

FORBUS, W. D., and BESTEBREURTJE, A. M.: Coccidioidomycosis: A Study of 95 Cases of the Disseminated Type with Special Reference to the Pathogenesis of the Disease, Mil. Surgeon, *99*, 653, 1946.

FREEHAFER, A. A., FUREY, J. G., and PIERCE, D. S.: Pyogenic Osteomyelitis of the Spine Resulting in Spinal Paralysis, J. Bone & Joint Surg., *44–A*, 710, 1962.

FREIBERG, J. A., and PERLMAN, R.: Pelvic Abscesses Associated with Acute Purulent Infection of the Hip Joint, J. Bone & Joint Surg., *18*, 417, 1936.

FREUND, E.: Über Osteomyelitis und Gelenkseiterung, Virchows Arch. path. Anat., *283*, 325, 1932.

GANADO, W., and CRAIG, A. J.: Brucellosis Myelopathy, J. Bone & Joint Surg., *40–A*, 1380, 1958.

GANGOLPHE, M.: *Kystes hydatiques des os*, Paris, O. Doin, 1886.

GARCIA, A., JR., and GRANTHAM, S. A.: Hematogenous Pyogenic Vertebral Osteomyelitis, J. Bone & Joint Surg., *42–A*, 429, 1960.

GARRÈ, C.: Ueber besondere Formen und Folgezustände der akuten infektiösen Osteomyelitis, Beitr. klin. Chir., *10*, 241, 1893.

GEHWEILER, J. A., CAPP, M. P., and CHICK, E. W.: Observations on the Roentgen Patterns in Blastomycosis of Bone, Am. J. Roentgenol., *108*, 497, 1970.

GILMOUR, W. N.: Acute Haematogenous Osteomyelitis, J. Bone & Joint Surg., *44–B*, 841, 1962.

GOSLING, H. R., and GILMER, W. S., JR.: Skeletal Cryptococcosis (Torulosis), J. Bone & Joint Surg., *38–A*, 660, 1956.

GREEN, W. T., and SHANNON, J. G.: Osteomyelitis of Infants. A Disease Different from Osteomyelitis of Older Children, Arch. Surg., *32*, 462, 1936.

GWYN, N. B.: A Case of General Infection by the Diplococcus Intracellularis of Weichselbaum, Johns Hopkins Hosp. Bull., *10*, 112, 1899.

HANSEN, G. A.: Spedalskhedens Arsager. (Causes of Leprosy), Internat. J. Leprosy, *23*, 307, 1955, translated from the Norsk mag. laegevidensk., *4*, 76, 1874.

HANZAWA, S., and SUDA, H.: Zur Statistik der hämatogenen, akuten, eitrigen Osteomyelitis mit besonderer Berücksichtigung ihres Erregers, Mitt. u. allg. Path. u. path. Anat., *6*, 317, 1930.

HARBITZ, F.: Trophoneurotic Changes in Bones and Joints in Leprosy, Arch. Int. Med., *6*, 147, 1910.

HARRIS, J. R., and BRAND, P. W.: Patterns of Disintegration of the Tarsus in the Anaesthetic Foot, J. Bone & Joint Surg., *48–B*, 4, 1966.

HARRIS, N. H.: Some Problems in the Diagnosis and Treatment of Acute Osteomyelitis, J. Bone & Joint Surg., *42–B*, 535, 1960.

———: *Salmonella typhi* Osteomyelitis, Proc. Roy. Soc. Med., *59*, 709, 1966.

HARRIS, N. H., and KIRKALDY-WILLIS, W. H.: Primary Subacute Pyogenic Osteomyelitis, J. Bone & Joint Surg., *47–B*, 526, 1965.

HARVEY, A. M.: Salmonella Suipestifer Infection in Human Beings, Arch. Int. Med., *59*, 118, 1937.

HEBERLING, J. A.: A Review of Two Hundred and One Cases of Suppurative Arthritis, J. Bone & Joint Surg., *23*, 917, 1941.

HERRICK, W. W., and PARKHURST, G. M.: Meningococcus Arthritis, Am. J. M. Sc., *158*, 473, 1919.

HIGHMAN, J. H.: Congenital Osseous Rubella, Clin. Radiol., *18*, 445, 1967.

HILLIS, J. D.: *Leprosy in British Guiana. An Account of West Indian Leprosy*, London, J. & A. Churchill, 1881.

HIRSCHBERG, M., and BIEHLER, R.: Lepra der Knochen, Dermat. Ztschr., *16*, 415 and 490, 1909.

HOGG, T. C., LAW, W. B., and McINTYRE, E. D.: Hydatid Disease of Bone in Tasmania, J. Bone & Joint Surg., *52–B*, 790, 1970.

HOGSHEAD, H. P., and STEIN, G. H.: Mycetoma Due to *Nocardia brasiliensis*, J. Bone & Joint Surg., *52–A*, 1229, 1970.

HOPKINS, R.: Bone Changes in Leprosy, Radiology, *11*, 470, 1928.

HOPKINS, R., and FAGET, G. H.: Recent Trends of Leprosy in the United States, J.A.M.A., *126*, 937, 1944.

HSIEH, C. K.: Echinococcus Involvement of the Bones, Radiology, *14*, 562, 1930.

HUENEKENS, E. J., and RIGLER, L. G.: Osteomyelitis Variolosa: Report of a Case Observed During the Acute Stage, J.A.M.A., *87*, 295, 1926.

HUNT, D. D.: Cervical Spondylitis Caused by *Salmonella oranienburg*, J. Bone & Joint Surg., *47–A*, 1243, 1965.

HUTCHISON, W. F., THOMPSON, W. B., and DERIAN, P. S.: Osseous Hydatid (Echinococcus) Disease, J.A.M.A., *182*, 81, 1962.

JAFFE, H. L.: The Vessel Canals in Normal and Pathological Bone, Am. J. Path., *5*, 323, 1929.

————: *Tumors and Tumorous Conditions of the Bones and Joints*, Philadelphia, Lea & Febiger, 1958.

JAFFE, H. L., and LICHTENSTEIN, L.: Osteoid-Osteoma: Further Experience with this Benign Tumor of Bone, J. Bone & Joint Surg., *22*, 645, 1940.

JONES, R., JR., and ROBERTS, L.: Acute Osteomyelitis of the Upper End of the Femur, Surg. Gynec. & Obst., *65*, 753, 1937.

JOSEFIAK, E. J., and KOKIKO, G. V.: Mycetoma of the Hand, Arch. Path., *67*, 55, 1959.

KASAKOW, M. M., and POKROWSKI, A. S.: Primäre chronische Herdosteomyelitis, Arch. klin. Chir., *174*, 417, 1933.

KEEFER, C. S., PARKER, F., JR., and MYERS, W. K.: Histologic Changes in the Knee Joint in Various Infections, Arch. Path., *18*, 199, 1934.

KEEFER, C. S., and SPINK, W. W.: Gonococcic Arthritis: Pathogenesis, Mechanism of Recovery and Treatment, J.A.M.A., *109*, 1448, 1937.

KELLY, P. J., MARTIN, W. J., and COVENTRY, M. B.: Bacterial (Suppurative) Arthritis in the Adult, J. Bone & Joint Surg., *52–A*, 1595, 1970.

KEY, J. A., and LARGE, A. M.: Histoplasmosis of the Knee, J. Bone & Joint Surg., *24*, 281, 1942.

KINNMAN, J. E. G., and LEE, H. S.: Chronic Osteomyelitis of the Mandible, Oral Surg., *25*, 6, 1968.

KLAGES, F.: Der alveoläre Echinokokkus in Genf, insbesondere sein Auftreten im Knochen, Virchows Arch. path. Anat., *278*, 125, 1930.

————: Nichttuberkulöse Psoaserkrankungen im Kindesalter, Bruns' Beitr. klin. Chir., *158*, 171, 1933.

KLEIN, E. W., and GRIFFIN, J. P.: Coccidioidomycosis (Diagnosis Outside the Sonoran Zone), Am. J. Roentgenol., *94*, 653, 1965.

KLEIN, H. M.: Acute Osteomyelitis of the Vertebrae, Arch. Surg., *26*, 169, 1933.

KLEMM, P.: Ueber die Gelenkosteomyelitis, speciell die osteomyelitische Coxitis, Arch. klin. Chir., *97*, 414, 1912.

KULOWSKI, J.: Pyogenic Osteomyelitis of the Spine, J. Bone & Joint Surg., *18*, 343, 1936.

KULOWSKI, J., and STOVALL, S.: Maduramycosis of Tibia in a Native American, J.A.M.A., *135*, 429, 1947.

LADEWIG, W.: Über eine intrauterin entstandene umschriebene Osteomyelitis des Schädeldaches, Virchows Arch. path. Anat., *289*, 395, 1933.

LIGGETT, A. S., and SILBERMAN, Z.: Blastomycosis of the Knee Joint, J. Bone & Joint Surg., *52–A*, 1445, 1970.

LOUW, J. H., and SHANDLING, B.: Acute Haematogenous Osteomyelitis with Special Reference to Osteitis of the Neck of the Femur, Arch. Dis. Childhood, *36*, 117, 1961.

LOWBEER, L.: Brucellotic Osteomyelitis of Man and Animal, Proc. Staff Meet. Hillcrest Memorial Hosp., *6*, 1, 1949.

————: Skeletal and Articular Involvement in Brucellosis of Animals, Lab. Invest., *8*, 1448, 1959.

MACCALLUM, W. G.: *A Text-Book of Pathology*, 5th ed., Philadelphia, W. B. Saunders Company, 1932 (p. 595).

MACEWAN, D. W., and DUNBAR, J. S.: Early Radiologic Recognition of Pus in the Joints of Children, J. Canad. A. Radiol., *12*, 72, 1961.

MADGWICK, J. C.: Infective Arthritis of the Hip in Infancy, J. Bone & Joint Surg., *48–B*, 181, 1966.

MAJID, M. A., MATHIAS, P. F., SETH, H. N., and THIRUMALACHAR, M. J.: Primary Mycetoma of the Patella, J. Bone & Joint Surg., *46–A*, 1283, 1964.

MAKIN, M., ALKALAJ, I., and ROZANSKY, R.: Mono-Articular Brucellar Arthritis, J. Bone & Joint Surg., *39–A*, 1183, 1957.

MARBURY, W. B., and PECKHAM, H. L.: Brodie's Abscess of Radius, Due to Typhoid, J.A.M.A., *107*, 1284, 1936.

MAREK, F.: Über postoperative Schädelosteomyelitis, Arch. klin. Chir., *181*, 78, 1934.

MARTINELLI, B., and TAGLIAPIETRA, E. A.: Actinomycosis of the Arm, Bull. Hosp. Joint Dis., *31*, 31, 1970.

MCNAE, J.: An Unusual Case of Clostridium Welchii Infection, J. Bone & Joint Surg., *48–B*, 512, 1966.

MELCHIOR, E.: Zur Kenntnis der nichtspezifischen hämatogenen Knochenabszesse, Bruns' Beitr. klin. Chir., *163*, 425, 1936.

MENDELSOHN, B. G.: Actinomycosis of a Metacarpal Bone, J. Bone & Joint Surg., *47–B*, 739, 1965.

MILLARD, D. G.: Displacement of the Linear Thoracic Paraspinal Shadow of Brailsford; An Early Sign in Osteomyelitis of the Thoracic Spine, Am. J. Roentgenol., *90*, 1231, 1963.

MILLS, T. J.: Paraplegia Due to Hydatid Disease, J. Bone & Joint Surg., *38–B*, 884, 1956.

MURRAY, R. O., and HADDAD, F.: Hydatid Disease of the Spine, J. Bone & Joint Surg., *41–B*, 499, 1959.

MUSGRAVE, W. E., and SISON, A. G.: The Bone Lesions of Smallpox, Philippine J. Sc., *5*, 553, 1910.

————: The Bone Lesions of Smallpox, Philippine J. Sc., *8*, 67, 1913.

NATHAN, M. H., RADMAN, W. P., and BARTON, H. L.: Osseous Actinomycosis of the Head and Neck, Am. J. Roentgenol., *87*, 1048, 1962.

O'DONOGHUE, A. F.: Septic Arthritis in the Hip Caused by Brucella Melitensis, J. Bone & Joint Surg., *15*, 506, 1933.

OSLER, W.: The Etiology and Diagnosis of Cerebro-spinal Fever: Arthritis, Brit. M. J., *1*, 1517, 1899 (see p. 1521).

OYSTON, J. K.: Madura Foot, J. Bone & Joint Surg., *43–B*, 259, 1961.

PASQUALI, E.: Sulla localizzazione ossea dell'echinococco, Chir. org. movimento, *15*, 355, 1930.

PATERSON, D. C.: Acute Suppurative Arthritis in Infancy and Childhood, J. Bone & Joint Surg., *52–B*, 474, 1970.

PATTERSON, R. L., JR., and LEVINE, D. B.: *Hemophilus influenzae* Pyarthrosis in an Adult, J. Bone & Joint Surg., *47–A*, 1250, 1965.

POLLOCK, S. F., MORRIS, J. M., and MURRAY, W. R.: Coccidioidal Synovitis of the Knee, J. Bone & Joint Surg., *49–A*, 1397, 1967.

POWELL, C. S., and SWAN, L. L.: Leprosy: Pathologic Changes Observed in Fifty Consecutive Necropsies, Am. J. Path., *31*, 1131, 1955.

PRITCHARD, A. E., and THOMPSON, W. A. L.: Acute Pyogenic Infections of the Spine in Children, J. Bone & Joint Surg., *42–B*, 86, 1960.

PYRAH, L. N., and PAIN, A. B.: Acute Infective Osteomyelitis, Brit. J. Surg., *20*, 590, 1933.

RABINOWITZ, J. G., WOLF, B. S., GREENBERG, E. I., and RAUSEN, A. R.: Osseous Changes in Rubella Embryopathy, Radiology, *85*, 494, 1965.

RALSTON, E. L.: Osteomyelitis of the Spine Due to *Salmonella cholerae suis*, J. Bone & Joint Surg., *37–A*, 580, 1955.

RASK, M. R., and LATTIG, G. J.: Primary Intramuscular Hydatidosis of the Sartorius, J. Bone & Joint Surg., *52–A*, 582, 1970.

RAZIM, E. A., and FRIEDBERG, S. A.: Frontal, Maxillary, and Mandibular Bone Infections, Arch. Otolaryng., *82*, 67, 1965.

REES, R. J. W., WEDDELL, A. G. M., PALMER, E., and PEARSON, J. M. H.: Human Leprosy in Normal Mice, Brit. M. J., *3*, 216, 1969.

REMKY, E.: Zur Osteomyelitis des Oberkiefers beim Säugling, Ztschr. Augenheilk., *75*, 240, 1931.

RIORDAN, D. C.: The Hand in Leprosy. Part I. General Aspects of Leprosy, J. Bone & Joint Surg., *42–A*, 661, 1960.

————: The Hand in Leprosy. Part II. Orthopaedic Aspects of Leprosy, J. Bone & Joint Surg., *42–A*, 683, 1960.

ROBERTS, P. H.: Disturbed Epiphysial Growth at the Knee After Osteomyelitis in Infancy, J. Bone & Joint Surg., *52–B*, 692, 1970.

SAROSI, G. A., PARKER, J. D., DOTO, I. L., and TOSH, F. E.: Chronic Pulmonary Coccidioidomycosis, New England J. Med., *283*, 325, 1970.

SAWTSCHENKO, J.: Zur Frage über die Veränderungen der Knochen beim Aussatze (Osteitis et Osteomyelitis leprosa), Beitr. path. Anat., *9*, 241, 1891.

SCHEIN, A. J.: Articular Manifestations of Meningococcic Infections, Arch. Int. Med., *62*, 963, 1938.

SCHENKEN, J. R., and PALIK, E. E.: Coccidioidomycosis in States Other Than California, with Report of a Case in Louisiana, Arch. Path., *34*, 484, 1942.

SERRE, H., SIMON, L., and CLAUSTRE, J.: Les sacro-iléites mélitococciques, Semaine hôp. Paris, *46*, 3311, 1970.

SEWALL, S.: Vaccinia Osteomyelitis. Report of a Case with Isolation of the Vaccinia Virus, Bull. Hosp. Joint Dis., *10*, 59, 1949.

SIMPSON, W. M., and McINTOSH, C. A.: Actinomycosis of the Vertebrae (Actinomycotic Pott's Disease), Arch. Surg., *14*, 1166, 1927.

SINGLETON, E. B., RUDOLPH, A. J., ROSENBERG, H. S., and SINGER, D. B.: The Roentgenographic Manifestations of the Rubella Syndrome in Newborn Infants, Am. J. Roentgenol., *97*, 82, 1966.

SKINSNES, O. K.: The Immunological Spectrum of Leprosy, in *Leprosy in Theory and Practice*, 2nd ed., edited by R. G. Cochrane and T. F. Davey, Bristol, John Wright & Sons Ltd., 1964. (See p. 156.)

SOEUR, R.: Ostéomyélite de la hanche, Rev. chir., *50*, 377, 1931.

SRINIVASAN, H., and DESIKAN, K. V.: Cauliflower Growths in Neuropathic Plantar Ulcers in Leprosy Patients, J. Bone & Joint Surg., *53–A*, 123, 1971.

SRIVASTAVA, A. N.: Orthopaedic Complications of Smallpox, J. Bone & Joint Surg., *48–B*, 183, 1966.

STEINBERG, C. L.: Brucellosis as a Cause of Sacroiliac Arthritis, J.A.M.A., *138*, 15, 1948.

STEWART, G. A.: The Report of Five Cases of Subacute Osteomyelitis of the Femur Resembling Sarcoma, Radiology, *16*, 271, 1931.

SYMMERS, D., and SPORER, A.: Maduromycosis of the Hand, Arch. Path., *37*, 309, 1944.

THOMPSON, R. H. S., and DUBOS, R. J.: Production of Experimental Osteomyelitis in Rabbits by Intravenous Injection of Staphylococcus aureus, J. Exper. Med., *68*, 191, 1938.

TORG, J. S., and LAMMOT, T. R., III: Septic Arthritis of the Knee due to *Clostridium welchii*, J. Bone & Joint Surg., *50–A*, 1233, 1968.

TORGERSON, W. R., and HAMMOND, G.: Osteomyelitis of the Sesamoid Bones of the First Metatarsophalangeal Joint, J. Bone & Joint Surg., *51–A*, 1420, 1969.

TRUETA, J.: The Three Types of Acute Haematogenous Osteomyelitis, J. Bone & Joint Surg., *41–B*, 671, 1959.

VARADARAJAN, M. G.: Actinomycosis of Bone, Punjab M. J., *10*, 321, 1961.

VOLKMANN, R.: Zur Histologie der Caries und Ostitis, Arch. klin. Chir., *4*, 437, 1863.

WALL, J. J., and HUNT, D. D.: Acute Hematogenous Pyarthrosis Caused by *Hemophilus influenzae*, J. Bone & Joint Surg., *50–A*, 1657, 1968.

WARD, J. R., and BISHOP, B.: Varicella Arthritis, J.A.M.A., *212*, 1954, 1970.

WEARNE, W. M.: Actinomycosis of the Finger, Proc. Roy. Soc. Med., *53*, 884, 1960.

WEAVER, J. B., and SHERWOOD, L.: Hematogenous Osteomyelitis and Pyarthrosis Due to Salmonella suipestifer, J.A.M.A., *105*, 1188, 1935.

WEHNER, K.: Beobachtungen über die blande Osteomyelitis, Ztschr. orthop. Chir., *57*, 211, 1932.

WESTERLUND, N. C., and BIERMAN, A. H.: Salmonellosis, Am. J. Clin. Path., *53*, 92, 1970.

WILENSKY, A. O.: Osteomyelitis of the Skull, Arch. Surg., *27*, 83, 1933.

WILEY, A. M., and TRUETA, J.: The Vascular Anatomy of the Spine and Its Relationship to Pyogenic Vertebral Osteomyelitis, J. Bone & Joint Surg., *41–B*, 796, 1959.

WILLIAMS, H. J., and CAREY, L. S.: Rubella Embryopathy, Am. J. Roentgenol., *97*, 92, 1966.

WILSON, J. W., and PLUNKETT, O. A.: *The Fungous Diseases of Man*, Berkeley, University of California Press, 1965 (see p. 84).

YAMATO, S.: Über den Echinokokkus der Wirbelsäule und der Pleura mediastinalis, Virchows Arch. path. Anat., *253*, 364, 1924.

YOUNG, W. B.: Actinomycosis with Involvement of the Vertebral Column, Clin. Radiol. *11*, 175, 1960.

ZADEK, I.: Acute Osteomyelitis of the Long Bones of Adults, Arch. Surg., *37*, 531, 1938.

Index

Page numbers in **bold** indicate principal discussion.